ear

DISEASES, DEAFNESS, AND DIZZINESS

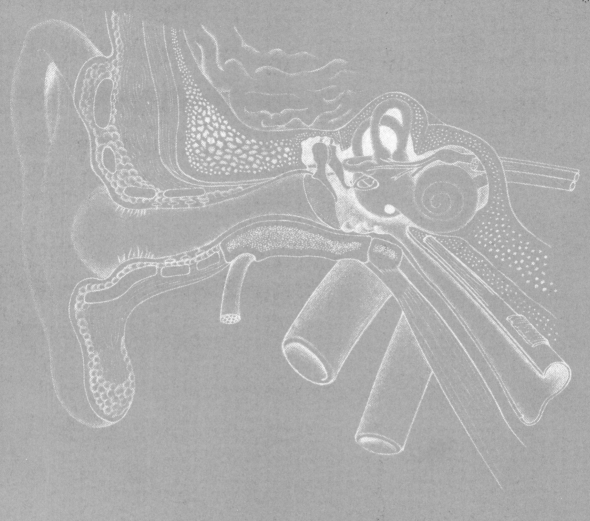

MEDICAL DEPARTMENT
HARPER & ROW, PUBLISHERS
HAGERSTOWN, MARYLAND
NEW YORK, SAN FRANCISCO, LONDON

ear

DISEASES, DEAFNESS, AND DIZZINESS

with 16 color illustrations

VICTOR GOODHILL, M.D., F.A.C.S.

PROFESSOR OF SURGERY (ADJUNCT-OTOLOGIC SURGERY),
DIVISION OF HEAD AND NECK SURGERY,
UCLA SCHOOL OF MEDICINE, LOS ANGELES, CALIFORNIA

WITH 14 CONTRIBUTORS

EAR DISEASES, DEAFNESS, AND DIZZINESS. Copyright © 1979 by Harper & Row, Publishers, Inc. All rights reserved. No part of this book may be used or reproduced in any manner whatsoever without written permission except in the case of brief quotations embodied in critical articles and reviews. Printed in the United States of America. For information address Medical Department, Harper & Row, Publishers, Inc., 2350 Virginia Avenue, Hagerstown, Maryland 21740.

Library of Congress Cataloging in Publication Data
Main entry under title:
Ear diseases, deafness, and dizziness.
    Includes bibliographies and index.
    1. Ear—Diseases. 2. Deafness. 3. Vertigo.
I. Goodhill, Victor. [DNLM: 1. Ear diseases.
2. Deafness. 3. Vertigo. WV200 G652e]
RF121.E37   617.8   78-6766
ISBN 0-06-140981-2

The authors and publisher have exerted every effort to ensure that drug selection and dosage set forth in this text are in accord with current recommendations and practice at the time of publication. However, in view of ongoing research, changes in government regulations, and the constant flow of information relating to drug therapy and drug reactions, the reader is urged to check the package insert for each drug for any change in indications and dosage and for added warnings and precautions. This is particularly important when the recommended agent is a new and/or infrequently employed drug.

80 81 82 83 84   10 9 8 7 6 5 4 3 2

TO MY WIFE, RUTH,
WHOSE DEVOTION, UNDERSTANDING, AND ENCOURAGEMENT
MADE THIS BOOK POSSIBLE

CONTENTS

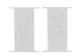

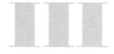

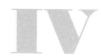

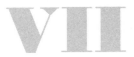
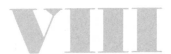
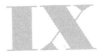

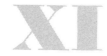

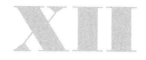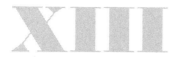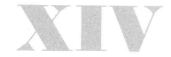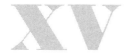

CONTRIBUTORS

SEYMOUR J. BROCKMAN, M.D., F.A.C.S.

chapters 15, 17, 29

ASSOCIATE CLINICAL PROFESSOR, DIVISION OF HEAD AND NECK SURGERY,
UCLA SCHOOL OF MEDICINE, LOS ANGELES, CALIFORNIA

STEPHEN H. COOPER, M.D.

chapter 17

CLINICAL INSTRUCTOR, DIVISION OF HEAD AND NECK SURGERY,
UCLA SCHOOL OF MEDICINE, LOS ANGELES, CALIFORNIA

BARRY S. ELPERN, Ph.D.

chapter 43

PRESIDENT, VALLEY HEARING AID SERVICES, INC., SHERMAN OAKS,
CALIFORNIA

RUTH GUSSEN, M.D.

chapter 32

ADJUNCT ASSOCIATE PROFESSOR, DEPARTMENT OF PATHOLOGY, AND
DIVISION OF HEAD AND NECK SURGERY, UCLA SCHOOL OF MEDICINE,
LOS ANGELES, CALIFORNIA

WILLIAM N. HANAFEE, M.D.

chapter 4

PROFESSOR, DEPARTMENT OF RADIOLOGY, UCLA SCHOOL OF MEDICINE,
LOS ANGELES, CALIFORNIA

IRWIN HARRIS, M.D., F.A.C.S.

chapters 10, 17, 26, 37

ASSOCIATE CLINICAL PROFESSOR, DIVISION OF HEAD AND NECK SURGERY,
UCLA SCHOOL OF MEDICINE, LOS ANGELES, CALIFORNIA

H. PATRICIA HEFFERNAN, M.A.

chapters 6, 8, 36

DIRECTOR, AUDIOLOGIC SERVICES, OTOSURGICAL GROUP MEDICAL CLINIC,
BEVERLY HILLS; ADJUNCT ASSISTANT PROFESSOR, SPECIAL EDUCATION,
CALIFORNIA STATE UNIVERSITY, LOS ANGELES, CALIFORNIA

VICENTE HONRUBIA, M.D.

chapter 1

PROFESSOR, DIVISION OF HEAD AND NECK SURGERY, UCLA SCHOOL OF MEDICINE,
LOS ANGELES, CALIFORNIA

RICHARD G. LEWIS, Ph.D.

chapter 35

ASSISTANT PROFESSOR, SPECIAL EDUCATION, CALIFORNIA STATE UNIVERSITY,
LOS ANGELES, CALIFORNIA

EDGAR L. LOWELL, Ph.D.
chapter 44
DIRECTOR, JOHN TRACY CLINIC, LOS ANGELES, CALIFORNIA

R. LORENTE DE NÓ, M.D.
chapter 2
VISITING PROFESSOR, DIVISION OF HEAD AND NECK SURGERY,
AND DEPARTMENT OF ANATOMY, UCLA SCHOOL OF MEDICINE,
LOS ANGELES, CALIFORNIA

JOEL B. SHULMAN, M.D.
chapters 24, 38, 39
RESEARCH OTOLOGIST, DIVISION OF HEAD AND NECK SURGERY,
UCLA SCHOOL OF MEDICINE, LOS ANGELES, CALIFORNIA

MARSHA R. SIMONS, M.A.
chapters 6, 7, 8, 36
AUDIOLOGIST, OTOSURGICAL GROUP MEDICAL CLINIC, BEVERLY HILLS;
ADJUNCT ASSISTANT PROFESSOR, SPECIAL EDUCATION,
CALIFORNIA STATE UNIVERSITY, LOS ANGELES, CALIFORNIA

D. M. STEIN, M.A.
chapter 34
EDUCATIONAL AUDIOLOGIST, DIVISION OF SPECIAL EDUCATION,
OFFICE OF LOS ANGELES COUNTY SUPERINTENDENT OF SCHOOLS,
DOWNEY, CALIFORNIA

PREFACE

Ear diseases produce human problems which are unique. To be sure, the innumerable lesions of the temporal bone encompass almost every type of pathology—congenital malformations, infections, degenerations, tumors—and in this respect, temporal bone changes mirror those in other parts of the body. Unique to ear lesions, however, are the involvements of two cranial nerves, the eighth nerve (auditory and vestibular) and the seventh nerve (facial nerve function). Hearing and human communication through language and speech are dependent on auditory function. Thus, communicative disorders (hearing loss and deafness) due to auditory malfunction can seriously influence human–societal relationships. Vestibular nerve functions relate to human equilibrium and thus cause many forms of "dizziness." Facial nerve lesions can cause facial paralyses with serious functional and cosmetic sequelae.

Some 25 years ago, the late Dr. George von Bekesy, the physicist who received the 1961 Nobel prize in Medicine for his contributions to our knowledge of the ear and hearing, asked me to recommend to him a textbook on clinical otology. After much reflection I had to tell him that I knew of no better work on basic otology than the "Lehrbuch der Ohrenheilkunde" written in 1878 by Prof. Dr. Adam Politzer. Dr. von Bekesy used my copy of Politzer as his clinical reference text for a number of years.

I was inspired to write this present book on otology by Politzer's masterpiece, which is still a classic in basic conception and content. Much has happened to the knowledge of otology in these 100 years, but the solid scientific thinking and the countless wise clinical observations of Politzer remain my models. His book was written for all physicians, not only for otolaryngologists. This book follows the same pattern.

A century ago, diseases of the ear and the temporal bone were responsible for many common life-threatening conditions, especially otomastoiditis and its complications. The dawn of chemotherapy and the antibiotic era changed this state of affairs drastically. This fortunate event in medical history (in the 1940s) caused prophetic predictions of the virtual demise of otology as a necessary medical specialty. However, the radical shift away from the then common problems of otogenic meningitis, temporal lobe and cerebellar abscesses, lateral sinus thrombophlebitis with septicemia, and the other dangerous otologic complications, brought a striking change in the emphasis of otology. As these complications became less common, otologists were able to turn to other facets of ear diseases, including new surgery for hearing loss, new insights into the problems of dizziness, new approaches to facial nerve paralysis and to the many other aspects of otology covered in the 44 chapters of this book.

Thus, otology has become a special medical discipline, as comprehensive in scope as ophthalmology. While otolaryngologists are especially trained to deal with otologic lesions, many other physicians must deal with ear problems. Practitioners of pediatrics, internal medicine, family–primary care medicine, neurology, emergency medicine, and other specialties are frequently confronted by ear diseases, deafness and dizziness. Audiologists and speech pathologists must also have a familiarity with many aspects of otology.

Ear infections and hearing losses in infants, children, and adolescents are common problems seen by pediatricians and family (primary care) practitioners, and it has been estimated that 20%–30% of a pediatric practice may involve otologic problems.

The Biblical phrase "do not curse the deaf" (Leviticus 19:14) is strange, but can be understood clearly by millions of hard of hearing and deaf children and adults in the world. A great "curse" is non-recognition of auditory handicaps. Hearing losses of moderate degree frequently escape recognition by families and by primary physicians. Much can now be done to improve early diagnosis which will lead to proper management. Increased knowledge of modern otologic techniques will do much to remove the "curse" of hearing losses and deafness.

Hearing losses in adults are also common, and the growing geriatric population creates a need for awareness of communication handicaps, which may be subtle, and which require an understanding of basic auditory lesions and their rehabilitation aspects. The physician (and not the hearing-aid dealer) has the responsibility for proper diagnosis, evaluation and guidance of such patients, especially since many lesions causing hearing loss and deafness are treatable medically or surgically.

The "dizzy patient" constitutes a diagnostic and therapeutic challenge to most physicians. The otologist may be the final physician in some cases, but in the vast majority of patients the nonotologist can competently deal with "dizziness." However, a working knowledge of the neurootologic aspects of vertigo, motion sickness and dysequilibrium is essential.

Many otologists and basic scientists have contributed greatly to this expanding branch of medicine during the past three decades. References are made to the contributions of authors throughout the world. However, this book represents the consensus of a small clinical otosurgical group working closely together. In many controversial areas, we clearly share our experiences with the reader and express our opinions. In a sense, therefore, this is a personal document, and not the work of disparate contributors.

While broadly directed to the entire medical profession, and to audiologic and related paramedical professionals, this book also contains specific details for our colleagues in otolaryngology. Thus, it is hoped that it will be of value to medical students and to house officers in otolaryngology, head and neck surgery, and related fields. Since this book is broadly based, the essential text is printed in regular type, with an indented smaller type format for description of scientific and/or technical details.

Most of the photographs, drawings, charts and radiographs reflect my experiences and those of my co-workers. A significant number of unique illustrations and tables have been reprinted with the generous and gracious permissions of colleagues throughout the world. In order to facilitate illustrative examples, the format has been directed to the right ear. Wherever possible, the right ear, the right temporal bone, the right side of skull, the right neck and the right side of the face have been used in drawings and photographs for consistency.

V.G.

ACKNOWLEDGMENTS

I am deeply indebted to my otologic colleagues, Dr. Seymour J. Brockman, Dr. Irwin Harris, Dr. Joel B. Shulman, and Dr. Stephen H. Cooper, for their participation and collaboration in many chapters. Other faculty members of the Division of Head and Neck Surgery at UCLA (Dr. Paul H. Ward, Chief) have been very helpful.

Advances in audiology during the past few decades have been incalculable to the growth of otology. H. Patricia Heffernan, M.A., and Marsha Simons, M.A., of our clinic have not only co-authored several chapters, but were responsible for audiologic guidance. Dorothy Stein, M.A., Richard Lewis, Ph.D., Edgar Lowell, Ph.D., and Barry Elpern, Ph.D., contributed valuable chapters on the rehabilitation of hard of hearing and deaf children. These audiologic chapters are models of collaboration between the two disciplines of otology and audiology and demonstrate the value to patients of such close clinical relationships.

Dr. William Hanafee is responsible for an indispensable contribution on radiographic approaches to otology. The diagnostic values of plain films, polytomography and computerized scanning techniques are lucidly presented and brilliantly illustrated in his chapter on Otoradiology.

Dr. Vicente Honrubia and I have collaborated on the introductory clinical anatomy and physiology chapter, a presentation of contemporary otologic morphology and physiology combined with clinical significance.

The unique description of VIII N. pathways by Dr. Rafael Lorente de Nó focuses on the remarkable complexity of these pathways. Thus, the cochlear nucleus, in itself, is shown to constitute an "auditory brain." His contribution (Chapter 2) contains much previously unpublished material, which is indispensable to an understanding of auditory and vestibular function.

Dr. Ruth Gussen, who has brought the unusual expertise of a general pathologist to the specialized field of temporal bone pathology, has contributed wise advice and many valuable photomicrographs (some previously unpublished) to almost every chapter of this book. I am very grateful to her for these basic contributions and for her many kindnesses.

The writing of this book required extraordinary collaboration for which I am especially grateful to three people. Ms. Christine Davis, M.A., has been a devoted, enthusiastic and tireless assistant, dealing with the innumerable secretarial, bibliographic and logistic responsibilities involved. Mrs. Loretta Douglass, B. A., a gifted medical artist, was responsible for virtually all of the original drawings in this book. Ms. Ann Marie Westerbergh, R.N., my surgical assistant for almost two decades, was of invaluable help in meticulous collation of illustrative material.

Finally, I should like to express my personal thanks to the Harper and Row Medical Department for patient encouragement over a long period of time. These talented associates have been extremely helpful.

ear

DISEASES, DEAFNESS, AND DIZZINESS

Color Fig. 1. Large osteoma, external auditory canal.

Color Fig. 2. Superior and posterior osteophytes and infero-anterior osteoma.

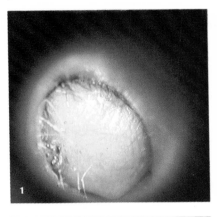
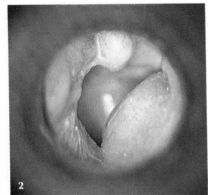

Color Fig. 3. Suppuration external canal.

Color Fig. 4. Otomycosis external canal.

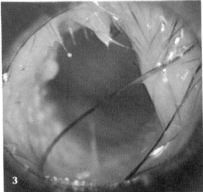
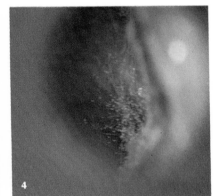

Color Fig. 5. Bullous myringitis (viral).

Color Fig. 6. Acute secretory otitis media with air bubbles.

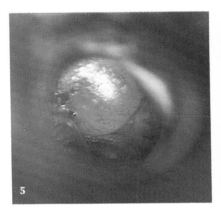
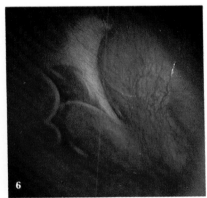

Color Fig. 7. Chronic secretory otitis media "blue drum."

Color Fig. 8. Secretory otitis media, postmyringostomy, with middle ear ventilation tube.

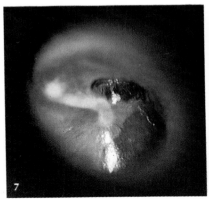
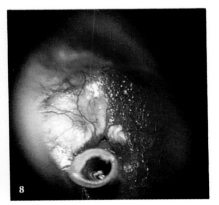

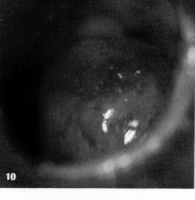

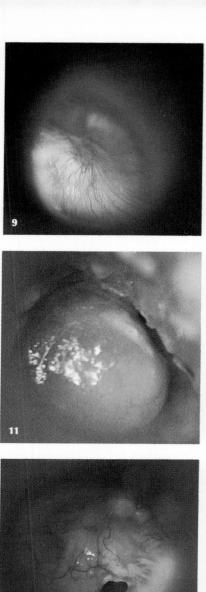

Color Fig. 9. Recurrent acute otitis media with bulging tympanic membrane.

Color Fig. 10. Polypoid granuloma in external auditory canal.

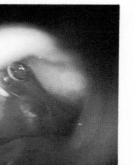

Color Fig. 11. Middle-ear polyp projecting into external canal.

Color Fig. 12. Recurrent keratoma with pus in external canal.

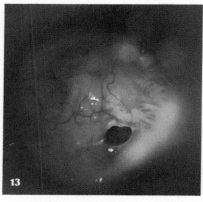

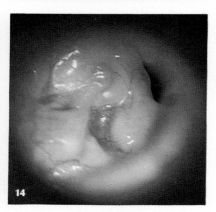

Color Fig. 13. Small central perforation and tympanosclerosis.

Color Fig. 14. Obliterative tympanosclerosis (tympanic membrane and middle ear).

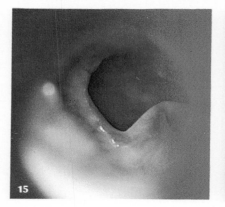

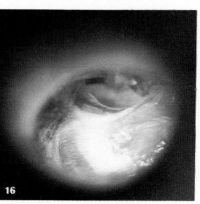

Color Fig. 15. Posterosuperior perforation, inferior middle ear keratoma.

Color Fig. 16. Attic (epitympanic) perforation of tympanic membrane with calcific plaques.

I

ANATOMY
AND PHYSIOLOGY

1

CLINICAL ANATOMY AND PHYSIOLOGY OF THE PERIPHERAL EAR

VICENTE HONRUBIA
VICTOR GOODHILL

DEVELOPMENTAL ASPECTS OF THE HUMAN EAR

The cartilaginous auricle and the temporal bone are the basic structures involved in ear diseases. Temporal bone relationships with the other skull bones and their contents are crucial in evaluating otologic problems.

The complex and interrelated hearing and equilibrium systems and their end-organs provide sensory inputs for the eighth (auditory-vestibular) cranial nerve. Since the seventh (facial) cranial nerve accompanies the eighth nerve through much of its intracranial course, these two cranial nerves are significantly interrelated clinically.

CONTRIBUTIONS OF THE THREE PRIMITIVE GERMINAL LAYERS

The human ear can be divided into three parts for clinical purposes, external, middle, and inner. The three primitive germ layers contribute in different ways to the three parts of the ear (Fig. 1–1).

Ectoderm contributes to external and internal ear developments. External ear derivatives include auricular, meatal, and tympanic membrane epithelial components. In the internal ear, the complex membranous labyrinth is of ectodermal origin.

Mesoderm contributes to all three parts of the ear. In the external ear, the auricular cartilages and muscles are of mesodermal origin. In the middle ear, mesodermal derivatives include the three ossicles, the two muscles, and the mucosal elements of the tympanic membrane and the middle ear space. The periotic labyrinth and the otic capsule are of inner-ear mesodermal origin.

Entoderm contributes only to middle-ear developments, giving rise to the total tubotympanic air-cell system from the eustachian tube orifice to the most distant mastoid air cell.

DEVELOPMENTAL INTERRELATIONS

The three divisions of the tripartite human ear, which arise from separate primordia, have a number of important interrelationships and timing differences. A variety of congenital developmental defects can occur in any of the three divisions, external, middle, or inner ear, singly or combined.

At the end of the third week of embryonic development, the auditory placode appears as an ectodermal thickening adjacent to the neural tube and lateral to the acousticofacial ganglion (Fig. 1–2). The auditory placode, which will contribute to inner ear development, and the primitive gut endoderm, which will form the middle ear cavity, are growing simultaneously.

The ectodermal auditory placode rapidly invaginates, forming the otic pit (Fig. 1–3), and soon closes to form the early otocyst (otic vesicle). Simultaneously, there is beginning development of the first branchial groove (Fig. 1–4) and condensation of mesenchyme between the groove and the endodermal pouch. This mesenchymal condensation represents the anlage of future middle-ear components, including the middle-ear ossicles, which will occupy the tympanic portion of the tubotympanic air-cell system.

As the otocyst and acousticofacial ganglion begin to form labyrinthine endolymph-system components (Fig. 1–5), the first branchial arch (mandibular), the second branchial arch (hyoid), and the maxillary processes are developing (Fig. 1–6).

By the sixth week hillock formations (Fig. 1–7) for auricle development have appeared. The first branchial groove accompanied by first and second branchial arch derivatives will form the external auditory meatus.

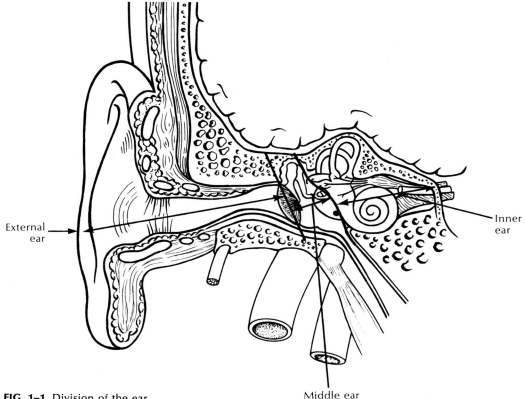

FIG. 1–1. Division of the ear.

External ear

Middle ear

Inner ear

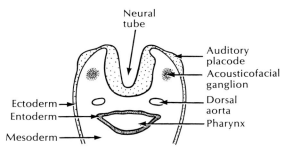

FIG. 1–2. Auditory placode stage in development of the ear. (Adapted from Pearson AA: The Development of the Ear: A Manual. Rochester, Minn, American Academy of Ophthalmology and Otolaryngology, 1967)

Neural tube

Auditory placode

Acousticofacial ganglion

Dorsal aorta

Pharynx

Ectoderm

Entoderm

Mesoderm

FIG. 1–3. Otic pit stage in development of the ear. (Adapted from Pearson AA: The Development of the Ear: A Manual. Rochester, Minn, American Academy of Ophthalmology and Otolaryngology, 1967)

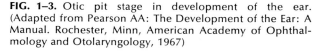

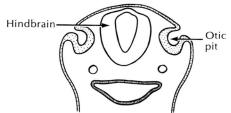

Hindbrain

Otic pit

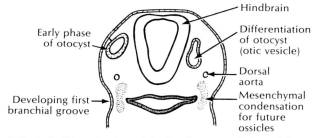

FIG. 1–4. Otocyst-otic vesicle development. (Adapted from Pearson AA: The Development of the Ear: A Manual. Rochester, Minn, American Academy of Ophthalmology and Otolaryngology, 1967)

Hindbrain

Early phase of otocyst

Differentiation of otocyst (otic vesicle)

Dorsal aorta

Developing first branchial groove

Mesenchymal condensation for future ossicles

FIG. 1–5. Primitive endolymphatic system stage in development of the ear, accompanied by branchial arch differentiation from primitive entoderm. (Adapted from Pearson AA: The Development of the Ear: A Manual. Rochester, Minn, American Academy of Ophthalmology and Otolaryngology, 1967)

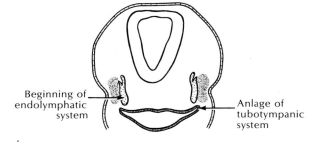

Beginning of endolymphatic system

Anlage of tubotympanic system

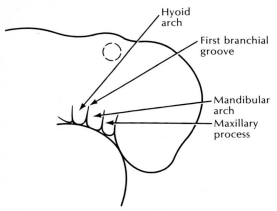

FIG. 1–6. Primitive branchial arch relations in development of the ear.

FIG. 1–7. Hillock formations surround first branchial groove, which will become external auditory meatus.

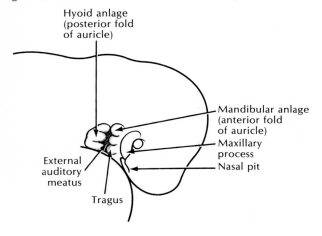

EXTERNAL EAR DEVELOPMENT

The development of the auricle will proceed from the six hillocks coming from mandibular and hyoid arch anlages to coalesce by the third fetal month. The tragus develops from the first (mandibular) arch and the rest of the auricle from the remaining five hillocks which are of second (hyoid) arch origin. Invagination of the branchial groove (Fig. 1–8) at first meets the primitive entodermal pharyngeal pouch. A brief ectodermal–entodermal apposition is followed by mesodermal encroachment from mesodermal elements above and below to separate the brief union (Fig. 1–9). These mesodermal anlages will form ossicle components as the pouch begins to form the primitive tubotympanum.

The mesodermal elements will form dorsal and ventral cartilaginous wall anlages around the funnel shaped primitive future cartilaginous external auditory meatus and lateral external auditory canal. A solid core of epithelial cells remains, the meatal plate, which medially approaches the entodermal pharyngeal tube anlage (Fig. 1–10).

Medial mesodermal elements begin to ossify at the third month to form the tympanic ring (annulus) for tympanic membrane support. Not until the seventh fetal month does the ectodermal solid epithelial core (tympanic plate) finally split to form the lateral squamous tympanic membrane epithelium and the skin of the medial bony external auditory canal that is arising simultaneously from the tympanic ring (Fig. 1–11).

The floor of the external auditory canal in newborns is short, flaccid, and fibrocartilaginous in structure. Malformations of the auricle are due to failure in differentiation of the first and second branchial arches and may include anotia, microtia, and various auricular cartilage malformations, as well as malposition of the auricle (e.g., low-set auricles).

Failure of first branchial groove development is responsible for congenital external meatus atresia, which may occur with a normally differentiated and functioning tympanic membrane and ossicular chain.

MIDDLE EAR DEVELOPMENT

As the first (ectodermal) branchial groove invaginates to approach the primitive entodermal tubotympanic recess, mesodermal aggregations appear above and below to separate the primitive junction. Tympanic membrane and middle-ear structures will develop from them, including ossicles, muscles, and tendons.

The first pharyngeal pouch, which is entoderm lined, expands to form the eustachian tube and middle-ear cavity.

The ossicles have multiple origins (Fig. 1–12). The superior aspects of incus and malleus (forming the incudomalleal joint) will arise from the first (mandibular) arch (Meckel's cartilage). The lower aspects of the incus and malleus and the arch of the stapes will arise from the second (hyoid) arch (Reichert's cartilage). The stapes footplate will arise from the otic capsule.

The dorsal malleal manubrium anlage is above the meatal plate, which is lateral to the primitive middle-ear air space. Superior to the middle-ear

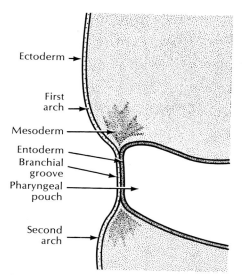

FIG. 1–8. Brief ectodermal-entodermal apposition.

FIG. 1–9. Mesodermal anlages of ossicles encroach on apposition area.

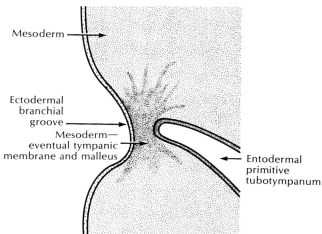

space is the cartilaginous anlage for the incus, and medial to it is that for the stapes arch, the latter in close proximity to the otic capsule.

As the ossicles develop and assume their relationships within the mesotympanum, the eustachian tube remains as an air-filled space, whereas tympanic mesenchyme still occupies the region of the future middle ear. Clinically, it is not unusual for mesenchyme to persist in the infant middle ear.

The eustachian tube primordium from primitive gut entoderm provides ciliated epithelium for cellular air-space temporal bone development—*i.e.*, the middle-ear tympanic cavity, the attic (epitympanic recess), the major mastoid air cell (antrum), and finally, the entire mastoid air-cell system.

Differentiation problems in the first pharyngeal pouch may be responsible for maldevelopment of the eustachian tube, the middle ear, and defects in mastoid process pneumatization. Thus, there are obvious prenatal anatomic possibilities for malformations, such as those associated with cleft palate–tubotympanic problems and more subtle abnormalities that may result in air-space and mucosal malfunctions. The predisposition of some children to recurrent secretory otitis media may be due to such maldevelopments and may not be entirely attributable to immunologic problems.

INNER EAR DEVELOPMENT

The inner ear, the complex neuroepithelial-fluid-filled structure within the bony labyrinth, begins to develop 3 weeks after conception, with appearance of the auditory placode, a thickening of head ectoderm on either side of the rhombencephalon.

FIG. 1–10. Primitive external auditory canal, meatal plate, and middle ear.

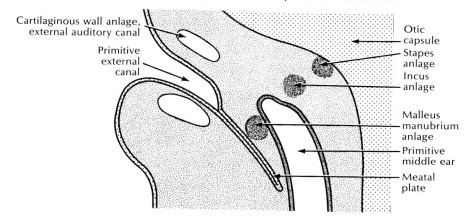

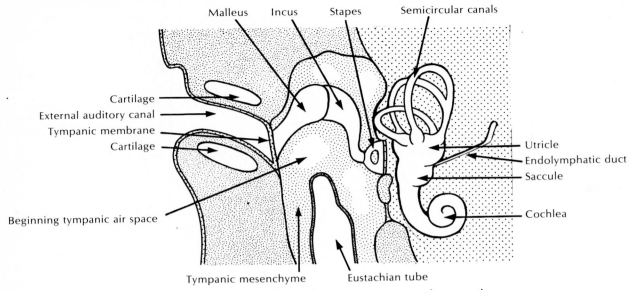

FIG. 1–11. Development of definite external, middle, and inner ear structures by seventh fetal month.

FIG. 1–12. Multiple origins for the three ossicles.

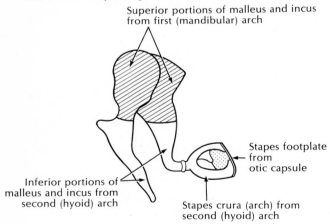

The auditory placode rapidly undergoes invagination into a pit, which closes off at the surface to form the otocyst or otic (auditory) vesicle. Invaginations within the vesicular wall divide it into vestibular and cochlear components.

Concurrent with the auditory placode–pit–vesicle development, the statoacousticofacial ganglion forms from the neural crest at the end of the third week. The developmental contributions of this ganglion to seventh and eighth nerve developments are still under study.

Van de Water (30) reported that hair cells in mouse otocyst (studied by *in vitro* organ cultures)

can differentiate in the complete absence of the statoacoustic ganglion complex. Thus, a neurotrophic effect does not appear to be essential for sensory cell differentiation.

These new studies will throw much light on the complexities of inner ear malformation encountered in neonates (see Ch. 31, Congenital Hearing Losses; and Ch. 32, Hereditary Congenital Ear Syndromes).

The primitive otocyst develops into the vestibular duct from which an anteroinferior cochlear diverticulum appears (Fig. 1–13A). The vestibular duct differentiates into the three semicircular canals as the cochlear duct begins to develop from its saccular (inferior) portion (Fig. 1–13).

Very early in development (on the 12th postcoital day), the neuroepithelium in the otocyst has progressed to formation of microvilli and begins to form the cochlear turns by the sixth to seventh week, with completion of 2.5 turns by the eighth week. By the fifth month, the primitive organ of Corti has formed within the cochlear duct (Fig. 1–14).

The statoacoustic facial ganglion divides into a superior portion which sends fibers to the utricle, to superior and lateral ampullas, and into an inferior portion, from which fibers go to the saccule and posterior ampulla. The remainder of the acoustic ganglion becomes the spiral ganglion of the cochlea. Facial nerve differentiation from the facial ganglion occurs simultaneously.

The primitive mesodermal anlage of the otic capsule, which forms the framework of the membranous labyrinth, is related laterally to the middle ear by oval-window formation, including the mobile stapedial footplate and ligament, which seal the scala vestibuli. Similarly, the round-window niche develops from mesoderm, and the round window membrane acts as a mobile seal for the scala tympani.

Medial inner-ear development relates to vestibular and cochlear aqueduct connections to the dura and subarachnoid space. Ectodermal otocyst components that form the neural elements of the inner ear interact with mesodermal plates to form these aqueducts. The "blind" ending of the closed vestibular duct and sac in contact with the dura contrasts with the open communication of the cochlear aqueduct, providing hydraulic contiguity between scala tympani perilymph and subarachnoid space CSF.

A number of clinical lesions involving these two aqueducts, such as Meniere's disease (see Ch. 26, Peripheral Vertigo, Labyrinthitis, and Meniere's Disease) and the labyrinthine membrane rupture syndrome (see Ch. 37, Sudden Hearing Loss Syndrome) may be related to congenital malformations between such developmental relationships.

In the late fetal state the semicircular canals, the saccule, and the utricle are fully formed, and the cochlear duct has reached its final development (Fig. 1–15).

Since the membranous labyrinth derives from the ectodermal otocyst independently from the rest of the ear, which is primarily a branchial system apparatus, combined malformations of the inner ear and external and middle ear are relatively infrequent, but they do occur.

TEMPORAL BONE DEVELOPMENT

Temporal bone development as part of the fetal skull arises in three parts. The **petrous** part arises

FIG. 1–13. A. Cochlear diverticulum appears from otic vesicle. **B.** Semicircular canal and cochlear primordia. **C.** Canals, utricle, and saccule are developed; cochlea is still primitive. **D.** At 30-mm stage full cochlear development is present.

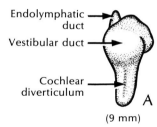

(9 mm)

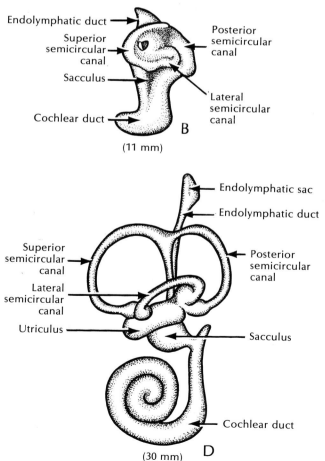

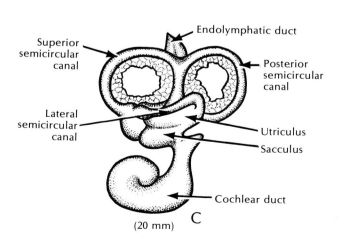

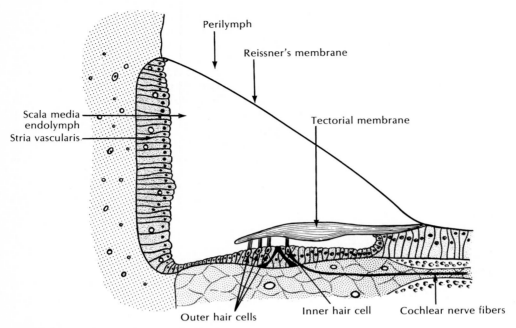

FIG. 1–14. Primitive cochlear development: organ of Corti.

FIG. 1–15. Late fetal stage of inner ear development.

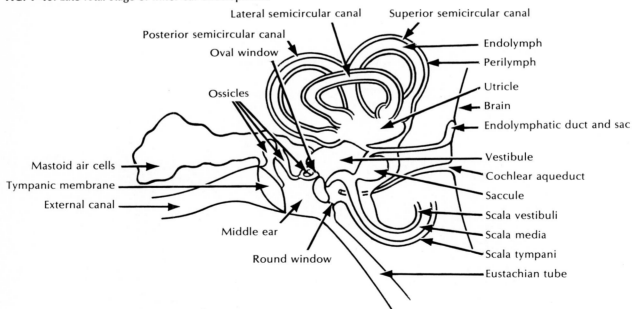

FIG. 1–16. A. Components of infant temporal bone. **B.** Infant temporal bone. **C.** Adult temporal bone.

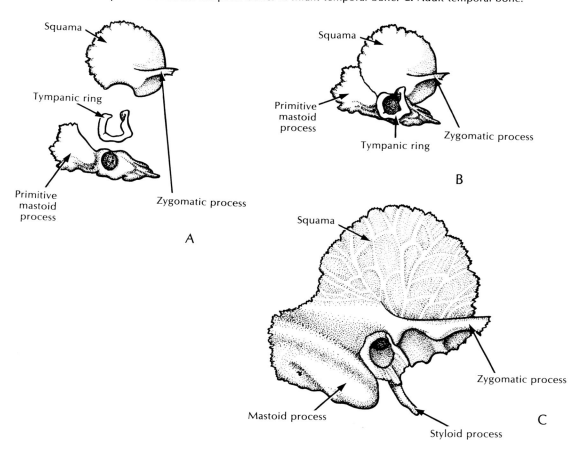

FIG. 1–17. A. Fetal skull. **B.** Adult skull.

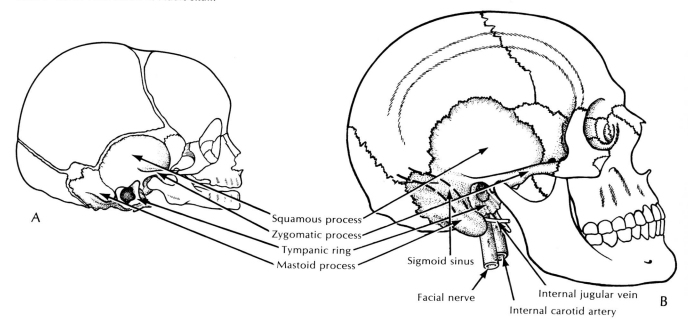

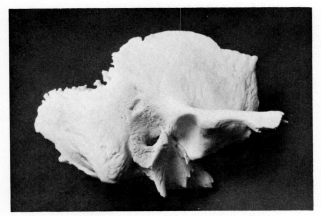

FIG. 1–18. Right temporal bone, lateral view.

from cartilage, but the **squamous** and **tympanic** parts arise from membrane bone. The three-part formation is well along by the 8th to 12th weeks.

The squama with its zygomatic process, the tympanic ring, and the primitive mastoid process of the infant temporal bone provide all the basic components of the future adult temporal bone by the end of the fourth month (Fig. 1–16).

The primitive tympanic air space, which develops into the first mastoid cell, the antrum cell, constitutes a very small air space within the temporal bone. It is eventually followed by the development of the entire mastoid air-cell system.

TEMPORAL BONE AND SKULL

ANATOMY

The temporal bone forms a large portion of the lateral aspect of the skull, with intimate suture-line connections to the other skull bones (Fig. 1–17).

Laterally (Fig. 1–18), the large superior **squamous part** articulates with the occipital bone, the parietal bone, and with the sphenoid bone. It forms part of the lateral bony wall of the middle cranial fossa. Its anterior zygomatic portion (process) articulates with the zygoma and forms the roof of the temporomandibular fossa for mandibular articulation. The small lateral **tympanic part** forms the bony external auditory canal. The posterior **mastoid part** articulates laterally with the parietal and occipital bones and houses a major portion of the complex mastoid air-cell system, which communicates with the nasopharynx through the middle ear and eustachian tube. Medially this air-cell

system is also in continuity with petrous pyramid air cells. The medial **petrous part** is intimately related to the internal carotid artery, the sigmoid venous sinus, and the facial nerve. It surrounds the bony labyrinth with its neural aperture, the internal auditory canal, and contains the vestibular and cochlear fossulas.

Medially (Figs. 1–19, 1–20), the anterior surface of the temporal bone contributes to the floor of the middle cranial fossa, and is thus in contact with temporal lobe dura. The posterior surface is almost at right angles to the anterior surface, separated by the superior petrosal sulcus, and contributes to the floor of the posterior fossa. The posterior surface landmarks include the depression for the sigmoid (lateral) sinus, the vestibular and cochlear aqueduct fossulas, the internal auditory meatus, and the jugular foramen. It is in contact with cerebellar dura.

The internal auditory meatus is the major access route for the seventh and eighth cranial nerves from the cerebellopontine angle into the temporal bone. The meatus is divided into superior and inferior portions by a transverse bony crest. The inferior portion serves as conduit for the cochlear division of the eighth nerve anteriorly and for the inferior vestibular nerve posteriorly. The latter also contains the foramen singulare for the nerve to the posterior semicircular canal and also the saccular nerve. The superior portion is divided by a vertical crest into the anterior channel for the seventh nerve and the posterior channel for the superior vestibular nerve innervating the superior and lateral semicircular canals, utricle, and a portion of the saccule (Fig. 1–21).

The seventh and eighth nerves in the cerebellopontine angle are in a superomedial relationship with the fifth nerve. Inferomedially they are in fairly close proximity to the jugular foramen with its contents, e.g., the ninth, tenth, and eleventh nerves (Fig. 1–22).

The mastoid process is the posterior part of the temporal bone visible as a bony protuberance behind, above, and below the auricle. In clinical terminology, the term **mastoid** refers not only to the anatomic mastoid process but to the entire interconnecting system of air cells with which the temporal bone is normally honeycombed. The petrous apex, which is at the base of the skull, has an air-cell system that is usually also in contiguity with the mastoid air cell system (Figs. 1–23, 1–24).

The periantral triangle within the mastoid has boundaries defined by the posterior fossa plate and sigmoid sinus plate posteromedially, the middle

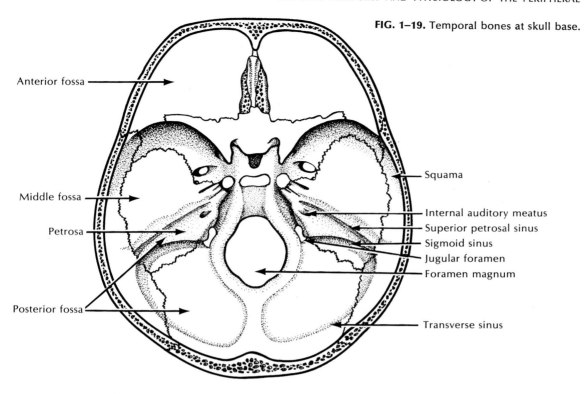

FIG. 1–19. Temporal bones at skull base.

Anterior fossa

Middle fossa

Petrosa

Posterior fossa

Squama

Internal auditory meatus

Superior petrosal sinus

Sigmoid sinus

Jugular foramen

Foramen magnum

Transverse sinus

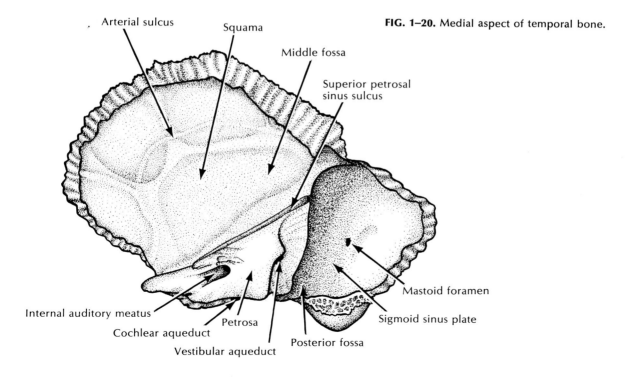

FIG. 1–20. Medial aspect of temporal bone.

Arterial sulcus

Squama

Middle fossa

Superior petrosal sinus sulcus

Mastoid foramen

Sigmoid sinus plate

Internal auditory meatus

Cochlear aqueduct

Petrosa

Posterior fossa

Vestibular aqueduct

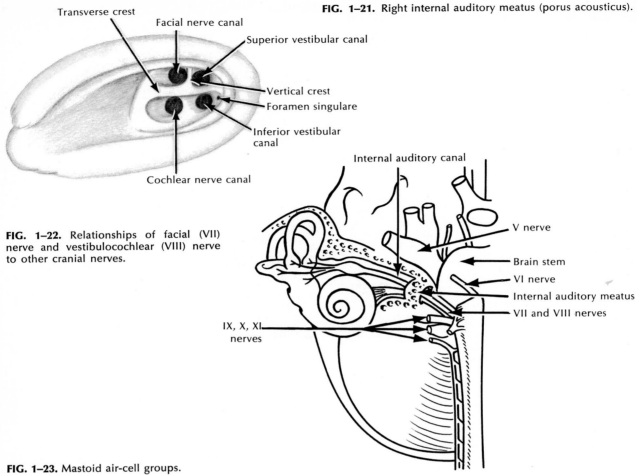

Transverse crest

Facial nerve canal

Superior vestibular canal

Vertical crest

Foramen singulare

Inferior vestibular canal

Cochlear nerve canal

FIG. 1–21. Right internal auditory meatus (porus acousticus).

Internal auditory canal

V nerve

Brain stem

VI nerve

Internal auditory meatus

VII and VIII nerves

IX, X, XI nerves

FIG. 1–22. Relationships of facial (VII) nerve and vestibulocochlear (VIII) nerve to other cranial nerves.

FIG. 1–23. Mastoid air-cell groups.

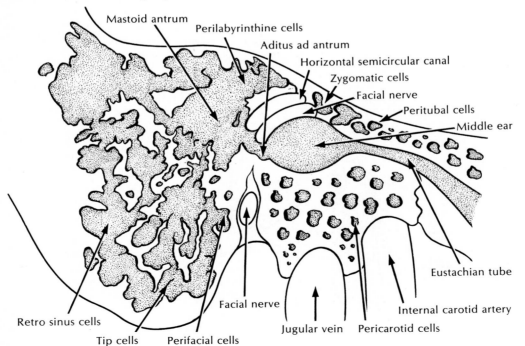

Mastoid antrum

Perilabyrinthine cells

Aditus ad antrum

Horizontal semicircular canal

Zygomatic cells

Facial nerve

Peritubal cells

Middle ear

Retro sinus cells

Tip cells

Perifacial cells

Facial nerve

Jugular vein

Pericarotid cells

Internal carotid artery

Eustachian tube

fossa plate (tegmen) superiorly, and the posterior bony canal wall (anterior mastoid cortex) anteriorly. Normally, cellular pneumatization areas occur throughout the temporal bone and may even extend beyond the temporal bone into parietal, occipital, and zygoma bones. This air-cell system is created by an embryologic process in which a primitive connective tissue (embryonic mesenchyme) disappears upon the invasion of mucosal epithelium from the first branchial pouch (via the eustachian tube anlage). As the mesenchyme disappears, many of its cells contribute to the epithelialization of the various components of the tympanomastoid air space. The mastoid cell mucosa lining is derived partly from mesenchyme and partly from first pharyngeal pouch gut endoderm. There are variations in degree of air-cell development (pneumatization) (Figs. 1–25 to 1–28).

Within the mastoid air-cell system a number of important "viscera" are located. These include the horizontal, posterior genu, and vertical portion of the facial (VII) nerve, the chorda tympani nerve, and the nerve to the stapedius muscle, the bony labyrinth capsule and its contents, and the sigmoid sinus. The internal carotid artery is in anterior relationship to the middle ear, and to the eustachian tube and petrous apex.

The mucosa of the mastoid air-cell system is in anatomic mucosal continuity with the middle ear, the eustachian tube, and the nasopharynx and its adnexas.

FIG. 1–24. Air cells have been extensively removed in a "radical" mastoidectomy. Right temporal bone (lateral view).

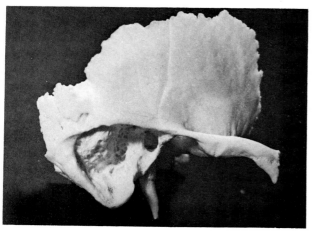

The infant temporal bone varies from that of the adult just as the infant skull differs from the adult skull. All major components are formed. There is a rudimentary bony external canal, consisting only of the bony tympanic ring; thus the external auditory canal of the infant is almost entirely cartilaginous.

The petromastoid portion of the infant temporal bone contains at least one major air cell, the mastoid "antrum," a primordium for development of the rest of the mastoid air-cell system. The lateral bony margin of this primordial mastoid cell at birth is formed by the squama.

CLINICAL ASPECTS

The common disease, otomastoiditis, can involve all or any part of the temporal bone, in the complex tympanomastoid air-cell system. Infections of the mastoid cell system are due to tubotympanic disease. Almost every case of mastoiditis starts with a middle-ear infection.

Middle-ear infections and eustachian tube blockage in childhood may interfere with mastoid antrum ventilation, thus blocking normal mastoid pneumatization patterns. Thus, the adult size of an air-cell system may well be a clue to the time of onset of an otomastoid infection (Figs. 1–29, 1–30).

Since the primordial air cell (the so-called mastoid antrum) is bounded by the squama laterally, in infantile mastoidectomy it is actually necessary to uncover a portion of the posterior squamal process to reach this primary mastoid cell. In postauricular incisions in infant mastoidectomy, the incision is more superior and slopes in a posterior direction for adequate surgical exposure of the mastoid antrum and to avoid injury to the superficial portion of the seventh nerve as it exits from the stylomastoid foramen (see Ch. 12, Basic Otosurgical Procedures).

The infant stylomastoid foramen is very superficial, thus the seventh (facial) nerve may also be traumatized by forceps delivery and by physical trauma.

EXTERNAL EAR

The external ear includes the cartilaginous auricle (pinna), external auditory meatus, and cartilaginous and bony portions of the external auditory canal, terminating at the tympanic membrane (eardrum).

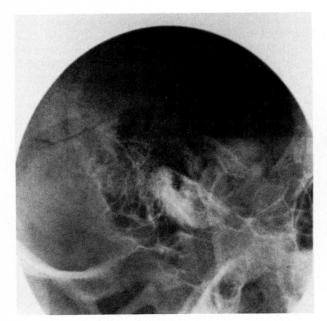

FIG. 1–25. Extensively pneumatized normal mastoid in an adult.

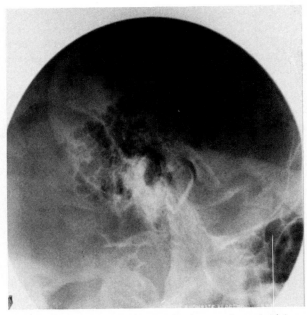
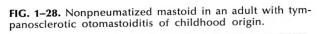

FIG. 1–26. Moderately pneumatized normal mastoid in an adult.

FIG. 1–27. Poor pneumatization; healed childhood otomastoiditis in an adult.

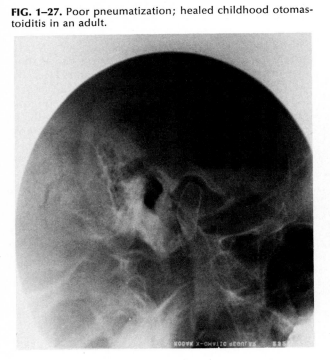

FIG. 1–28. Nonpneumatized mastoid in an adult with tympanosclerotic otomastoiditis of childhood origin.

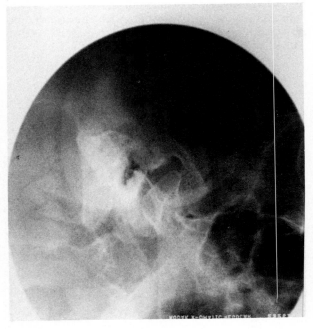

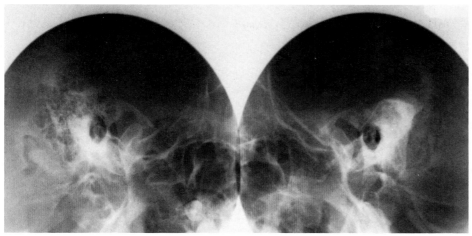

FIG. 1–29. Normal right mastoid cells (Schuller view) and petrosa.

FIG. 1–30. Sclerotic left mastoid and petrosa (Stenver view) in a 12-year-old child with recurrent left otomastoiditis.

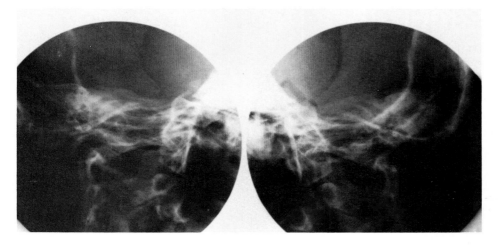

AURICLE AND EXTERNAL AUDITORY MEATUS

ANATOMY

The auricle is formed on the framework of a complex auricular cartilage structure (Fig. 1–31). In the infant and young child the auricle is soft, elastic, and shallow. The helix, and the central portion of the auricle, especially the concha, is relatively large compared to the adult auricle. The lobule is small by comparison (Fig. 1–32).

The lateral superior margin is the helix, which acts as boundary to the enclosure, includes (from posterior to anterior) the scapha, antihelix, triangular fossa, antitragus, concha, and is apposed anteriorly to the external auditory meatus by the tragus. The lobule (noncartilaginous) is the inferior appendage of the auricle. The intertragic notch separates the antitragus from the tragus.

PHYSIOLOGY

The auricle "collects" air-borne sound waves and funnels them with some degree of auditory focusing via the external auditory meatus to the external auditory canal and to the tympanic membrane (TM). Early acousticians recognized the importance of the auricle to human hearing, along with the observations of comparative anatomists. The size of the auricle and its geometric facets were appreciated by the inventors of ancient horns and similar devices. Simple ear cupping, which

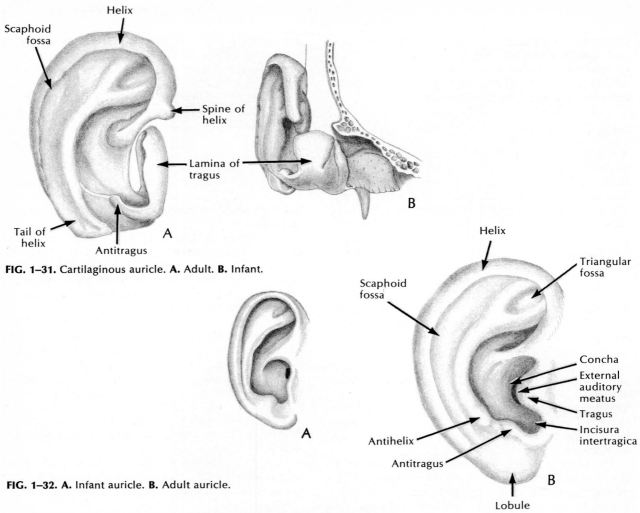

FIG. 1–31. Cartilaginous auricle. **A.** Adult. **B.** Infant.

FIG. 1–32. **A.** Infant auricle. **B.** Adult auricle.

FIG. 1–33. Frontal view of auricle and external auditory meatus and canal.

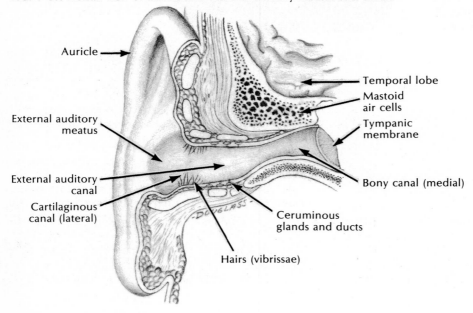

effectively increases the acoustic receptive area and directionality of the auricle, thus improves reception of acoustic energy with varied frequency emphases and is still an important rehabilitation adjunct for several types of hearing loss.

CLINICAL ASPECTS

A number of skin and cartilage lesions can involve auricle and external auditory meatus. These include malformations and dermatologic, neoplastic and traumatic problems, such as eczema, dermatitus, carcinoma, burns, lightning injuries, and other lesions (see Ch. 13, External Ear Diseases).

THE EXTERNAL EAR CANAL

ANATOMY

The cartilaginous external ear canal is the lateral aspect of the external auditory canal (EAC) and is contiguous with the external auditory meatus (Fig. 1–33). This portion contains a thick epithelium and subepithelial stroma with a very rich blood supply, hairs (vibrissas), and a variable number of subcutaneous ceruminal glands (Fig. 1–34). There are significant variations in diameter and shape of the infant and the adult cartilaginous canals, and in the distribution and density of hairs and ceruminal glands.

The bony external canal is basically a portion of the temporal bone. The thin skin lining is intimately attached to the periosteum of the bony canal. In contrast to the cartilaginous canal the bony canal is extremely sensitive to touch. It contains no hairs and no glands. The epithelium of the auricle and the external canal are in contiguity with the epidermal (squamous) layer of the tympanic membrane.

PHYSIOLOGY

Acoustically the external canal can be thought of as similar to a rigid tube 2.5–3 cm long, closed on one end by the tympanic membrane. Part of the acoustic energy reaching the tympanic membrane is reflected, with the consequence that acoustic pressure in the canal is greater than that around the external ear. In the tubelike external canal a resonance similar to that in musical pipes takes place, so that sound pressures are greater for certain frequencies, *i.e.*, those whose wave lengths are multiples of the length of the external ear canal. Comparisons of sound pressures at the external auditory meatus and at the tympanic

membrane show (as predictable by the physical properties of the external canal) that there is a resonance frequency of 3000 Hz, for which there is an increase of more than 10 dB in sound pressure. This increase is the first in a series of transformations made by different parts of the ear in the transmission of sound energy.

CLINICAL ASPECTS

Physical blockade of the EAC by cerumen, foreign bodies, or infectious or neoplastic lesions can produce conductive hearing losses if obstruction is complete.

Differences in elasticity and contour that are present in the auricle also occur in the cartilaginous EAC. Examination of the infant and young child to visualize the bony EAC and tympanic membrane requires posterosuperior elevation of the flexible auricle.

The hairs, wax, and ceruminal glands of the cartilaginous EAC contribute to a number of forms of external otitis (see Ch. 11, Head and Neck Problems and Ear Diseases). Contiguity of the bony EAC posteriorly with the anterior mastoid cortex is responsible for occasional fistulas from mastoid to medial EAC. Contiguity of the bony EAC with the temporomandibular joint anteriorly is related to ear symptoms from temporomandibular joint lesions.

Congenital branchial cleft fistulas and tracts frequently involve both cartilaginous and bony portions of the EAC.

TYMPANIC MEMBRANE, OSSICLES, AND MIDDLE EAR

The tympanic membrane separates the EAC from the middle ear (ME). The middle ear (tympanum) is an air-containing space within the temporal bone, contiguous anteroinferiorly with the eustachian tube and nasopharynx, and posteriorly with the air cell systems of the mastoid and petrous portions of the temporal bone.

TYMPANIC MEMBRANE

ANATOMY

The tympanic membrane (eardrum; membrana tympani) is a membranous structure with two bony attachments (Fig. 1–35). This cone-shaped membrane has 1) a fixed circumferential annular attachment to the bony tympanic ring, and 2) a

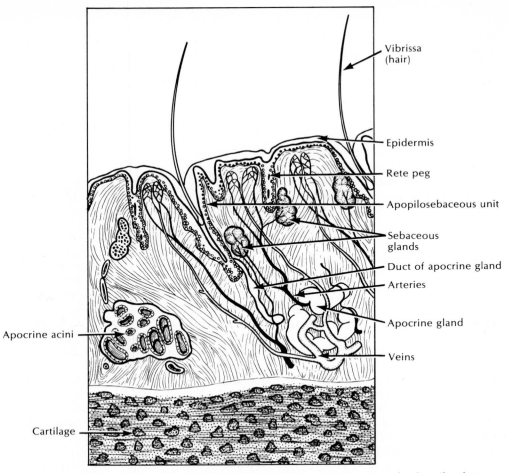

FIG. 1–34. Cartilaginous external canal skin with apocrine and sebaceous glands, pilosebaceous units, and vibrissas (hairs). (Adapted from Senturia BH: Diseases of the External Ear. Springfield, Ill, Charles C Thomas, 1957)

FIG. 1–35. Tympanic membrane landmarks. The long crus of the incus **(left)** is visible only through a translucent TM.

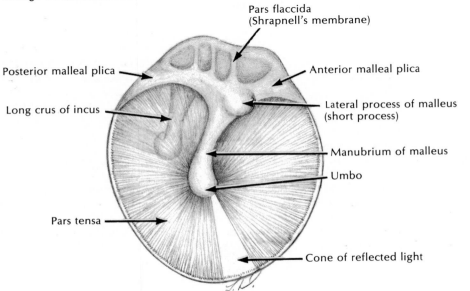

FIG. 1–36. Frontal view of tympanic membrane and middle ear relationships. The **heavy dashes** demarcate the mesotympanum.

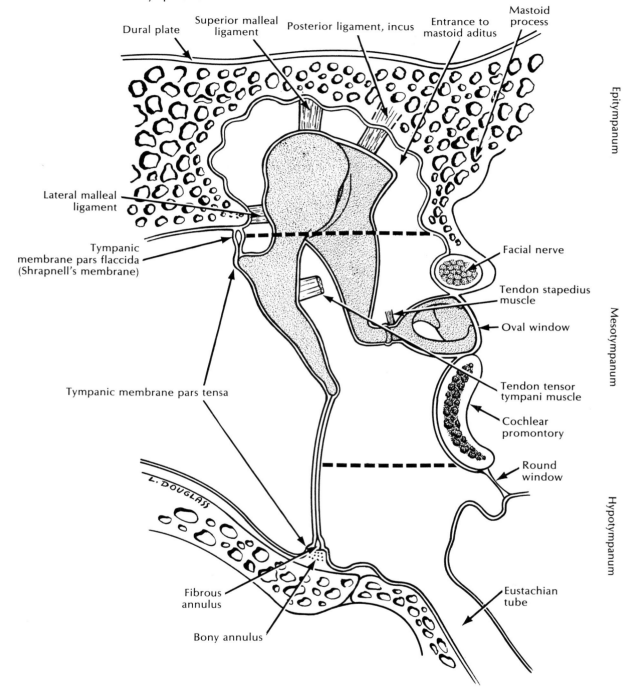

Dural plate

Superior malleal ligament

Posterior ligament, incus

Entrance to mastoid aditus

Mastoid process

Epitympanum

Lateral malleal ligament

Tympanic membrane pars flaccida (Shrapnell's membrane)

Facial nerve

Tendon stapedius muscle

Oval window

Mesotympanum

Tympanic membrane pars tensa

Tendon tensor tympani muscle

Cochlear promontory

Round window

L. DOUGLASS

Hypotympanum

Fibrous annulus

Eustachian tube

Bony annulus

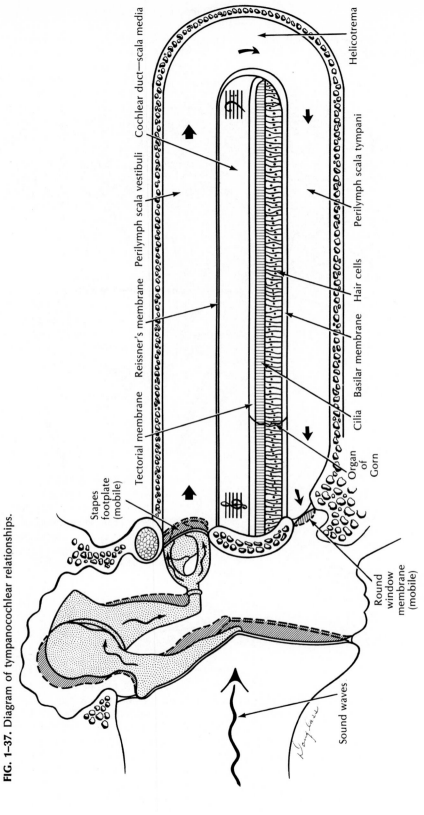

FIG. 1-37. Diagram of tympanocochlear relationships.

Helicotrema

Cochlear duct—scala media

Perilymph scala tympani

Perilymph scala vestibuli

Reissner's membrane

Hair cells

Tectorial membrane

Basilar membrane

Cilia

Organ
of
Gorn

Stapes
footplate
(mobile)

Round
window
membrane
(mobile)

Sound waves

central attachment to the manubrium and short process of the malleus. The umbo of the malleal manubrium is the medial apex of the tympanic membrane (TM) cone (Fig. 1–36).

The major portion of the TM is the pars tensa, which is separated from the small superior portion known as pars flaccida (Shrapnell's membrane) by an anterior malleal plica (fold) and a posterior malleal plica that extend laterally from the malleal short (lateral) process. The malleal short process and umbo are the two chief clinical TM landmarks.

The pars tensa is normally translucent, occasionally permitting visualization of the incus long process and the incudostapedial joint through the posterior TM region. Three histologic layers comprise the TM: an outer (squamous), a middle (fibrous), and a medial (mucous membrane) layer.

The TM measures approximately 9 mm in diameter with radii varying from 4–5 mm. The large tensor tympani muscle attaches to the malleal manubrium and maintains a variable tension on the tympanic membrane. In addition, there are superior, anterior, posterior, and mediolateral suspensory ligamentous attachments to the malleus and incus.

PHYSIOLOGY

The many complex functions of the tympanic membrane constitute facets of numerous physiological measurements. It is not only a conelike lateral acoustic receptive diaphragm, but it is also balanced medially by the "loading force" of the intravestibular fluid system (Fig. 1–37) as transmitted from perilymph in the scala vestibuli through the stapes footplate, crura, incudostapedial joint, incus, incudomalleal joint, and malleal manubrium to the TM. The tension of the tensor tympani muscle and, to a lesser degree, that of the stapedius muscle contribute regulatory roles to TM mobility.

The most sensitive region of the TM is located below the insertion of the umbo—the area that starts vibrating in response to the faintest sound. As the sound pressure increases, the vibration amplitude increases, and the vibration area of the TM increases also, in a concentric manner (Fig. 1–38). The pattern of motion is more complex during vibrations induced by high-frequency sounds. The membrane vibrates in sections, each one vibrating at the same frequency but with different patterns. All frequency vibrations are transmitted to the long process of the malleus

(manubrium), to the incus, and finally to the stapes, which transmits airborne acoustic energy to the inner ear fluid system.

An area of 55 sq mm out of the total 85 sq mm of the TM is tightly connected to the manubrium. The surface area of the stapedial footplate is 3.2 sq mm. Thus there is a pressure increase of approximately 17 times as a result of differences in areas.

Recent advances in impedance audiometry and tympanometry make it possible to measure and record TM mobility, and other important physical characteristics of the tympanic membrane and the ME for the transmission of sound.

CLINICAL ASPECTS

Tympanic membrane perforations produce variable conductive hearing losses, depending upon size, location, and relationship to ME structures. Tympanic membrane fixations, retractions, atelectases, and many other lesions constitute components of a number of tympanomastoid diseases.

THE OSSICLES

MALLEUS

The malleus consists of a head, neck, and three processes: the manubrium into which the TM is inserted (Fig. 1–39), the anterior process (usually vestigial), and the lateral (short) process. The lateral process constitutes a diagnostic landmark in otoscopy. The malleal head, which occupies a major portion of the epitympanum (attic), is supported by ligaments, which may become ossified and create primary fixation of the malleus and the TM (see Ch. 20, Lateral Ossicular Fixation).

INCUS

The incus consists of a body, a long process, and a short process. The body articulates with the head of the malleus, forming the incudomalleal joint. The short process projects into the posteroinferior portion of the epitympanic recess. In this position it can be seen from a mastoid view as a landmark in mastoidectomy. The long process descends behind (posterior) and parallel to the malleal manubrium and, turning medially, ends in a rounded termination, the lenticular process, which articulates with the head (capitulum) of the stapes (the incudostapedial joint). This lenticular process frequently atrophies or becomes necrotic in chronic otitis media, producing ossicular discontinuity and a conductive hearing loss.

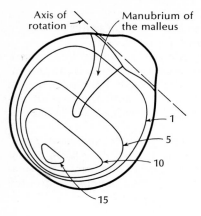

FIG. 1–38. Equal amplitude curves for eardrum vibrations at frequencies below 2000 cps. (Bekesy G von: Experiments in Hearing. New York, McGraw-Hill Book Company, 1960. Used with permission of McGraw-Hill Book Company)

FIG. 1–39. Morphologic features of the three ossicles. **A.** Malleus (two views). **B.** Incus (two views). **C.** Stapes. **D.** The three ossicles in relation to each other.

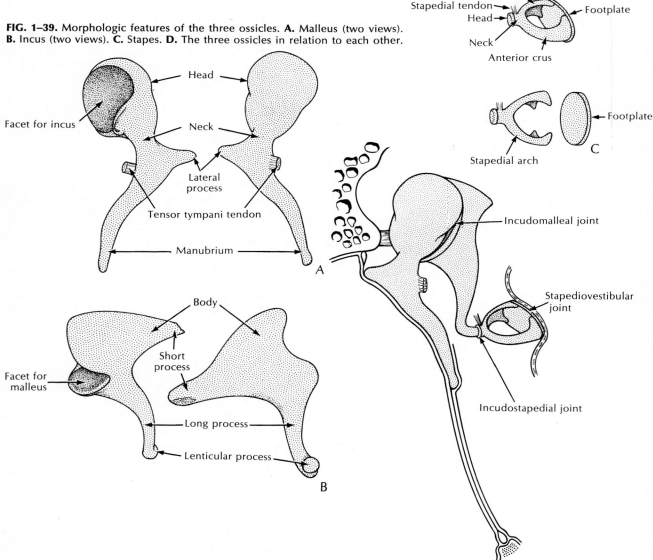

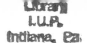
STAPES

The stapes, the smallest bone in the body, consists of a head (capitulum), which articulates with the incus at the incudostapedial joint, a neck, two crura or legs, and the footplate. The head, neck, and crura form the stapedial arch (sometimes inaccurately called "superstructure"), which is attached to the footplate. The stapedial footplate becomes fixed in otosclerosis, a very common cause of conductive hearing loss (see Ch. 19, Otosclerosis).

The head and neck of the arch resemble malleus and incus and consist of marrow bone. The somewhat fragile crura consist of semicylindrical shells of cortical bone. The partly hollow crura form the boundaries of the obturator (stapedial) artery, which occupies this space in fetal life but which occasionally persists, producing a conductive hearing loss and tinnitus. It may coexist with otosclerosis.

PHYSIOLOGY

The ossicular chain functions normally as a unit (the ossicular joints remaining relatively immobile) (Figs. 1–40, 1–41), as the component of a loaded lever system, communicating energy from the TM to the oval window via the stapedial footplate. During motion, the stapes (placed at a relative right-angle position to the long process of the incus) moves like a piston over the oval window. The displacement of the manubrium at the tympanic membrane sets the rest of the ossicular chain, working as a unit, into vibration. The motion of the ossicular chain can be thought of as

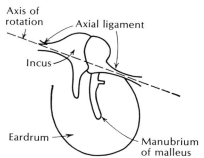

FIG. 1–41. Lateral view of eardrum and ossicles, showing axis of rotation. (From Bekesy G von: Experiments in Hearing. New York, McGraw-Hill Book Company, 1960, p 102. Used with permission of McGraw-Hill Book Company)

being identical to that of a rigid angled bar pivoted to the walls of the ME by the anterior malleal and the posterior incudal ligaments. It works in a manner similar to that of a mechanical lever, with the characteristic that the malleal arm is shorter than the arm formed by the long process of the incus and stapes (Fig. 1–42). An advantageous ratio in the length of the lever arms produces a mechanical gain, making the force at the stapes 1.3 times greater than at the manubrium. The total pressure transformation in the middle ear is the sum of that due to the difference in areas of the tympanic membrane and the stapedial footplate (piston mechanism) and the lever ratio mechanism. This has a total value of 20–25, corresponding to an increase in the intensity of sound to almost 30 dB. This gain, however, is necessary to overcome the loss of acoustic energy resulting from the transfer of energy from air to the fluids in the inner ear.

THE TYMPANUM

ANATOMY

The tympanum (tympanic cavity, middle ear) is divided topographically into the epitympanum, the mesotympanum, and hypotympanum. These anatomic divisions relate to many clinical lesions.

Epitympanum (Attic)

The epitympanum houses the incudomalleal joint, the head of the malleus, and the body of the incus with their suspensory ligaments. The epitympanic air space is in direct contiguity anteriorly with the zygomatic air-cell system and is bounded superiorly by the tegmen tympani, the relatively thin bony plate separating the middle ear from temporal lobe dura in the middle cranial fossa. The

FIG. 1–40. Cross-sectional view of eardrum. (Bekesy G von: Experiments in Hearing. New York, McGraw-Hill Book Company, 1960, p 101. Used with permission of McGraw-Hill Book Company)

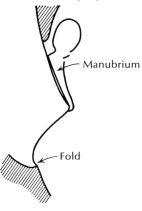

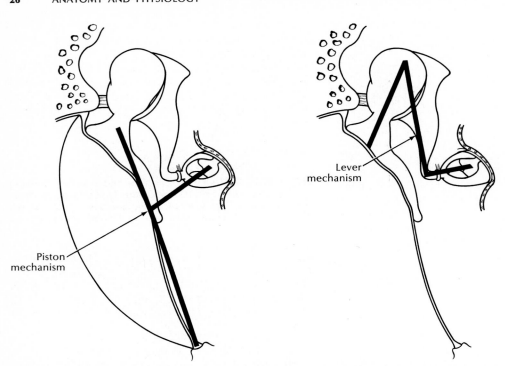

Piston
mechanism

Lever
mechanism

FIG. 1–42. Middle ear function is to conduct airborne sound energy to inner-ear fluid system. The piston mechanism and lever mechanism combine to increase sound intensity by as much as 30 dB. Schematic views.

FIG. 1–43. Section of right ear at epitympanum (attic level); note malleus, horizontal seventh nerve course, cochlea, and contents of vestibule. **1.** Mastoid air cells and trabeculas. **2.** Malleus in epitympanum. **3.** Facial (VII) nerve in horizontal course. **4.** Cochlea. **5.** Cochlear nerve. **6.** Vestibule, containing utricle, horizontal ampulla, and canal; saccule; posterior semicircular canal. **7.** Internal auditory canal. **8.** Vestibular nerve. **9.** Endolymphatic sac in vestibular duct. (Courtesy of Dr. R. Gussen)

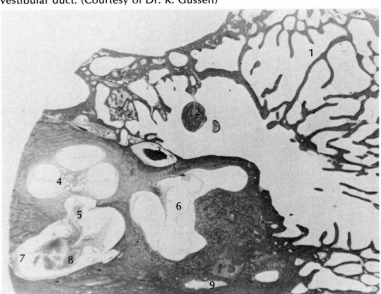

epitympanic air space communicates posteriorly through the aditus ad antrum with the mastoid air cell system via the primary major cell—the mastoid "antrum." The superior semicircular canal is in medial wall relationship, and the anterior portions of horizontal semicircular canal and the horizontal portion of the facial bony canal constitute medioposterior limits (Fig. 1–43). Laterally, it is bounded by pars flaccida (Shrapnell's membrane) of the TM, and by the external bony attic wall (scutum). The epitympanum is frequently the location of keratoma (cholesteatoma), a special form of chronic otomastoiditis.

Mesotympanum (Middle Ear)

The mesotympanum is the major part of the ME space. Laterally the TM pars tensa separates it from the external auditory canal. Contained within the mesotympanum are the neck and manubrium of the malleus, the long process of the incus, the stapes and its oval window, and the round window niche. The horizontal portion of the facial nerve (VII N.), which is usually but not always protected by a bony canal, forms the superomedial boundary of the mesotympanum; it is also the superior boundary of the oval window niche.

The oval window niche is normally occupied by the stapes (Fig. 1–44). The medial boundary of the oval window niche is the stapedial footplate and its annular ligament, providing normally a sealed and mobile communication between the mesotympanic ME space and the perilymph-filled vestibule (scala vestibuli) of the labyrinth. The normally mobile bony stapedial footplate (1.75 × 3.75 mm) (Fig. 1–45), framed by a flexible "water tight" annular ligament, is the medial end of the ossicular system that conducts amplified acoustic energy from the TM to the perilymph system of the cochlea. Airborne sound is thus converted to "water-borne" sound to proceed as a traveling wave through the perilymph system of the cochlea. Acoustic information is thus transmitted to the organ of Corti and its hair cells, to be further processed in the form of bioelectric signals to cochlear nuclei and to components of the central auditory nervous system.

The cochlear promontory of the otic capsule is a rounded, smooth, bony surface forming one-third of the medial wall of the mesotympanum, and separates the oval window niche from the round window niche. The lower portion of the promontory forms the lower level of the mesotympanum, and the upper part of the hypotympanum.

The anterior portion of the mesotympanum joins with the anterior epitympanum to form the protympanum (Fig. 1–46) the tubotympanic funnel, to communicate with the cartilaginous eustachian tube (Fig. 1–47).

Hypotympanum—Floor of Middle Ear Space

The hypotympanum is the lowest level or floor of the ME space, which communicates with hypotympanic and retrofacial pneumatic cell systems anteriorly and posteriorly. Its floor is the bony dome of the jugular bulb.

The round window niche is inferoposterior to the promontory, a somewhat tortuous cavelike structure, in which is inserted the round-window membrane (secondary TM) in its anterosuperior portion. The round-window membrane is a cone-shaped vibratile structure, well protected deep within the upper part of its bony niche (Fig. 1–48). It has no ossicular connections but is in contact laterally with ME air space, and medially with scala tympani perilymph. It is in close proximity to the labyrinthine opening of the cochlear aqueduct, a partly open conduit for cerebrospinal fluid (CSF) from the subarachnoid space to a variable interface relationship with scala tympani perilymph (see Ch. 37, Sudden Hearing Loss Syndrome). These intricate relationships between middle ear, round-window membrane, perilymph

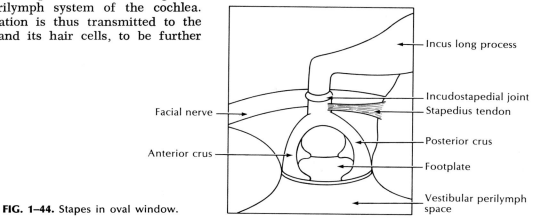

FIG. 1–44. Stapes in oval window.

- Incus long process
- Incudostapedial joint
- Stapedius tendon
- Facial nerve
- Posterior crus
- Anterior crus
- Footplate
- Vestibular perilymph space

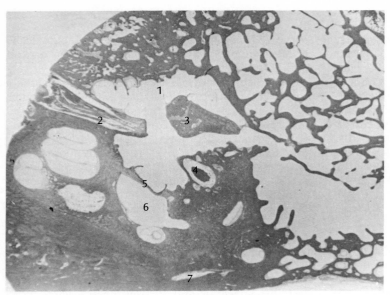

FIG. 1–45. Section of right ear with stapes footplate, incudomalleal joint, facial (VII) nerve, vestibule, and mesotympanic relationships. **1.** Middle ear. **2.** Tensor tympani muscle. **3.** Incudomalleal joint. **4.** Facial nerve. **5.** Stapes footplate with crural stumps. **6.** Vestibule. **7.** Endolymphatic sac in vestibular aqueduct. (Courtesy of Dr. R. Gussen)

FIG. 1–46. Section of left ear, showing relationship of parts. **1.** External auditory canal. **2.** Middle ear. **3.** Protympanum. **4.** Eustachian tube at entrance to middle ear. **5.** Tympanic membrane attached to malleal manubrium. **6.** Internal carotid artery. **7.** Chorda tympani. **8.** Cochlea. **9.** Stapedius tendon, attaching to posterior stapes crus. **10.** Facial nerve. **11.** Vestibule. **12.** Mastoid antrum. **13.** Internal auditory canal. Note proximity of eustachian tube to carotid. (Courtesy of Dr. R. Gussen)

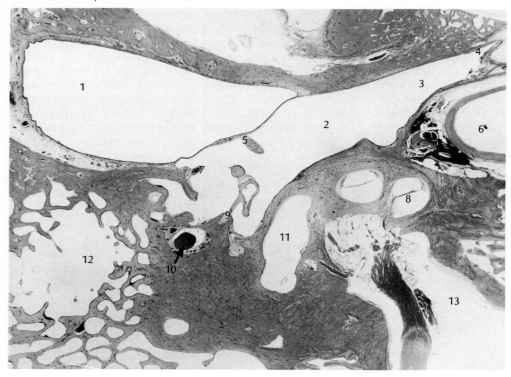

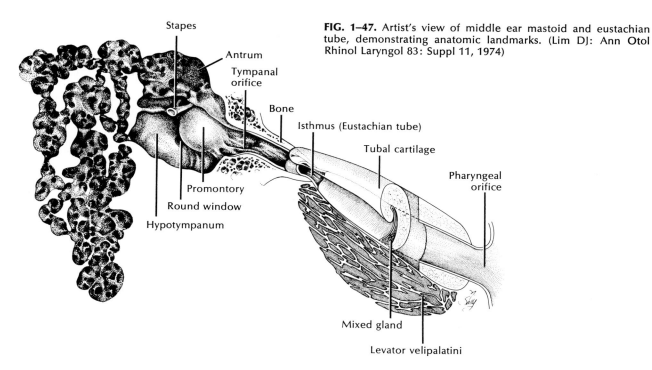

FIG. 1–47. Artist's view of middle ear mastoid and eustachian tube, demonstrating anatomic landmarks. (Lim DJ: Ann Otol Rhinol Laryngol 83: Suppl 11, 1974)

Stapes

Antrum

Tympanal orifice

Bone

Isthmus (Eustachian tube)

Tubal cartilage

Pharyngeal orifice

Promontory

Round window

Hypotympanum

Mixed gland

Levator velipalatini

FIG. 1–48. Section of right ear, emphasizing relationships of round window niche and membrane, scala tympani, and posterior semicircular canal and ampulla. **1.** External auditory canal. **2.** Ceruminal glands. **3.** Lower portion of tympanic membrane. **4.** Cochlear hook region. **5.** Scala tympani. **6.** Chorda tympani nerve. **7.** Round window membrane. **8.** Facial nerve recess. **9.** Cochlear aqueduct. **10.** Round window niche. **11.** Sinus tympani. **12.** Stapedius muscle. **13.** Facial nerve in its vertical course through mastoid. **14.** Posterior ampulla and semicircular canal. **15.** Mastoid antrum. **16.** Vestibular aqueduct with its endolymphatic sac. (Courtesy of Dr. R. Gussen)

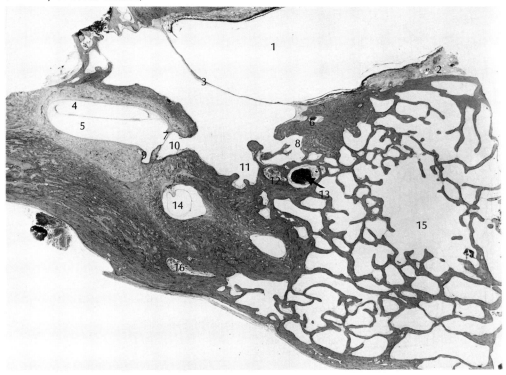

system, and the CSF system are of significant clinical importance (see Ch. 37).

Intratympanic Structures

The facial nerve (Fig. 1–49) enters the internal auditory meatus with the eighth nerve. The bony facial canal through which the facial (VII N) cranial nerve transverses the ME forms part of the medial ME wall above the oval window. The facial nerve (Fig. 1–50) in its bony canal leaves the geniculate region via the upper (anterior) genu, enters the upper mesotympanum and leaves the middle ear via the lower (posterior) genu to course through the vertical fallopian canal within the mastoid and finally emerge into the upper neck through the stylomastoid foramen. (For further details of seventh nerve anatomy, see Chapter 28, Seventh Nerve Diagnostic Techniques.)

The two tympanic muscles lie within the mesotympanum. The stapedius muscle, arising from the pyramidal eminence and attached to the neck of the stapes, is primarily responsible for the im-portant **acoustic reflex,** which can be elicited and measured for diagnostic purposes. Among its roles is a protective function, mitigating the effect of very loud sounds upon the cochlea. The tensor tympani muscle arises from within a canal parallel to the eustachian tube and courses posteriorly to a bony eminence, the *processus cochleariformis* (overlying the bony canal of the facial nerve in its intratympanic portion). At this point the tendon of the tensor tympani muscle makes a right-angle turn laterally to insert upon the base of malleal manubrium. It plays an important part in variations of TM tensions (Figs. 1–51, 1–52).

The eustachian tube connects the nasopharynx and all of its adenexas with the ME (Fig. 1–53). It's upper (tympanic) orifice lies within the mesotympanum, a rather spacious bony channel (protympanum) arising high on the anteromedial wall of the tympanic cavity. The tympanic portion of the eustachian tube is bony and rigid, shaped like a cone pointing inferoanteriorly. At the apex of the cone is the isthmus of the eustachian tube.

FIG. 1–49. Schematic drawing of facial (VII) nerve pathway from origins in precentral gyri to pontine nuclei, through internal auditory canal, middle ear, and mastoid to exit at stylomastoid foramen.

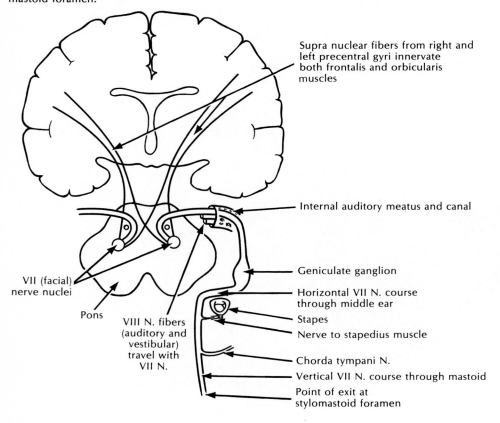

Supra nuclear fibers from right and left precentral gyri innervate both frontalis and orbicularis muscles

Internal auditory meatus and canal

VII (facial) nerve nuclei

Pons

VIII N. fibers (auditory and vestibular) travel with VII N.

Geniculate ganglion

Horizontal VII N. course through middle ear

Stapes

Nerve to stapedius muscle

Chorda tympani N.

Vertical VII N. course through mastoid

Point of exit at stylomastoid foramen

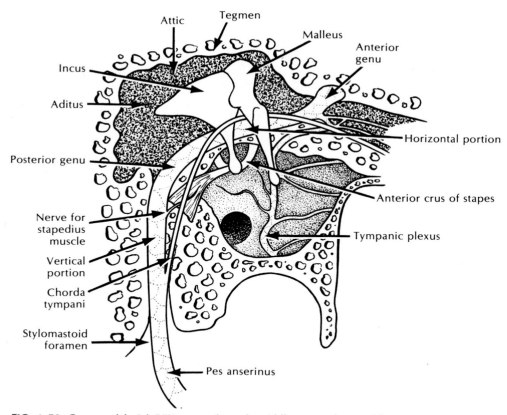

FIG. 1–50. Course of facial (VII) nerve through middle ear and mastoid.

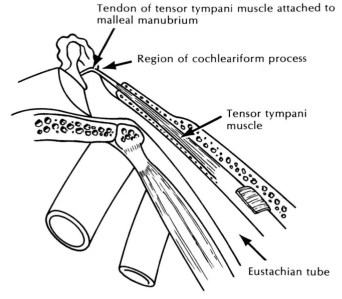

FIG. 1–51. Tensor tympani muscle and tendon.

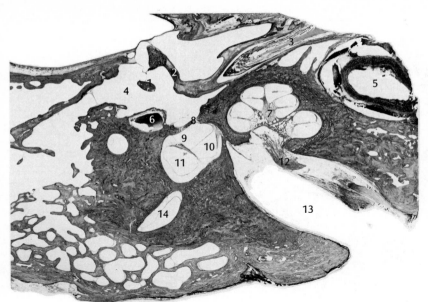

FIG. 1–52. Left ear section, showing mid-modiolar cochlear region with auditory branch of eighth nerve, internal auditory canal and meatus. Note saccular and utricular maculas and crus osseum commune. 1. Incus. 2. Tensor tympani tendon attached to malleus neck. 3. Tensor tympani muscle. 4. Middle ear. 5. Internal carotid artery. 6. Facial nerve. 7. Mid-modiolar cochlear region. 8. Stapes footplate. 9. Vestibule. 10. Saccule with macula. 11. Utricle with macula. 12. Cochlear (VIII) nerve. 13. Internal auditory canal and meatus. 14. Crus osseum commune. (Courtesy of Dr. R. Gussen)

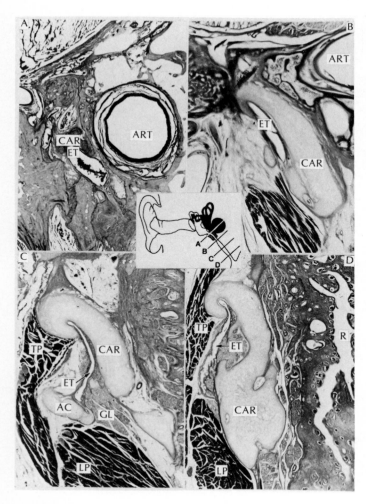

FIG. 1–53. A. Cross-sectional view of human eustachian tube (ET), showing bony part next to carotid artery (ART). Remnant of tubal cartilage (CAR) is still seen in this area. B. Near tubal isthmus at cartilaginous portion (CAR) of eustachian tube (ET). Carotid artery (ART). C. Cartilaginous portion of eustachian tube (ET), showing tubal cartilage (CAR), accessory cartilage (AC), and tubal glands (GL). Tensor velipalatini (TP); levator velipalatini (LP). D. Pharyngeal end of tube (ET) shows thickening of tubal cartilage (CAR). Rosenmuller's fossa (R). Insert. Level of histologic section represented by the four parts A, B, C, D. (Hematoxylin and eosin, × 6) (Lim DJ: Ann Otol Rhinol Laryngol 83: Suppl 11, 1974)

Inferior to the isthmus, the membranous and cartilaginous eustachian tube becomes slitlike in form. Superomedially, it is surrounded by a cartilage, to which are attached two important muscles, the tensor palati, laterally, and the levator palati, medially. These muscles, which are related to soft palate motion also function in regulation of the eustachian tube lumen. The eustachian tube is normally closed but opens with swallowing, yawning, and palatal elevation. In so doing, it acts periodically to equalize intratympanic and external air pressures.

The mucosa of the eustachian tube and ME represents a complex mucociliary mechanism of enormous significance in ME and mastoid disease, especially in secretory otitis media. Ciliated, secretory, and nonsecretory cells play major roles in middle ear physiology, with serious sequelae following cytologic malfunctions (Figs. 1–54, 1–55).

PHYSIOLOGY

The reception of sound in the inner ear is limited by the impedance (resistance) offered by the middle- and inner-ear structures to the transmission of pressure waves. Acoustic impedance is defined as the ratio of the pressure to the velocity of motion of the vibrating medium. Therefore, the greater the impedance, the more pressure is necessary to produce a displacement of the ear structures at a given velocity. Changes in the structures which change the acoustic impedance could result in specific changes in the ear function, depending on the frequency of sound.

The displacement of bodies is usually hindered by forces dependent on three properties of matter: elasticity, friction, and inertia. The influence of these forces is different for different sound frequencies. An elastic force (its springlike property) is proportional to the displacement of the body. Changes in the ear structures that increase stiffness affect the transmission of low frequencies much more than high frequencies. To maintain an equal velocity, the displacement of a body must increase as the frequency of oscillation is decreased. Changes resulting in an increase in mass produce an increase in the force necessary to overcome the opposing inertial force for the displacement of the body. The impedance change due to increase in mass is greater, the higher the frequency of sound, thus affecting high-frequency transmission. Frictional forces are proportional to the velocity of displacement and consequently the change in impedance due to increase in this force is independent of sound frequencies.

Absolute estimates of ME impedance have been obtained in experiments on animal and human temporal bones, where it has been found that the combined effect of the restraining forces of the ear structures for the transmission of sound is such that a constant sound pressure level at the tympanic membrane produces a constant stapes displacement for low frequencies of sound up to approximately 1000 Hz and then decays in proportion to the increase in frequency (27, 35). Unfortunately, techniques to evaluate absolute values of impedance are too complicated for clinical practical use. More successful has been the application of techniques using relative measures in impedance. Such techniques make a comparison of impedance at different frequencies of sound, with the objective of determining whether the relative contribution of any of the impedance components, *i.e.*, friction, elasticity, or inertia, have changed. Clinically, however, changes in impedance of the ear are due to a combination of changes in several of the restraining forces. Only exceptionally, as in ME ossicle fixation (malleoincudal ankylosis) is the result a definitive increase in stiffness. Opposite changes are seen in cases of ME discontinuity (incus or stapes necrosis), in which case the tympanic membrane becomes abnormally mobile.

The technique of dynamic ME impedance measurement takes advantage of impedance changes that result when 1) middle ear muscles contract, 2) the eustachian tube opens, or 3) the displacement of the tympanic membrane is modulated by changing the static pressure in the ME. These dynamic changes do not take place if the ME reflexes are absent, if the ME is filled with blood or serous fluid, or if there is reabsorption of air with resultant large negative pressure in the ME. These impedance measurement techniques have considerably increased the differential diagnostic capabilities of clinical audiometry (see Ch. 7, Acoustic Impedance Tests).

THE INNER EAR (COCHLEAR AND VESTIBULAR LABYRINTHS)

The inner ear is a neuromembranous labyrinthine structure within the osseous otic capsule of the petrous pyramid (Fig. 1–56). The bony labyrinth that houses the membranous labyrinth is in medial relationship to the medial bony wall of the ME, with which it communicates via two "windows" (Fig. 1–57): the oval window covered by the mobile stapedial footplate, and the round window

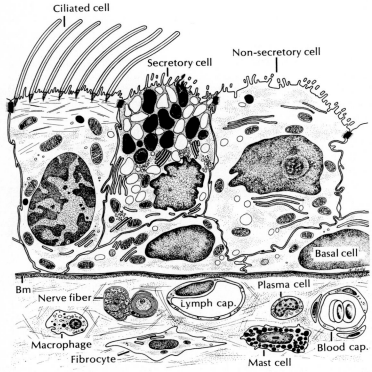

FIG. 1–54. Middle ear mucosal cells. (Lim D: Ann Otol Rhinol Laryngol 83: Suppl 11, 1974)

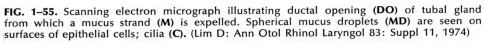

FIG. 1–55. Scanning electron micrograph illustrating ductal opening **(DO)** of tubal gland from which a mucus strand **(M)** is expelled. Spherical mucus droplets **(MD)** are seen on surfaces of epithelial cells; cilia **(C)**. (Lim D: Ann Otol Rhinol Laryngol 83: Suppl 11, 1974)

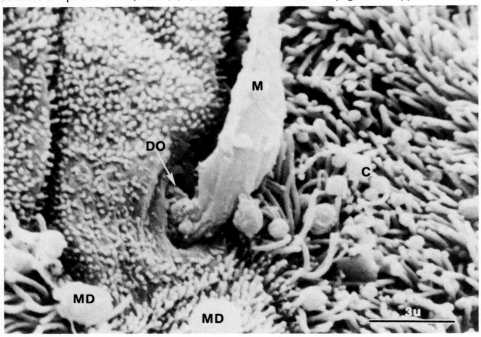

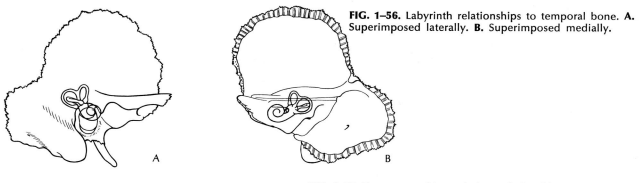

FIG. 1–56. Labyrinth relationships to temporal bone. **A.** Superimposed laterally. **B.** Superimposed medially.

A   B

FIG. 1–57. Tympanocochlear window relationships.

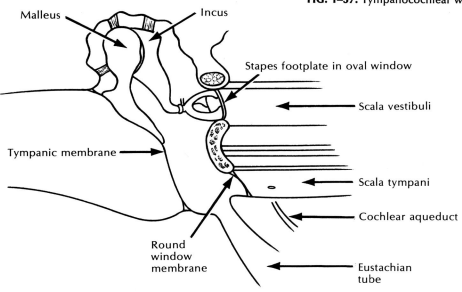

Malleus

Incus

Stapes footplate in oval window

Scala vestibuli

Tympanic membrane

Scala tympani

Cochlear aqueduct

Round window membrane

Eustachian tube

FIG. 1–58. Inner ear, schematic view.

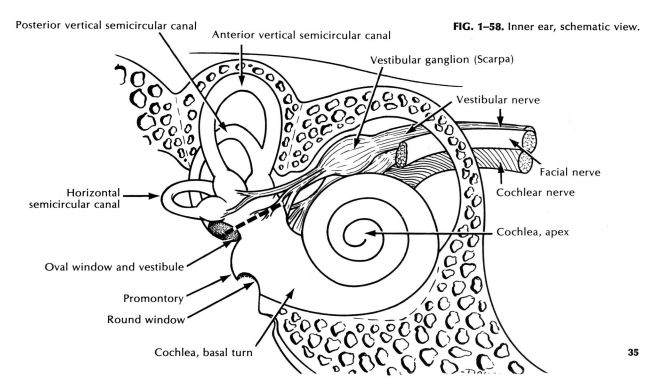

Posterior vertical semicircular canal

Anterior vertical semicircular canal

Vestibular ganglion (Scarpa)

Vestibular nerve

Horizontal semicircular canal

Facial nerve

Cochlear nerve

Cochlea, apex

Oval window and vestibule

Promontory

Round window

Cochlea, basal turn

35

covered by the round-window membrane (Fig. 1–58). The term **labyrinth** refers anatomically to the entire inner ear mechanism and includes two principal portions, the vestibule and semicircular canals superoposteriorly, and the cochlea inferoanteriorly (Fig. 1–59). It is common clinical practice to use the noun "labyrinth" and the adjective "labyrinthine," with special reference to the vestibular or equilibrium portion (pars superoposterior) of the inner ear.

The bony labyrinth is a complex of interconnected bony excavations within the ivory hard bone of the otic capsule (Fig. 1–60). Its central bony cavern is the vestibule, which connects with the semicircular canals above and posteriorly and the cochlea anteriorly.

The three semicircular hollow canals are arranged in three mutually perpendicular planes of space, horizontal (lateral), anterior vertical (superior), and posterior vertical (inferior). Each canal resembles a semicircular arc. The horizontal (lateral) canal joins the vestibule at each terminal end. The two vertical canals join to form a common duct, the crus commune, with individual anterior and posterior entrances. Thus, instead of six communications for the three canals with the vestibule, there are five. Each canal has one sense organ in its ampullary region, a total of three ampullas. Anteriorly, the bony vestibule connects with the bony snail-like excavations of the cochlea. The first (basal) portion of the cochlea, known as the "hook," begins immediately inferior to the vestibule. Its long course traverses anteriorly and

bends superiorly, rolled into a three-dimensional ascending spiral of 2.5 turns, around the central modiolus. These turns become smaller toward the apex, and the cochlear spiral points in an anterolateral direction (Figs. 1–61, 1–62).

Perilymph fills the three bony semicircular canals, the vestibule, the scala vestibuli, and scala tympani of the cochlea. Scala tympani perilymph is in intimate contiguity with the subarachnoid space CSF through the cochlear aqueduct, which in most instances is filled with a loose net of fibrous tissue.

Within the perilymphatic space there is another series of membranous cavities known as the endolymphatic system (Fig. 1–63), for the most part molded to the shape of the perilymphatic space. Three main areas are formed, the utricle and semicircular canals, the sacculus and cochlear duct, and lastly the endolymphatic duct and sac. The membranes of this system of cavities at different locations show areas of differentiation corresponding to the receptor organs. The membranous cochlea holds the organ of Corti for the transduction of sound energy. The utricle, semicircular canals and sacculus constitute the membranous vestibular labyrinth proper, which contains the receptor organs for sense of motion and position.

The fluids in the endolymphatic system have a high potassium concentration: $[K^+] = 144$ mEq/liter; and a low sodium concentration: $[Na^+] = 5$ mEq/liter. The opposite is true for the perilymphatic fluids, which have a low potassium concentration: $[K^+] = 10$ mEq/liter, and a high sodium concentration: $[Na^+] = 140$ mEq/liter.

The concentration of proteins in the endolymph is 127 mg/100 ml; in the perilymph it is approxi-

FIG. 1–59. Cochleovestibular system and basic innervation.

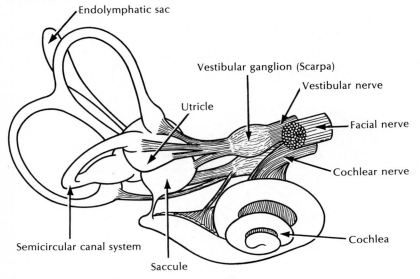

Endolymphatic sac

Vestibular ganglion (Scarpa)

Vestibular nerve

Utricle

Facial nerve

Cochlear nerve

Semicircular canal system

Cochlea

Saccule

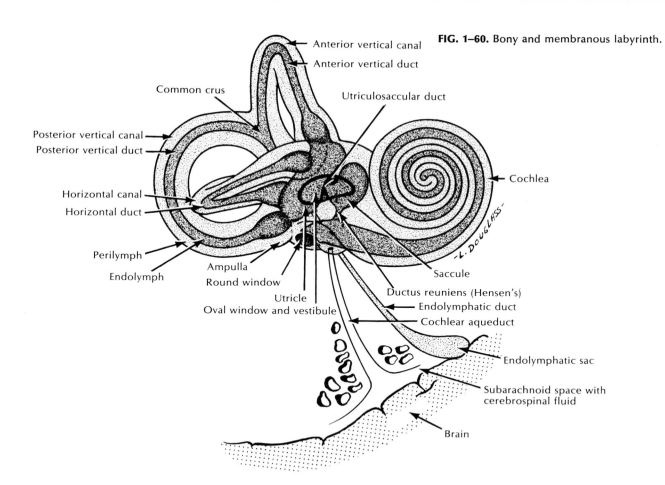

FIG. 1–60. Bony and membranous labyrinth.

Anterior vertical canal
Anterior vertical duct
Common crus
Utriculosaccular duct
Posterior vertical canal
Posterior vertical duct
Cochlea
Horizontal canal
Horizontal duct
-L. DOUGLASS-
Perilymph
Endolymph
Ampulla
Round window
Saccule
Utricle
Oval window and vestibule
Ductus reuniens (Hensen's)
Endolymphatic duct
Cochlear aqueduct
Endolymphatic sac
Subarachnoid space with cerebrospinal fluid
Brain

FIG. 1–61. Adult human cochlea, showing modiolus with osseous spiral lamina and myelinated nerve bundles. The bony capsule, spiral ligament, and Reissner's membrane have been removed. The basal end of osseous spiral lamina is set right, and the lower basal coil extends to left. Above it, the middle and apical coils are exposed. The cochlear aqueduct is shown lying opened. (× 13) (Bredberg G: Acta Otolaryngol Suppl 236:36, 1968)

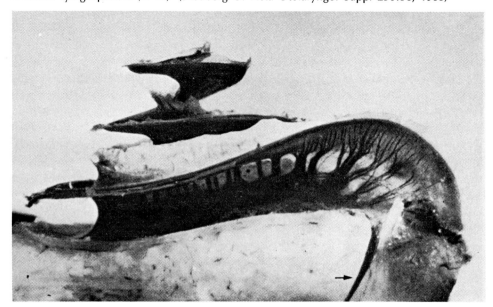

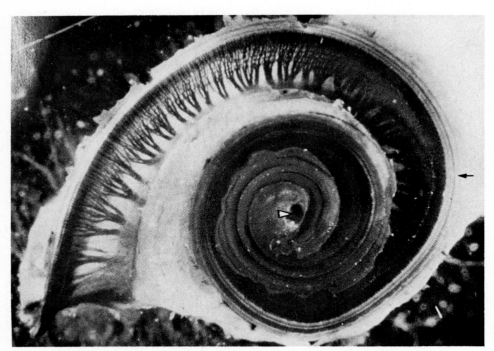

FIG. 1–62. Human cochlea seen from above. Myelinated nerve bundles within osseous spiral lamina are in lower basal coil. The organ of Corti **(black arrow)** is at peripheral margin of osseous spiral lamina. The helicotrema is at center **(white arrow).** ($\times$ 13) (Bredberg G: Acta Otolaryngol Suppl 236:37, 1968)

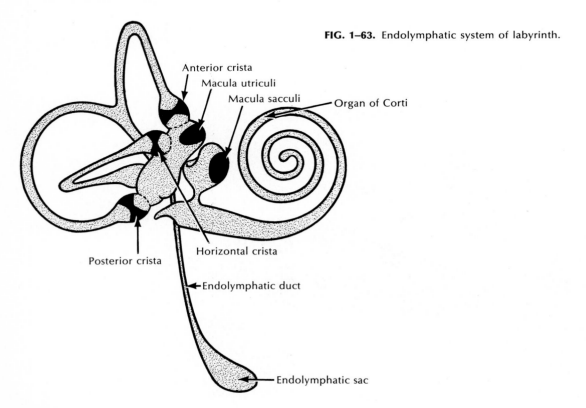

FIG. 1–63. Endolymphatic system of labyrinth.

Anterior crista
Macula utriculi
Macula sacculi
Organ of Corti
Posterior crista
Horizontal crista
Endolymphatic duct
Endolymphatic sac

mately 300 mg/160 ml. These figures are different from that of the concentration of protein in CSF, which is about 35 mg/100 ml.

The origin of the inner ear fluids is not yet well established. The perilymph is thought to represent in part a filtration of CSF and a secretory process from blood vessels in the ear. The most likely sources for the production of endolymph are the secretory cells in the stria vascularis and the dark cells of the vestibular labyrinth. The reabsorbtion of endolymph is generally thought to take place in the endolymphatic sac.

GENERAL CELLULAR CHARACTERISTICS OF LABYRINTHINE SENSORY RECEPTORS

The principal anatomic features of the sensory receptors, the hair cells, are already developed in invertebrates (33). They are found surrounded by supporting cells in specialized epithelial areas in the walls of the receptor organs. They have a distal flat portion that is provided with a hair bundle of nonmotile cilia which protrudes from its surface. The basal portion of the cell makes contact with many dendritic terminals of afferent nerve fibers, by means of which information is sent from the receptor to the central nervous system, and with dendrites of efferent fibers, which provide feedback to hair cells. These cells fall into two main classes, globular or flask-shaped (type I), and cylindrical (type II) (Fig. 1–64). The cylindrical type is most numerous in the ears of mammals. The globular type has the distinction of being

innervated by larger calciform dendrites that characteristically originate from large-diameter fibers (up to 20μ) found in the vestibular nerve. These fibers are among the largest in the CNS.

On the apical end of each receptor cell the bundle of stereocilia protrudes from the anchoring cuticular plate, distributed in a diagonal shape. The height of the stereocilia increases stepwise from one side to the other of the surface of the cell. Next to the tallest of the stereocilia there is a thicker, longer hair, the kinocilium, which protrudes from the cell's cytoplasm through a segment of cell membrane lacking the cuticular plate. It is anchored to the cell by a structure closely resembling that of the centriole, called the basal body. The kinocilium is absent from hair cells of the cochlea, but the basal body remains.

It was postulated by Bekesy that the stimulus for hair-cell excitation was the force acting parallel to the top of the cell, resulting in a displacement of the hairs. Recent experiments in the lateral line of the toad and in the labyrinth of squirrel monkeys have verified this proposal (2, 10).

The stimulation of the hair cells is considered to be maximal when the hairs are displaced along an axis that bisects the stereocilia and goes through the kinocilium. Deflection of the hairs in the direction of the kinocilium results in excitation of the sensory cells; there is inhibition when the bending is in the opposite direction. Therefore, excitation is minimized when the deflection of the hairs is perpendicular to the major excitation axis and increases in proportion to the cosine of the angle made by the line of displacement with the axis of functional polarization of the cell.

FIG. 1–64. Basic type I and type II labyrinthine hair cells.

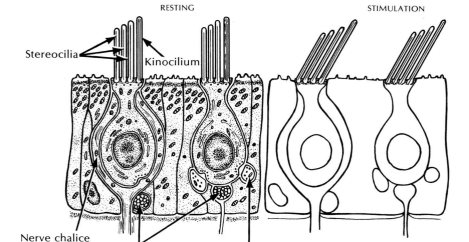

RESTING

STIMULATION

Stereocilia

Kinocilium

Nerve chalice

Efferent nerve endings

Afferent nerve endings

The overall magnitude of excitation is consequently a function of the direction of the force and of its magnitude (Fig. 1–65).

SPECIFIC MORPHOLOGIC CHARACTERISTICS OF THE COCHLEA

A cross section of the bony spiral canal in the cochlea shows that there are three compartments: an upper one called the scala vestibuli; a lower one, the scala tympani; and in the center, a triangular-shaped cavity, the cochlear duct, also known as the scala media (Fig. 1–66).

The scala vestibuli tapers as it proceeds from the vestibule at the level of the oval window towards the apex after almost three complete spiral turns. At the apex, it communicates through the helicotrema with the lower channel, the scala tympani, whose other end is at the round window.

The triangular scala media (Fig. 1–67) is separated from the scala vestibuli by the thin, obliquely lying, two-cell-layered Reissner's membrane. The important basilar membrane that separates the scala media from the scala tympani is located between a crest in the inner side of the cochlear wall, the osseous spiral lamina, and a crest in a moon-shaped ligament on the outside, the spiral ligament (Fig. 1–68). It is attached at right angles to the spiral ligament, which constitutes the third side of the scala media. The inner surface of the spiral ligament is covered by the stria vascularis, a three-layer membrane with secretory cells and a rich vascular bed. The basilar membrane, 30 mm long, varies in width from a maximum of 0.5 mm at the first turn to less than 0.1 mm at the apex. In the scala media rests the organ of Corti, containing the 13,000 receptor hair cells (Figs. 1–69, 1–70) for acoustic energy excitation. They are aligned in rows of four or five cells deep. The inner row of 3500 cells is anatomically different from the outer row. A globular type of cell (type I hair cell) characterizes the inner hair-cell group, separated from the outer hair-cell group by a spiral space, the tunnel of Corti. The outer hair cells (9500) are cylindrical and placed in rows of 3–4 cells each; their axis is at an angle with that of the inner hair cells. Several types of supporting cells complete the structure of the organ of Corti, which has a cross-sectional area of 0.005389 mm at its maximum. The top of the hair cells, the cuticular plate, is attached by rigid connections to the top of the neighboring supporting cells with the hairs (cilia) protruding from their surface. A gelatinous tectorial membrane rests over the organ of Corti, supported medially at the wall of the cochlear duct at the limbus, and laterally to the outer edge of the organ of Corti. Therefore, during vibrations of the basilar membrane, the tectorial membrane (fixed to the inner wall) is subjected to shear displacements (Fig. 1–71) in relationship to the motion of the hairs of the sensory cells. The displacements of the hairs relative to the tectorial membrane constitute the physiologic stimuli to the acoustic receptor organ.

The bipolar ganglion cells of the afferent acoustic fibers are located in the modiolus in its spiral course. The terminal dendrite of each cell enters the cochlea through the habenular opening after traveling in a straight course through the Rosenthal canal (spiral canal of the modiolus). Next to the spiral ganglion (also in a spiral course) is a group of nerve fibers belonging to the efferent system (Rasmussen's bundle).

The cochlear duct ends at the apex in a cul-de-sac, the cupular cecum, and at the base, in another narrow cul-de-sac, the vestibular cecum, at the

FIG. 1–65. Directional sensitivity of hair cell approximates a cosine function of stimulus direction; output varies as cosine of angle between direction of maximum sensitivity and applied displacement. (Flock A: Handbook of Sensory Physiology, Vol. I, Ch. 14. New York, Springer Verlag, 1971)

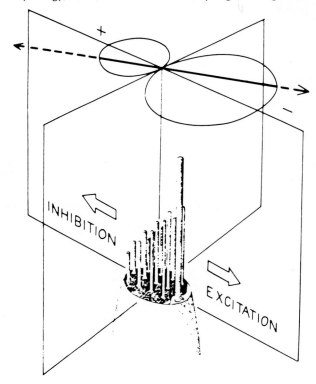

level of the vestibule. Here there is a communication with the sacculus through the narrow, short ductus reuniens, thereby establishing continuity between the endolymphatic spaces of the auditory and vestibular systems.

SPECIFIC MORPHOLOGIC CHARACTERISTICS OF THE VESTIBULAR LABYRINTH

The membranous labyrinth within the vestibule forms two globular cavities, the utricle and saccule. The saccule lies in the medial wall in a spherical recess inferior to the utricle, with which it is in contact but without communication. It communicates, however, with the endolymphatic duct via the saccular duct and with the cochlear duct via the ductus reuniens. The sensory area is

a differentiated patch of membrane in the medial wall, hook-shaped and predominantly in a vertical position.

The utricle, in a superior relation to the saccule, is oval in shape with communications for the membranous semicircular canals via five openings. The canals are aligned in such a way that they form a Cartesian system. The lateral semicircular canal makes a 30° angle with the horizontal plane and has two openings in the lateral wall of the utricle. The other two canals, in a position vertical to the horizontal, are orthogonal to each other. The superior canal is medial and lateral above the roof of the utricle, and the posterior canal is behind the utricle, in an inferior and lateral direction.

The macula of the utricle is located next to the

Fig. 1–66. Schematic midmodiolar section of cochlea.

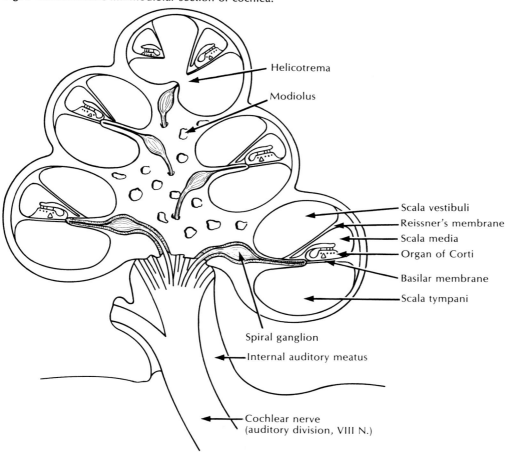

Helicotrema

Modiolus

Scala vestibuli
Reissner's membrane
Scala media
Organ of Corti
Basilar membrane
Scala tympani

Spiral ganglion
Internal auditory meatus

Cochlear nerve
(auditory division, VIII N.)

FIG. 1–67. The three cochlear compartments.

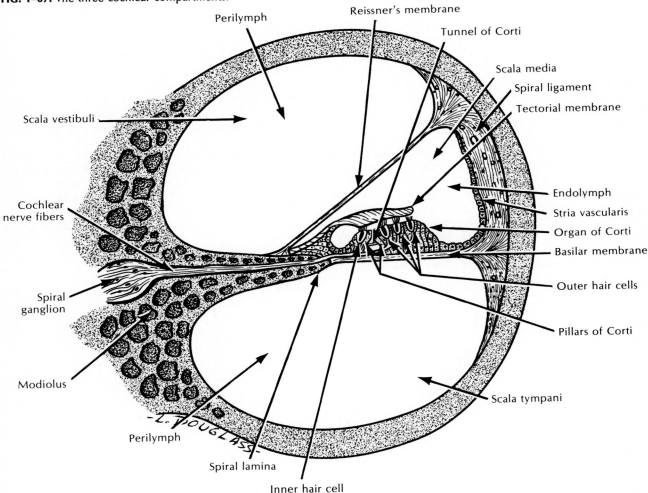

anterior opening of the horizontal semicircular canal and lies in a horizontal position on a recess of the anterior part of the utricle. The surface of the macula (Fig. 1–72) is covered by the otolithic membrane, a gelatinous structure consisting of a mesh of fibers embedded in a gel made of acid mucopolysaccharides. This membrane bears superficially calcareous deposits called otoconia. These are small crystals ranging from 0.5μ–30μ, of a density more than twice that of water, and composed of calcium carbonate (Fig. 1–73). The otoconial layer is thinner at the center than at the periphery.

Both maculas can be divided into two areas by an elevated curved line running through their centers named the striola. There is a higher proportion of type I hair cells near the striola than in the rest of the macula. It is characteristic that the hair cells in each side of the striola are oriented so as to place their kinocilia in opposite directions at each side of the center line. In addition, the hair cells in the utricle have their kinocilia closer to the striola while in the saccule the kinocilia are distal to the center line. As a consequence, displacement of the otolithic membrane in one direction in each of the maculas has an opposite physiological influence on the set of hair cells at each side of the striola. Furthermore, because of the curvature of the striola, there are hair cells oriented in different angles to the surface, making the macula multidirectionally sensitive. Since the two organs are almost perpendicular to each other, a given ear can detect head position in all planes of space.

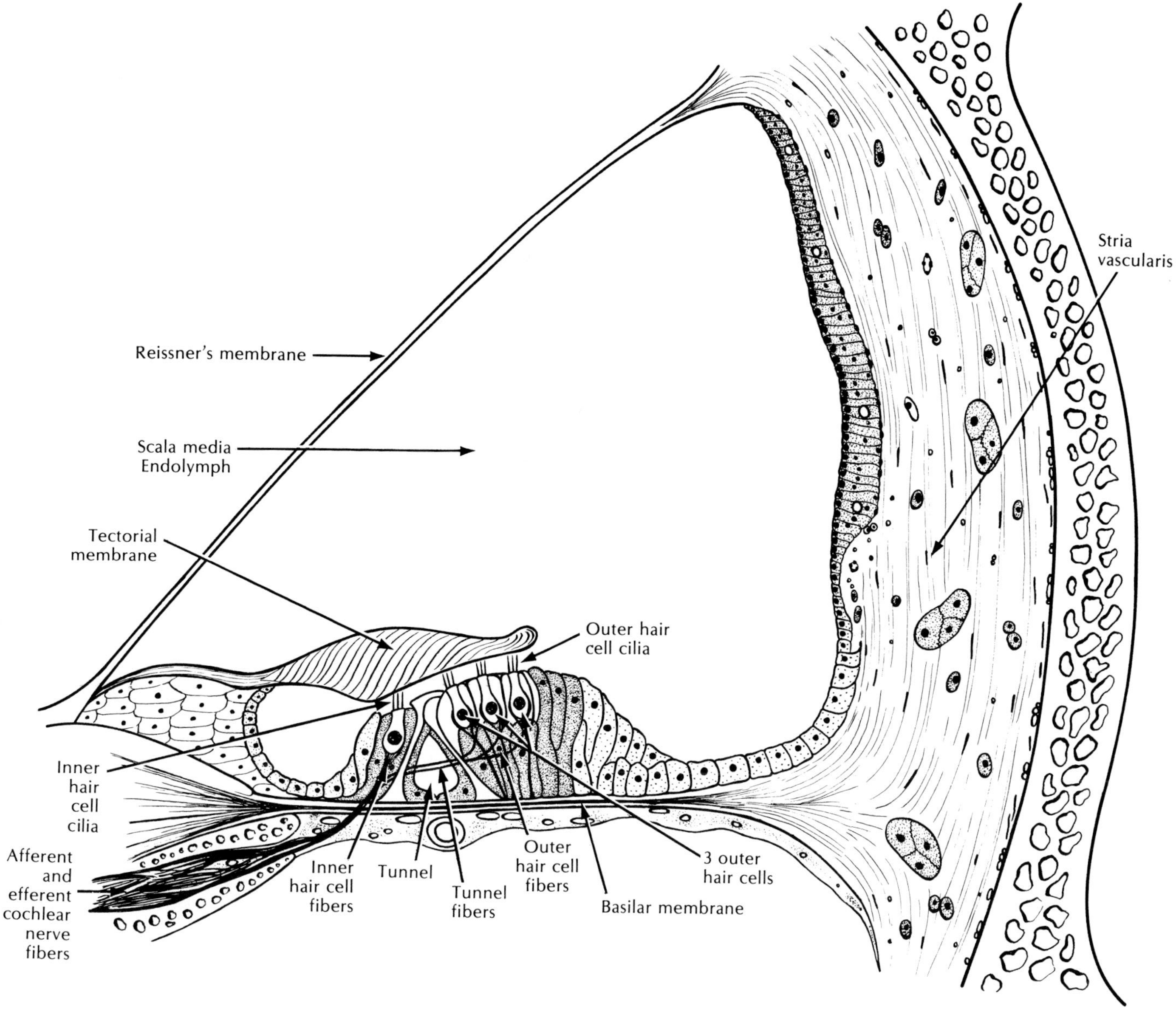

FIG. 1–68. Adult organ of Corti within scala media.

Stria vascularis

Outer hair cell cilia

3 outer hair cells

Basilar membrane

Outer hair cell fibers

Tunnel fibers

Tunnel

Inner hair cell fibers

Reissner's membrane

Scala media Endolymph

Tectorial membrane

Inner hair cell cilia

Afferent and efferent cochlear nerve fibers

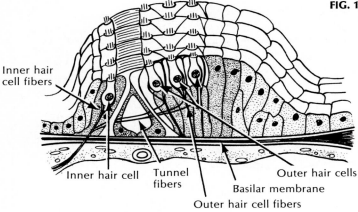

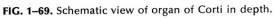

FIG. 1–69. Schematic view of organ of Corti in depth.

Inner hair
cell fibers

Inner hair cell   Tunnel
fibers

Outer hair cells

Basilar membrane

Outer hair cell fibers

FIG. 1–70. Schematic correlation between light and transmission electron microscopic details of organ of Corti.

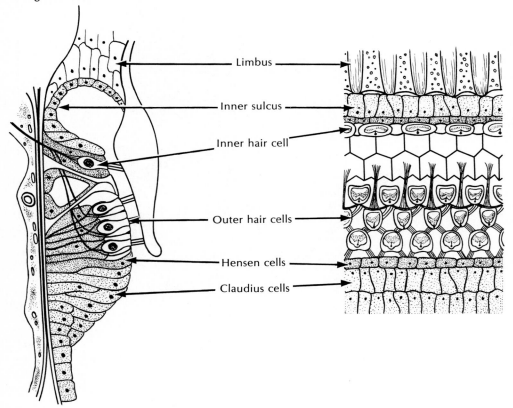

Limbus

Inner sulcus

Inner hair cell

Outer hair cells

Hensen cells

Claudius cells

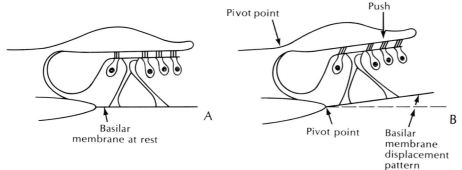

FIG. 1–71. A. Organ of Corti at rest. **B.** Basilar membrane displacement pattern in response to acoustic stimulation. (Adapted from Bekesy G von: Experiments in Hearing. New York, McGraw-Hill, 1960)

FIG. 1–72. Macular structure.

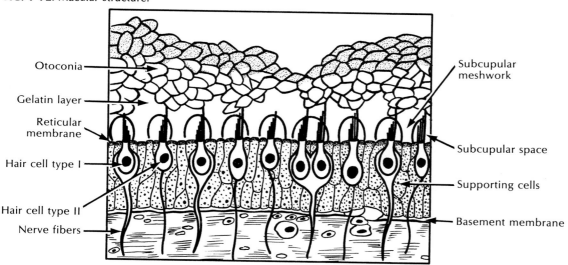

The utricular cavity communicates through the utricular duct with the sinus of the endolymphatic duct (Fig. 1–74). At this level in the walls of the duct, there is a reinforcement, which acts as a valve, probably limiting transmission of fluid and pressure back to the utricular cavity.

The membranous semicircular canals are three thin tubes inside the bony canals, each forming about two-thirds of a circle with a diameter of 6.5 mm and a cross section with a diameter of 0.4 mm. Next to the anterior opening of the horizontal and superior canals and to the inferior opening of the posterior canal, each tube enlarges to form an ampulla (Fig. 1–75). The tubes mostly occupy eccentric positions to the bony semicircular canals, from which they are restrained by strands of con-

nective tissue. The cavity outside this membranous tube is filled with perilymph while the inside contains endolymph, which is continuous with that of the utricle. A crestlike septum crosses the ampulla in a perpendicular direction to the longitudinal axis of the canal. It rests on the bone of the canal wall and is made up of sensory epithelium resting on a mound of connective tissue, where blood vessels and nerve fibers reach the sensory receptor area. On the surface of the crista are located the hair cells with their cilia protruding into the endolymphatic space. A gelatinous mass, the cupula, of the same composition as the otolithic membrane, extends from the ceiling of the ampulla to the surface of the crista, making what appears to be a water-tight seal. There is a higher proportion of

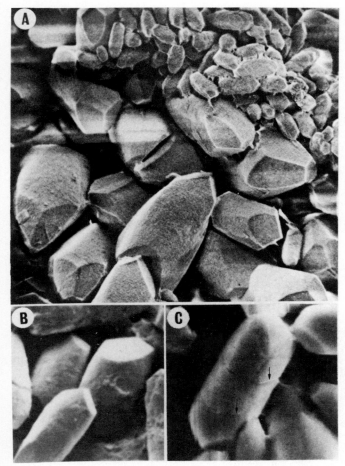

FIG. 1–73. A. Scanning photomicrograph of otoconia from utricle, showing differences in size between small and large crystals. Note cylindric form of lateral surface of otoconia. **B.** One crystal, showing typical cylindrical form. **C.** There are double bands on side of crystal **(arrows).** (Lim D: Trans Am Acad Ophthalmol Otolaryngol 73:863, 1969)

type I hair cells in the center of the crista than in the periphery. In the margins of the crista there are zones of transitional epithelium containing cells rich with infoldings and believed to have secretory functions (Figs. 1–76, 1–77).

BLOOD SUPPLY TO THE INNER EAR

The blood supply to the inner ear is independent of that of the otic capsule and tympanic cavity. The labyrinthine artery, which supplies the membranous labyrinth and nerve structures, originates within the cranial cavity. This vessel starts from the anterior inferior cerebellar artery, and in some cases directly from the basilar artery. As it enters the internal auditory meatus, it begins to branch out, supplying the ganglion cells, nerves, dura, and arachnoidal membranes. Shortly after entering the canal, the labyrinthine artery divides into two main branches: the common cochlear artery and the anterior vestibular artery (Fig. 1–78). The arteries course independently within the canal. Therefore, it is possible that alterations in one of the branches can result in changes only in that part of the inner ear that receives blood from a specific arteriole.

The common cochlear artery enters the central canal of the modiolus, where it gives off radiating arterioles, forming several plexuses within the cochlea, supplying the spiral ganglion, the structures in the basilar membrane, and stria vascularis. The capillaries in the stria vascularis constitute a serpentine meshwork, probably interconnected, and forming a compact strip that runs a spiral course

FIG. 1–74. Endolymphatic duct arising from utricular and saccular ducts and traveling through vestibular aqueduct to a blind contact with posterior fossa dura.

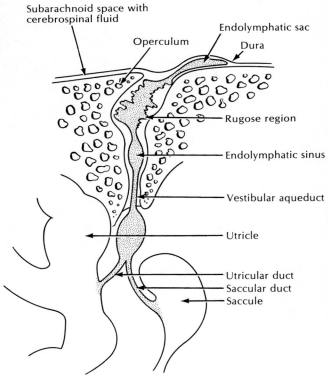

FIG. 1–75. Section of right ear through epitympanum with incudomalleal joint. **1.** Short process of incus extending from incudomalleal joint toward aditus. **2.** Cochlea. **3.** Facial (VII) nerve, horizontal portion. **4.** Vestibule with horizontal semicircular canal. **5.** Endolymphatic sac. (Courtesy of Dr. R. Gussen)

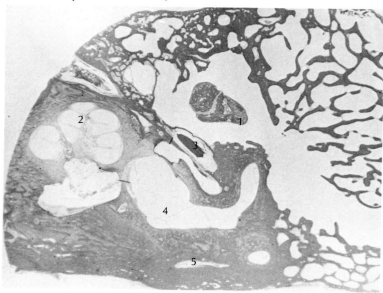

throughout the cochlea. The posterior vestibular artery, a branch of the common cochlear artery, supplies the inferior part of the saccule and the ampulla of the posterior semicircular canal.

The other primary branch of the labyrinthine artery, the anterior vestibular artery, provides circulation to the utricle and to the ampullas of the superior and horizontal semicircular canals, as well as to a small portion of the saccule.

Blood from the cochlea drains through the common modiolar vein, and blood from the utricle, the ampullas of the superior and lateral canals, and the saccule drains through the vein in the cochlear aqueduct into the inferior petrosal sinus. Blood from the inferior canal passes toward the vestibular aqueduct in a vein that accompanies the endolymphatic duct and drains into the lateral venous sinus.

Interruption of the blood supply in the internal auditory artery or in any of the branches seriously impairs the function of the inner ear, since these are terminal arteries without anastomoses with any other major vessel in the skull or in the middle ear. Within 15 sec of blood flow interruption, it has been experimentally shown that the auditory nerve fibers become inexcitable and the receptor

potentials in the ear abruptly diminish. If the interruption lasts for a prolonged period of time, the changes are irreversible and the loss of function is followed by degenerative changes, in which ganglion cells and sensory cells suffer autolysis and new bone growth fills the ear cavity.

INNERVATION OF THE INNER EAR

Afferent innervation of the cochlear receptors is provided by bipolar cells from the spiral ganglion of Corti. There are approximately 30,000 neurons whose dendrites have a different course along the organ of Corti. The majority of neurons (95%) innervate the inner hair cells, each neuron branching to only one or few hair cells. The rest of the neurons innervate several outer hair cells with fibers that have a radial or spiral type of trajectory on the basilar membrane (23).

In addition to afferent innervation, the hair cells of the cochlea also receive the efferent fibers of the olivo-cochlear bundle (26). There are approximately 500 of these fibers, which terminate in the inner but mostly in the outer hair cells (Fig. 1–79). By means of these fibers the CNS gates the activity of the receptor organs (15). The central

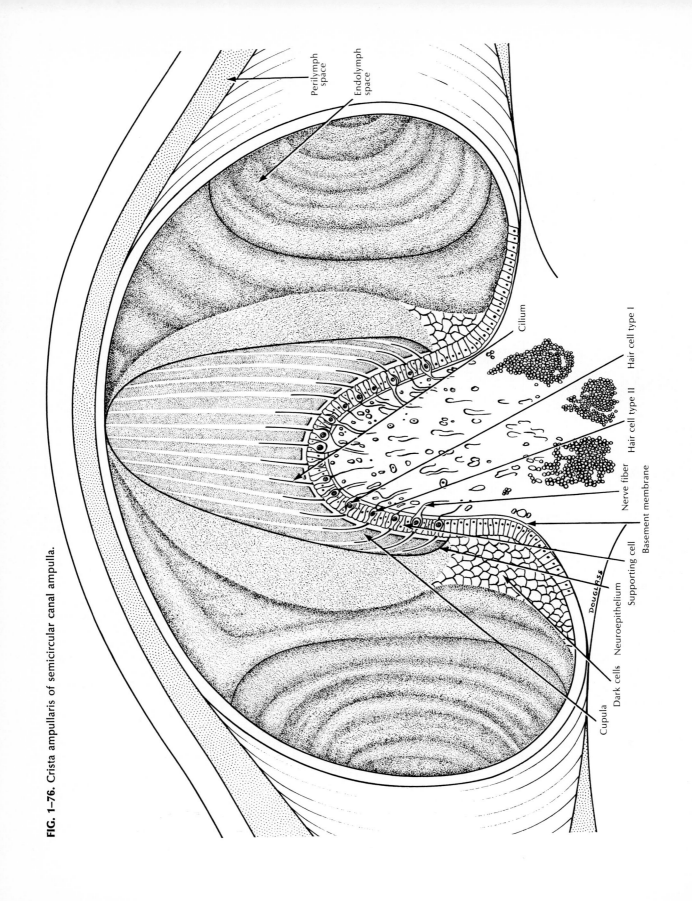

FIG. 1–76. Crista ampullaris of semicircular canal ampulla.

Perilymph space

Endolymph space

Cilium

Hair cell type I

Hair cell type II

Nerve fiber

Basement membrane

Supporting cell

Neuroepithelium

Dark cells

Cupula

Douglass

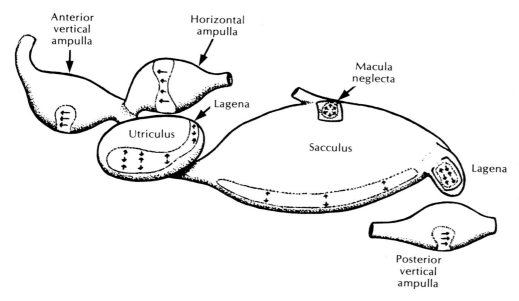

FIG. 1–77. Diagram of polarity of sensory hair bundles found in cristas and maculas of left labyrinth of the ray (*Raja clavata*). Part of dorsal wall of sacculus above macula neglecta and of the posterior wall of the lagena have been cut away to show their two sensory areas. In this schematic rendering, the orientation of the hair bundle is symbolized by an arrow, the arrow head indicating the position of the kinocilium. (Lowenstein O, Wersall J: Nature (Lond) 184:1807–1810, 1959)

FIG. 1–78. Diagram of arterial system of mammalian membranous labyrinth. (Schuknecht HF: Pathology of the Ear. Cambridge, Harvard University Press, 1974, p 62)

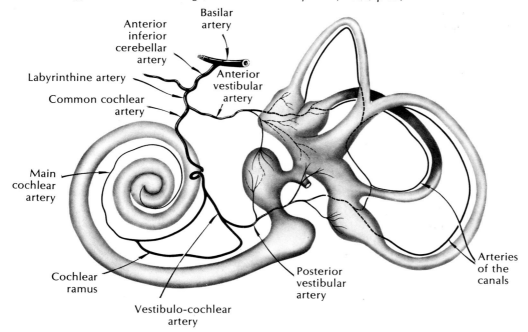

part of the afferent auditory fibers divide into two primary branches, which innervate the dorsal and ventral cochlear nuclei.

Afferent innervation of the vestibular labyrinthine organ is provided by bipolar ganglion cells located in the vestibular branch of the acoustic nerve in the internal auditory canal. The superior division of the vestibular nerve innervates the cristas of the superior and lateral canals, the macula of the utricle, and the anterior superior part of the macula of the saccule. The rest of the labyrinthine organ is innervated by the inferior division of the vestibular nerve. Approximately 20,000 ganglion cells provide different types of nerve fibers which differ in diameter sizes. The class of fibers with the largest diameter are found predominantly at the center of the crista and on the striola part of the maculas innervating type I hair cells with large chalice type endings. These large-diameter fibers have their ganglion cells located mostly in the caudal portion of the superior division of the vestibular nerve (Fig. 1–80) (14, 22).

There is also an efferent vestibular system. A few hundred efferent fibers run together with those for the cochlear system in the internal auditory canal. At the level of the saccular ganglion, the vestibular efferent fibers separate to innervate all of the crista and macula in each ear. They form boutons that synapse with hair cells directly or on nerve fibers. The cerebral origin of the efferent fibers is bilateral and from neurons located ventromedial to the lateral vestibular nuclei (13).

Upon entering the brainstem at the level of the cerebellopontine angle, the central projections of the ganglion cells consistently divide into ascending and descending branches that make synaptic contacts with neurons of the vestibular nuclei complex. Some of the fibers also send terminals to the cerebellum. No synaptic contacts from primary vestibular fibers have been described with the neurons of the reticular substance or with the vestibular nuclei of the opposite side.

The vestibular nuclei consist of a group of neurons located on the floor of the fourth ventricle medial to the entrance of the root of the vestibular nerve and bounded laterally by the restiform body, the descending root of the trigeminal nerve, and the pontine reticular formation. Four distinctive anatomic groups of neurons have traditionally been considered to constitute the vestibular nuclei although not all the neurons in these nuclei receive primary afferent vestibular nerve fibers. In addition, seven additional small groups of cells have been recognized in degeneration studies, either because of their singular morphologic characteristics or because of their specific anatomic connections. The main vestibular nuclei are the **superior** (also known as the angular or Bechterew) nucleus, the **lateral** (nucleus of Deiter), the **medial** (nucleus triangularis of Schwalbe), and the **descending** (spinal vestibular) (4).

BASIC PHYSIOLOGIC PROCESSES OF EXCITATION IN THE INNER EAR

All the sensory organs of the inner ear depend on the same elementary unit for their function—the hair cell. These sensory receptors have been shown to operate in the same manner regardless of the physiologic role of the organs in which they are found, ranging from the statocyst of the octopus and the lateral line of fish and amphibians to the acoustic and vestibular receptors of the mammalian inner ear.

The molecular process causing excitation in these receptors is believed to be that which results in a change in the electrical conductance of the cell membrane at the hair-bearing part of the sensory cells by the mechanical deformation of the hairs during their displacement (6, 19). It has been postulated that this section of the cell membrane, which is morphologically different from the rest, being thicker and more electron-dense, also has different physiologic properties: It is nonelectrogenic, and its ohmic resistance changes during physiologic stimulation in proportion to the magnitude of the hair deflection. The nonuniformity of the membrane results in local electric currents between other areas of the cell membrane and the membrane at the top (Fig. 1–81). These currents require for their maintenance a large amount of energy, which is available in the form of glycogen stores in the cell body. These changes in electric current act upon the synaptic contacts between the hair

FIG. 1–79. Eighth nerve fibers crossing tunnel of Corti.

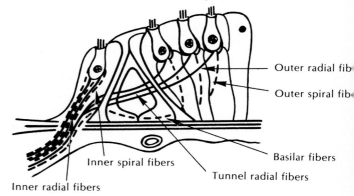

Outer radial fib

Outer spiral fib

Basilar fibers

Inner spiral fibers

Tunnel radial fibers

Inner radial fibers

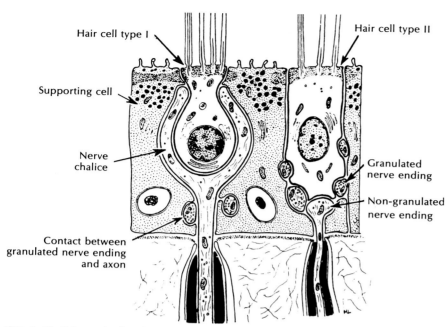

Hair cell type I

Hair cell type II

Supporting cell

Nerve chalice

Granulated nerve ending

Non-granulated nerve ending

Contact between granulated nerve ending and axon

FIG. 1–80. Schematic drawing of innervation of hair cells in vestibular sensory epithelium as it appears in cat, guinea pig, and rat. (Wersall J: In Rasmussen GL, Wendle WF (eds): Neural Mechanisms of the Auditory and Vestibular Systems. Springfield, Ill, Charles C Thomas, 1960, p 242)

FIG. 1–81. A. Hair cell model with nonuniform membrane properties. Apical (hair-bearing) end is assumed to be a purely passive (ohmic) resistance whose value, as indicated by the schematic variable resistor, is modulated during mechanical displacement of sensory hairs. Remainder of cell membrane is assumed to exhibit active ion transport and maintain a transmember potential, as indicated by schematic batteries. Nonuniformity of membrane's electrical properties results in local currents through hair cells **(arrows)**. **B.** Network model of cochlea, incorporating concepts of hair cell model of Figure 1–81A. Network branches represent lumped-equivalent electrical resistances between scala media **(SM)**, scala vestibuli **(SV)**, scala tympani **(ST)**, and neck muscles **(NE)**. Schematic batteries represent biochemical sources of electromotive force in stria vascularis and organ of Corti. (Honrubia V, Strelioff D, Sitko S: Ann Otol Rhinol Laryngol 85:697–701, 1976)

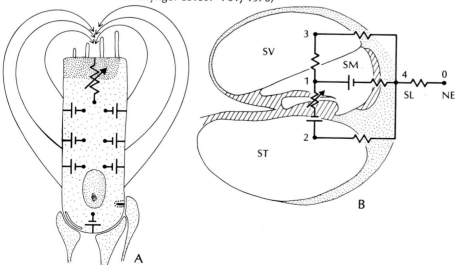

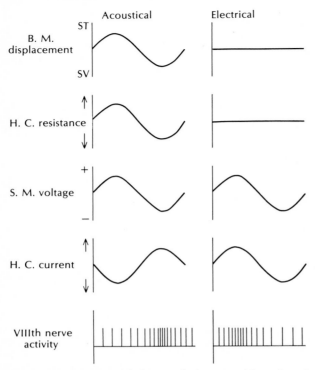

Acoustical   Electrical

B. M.
displacement

H. C. resistance

S. M. voltage

H. C. current

VIIIth nerve
activity

FIG. 1–82. Summary of theory of changes taking place in the peripheral auditory system at different stages in sequence of events culminating in modulation of impulse activity in eighth nerve fibers. **At left,** changes occurring during acoustic stimulation. **At right,** changes occurring during stimulation with extrinsic currents applied across organ of Corti. For acoustic stimuli the theory predicts an increase in hair-cell current and increased neural activity during the decrease of endocochleal potential, whereas during polarization with extrinsic currents, increased hair-cell current and increased neural activity is associated with increase in endocochlear potential. **BM,** basement membrane; **HC,** hair cell; **SM,** scala media. (Honrubia V, Strelioff D, Sitko S: Ann Otol Rhinol Laryngol 85:697–701, 1976)

cells and the dendrites. The stimulatory effect of the current is achieved either directly or by activating chemical transmitters that modulate the firing of action potentials by the afferent neurons (Fig. 1–82).

Interestingly, the hair cells in the cochlea have a special electrical arrangement with other elements of the inner ear, resulting in an increase of their sensitivity. The hair cells are situated between two fluid compartments: 1) the scala media, filled with endolymph and maintained at +80 mV (usually referred to as the stria vascularis generated endocochlear potential [EP]) with respect to the plasma; and 2) the spaces inside the organ of Corti, filled with perilymph at approximately +5 mV with respect to plasma. The +80 mV EP of the scala media, together with the −70

to −80 mV intracellular membrane potential, results in a 150–160 mV potential gradient across the mechanosensitive section of the membrane at the top of the sensory hair surface. This is the part of the membrane that changes the impedance during motion of the hairs. The action of the sensory cells, by the gating controls they have in this potential gradient, is to produce a greater current than would be possible otherwise, resulting in larger amplification of the transduction of mechanical into bio-electrical energy. However, the maintenance of this extracellular positive EP, generated by the cells of the stria vascularis for the increased sensitivity of the cochlea requires the utilization of considerable oxidative energy (approximately $0.2 \mu W/mm$), making the function of the organ of Corti extremely dependent on an adequate energy supply.

According to this theory of hair function, it should be possible to excite the hair cells and their synaptic contacts with the afferent fibers by means of electrical polarization with extrinsic current. In this case, increase in current through the hair cells is induced by making the top of the hair cell electrically more positive. This is the opposite of what happens during physiologic stimulation. In this case, the decreased resistance of the mechanically sensitive part of the hair cell produces a negative potential change in the endocochlear potential (Fig. 1–82). Most of these theoretical predictions have been verified in hair-cell systems of the lateral-line organs.

The voltages produced in the vicinity of the hair cells by the varying current are the microphonic potentials (CM). They are the generator potentials of these receptor organs. These potentials follow the frequency of the stimuli, increasing almost linearly in magnitude for a large range of stimuli. In contrast to nerve action potentials, the CM have no refractory periods. The potentials are highly resistant to anoxia and some remain after the animal's death (5, 18).

An important attribute of all these receptor organs is the existence of spontaneous action potentials firing in the afferent neurons. While the nature of this spontaneous activity is not known, it has important physiologic consequences (Figs. 1–83, 1–84). Basically, the response to neural stimulation consists of a modulation of the spontaneous activity either increasing or decreasing the frequency of spontaneous action potentials. Consequently, a stimulus can be excitatory by increasing the spontaneous activity, but it can also be inhibitory by decreasing the spontaneous firing rate. These effects are significant, particularly in the labyrinthine organs, where the spontaneous activity contributes to the creation of a labyrinthine tonus important for the maintenance of posture.

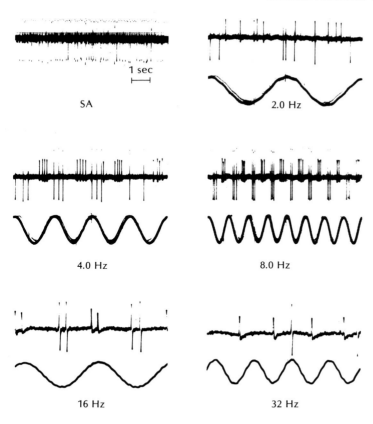

FIG. 1–83. Typical recordings of neural activity from a two-fiber preparation during spontaneous activity **(SA) (upper left)** and during stimulation with 165 μm of peak to peak (μp-p) water movements at indicated frequencies. Output of transducer recording water movement, shown below neural recordings, can be used to determine time scale for each record and to illustrate phase-locking and directional sensitivity. Action potentials of the two nerves can be readily distinguished by their different wave forms. (Bauknight RS, Strelioff D, Honrubia V: Laryngoscope 86: 1836–1844, 1976. Photo, courtesy of Dr. Strelioff)

SA

2.0 Hz

4.0 Hz

8.0 Hz

16 Hz

32 Hz

1. THE BASIS FOR PHYSIOLOGIC SPECIFICITY OF RECEPTOR ORGANS

The physiologic differentiation of the receptor organs is based mostly on anatomic characteristics of the structures that support the hair cells. The otoliths in the maculas of the utricle and the saccule, having a density greater than the surrounding fluid in the labyrinthine cavity, are displaced when the position of the head is changed in relation to the direction of gravitational force (*e.g.*, during head tilts). This displacement produces shearing forces over the surface of the cells displacing the hair and thus stimulating the organ.

When the surface of the macula is horizontal, the magnitude of the force (Fg) acting upon the hair cells is equal to the product of the otolith mass and the gravitational acceleration ($m \times g$) and is directed perpendicularly over the hair cells. These forces, as well as the compressional forces, are ineffective as hair cell stimuli (Fig. 1–85, A) (2, 10). After tilting, the magnitude of the force or weight does not change, but due to the new position of the head, the distribution of this force upon the surface of the hair cells is different. It can be represented by two vectors: one perpendicular to the hair cells (Fn), and one tangential to the surface of the sensory epithelium (Ft). The magnitude of Ft is that of the sine of the angle made by Fn with the gravitational vector (Fig. 1–85, B).

Likewise, if the head is subjected to a linear acceleration, the otoliths, due to their inertia, lag behind the displacement of the walls of the labyrinth, exerting a force over the otolithic membrane in a direction opposite to that of the displacement of the head. The effective force is that of the vector tangential to the surface of the macula. If the displacement is parallel to the plane of the macula, the effective force is directly proportional to the acceleration. This force, however, combines with the gravitational force in the direction of the center of the earth, resulting in a new vector ($F'g$), which is interpreted as the apparent direction of the gravity (Fig. 1–85, C). The angle of the resulting vector has a tangent equal to the ratio of Ft/Fg and can be calculated if $F(t)$ is known.

The hairs of the sensory cells in the semicircular canals are embedded in a jellylike substance, the cupula, which has approximately the same density as the fluid in its surroundings. Consequently, changing the positions of the cristas of the semicircular canals in space does not result in a relative

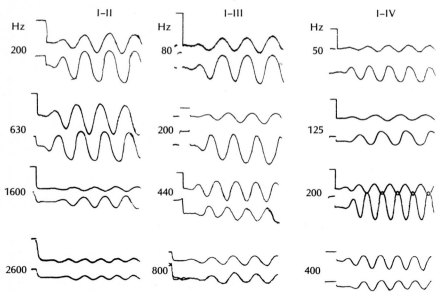

FIG. 1–84. Simultaneous recordings of cochlear potentials at two different turns of cochlear duct obtained from turns one and two, **first column;** turns one and three, **second column;** and turns one and four, **third column.** Frequency of sound stimulus is indicated at left of each pair of records. Calibration signal at beginning of each record, slightly retouched in some records, is 1 mV in amplitude. Frequencies chosen for this illustration are those demonstrating phase differences of approximately $\frac{1}{2}\pi$, π, $\frac{3}{2}\pi$, and between the first turn and each of the other turns. (Honrubia V, Strelioff D, Ward PH: J Acous Soc Am 54:600–609, 1973)

FIG. 1–85. Main anatomophysical elements of macular organ's function, otolithic membrane, sensory epithelium, and vector, upon sensing gravitational force **(Fg). A.** Head displacement due to linear accelerations. **B** and **C.** Changes in distribution of gravitational force **(Fg)** during head tilts **(B)** and linear acceleration **(C). F(t),** component of force tangential to surface of macula, resulting from head tilts. θ [t], angular displacement of head in tilt.

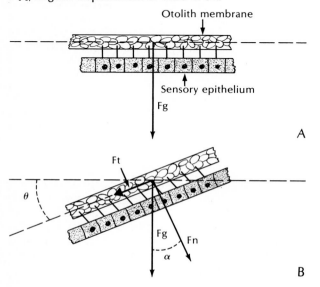
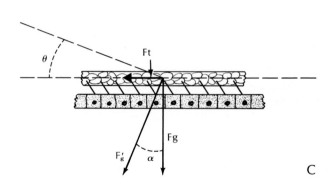

displacement of the cupula in relationship to the walls of the labyrinth. However, these displacements take place during angular accelerations of the head in the plane of the semicircular canal, with the center of motion at the center of the canal ring. The fluid in the cylindrical tubes, because of its mass, has an inertia that delays its displacement in relationship to the rigid walls of the labyrinth membranes. The force thus created, which is proportional to the endolymph inertia, acts over the cristas, resulting in a displacement of the hairs of the sensory cells, which are rigidly mounted on the walls of the labyrinth (Fig. 1–86) (34).

Changes in atmospheric pressure produced by sound sources at the tympanic membrane are transmitted to the scala vestibuli of the cochlea through the middle-ear ossicles, resulting in the creation of a pressure difference across the basilar membrane located between the scala vestibuli and tympani. Because of the variation of pressure difference, there is a displacement at the frequency of sound of this flexible membrane on which the organ of Corti with the hair cells is located (see Fig. 1–71).

In all cases, the effective stimuli for the sensory cells are the displacements of hairs produced by the application of mechanical force to their surroundings. However, since the supporting structures have different viscoelastic properties, the ranges of frequencies at which they can be moved with ease also differ. The otolith organs are sensitive to constant linear accelerations, such as those during steady head movements, but the otolith displacements diminish at frequencies greater than 0.1–0.5 Hz. Likewise, the semicircular canals respond maximally to constant angular acceleration. However, for sinusoidally changing acceleration, their sensitivity starts decreasing substantially above 0.05–0.1 Hz and is minimal after 5–10Hz. The cochlea is sensitive to pressure variations between 20 Hz and 20,000 Hz.

COCHLEAR PHYSIOLOGY

Central to the phenomenon of hearing is the role of the cochlea in the transduction of mechanical into bioelectric signals, which takes place with an unparalleled sensitivity and frequency resolution. These two important properties of cochlear function are determined by the characteristics of the motion of the basilar membrane during acoustic stimulation. The description of this movement is embodied in the concept of the "traveling wave" as developed by von Bekesy in his Nobel prize-winning experiments in the ears of animals and humans, dating back to the 1920's (3, 7). His profound influence on the science of hearing continued during his lifetime, extending to other aspects of biophysics, physiology, psychoacoustics, and otology.

Bekesy demonstrated that the pattern of vibration of the basilar membrane depends on the frequency and the sound pressure level of the stimulus. The cochlea behaves as a mechanical filter with each point of the basilar membrane vibrating with greater sensitivity at a particular frequency (Fig. 1–87). Low frequencies of sound (*e.g.*, 200 Hz) produce maximum displacement toward the apex of the basilar membrane and high

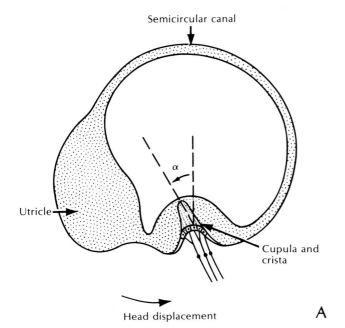

FIG. 1–86. A. Schematic drawing of semicircular canal, showing relationship between direction of head rotation and displacement of cupula. **B.** Curves showing relationship between sinusodial head displacement and its velocity and acceleration.

Semicircular canal

Utricle

α

Cupula and crista

Head displacement

A

Head displacement
Head velocity
Head acceleration

B

frequencies (*e.g.*, 8–10 kHz) produce maximum displacement close to the location of the stapes. This spacial property is such that the points of maximum stimulation change by approximately 4–5 mm for a change of an octave (doubling) in the sound frequency in the human cochlea. The pattern of the basilar membrane motion is such that the maximum displacement occurs with a certain delay after the maximum of the stapes displacement and is dependent on the sound frequency. Contrary to what would be expected if the basilar membrane worked as a simple resonator (showing a simple up-and-down motion along its entire length), different sections of the basilar membrane have different phase relations with the

motion of the stapes. The point of maximum displacement shows a phase angle difference that has been found to increase with the frequency of sound, the smallest being approximately $3/2\pi$ radians for 200 Hz sound. This corresponds to a delay of 3/4 of a cycle, equivalent to 3.75 msec. Thereafter, the amplitude of the basilar membrane displacement decreases for an additional two or more cycles of vibration at an exceedingly high rate (Fig. 1–88).

Intensive research in this field has provided quantitative information about the relationship between the frequency and magnitude of sound and 1) the amplitude of the vibration of the middle-ear ossicles; 2) basilar membrane displacement; 3) characteristics of the bioelectric potential in the ear during transduction; and 4) the coding of sound by the eighth nerve as reflected in the frequency of action potential firing in single nerve fibers. These investigations, in addition to providing a substantial body of evidence for understanding hearing processes, have revealed new aspects of sensory and nervous system functions that are significant for the understanding of the physiology of other sensory receptors in addition to the ones in the cochlea.

By means of special methods, such as the application of the Mossbauer effect (20) or very sensitive capacitative probes (32), the displacements of the stapes and basilar membrane have been measured in several species of animals. Of particular interest are the data obtained from experiments in the cochlea of the squirrel monkey (27), where measurements have been obtained on each of the four aspects of auditory function mentioned in the foregoing paragraph.

Figure 1–89 shows the relationships between the displacement of one of the middle ear ossicles (malleus) and that of the basilar membrane for different frequencies of sound with equal sound pressure level. The malleus displacement is independent of the frequency of stimulation within a range of 200–2000 Hz. For higher frequencies, it appears to decrease by a factor of ten for each change of one octave in the frequency of the stimulus. The same plot shows simultaneous measurements of basilar membrane displacement in the basal region of the cochlea in a zone that has the maximum resonance for sound of 7–8 KHz. When the amplitude of the basilar membrane is compared with that of the malleus (Fig. 1–89, B), the following relationship applies: The magnitude of the vibration of the basilar membrane increases with the frequency of the sound up to the most sensitive frequency, which is usually referred to as the characteristic frequency (CF), and thereafter decreases at an exceedingly high rate. It diminishes by a factor of 100,000 for each change in sound frequency of one octave. The decrease in amplitude expressed in a logarithmic scale is equivalent to 100 dB per octave. Before the maximum, the curve shows two distinctive

FIG. 1–87. Patterns of vibration of cochlear partition of cadaver specimen for various frequencies. (Bekesy G von: Experiments in Hearing. New York, McGraw-Hill Book Company, 1960. Used with permission of McGraw-Hill Book Company)

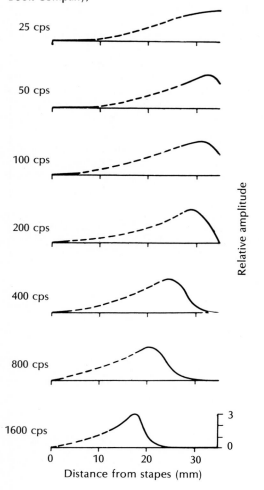

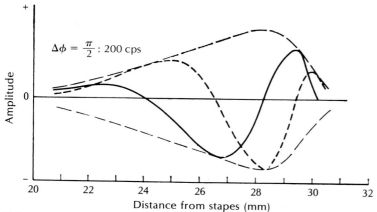

FIG. 1–88. Detail of form of vibration of cochlear partition for 200 cps at two instants within a cycle. The symbols $\Delta\phi$ = phase angle difference, and π_2 = half pi. (Bekesy G von: Experiments in Hearing. New York, McGraw-Hill Book Company, 1960. Used with permission of McGraw-Hill Book Company)

regions: In the first one, at the lowest frequency, the amplitude of the vibration increases at the rate of approximately 6 dB per octave; and for frequencies immediately before the CF, the basilar membrane displacement increases at about three or four times that rate (18–24 dB) per octave.

These relationships suggest the following characteristics of middle ear and basilar membrane motion: 1) The impedance of the middle ear for low frequencies is inversely proportional to the sound frequency, behaving as if controlled by elastic forces, so that if the amplitude of the stimulus is kept constant, the velocity of the middle-ear ossicles will increase by increasing frequency, or similarly, the magnitude of the displacement will remain constant. 2) Since the amplitude of the basilar membrane displacement increases linearly with the frequency of the sound, and furthermore, since at low frequencies the basilar membrane displacement is 90° ahead of the middle-ear ossicles, the displacement of the basilar membrane is proportional to the velocity of the stapes and to the difference in pressure between the scala vestibuli and the scala tympani. The basilar membrane position would be down (toward scala tympani) during displacement of the stapes from the scala vestibuli to the scala tympani, and vice versa.

The magnitude of basilar membrane displacement is exceedingly small, being measured in angstroms (Å) for most physiologic acoustic stimuli. If the assumption is accepted that the displacement of the basilar membrane is a linear function of sound pressure level, the threshold for hearing in this part of the basilar membrane for this most sensitive frequency is reached with a displacement of only 0.1–0.3 Å.

Some interesting results are provided by comparison of measurements of the cochlear microphonics at this level of the cochlear duct and the basilar membrane displacement in this animal. During constant sound pressure level stimulation, it was found that the voltage of the microphonics is linearly related to the frequency of sound up to 2000 Hz (Fig. 1–90). That is, the magnitude of the microphonics is linearly related to the basilar membrane vibration amplitude, suggesting that they are proportional to the displacement of the basilar membrane and are produced by the displacement of the hair cells. Quantitative comparison of the microphonic data with those of the basilar membrane displacement indicate that one mV of microphonics corresponds to a basilar membrane displacement of 0.1μ. At threshold, the magnitude of microphonics is estimated to be of the order of 10^{-4} mV.

The role of the microphonics in the excitation process in the cochlea has not yet been completely elucidated. Their measurements provide an indirect method to evaluate basilar membrane motion throughout the length of the cochlea in all other points along the membrane, which could not be visualized. By introducing microelectrodes in the fluid spaces of the cochlea, for example, simultaneous recording of the microphonics at different locations of the cochlear duct did provide an earlier evidence for the traveling wave motion of the basilar membrane, giving a measure of the relative displacement of different parts for a given stimulus. These measurements allowed the computation of the velocity of propagation of the basilar membrane disturbance, approximately 114 msec at the origin and decaying exponentially, decreasing to one-third every 4 mm along the cochlea (Fig. 1–84) (18).

The microphonics furnish a rather simple, widely used method of experimentally evaluating the state of the organ of Corti. Unfortunately, the very rapid phase change of the basilar membrane motion near the point

FIG. 1–89. A. Amplitude of vibration of malleus and of basilar membrane as a function of frequency. Measurements in vicinity of maximum ratio were made at 80 dB SPL; those at lower frequencies were made at higher intensities and have been linearly extrapolated for a stimulus of 80 dB SPL. In this figure and in parts B and C, each point is an experimentally determined value, and each line is a free-hand fit to these points. **B.** Input-output ratio, in decibels, for malleus and basilar membrane. **C.** Phase differences between motion of basilar membrane and motion of malleus. Negative numbers signify that basilar membrane motion lags behind that of malleus. **Arrows,** values of curves at maximally effective frequency. Note that value of the phase difference is 1.6 radians (about 90°) at frequencies less than 300 Hz θd = angle difference. (Rhode WS: Ann Otol Rhinol Laryngol 86:610–6126, 1974)

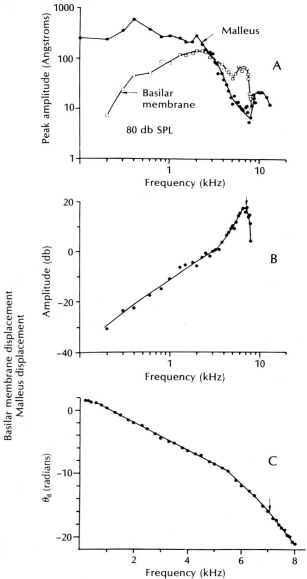

of maximum displacement results in a cancellation of the voltages produced by the out-of-phase cochlear microphonic generator in this part of the traveling wave, imposing severe limitations in the usefulness of this technique.

The most startling findings concerning the function of the cochlea have been obtained from measurements of the action potentials in single fibers of the acoustic nerve (21, 29). The fibers show frequency-dependent excitability, which resembles the filter properties of the basilar membrane. Each fiber has a characteristic frequency at which it is most sensitive. For frequencies different from the CF, the sensitivity decays very rapidly on either side of the CF (Fig. 1–91). For higher frequencies than the CF, changes in sensitivity as great as 200–400 dB per octave have been measured. At lower frequencies the change in sensitivity as a function of frequency is smaller but still has been shown to be greater than the change in amplitude of the basilar membrane.

Careful comparison of the results of basilar membrane vibration amplitude and responses of acoustic nerve fibers in the squirrel monkey has shown that the difference in sensitivity lies mostly in sounds whose frequency is close to the CF. Furthermore, it appears that this increased sensitivity of the nerve fiber in comparison with basilar membrane motion is a function of several variables; such as the physiologic state of the preparation, the availability of oxygen and adequate blood supply to the ear, electrolytic composition of the fluids in the inner ear, etc., indicating that a substantial sharpening of the fiber response is not related to mechanical tuning. It has always been understood that tuning must depend on biologic processes, such as synaptic activity or innervation patterns, but it appears that the contribution of these physiological variables is indeed crucial to obtain the frequency resolution achieved by cochlear nerve fibers. Although the precise mechanisms involved in the excitation of acoustic nerve fibers are not yet understood, recent experimental evidence suggests that the electrical current in the cochlea responsible for the production of cochlear microphonics and nonlinear processes involved in the excitation of hair cells may be responsible for the remarkable sensitivity of nerve fibers to basilar membrane displacement.

In summary, the function of the cochlea in the perception of acoustic energy depends on its ability to perform a frequency analysis of sound, transforming mechanical energy delivered to a section of the cochlea into biologic energy, which produces a change in the frequency of action potentials in fibers innervating that section of the basilar membrane. The coding of acoustic information depends on three properties of the basilar membrane: 1) the distinctive localization of the maximum of stimulation for different frequencies (place principle); 2) the ability to modulate the frequency of

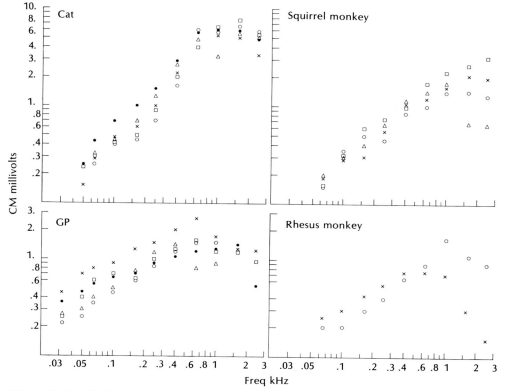

FIG. 1–90. Amplitude of cochlear microphonics produced by different frequencies with 95 dB constant SPL at eardrum. Recordings made inside scala media at level of round window. Closed-system stimulation. Each symbol represents a different animal. (Honrubia V, Strelioff D, Ward PH: J Acoust Soc Am 54:600–609, 1973)

action potentials firing with the periods of the basilar membrane vibration (periodicity principle); and 3) the ability to spatially distribute the energy of sound over a relatively wide area of the basilar membrane, whereby fibers other than those of the characteristic frequencies are affected by sound and propagate action potentials to the CNS with different degrees of excitation and phase relationships (spatial distribution principle).

SEMICIRCULAR CANAL PHYSIOLOGY

The physiologic characteristics of the semicircular canals depend on the manner in which the cupula, during head movements, transmits to the hair cells the degree of endolymph displacement in relation to the walls of the membranous labyrinth. The cupula works as a swinging door, transmitting mechanical forces to the sensory cells, and effectively acting as the coupler between the external world (for force due to angular acceleration of the head) and the hair cells (the transducer of

mechanical to biologic energy), leading to the production of action potentials in the vestibular nerve.

The displacement of the endolymph inside the canal is opposed by three restraining forces: 1) an elastic force (K) due to the cupular springlike property, which is proportional to the magnitude of cupular displacement; 2) an inertial force due to the fluid-cupula mass (M), proportional to the acceleration of the fluid; and 3) the most significant within the range of natural head movements, a force due to viscosity (C) of the fluid, whose magnitude is proportional to the velocity of fluid motion. The force (F) acting upon the endolymph-cupula system is equal (by Newton's second principle) to the product of the mass (M) and its acceleration ($\ddot{\theta}h$ [t]) or $F = M\,\ddot{\theta}h\,(t)$, where $\ddot{\theta}h\,(t)$ is actually the acceleration of the head. Mathematically, the displacement of the cupula-endolymph system can be simply expressed by equating the total force applied to the cupula (F) to the sum of the restraining forces, which tend to maintain the cupula in a stationary position:

Equation 1: $F = M\,\ddot{\theta}_c(t) + C\,\dot{\theta}_c(t) + K\,\theta_c(t)$

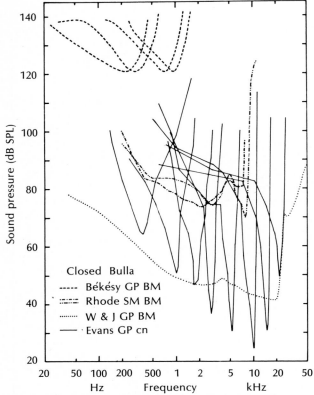

FIG. 1–91. Mechanical and fiber thresholds. (Wilson JP: In Zwicker E, Terhardt E (eds): Facts and Models in Hearing. New York, Springer Verlag, 1974, p 59)

FIG. 1–92. Cupula deflection during constant angular accelerations according to the TP model. TP = "torsion pendulum" model, "Chi" No-X = distance, alpha₁, alpha₂ = two different acceleration magnitudes, T = time. (Guedry FE: Handbook of Sensory Physiology. New York, Springer Verlag, 1974)

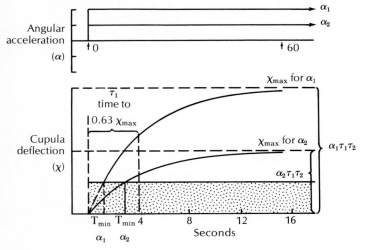

where $\theta_c(t)$, $\dot{\theta}_c(t)$, and $\ddot{\theta}_c(t)$ indicate the deviation of the cupula and its first (velocity) and second (acceleration) time derivatives.

The above equation is similar to that describing the displacement of a pendulum moving in a viscous medium and is usually referred to as the equation pendulum of model cupular motion (31, 34).

On the basis of experimental observation and physicomathematical treatment of the model, the following generalizations can be made in the description of the major characteristics of cupular motion during head rotations:

During most of natural head movements, viscous restraining forces control the displacement of the cupula in such a way that the cupular deviation is proportional to the velocity of head rotation, since there is a minimum contribution by other than viscosity forces in restraining the cupula. Therefore, the following approximation holds for the description of cupular motion.

Equation 2: $\theta_c(t) \approx \dot{\theta}_h(t)$

Accordingly, even if the natural stimulus is head acceleration, the deviation of the cupula ($\theta_c[t]$) during sinusoidal head rotation at frequencies between 0.1–1 Hz is in phase with the velocity of the head ($\dot{\theta}_h[t]$). This is an important relationship because most vestibular reflexes originating in the semicircular canals depend on the cupular deviation, and therefore they reflect the influence of this relationship to the head movements. These relationships are illustrated in Figure 1–86, B. The curves describing the velocity of the head can all be interpreted as representing the deviation of the cupula.

Mathematical treatment of equation 1, in addition to verifying the above generalization, provides a more detailed visualization of the kinematics of the cupula, allowing complete description of its movement following application of different force inputs.

Graphs showing the temporal course of the displacement of the cupula following two different magnitudes a_1 and a_2 of constant angular accelerations are shown in Figure 1–92 (17). According to the pendulum model, 63% of the total cupula deviation, regardless of its final value, takes place always after a delay, determined by what is known as the slow time constant (T_1) of the system, which has been estimated to be 4 sec. The subsequent deviation of the cupula increases at the same rate (63% of the remainder every 4 sec) so that 95% of the final deviation will take place after approximately 12 sec.

According to the model, not only the maximum deviation of the cupula is delayed in relationship to the start of the acceleration, but after the stimulus is terminated, the cupula returns with the same exponential time course to the resting position. It was precisely the observation by Steinhausen (28) of the slow return of the deviated cupula to the resting position on isolated labyrinth experiments which led to the formulation of the pendulum model.

At the time of maximum deviation of the cupula following a constant acceleration, a balance is established between the applied and restraining forces and the cupula-endolymph complex moves simultaneously with the walls of the labyrinth facilitating the calculation of the magnitude of the cupular displacement. Once the endolymph is stationary as a result of the balance of forces, the cupula velocity $\dot{\theta}_c(t)$ and its acceleration $\ddot{\theta}_c(t)$ in relation to the walls are equal to zero, and consequently the terms for viscous and inertial restraining forces vanish in the equation 1, which now is reduced to:

$$\text{Equation 3: } K\,\theta_c(t) = M\,\ddot{\theta}_h(t)$$

or

$$\text{Equation 4: } \theta_c(t) = M/K \times \ddot{\theta}_h(t)$$

The final displacement of the cupula depends on a proportionate constant (M/K) and on the magnitude of the constant angular acceleration $(\ddot{\theta}_h[t])$.

The relationships embodied in equations 2 and 4 are two of the fundamental concepts of cupula function. To restate them: the deviation of the cupula increases proportionately to the magnitude of the velocity of the head during sinusoidal head rotations or to the magnitude of the acceleration during rotations with constant angular acceleration. They are the basis for evaluation of several tests of vestibular function used experimentally and in clinical practice.

Measurements of the firing of action potentials in the vestibular nerve and in neurons within the vestibular nuclei support the above conclusions made on theoretical grounds (8, 16, 25). Most important, the measurements of eye velocity during vestibulooocular reflexes (*i.e.*, velocity of the slow component of nystagmus) show the same type of relationships (34). Because of these similarities, functional tests of semicircular canal function generally use measurements of the velocity of the eye during the slow component of nystagmus as an estimation of cupular function, even when the nystagmus is not induced by physiological methods, as with the caloric test.

It is worth while to anticipate now that during vestibular reflexes, gaze stabilization is properly achieved regardless of the magnitude of the angle of head rotation. By means of nystagmus, fixation and clear vision are possible, even though this angle may be larger than the maximum possible displacement of the eye in the orbit. During the slow component of nystagmus, the eyes have the same speed as the head, but in the opposite direction. Therefore, they remain fixed in the horizontal while the head is moving.

OTOLITH PHYSIOLOGY

Whenever a tangential force, regardless of its origin, is applied over the maculas, the otoconia slide over the surface of the sensory epithelium, stimulating the hair cells. Because of its mass, the otolithic membrane always exerts a force upon the macula, as a result of the action of the gravitational pull. When a force is applied to the organ, the otoliths would slide over the sensory epithelium if the viscoelastic restraining forces of the supporting ligaments did not balance the otoconia. The position of the otoliths changes whenever the head position is changed or during head displacements, with a component of linear acceleration, reflecting the interaction of gravitational and applied forces. The viscoelastic properties of the otolith membrane cause the displacement of the otoliths during sinusoidal linear accelerations to diminish as the frequency of the stimuli increases. The dynamics of the otoliths can be thought of as those of a low-pass filter, *i.e.*, the displacement due to linear acceleration is greater for low frequencies, including stimulation with constant acceleration (*i.e.*, head tilts) than for high frequencies. For frequencies greater than 0.5 Hz the displacement of the otoliths decreases to half every time the frequency doubles (1, 9, 34).

The nerve fibers innervating the macular organs of the labyrinth are sensitive to changes in position of the head. Each one has a preferred direction of tilt to which it responds in such a way that the maximum response is obtained by head positions along a vector in a three-dimensional space whose coordinates are drawn in relationship to the earth's gravitational pull. It is as if the nerve fibers innervate only hair cells that have their kinocilia oriented in a given direction in space. Interestingly, the vestibular nerve branch innervating the macula sacculi appears to have the largest number of fibers sensitive to both forward and backward pitches. This is as would be expected because of the vertical orientation of the macula and because of the superior-inferior direction of the striola dividing the macula in two main fields, with the majority of hair cells aligned with the polarization vector normal to the striola. Nerves innervating the macula utriculi, on the other hand, have a larger number of fibers (70%) sensitive to ipsilateral tilts. Here the macula is horizontal and the striola is directed mostly in a lateral-medial direction. However, for every head tilt there is some responsive fiber in the nerves of the two maculas (9, 10).

Although the two maculas of each ear are capable of detecting acceleration forces in all planes of space, electrical stimulation experiments have suggested that the connection of each macula is rather limited to a small group of eye motor neurons. Electrical stimulation limited to a given small area of the macula produces contraction of only one of the extrinsic eye muscles (12). Therefore, all eye muscles must be activated during otolithic organ stimulations in different degrees to result in coordinated eye movements that are specific with reference to the stimuli that induce the reflex.

Physiologically, the eye movements resulting from otolithic stimulation have as their objective the stabilization of gaze by compensating the displacement of the head from the gravitational vector. This is accomplished by rotating the eye at an angle proportional to the angle formed by the axis of the head and an imaginary line perpendicular to the surface of the earth.

Intuitively, it can be expected that if the head is tilted forward, the eyes will execute a vertical angular movement within the orbit. If the head is tilted sideways, the eyes will counter-rotate to position themselves in the same spatial relationship to the earth's gravitational vector. What happens during head motion with a linear acceleration vector? Two methods have often been used to study this type of eye movement: a parallel swing or a horizontal track. Two distinctive types of eye movement similar to the two described are produced: either a vertical angular deviation or a counter torsion, depending on the direction of the resulting vector force during motion. Transverse displacement along a longitudinal track (the acceleration vector going through the bitemporal axis) results in torsional eye movement. Displacement along the sagittal axis of the subject in the track (the acceleration vector passing anteroposteriorly in the head) results in vertical eye movements. Unfortunately, human data are limited, and our understanding of maculoocular reflexes is based mainly on results obtained in animal experiments (1).

REFERENCES

1. Baarsma EA, Collewijn H: Eye movements due to linear acceleration in the rabbit. J Physiol (Lond) 245:227–247, 1975

2. Bauknight RS, Strelioff D, Honrubia V: Effective stimulus for the *Xenopus laevis* lateral-line hair-cell system. Laryngoscope 86:1836–1844, 1976

3. Bekesy G von: Experiments in Hearing. New York, McGraw-Hill, 1960, 635–710

4. Brodal A: Anatomy of the vestibular nuclei and their connections. In Handbook of Sensory Physiology, Vol VI. New York, Springer Verlag, 1974

5. Butler RA, Honrubia V, Johnstone BM, Fernandez C: Cochlear function under metabolic impairment. Ann Otol Rhinol Laryngol 71:648–656, 1962

6. Davis H: A model for transducer action in the cochlea. Cold Springs Harbor Symp, Quant Biol 30:181–190, 1965

7. Eldredge HE: Inner ear cochlear mechanics and cochlear potentials. In Handbook of Sensory Physiology, Vol V. New York, Springer Verlag, 1974

8. Fernandez C, Goldberg JM: Physiology of peripheral neurons innervating semicircular canals of the squirrel monkey. I. Resting discharge and response to constant accelerations. J Neurophysiol 34:661–676, 1971

9. Fernandez C, Goldberg JM: Physiology of peripheral neurons innervating otolith organs of the squirrel monkey. I. J Neurophysiol 39:970–984, 1976

10. Fernandez C, Goldberg JM: Physiology of peripheral neurons innervating otolith organs of the squirrel monkey. II. Directional selectivity and force-response relations. J Neurophysiol 39:985–995, 1976

11. Flock A: Sensory transduction in hair cells. In Handbook of Sensory Physiology, Vol I, Ch 14. New York, Springer Verlag, 1971

12. Fluur E, Mellstrom A: Sacular stimulation and oculomotor reactions. Laryngoscope 80:1713–1721, 1970

13. Gacek R: Efferent component of the vestibular nerve. In Rasmussen G, Windle W (ed): Neural Mechanisms of the Auditory and Vestibular Systems. Springfield, Ill, Charles C Thomas, Publishers, 1960

14. Gacek R: The innervation of the vestibular labyrinth. Ann Otol Rhinol Laryngol 77:676–685, 1968

15. Galambos R: Suppression of auditory nerve activity by stimulation of efferent fiber to cochlea. J Neurophysiol 19:424–437, 1956

16. Groen JJ, Lowenstein O, Vendrik AJ: The mechanical analysis of the responses from end organs of the horizontal semicircular canals in the isolated elasmobranch labyrinth. J Physiol 117:329, 1952

17. Guedry FE: Psychophysics of vestibular sensation. In Handbook of Sensory Physiology, Vol VI. New York, Springer Verlag, 1974

18. Honrubia V, Strelioff D, Ward PH: A quantitative study of cochlear potentials along the scala media of the guinea pig. J Acoust Soc Am. 54:600–609, 1973

19. Honrubia V, Strelioff D, Sitko ST: Physiological basis of cochlear transduction and sensitivity. Ann Otol Rhinol Laryngol 85:697–701, 1976

20. Johnstone BM, Boyle AJF: Basilar membrane vibration examined with the Mossbauer technique. Science 158:389–390, 1967

21. Kiang NYS, Watanabe T, Thomas EC, Clark LF: Discharge Patterns of Single Fibers in the Cat's Auditory Nerve. Research Monograph No. 35. Cambridge, Massachusetts Institute of Technology Press, 1965

22. Lorente de Nó R: Études sur l'anatomie et la physiologie du labyrinthe de l'oreille et du VIIIe nerf deuxieme partie. Quelques données au sujet de l'anatomie des organes sensoriels du labyrinthe. Trav Lab Rech Biol Univ Madrid 24:53, 1926

23. Lorente de No R: The sensory endings in the cochlea. Laryngoscope 47:373–377, 1937

24. Lowenstein O, Wersall J: A functional interpretation of the electron microscopic structure of the sensory hairs in the cristae of the elasmobranch, *Raja clavata*, in terms of directional sensitivity. Nature (Lond) 184:1807–1810, 1959

25. Melvill JG, Milsum JH: Frequency-response analysis of central vestibular unit activity resulting from rotational stimulation of the semicircular canals. J Physiol 219:191–215, 1971

26. Rasmussen G: Anatomic relationships of the ascending and descending auditory systems. In Fields W, Alford B (ed): Neurological Aspects of Auditory and Vestibular Disorders. Springfield, Ill, Charles C Thomas, Publishers, 1964

27. Rhode WS: Measurements of vibration of the basilar membrane in the squirrel monkey. Ann Otol Rhinol Laryngol 83:619–626, 1974

28. Steinhausen W: Uber den Nachweis der Bewegung der Cupula in der Intakten Bogengangsampulle des Labyrinths Bei der Naturlichen Rotatorischen und Kalorischen Reizung. Pfluegers Arch 228:322–328, 1931

29. Tasaki I: Afferent impulses in auditory nerve fibers and the mechanism of impulse initiation in the cochlea. In Rasmussen G, Windle W (ed): Neural Mechanisms of the Auditory and Vestibular System. Springfield, Ill, Charles C Thomas, Publishers, 1960

30. Van de Water T: Effects of removal of the statoacoustic ganglion complex upon the growing otocyst. Ann Otol Rhinol Laryngol 85 (Suppl 33), 1976

31. Van Edmond AAJ, Groen JJ, Jongkees LBW: The mechanics of the semicircular canal. J Physiol 110:1–17, 1949

32. Wilson JP: Basilar membrane vibration data and their relation to theories of frequency analysis. In Zwicker E, Terhardt E (ed): Facts and Models in Hearing. New York, Springer Verlag, 1974

33. Wolff HG: Efferente Aktivitat in den Statonerven einiger Landpulmonaten (Gastropoda). Z vergl Physiol 70:401–409, 1970

34. Young LR: The current status of vestibular system models. Automatica (Oxf.) 5:369–383, 1969

35. Zwislocki JJ: Analysis of some auditory characteristics. In Luce RS, Galante E: Handbook of Mathematical Psychology, Vol. III. New York: John Wiley & Sons, 1965

CENTRAL REPRESENTATION OF THE EIGHTH NERVE*

R. LORENTE DE NÓ

GENERAL PLAN OF THE ACOUSTIC SYSTEM

The centripetal acoustic system begins in the organ of Corti (Fig. 2–1). The bipolar cells of Corti's ganglion send their peripheral processes (usually called peripheral acoustic fibers or dendrites) to the organ of Corti, where they form endings in contact with the hair cells (external and internal). The central processes of the ganglion cells form the cochlear nerve.

According to classic concepts, there are three main primary cochlear nuclei: 1) the ventral nucleus, 2) the posterior nucleus (which, in fact, has two distinct parts, the posterior lateral nucleus and the posterior medial or interfascicular nucleus), and 3) the dorsal nucleus, which is often called the *tuberculum acusticum* (Tac). All central cochlear fibers divide into two branches, the anterior branch, which ends in the ventral nucleus (NuV), and the posterior branch, which, after crossing successively through the posterior lateral and interfascicular nuclei, ends in the Tac. In turn an important fraction of the axons of the neurons of the primary nuclei form the efferent pathways.

Three main pathways leave the primary acoustic nuclei. Two of them, often called the acoustic striae, are generally believed to be entirely crossed. They are the dorsal stria (of von Monakow),

* This chapter is a brief and partial summary of a forthcoming monograph.

which arises from the dorsal acoustic nucleus, and the intermediate stria (of Held), which arises chiefly from a particular part of the posterior nucleus (for a recent presentation, see Adams and Warr [1]). The most powerful efferent pathway is the trapezoid body. The view has frequently been presented that the trapezoid body supplies fibers only to the contralateral lemniscus, it is likely, however, that the trapezoid body also supplies a smaller number of fibers (indicated in Figure 2–1 by dashed line at lower left) to the homolateral lemniscus.

All three efferent paths, particularly the trapezoid body, give branches to the exceedingly complex system of nuclei of the superior olivary complex as well as to the reticular formation. One of the reasons the superior olivary complex has received much attention is that this complex is the first part of the brain stem in which fibers from the primary acoustic nuclei of the two sides may act simultaneously or in quick succession upon one and the same group of neurons. It therefore seems reasonable to assume that the superior olivary complex plays a role in the localization of the source of sound. An interesting diagram, based upon an idea of Bekesy, as to how localization of sound may be perceived, was published by Bergeijk (2). A more elaborate diagram of a similar nature has been recently published by Kiang (5).

For the reason that the exact composition of the main ascending path, the lateral lemniscus, is not known in detail, the path has been represented in Figure 2–1 by a single line. After it has given collateral branches to establish contacts with neurons located between its fibers (these neurons are said to be the nuclei of the lateral lemniscus), the lateral lemniscus ends in the nucleus of the inferior colliculus. This nucleus is the origin of a new ascending pathway, the quadrigeminal brachium, which ends in the medial geniculate body.

Fibers given off by the lateral lemniscus also end in more medial parts of the posterior colliculus, where the identities of the two colliculi become indistinct. Indeed, a determination of the boundaries in the collicular region of the distribution of the optic, acoustic, and spinotectal fibers is not possible because there are partial overlappings. The impulses initiated by the interaction of the activities of those three groups of fibers (for the sake of simplicity, optic and spinal afferents have not been included in the diagram) are carried downward by the tectospinal tracts as well as forward, by means of short fibers, into the thalamic reticular substance.

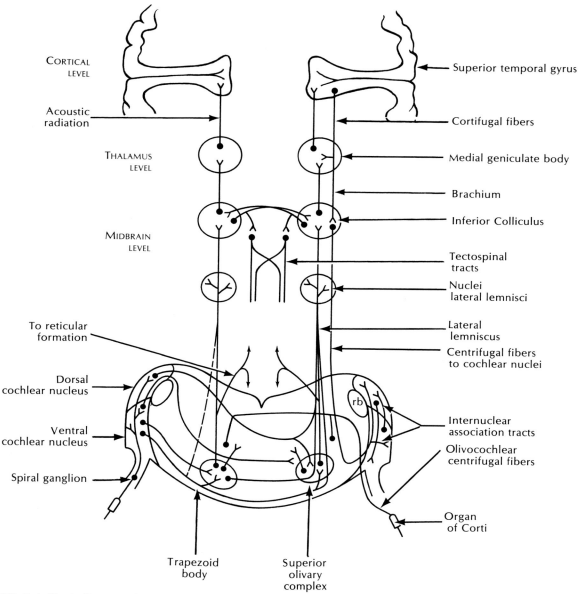

FIG. 2–1. Block diagram of acoustic system. **At left,** only uncrossed ascending or centripetal pathways are presented; **at right,** in addition to crossed centripetal pathways, there are also descending or centrifugal pathways. **Dashed line,** probable supply of fibers from trapezoid body to homolateral lemniscus; **rb,** restiform body.

The medial geniculate body is the origin of the acoustic radiation, which in man is believed to end in the superior temporal gyrus (convolution of Heschl). Animal experimentation has shown that acoustic responses may be recorded from several adjacent parts of the cerebral cortex (25).

The descending or centrifugal path begins in the cerebral cortex. The existence of corticofugal fibers, which end in thalamic nuclei, was first established by S. R. Cajal in 1900 (3), and it is at present believed that such corticofugal fibers exist in all thalamic nuclei. Whether corticofugal fibers descend beyond the internal geniculate body has not been ascertained, but there is experimental evidence, obtained by Rasmussen (19), that lesions in the collicular region cause the degeneration of centrifugal fibers that run peripherally to end in both primary acoustic nuclei (ventral and dorsal). A powerful bundle of centrifugal fibers for the Tac had already been identified in Golgi sections (Fig. 2–3, **CF**). Remarkably enough, in the Tac, both the cochlear afferent fibers and the centrifugal fibers establish much the same type of synaptic connections. In 1934, I found, during the study of Golgi sections that a remarkable situation existed. In spite of persistent search, no centrifugal fiber was found to arrive in the trapezoid body to enter into the oral part of the ventral nucleus (NuV=III), but a number of centrifugal fibers were found to arrive in the trapezoid body to end in the central and caudal parts of the ventral nucleus (NuV=II and NuV=I) by means of extensive arborizations.

As the last centrifugal path, Figure 2–1 presents Rasmussen's bundle, which has its origin in the retro-olivary reticular substance of the same side and of the contralateral side. Recently, with the use of an axonal transport method, the location of the cells of origin of the centrifugal fibers has been accurately ascertained by Warr (23). The fibers of Rasmussen's bundle end in the organ of Corti underneath the hair cells, both internal and external.

Finally, the right-hand side of the diagram in Figure 2–1 illustrates the existence of powerful internuclear association tracts that run as well from the NuV into the Tac as from the Tac into the NuV. In view of the presence of powerful internal association tracts, it is evident that the three main classic divisions of the acoustic nuclei, the NuV, the posterior nucleus, and the Tac, could never perform work independently from one another. Indeed, detailed anatomic analysis has shown that the *primary acoustic nuclei constitute a miniature brain,* which possesses a "cerebellum" of its own, the Tac. The essential features of the role played by that miniature brain are not difficult to ascertain.

Upon its arrival at the primary nuclei, any nerve impulse (i) initiated in the cochlea finds a large number of alternate anatomic paths into which it could enter to continue its propagation. The function of the miniature brain is to decide which paths should be open and which ones should be closed to cochlear impulse (i), depending upon the constellation of impulses that accompany (i) and upon the constellations of impulses that have preceded i. The existence of centrifugal fibers end-

ing in the primary nuclei insures that the decisions made in the primary nuclei match the instantaneous state of the upper acoustic stations.

Consideration of the block diagram in Figure 2–1 may serve to provide a general concept of the location of the acoustic pathways; consequently, if additional information on the anatomy of the brain is taken into account, the diagram may help in the interpretation of acoustic symptoms accompanying neurologic disorders. Problems of this kind, however, belong to specialized treatises such as the recent, well-documented book by Dublin (4).

PERIPHERAL ENDINGS IN THE COCHLEA

The types of fibers that innervate the organ of Corti are illustrated in Figure 2–2. To simplify the description, let the upper part of the figure be regarded as divided into fourths. In the first (right) quarter there are radial bundles (**1–6**) that innervate internal hair cells. These afferent fibers may be called specific radial fibers. In the second quarter of Figure 2–2 are radial bundles (**7–11**) that reach the level of the external hair cells and bend at sharp angles to form spiral fibers oriented toward the base. Each of these fibers establishes contacts with a number of hair cells. The maximal length of the baseward course of a spiral fiber may be as long as one-third of a spiral. These afferent fibers may be called spiral fibers.

In the third quarter there also are radial bundles containing thin fibers resulting from successive division of thick ones. In the ganglion of Corti there is a particular type of ganglion cell, which is represented in Figure 2–2 by two ganglion cells, one above the lower **b** and the other below the upper **b,** which send their peripheral processes toward the margin of the ganglion where they divide to form several thin radial fibers that reach the internal hair cells. Similar behavior is shown by fibers **13** and **14** (**12** is the peripheral process of a **b** ganglion cell). Thus it appears that there is a particular category of peripheral branches of Corti ganglion cells that divide into several thin fibers and innervate internal hair cells located at considerable distances from each other. These afferent fibers may be called unspecific radial fibers.

The last quarter of Figure 2–2 is difficult to analyze. It undoubtedly contains an admixture of unspecific radial afferents and of Rasmussen's efferents. Probably bundles **16** and **17** belong to the efferent system.

CENTRAL ENDINGS IN THE COCHLEAR NUCLEI

Although from time to time it has been reported that cochlear fibers may end outside the primary cochlear nuclei, reexamination of the problem (for a recent discussion, see Powell and Cowan [16]) has always led to the conclusion that the opinion of the classic investi-

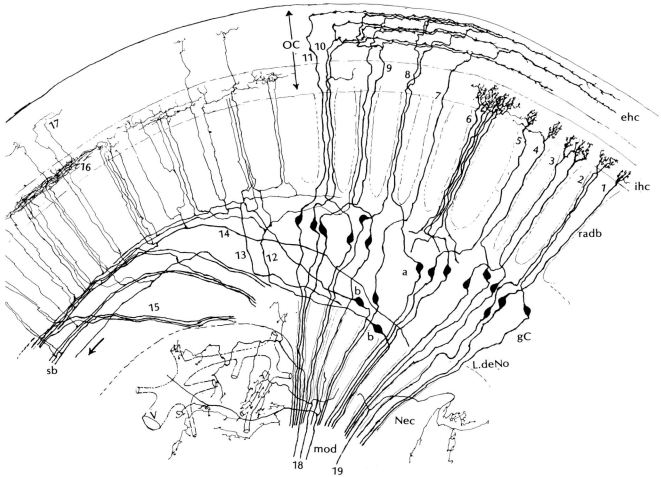

FIG. 2–2. Except for fibers **18** and **19** that innervate blood vessels (**V**), the drawing presents nerve cells and fibers found in a single section passing through the basal spiral turn of the cochlea. Eight-day-old mouse, Golgi rapid method. **gC,** ganglion of Corti; **Nec,** cochlear nerve; **mod,** modiolus; **OC,** organ of Corti. Ganglion cells (**a**) give rise to specific radial fibers (**1–6**) for internal hair cells (**ihc**) and to external spiral fibers (**7–11**) for external hair cells (**ehc**). Ganglion cells (**b**) give rise to unspecific radial fibers for internal hair cells (note ramified fibers **12, 13,** and **14**); **radb,** radial bundles; **sb,** spiral bundles (**arrow** points toward apex of cochlea); **15,** bundle of fibers joining the spiral system; **16** and **17,** bundles of fibers probably belonging to Rasmussen's efferent system.

gators (cf. Cajal [3]) was correct and that consequently all the cochlear fibers end within the boundaries of the primary nuclei.

These nuclei occupy a small volume, about 100–150 cu mm, but the cells that they contain have many times smaller volumes. For example, the largest neurons in the acoustic nuclei are the spherical cells, the body of which may have a diameter of 0.03 mm and consequently a volume of about 3.6×10^{-5} cu mm. In addition, the acoustic nuclei contain very numerous neurons with much smaller cell bodies (diameter as small as 3 or 4μm). Therefore, the facts cannot be surprising that the acoustic nuclei contain several hundreds of thousands of neurons and that the number of neurons in the acoustic nuclei is several times greater than the number of fibers in the acoustic nerve (about 50,000).

As was established by the classic investigators (see Koelliker [6] and Cajal [3] with extensive references to the classic literature), shortly after entering into the medulla, the cochlear fibers divide into two branches. These have been variously termed, but here they are called anterior and posterior branches. The division occurs with great regularity, and the points of division

FIG. 2–3. Parasagittal section through primary acoustic nuclei of a 4-day-old cat. Root fibers of the cochlear nerve **(NeC)** bifurcate to yield anterior **(ant)** and posterior **(po)** branches. The anterior branches cross through the three subdivisions **(I, II, III)** of ventral nucleus **(NuV)**. The posterior branches cross through interfascicular nucleus **(NuIntf)** to reach acoustic tubercle **(Tav)**; **CF,** bundle of centrifugal fibers ending in cortex of **Tac; CZ,** confluence zone of anterior and posterior lateral nuclei. Golgi rapid method. (Lorente de Nó R: Laryngoscope 47:373–377, 1937)

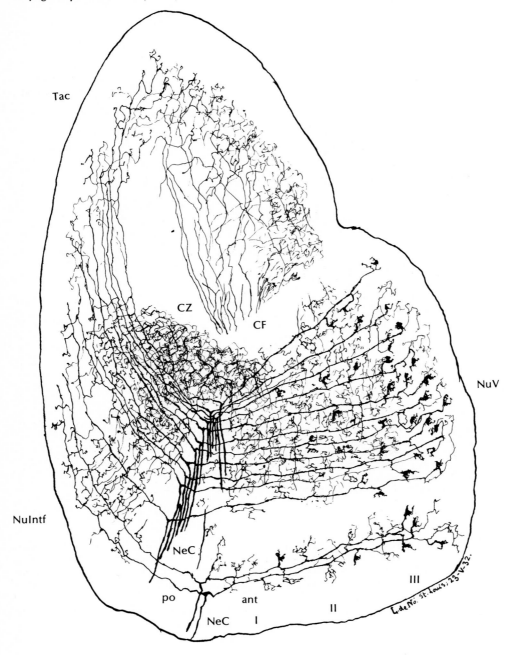

FIG. 2–4. Parasagittal section through cochlear root and neighboring parts of **NuV** and interfascicular nucleus (**NuIntf**). The endogenous fiber (**a**) forms an extensive ramification in caudal part of **NuV**. The cochlear root fibers (**1–19**) display a very regular arrangement of their points of division into anterior and posterior branches. Fiber **1** is supposed to belong to the apical end, and fiber **19** to the basal end, of the ganglion of Corti. A number of root fibers give off collateral branches (**b**) at variable distances from their points of division. Cat, a few days of age. Golgi rapid method. (Lorente de Nó R: Laryngoscope 43:1–38, 1933)

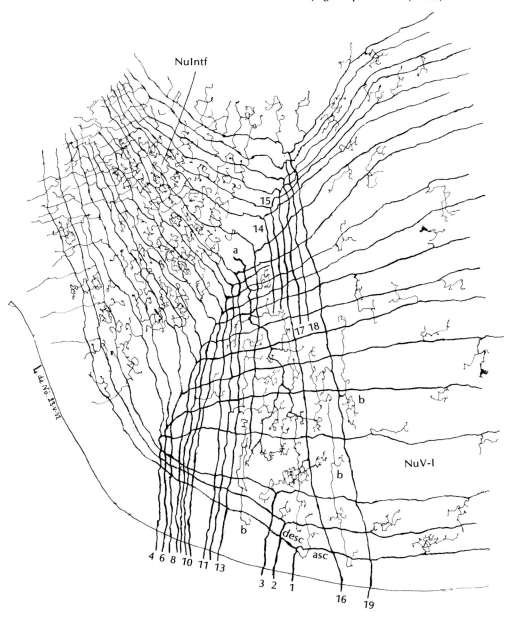

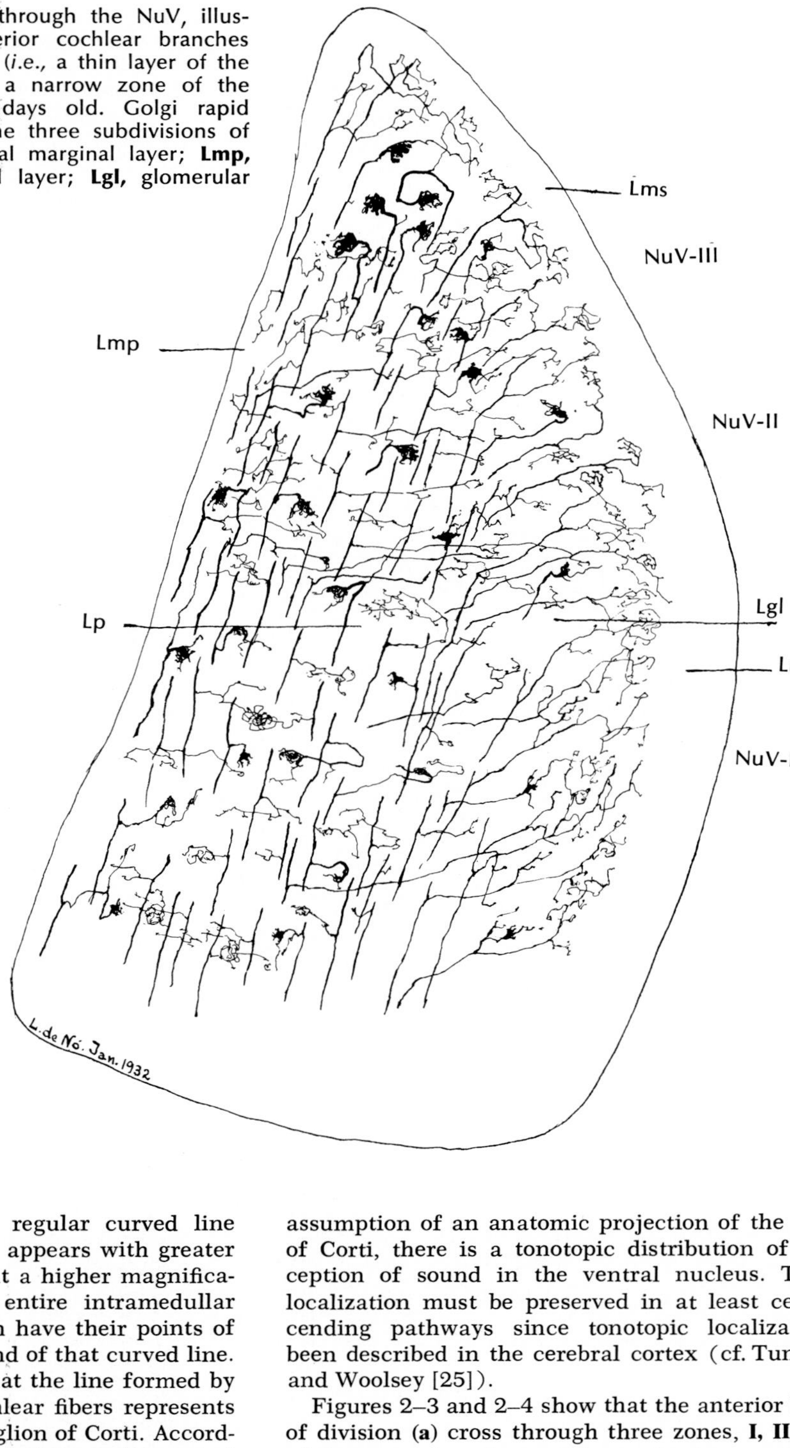

FIG. 2–5. Oblique frontal section through the NuV, illustrating the three streams of anterior cochlear branches present in each elementary lamella (*i.e.*, a thin layer of the nucleus that receives fibers from a narrow zone of the ganglion of Corti). Cat, several days old. Golgi rapid method. **NuV-I, NuV-II, NuV-III,** the three subdivisions of the ventral nucleus; **Lms,** superficial marginal layer; **Lmp,** deep marginal layer; **Lp,** principal layer; **Lgl,** glomerular layer; **Lmol,** molecular layer.

of the individual fibers form a regular curved line (Fig. 2–3). This important detail appears with greater clarity in Figure 2–4 (prepared at a higher magnification). Figure 2–4 includes the entire intramedullar course of fibers 16 and 19, which have their points of division near to or at the dorsal end of that curved line. At present it is widely believed that the line formed by the points of division of the cochlear fibers represents the projection of an uncoiled ganglion of Corti. According to the observations of Levy and Kobrak (8) and of Sando (21), the lowest (ventral) points of that line correspond to the apex of the cochlea. As was described by Rose and associates (20), in agreement with the assumption of an anatomic projection of the ganglion of Corti, there is a tonotopic distribution of the perception of sound in the ventral nucleus. Tonotopic localization must be preserved in at least certain ascending pathways since tonotopic localization has been described in the cerebral cortex (cf. Tunturi [22] and Woolsey [25]).

Figures 2–3 and 2–4 show that the anterior branches of division (a) cross through three zones, **I, II,** and **III,** of the ventral nucleus, each one having specific structural traits. For example, the size of the Held endings increases progressively from NuV-I to NuV-III. The posterior branches of division, after having left collaterals in the interfascicular nucleus reach the Tac, where they end intermingled with centrifugal fibers. Above the highest point of division of the cochlear fibers there is the dense fibrillar plexus of an association nucleus, the confluence zone (Fig. 2–3, **CZ**), where the anterior and posterior lateral nuclei become continuous. Although the confluence zone receives branches from cochlear fibers, its main sources of supply of nerve fibers are endogenous association tracts.

As it appears in Figure 2–3, the situation offered by the NuV seems to be quite simple, because the anterior cochlear branches cross through the entire ventral nucleus in more or less parallel bundles, which form nearly 90° angles with the cochlear root fibers. When reference is made to Golgi-stained longitudinal sections through the ventral nucleus of a cat a few days old, it does not seem improper to speak of the "line" formed by the points of division of the cochlear fibers, even though in each section the line is about 100 μm thick and the line may be present in two or even in part in three successive sections. To do so, however, is no longer possible in the analysis of the acoustic nuclei of adult cats. In reference to adult nuclei, when speaking about projection of the ganglion, the correct procedure suggested by Osen (15) is to state that to each small segment of the ganglion corresponds a layer (*lamella*) of anterior cochlear fibers. Exact information is not available as to whether the elementary layers are plane or—what is more likely—curved, nor is there any information upon the angle that each elementary layer forms with the "surface" created by the points of division of the cochlear root fibers. However, since histologic sections that are parallel (or nearly so) to the anterior cochlear branches can include only parts of closely neighboring layers, in a first approximation, it is permissible to regard such sections as exhibiting the composition of each elementary layer.

Figure 2–5 reproduces an oblique frontal section through the NuV in which long segments of the individual anterior cochlear branches are included. Therefore, the section may be said to illustrate the behavior of the anterior cochlear branches in an elementary layer of the nucleus.

The section illustrated in Figure 2–5 passed through that part of the NuV that belongs to the base of the cochlea; NuV-III with its large Held chalices, therefore, had a much shallower depth than in the rest of NuV. The anterior cochlear branches form three parallel streams, the widest of which, by far, is the central stream (Fig. 2–5). This stream carries the fibers that form the majority of Held endings. The fibers of the central stream also give off short and long collaterals; the short ones form synaptic endings (boutons of various sizes) in the neighborhood of the fiber of origin, while the long ones reach the glomerular layer of the anterior lateral nucleus. The fibers of the lateral stream do not reach the zone (NuV-III) where large Held chalices are present. They cross only through NuV-I and NuV-II, where they form a discrete number of small Held bulbs, while they supply numerous collaterals and even terminal fibers to the anterior lateral nucleus. In all probability, at least a significant part of the fibers of the lateral stream correspond to the cochlear spiral afferents. In Figure 2–5 only a minute part of the medial stream is present, the two lax ramifications above the line labeled **lmp** that ends in the deep marginal lamina. Further details on anterior cochlear branches can be found in reference 12.

PARCELING OF THE PRIMARY ACOUSTIC TERRITORY

On further analysis I found it advisable to improve details of the parceling originally made (10), chiefly by removing the designation *nucleus interstitialis*. The presence of bundles of myelinated root fibers between the neurons does not convert the interstitial nucleus into an anatomic entity. According to its structure, the anterior (oral) part of the interstitial nucleus belongs to zone I of the ventral nucleus while the posterior (caudal) part belongs to the principal layer of the lateral posterior nucleus. Nevertheless, the fact may not be ignored that in the part of NuV-I included within the bundles of root fibers, collaterals may be seen arising directly from the root fibers at considerable distances from the points at which those fibers divide into anterior and posterior branches. Examples of such situations can be found in Figure 2–4 (**12, 13, 16, 19**). In Figure 2–6 the cells that receive endings from root collaterals have been labeled "irregular neurons."

Elaborations introduced in the new parceling (Fig. 2–6) are as follows: The lateral layers of NuV-I and NuV-II have been grouped into a lateral anterior nucleus (*nucleus lateralis anterior*), because they contain neurons that make contributions to an important association bundle, the lateral ventrotubercular tract (*tractus ventrotubercularis lateralis*). Similarly, part **a** of the old posterior nucleus has been joined with the old lateral nucleus to form a new posterior lateral nucleus (*nucleus lateralis posterior*), which is the origin of an important association bundle the posterotubercular tract (*tractus posterotubercularis*). Parts **b** and **c** of the old posterior nucleus have now become the lax and dense zones of the interfascicular nucleus. Probably, at least part of the lax zone of the interfascicular nucleus corresponds to Osen's region of octopus cells. The fibrillar and dendritic plexuses of the anterior and posterior lateral nuclei become continuous in a zone located above the highest points of division of the cochlear root fibers called the confluence zone (Fig. 2–3, **CZ**). In the dorsal direction this zone extends up to the central nucleus of the Tac.

In Figure 2–6 the nuclei at the left have been labeled **primary** because they receive comparable numbers of cochlear afferents and of endogenous association fibers. The nuclei on the right have been labeled **association** because they receive mainly fibers of endogenous

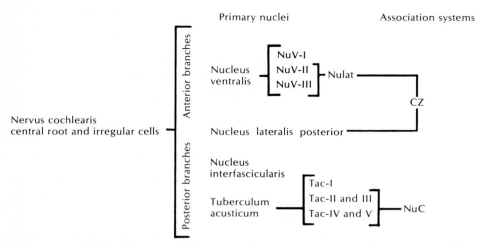

FIG. 2–6. Parceling of primary nuclei of cochlear nerve **(NeC). NuV-I, NuV-II, NuV-III,** the three subdivisions of the ventral nucleus; **Nula,** anterior lateral nucleus; **Nulp,** posterior lateral nucleus; **NuIntf,** interfascicular nucleus; **NuC,** central nucleus; **Tac,** acoustic tubercle; **CZ,** confluence zone.

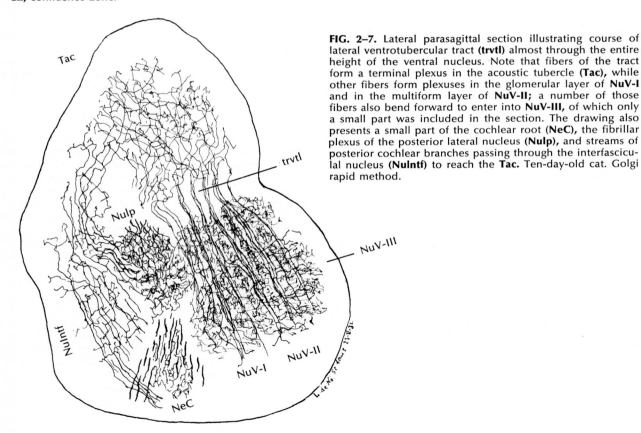

FIG. 2–7. Lateral parasagittal section illustrating course of lateral ventrotubercular tract **(trvtl)** almost through the entire height of the ventral nucleus. Note that fibers of the tract form a terminal plexus in the acoustic tubercle **(Tac),** while other fibers form plexuses in the glomerular layer of **NuV-I** and in the multiform layer of **NuV-II;** a number of those fibers also bend forward to enter into **NuV-III,** of which only a small part was included in the section. The drawing also presents a small part of the cochlear root **(NeC),** the fibrillar plexus of the posterior lateral nucleus **(Nulp),** and streams of posterior cochlear branches passing through the interfascicular nucleus **(NuIntf)** to reach the **Tac.** Ten-day-old cat. Golgi rapid method.

origin. Indeed, the central nucleus of the Tac does not receive either cochlear afferents or centrifugal fibers.

There are five association tracts. The marginal tract (*tractus marginalis*) of the ventral nucleus, the lateral ventrotubercular tract (*tractus ventrotubercularis lateralis*, Fig. 2–7, **trvtl**), the central ventrotubercular tract (*tractus ventrotubercularis centralis*), the medial ventrotubercular tract (*tractus ventrotubercularis medialis*) and the posterotubercular tract (*tractus posterotubercularis*). Except for the medial ventrotubercular tract, which consists solely of fibers from NuV-I and NuV-II to the Tac (Fig. 2–8) all the other tracts include fibers going in the two opposite directions.

The available space allows only consideration of the most prominent structural features of the NuV and of the Tac. Nevertheless, the information will be sufficient to justify significant theoretic arguments.

DETAILS OF STRUCTURE OF THE VENTRAL NUCLEUS

In the principal layer of the NuV (Fig. 2–5, **Lp**) there are two classes of neurons. Neurons with long efferent axons that leave the NuV in the trapezoid body (Fig. 2–8, **2–6, 9**) and neurons with short axons that form more or less extensive ramifications within the NuV itself (Fig. 2–8, **1, 7, 8, A, A**).

There are two main types of neurons with efferent axons: 1) brush cells (spherical cells of Osen) that have a more or less spherical body from which one or two, rarely three, short dendrites arise; by repeated division each dendrite generates a large number of slender branches (Fig. 2–10, **1–17**; Fig. 2–11, **A**); 2) multipolar or polygonal neurons that have cell bodies of variable shape and several long and discreetly ramified dendrites (Fig. 2–10, **p, p**). The multipolar cells located in the oral part of NuV may also be called basket cells because their terminal branches form baskets surrounding bodies of brush cells (Fig. 2–8, **2, 8, 9**; Fig. 2–11, **G, d, d′**). An important difference between brush cells and all other types of cells consists in that the so-called Held endings (chalices or bulbs) of cochlear fibers make contact only with brush cells. In NuV-III each cochlear fiber forms only one Held chalice, and no brush cell receives more than one chalice. In more caudal parts of the NuV brush cells may receive two or even three Held bulbs formed by different cochlear fibers (Fig. 2–11, **D**).

In the principal lamina of NuV-III that corresponds to Osen's zone of large spherical cells, the brush cells greatly outnumber the multipolar neurons; the relative number of multipolar neurons progressively increases throughout NuV-II, and in NuV-I the number of multipolar cells becomes greater than that of brush cells. In addition, the behaviors of the efferent axons establish an essential difference between NuV-III on one hand and NuV-II and NuV-I on the other. In NuV-III the efferent axons (Fig. 2–9, **1–8**) give off recurrent collaterals, and as a rule, after having joined the trapezoid

body (Fig. 2–9, **ctr**), they give off one or two branches that, after a course parallel to the medial marginal lamina, re-enter NuV-III as U-fibers to form extensive ramifications. With advancing maturation, the plexus formed by recurrent collaterals and U-fibers becomes an important fraction of the total fibrillar plexus in NuV-III (cf. Figure 11 in reference 12). No branch of an efferent axon of NuV-III has ever been observed joining one of the ventrotubercular tracts.

In NuV-II and in NuV-I the efferent axons give off, if any, only one or, exceptionally, two poorly ramified recurrent collaterals, but all or at least by far the majority of the efferent axons give off a thick branch that joins a ventrotubercular tract. The axons of multipolar cells always send their association branches to the medial ventrotubercular tract. As a rule, the axon divides into efferent and association branches after having reached the trapezoid body (Fig. 2–8, **4, 6, 9**) but earlier divisions of the axon also take place (Fig. 2–8, **2**). The axons of brush cells send their association branches to the central or to the lateral ventrotubercular tract. For example, Figure 2–8 illustrates two brush cells (**3, 5**). The axon of cell **3**, after division within the trapezoid body, sent its association branch back into the NuV to reach either the central or the lateral ventrotubercular tract, while the axon of cell **5** divided in the neighborhood of the cell body into an efferent branch for the trapezoid body and an association branch for the lateral ventrotubercular tract.

DETAILS OF SYNAPTIC ARTICULATIONS IN NuV-III

Synaptic articulations are established between two plexuses: the receptor plexus formed by the bodies and dendritic arborizations of the neurons and the transmitter or fibrillar plexus formed by the terminal arborizations of several kinds of fibers—cochlear afferents; collaterals and U-fibers arising from efferent axons; association fibers originating in other subdivisions of the acoustic nuclei; and arborizations of short axons. In other subdivisions of the acoustic nuclei a fifth component has to be considered: centrifugal fibers descending from upper centers.

In NuV-III, where the brush cells constitute by far the largest fraction of the cell population, it is often found that the cell bodies are collected in groups outside the dense plexus formed by the confluence of dendritic branches from a number of brush cells. For example, it can be seen in Figure 2–10 that dendrites of cells **2** and **4–7** converge to form a dense local plexus and that the dendrites of cells **8, 9,** and **11–13** also converge to form another local plexus. Often, brush cells that have several dendrites contribute to several local plexuses; such is the case, for example, with cells **2** and **10–12** in Figure 2–10. The bodies of multipolar cells with efferent axons and of cells with short axons are always located within local dendritic plexuses of brush cells and their dendrites cross between and through a number of local plexuses.

FIG. 2–8. Frontal section through NuV-II immediately adjacent to caudal end of NuV-III, containing cells with long or efferent axon of two different types—brush cells **(3, 5)** and multipolar or basket cells **(2, 4, 6, 9)**—and cells with short axons **(1, 7, 8); A, A,** end arborizations of short axons. Only the initial parts of the dendrites of cell **4** have been reproduced. **Arrows** at bottom indicate that the efferent axons divide into two branches going in different directions, toward trapezoid body **(to trb)** and toward Tac **(to Tac).** Cat, a few days old. Golgi rapid method.

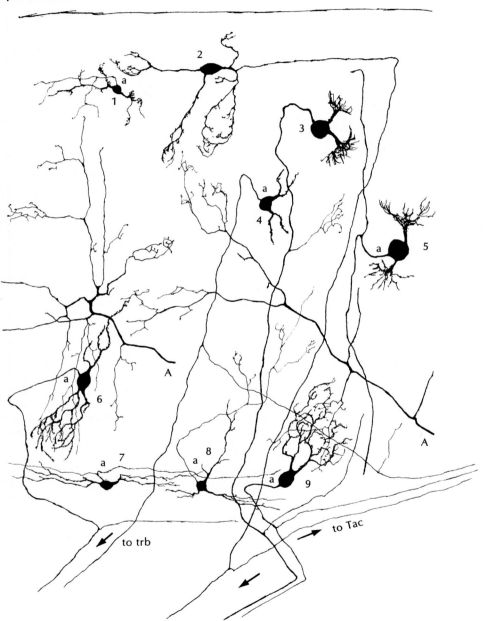

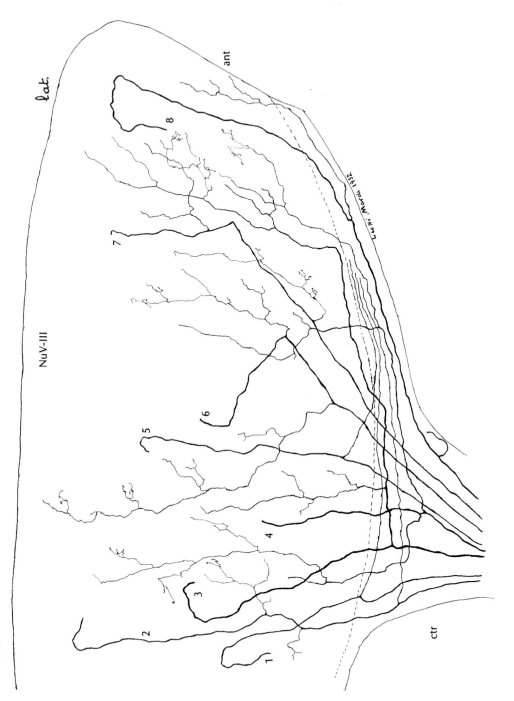

FIG. 2–9. Types of efferent axons of **NuV-III** observed in several rapid Golgi-stained sections, presented in semidiagrammatic fashion. **ant,** anterior; **lat,** lateral; **ctr,** trapezoid body. Newborn cats.

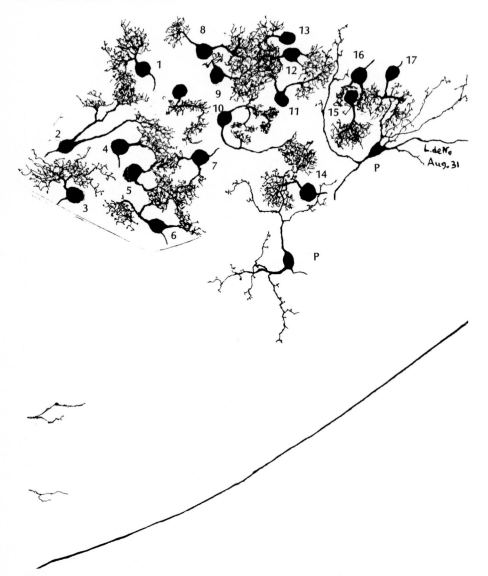

FIG. 2–10. Longitudinal section through the part of NuV-III, that belongs to central part of Corti's ganglion. All cells **(1–17)** are brush cells; **P,** polygonal neurons, presumably with efferent axons. Adult cat. Golgi-Cox method.

Owing to the complexity of the dendritic and fibrillar plexuses in the NuV, it is practically impossible to ascertain, with the use of present-day techniques the distribution of synapses of different kinds along the dendritic branches. However, no major difficulty is encountered in ascertaining the main features of the synaptic junctions on the bodies and initial segments of dendrites. It is always found that a number of fibers contribute to the formation of a synaptic shell that covers the cell body and the initial segments of the dendrites.

The constitution of the synaptic shells of brush cells in the NuV is illustrated in Figure 2–11. As it appears in **B,** the Held chalice does not form a continuous layer covering nearly one hemisphere of the brush cell. In the chalice itself there are wide holes, and empty spaces are present between the irregular processes that arise from the ragged contour of the chalice. However, the holes and other empty spaces (Fig. 2–11, **B**) are filled by synaptic boutons formed by fibers that in part are collaterals of cochlear fibers while the rest have one of the endogenous origins mentioned previously. In

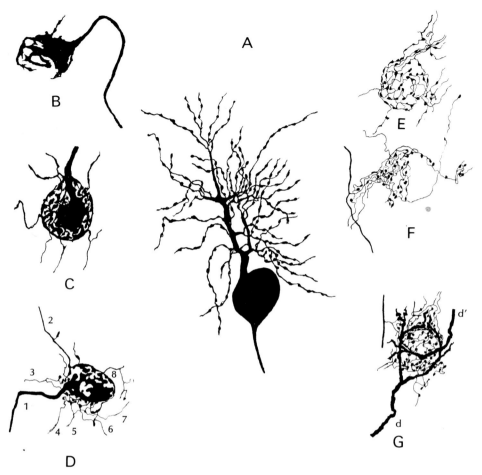

FIG. 2–11. A, spheroidal brush cell of NuV-II. Arborization of the single dendrite has been reproduced as accurately as possible. **B, C, D** illustrate the fact that a Held Chalice (**B, C**) or two articulated Held bulbs (**D, 1, 2**) cannot cover more than one hemisphere of the cell body, as well as the fact that synaptic boutons formed by other fibers (**D, 3–8**) are present in the "holes" of the Held endings. The other hemisphere of the synaptic shell is formed by synaptic boutons of ordinary sizes. **d, d',** terminal dendritic branches of a basket cell surrounding the synaptic shell of a brush cell. **A,** adult cat; Golgi-Cox method; **B–G,** synaptic shells from cats a few days old. Golgi rapid method.

Figure 2–11, **D,** the fact is illustrated that two different cochlear fibers (**1, 2**), one forming a large Held bulb and the other a small bulb, may create a perforated synaptic shell covering nearly one hemisphere of the cell body. Fibers **3–8** formed synaptic boutons to fill empty spaces within and between the two two Held bulbs. The other hemisphere of the brush cell is covered by interlacing clusters of synaptic boutons (Fig. 2–11, **E–G**) a number of which are formed by fibers that also deposit boutons along a dendrite. The axon of the brush cell always has its origin in the hemisphere of the cell body that is covered by synaptic boutons; to be more specific, the axon never has its origin in that part of the cell body covered by the chalice or the bulbs.

DETAILS OF STRUCTURE OF THE ACOUSTIC TUBERCLE

The acoustic tubercle (Tac) must be divided into cortex and central nucleus. Although in the cortex several zones must be considered, Tac I, Tac II and III, and Tac IV and V, in this brief summary only the structure of Tac II will be analyzed.

In Figure 2–12 **(B)** the stratification of Tac II has been indicated by means of a few representative elements: **gr** is a dwarf cell (granule) with a short axon that forms a horizontal fiber in the plexiform layer; **sc** is a cell with a short axon of the plexiform layer, which may be called a basket cell because its axon form an arborization surrounding the bodies of bipolar cells;

bc is a bipolar cell with axon **a** that descends to join Monakow's stria. To the left of the same bipolar cell body **(bc)** there are the dendritic and axonal arborizations of a cell with short axon belonging to layer II; **cc** is a vertical or fusiform cell of layer III, having its axon ramified within layers II and III; **pc** is a cell with efferent axon of the polymorphic layer **(IV)**. To the right of it a small cell of the polymorphic layer has an ascending axon **(a)** which reaches the plexiform layer.

Segment **A** of Figure 2-12 illustrates the innervation of Tac II by cochlear fibers **(cf)**. Since these fibers cross through layer IV without leaving in it terminal branches and since they do not reach layer I, it is evident that cochlear fibers can establish synaptic contacts only with bodies and dendrites located in layers II and III. The majority of the synapses must be established in layer III, where the terminal plexus has the greater density. It is a remarkable fact that the mode of termination of cochlear afferents is very similiar to the mode of termination of the centrifugal fibers (Fig. 2–3, **CF**) and to the mode of termination of collateral branches of axons of vertical cells (Fig. 2–15, **a** and **b–d**). Also worthy of mention is the fact that, in the Tac, the contribution to the presynaptic plexus made by cochlear afferents is small in relation to the total contribution made by fibers of endogenous origins.

An important component of the plexiform layer is a wealthy system of parallel fibers. Figure 2–13 presents the Tac of a 16-day-old mouse as it appeared in a rapid Golgi parasagittal section. The density of the stream of parallel fibers is comparable to that found in the molecular layer of the cerebellar cortex. In the Tac, however, the parallel fibers have more varied origins: cells with horizontal axon of layer I (Fig. 2–14, **3, 4**), cells with ascending axon of layers III and IV (Fig. 2–12; Fig. 2–14, **10, 11**) and probably also small cells of the central nucleus.

Layer II, besides numerous small cells with short axons of different types (Fig. 2–12; Fig. 2–15, **2**), contains the cell bodies of the bipolar cells and the end ramifications of dendrites of a number of cell types of layers III and IV (Fig. 2–14, **6, 12**; Fig. 2–15, **1, 2, 4**).

The most numerous elements of layer III are the vertical or fusiform cells (Fig. 2–14, **5, 8**; Fig. 2–15, **4**). the dendrites of which run chiefly in vertical directions, *i.e.*, perpendicular to the surface of the Tac. The ascending dendrites never reach the plexiform layer (I). When they are present, the descending dendrites do not penetrate into layer IV. The small vertical cells are typical short axon cells; their axons may be ramified either in layers III and IV (Fig. 2–14, **5**) or only within layer IV (Fig. 2–14, **8**). The large vertical cells (Fig. 2–15, **4**) have semilong axons that, after having given off a number of branches, leave the Tac and join the lateral ventrotubercular tract, ultimately to reach the ventral nucleus. In layer III there also are polygonal cells having short ascending axons that form arborizations in layer II (Fig. 2–14, **1**).

In layer III, as well as in layer IV, there are certain large or medium-sized multipolar neurons (Fig. 2–14, **6, 12**) with efferent axons, that without having given off any collateral branch join the stria of von Monakow. The dendrites of those multipolar cells ramify themselves in layers IV, III and II, but their branches never reach the plexiform layer (I).

In layer IV, besides the multipolar neurons with efferent axons, there are numerous cells with short axons ramified within layer IV (Fig. 2–14, **9**, Fig. 2–15, **6, 7**), or with axon ascending to layer III (Fig. 2–15, **3, 5**), or with axon ascending to layer I (Fig. 2–14, **10, 11**).

In the central nucleus, besides large multipolar neurons with efferent axons that join von Monakow's stria, there are medium sized multipolar neurons that have axons joining ventrotubercular tracts and small neurons having axons that probably ascend to reach upper layers of the cortex of the Tac.

FUNCTIONAL PROBLEMS RELATED TO STRUCTURE

At present the mechanism of synaptic transmission is still far from being understood. Consideration of the anatomic arrangements leaves no doubt that each neuron is a summation apparatus that discharges an impulse into its axon only in response to activation of a number of synapses. In a few cases that include the bipolar cells of the Tac, the anatomic information (Figs. 2–11 to 2–14) is sufficient to ascertain the location of the synapses with different kinds of fibers. In general, however, the distribution of synapses of various kinds on dendrites cannot be ascertained because even in 120-μm thick histologic sections, dendrites and presynaptic fibers of different kinds are mixed in a seemingly haphazard manner. For this reason, although the dendritic arborization includes by far the larger part of the surface of each brush cell (Figs. 2–10 and 2–11,**A**), the question must remain open as to how those dendrites participate in the process of summation of synaptic stimuli. Nevertheless, concerning the brush cells, in particular those of NuV-III, the assumptions seem to be reasonable that 1) synaptic inputs to dendrites serve only to regulate the stimulation threshold of the body of the neuron, and 2) a similar role is played by the synaptic boutons that make contact with the cell body. According to those assumptions, the brush cells discharge only in response to impulses arriving at a Held chalice.

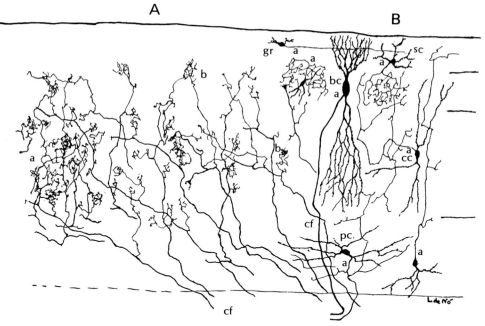

FIG. 2–12. In **A,** ramifications of cochlear fibers **(cf)** in layers II and III are presented. At **a** is the zone where the terminal plexus has greatest density; **b, b,** cochlear endings for bodies of bipolar cells of layer II or of large multipolar cells of layer III. **B** is a diagram of important structural features of the Tac. Approximate boundaries between layers are indicated by horizontal lines at right. **gr,** granule of molecular layer (layer I) giving rise to a parallel fiber; **sc,** cell of molecular layer, having a short axon ramified in the layer of bodies of bipolar cells (layer II); **bc** bipolar cell, with ascending dendrites ramified in layer I, descending dendrites ramified in layer III and an axon **(a)** that, without giving off collaterals, reaches the white matter. To the left of the body of that cell is a small cell with short axon **(a)** ramified within layer II. **cc,** a cell with short axon of the layer of vertical cells (layer III); **pc,** a cell of layer IV (of polymorphic cells), with axon reaching white substance. To the right of that cell is one with ascending axon that reaches the molecular layer. Cat, 12 days old. Golgi rapid method. (Lorente de Nó R: Laryngoscope 43:327–350, 1933)

FIG. 2–13. Parasagittal section through acoustic tubercle of a 16-day-old mouse, showing dense array of parallel fibers in plexiform **(pl)** or molecular layer, the seemingly empty layer of the bodies of bipolar cells **(b),** and the dense fibrilar plexus in the deeper layers and in the central nucleus **(NuC); o,** oral; **c,** caudal; **a,** axon. Golgi rapid method.

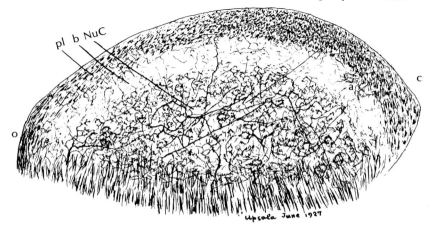

Whether an impulse arriving at the chalice will be sufficient to initiate an impulse in the underlying cell body will depend upon the instantaneous value of the stimulation threshold, and if the threshold is high the impulse in the chalice may fail to effect postsynaptic stimulation unless excitatory impulses have arrived simultaneously or nearly so at synaptic boutons located in a hole, or near the margin, of the chalice. At any rate, the nascent impulse must be initiated underneath the chalice and it must propagate itself incrementally, along one or more narrow paths, through nearly one hemisphere of the cell membrane, to reach the axon. If inhibitory impulses are delivered to boutons located outside the chalice and near the axon, the nascent impulse will be conducted decrementally, and it will become extinguished before reaching the axon.

Similar conditions must apply to the initiation of impulses in the bodies of multipolar neurons. The postsynaptic impulse will be initiated in a discrete zone of the body membrane covered by synaptic boutons that happen to be active simultaneously or nearly so. The nascent impulse will propagate itself incrementally through narrow paths in the membrane of the cell body, ultimately to reach the axon, unless the propagation is caused to be decremental by the activity of inhibitory boutons. However, in the case of multipolar neurons with long dendrites and especially in the case of the giant neurons with short axons of NuV the possibility must undoubtedly exist of initiation of postsynaptic impulses in discrete zones of dendrites.

Among the many important facts brought to light by electrophysiological research, a few may be singled out for consideration. In the absence of peripheral stimulation, the acoustic nuclei are the site of continuous activity maintained by the arrival of nerve impulses spontaneously initiated in the cochlea. The activity is necessarily accompanied by circulation of impulses in chains of neurons. Since spontaneous activity in the cochlea and in the acoustic centers is perceived by humans as silence, it must be concluded that the spontaneous activity serves to determine the background states of the various subdivisions of the acoustic nuclei, to which deviations caused by

FIG. 2–14. Transverse section through the acoustic tubercle (Tac-II). Note that only the ascending dendrites of the bipolar cells are ramified in the plexiform or molecular layer; the ascending dendrites of vertical or multipolar neurons of layers III and IV end within the layer of the bodies of bipolar cells (II). **1, 2,** bipolar cells, whose axons, without giving off collaterals, join von Monakow's stria; **3, 4,** cells of the plexiform layer with axons **(a)** joining the stream of parallel fibers; **5, 7, 8, 9,** cells with short axons ramified either within one layer **(8, 9)** or in both layers III and IV **(5, 7)**; **10, 11,** cells with axons that ascend to the plexiform layer and form parallel fibers; **6, 12,** multipolar neurons. Cat, several days old. Golgi rapid method.

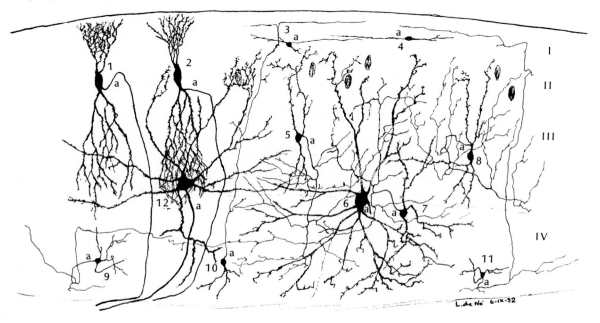

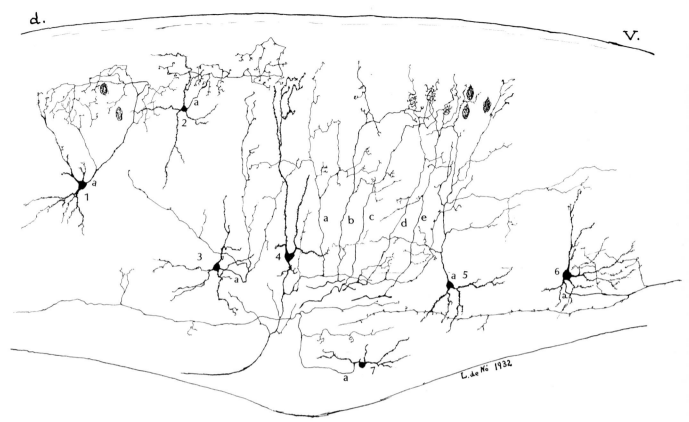

FIG. 2–15. Transverse section through acoustic tubercle (Tac-II). **1, 2,** cells of layers III and II with short axons **(a)** forming terminal arborizations chiefly in the layer of the bodies of the bipolar cells; **3, 5,** cells of layer IV with short ascending axons **(a)** ramified in layers II and III. **6, 7,** cells of layer IV with short axons **(a)** ramified within the same layer. **4,** a large vertical cell with axon that after having given off a number of collateral branches joined an association tract. The end arborization of one of the collaterals **(a)** was entirely contained in the histologic section. This arborization is remarkably similar to the end arborizations **(b-e)** of cochlear fibers that were observed in a different section. Cats, 12 days old. Golgi rapid method.

sound stimuli are referred. In other words, what we hear is the result of those deviations from the ground states of the acoustic nuclei, which are caused by external sources of sound.

According to Koerber and co-workers (7), destruction of the cochlea practically abolished the spontaneous activity in the NuV while the spontaneous activity in the Tac changed but little. From those two fundamental facts both a particular and a general conclusion may be drawn.

The particular conclusion is easily reached: In the Tac important association pathways arise, which end in the NuV. Since by itself, spontaneous activity in the Tac cannot elicit neuronal discharges in the NuV, it is clear that the role of

impulses conducted by those association paths consists chiefly of modifying the effects that cochlear impulses may produce in the neurons of the ventral and posterior nuclei. The general conclusion (or rather, assumption) is that activity in the Tac and upper centers serves to maintain in the acoustic nuclei the engram of the background state of "active silence" to which the perception of sound is referred.

To emphasize the important role that chains of neurons play in the transmission of cochlear impulses through the primary nuclei, let us consider the responses of brush cells of NuV-III to volleys of cochlear impulses arriving at Held chalices. As already mentioned, the response of those neurons is determined by activities both in the chalices and in synaptic boutons (Fig. 2–11). Consequently, the response to a given volley of cochlear impulses must depend upon the effects that previous volleys have produced in a variety of neurons. In the first place, since the axons of the brush cells of NuV-III give off recurrent collaterals and U-fibers (Fig. 2–9), the response of any one brush cell must depend upon previous discharges of neighboring and distant brush cells of NuV-III, as well as upon discharges of neurons with short axons. On the other hand, since through the ventrotubercular association tracts the neurons with efferent axon of NuV-I and NuV-II send impulses to the Tac, and since in turn the Tac, through the ventrotubercular tracts, sends impulses to NuV-III (see ref. 12, Fig. 12), it is evident that the responses of the brush cells of NuV-III must depend upon the effects that previous discharges of neurons of NuV-I and NuV-II have caused in the Tac. Similarly, the effects that impulses arriving from NuV-I and NuV-II may produce in the Tac must depend upon the constellation of impulses initiated in upper centers that are arriving at the Tac through the powerful centrifugal tract (Fig. 2–2, **CF**). As was mentioned early in this chapter, no centifugal fiber enters into NuV-III, but centrifugal fibers enter into NuV-II and NuV-I. Consequently, upper acoustic centers can influence the activity in NuV-III only by modifying either the activity in NuV-II and NuV-I or the activity in Tac.

Thus, it appears that the role played by the primary nuclei in the transmission of cochlear impulses is essentially different from, and far more complex than the role that would be played by an assembly of mutually independent neurons, each one acting as a relay that converts trains of afferent cochlear impulses having given frequency and duration into trains of efferent impulses having either the same or different frequency and duration. In the primary acoustic nuclei, as a result of the activity of superimposed short and long chains of neurons, determination is made of what cochlear impulses should be transmitted and how the transmission should be made. Figuratively speaking, as stated earlier in this chapter, transmission of impulses through the primary acoustic nuclei involves the operation of a miniature brain that possesses a cerebellum of its own—the acoustic tubercle.

There is an important, theoretic reason to believe that the Tac is the "cerebellum" of the acoustic system. In the course of phylogenetic evolution, the cochlea appeared at a very late stage, after the structure and connections of the cerebellum had been developed in manners exquisitely suitable for functions such as the regulation of body posture and motion. Consequently, when the cochlea and the acoustic system made their late phylogenetic appearance, no addition could be made to the old cerebellum that would suit the needs of the newly created acoustic function. For this compelling reason, a new cerebellum—the Tac—had to be developed. In view of its recent phylogenetic origin, it should not be surprising that the acoustic "cerebellum" has a similar but far more elaborate structure than the motor cerebellum.

To avoid misunderstandings, it should be emphasized that although the cochlear nerve and the primary acoustic nuclei have no direct connection at all with the cerebellum, other parcels of the acoustic system may have cerebellar connections. To be more specific, there are, in the reticular substance, parcels that are related to the superior olive complex and that participate in the regulation of motor actions. Such parcels must be expected to have their own cerebellar connections.

REFERENCES

1. Adams JC, Warr WB: Origins of the axons in the cat's acoustic striae determined by injection of horseradish peroxidase into several tracts. J Comp Neurol 170:107–122, 1976

2. Bergeijk WA Van: Variations on a theme of Bekesy: a model of binaural interaction. J Acoust Soc Am 34:1431–1437, 1962

3. Cajal SR: Histologie du Systeme Nerveux de l'Homme et des Vertebres, Vol I, II. Paris, A Maloine, 1909, 1911

4. Dublin WB: Fundamentals of Sensorineural Auditory Pathology. Springfield, IL, CC Thomas, 1976

5. Kiang NYS: Stimulus representation in the discharge patterns of auditory neurons. In Tower DB (ed): The Nervous System, Vol 3. New York, Raven Press, 1975, pp 81–96

6. Koelliker A: Handbuch der Gewebelehre des Menschen. Leipzig, Engelmann, 1896

7. Koerber KC, Pfeiffer RR, Warr WB, Kiang NYS: Spontaneous spike discharges from single units in the cochlear nucleus after destruction of the cochlear. Exp Neurol 16:119–130, 1966

8. Levy FH, Kobrak H: The neural projection of the cochlear spirals in the primary acoustic centers. Arch Neurol Psychiatry 35:839–852, 1936

9. Lorente de Nó R: Anatomy of the eighth nerve. The central projection of the nerve endings of the internal ear. Laryngoscope 43:1–38, 1933

10. Lorente de Nó R: Anatomy of the eighth nerve. III. General plan of structure of the primary cochlear nuclei. Laryngoscope 43:327–350, 1933

11. Lorente de Nó R: The neural mechanism of hearing. I. Anatomy and physiology. B. The sensory endings in the cochlea. Laryngoscope 47:373–377, 1937

12. Lorente de Nó R: Some unresolved problems concerning the cochlear nerve. Ann Otol Rhinol Laryngol [Suppl] 85 (34):1–28, 1976

13. Morest DK: Structural organization of the auditory pathways. In Tower DB (ed): The Nervous System, Vol 3. New York, Raven Press, 1975, pp 19–29

14. Osen KK: Cytoarchitecture of the cochlear nuclei in the cat. J Comp Neurol 136:453–483, 1969

15. Osen KK: Course and termination of the primary afferents in the cochlear nuclei of the cat. Arch Ital Biol 108:21–51, 1970

16. Powell TPS, Cowan WM: An experimental study of the projection of the cochlea. J Anat 96:269–284, 1962

17. Rasmussen GL: Efferent fibers of the cochlear nerve and cochlear nuclei. In Rasmussen GL, Windle WF (eds): Neural Mechanisms of the Auditory and Vestibular Pathways. Springfield, Ill, CC Thomas, 1960, pp 105–115

18. Rasmussen GL: Anatomical relationships of the ascending and descending auditory systems. In Fields WS, Alford BR (eds): Neurological Aspects of Auditory and Vestibular Disorders. Springfield, Ill, CC Thomas, 1966, pp 5–19

19. Rasmussen GL: Efferent connection of the cochlear nucleus. In Graham AB (ed): Sensorineural Hearing Processes and Disorders. Boston, Little, Brown, 1967, pp 61–75

20. Rose JE, Galambos R, Hughes J: Organization of frequency sensitive neurons in the cochlear nuclear complex of the cat. In Rasmussen GL, Windle WF (eds): Neural Mechanisms of the Auditory and Vestibular Systems. Springfield, Ill, CC Thomas, 1960, pp 116–136

21. Sando I: The anatomical interrelationships of the cochlear nerve fibers. Acta Otolaryngol (Stockh) 59:417–436, 1965

22. Tunturi AR: Physiological determination of the arrangement of the afferent connections to the middle ectosylvian auditory area of the dog. Am J Physiol 162:489–502, 1950

23. Warr WB: Olivocochlear and vestibular efferent neurons of the feline brain stem: their location, morphology and number determined by retrograde axonal transport and acetylcholinesterase histochemistry. J Comp Neurol 161:159–182, 1975

24. Whitfield IC: The Auditory Pathway. Baltimore, Williams & Wilkins, 1967

25. Woolsey CN: Organization of cortical auditory system: a review and synthesis. In Rasmussen GL, Windle WF (eds): Neural Mechanisms of the Auditory and Vestibular Systems. Springfield, Ill, CC Thomas, 1960, pp 165–200

VESTIBULO-OCULAR REFLEX ARC IN THE VESTIBULAR SYSTEM

In a simplified form, the pathways involved in the production of eye movements are indicated in Figure 2–16. The vestibular pathway begins in the three semicircular canals and in the two otolithic maculas. Two cells of Scarpa's ganglion have been included in the diagram to indicate that all the vestibular fibers innervating the three cristas and the two maculas end in the vestibular nuclei, where they have partly overlapping distributions. From the primary vestibular nuclei several pathways arise; some of them carry nerve fibers directly to the oculomotor nuclei while others end in the reticular substance. In this substance new paths arise that supply terminal fibers to the oculomotor nuclei. The diagram illustrates this situation by presenting in the vestibular nuclei a hypothetical neuron with an axon (a) that after having left recurrent collaterals (c) in the vestibular nuclei forms the efferent path V. This path divides into two branches: one branch (V_1) goes directly to the oculomotor nuclei and the other (V_2) ends in the reticular substance where a new path (V_2) arises.

Visual stimuli initiate impulses in the retina which are carried by the optic nerve (Fig. 2–16 **on**) to the external geniculate body (**egb**) and to the superior colliculus (**scol**). The geniculate body is the origin of the optic radiation to the primary visual cortex (Fig. 2–16, C_1) that has connections with other cortical areas (C_2), electrical stimulation of which causes eye movements. Besides C_1 other cortical areas (C_3) may cause eye movements operating through area C_2 that give rise to the oculomotor pathway (**omp**).

It is quite possible that in primates fibers of the oculomotor path reach the oculomotor nuclei, but as far as is known in rodents, the cortical pathway ends in the reticular substance. In those animals the optic path through the superior colliculus plays the more important role. Indeed, with rabbits, after removal of the cerebral cortex, combinations of labyrinthine stimuli (angular accelerations) and optic stimuli elicit a nystagmus that is undistinguishable from the nystagmus observed before decortication. On the other hand, as was first observed by Bechterew early in the present century, electrical stimulation (trains of brief shocks at about 60/sec) delivered through bipolar electrodes placed on the anterolateral surface of the superior colliculus, results in the appearance of a nystagmus that outlasts the stimulation period. This nystagmus involves chiefly the horizontal eye

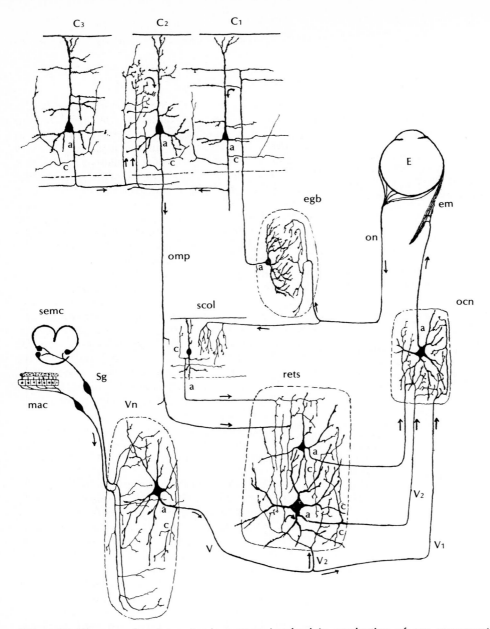

FIG. 2–16. Diagram of main anatomic systems involved in production of eye movements. Optic arc includes: retina; optic nerve **(on)**; external geniculate body **(egb)**; optic radiation; primary optic cortex (area 17) **(C₁)**; occipital motor center of eye movements in angular gyrus (area 18) **(C₂)**; descending oculomotor path **(omp)**; correlation nuclei in reticular substance of midbrain, pons and medulla **(rets)**; oculomotor nuclei **(ocn)**; and eye muscles **(em)**. Other zones of the brain **(C₃)** may produce eye movements through **C₂** (voluntary movements). Note that no cortical fiber reaches the oculomotor nuclei; these fibers end in the correlation nuclei. Another optic reflex arc is closed through the superior colliculus **(scol)**. Vestibular arc includes: semicircular canals **(semc)** and maculas **(mac)**; vestibular nerve with Scarpa's ganglion **(Sg)**; primary vestibular nuclei **(Vn)**, secondary vestibular paths **(V)**, dividing into two pathways: one **(v₁)** reaches the oculomotor nuclei without interruption; the other **(v₂)** is interrupted in the correlation nuclei **(rets)**. Note that correlation nuclei receive both optic and vestibular impulses. In each nucleus one or two representative nerve cells have been drawn as accurately as possible. **a,** axon of each cell; **c,** collateral branches. (Lorente de Nó R, Berens C: Nystagmus. In Piersol (ed): The Cyclopedia of Medicine. Philadelphia, FA Davis Co, 1936, pp 684–706)

FIG. 2–17. Diagram of main connections of vestibular nerve. **M**, medulla; **P**, pons; **Mb**, midbrain; **Lab**, labyrinth; **Cer**, cerebellum; **Cortex**, cerebral cortex; **Sg**, Scarpa's ganglion; **rets**, reticular substance. Vestibular nerve innervates cristas of semicircular canals **(c)**, utricular macula **(u)**, and saccular macula **(s)**. It ends in the primary vestibular nuclei, main divisions of which are: Bechterew's nucleus **(Bn)**; Deiter's nucleus **(Dn)**; and descending nucleus, **(desn)**; 1–5, cells of vestibular nuclei **(Vn)**: **1**, with axon reaching cerebellar cortex through vestibulocerebellar tracts **(vctr)**; **2**, with axon joining tractus vestibulomesencephalicus **(trvm)**; **3**, with axon joining posterior longitudinal bundle **(plb)**; **4**, with axon ending in reticular substance; **5**, with axon joining tractus Deiterospinalis; **vsp**, thin branches of vestibular nerve reaching cervical segments of spinal cord. Part of reticular substance **(rets)** having vestibular connections contains various types of cells **(6, 7, 8,** and **9)**, axons of which form either short pathways **(6, 8)** or join tractus predorsalis **trpd**, and descend to spinal cord **(6, 7, 8, 9)**. Note that reticular formation receives many vestibular fibers and also sends branches to vestibular nuclei. Cerebellum establishes connections with vestibular nuclei by means of axons of Purkinje cells, **cvtr**, and by means of axons of cells of *nucleus tecti* **(nt)**, which form tractus uncinatus **(tru)**. Note that this tract also has connections with reticular substance. Superior cerebellar peduncle **(scp)**, which arises from *nucleus dentatus* **(nd)**, gives branches to reticular formation in oral portion of midbrain **(Mb)**. The cerebral cortex, establishes connections with reticular formation by means of descending cortical paths **(cp)**. Motor nuclei of eye muscles **(III, IV,** and **VI)** receive branches from vestibular and reticular tracts. (Lorente de Nó R, Berens C: Nystagmus. In Piersol (ed): The Cyclopedia of Medicine. Philadelphia, FA Davis Co, 1938, pp 684–706)

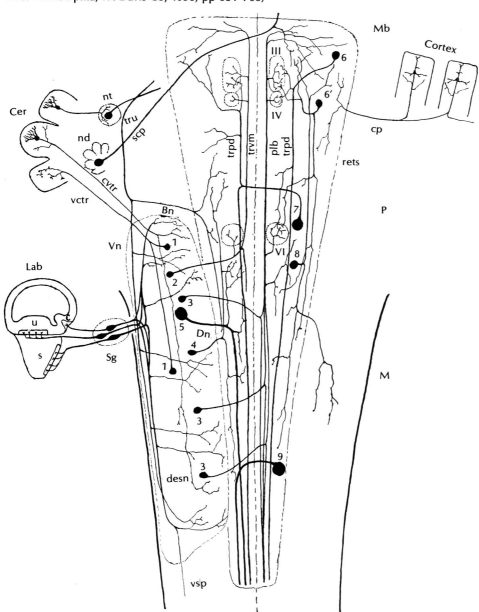

muscles. According to observations made by Blohmke, under the supervision of Lorente de Nó, destruction of the reticular substance underneath the stimulating electrodes prevents initiation of nystagmus by electrical stimulation even though vestibular nystagmus still can be produced.

The block diagram (Fig. 2–16) shows that fibers of several pathways establish connections with the motoneurons of the oculomotor nucleus. Physiological experimentation has proved that the motoneurons are stimulated above threshold to discharge impulses into their own axons only when volleys of presynaptic impulses activate, simultaneously or nearly so, at least the majority of the synaptic boutons present in a discrete zone of the synaptic shell. By itself, conduction of impulses by a single type of afferents cannot be expected to initiate motor discharges. To be sure, selective electrical stimulation of a part of V_1 (Fig. 2–16), the so-called posterior or medial longitudinal bundle, may cause motor discharges, but it does so only in the presence of subliminal bombardment of the motoneurons by internuncial impulses. On the other hand it should be emphasized that the production of the rapid component of vestibular nystagmus requires the integrity of the reticular pathways in the pons and oral part of the medulla. If the operation of the reticular substance is impaired by the severance of reticular commissural pathways, the nystagmus loses its fast component and it becomes a monophasic eye movement which is established by uninterrupted contraction or relaxation of the external rectus muscle.

Figure 2–16 presents the vestibular nuclei as receiving only vestibular afferents. In fact, however, the vestibular nuclei receive other afferents. Figure 2–17 illustrates the fact that the vestibular nuclei receive important streams of fibers originating in the cortex as well as in the central nuclei of the cerebellum. In addition, the vestibular nuclei receive numerous collaterals from the fibers of the restiform body and probably also from the dorsal roots of the first three cervical nerves (these connections are not included in the diagram). The vestibular nuclei also receive a considerable input from the reticular substance, and modern research has shown that the vestibular nuclei of the two labyrinths are cross-linked by commisural fibers. Further information is contained in the legend for Figure 2–17.

As a whole, the vestibular nuclei and the reticular substance constitute a gigantic system of cross-linked chains of neurons, and superimposed upon that system are parallel chains that include cerebellar neurons. The fact that vestibular reflexes can still be elicited after destruction of parts of the vestibular nuclei or of the reticular substance, and after removal of the cerebellum, does not indicate that the destroyed structures do not participate in, or are not essential for the establishment of labyrinthine function. All parts of the vestibular system are necessary for normal function, even though at times, abnormalities in function may be difficult to detect.

Information on reports by classic investigators may be found in:

Lorente de Nó R: Ausgewaehlte Kapiteln aus der vergleichende Physiologie des Labyrinths. Ergeb Physiol 32:73–242, 1931

Lorente de Nó R: Vestibulo-ocular reflex arc. Arch Neurol Psychiatry 30:245–291, 1933

Lorente de Nó R, Berens C: Nystagmus. In Piersol (ed): The Cyclopedia of Medicine. Philadelphia, FA Davis, 1938, pp 684–706

Information on reports on later work may be found in:

Brodal A: Anatomy of the vestibular nuclei and their connections. In Handbook of Sensory Physiology, Vol VI/I. New York, Springer Verlag, 1974, pp 240–352

Brodal A, Pompeiano O (eds): Progress in Brain Research, Vol 37. Basic Aspects of Central Vestibular Mechanisms XI. Amsterdam, Elsevier, 1972, 656 pp

Pompeiano O: Cerebello-vestibular interrelations. In Handbook of Sensory Physiology, Vol VI/I. New York, Springer Verlag, 1974, pp 417–476

Precht W: The physiology of the vestibular nuclei. In Handbook of Sensory Physiology, Vol VI/I. New York, Springer Verlag, 1974, pp 353–416

EXAMINATION
TECHNIQUES

3

EAR EXAMINATION*

The patient complaining of ear pain, discharge, hearing loss, dizziness, tinnitus, or any other ear symptom may have a significant related or unrelated general medical problem that plays a role in the presenting otologic complaint. Therefore, the oto-audiologic examination should be undertaken with recognition of the need for either prior or subsequent general medical examination.

EAR HISTORY

A questionnaire does not replace a thorough history, but it does help in channeling the attention of both physician and patient to specific otologic details. Skill in history-taking is as crucial in otology as in any facet of medicine. The fact that an ear problem is frequently accompanied by a communication disability makes the use of a questionnaire valuable as an adjunct. The adult ear–hearing questionnaire (Appendix A) has been found useful as a guide, but it does not replace the oral history. The dialogue between the patient (a person) and the physician (a person) cannot be replaced by a questionnaire or by a computer. A special pediatric questionnaire is essential in pediatric otologic problem investigations (Appendix B).

BASIC HEAD AND NECK EXAMINATION

The ear physical examination begins with a basic head and neck examination (Ch. 12) and is conveniently recorded (Fig. 3–1A). This includes examination and palpation of the neck, mandible, maxilla, and skull. Special attention is directed to

* Appendices A and B can be found at the end of the chapter.

the temporomandibular joint area in open and closed bite positions. A screening examination of the eyes includes examination of the orbit, globe movement, pupillary responses to light and accommodation, palpation for tension, manifest nystagmus, ophthalmoplegias, and corneal reflex sensitivity. Facial nerve function is examined. Auscultation for neck, skull, and ear bruits is important.

The mucosa of the eustachian tube, the middle ear, and the temporal bone air cell system is a direct anatomic and physiological continuum of the mucosa of the nasopharynx, nose, and paranasal sinuses. Minor cytologic variations occur in this long and tortuous mucosal tract, but the continuum from nose and throat (Fig. 3–1B) to the most remote petrosal apex or retrosinus air cell has great pathologic significance.

Diseases of the faucial tonsils, lingual tonsils, and the nasopharyngeal adenoid area—indeed, all of the lymphoid components of Waldeyer's ring—are in mucosal, vascular, and lymphatic contiguity with the middle ear and with all the extensions of the middle-ear air spaces into the temporal bone. The pharyngeal orifice of the eustachian tube is analogous to the ostium of a paranasal sinus. Thus, in effect, the middle ear and mastoid can be considered a paranasal sinus in terms of intimate physiopathologic relationships.

Many diseases of the middle ear and some diseases of the inner ear are etiologically related to diseases and anomalies of the nose, paranasal sinuses, and nasopharynx.

No examination of the ear is complete without an examination of the nose, throat, head, and neck. No evaluation of an infection in the middle ear is complete without an evaluation of possible related problems in the nose, sinuses, and nasopharynx.

The nasal septum forms the midline of the nasal chamber. There are close relationships between septal deformations and disturbed intranasal physiology. Deformities of the external nose (bony and cartilaginous) and the nasal lobule also contribute substantially to nasal malfunction. Malformations and diseases of the turbinates produce abnormal sequelae in nasal physiology and in sinus and eustachian tube ventilation.

Abnormal positive or negative intranasal pressures produced by lesions of the alae, septum, and turbinates produce ciliary and secretory cellular dysfunction. Changes in temperature, humidity, and ciliary function will result in disturbed eustachian tube function.

Careful nasal examination by anterior rhinoscopy involves inspection of the lobule, septum, turbinates,

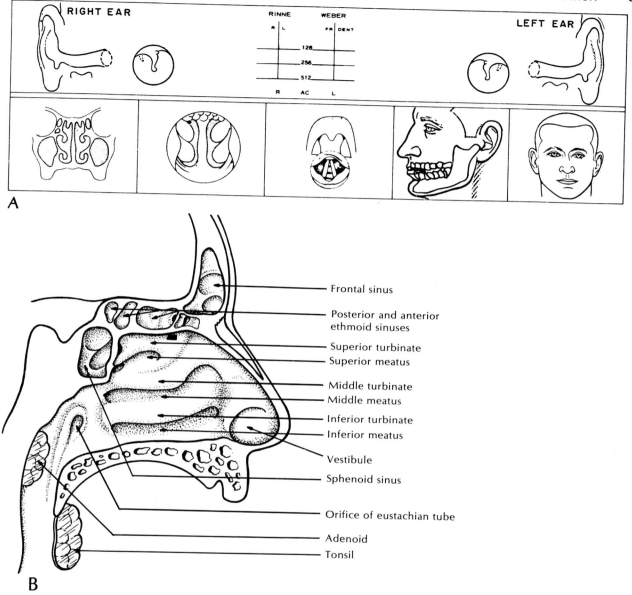

FIG. 3–1. A. Chart for recording ENT findings. **B.** Nasal and nasopharyngeal structures.

lateral meatuses, and upper nasopharyngeal vault. Nasal edema may prevent adequate rhinoscopy, unless the nose is adequately decongested by serial use of a mild, nasal, topical, decongestant spray. The most effective method is to warm the atomizer and spray the nasal mucosa in two stages. Preliminary spraying will usually "open" the anterior half of the nose. After a few minutes, a second spray will result in adequate decongestion of the entire airway to the posterior choanae. Such nasal "shrinkage" will allow visual-

ization of the upper part of the nasopharynx through anterior rhinoscopy in many patients.

Rhinologic examination frequently discloses crusts and purulent or mucoid secretions. Hypertrophic nasal mucosa may not respond to topical decongestants. Nasal and nasopharyngeal direct smears (cytology, yeasts, and fungi) and microbiologic (bacterial) cultures are important in differential diagnosis. Granulomatous or polypoid changes are significant. Posterior nasal tumors are occasionally found that were unsuspected as etiologic factors in chronic otitis media. Biopsy may reveal a carcinoma as a cause of so-called "serous" (secretory) otitis. Obstructive benign polyps occur not only in allergy, but also in chronic maxillary or ethmoid sinusitis.

Palpations of maxillary, ethmoid, and frontal regions for tenderness should precede definitive sinus studies. Peroral transillumination of the maxillary sinuses is useful, but it does not provide conclusive evidence of the presence or absence of significant maxillary sinus (antral) disease.

Quiescent chronic maxillary sinus disease of long standing is not infrequently characterized by poor ipsilateral transillumination. Such a "dark antrum" may be purely of "historic" significance and need not reflect current significant disease relating to the middle ear. Subacute maxillary sinusitis with active purulent discharge through the middle meatus into the nose may elude transillumination diagnosis.

Radiography of the sinuses is extremely important in cases of otomastoid disease. Very frequently, either secretory otitis media or chronic otomastoiditis is related to an ipsilateral active maxillary sinusitis, which will show up only on x-ray. Related sinusitis may be bilateral and can be contralateral. Ethmoiditis may accompany maxillary sinusitis or may occur alone.

Radiography of the maxillary sinuses (Water's views) along with appropriate temporal bone x-rays (Schuller's and Stenver's views) are indicated in cases of secretory and chronic otitis media.

When radiographic evidence of maxillary sinus disease is found in a patient with otomastoiditis, final determination of the possible etiologic role may require diagnostic irrigation of the antrum. Direct (inferior meatal) puncture or cannulation and irrigation of the middle meatus will usually result in the recovery of mucus, pus, or a combination. Cytologic and bacteriologic studies of such secretions are helpful in assaying the relationships between the nose and throat and otomastoiditis.

The ethmoid sinuses are less commonly related to ear and mastoid disease. This is also true of the sphenoid and frontal sinuses. The maxillary sinus is the chief sinus source of primary or repetitive infection in many patients with recurring otomastoid disease.

Examination of the upper nasopharynx is frequently possible by anterior rhinoscopy after adequate nasal mucosal decongestion. The use of a nasopharyngeal mirror should be part of the nose and throat examination wherever possible. In very young children or in sensitive "gagging" adults, the use of a small mirror may not be possible. When it is not possible to adequately examine the entire nasopharynx with a mirror, the only alternative is through the use of a nasopharyngoscope. The classic transnasal nasopharyngoscope is a useful instrument. Topical anesthesia of the nasal mucosa is usually advisable to facilitate atraumatic and comfortable examination. The recent introduction of the Hopkins nasopharyngoscope has been of great

value. (Fig. 3–2). This peroral endoscope makes possible not only examination of the nasopharynx through the mouth in a brilliantly illuminated optical system, but also concomitant examination of the lateral pharynx and larynx. This new endoscope is of great value in nasopharyngeal diagnosis (Fig. 3–3) of such lesions as nasopharyngeal fibroma, nasopharyngeal carcinoma, chordomas, and other tumors. Secretory otitis media may be secondary to such tumors.

Examination of the oral cavity is an intrinsic part of the otologic workup. It is part of the cranial nerve survey in neurootologic problems. Motor function of the lips, examination of the oral cavity for tumors of the soft and hard palate, inspection of the tongue, dentition, and salivary gland orifices are part of the nose and throat survey.

Status of upper and lower jaw dentition and temporomandibular joint function are very important in the patient with otalgia. Motor function disturbances of the tongue, soft palate, and vocal cords may have diagnostic significance in neurootologic problems.

The tonsils and the adenoid portions of Waldeyer's lymphatic ring may be of basic etiologic importance in the patient with secretory otitis media or chronic otomastoiditis. Examination of the tonsils and adenoids may reveal purulent exudate requiring microbiologic studies by smears and cultures.

EAR EXAMINATION

The examination of the ear begins with the auricle and periauricular region, with special attention to skin and cartilage lesions and to possible tenderness of tragus, concha, and helix. The mastoid process, the tip, the squama, and zygomatic areas are methodically inspected and palpated.

Examination of the ear requires suitable illumination. The conventional head mirror, although useful for screening, is inadequate because it limits the examiner to monocular vision and thus fails to provide binocular depth perception. An adjustable electric headlight is superior, for it allows binocular vision, depth perception, and the use of a magnifying binocular loupe. Such loupes are available with 2.5× to 6× magnification (Fig. 3–4). The combination of headlight and loupe allow for bimanual flexibility in the use of an ear speculum and for precise instrumentation in examination of the auricle, external auditory canal, and the tympanic membrane. Otoscopic examination of the tympanic membrane is impossible in the presence of obstructive cerumen, epithelial debris, otorrhea, and pathologic lesions such as polypi, cholesteatomas, and granulomas. With headlight and loupe, the examiner has one hand free for speculum manipulation. The other hand is then used for instrumentation—*i.e.*, suction tip, cerumen, curet, ear forceps, etc. Adequate visualization is possible following removal of cerumen

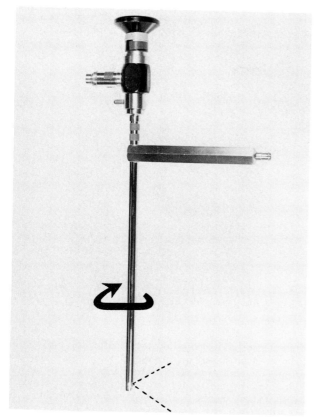

FIG. 3–2. Nasopharyngoscope. (Ward P, Berci G, Calcaterra T: Ann Otol Rhinol Laryngol 83:754, 1977)

FIG. 3–3. Nasopharyngeal photograph taken through nasopharyngoscope. (Courtesy of Dr. George Berci)

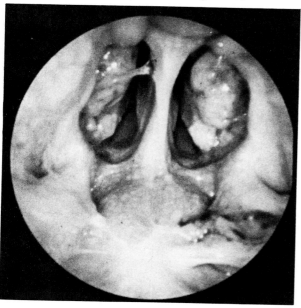

and epithelial and other obstructive material, allowing complete access to the external auditory canal and the tympanic membrane.

The electric otoscope is a very useful instrument and is not replaced by the headlight-loupe combination. The otoscope should be equipped with a clear bright light (such as the "halogen" bulb), a large lens, and a pneumatic bulb for pneumatic otoscopy (Fig. 3–5). An assortment of round and oval plastic and metal speculums makes examination convenient. As a screening instrument, it is quite adequate for many patients. In the absence of cerumen, epithelial debris, and foreign bodies, the electric otoscope is sufficient by itself for static and pneumatic examination. However, it is not the instrument of choice for primary otoscopy if removal of obstructive external ear canal material is necessary. The electric otoscope monopolizes one hand of the examiner. Attempts at cerumen removal and other instrumentation through an otoscope are frequently frustrating and occasionally traumatic to external ear canal, tympanic membrane, and possibly to the middle ear. The ideal combination is that of 1) the electric headlight-loupe combination, and 2) the electric otoscope.

The ultimate in ear examination is the use of the ear microscope. It is not essential in the basic otologic examination, but it is valuable in surgery (Fig. 3–6).

Following adequate cleansing and visualization of the external canal with the headlight and the magnifying loupe, the otoscope is brought into use. In suspected secretory otitis media, it may be helpful to move the patient's head up and down and from side to side during the observation with the otoscope, to elicit the presence of an air bubble or a meniscus line. The pneumatic otoscope allows for positive and negative pressures in observation of tympanic membrane and malleus mobility. Such rarefaction—compression observations are of great importance in recognizing problems such as latent secretory otitis media, ossicular fixation, and determination of areas of tympanic membrane atelectasis. Compressional otoscopy may also give information regarding the presence of a labyrinthine fistula. A positive "fistula test" can occur in positive—negative pneumatic otoscopy in the presence of a perforated tympanic membrane and a labyrinthine fistula. It will be manifested by evoked nystagmus and/or sudden vertigo. A response to the fistula test may be evoked even through an intact tympanic membrane in some cases.

Abnormal findings on otoscopy should be charted on a sketch of the ear drum using the quadrant system for recording lesions (Fig. 3–7).

The intimate relationships between tympanomastoid area disease and the nasopharynx are based on the physiopathology of the eustachian tube. A number of major otologic conditions are related intimately to tubotympanic problems. Eu-

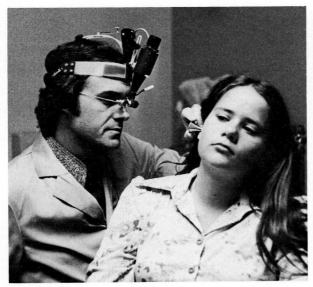

FIG. 3–4. Use of electric headlight with binocular loupe.

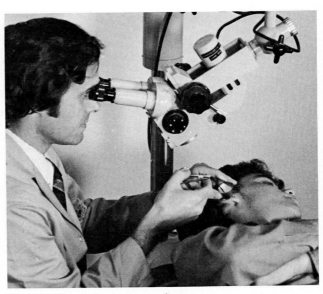

FIG. 3–6. Surgical microscope in use.

FIG. 3–5. Electric pneumatic otoscope in use.

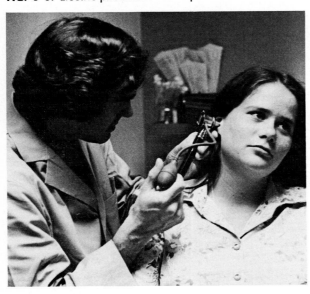

stachian tube examination is an indispensable part of the ear examination.

Visualization of tubal orifices in the nasopharynx is possible by transnasal and by peroral nasopharyngeal examinations, as previously described. Indirect information regarding certain aspects of eustachian tube physiopathology may be obtained by otoscopic visualization and by transcanal auscultation.

Presumptive information concerning the eustachian tube may be based on otoscopic observation. For example, the condition of abnormal tubal patency may be diagnosed by otoscopic observation of a hypermobile drum, which moves with respiratory movements. At the other end of the spectrum, in some cases of complete eustachian tube obstruction, atelectatic drum changes will be noted.

Transcanal auscultation will yield information regarding tubal patency. Ear auscultation tubes (modified from a stethoscope), which may be monaural or binaural, will allow the examiner to hear auditory signals produced by positive inflation of the eustachian tubes. Several methods of simultaneous bi-tubal inflation and a method of unilateral inflation are available to the examiner.

Two methods are based on the principle of simultaneous bi-tubal mass inflation: the Valsalva method and the Politzer method. The Valsalva method of self-inflation is based upon forced nasal expiration, by instructing the patient to hold both nostrils and lips closed tightly and then attempt to blow his nose. The sealed nasopharynx, glottis, and the splinted diaphragm make possible a sudden pressure increase through both eustachian tubes (if patency exists) to both middle ears, allowing either visualization or auscultation for monitoring these pressure changes.

The Politzer method of mass inflation is based upon the physician's use of positive pressure through one nostril while the other is held closed tightly. The positive pressure may be obtained by the use of a rubber bulb or by monitored compressed air delivered through an olive-tip nebulizer or insufflator while the patient says "KKK" or swallows a sip of water. Here again,

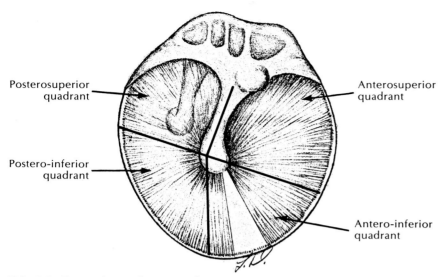

Posterosuperior quadrant

Anterosuperior quadrant

Postero-inferior quadrant

Antero-inferior quadrant

FIG. 3–7. Tympanic membrane quadrants.

FIG. 3–8. Otoscopic observation of tympanic membrane changes during inflation.

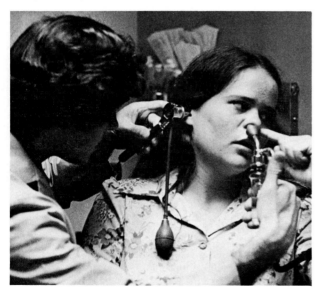

visualization and/or auscultation can be used for monitoring purposes.

These two mass, simultaneous bi-tubal methods are of value as gross tests. Practice in ear auscultation is necessary for acquisition of fine auditory discrimination for differentiating the characteristics of open, partially open, and closed eustachian tubes. With practice, the physician will learn to recognize, for example, the special squeak of a constricted tube, the hollow loud sound of a hyperpatent tube or of an excessively mobile tympanic membrane, or the gurgling sound of fluid, which can be heard in some cases of secretory otitis media. The recognition of auscultatory information in the otologic examination is an art comparable to that of cardiac, pulmonary, and abdominal stethoscopy. It can be acquired only through practice.

There are some drawbacks and hazards associated with "mass inflation" attempts. The contralateral ear may be traumatized unwittingly because of unsuspected problems, such as a delicately healed neomembrane, which may be stretched or ruptured by great positive pressure. It is conceivable that such pressure might also damage a round window membrane or a poststapedectomy oval-window seal.

Unilateral inflation that avoids mass bi-tubal nasopharyngeal pressure is possible through the use of a eustachian cathether. Skillful passage of such a catheter usually requires local anesthesia to the nasal membranes. Tubal patency is usually estimated by the auscultation technique in the use of the eustachian catheter. It is difficult to combine visual otoscopy with eustachian catheter inflation techniques unless the procedure is performed jointly by two examiners.

Otoscopic observation (Fig. 3–8) during mass inflation by the Valsalva or Politzer techniques yields information regarding tympanic membrane mobility characteristics in addition to information regarding specific tubal characteristics. The tympanic membrane findings may include differences in quadrantal mobilities, neomembranes, intratympanic fluid movements, or air escape through a small, previously unrecognized perforation. If the latter is suspected, the mass inflation may be repeated using simple oil (mineral oil) in a nebulizer. The very small amount of nebulized oil suspension is harmless and can be seen to escape visibly from the midde ear through a small perforation. As mentioned before, special care must be taken to avoid inordinate force in the Valsalva or Politzer inflation techniques.

Such visual examination can also be performed by the use of a headlight and magnifying loupe.

Special warning is necessary regarding one method of examination (or treatment) that has been used by some physicians. This is the attempt to force a diagnostic fluid or liquid medication by transcanal pressure through a perforated eardrum into the middle ear and down through the eustachian tube into the nasopharynx. Usually this has been done by application of positive pressure through a pneumatic otoscope in a patient with a tympanic membrane perforation. Occasionally it has been attempted by transtympanic-membrane needle puncture and forceful introduction of a test fluid. Although there is some physiological rationale for such an approach in diagnosis and treatment, there are significant risks to such procedures.

Attempts have been made to inspect the middle ear by transtympanic-membrane passage of a mini-endoscope. This approach is not recommended as an office examination procedure. It may be occasionally of value in special instances as a sterile operating-room procedure, but more definitive information may be obtained by the less traumatic exploratory tympanotomy operation.

Transtympanic needle puncture (tympanocentesis) for diagnostic aspiration of intratympanic fluid is necessary in some cases (see Ch. 15, Secretory Otitis Media) and is performed with either headlight–magnifying-loupe visualization or with the ear microscope. It should not be attempted through the speculum of a conventional otoscope.

SCREENING HEARING EXAMINATION

At the present state of our knowledge, it is inadvisable to rely on uncontrolled hearing tests such as the use of whispered voice or spoken voice, with inadequate and frequently misleading attempts to mask the opposite ear. Precise diagnoses of otologic diseases require definitive audiologic techniques. Although it is possible to get some crude information by whispered and spoken voice tests, undue reliance upon such tests may indeed lead to wrong diagnosis.

The general term **conductive hearing loss** is customarily attributed to a lesion in the external or middle ear. The general term **sensorineural hearing loss** is attributed to a lesion either of cochlear, retrocochlear, or of central auditory pathway origin.

Tuning-fork tests assist in differential diagnosis between conductive and sensorineural hearing

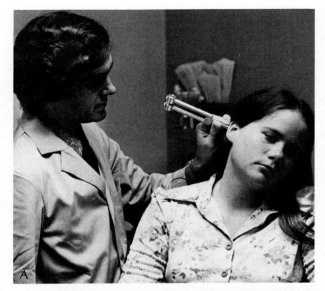

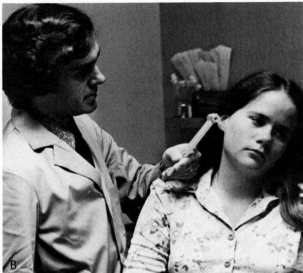

FIG. 3–9. Rinne test with 128-Hz tuning fork placed on mastoid tip. **A.** Bone conduction response as compared with air conduction response. **B.** Air conduction.

loss. Tuning fork tests should be used only for screening or confirmatory purposes. Low frequency tuning forks (128 Hz, 256 Hz, and 512 Hz) for the Rinne and Weber tests are recommended.

The Rinne test is performed by comparing mastoid bone conduction with external ear air conduction for duration and loudness (Fig. 3–9, A and B).

A **positive Rinne response** is that obtained when air conduction is greater than bone conduction, suggesting

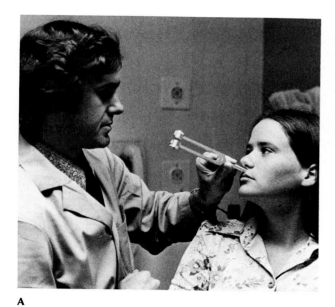
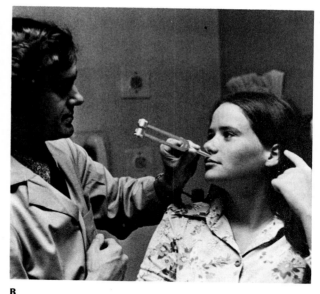

A   B

FIG. 3–10. A. Weber test on upper lip. Response is midline (nonlateralized). **B.** Response is toward left ear.

either a sensorineural hearing loss or normal hearing. A **negative Rinne response** is that obtained when bone conduction is greater than air conduction, suggesting a conductive hearing loss. The most informative responses for the Rinne test (bone versus air conduction) are obtained with low-frequency tuning forks.

Because the patient is sometimes confused as to bone conduction responses when the hearing loss is unilateral, masking is important in performing the Rinne test. A small Bárány noisemaker is used in the "healthy" ear to mask it and thus avoid confusion due to contralateral bone conduction responses.

The Weber test, traditionally performed by placing a tuning fork on the forehead, is more advantageously performed by placement on the upper incisor teeth or upper lip. The Weber test is designed to elicit lateralization or referral of the tuning-fork sound from the midline of the skull (forehead or upper incisor teeth) either to the right ear or to the left ear, or nonlateralized (in the midline) (Fig. 3–10, A and B).

The Weber test (stem of fork on upper central incisor teeth or on the medial plane of the maxilla) for lateralization is frequently a sensitive and useful diagnostic procedure. In normal ears, or in ears with symmetrical hearing losses, lateralization does not occur. In a unilateral hearing loss, lateralization toward the poorer ear suggests a conductive lesion, but lateralization toward the opposite (better hearing ear) suggests a sensorineural lesion.

A serious problem encountered in administering the Weber test is that patients are hesitant to report hearing the tone in their "poorer" ear. They may, in fact, indicate hearing the tone in the "better" ear, certain that their judgment of hearing in the poorer ear was in error.

Both Weber and Rinne tuning-fork tests are valuable ancillary techniques, particularly in certain mixed conductive-cochlear hearing losses. At best, however, they are adjunctive and not fully diagnostic in themselves. It is no more justifiable to rely on tuning-fork tests and voice tests in otology today than it would be to make a cardiac diagnosis without an electrocardiogram. Thus, *the audiometric examination is an indispensable part of the ear examination* (see Ch. 6, Audiologic Assessment, Functional Hearing Loss, and Objective Audiometry, for definitive audiologic evaluation test procedures and interpretation).

SCREENING VESTIBULAR EXAMINATION

The basic otologic examination should include a screening vestibular study. This includes detection of gross positional nystagmus, gaze nystagmus, the Romberg test, and gait examination.

More precise information regarding the vestibular system is indicated in all patients with vertigo or ataxia and in many patients without vertigo or ataxia who have complex or asymmetrical sensorineural hearing problems or unilateral persistent tinnitus. A definitive vestibular examination begins with a detailed history of dizziness and

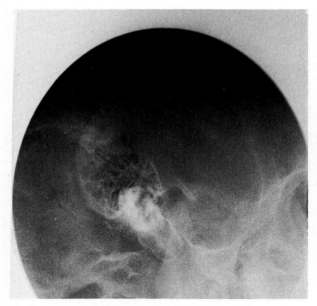

FIG. 3–11. Radiograph, Schuller view. Normal pneumatization in a 3-year-old child.

FIG. 3–12. Radiograph, Schuller view. Normal, well-pneumatized mastoid **(arrow)** in adult.

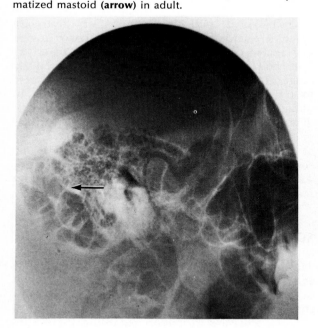

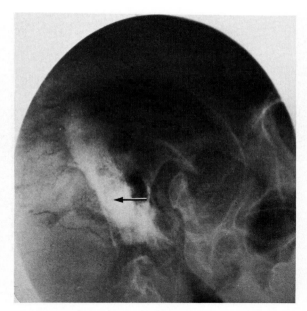

FIG. 3–13. Radiograph, Schuller view. Sclerotic, nonpneumatized mastoid **(arrow).**

FIG. 3–14. Radiograph, Stenver view. Normal internal auditory canal **(arrow)** and petrous apex.

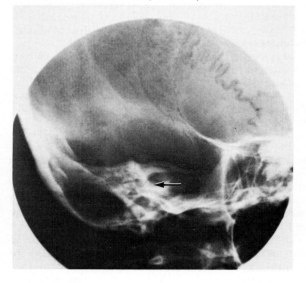

includes a neurootologic examination, and an electronystagmographic vestibular system examination (see Ch. 9, Equilibrium and Dizziness, and Ch. 10, Examination of the Dizzy Patient, for detailed vestibular studies).

RADIOGRAPHIC EXAMINATION

An otologic examination is incomplete without at least two screening radiographic views of the temporal bone: 1) the Schuller view of the lateral mastoid cellular complex, and 2) the Stenver view of the petrous pyramid, labyrinth, and internal auditory meatus. It is no more possible to make a definitive diagnosis of an otologic problem without such radiographs than it is to make a definitive diagnosis of a pulmonary condition without a chest radiograph (Figs. 3–11 to 3–14) (see Ch. 4, Otoradiology, for greater details on otoradiologic diagnostic techniques).

CLINICAL LABORATORY STUDIES

In dealing with infections of the auricle, external auditory canal, and/or middle ear, smears and cultures of secretions and scrapings are essential for definitive microbiologic diagnosis. Sterile, fine metal, cotton-wrapped applicators are used through a sterile speculum to obtain material for smears for cytology, yeasts, and fungi, and cultures for bacterial flora and antibiotic sensitivity tests.

Exudate may be present in the external auditory canal as a result of either external canal disease or as a result of middle ear disease in the presence of a tympanic membrane perforation. In certain specific instances, it may be necessary to obtain exudate from the middle ear either through needle aspiration (tympanocentesis) or through aspiration with a sterile suction tip via a myringostomy incision or an existing perforation. Ear specimens are studied for the presence of bacteria, fungi, or yeasts. Gram stains are used for gross differentiation of bacterial flora. Hansel's stains are used for cytologic detail—polymorphonuclear leukocytes, eosinophils, and lymphocytes. Such studies are very valuable in assessing the relative roles of allergy and infection in exudates. Material for bacteriologic culture is implanted under both aerobic and anaerobic conditions. Sensitivity tests for antibiotics and chemotherapeutic agents are carried out.

Exudate is frequently obtained from the nasopharynx or the pharynx particularly in instances of otomastoiditis with an intact tympanic membrane. Pathogenic organisms in middle-ear infections are correlated with nasopharyngeal flora in only 60% of cases; therefore, it cannot simply be assumed that identification of pathogenic microorganisms in the nose or throat will necessarily give sufficient information for adequate treatment of an ear infection. However, the information is valuable as a corroborative finding in many cases.

Laboratory examinations of blood and urine may be crucial to an otologic diagnosis in some cases. Fluorescent treponemal antibody absorption tests to rule out syphilis are frequently required. Leukemia, anemia, and polycythemia, as well as other blood dyscrasias, may produce otologic disturbances and require proper hematologic studies.

When central nervous system (CNS) complications occur in the course of ear disease, it frequently becomes necessary to study cerebrospinal fluid (CSF) by lumbar puncture, not only to obtain fluid for chemical, serologic, and cytologic examinations, but for definitive CSF pressure studies. In suspected sigmoid sinus or jugular bulb thrombophlebitis, jugular compression studies (Queckenstedt, Tobey-Ayer) studies for comparative right and left CSF dynamics are necessary.

In some diagnostic problems, biochemical studies of vestibular perilymph obtained through the stapedial footplate by puncture and aspiration may have important diagnostic implications.

PEDIATRIC EAR EXAMINATION

Examination of the infant or very young child will require competent assistance and careful use of restraints to prevent trauma to the ear during otoscopy. This is particularly important in the removal of cerumen or epithelial debris. A number of small oval and round otoscopic speculums should be available to conform to the varying external auditory canal sizes encountered clinically. Removal of cerumen or desquamated epithelium is occasionally accompanied by discovery of unexpected foreign bodies in the ear canals of infants and children.

The use of a fine suction cannula is of great help in avoiding traumatization of canal wall skin.

The availability of the examiner's two hands is essential in the examination of the infant or the small child. The use of an electric headlight and a binocular loupe is recommended, prior to the use of the otoscope. Adequate illumination and magnification and immobilization of the patient are essential. The pneumatic electric otoscope may suffice in a child with a wide ear canal without cerumen or debris.

Ear irrigation for removal of cerumen or debris is not advisable in a patient seen for the first time when the presence of an intact tympanic membrane is unknown. The "cerumen" may hide a tympanic membrane perforation, cholesteatoma (keratoma), a mycotic epithelial cast, or a foreign body. This is especially important with children. Meticulous bimanual ear cleansing technique with a blunt spoon curet and suction is necessary as a preliminary approach.

In examining the pharynx of an infant or young child, the conventional wooden tongue depressor is not advisable. A delicate slightly curved metal tongue depressor provides better control and minimizes gag reflexes. It allows a far more complete examination in a shorter period of time.

Examination of the nasopharynx in the child usually presents a problem. It is not always possible to visualize the nasopharynx in the infant or the very young child. Digital palpation of the nasopharynx is occasionally necessary, but it should be avoided if adequate information can be obtained from other sources, such as anterior rhinoscopy. Examination of the nasopharynx with a small nasopharyngeal mirror and a headlight is possible in older children, if care is taken in gentle use of the delicate tongue depressor.

In some infant ear problems, general anesthesia may be necessary to acquire definitive nasopharyngeal information. Adequate illumination, soft palate elevation, and mirror examination usually suffice, although there are occasions when a transnasal or peroral endoscope may be necessary.

Appendix A. Adult Ear Hearing Questionnaire

A. CHECK (√) RIGHT, LEFT, OR BOTH, AND GIVE DURATION (**Weeks, Months, Years**)

	Right	Left	Both	Duration
Hearing loss?				
Ringing, roaring, or buzzing in ear?				
Fullness or pressure in ear?				
Pain or discomfort in ear?				
Itching in ear?				
Discharge or drainage from ear?				
Do you wear a hearing aid?				

B. ANSWER NO OR YES AND GIVE DATES AND DETAILS

	No	Yes	Dates and Details
Have you had dizzy spells, loss of balance or lightheadedness?			
Have you had any ear operations?			
Have you had tonsil, adenoid, or other nose or throat surgery?			
Have you consulted an ear specialist?			
Are you taking any medication?			
Are you allergic or sensitive to any drugs?			Which ones?
Have you ever taken large doses of aspirin, Anacin, Bufferin, Empirin, or quinine?			
Have you ever received antibiotic injections? (Coly-mycin, streptomycin, kanamycin, or gentamicin?)			
Do you drink coffee and/or tea?			How much?
Do you smoke?			How much?
Have you been exposed to loud noises? (machinery, gunfire, rock music)			
Is there a history of hearing difficulties in your immediate family?			
Is your general health good?			

Appendix B. Pediatric Hearing—Problem Questionnaire

Child's name _____   Date of this visit? _____
Birth date _____   Age _____
Mother's age _____
Father's age _____

I. ONSET
   1. At what age did you first suspect your child might have a hearing loss?
   2. What were the circumstances that led you to think your child was not hearing normally?
   3. What are your own ideas as to what may have caused the hearing loss?
   4. As far as you know, did the hearing loss exist from birth? _____
     A. Could you awaken him by calling his name? _____ If not, how did you awaken him?
     B. What things disturbed his sleep?
   5. Has his hearing loss remained the same?
   6. If you think his hearing has improved, at what age did this improvement take place?
     A. What things does he hear now that he did not hear before the improvement?
     B. To what do you attribute the improvement?
   7. If you think his hearing has become worse, at what age did it become worse?
     A. Describe the kinds of things your child heard previously, and does not seem to hear at present.
     B. What event or illness do you think may have caused his hearing to become worse?
   8. If your child's hearing loss came on after the age of 2 years, was there any change in his speech?   Describe.
   9. Does your child's hearing seem better at certain times than at other times?   Describe.
  10. Does your child have any other handicapping conditions in addition to the hearing loss, such as poor eyesight, heart disease, muscular incoordination, mental retardation?

II. GENETIC FACTORS
   1. Is there hearing loss in any of your other children? _____
   2. Is there hearing loss in either father or mother? _____
   3. Is there hearing loss in the immediate family of the father or mother? _____
     In remote relatives? _____
   4. Are father and mother blood relatives? _____
   5. Do any of your children have handicapped conditions such as heart disease, muscle incoordination, mental retardation, poor eyesight, etc?

III. INTRAUTERINE FACTORS
   1. Rubella
     A. Did you have German measles or any other rash during your pregnancy? _____
     B. If so, give details regarding type of rash and exact month of pregnancy in which it occurred.
   2. If you had any of the following illnesses during pregnancy, please check and give the exact month in which it occurred.
     A. Mumps _____
     B. Measles _____
     C. Influenza (flu) _____
     D. Grippe _____
     E. Severe virus infection _____
     F. Toxemia _____
     G. Any other illnesses _____
   3. Did you receive quinine, streptomycin, salicylates, antibiotics, or other drugs during your pregnancy?
   4. How much do you smoke?
   5. How much alcohol do you use?

IV. NATAL FACTORS
   1. Rh Factor
     A. What is your Rh blood type? _____
     B. What is your husband's Rh blood type? _____
     C. How many miscarriages have you had? _____
     D. Did your child receive a blood transfusion after birth? _____
     E. Was your child yellow or jaundiced after birth? _____
     F. Was a blood transfusion ever necessary for any of your other children? _____
     G. Were any of your other children yellow or jaundiced after birth? _____
     H. Did any of your other children die shortly after birth? _____
   2. Birth Injury and/or Anoxia
     A. Was there any birth injury followed by paralysis or convulsions at the time of delivery of this child? _____
     B. Was the baby full term? _____
       Premature? _____
       What was the child's birth weight? _____
       Was the child in an incubator? _____
       If so, how long? _____

(continued)

C. Was the birth normal? _____
Caesarean? _____
Breech? _____
Instrumental? _____
D. Did your baby require oxygen at birth? _____
For how long? _____
E. Did any of your other children require oxygen at birth? _____
For how long? _____

V. POSTNATAL FACTORS
1. Meningitis
   A. Did your child ever have meningitis? _____
   B. If so, was it meningococcic (epidemic)? _____
   C. Other types of meningitis, such as pneumococcic? _____
      Tuberculous? _____ Etc.
   D. Did your child receive streptomycin or neomycin, or other antibiotics during the meningitis? _____
2. Encephalitis
   A. Did your child ever have encephalitis? _____
   B. If so, was it due to measles? _____
      Or other disease? _____
3. Other diseases
   Please check any of the following diseases which your child has had and give his age at the time of the illness.
   A. Mumps _____
   B. Whooping cough _____
   C. Measles _____
   D. Chicken pox _____
   E. Scarlet fever _____
   F. Diphtheria _____
   G. Polio _____
   H. Rubella (German measles) _____
4. Unusual high fever
   Has your child had any unusually high fevers? _____ If so, describe; give duration of fever, cause, treatment, and age of child. _____
5. Other
   A. Did your child ever have convulsions? _____
   B. Did your child ever have muscle weakness? _____
   C. Did your child ever have poor coordination? _____
   D. Has your child received antibiotics by injections? _____
      If so, give details: _____

VI. OTITIS MEDIA AND RELATED CONDUCTIVE LESIONS
1. Does your child have frequent colds? _____ How long do they usually last? _____
   Is it necessary for you to have your child under a doctor's care before the cold clears up? _____
2. Has your child had ear abscesses which either opened spontaneously or required lancing? _____
3. Has your child required penicillin, sulfa, or other antibiotic drugs for earaches? _____
   Give details: _____
4. Does your child snore at night? _____
5. Does your child sleep with mouth open? _____
6. Does your child have a sore throat frequently—with or without fever? _____
7. Does your child sneeze often every day? _____ especially in morning? _____
8. Does your child complain of a blocked nose frequently? _____
9. Does your child have enlarged or tender swellings in the neck? _____
10. Does your child seem to have excessive ear wax or other secretion from ears? _____
    Does secretion have an odor? _____
11. Does your child's nose discharge mucus or pus frequently? _____

VII. INJURIES
1. Has your child ever suffered a severe head injury? _____
   If so, describe the accident. _____

2. Are there any other pertinent facts that may relate to the cause of the child's deafness? _____ Give details:
   _____

(continued)

VIII. RESIDUAL HEARING
    1. How do you get his attention when his back is turned to you? _____
    2. Do you think he hears your voice? _____ How do you know? _____
    3. Does he turn around if you call his name? _____ How close must you be? _____
       Do you use a soft, loud, or normal speaking voice? _____
    4. What sounds does he seem to hear? List them and describe how he shows you he heard the sound. (This may include such things as the doorbell, water running in the bathtub, car in the driveway, alarm clock, radio, telephone, dog barking, baby crying, toys which make noise, Good Humor Man.)

SOUND	HEARD AT WHAT DISTANCE	CHILD'S REACTION

    5. Are there particular sounds your child *likes* to hear and to which he spends time in listening? _____
    6. Does he seem to know from what direction the sound came? _____
    7. If several persons are in a room, does he know which person spoke to him? _____
    8. Does he seem to hear better with one ear than the other? _____
       What makes you think so? _____

IX. UNDERSTANDING FOR SPEECH
    1. Do you use gestures when you speak to him? _____
    2. Does he seem to hear better if you talk louder? _____
    3. Does he follow your spoken direction when he is not looking at you? _____
       Give examples: _____
    4. Are there single words he *understands* (such as: Bye-bye; Baby; No; Cookie; Bath?) If so, list them, describe what he does to show you he understands the word. _____
    5. Do you think your child is doing any lip reading? _____
       What makes you think so? _____

X. SPEECH
    1. Did your child make the usual babbling sounds that babies make? _____
    2. Did these babbling sounds continue? _____
    3. At what age did he say his first words? _____
       What were they? _____
    4. Approximately how many words does he say now? _____ List as many of them as you can. _____
    5. Does he pronounce the words correctly? _____ Describe: _____
    6. Does your child talk in sentences? _____ If so, give four or five examples. _____
    7. Does your child imitate or repeat what you say? _____
       If he does try to imitate, does he use his voice, or does he move his lips without voice? _____
    8. How does he tell you what he wants—*i.e.*, does he use sentences, words, sounds or gestures? _____
       If he uses gestures mainly, does he usually make sounds along with the gestures? _____ What sounds does he make? _____
    9. How does he attract your attention? _____

XI. HEARING AID
    1. Is your child wearing a hearing aid? _____ If so, what ear? _____
    2. When did he first start wearing an aid? _____
    3. How long per day does he wear it? _____
    4. What make and model of aid is he wearing? _____
    5. What sounds do you think he hears when he wears the aid that he does not hear when not wearing it? _____
    6. Does he enjoy the aid? _____

XII. SCHOOL
    1. Is your child in school? _____
       Please give name and address of school and duration of attendance. _____
    2. What grade is he in? _____
    3. How many children are in his classroom? _____
    4. Is this a regular public school classroom of children who hear normally? _____
    5. Is he in a class with only deaf children, only hard of hearing children, or both deaf and hard of hearing children? ___
    6. Is he attending regular classes with hearing children, but is taken out for special help? _____
       A. Is the special help individual or group? _____
       B. What kind of special help? _____
       C. How often does he have the special class? _____
       D. How long is the special class? _____
    7. If your child is not in school, what are your plans for his education? _____

(continued)

XIII. GENERAL DEVELOPMENT

    1. List all children in the family (including this child) in order of birth, and give ages of the children. _____

    2. A. In your opinion, has your child's general development been more rapid _____ slower _____ or average _____ as judged by your other children or children you have known.

        B. If his development had been different, please explain in what ways. _____

    3. At what age did he sit alone? _____ Stand up? _____

    4. At what age did he begin to crawl? _____

    5. When did he walk alone? _____

    6. At what age did his first tooth appear? _____

    7. Is he toilet trained? _____

    8. Can he dress himself? _____ Attempts to help? _____

    9. Can he feed himself? _____ Attempts to help? _____

    10. At what age did he begin to eat solid foods? _____

    11. What languages are spoken in the home? _____

    12. Does mother work outside the home? _____ If so, what arrangements are made for care of the child? _____

    13. Has your child had nursery school experience? _____ For how long? _____ Where? _____

    14. Does your child have other children in his family (or in neighborhood) with whom he plays? _____ What are their ages? _____.

        Do you feel your child's general behavior (other than the suspected hearing problem) is similar to that of other children his age? _____

    15. What kind of play activities or toys does he enjoy? _____

    16. In what types of activity does he spend most of his day? _____

XIV. INFORMATION

    1. What agencies or clinics have you consulted regarding your child? *What were you told?* _____

    2. Has your child had other hearing tests? _____ Where? _____ *What were your told?* _____

XV. SPECIAL QUESTIONS

    1. List any special questions you may have concerning your child's hearing loss, speech, hearing aid, schooling, etc.

4

OTORADIOLOGY

WILLIAM N. HANAFEE

Developments in otoradiology have paralleled the rapid advances in otologic diagnosis and surgery of the past two decades. These have occurred in the three areas of plain films, tomography, and computerized tomography.

PLAIN FILMS

The problems of the vast majority of patients referred for radiologic examination of the mastoids comprise two main groups: inflammatory disease and sensorineural hearing loss. The routine projections required for the inner ear structures—*i.e.*, the sensorineural lesions—are quite different from those necessary for cases of inflammatory diseases of the middle ear and mastoid processes and their complications. The anatomy of the temporal bone further emphasizes this dichotomy because of the very dense nature of the otic capsule surrounding the cochlea and semicircular canals. Investigations of the internal auditory canal in patients with sensorineural hearing loss require a more penetrating x-ray beam for fine details. Usually, with this exposure, the delicate details of the mastoid air cells are overpenetrated on the film. Conversely, when visualization of the middle ear cavity and mastoid air cells is required, care must be taken to prevent superimposition of the dense otic capsule on the desired structures.

To accomplish these goals, over 50 projections of the temporal bone have been recommended, but basically they are all variations of anteroposterior, lateral, or oblique projections.

The simplest to consider in the sensorineural hearing loss series is the investigation for acoustic neurinoma. When the patient lies supine on the radiographic table, the internal auditory canal is parallel to the table top. The true length and dimensions of the internal auditory canal are best demonstrated by the avoidance of any oblique projections. A clear visualization of the internal auditory canal is usually possible by projecting the internal auditory canal through the orbit or projecting the canal over the basiocciput by a Towne projection. At times the subbasal projection may give additional anatomic detail.

For the anteroposterior transorbital view, the chin is flexed. A line connecting the lateral palpebral fissure of the eye with the external auditory meatus (canthomeatal line) is placed perpendicular to the film (Fig. 4–1). Two exposures are made, one with the tube angled 5° caudally and one with the tube 5° cranially. The resultant stereographic pair of films will usually provide one view of the internal auditory canals free of supraimposed bony plates, such as the orbital roof or floor of the middle cranial fossa. At times, air cells in the petrous tip may be confusing. Good penetration is emphasized to see through the dense otic capsule.

The Towne projection is made by angulating 30° caudally to the orbitomeatal line with the x-ray beam entering anteriorly at about the hairline and passing through the external auditory canal (Fig. 4–2). If the patient's chin is kept well flexed, the x-ray beam will tend to be more perpendicular to the film, and greater detail is possible with less magnification. The cortical margins of the posterior superior wall of the *porus acusticus* is best seen in this view.

The subbasal projection (5) is not a true submentovertical (Hertz) projection but is angulated approximately 75° to the orbitomeatal line (Fig. 4–3). If a true submentovertical projection is obtained, the transverse foramen of the first cervical vertebra will frequently superimpose on the internal auditory canal.

As mentioned earlier, the projections used for inflammatory disease are designed to give information concerning the middle-ear cavity and periantral air cells. Although plain films will not record detailed anatomy, such as the condition of the long process of the incus and incudostapedial joint, nevertheless, some exceedingly useful information for the otologic surgeon is possible. In our routine we use a lateral projection (Schuller's view), Owen's modification of the Mayer projection, a Stenver view, and a Guillen projection.

The Schuller projection (8) is obtained by placing the patient in the lateral position and angling the x-ray tube 25° toward the feet to prevent supraimposition of the two mastoid bones (Fig. 4–4). Another lateral projection is Law's view, which is obtained by angling the patient's face 15° toward the table when the patient is in the lateral position and angling the x-ray tube 15°

FIG. 4–1. Acoustic neurinoma, anteroposterior transorbital view. **A.** The chin is flexed so that a line connecting the lateral canthus of the eye and superior margin of the external auditory canal is made perpendicular to the table top. The x-ray beam enters anteriorly at approximately the level of the junction of the superior margin of the iris with the sclera. This stereographic pair of films is obtained by angling the tube, first 5° caudally and then 5° cranially. **B.** Line drawing of representative roentgenogram **(C)** in a patient with a right acoustic neurinoma. The vertical height of the internal auditory canal measures 2 mm greater on the right (↑↓) than on the left (↓↑) at the level of the posterior wall of the internal auditory canal. The groove on the petrous apex may appear constricted or flared in the normal patient and should not be used as a criterion of pathology in the *porus acusticus.*

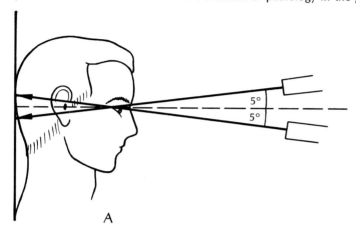

A

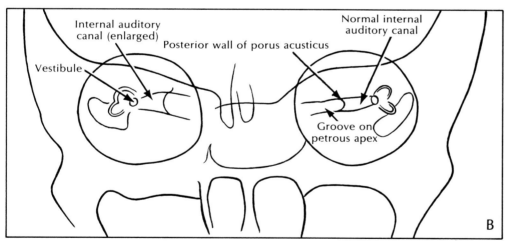

B

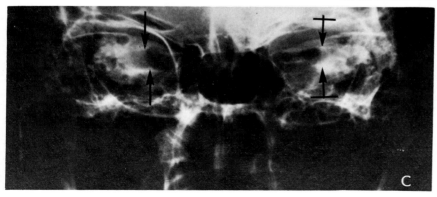

C

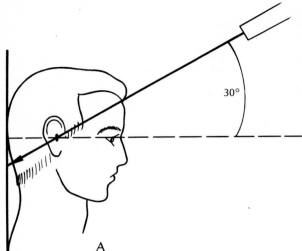

A

FIG. 4–2. Acoustic neurinoma—Towne projection. **A.** The patient is positioned with the orbital meatal line perpendicular to table top. The x-ray tube is angled so that the central ray enters at approximately the hairline and exits through the external auditory canal. Too steep an angulation will project the internal auditory canal over very dense bone adjacent to the foramen magnum **B** and **C.** Enlargement of the internal auditory canal by an acoustic neurinoma is present at right (↓ ↑). Left is normal (↓ ↑). At times, early erosion of the posterior-superior lip of the *porus acusticus* can best be demonstrated in this projection. Note that the orbits and floors of the middle cranial fossa are projected below the petrous pyramids, while the margins of the foramen magnum are not superimposed on the otic capsules.

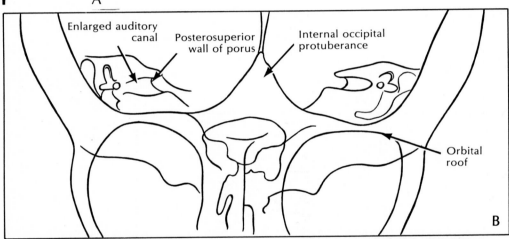

B

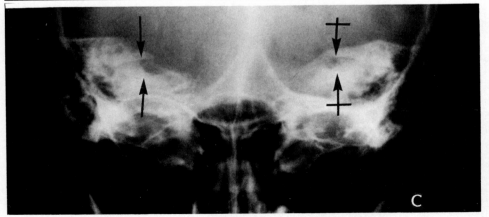

C

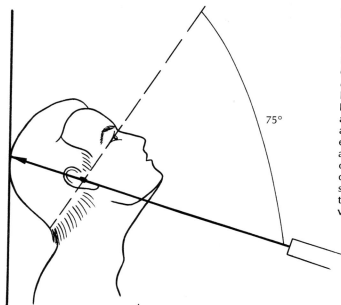

FIG. 4–3. Acoustic neurinoma, subbasal projection. **A.** The patient may be either erect or recumbent. The purpose of the projection is to visualize internal auditory canals with the petrous pyramids projected posterior to the mandibular angles and anterior to the transverse foramens of C–1 vertebra. Angulation of approximately 75° to the orbital meatal line is selected, and the x-ray tube central beam is made to pass through the external auditory canal. **B.** Line drawing of roentgenogram **(C).** This projection allows evaluation of the posterior wall of the internal auditory canal. There is posterior displacement and erosion of this wall at right (↑) compared to the normal at left (↑). At times, the internal auditory canals may be oval in shape, with the long axis of the oval in opposite directions on the two sides. The base projection gives a second dimension to radiologic measurement of the internal auditory canal. **C–1,** transverse foramen of C–1 vertebra.

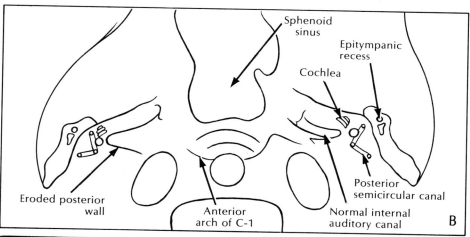

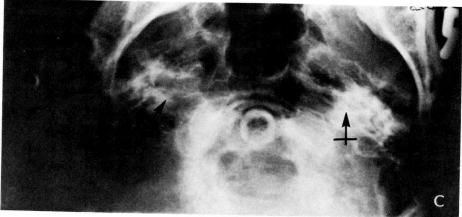

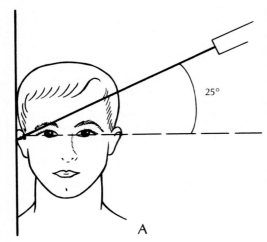

FIG. 4–4. Schuller's projection, normal mastoid. **A.** The patient is placed in a true lateral position with respect to the film. The x-ray tube is angled 25° toward the feet to prevent superimposition of the two temporal bones. This angulation also projects the very dense otic capsule inferiorly to the structures of the middle cavity and mastoid air cells. **B.** Line diagram of roentgenogram **(C).** The cortical bone of the tegmen of the mastoid antrum and tegmen of the epitympanic recesses cast a shadow through superimposed air cells. The tegmen forms an angle of approximately 90°, with the sigmoid plate in a well-developed mastoid. In lesser degrees of mastoid development, this angle may be reduced to 60–65°.

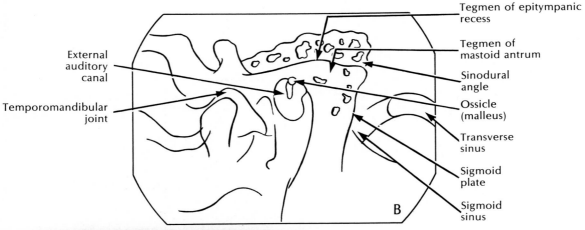

External auditory canal

Temporomandibular joint

Tegmen of epitympanic recess

Tegmen of mastoid antrum

Sinodural angle

Ossicle (malleus)

Transverse sinus

Sigmoid plate

Sigmoid sinus

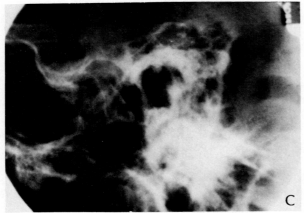

toward the feet. Either view gives essentially the same information concerning the development of the mastoid bone and the aeration of the mastoid air cells. The sigmoid plate should form an angle approximating 90° with the roof of the epitympanic recess and mastoid antrum, thus forming a sinodural angle closely approximating 90°. Lesser degrees of angle formation at the sinodural angle indicate underdevelopment of the mastoid. Deficiencies of the tegmen of the epitympanic recess and destruction of the sigmoid plate by inflammatory disease can also be approximated.

The Owen modification of the Mayer view is best understood by the otologic surgeon, as the patient is positioned so that the resultant radiograph approximates the same anatomic relationships that the surgeon will encounter during the classic approach to mastoidectomy (3). The patient is so positioned that his mastoid process is in firm contact with the x-ray grid. The face is turned away from the film 30°, and the x-ray tube is angulated 30° toward the feet (Fig. 4–5). In this projection, the otic capsule is displayed below the level of the epitympanic recess and mastoid

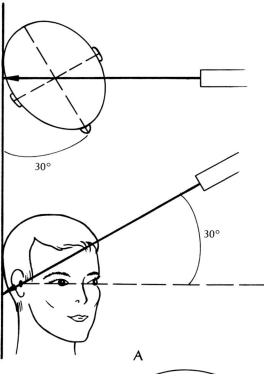

FIG. 4–5. Owens view, normal mastoid. **A.** As viewed from above, the patient's face is turned 30° away from the film, and the tube is angled 30° toward the feet. The patient is so positioned to the film that the central beam exits through external auditory canal. **B.** Line diagram of roentgenogram **(C).** There is some elongation of the "key area" (epitympanic recess, *aditus ad antrum,* and mastoid antrum) because the structures are projected above the level of the very dense otic capsule. The short process of the incus is faintly visible.

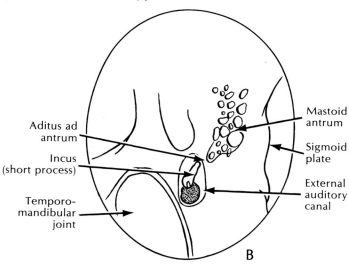

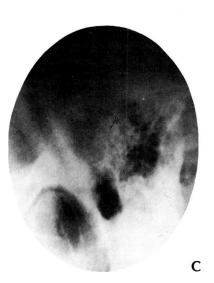

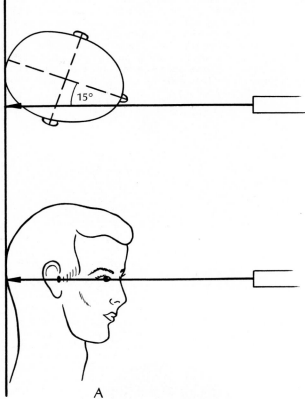

FIG. 4–6. Guillen projection, normal mastoid. **A.** Positioning begins by first placing the patient on the table or erect, with the chin well flexed. The orbital meatal line is made perpendicular to the film. The central beam is directed to the superior margin of the iris at its junction with the sclera, immediately above the pupil. The patient's head is then turned 15° toward the side under investigation. By this maneuver the x-ray beam will enter the upper medial quadrant of the orbit just beneath the brow. **B.** Line drawing of roentgenogram **(C).** The central beam passes tangent to the promontory. The space between the horizontal semicircular canal and scutum are well visualized. The combined shadow of malleus and incus can be seen in this space. The internal auditory canal is visualized through the orbit but the canal itself is somewhat foreshortened.

A

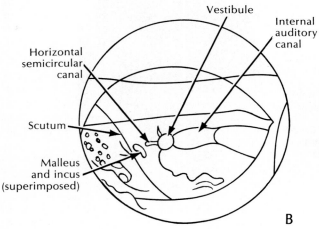

Vestibule

Internal
auditory
canal

Horizontal
semicircular
canal

Scutum

Malleus
and incus
(superimposed)

B

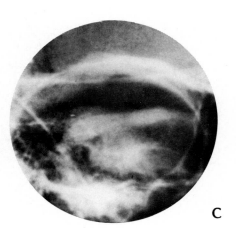

C

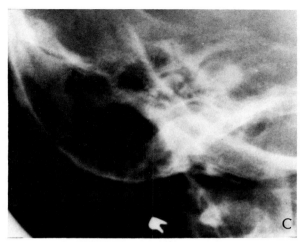

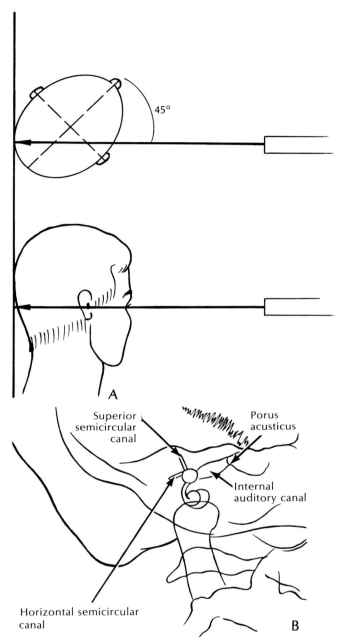

Superior semicircular canal

Porus acusticus

Internal auditory canal

Horizontal semicircular canal

FIG. 4–7. Stenver projection—normal mastoid. **A.** In the Stenver projection, the purpose is to visualize the mastoid air cells with the x-ray beam perpendicular to the posterior surface of the petrous bone. The chin is well flexed, with the orbital meatal line perpendicular to the film. The positioning is begun by having the patient's head perpendicular to the x-ray film. The central x-ray beam is directed to the junction of iris and sclera immediately above the pupil. After centering, the patient's head is rotated 45° away from the side under investigation. **B.** Line drawing of roentgenogram **(C).** The internal auditory canal is considerably foreshortened in this projection; however, the *porus acusticus* is fairly visible. The horizontal semicircular canal and superior semicircular canals are readily identified. Lateral to these structures are the cavity of the mastoid antrum and the periantral air cells. Somewhat lateral and inferior to the horizontal semicircular canals, ossicles can be identified in the epitympanic recess.

antral area. At times the ossicles can be visualized in the shadow of the auditory canal, although fine detail of the integrity of the incudostapedial joint is not possible. Erosive changes about the epitypmanic recess, *aditus ad antrum* or mastoid antrum are clearly delineated in this Owen projection.

The Guillen projection is an oblique view of the middle-ear cavity and mastoid antrum through the orbit. The chin is comfortably flexed on the chest so that the outer canthus of the eye projects at the inferior margins of the external auditory canal. The patient's face is rotated 15° toward the side under investigation. With the patient lying on his back, the middle ear cavity can be clearly delineated through the orbit (Fig. 4–6). The central axis of the x-ray beam is tangent to the lateral wall of the epitympanic recess and visualizes the incus and malleus surrounded by air in the epitympanic recess. There is no superimposition of dense otic capsule over the long process of the incus or stapes arch. In relatively normal patients, the horizontal portion of the facial nerve can be seen under the horizontal semicircular canal. Unfortunately, no statement can be made regarding localized dehiscences of the bony margins of the facial canal. Dehiscences of the horizontal semicircular canal will probably escape detection (unless they are far advanced) because of the superimposition of remaining portions of otic capsule.

The Stenver projection (9) is essentially a view with the central beam perpendicular to the posterior surface of the petrous bone. The patient's chin is well flexed on the chest, which places the orbitomeatal line almost perpendicular to the film. The patient's face is rotated 45° away from the side under investigation. The resultant radiograph projects the periantral air cells and petrous tip free of overlapping bone (Fig. 4–7). Excellent detail of the cellular structures of the periantral region can be obtained. Unfortunately, the ossicular mass and major portion of the middle ear cavity will overlap the very dense otic capsule. The visualization of the internal auditory canal is somewhat distorted since the canal is greatly foreshortened. On the other hand, the *porus acusticus* is parallel to the plane of the film and the fine detail of its cortical margin is clearly visible. The semicircular and vestibular regions will usually overlap the internal occipital crest and torcular Herophili.

At times, other projections will be required, depending on the clinical problem under investigation. For example, the submentovertical projection in the newborn is extremely helpful in the diagnosis of congenital malformations.

Trauma patients require a great deal of personalization of the plain film examination, depending on the presence or absence of fractures of the calvarium. With parietal fractures, multiple variations of the lateral projection may prove quite useful. If the patient has a basal fracture that extends into the petrous bone, multiple variations of the anteroposterior or oblique views may be required to show the fracture line extending across the long axis of the petrous bone.

In all probability, the fine detail required for these special situations can be achieved better by the judicious use of tomography.

TOMOGRAPHY

The field of otoradiology has changed radically with the advent of thin-section tomography. One must reassess the role of routine films in the light of the precision of anatomic details available by pluridirectional tomography. This new modality has introduced a criterion of diagnosis that is only occasionally seen in other fields of roentgen interpretation; that is, the diagnosis is made by the absence of visualization of an anatomic structure. This makes interpretation exceedingly difficult, as

one must be assured of high quality techniques through all phases of the radiographic examination, starting with patient immobilization and x-ray equipment function, all the way through film-intensifying screen combinations and x-ray film processing.

HISTORY

Patent applications for tomographic devices began to appear throughout the period 1920–1930. In the ensuing years, multiple terminologies were introduced, such as laminagraphy, tomography, planography, stratography, and others, depending on the mechanical arrangements of x-ray tubes and film. More importantly they reflected an individual inventor placing his own name on a particular x-ray apparatus. Ziedses des Plantes (14) first published research on tomography in 1931 and pointed out that a spiral motion of the x-ray tube and film would give a better image than circular or linear motion. Thus the advent of the polytome by the Phillips X-Ray Company in 1950 and the Stratomat by the CGR X-Ray Company added a new dimension of tomography. The hypocycloidal movement of the tube by the Phillips unit and the trispiral movement by the CGR unit have been termed pluridirectional motions. This means that the x-ray tube and film have a movement pattern beyond one that is merely linear, circular, or elliptical. The completeness of the blurring of unwanted superimposed anatomic structures has allowed considerable refinements of interpretation.

TECHNIQUE

Whether hypocycloidal or trispiral blurring patterns are utilized in performing tomography, accurate coning and positioning are essential. We utilize a lead diaphragm that produces a 5.5-cm circular image on the film. Each side of the mastoid is exposed separately. Optimum contrast is obtained when the exposures are made at 55–58 kV, 40 mamp for a 6-sec exposure. For a very dense sclerotic mastoid, one may have to increase the penetration to 65 or 66 kV.

For visualization of the internal auditory canal, the patient is placed supine, with the canthomeatal line perpendicular to the table top. The central beam is directed at the level of the median of the pupil at the medial junction of the iris with the sclera.

For the Guillen projection, the patient is placed supine with the chin flexed approximately 5° and the central beam is centered at the superior margin of the junction of iris with the sclera. After the central beam has been positioned, the patient's head is turned 15° toward the side under investigation.

Tomographic cuts are taken at 1-mm intervals, starting with the anterior margin of the cochlea and carried through to the posterior limb of the horizontal semicircular canal for a total of 10 "cuts." This technique

FIG. 4–8. A. Hollow glass rods in a test-tube rack. At left, the first rod is perpendicular to the table top, while the remaining glass rods are placed at increased angles to the table top. Roentgenograms are then made by taking a "tomographic cut" through the center of the glass rods. Note that the perpendicular rod casts a shadow of a perfect circle **(left)** with "intact" walls. The shadows of the remaining glass rods range from the appearance of an eclipse to horizontally placed parentheses. The disappearance of a portion of the wall of the glass rod at the steeper angles is highly significant when one considers tomography of bony canals. Apparently, in the hollow glass rods, the walls on the superior and inferior surfaces of the inclined rods are too thin to cast a shadow. Along the lateral margins, although some density is lost because of curvature, there is a sufficient buildup of wall thickness to cast a shadow. **B.** Hypocycloidal tomography. **C.** Trispiral tomography.

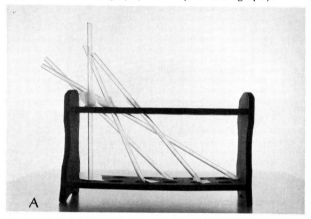

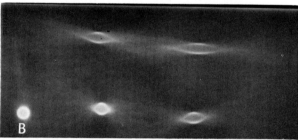

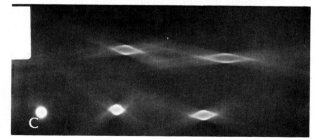

may be altered in accordance with the clinical problems.

Pluridirectional tomography, with sections ranging from 1–1.5 mm in thickness also creates some image peculiarities that must be thoroughly understood for a meaningful interpretation of the roentgenograms. One in particular is the "45 degree angle effect" described by Vignaud (11, 12) (Fig. 4–8). This effect explains why at times there will appear to be a deficiency in the bony covering of the promontory or facial nerve when the tangent of a plate of bone is at a 45° angle to the central axis of the x-ray beam.

The thickness of the cut is profoundly affected by the angle of sweep of the x-ray tube, and the sharpness of image is affected by the degree of blurring of unwanted structures. If one places a sheet of lead with a pinpoint hole between the x-ray tube and the film and makes a continuous exposure, the pattern of movement of the x-ray tube is then recorded (Fig. 4–9). The two patterns displayed represent the widely used pluridirectional x-ray units. Undoubtedly others will be added to the marketplace with time. One will notice, with the trispiral pattern, that the x-ray film is "blackened" most near the central portion of the spiral. This occurs when the tube slows near the center of its sweep and the angulation of the tube is less. The effect is evidenced in the glass rods by greater contrast because the section is thicker than with the hypocycloidal movement (Fig. 4–8). Both advantages and disadvantages in mastoid tomography are created by this phenomenon. At times, evidence of bone destruction can be better evaluated because of the improved contrast with a slightly thicker section. On the other hand, delineating extremely slender ossicles, such as the long process of the incus, is best with the thinner section.

All the above factors are greatly influenced by the judicious use of techniques in the range of 55–58 kV in the average mastoid, with proper selection of film–screen combinations and optimal processing of film.

ANATOMY

If one systematically "builds up" the anatomy of the temporal bone, the reasons for selecting various projections becomes clearer. If one begins by looking down on top of a skull with the bony calvarium removed, an X-like pattern is presented by the lateral walls of the orbit and the posterior surfaces of the 2 temporal bones (Fig. 4–10). In the center of the X is the fossa for the pituitary gland. The angle between the limbs of the X may vary from 80°–120° in a normal patient. To make up the roentgen image, one must think of the film being placed behind the head and the x-ray beam coming directly into the face from anterior to posterior. As shown in Figure 4–11, the internal auditory canal is parallel to the plane of the x-ray film, and the external auditory canal is almost parallel to the plane of the film. The semicircular canals can be drawn in, with the posterior semicircular canal parallel to the posterior

FIG. 4–9. Movement patterns of x-ray tubes during tomography. By placing a lead sheet with a pinhole between the x-ray tube and film during exposure, considerable information can be obtained regarding the movement pattern of the x-ray tube, focal spot size, angle of sweep, and many other technical factors. **A.** Trispiral movement of the stratomatic made by CGR X-ray Company. **B.** Hypocycloidal pattern of the polytome made by the Phillips X-ray Company.

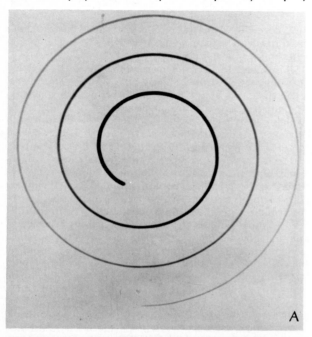

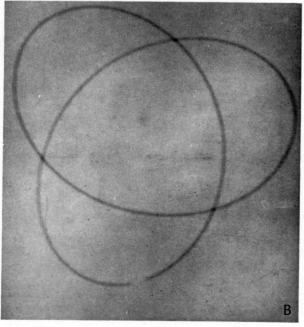

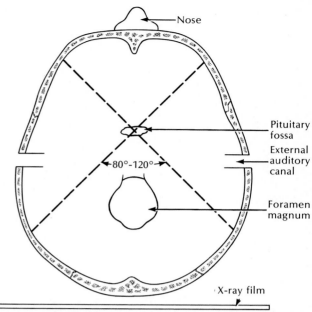

FIG. 4–10. Diagrammatic representation of the skull base as viewed from above with the calvarium removed. The X-like pattern consists of the lateral walls of the two orbits and the posterior walls of the two temporal bones. The angle of the two limbs of the X will vary, depending on the skull configuration.

surface of the petrous bone, the superior semicircular canal perpendicular to the posterior surface of the petrous bone, and the horizontal semicircular canal perpendicular to the x-ray film (Fig. 4–12). The cochlea is directed anteriorly in such a fashion that its long axis is perpendicular to the plane of the posterior surface of the petrous bone. In tomography, because the cochlea is anterior, those cuts that are anterior and include the cochlea are called the cochlear planes. Those that are more posterior and go through the semicircular canals are called the vestibular planes. An easy way to remember these relationships involves the anatomic relationships of the nerves in the internal auditory canal. If one cuts across the internal auditory canal in its more lateral portion (Fig. 4–13), the canal is divided into quadrants, with the facial nerve in the anterosuperior quadrant, the cochlear nerve in the anteroinferior quadrant, and the superior vestibular nerves in the two posterior quadrants. Naturally, the cochlear nerve is in the anterior quadrant to serve the anteriorly placed cochlea, whereas the two vestibular nerves are in the posterior quadrants to supply the vestibular apparatus.

The facial nerve, which is superior to the cochlear nerve, exits from the internal auditory canal superior to the cochlea then courses anteriorly for a short distance to form the anterior genu (Fig. 4–14). It abruptly turns posteriorly beneath the horizontal semi-

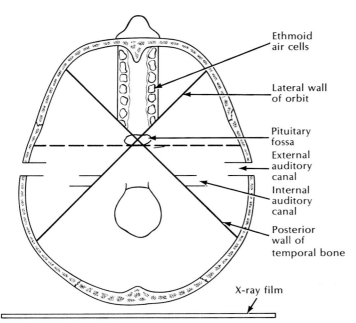

Ethmoid air cells

Lateral wall of orbit

Pituitary fossa

External auditory canal

Internal auditory canal

Posterior wall of temporal bone

X-ray film

FIG. 4–11. Diagrammatic representation of the skull base with the calvarium removed. As more structures are added, the upper limbs of the X can be identified more clearly as the lateral walls of the orbits, with the more medially placed ethmoid air cells and *lamina papyracea* forming the medial wall of the orbit. The lower limbs of the X form the posterior walls of the petrous portions of the temporal bone. The anterior portions of the petrous portion of the temporal bone form almost a straight line across the base of the skull. The internal auditory canals are approximately parallel to the x-ray film that is placed behind the patient's head. The external auditory canals are also approximately parallel to that same x-ray film.

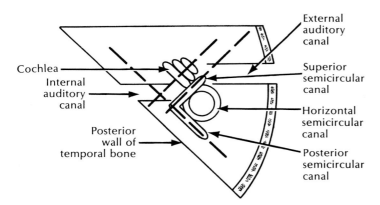

Cochlea

Internal auditory canal

Posterior wall of temporal bone

External auditory canal

Superior semicircular canal

Horizontal semicircular canal

Posterior semicircular canal

FIG. 4–12. Diagrammatic representation of the petrous portion of the right temporal bone as viewed from above. For orientation, the posterior wall of the temporal bone is the crucial surface. The axis of the posterior semicircular canal is parallel to the posterior wall, and the axis of the cochlea and axis of the superior semicircular canals are perpendicular to the posterior wall. The horizontal semicircular canal lies in the plane of the paper, and its axis would be perpendicular to an x-ray film placed behind the patient's head. The posterior semicircular canal and the superior semicircular canal share a common limb—hence the name, common crus.

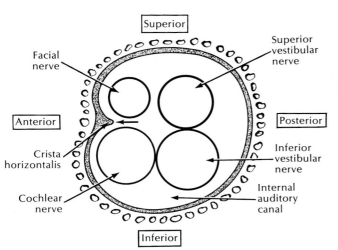

Superior

Facial nerve

Anterior

Crista horizontalis

Cochlear nerve

Inferior

Superior vestibular nerve

Posterior

Inferior vestibular nerve

Internal auditory canal

FIG. 4–13. Cross section of the internal auditory canal immediately medial to the cochlea. The *crista horizontalis,* separating the facial nerve from the cochlear nerve, lies at approximately the junction of the middle and upper thirds of the vertical height of the internal auditory canal. A dense margin of cortical bone surrounds the entire internal auditory canal at this point.

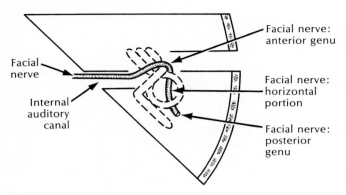

Facial nerve

Internal auditory canal

Facial nerve: anterior genu

Facial nerve: horizontal portion

Facial nerve: posterior genu

FIG. 4–14. Course of the facial nerve. The facial nerve enters the internal auditory canal and courses to the anterior upper quadrant of the canal as it passes peripherally. The facial nerve makes a sharp hairpin turn after leaving the internal auditory canal. This anterior bend (anterior genu) lies above the level of the cochlea and anteriorly to the superior semicircular canal. The facial nerve then dips down, to pass on the under surface of the horizontal semicircular canal—hence the name horizontal portion. At the level of the posterior limb of the horizontal semicircular canal, the facial nerve makes a distinct bend downward (posterior genu) to exit eventually from the temporal bone through the stylomastoid foramen. The portion from the posterior genu to the stylomastoid foramen is called the descending portion of the facial nerve.

FIG. 4–15. Middle-ear cavity and mastoid antrum. The footplate of the stapes rests in the oval window. The footplate lies at an angle approximately 15° to the midsagittal plane. Projecting laterally from the footplate are the stapes crura and head (arch), which articulate with the long process of the incus. This ossicular chain lies in a plane that is perpendicular to the 15° angle plane. Note the hourglass type of configuration of the epitympanic recess, with the narrow aditus and the lower portion of the hourglass being formed by the mastoid antrum. The axis of the hourglass also lines up on the 15° plane.

circular canal; this is called its horizontal portion. This horizontal portion lies at an angle of 15° to the sagittal plane of the skull. At approximately the level of the posterior limb of the horizontal semicircular canal, the facial canal undergoes a posterior turn or genu to descend (the descending portion) and to exit from the mastoid through the stylomastoid foramen.

Other important angulated structures also "line up" on this same 15° angle to the sagittal plane, such as the articulation of the head of the malleus with the arch of the stapes, and the cavities of the epitympanic recess, *aditus ad antrum,* and mastoid antrum (Fig. 4–15). This 15° angle plane is also important because the long process of the incus is directed inferomedially to articulate with the stapes arch. The angulated structures lie perpendicular to this plane. The incudostapedial joint can be visualized as a "V" if the central beam passes along the 15° axis. The oval window niche lies parallel to the 15° angle line.

The illustration of the glass rods (Fig. 4–8) makes it easy to understand why the best visualization of the horizontal portion of the facial nerve will occur when the planographic cuts are made perpendicular to this 15° angle line. Similarly, the margins of the oval window will be more sharply delineated and there is a greater chance of including the long process of the incus and the stapes arch in one tomographic cut if the head is turned 15° toward the side under investigation (Guillen projection, Fig. 4–6).

A precise understanding of the temporal bone anatomy on a three-dimensional basis is essential for the diagnosis of pathologic conditions. The basal projection will be used because it is simpler to correlate with histologic sections and because there is a distinct advantage of being able to view the maximum number of anatomic structures without overlap. Many investigators have expressed a preference for basal tomography in the investigation of some specific areas. In the newborn, a plain film basal projection of the skull is so revealing that usually tomography is not necessary to outline the inner ear structures. This single projection should be a must for any newborn with external canal atresia.

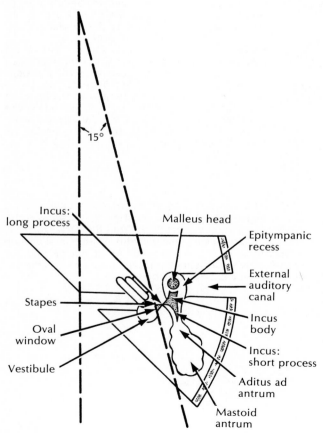

15°

Incus: long process

Malleus head

Epitympanic recess

External auditory canal

Incus body

Incus: short process

Aditus ad antrum

Mastoid antrum

Stapes

Oval window

Vestibule

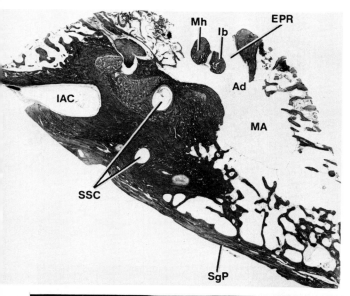

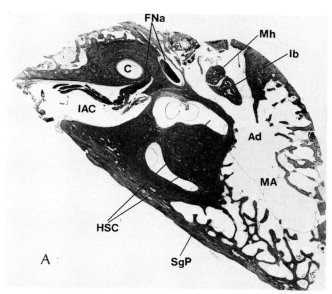

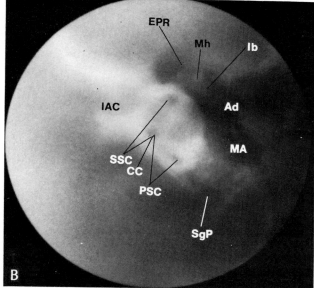

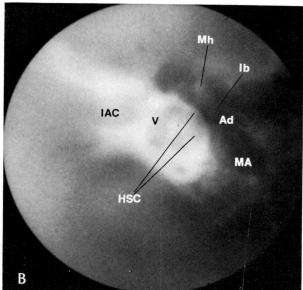

FIG. 4–16. Upper level of semicircular canals and epitympanic recess **(EPR).** The superior semicircular canal **(SSC)** has a larger diameter anteriorly than posteriorly, an indication of the anterior location of the ampulla. The more slender posterior limb is the common crus **(CC)** for the superior semicircular canal and posterior semicircular canal **(PSC). IAC,** internal auditory canal; **Mh,** malleus head; **Ib,** incus body. **A.** Histologic section. **B.** Roentgenogram. The cavities of the epitympanic recess, aditus **(Ad),** and mastoid antrum **(MA)** are better appreciated on the roentgenograms than on the sections. The fact that the sigmoid plate **(SgP)** appears as a thick bone on the sections, but casts very little shadow on the roentgenograms is presumably related to the angle that the posterior surface of the mastoid makes when the patient is in the basal projection. Patients with well-developed mastoid air cells have thinner sigmoid plates.

FIG. 4–17. Section through the horizontal semicircular canal **(HSC)** and internal auditory canal **(IAC).** Both the histologic section and the tomographic firm are through the horizontal semicircular canal. **A.** Histologic section. **B.** Roentgenogram. The histologic section shows the anterior genu of the facial nerve **(FNa)** and extreme upper portion of the cochlea **(C).** The internal auditory canal is well demonstrated on both histologic section and roentgenogram. The middle ear structures are cut at a more caudad level than the previous section, and the joint space between the head of the malleus **(Mh)** and body of the incus **(Ib)** are better demonstrated on both the histologic section and tomogram. The anterior placement of the cochlea **(C)** as compared to the posteriorly placed semicircular canal system becomes very evident in this and the following sections. **SgP,** sigmoid plate; **V,** vestibule; **MA,** mastoid antrum; **Ad,** aditus.

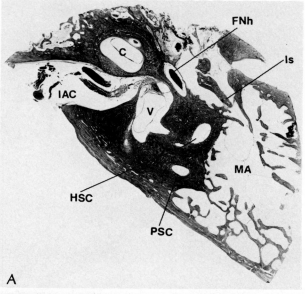

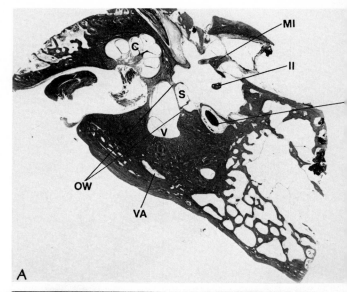

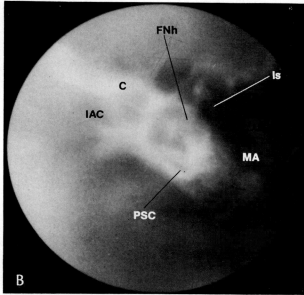

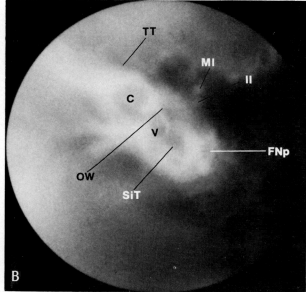

FIG. 4–18. Section through cochlea **(C)** and immediately below the horizontal semicircular canal **(HSC). A.** Histologic section. **B.** Roentgenographic section. In the histologic section the facial nerve **(FNh)** has completed the anterior genu and is turning posteriorly to pass beneath the horizontal semicircular canal. The histologic section shows principally the vestibule **(V)** whereas the radiographic section contains portions of the horizontal semicircular canal. Also in the radiograph, the facial nerve is not clearly visible and may represent only a summation of shadows. The short process of the incus **(Is)** is clearly visible on both the histologic section and tomographic cut. The relationship of the short process of the incus to the aditus is a constant finding, and any displacement is readily apparent in expensive processes or in trauma. **MA**, mastoid antrum.

FIG. 4–19. Section through the midcochlear **(C)** and oval window **(OW). A.** Histologic section. **B.** Roentgenographic section. In the histologic section the individual turns of the cochlea are distinctly visible. On the roentgenogram the lobulated pattern of the outline of the cochlea is visible but the delicate spiral ligament does not cast a shadow. Similarly, the anterior and posterior crura of the stapes **(S)** can be demonstrated on the histologic section but not on the roentgenogram. Because of the thicker section on the roentgenogram, the cavity of the tympanic sinus *(sinus tympani—SiT)* becomes clearly visible. This recess of the middle-ear cavity is demonstrated lying posteriorly and slightly lateral to the vestibule and basal turn of the cochlea. Its lateral border is formed by the pyramidal eminence **(PE)** and posterior genu of the facial nerve **(FNp). MI**, malleus; **Il**, incus long process; **Va**, vestibular aqueduct; **TT**, tensor tympani.

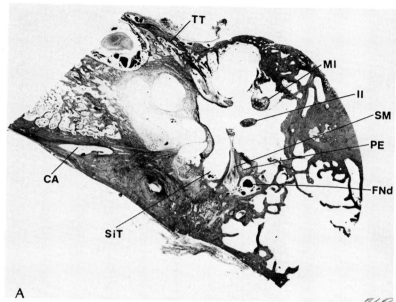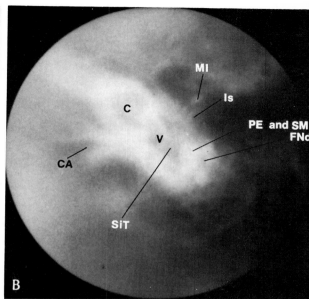

FIG. 4–20. Section through lower half of cochlea **(C)** and lower vestibule **(V). A.** Histologic section. **B.** Roentgenographic section. On both the histologic section and the roentgenogram, the basal turn of the cochlea can be seen entering the vestibule. The section is taken below the level of the oval window **(OW).** On the histologic section the pyramidal eminence **(PE)** is well demonstrated, together with the origin of the stapedius muscle **(SM).** Its tendon is visible, protruding from the opening of the pyramidal eminence. Lateral and posterior to the stapedius muscle is the descending portion of the facial nerve **(FNd).** The tympanic sinus **(SiT)** is well demonstrated on both the histologic section and roentgenogram. Medially, the opening of the cochlear aqueduct **(CA)** is visible on the roentgenogram, but in the histologic section, the cochlear aqueduct is seen extending more laterally, because of slight differences in angle. The terminal portions of the long process of the malleus **(MI)** and the long process of the incus **(II)** are visible on both the section and the tomogram.

In Figures 4–16 through 4–21 an attempt has been made to select histologic sections that correlate with tomography of the skull in the base projection as performed in a clinical setting. Because of the thickness of the radiographic sections (approximately 1 mm), as compared to the histologic sections (15 µ), considerably more anatomic structures will be in focus than in each of the radiographs. In addition, some of the denser structures cast "ghost shadows" on the radiographs. Figure 4–16 begins in the most cephalad portion of the temporal bone, and subsequent sections extend toward the feet. All illustrations have been printed to correspond to the right temporal bone as visualized from above. Because of the greater thickness of the radiographic section, the mastoid antrum appears as a much more clearly outlined cavity than on the thin histologic sections. This type of discrepancy will be evident throughout the comparison illustrations.

At times, the detail available on the radiographic section is not sufficient to be certain of anatomic correlation. For example, in Figure 4–18 B, the facial nerve in its horizontal portion **(FNh)** is labeled, but this negative shadow may well represent a portion of the middle-ear cavity being superimposed on the horizontal semicircular canal. On the other hand, its course should be directly beneath the horizontal semicircular canal and 2–3 mm lateral to the oval window niche.

As the reader proceeds from Figures 4–16 through 4–21, some important relationships should be noted. The cochlea is anteriorly placed with respect to the semicircular canal system. In addition, the semicircular canals lie more cephalad than the more caudad cochlea and middle-ear structures. The very dense nature of the otic capsule surrounding the cochlea and semicircular canals plays an important role in all radiographic procedures. From the histologic sections and tomograms in the base projection, one can see how the otic capsule would superimpose on the more delicate middle-ear structures if the x-ray beam entered the head either in an anteroposterior direction or in a lateral projection. The horizontal semicircular canal with its dense otic capsule and the promontory also bulge into the middle ear cavity, making ready access to roentgen demonstration extremely difficult.

By viewing the hypotympanum from above, it is easy to see how a recess such as the tympanic sinus (1) is

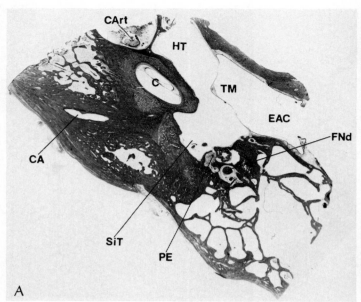

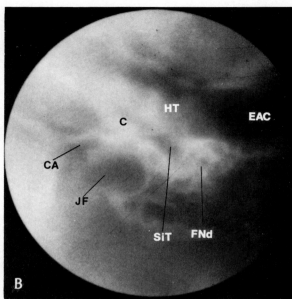

FIG. 4–21. Section through the lower cochlea **(C)** and lower hypotympanum **(HT)**. **A.** Histologic section. **B.** Roentgenographic section. The inferior sweep of the basal turn of the cochlea is visible on both the histologic section and tomogram. Because of a slightly different angle of the tomogram and the greater thickness of the cut, the jugular foramen **(JF)** can be visualized lying immediately posterior to the opening of the cochlear aqueduct **(CA).** The close proximity of the jugular foramen **(JF)** to the tympanic sinus **(SiT)** is evident. On the histologic section the tympanic membrane **(TM)** is well demonstrated, extending anteriorly and inferiorly, emphasizing the low position of the medial portion of the external auditory canal **(EAC).** The tympanic membrane **(TM)** cannot be demonstrated on the roentgenogram. The descending portion of the facial nerve **(FNd)** shows a clear relationship to the external auditory canal and mastoid air cells.

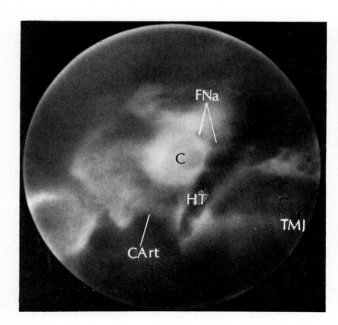

FIG. 4–22. Apical and intermediate coil of the cochlea **(C).** In this Guillen projection of the left ear, the external auditory canal **(EAC)** and ghost of the temporal mandibular joint **(TMJ)** are at the reader's right. The midline of the patient would be at the reader's left. The carotid artery **(CArt)** enters the skull at the level of the cochlea and then passes medially and anteriorly. Only the foramen is visible on this projection, but a distinct bony septum separates the carotid artery from the hypotympanum **(HT).** The delicate inner septums (spiral ligaments) of the cochlea are not visible. One must remember that the apical and intermediate coils occupy the central spherical lucent area of the cochlea, while the entire peripheral canal is the basal turn of the cochlea. The facial nerve in its anterior genu **(FNa)** courses rather far forward so that on frontal tomograms two distinct "holes" are visible. The medially placed hole is the facial nerve as it is coursing forward, and the laterally placed hole is the facial nerve coursing posteriorly to go beneath the horizontal semicircular canal.

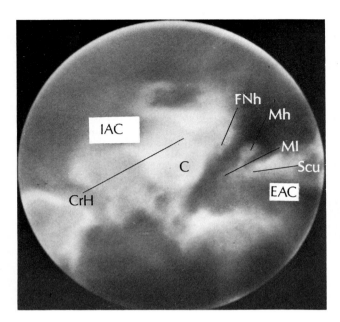

FIG. 4–23. Midcochlea **(C)**. In a tomogram 2 mm posterior to the one in Figure 2–22, the malleus is in clear focus, with the head of the malleus **(Mh)** lying within the epitympanic recess and the long process of the malleus **(Ml)** indicating the plane of the invisible tympanic membrane. The very important scutum **(Scu)** is made up by the posterior wall of the external auditory canal and the lateral wall of the epitympanic recess. The medial margin of the scutum supports the tympanic membrane and it becomes blunted when partially destroyed by the erosive process of cholesteatoma. The laterally placed "hole" of the anterior genu of the facial nerve **(FNa)** has continued posteriorly and is visible beneath the ghost shadow of the horizontal semicircular canal. The more medially placed "hole" has continued into the internal auditory canal **(IAC)**. In the Guillen projection the internal auditory canal is slightly foreshortened because of the 15° angulation. Within the internal auditory canal the facial nerve, lying superiorly, is separated from the cochlear nerve, lying inferiorly, by the crista horizontalis **(CrH)**. **EAC,** external auditory canal.

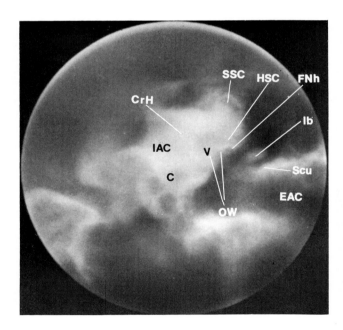

FIG. 4–24. Level of oval window **(OW)** and basal turn of cochlea. In a section 1 mm more posterior to the section in Figure 4–23 lies the oval window niche and the termination of the basal turn in the vestibule. At this level are also the ampullary or anterior limb of the horizontal semicircular canal **(HSC)** and the superior semicircular canals **(SSC)**. The facial nerve in its horizontal portion **(FNh)** lies immediately beneath the horizontal semicircular canal and is shown to have an intact bony covering. The nerve should lie at least 2 mm lateral to the opening of the oval window niche into the vestibule. On this same level lies the body of the incus **(Ib)**. In a medial direction from the body of the incus, the long process can be traced. On the original films, the incudostapedial joint was clearly visible, but it is extremely difficult to reproduce. An important relationship exists between the body of the incus and the margins of the epitympanic recess. If one draws a line from the lateral margin of the horizontal semicircular canal to approximately half way up the lateral wall of the epitympanic recess, this line should touch the very top of the body of the incus. The body of the incus should touch the line at the midpoint or slightly lateral to the midpoint of the line. Dislocations of the incus by cholesteatomas or trauma can be accurately evaluated by this relationship. **CrH,** crista horizontalis; **IAC,** internal auditory canal; **C,** cochlea; **V,** vestibule.

practically surrounded by dense bony otic capsule and cortical bone. The recess is open anterolaterally, but even this opening is partially obscured by the overlying stapedius tendon and stapes arch.

The anatomic relationships previously discussed apply also in examining anteroposterior tomography (Figs. 4–22 through 4–27). In the more anterior cuts, the cochlea, hypotympanum, and ossicular chains can

be visualized to a large extent. In the more posterior portions of the sections, the semicircular canals, aditus, and mastoid antrum can be seen. The internal auditory canal is midway in the sections, a logical site as nerves are being supplied to the anteriorly placed cochlea and the posteriorly placed semicircular canals. To visualize the middle-ear structures, such as the ossicular chain, and some of the bony canals, such as the facial canal,

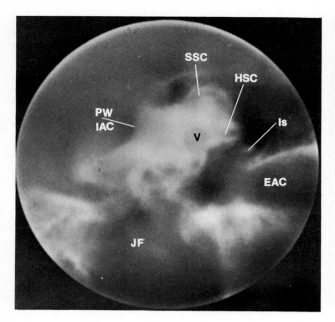

FIG. 4–25. Midhorizontal semicircular canal **(HSC)** and posterior wall of the internal auditory canal **(IAC).** This section, 2 mm more posterior than the preceding one, is beyond the level of the oval window niche. The lateral-most portion of the horizontal semicircular canal **(HSC)** is in sharp focus. The short process of the incus **(Is)** is also in sharp focus, an indication that the cut is in the posterior portion of the epitympanic recess. The posterior wall **(PW)** of the internal auditory canal **(IAC)** lies in the plane of the cut and indicates the level of the *porus acusticus.* At the inferior margin of the section, the jugular foramen is evident. Because of the obliquity of the wall, the separation between hypotympanum and jugular foramen **(JF)** appears almost fibrous. **EAC,** external auditory canal; **V,** vestibule.

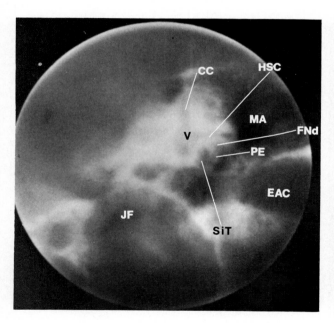

FIG. 4–26. Level of posterior limb of the horizontal semicircular canal **(HSC)** and the common crus **(CC).** A section 3 mm more posterior than the preceding one is at the level of the posterior limb of the horizontal semicircular canal. Lateral to this structure lies the mastoid antrum **(MA).** Inferior to the horizontal semicircular canal, the facial nerve is making its posterior genu, to become the descending portion of the facial nerve **(FNd).** Projected immediately below and medial to the shadow of the facial nerve is the pinpoint opening in the pyramidal eminence **(PE)** for the exit of the tendon of the stapedius muscle. The combination of pyramidal eminence and canal for the descending portion of the facial nerve forms the lateral boundary of the tympanic sinus **(SiT).** The dense otic capsule covering the lateral wall of the vestibule **(V)** forms a portion of its medial and superior wall. The common crus **(CC)** represents the posterior limb of the superior semicircular canal, sharing a common bony canal with the superior limb of the posterior semicircular canal. In special problems, the examination can be carried posteriorly for another 3 or 4 mm to demonstrate the more posterior portions of the mastoid antrum and posterior semicircular canals. **JF,** jugular foramen; **EAC,** external auditory canal.

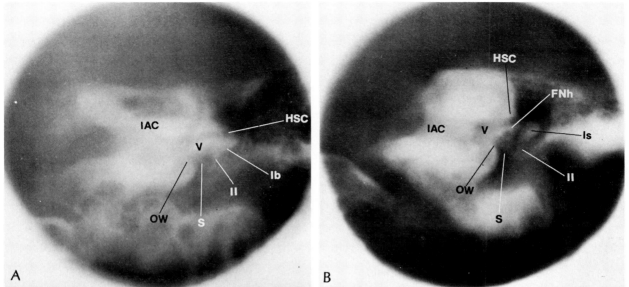

FIG. 4–27. Comparison views of the oval window (**OW**) and the epitympanic recess (**EpR**). **A.** Anteroposterior projection. **B.** Guillen projection. Comparison of the two projections shows the entire V-shaped ossicular chain all the way to the oval window niche in the Guillen projection. The stapes (**S**) arch is clearly visible on the anteroposterior projection as well. As indicated earlier the 15° angle projection of the Guillen view "opens up" the epitympanic recess and visualizes the ossicular chain without superimposition of otic capsule. In addition, the plane of the long process of the incus (**Il**) and head of the stapes arch lies in the plane of the x-ray film. On the other hand, the straight anteroposterior projection shows the true length of the internal auditory canal and is superior for the investigation of acoustic neurinoma, as the canal is not foreshortened. For these reasons we recommend the anteroposterior view for problems of the internal auditory canal and inner-ear structures, whereas the Guillen projection is superior for mastoid air-cell disease and disease processes involving the tympanic cavity and ossicular chain. **HSC,** horizontal semicircular canal; **FNh,** histologic section, facial nerve; **V,** vestibule; **IAC,** internal auditory canal; **OW,** oval window; **Is,** incus, short process; **Ib,** incus body.

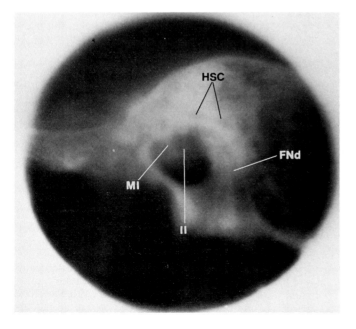

FIG. 4–28. Lateral tomogram through the epitympanic recess (**EpR**) and descending portion of the facial nerve (**FNd**). The lateral projection is useful to show the posterior genu of the facial nerve as it reaches the posterior limb of the horizontal semicircular canal (**HSC**). The facial nerve descends posterior to the external auditory canal and exits through the stylomastoid foramen. At times the bony margins may be somewhat indistinct because of the adjacent mastoid air cells. The venous plexus accompanying the facial nerve may also contribute to slight irregularities of the bony margins of the facial canal. The long process of the malleus (**MI**) and the long process of the incus (**Il**) descend from the epitympanic recess.

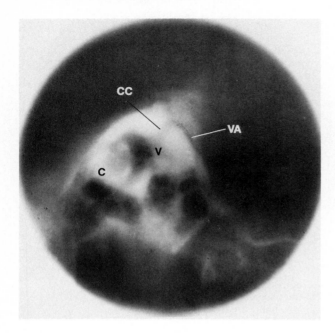

FIG. 4–29. Plane of the common crus **(CC)** and vestibule **(V)**. Five millimeters medial to the previous section is the entrance of the common crus into the vestibule. The common crus is formed by the posterior limb of the superior semicircular canal and the superior limb of the posterior semicircular canal sharing a common crus that unites with the vestibule. At this same level the turn of the cochlea enters the vestibule inferiorly. The apical and intermediate coils of the cochlear appear somewhat as a round lucency, for the spiral ligaments are not visible on the roentgenogram. In the posterior wall of the temporal bone is the vestibular aqueduct **(VA)**. The illustration has been retouched for clarity. From the posterior wall of the mastoid the vestibular aqueduct courses superiorly and medially to the common crus, then forms a right angle and descends into the vestibule. **C,** cochlea.

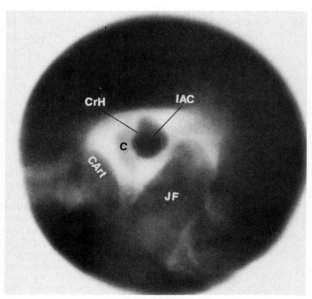

FIG. 4–30. Level of the internal auditory canal **(IAC)** and crista horizontalis **(CrH)**. This section is 2 mm medial to the preceding one and shows that the cochlea has now all but "disappeared." The medial portion of the basal turn of the cochlea casts a shadow anterior to the internal auditory canal **(IAC)**. The groove for the carotid artery **(CArt)** is anterior to the dense bony capsule, and the jugular foramen **(JF)** is visible posteriorly. Considerable variation will occur in the height of the jugular foramen in the mastoid. The *crista horizontalis* separates the facial nerve superiorly from the cochlear nerve inferiorly. This very important structure may be eroded or displaced by slowly growing expansive processes in the internal auditory canal. Note the dense cortical bone surrounding the internal auditory canal; local erosions may be the first sign of an acoustic neurinoma.

a series of tomograms is presented. These are in the Guillen projection—15° angulation of the face toward the side under investigation (Fig. 4–27).

One must constantly remember the 45° angle effect (Fig. 4–8) because many of the thin bony plates are not visible on tomography. It will be immediately apparent that there seems to be no bony roof to the epitympanic recess, yet anatomically, the tegmen is present only 1 or 2 mm above the level of the head of the malleus. Similarly, there is clearly a bony medial wall to the hypotympanum, but this will disappear at times between the hypotympanum and the jugular fossa. The lateral wall of the horizontal semicircular canal may, at times, appear deficient simply because of the angle of the lumen. In a clinical situation, one would be very concerned that a semicircular canal fistula had occurred secondary to an inflammatory process, if one did not remember its course as visual-

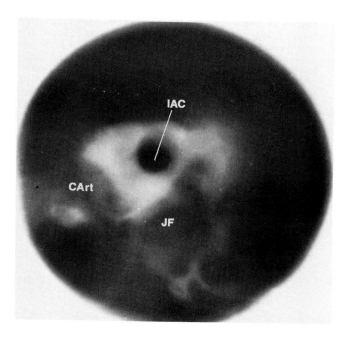

FIG. 4–31. Internal auditory canal (**IAC**) at the level of the porus acusticus (**PA**). Four millimeters medial to the previous section lies the porus acusticus. The *crista horizontalis* has disappeared. The posterior wall of the internal auditory canal is becoming indistinct and losing the dense cortical margin. The canal for the carotid artery (**CArt**) is beginning to turn more anteriorly. The very variable jugular foramen is disappearing, and its margins are becoming indistinct and out of focus, an indication that the tomographic cut is passing medial to the major portion of the jugular foramen (**JF**).

ized on the base projection (an excellent way to show the integrity of the wall of the horizontal semicircular canal throughout its course).

Figures 4–28 through 4–31 are lateral projections extending from the epitympanic recess to the *porus acusticus*. Fractures that extend through the long axis of the petrous bones are best evaluated in the lateral projection. The important parallel relationships between the long processes of the malleus and long process of the incus becomes distorted if there is disruption of the ossicular chain—in particular, displacement of the incus.

At times, the internal auditory canals may appear asymmetrical on anteroposterior projections, but yet the discrepancy between the two sides is not sufficient for a diagnosis of acoustic neurinoma. The lateral or possibly the base projection may show localized erosive changes of the cortex. Anatomic variations can be confirmed when the cross-section of the internal auditory canal is elliptical with the long axis of the ellipse being directed vertically on one side and horizontally on the opposite side.

COMPUTERIZED TOMOGRAPHY

Computerized tomography has created a new era of noninvasive radiologic diagnosis. Whereas the conventional roentgenogram represents the shadow of opaque and semiopaque structures recorded on photographic film, computerized tomography (CT) is a mathematically calculated image. The basic principles of computerized tomography can best be understood by the simplistic illustration in Figure 4–32.

Imagine that you are looking at a kind of box with numbers in the nine squares (Fig. 4–32A). An x-ray tube projects a constant, pencil fine, x-ray beam through the squares and strikes a sensing device on the opposite side of the squares. The sensing device is not recording an image but merely identifying the number of x-ray photons that have not been stopped by the numbers and have been able to penetrate the squares. Think of the numbers as increasing densities.

The x-ray tube is rigidly held to keep its beam focused to the sensing device, as the beam is moved across the squares (Fig. 4–32A, **arrows**). After all the squares have been "viewed" by the x-ray beam, the entire apparatus is rotated, and the numbers are "looked at" from a slightly different angle. The sensing device will now detect a different group of numbers that can be added up obliquely (Fig. 4–32B). After all the numbers have been viewed, the x-ray tube and sensing device are rotated again, and the numbers viewed from top to bottom. Now imagine, as shown in Figure 4–32C that someone has erased the numbers in the squares. Only the totals are known as the sensor has seen through the three different positions of x-ray tube and sensor. With proper mathematical calculations, one can determine what the sequence of numbers had to be, in each of the squares, to give the proper totals. This latter step is the function of the computer and hence the name computerized tomography. The computer will reconstruct the original grid of nine squares and place numbers in the squares. For a more pictorial representation, dots or symbols corre-

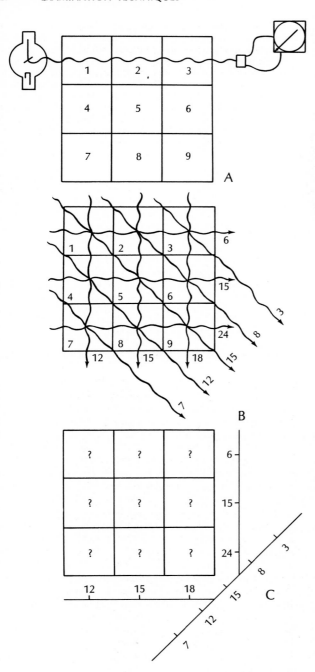

FIG. 4–32. Principles of computerized tomography. **A.** X-rays being generated by an x-ray tube **(at reader's left)** and passing through a patient, as represented by the box with nine squares. Opposite the x-ray tube is a sensing device telling how many x-rays have been attenuated by the numbers within the square. The sensing device does not record an image but merely measures the number of x-ray photons passing through the box. **B.** In the same situation the x-ray tube and sensing device are connected by a U-type of support mechanism that allows the x-ray tube and the sensing device to scan the entire box in a horizontal summation. A support mechanism will rotate and then again view the numbers in their oblique plane. Lastly, the system of x-ray tube and sensing device will add the numbers in a vertical column. **C.** Within the computer, the totals of the numbers in the boxes as viewed by the three different angles have been recorded. The computer knows only the totals and not which numbers were in individual squares. By a system of mathematical calculations, the probabilities of number arrangements are reconstructed to constitute the most likely distribution of numbers that will account for the totals recorded by the sensing device.

sponding to density can be substituted for numbers.

In an average scan, over 20,000 computations are made for each section. The numbers of squares involved may be varied and computer programming obviously plays a vital role in the final image. Suffice it to say, the field is in its infancy and is undergoing explosive technologic progress (2).

At the present state of the art, detail within bony structures, such as the temporal bone, is not sufficient for the refined type of diagnosis obtainable with routine films and tomography. Of particular interest to the radiologist and otologist has been the study of the adjacent brain and subarachnoid cisterns. Computerized tomography can give detailed information regarding the presence or absence of acoustic neurinoma (Figs. 4–33, 4–34). At times, a differential diagnosis of tumors in the cerebellopontine angle is possible (6).

Inflammatory processes within the mastoid and middle ear cavity will occasionally be accompanied by central nervous system symptoms. Computerized tomography can give valuable information concerning the adjacent brain, as scanning may show edematous changes or cerebritis. Brain abscess will closely mimic cerebritis except for central liquefaction.

All these differential diagnoses are possible, on the basis of the ability of the computerized scanner to compare the density of structures to a unit density. In other words, if a lesion is found in the cerebellopontine angle that is of less density than the arbitrary unit, one would suspect a lipoid-containing tumor, such as an epidermoid. On the other hand, meningiomas containing psammoma bodies with calcifications will appear quite dense on the CT scan.

The density of a tumor can be altered by the intravenous injection of contrast material that will stay as a "stain" within the tumor or adjacent brain. In the

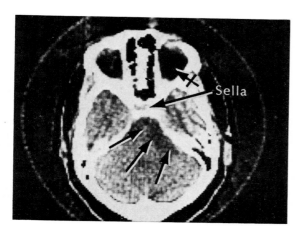

FIG. 4–33. Computerized tomography of a left acoustic neurinoma. The section extends through the mid-orbit and superior portion of the petrous bone. The patient is viewed as if the cut section were seen from below. In the lower half of the illustration is the posterior fossa with the two cerebellar hemispheres near the bottom, connected with the pons, near the middle of the illustration. A somewhat blacker area **(arrow)** is visible adjacent to the left petrous bone. This represents edema in the brain adjacent to a 1.5-cm acoustic neurinoma. The patient was later given contrast material intravenously (1.5 mg/kg of body weight), but no change in the density could be identified. In the illustration, the bones appear white and the fat in the orbit appears black **(crossed arrow)**. The brain substance is an intermediate gray. The blackened area of brain adjacent to the tumor and its accompanying edema is due to lessening density of the brain.

FIG. 4–34. Left acoustic neurinoma with contrast staining. A and B are computerized scans without the injection of contrast material. **A.** Approximately the level of the internal auditory canal. **B.** Near the upper portion of the petrous bone. The fourth ventricle **(crossed arrow)** is visible in midline position. No definite abnormalities within the cerebellopontine angles can be identified. **C** and **D.** Computerized tomography scans of the same patient taken approximately 5 min after the infusion of meglumine (Renografin) 1.5 mg/kg of body weight. As viewed from below, intense staining of an acoustic neurinoma can be seen on the left cerebellopontine angle **(arrows)**. A previous vertebral angiogram had failed to demonstrate any significant hypervascularity within the tumor, yet the intense uptake of contrast material is evident on the CT Scan.

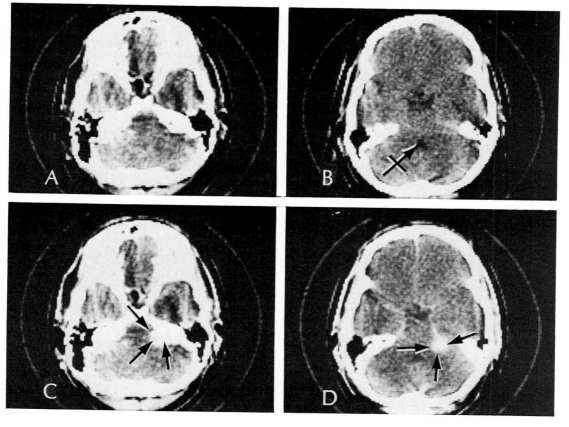

average adult 300 ml of 30% meglumine diatrizoate solution for contrast has greatly enhanced the accuracy of diagnosing acoustic neurinoma.

Although experience is limited, all investigators agree that computerized tomography is the radiologic procedure of choice after plain films and/or tomography (4, 9, 10). Recently, Witten (13) reported a 96% accuracy in identifying acoustic neurinomas in a group of 40 patients undergoing operation.

The accuracy of CT scanning is above 95% in lesions greater than 2 cm in diameter. Lesions 0.7–1.5 cm in diameter are an intermediate group and at times may be mimicked by bony thickenings and protuberances from the posterior surface of the petrous bone. On the other hand, Witten has found tumors 5 mm in diameter and has been able to pick up early changes about the *porus acusticus.*

As equipment improvements occur, it may well be possible to trace the nerves into the internal auditory canal and identify localized swellings. This is a far cry from the early disappointing results of CT scanning prior to the use of contrast enhancement.

REFERENCES

1. Anson BJ, Donaldson JA: The Surgical Anatomy of the Temporal Bone and Ear. Philadelphia, WB Saunders, 1967, pp 23, 28–29
2. Babin RW, Hanafee WN, Ward PH: Anatomic and radiographic correlates in the middle ear. Arch Otolaryngol 101:474–477, 1975
3. Compere WE: The roentgenologic aspects of tympanoplasty. Am J Roentgenol 81:956–963, 1959
4. Gyldensted C, Lester J, Thomsen J: Computer tomography in the diagnosis of cerebellopontine angle tumors. Neuroradiology 11:191–197, 1976
5. Movrell V: Atlas of Roentgenographic Positions, Vol 2, 3rd Ed. St. Louis, CV Mosby, 1967
6. Naidich TP, Lin J, Leeds N, Kricheff II, George AE, Chase N, Pudlowski R, Passalagua A: Computerized tomography in the diagnosis of extra-axial posterior fossa masses. Radiology 120:333–339, 1976
7. Schaefer RE: Roentgen anatomy of the temporal bone-tomographic studies. Medical Radiography and Photography 48(1):2–22. Rochester, NY, Eastman Kodak, 1972
8. Schuller A: Die Schadebasis im Rontgenbild. Hamburg, Tucas Grafe U. Sillem, 1905
9. Stenver HW: Roentgenology of the os petrosum. Arch Radiodiagn Electroradiol 22:97–119, 1917
10. Thomsen J, Gyldensted C, Lester J: Computerized tomography of cerebellopontine angle lesions. Arch Otolaryngol 103:65–69, 1977
11. Vignaud J: Personal communication
12. Vignaud J, Korach G: Exploration radiologique du rucher. Radiodiagn J Electroradiologie 51:1–17, 1969
13. Witten R: Workshop of the Midwinter Radiology Society. Los Angeles, January 28, 1977
14. Ziedses Des Plantes: B. G Een Byzondere Methode Voor bet Maken Van Roentgnfot's Van Schedel en Inverrelkolom. Med T Geneesk 75:5219, 1931

BASIC AUDIOLOGY

5

"HEARING LOSS" AND "DEAFNESS"

Normal hearing represents a range in auditory sensitivity rather than an absolutely fixed quantum. The use of the term normal is relative, as it is in other human physiological measurements. It is an average derived from population surveys and hearing examinations. According to the American National Standards Institute (ANSI), 1969, it is measured as a zero decibel hearing loss (level) on a pure-tone audiogram.

Hearing loss is used in this book to describe a loss in hearing expressed in decibels. An ear with even major hearing losses can respond to amplified sound.

Deafness describes an absolute lack of response to amplified sound. A person with bilateral hearing loss of any level is therefore potentially capable of hearing and understanding the spoken voice to some degree either as a result of medical or surgical treatment, or as a result of assistance by amplified sound (*i.e.*, use of a hearing aid). The person with bilaterally deaf ears is wholly incapable of receiving and reacting to human speech even with maximum acoustic amplification. Such a person may be described as deaf or a **deaf patient.** A patient may have one deaf ear, but will not be considered as deaf. A deaf patient is one who has two deaf ears.

Hypacusis is a synonym for hearing loss. The patient with hearing loss may be described as a patient with hypacusis. In descriptive terms, such a patient may be described as hard of hearing, or hypacusic. Similarly, an ear may be described as hard of hearing, or hypacusic.

Anacusis is a synonym for the term deafness. The patient with unilateral anacusis (unilateral deafness) and normal hearing in the opposite ear is not hard of hearing. The patient with bilateral anacusis is anacusic or deaf. Bilateral deafness—

anacusis—is a total auditory communication deficit and preferably should not be used as a synonym for hearing loss. However, common usage of "deafness" and "hearing loss" as synonyms will probably continue and thus will prolong confusion.

Dysacusis is a term describing a hearing abnormality other than that due to a quantitive decibel hearing loss. It may include auditory distortion problems, displacusis (bilateral pitch asymmetry), or abnormal recruitment (collection) of loudness. Most commonly, however, the term dysacusis is used to describe auditory perception problems due to lesions in the central nervous system. Dysacusis may be on an integrative or an interpretive level; it may be retrocochlear or involve lesions of the central nervous system (CNS) auditory system.

Autism is frequently confused with dysacusis, and is not truly an auditory disability, in that the auditory system (peripheral and central) may be completely intact physiologically.

AUDIOLOGIC TERMINOLOGY

In qualitative audiologic tests additional terms are used to quantify and describe hearing loss, such as **hearing level, threshold, threshold shift, threshold elevation,** etc. These audiologic terms are further separated into **pure tone** and **speech** hearing-level terms and are defined in **decibel levels** and in **percentage scores.** Other auditory profiles are also necessary in differential diagnosis and are further divided and described under separate headings depending upon the special test technique employed.

HEARING LOSS—CONDUCTIVE AND NERVE

For many decades, hearing loss was divided into two anatomic, physiological types, middle ear (conductive) and inner ear (nerve). For practical purposes this division was adequate. The classic tuning-fork tests, especially the Rinne and the Weber tests, were based on these two basic types.

At the present time (1978) the terms **conductive hearing loss** and **nerve hearing loss,** while useful, are inadequate and simplistic. The borderline between conductive system, anatomically and physiologically, and the nerve system has become more complex. We can no longer equate "conductive" with the middle ear alone and "nerve" with the inner ear alone.

The term **conductive** has been applied to any hearing loss resulting from a lesion involving the external ear and/or the middle ear. The limiting anatomic structure is the stapes footplate at the oval window. Thus, for example, the hearing losses of external ear congenital atresias are described as conductive. All otitis media–mastoiditis hearing losses are primarily conductive. Otosclerosis, the major adult cause of hearing loss is a classic conductive lesion. All of these lesions involve physiological disturbances lateral to the stapedial footplate in the oval window. Recent audiosurgical research, however, has broadened the conductive hearing loss category and will be detailed later in this chapter.

The term **nerve deafness** has been applied to all conditions involving the inner ear (cochlea), and also applied to lesions of the auditory nerve, the cochlear nuclei, the central auditory nervous system pathways, and the auditory cortex. The old term nerve deafness later acquired the synonym **perceptive deafness**. The new term **sensorineural** in modern audiology is a replacement for the terms nerve and perceptive. However, the term **sensorineural hearing loss** is no longer an adequate broad-group designation for nonconductive lesions. Recent audiologic, vestibular, radiologic, and otopathologic observations now permit us to separate purely cochlear (sensory) lesions from neural (eighth nerve) lesions, and from CNS (auditory pathway) lesions. We are now able to differentiate within the term sensorineural hearing loss the specific localizations of cochlear, retrocochlear internal auditory meatal lesions, cochlear nuclear lesions, brain-stem lesions, midbrain lesions, and cortical lesions.

OTO-AUDIOLOGIC CHARACTERISTICS OF CONDUCTIVE HEARING LOSSES

Tuning-Fork Tests (128 Hz, 256 Hz, and 512 Hz Forks)

The Rinne test is negative. Bone conduction responses are heard longer (and possibly "louder") than air conduction responses. The Weber test (central—forehead or teeth) is lateralized to the poorer ear (see Ch. 6, Audiologic Assessment, Functional Hearing Loss, and Objective Audiometry).

Pure-Tone Audiometric Characteristics

Pure-tone audiometric hearing losses may vary from a mild to a complete conductive hearing loss (10–70 dB). Hearing losses greater than 71 dB usually indicate either a recognized or unrecognized concomitant sensorineural hearing loss superimposed upon the conductive loss.

Bone conduction losses are nil or very slight in uncomplicated conductive hearing losses. There is always an air–bone gap. The air–bone gap, however, may require special techniques, such as a conductive loss battery, for determination (see Ch. 6, Audiologic Assessment, Functional Hearing Loss, and Objective Audiometry).

Speech-Reception Threshold

There is a very close agreement between pure-tone average and speech reception thresholds (see Ch. 6).

Speech-Discrimination Score

Intelligibility for speech as determined by monosyllabic word lists presented at a recommended sensation level will usually yield very high scores (86–100%) (see Ch. 6).

Recruitment of Loudness

There is no recruitment of loudness in conductive hearing losses.

Response to Amplification

In conductive hearing losses, amplification of speech usually yields excellent results. The patient with a conductive hearing loss should have virtually normal hearing with the use of a hearing aid (see Ch. 43, Hearing Aids).

CONDUCTIVE HEARING-LOSS CLASSIFICATION

In the past, the classic diagnostic concept of a conductive hearing loss has been based on audiometric evidence of an air-bone gap (normal bone conduction hearing with a hearing loss by air conduction), which is an outgrowth of the earlier concept of the negative Rinne tuning-fork test (BC hearing better and of longer duration than AC).

With the advent of recent, more precise audiometric techniques, including acoustic impedance measurements (stapedius and tensor tympani reflex measurements), the sensorineural acuity level test, and the frontal bone conduction test, it has become possible to differentiate conductive hearing losses into more specific patterns based upon current developments in physiologic acoustics. Precise microsurgical observations have also broadened our conceptions of conductive hearing loss. One example of such recent developments is the recognition of fixation of the tympanic membrane and malleus as a unit, as a physiologic problem quite different from other middle-ear conductive lesions such as otosclerotic stapes fixation.

The classic simple concepts of conductive hearing loss were based entirely upon conduction of sound waves through air (*i.e.*, through the tympanic system) only. Thus, a conductive loss would be attributed to lesions anywhere from the auricle, external auditory canal, tympanic membrane, ossicles, middle ear air space, to the medial aspect of the stapedial footplate (at the interface between the footplate and the scala vestibuli perilymph). This concept is now a simplistic one, as we recognize the additional characteristics of acoustic energy transmissions through cochlear fluids. Thus, conductive hearing losses may occur as a result of a failure in transmission of acoustic energy anywhere from the auricle to the organ of Corti hair cells. Conductive hearing loss, therefore, may result from defective transmission of acoustic energy from the collecting auricle to the bioelectric receptors in the organ of Corti hair cells. Both the tympanoossicular and the fluid-propagation-media systems must be considered in the total concept of conductive hearing loss.

Two extreme examples may be used for illustration. At the lateral end of the conductive systems is the example of conductive hearing loss due to congenital atresia of the auricle (see Ch. 32, Hereditary Congenital Ear Syndromes). At the medial end of the conductive system may be the example of early poststapedectomy oval window fistula with purely conductive hearing loss (see Ch. 19, Otosclerosis). The first example is due entirely to tympanic transmission blockade. The second example is due entirely to decompression of the cochlear fluid system resulting from loss of perilymph.

Conductive hearing losses may be due either to transmission fixations or to transmission discontinuities anywhere in the transmission system. Five anatomic groups of lesions may produce conductive hearing losses: 1) external ear; 2) myringomalleal; 3) intratympanic; 4) tympanocochlear interface; and 5) intracochlear fixations and discontinuities.

EXTERNAL-EAR CONDUCTIVE LESIONS

EXTERNAL-EAR FIXATIONS (CONDUCTIVE HEARING LOSSES)

These lesions include auricular aplasia, congenital or acquired atresia of cartilaginous and/or bony ear canal, acquired canal obstructions by tumors, webs, foreign bodies, and cerumen masses.

EXTERNAL EAR DEFECTS (NOT ORDINARY HEARING LOSS)

These defects are the hearing distortions due to abnormal resonance problems that can occur in auricle absence, in the abnormally wide external ear–mastoidostomy cavity, resulting from modified radical mastoidectomy with intact tympanic-membrane-ossicular system.

TYMPANIC MEMBRANE AND MYRINGOMALLEAL CONDUCTIVE LESIONS

TYMPANIC MEMBRANE LESIONS

These lesions include tympanic membrane fixations (partial or complete), such as immobilization by tympanosclerosis (Fig. 5–1); tympanic membrane flaccidity, such as atelactasis or atrophy (Fig. 5–2); and tympanic membrane perforations (Fig. 5–3).

MYRINGOMALLEAL LESIONS

Myringomalleal Fixations

The fixed-malleus syndrome in its early stages involves only the tympanic membrane and malleus, without secondary involvement of the incus and stapes; partial degrees of myringomalleal fixation occur in tensor tympani tendon contractures and/or in calcifications of malleal ligaments (congenital or acquired) (Fig. 5–4).

Myringomalleal Discontinuities

Examples are fracture of the malleal manubrium (Fig. 5–5), or necrosis of malleal neck.

INTRATYMPANIC LESIONS

TYMPANIC CAVITY LESIONS

Intratympanic Positive-Pressure Increase

This may follow acute infections with early intratympanic increased gas pressures or may follow sudden atmospheric pressure changes such as in diving or in other barotrauma (Fig. 5–6).

Intratympanic Negative-Pressure Changes

Negative intratympanic pressures may occur in otitis media and in atelectatic conditions of the tympanic membrane (Fig. 5–7).

Intratympanic Fluid Collections

Intratympanic fluid collections are seen in otitis media and may be partial or complete. The vis-

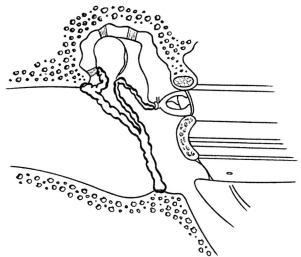

FIG. 5–1. Tympanic membrane tympanosclerosis producing fixation.

FIG. 5–2. Tympanic membrane flaccidity with atelectasis.

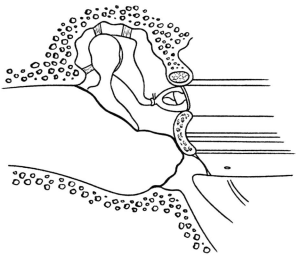

FIG. 5–3. Tympanic membrane perforation.

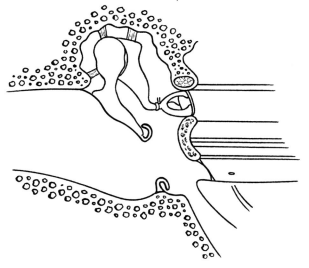

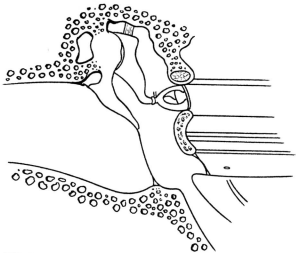

FIG. 5–4. Myringomalleal fixation.

FIG. 5–5. Malleal manubrial fracture.

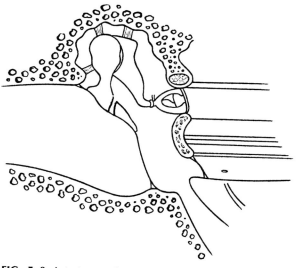

FIG. 5–6. Intratympanic pressure increased by barotrauma.

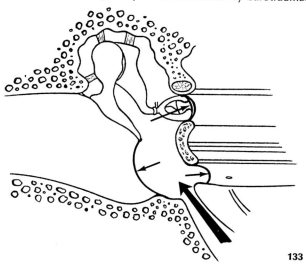

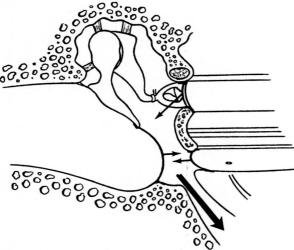

FIG. 5–7. Intratympanic pressure decreased by eustachian tube obstruction.

FIG. 5–8. Intratympanic fluid in secretory otitis media.

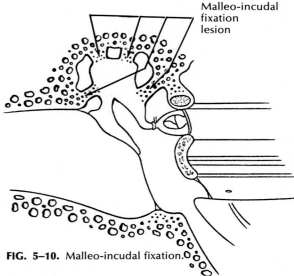

FIG. 5–10. Malleo-incudal fixation.

FIG. 5–11. Incus fixation.

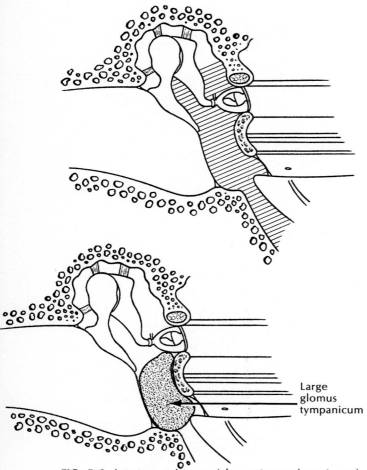

FIG. 5–9. Intratympanic mass (glomus tympanicum tumor).

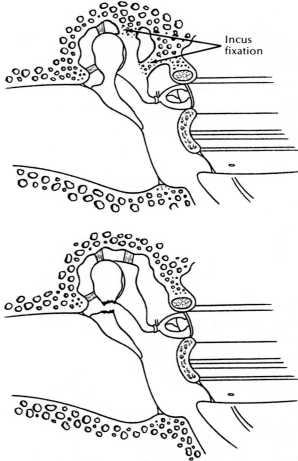

FIG. 5–12. Malleal neck fracture producing malleo-incudal discontinuity.

cosity of the fluid may vary from aqueous to extremely thick, as in the "glue ear" (Fig. 5–8).

Tympanic Cavity Masses

Tympanic air-space problems may be due to masses. A glomus tympanicum may partially or completely fill the middle ear, as may an abnormal jugular bulb or internal carotid artery. A facial nerve neurinoma may do the same (Fig. 5–9).

OSSICULAR CHAIN LESIONS

MALLEO-INCUDAL LESIONS

Malleo-incudal Fixations

The incus frequently becomes fixed, in the fixed malleus syndrome, as a result of secondary fixation to a special joint relationship that exists between malleus and incus (Fig. 5–10). Incus fixation, however, can also be primary, as a result of ossification of epitympanic incudal ligaments or of fixating lesions in the aditus due to mastoid fibrous-tissue lesions (Fig. 5–11).

Malleo-incudal Discontinuity

Discontinuity of the malleo-incudal joint is usually the result of necrotizing type B otomastoiditis lesions, such as keratoma or tympanosclerosis (Fig. 5–12). Occasionally polypoid granulomatous type A lesions may also produce partial incudal body necrosis (Fig. 5–13). However, the most common incudal lesion producing discontinuity involves the long process described in the section on incudostapedial discontinuities.

INCUDOSTAPEDIAL LESIONS

Incudostapedial Fixations

A mobile tympanic membrane and malleus become secondarily fixed by lesions of the incus, incudostapedial joint, and/or stapes. The incus may become fixed to the bony annulus as a result of inflammatory disease. Fixation can occur in stapedius muscle calcification (Fig. 5–14). Fixating lesions may also occur in the incudostapedial joint and in the crura (Fig. 5–15). The stapedial footplate may become fixed, as in otosclerosis (Fig. 5–16). Bony and fibrous fixating lesions may occur between the stapedial arch and the cochlear promontory (Fig. 5–17). Such fixations may also be due to tumors (glomus), or to such congenital abnormalities as persistent obturator foramen stapedial artery. Posterior stapedial crus–ponticulus fixations may occur as result of congenital or acquired lesions.

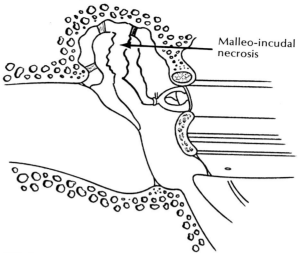

FIG. 5–13. Malleo-incudal discontinuity due to necrosis in joint.

FIG. 5–14. Ossification of stapedius muscle or tendon.

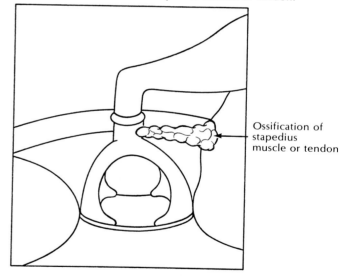

Ossification of stapedius muscle or tendon

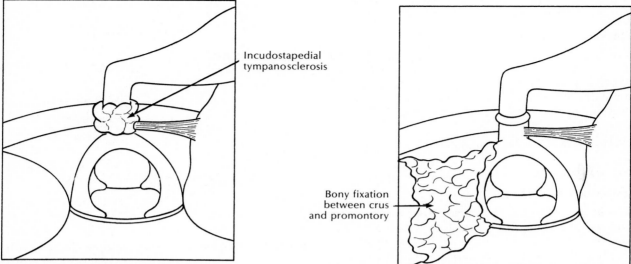

FIG. 5–15. Incudostapedial joint fixation.

FIG. 5–17. Bony fixation between crura and promontory.

FIG. 5–16. Crural fixation by anterior and posterior oto-sclerosis.

FIG. 5–18. Incudostapedial discontinuity due to necrosis of incus long process.

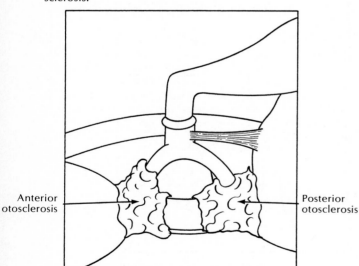

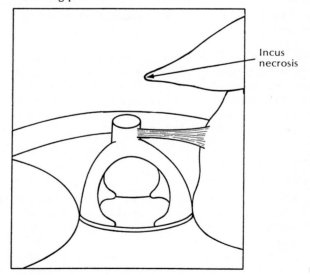

Incudostapedial Discontinuities

The most common discontinuity encountered in the ossicular chain is that of necrosis or atrophy of the long or lenticular process of the incus (Fig. 5–18). Incudostapedial joint discontinuity may be a result of trauma or contracture of the stapedius muscle. Crural necroses (Fig. 5–19) may follow long-standing middle ear infections, or atrophy may result from loss of blood supply, as in advanced obliterative otosclerosis of the oval window niche. Footplate fractures may occur as a result of trauma and occasionally as a result of demineralizing diseases, such as van der Hoeve's syndrome, tympanosclerosis, or keratoma (cholesteatoma).

TYMPANOCOCHLEAR HEARING LOSS

OVAL-WINDOW LESIONS

Oval-Window Fixations

The most common cause of this lesion is stapedial fixation in otosclerosis (Fig. 5–20). Similar fixations may be due to osteoarthritis, van der Hoeve's syndrome, Paget's disease, syphilis, tympanosclerosis, and other diseases.

Oval-Window Fistulas

The most common oval window fistula is that seen following stapedectomy. However, trauma or sudden increases in intracochlear pressures may cause ruptures of the footplate or of the annular liga-ment, producing fistulas and perilymph losses (Figs. 5–21, 5–22).

ROUND-WINDOW LESIONS

Round-Window Fixation

Cochlear otosclerosis is the most common cause of round-window fixation (Fig. 5–23). Less common causes are temporal bone tumors, tympanosclerosis, keratoma (cholesteatoma), and glomus jugulare.

Round-Window Fistulas

A round-window fistula may occur as a result of direct trauma, barotrauma, or increased perilymph pressure changes due to a patent cochlear aqueduct (Fig. 5–24).

INTRALABYRINTHINE CONDUCTIVE HEARING LOSSES

INTRACOCHLEAR HEARING LOSS

Membranous Lesions

Stiffness lesions may occur in "mechanical" presbycusis (hyalinization and calcium deposition in basilar membrane). Excessive compliances may occur, such as seen in hydrops with distended scala media with ectasia of Reissner's membrane (Fig. 5–25).

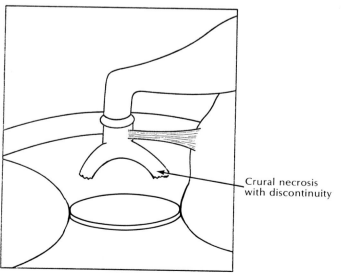

FIG. 5–19. Stapedial footplate discontinuity due to crural necrosis.

Crural necrosis with discontinuity

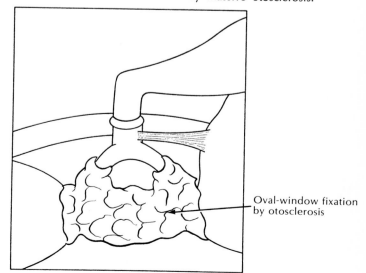

FIG. 5–20. Oval-window fixation by massive otosclerosis.

Oval-window fixation by otosclerosis

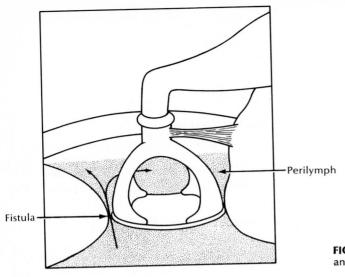

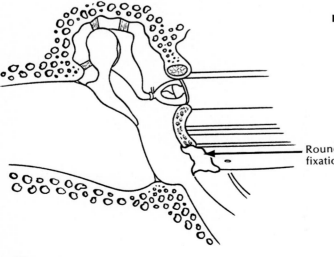

Fistula

Perilymph

FIG. 5–21. Traumatic disruption of oval-window footplate and annular ligament with perilymph fistula.

FIG. 5–22. Footplate fracture causing perilymph fistula and cerebrospinal fluid "gusher."

Footplate fracture with perilymph fistula

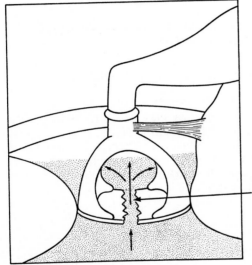
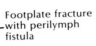

FIG. 5–23. Round-window fixation due to otosclerosis.

Round-window fixation

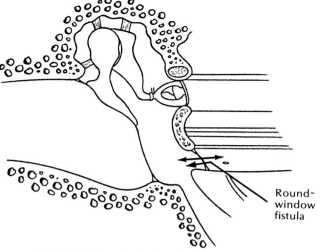

FIG. 5–24. Round-window fistula due to barotrauma.

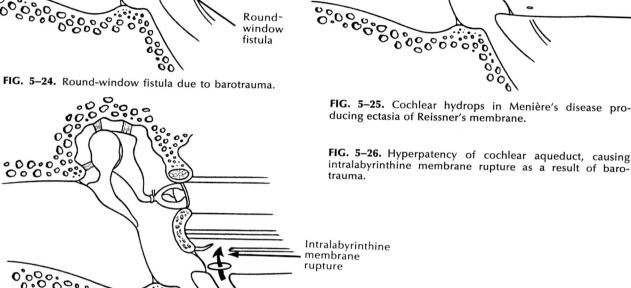

FIG. 5–25. Cochlear hydrops in Menière's disease producing ectasia of Reissner's membrane.

FIG. 5–26. Hyperpatency of cochlear aqueduct, causing intralabyrinthine membrane rupture as a result of barotrauma.

Dynamic Changes in Intracochlear Fluid

Chemical changes in intracochlear fluids may occur either in perilymph or in endolymph. Rheologic changes may be due to sodium/potassium ratio problems. Viscosity changes may be due to various ototoxic agents.

INTRALABYRINTHINE AQUEDUCTS

Vestibular Aqueduct

The vestibular aqueduct, and/or sac may be involved with various lesions that have been considered etiologic in Meniere's syndrome (labyrinthine hydrops).

Cochlear Aqueduct

The cochlear aqueduct in a state of hyperpatency may be responsible for sudden hearing losses due to stress, as recently demonstrated in the labyrinthine-membrane-rupture syndrome (Fig. 5–26).

It is possible that intraductal and extraductal vascular shunts and "lakes" may occur in the vestibular and/or cochlear aqueduct, as recently observed in temporal-bone studies in patients with Meniere's syndrome and in other types of sensorineural hearing losses (1).

INTRALABYRINTHINE CONGENITAL ANOMALIES

Scala communis in some congenital lesions may contribute an intracochlear conductive component to the overall hearing loss which is primarily sensorineural. In essence, such congenital anomalies probably are complex combinations of conductive, receptive, and transmissive lesions within the cochlea, involving the intracochlear partitions, the hair cells, the afferent nerves, and the cochlear spiral ganglion complex.

SUMMARY OF CLASSIFICATION OF CONDUCTIVE HEARING LOSS

This new conceptual approach to conductive hearing losses suggests that such losses may range in magnitude and complexity from a simple accumulation of cerumen laterally to labyrinthine window fistula medially, and even to intralabyrinthine conductive hearing loss lesions (either without damage or prior to damage to the organ of Corti hair cells).

SENSORINEURAL HEARING-LOSS CLASSIFICATION

In the past, the classic diagnostic concept of a sensorineural hearing loss was based on audiometric absence of an air–bone gap (equal loss of bone conduction and air conduction) an outgrowth of the earlier positive Rinne tuning-fork tests (air-conduction hearing "better" and of longer duration than bone conduction hearing).

With the growth of information regarding differences between inner and outer lesions of the organ of Corti hair cell and lesions of auditory neurons, spiral ganglia, eighth nerve (auditory division), cochlear nuclei, brain stem, midbrain, and cortex, the simplistic concepts of an air–bone gap absence and of positive Rinne tests have been replaced. This does not negate the screening value of these early diagnostic approaches. Many complex tests for the specific differential diagnosis of sensorineural hearing loss are now in use and are described in detail later in this chapter.

There are certain basic tests, however, which should be done beyond fork tests and beyond pure-tone bone conduction and air conduction audiometry in differentiating cochlear from retrocochlear lesions, and in pointing to differences between retrocochlear and auditory CNS lesions.

BASIC CHARACTERISTICS OF SENSORINEURAL LESIONS

DIAGNOSTIC ASPECTS OF ENTIRE GROUP

Sensorineural hearing loss, neural hypacusis, nerve "deafness," or perceptive "deafness" is characterized by the following oto-audiologic findings:

Tuning-Fork Tests

The Rinne test is positive and the Weber test lateralizes to the better ear (see Ch. 6, Audiologic Assessment, Functional Hearing Loss, and Objective Audiometry).

Pure-Tone Audiometric Characteristics

Pure-tone audiometric threshold losses may vary from mild hypacusis to profound hypacusis and anacusis. Bone-conduction threshold losses are usually equal to air-conduction threshold losses (within ±10 dB). There is no air–bone gap (see Ch. 6).

Speech-Reception Threshold

In contrast to conductive lesions, sensorineural lesions do not always show close agreement between pure-tone air-conduction threshold losses and speech-reception thresholds. In some types of sensorineural hypacusis, the agreement may be close, and in other types, the agreement may be poor. If the clarity (discrimination) of speech received is severely impaired (for example in the abrupt high-frequency loss), the speech-reception threshold may deviate much more than ±5 dB from the pure-tone average of the speech frequencies (500–2000 Hz) (see Ch. 6).

Speech-Discrimination Score

Speech discrimination may be good in some types of sensorineural lesions but may be poor or even completely absent in other types of sensorineural lesions. Various parameters of speech are affected so that loudness distortion, pitch distortion, and asynchronous time relationships may all contribute to the poor perception of speech (see Ch. 6).

Recruitment of Loudness

Recruitment of loudness is frequently found in sensorineural hypacusis, particularly in peripheral or organ of Corti lesions (see Ch. 6).

Response to Amplification

In sensorineural hypacusis, amplification of speech will yield variable results, with frequent examples of poor response to amplification (see Ch. 43, Hearing Aids).

Short-Increment Sensitivity Index

Cochlear lesions involving hair cell damage will be characterized by a high score on the short-increment sensitivity index. It will be high in conductive hearing loss and low in retrocochlear sensorineural hearing loss (see Ch. 6, Audiologic

Assessment, Functional Hearing Loss, and Objective Audiometry).

Bekesy Audiometry

In automatic Bekesy audiometry in which responses for continuous and interrupted signals are compared, cochlear lesions will usually result in type II patterns, in contrast to type I patterns in conductive hearing loss, and type III and type IV patterns in retrocochlear lesions.

Details of administration and interpretation of the cited tests appear in Chapter 6, Auditory Assessment, Functional Hearing Loss, and Objective Audiometry. Basic audiologic differential diagnosis is presented in Table 5–1.

DEAFNESS, DEAF-MUTE, DEAF AND DUMB

Society has applied labels, some of which are centuries and millenia old, to describe people who have hearing losses. Many inaccuracies and trag-

ically harmful stigmas have been applied by society to people with communication defects.

A person with a moderate hearing loss may be incorrectly described as deaf.

The terms **deaf-mute** and **deaf-mutism** are intended to identify a person who was born with a severe cochlear hearing loss and who has not been able to develop speech.

The term **deaf and dumb**, an equivalent of the German word "taubstummheit," represents a pejorative term, since the word dumb also connotes stupidity. The term deaf and dumb has no logical place in a discussion of hearing loss problems at the present state of our knowledge.

REFERENCES

1. Gussen R: Meniere syndrome. Compensatory collateral venous drainage with endolymphatic sac fibrosis. Arch Otolaryngol 99:414–418, 1974

TABLE 5-1. Basic Audiologic Differential Diagnosis of Conductive and Sensorineural Deafness

| | | Type of response | | |
| | | Sensorineural lesions | | |
Type of measurement	Conductive lesions	Cochlear	Neural (retrocochlear)	CNS
Hearing losses	H* loss only	H loss or deafness	H loss or deafness	Slight H loss or distortion
BC/AC† relationship	Air–bone gap	No air–bone gap	No air–bone gap	No air–bone gap
Rinne fork test	Negative	Positive	Positive	Positive
Speech reception threshold and pure-tone air conduction agreement	Excellent	Variable	Variable	Variable
Speech discrimination score	Excellent	Variable	Variable	Variable
Recruitment of loudness	None	Variable, usually present	Variable, often absent	Absent
Response to amplification	Excellent	Variable	Variable, often poor	Poor
Short increment sensitivity index	High score	High score	Low score	Variable
Békésy audiometry	Type I	Predominantly Type II or Type IV	Predominantly Type III or Type IV	Variable

*Hearing
†Bone conduction/air conduction

AUDIOLOGIC ASSESSMENT, FUNCTIONAL HEARING LOSS, AND OBJECTIVE AUDIOMETRY

H. PATRICIA HEFFERNAN
MARSHA R. SIMONS
VICTOR GOODHILL

AUDIOLOGIC ASSESSMENT

Otologic diagnosis is based, at least in part, on the assumption that a reliable and valid hearing test has been performed. Medicolegal decisions are highly dependent on the accuracy of these test measurements. Habilitative measures, such as hearing-aid fitting, require competent audiometric assessment. Rehabilitative planning, such as educational placement or vocational considerations, requires compilation of much background material, but the cornerstone is the audiogram.

When one views the audiogram in light of any one of these applications, the need for competent and well-trained personnel becomes apparent. Training must focus on more than merely the movement of dials and the recording of responses. The professional responsible for audiometric evaluation must have knowledge of: 1) anatomy and physiology of the auditory system; 2) otologic aspects of hearing loss; 3) equipment and its limitations; and 4) the psychophysical premises on which test procedures are found. This professional must then be able appropriately to interpret quantitative and qualitative audiometric findings to aid in determining the site of lesion and to recognize the need for further evaluation procedures.

The majority of hearing tests in the United States in 1977 are performed by casually trained assistants, most without formal academic training. For example, some facilities are currently employing trained "audiometric assistants" to perform the "routine" hearing testing. As a consistent, uniform training procedure for such paraprofessional personnel is lacking, several factors must be considered before it can be assumed that their test results are valid and/or reliable:

1. Extent of training, including accuracy of testing techniques, ability to relate inconsistent audiometric findings to appropriate psychophysical factors, and level of sophistication in the use of equipment
2. Degree of professional audiologic supervision available.

In the absence of full-time qualified supervision, the diagnostic, habilitative, and rehabilitative considerations recommended may be inappropriate as a result of inaccurate auditory assessment.

The Certificate of Clinical Competence of the American Speech and Hearing Association (3) is one way of determining the qualifications of an audiologist. The requirements include a Master of Arts degree (or its equivalent) in audiology and/or speech pathology, a prescribed year of supervised professional experience, and satisfactory performance on a written test of competence. Many states in the United States now have (or are considering the institution of) licensing requirements that must be met before applicants can qualify for a state license to practice audiology and/or speech pathology.

TUNING-FORK TESTS VERSUS PURE-TONE AUDIOMETRY

The purposes of pure-tone testing are to quantify the degree of hearing loss and to determine the nature of the auditory disability. Tuning-fork tests assist in identifying a possible conductive lesion; however, their use is limited in that they fail to quantify the degree or configuration of the hearing loss, and even identification results are occasionally incorrect. In contrast, standard audiometric results are easily quantified and, when performed in compliance with recommended psychophysical methods, are reliable indicators of hearing threshold levels.

When disagreement exists between tuning-fork test results and audiometric findings, the audiometric Weber test should be performed. If it fails to confirm the pure-tone results, one must investigate the probable mechanical or procedural problems that are influencing audiometric results. Conversely, if the audiometric Weber test confirms the audiometric findings, the validity of the original tuning-fork tests is in doubt, and these tests can probably be ruled out.

THE BASIC AUDITORY ASSESSMENT BATTERY FOR ADULTS

The basic hearing test battery should *always* include (but not be limited to): 1) pure-tone testing of thresholds both by air conduction and bone conduction, with masking employed where appropriate; 2) speech reception threshold (SRT), with masking employed where appropriate; 3) speech discrimination score (SDS), with masking employed where appropriate; and 4) acoustic impedance evaluation (see Ch. 7, Acoustic Impedance Tests).

THE AUDIOMETER AND THE TEST-ROOM FACILITY

Audiometric equipment, to assist minimally in medical diagnosis and recommendations, must offer the following facilities:

1. Air-conduction and bone-conduction pure-tone capabilities
2. A masking generator for wide-band white noise and/or narrow-band white-noise masking
3. A speech circuit for delivering speech materials via live-voice presentation, taped word list, and/or phonograph record word list presentation

Acoustically shielded ("sound-proof") booths are mandatory. Testing can be performed in either single-room or two-room test suite arrangements. Regardless of the setup, two factors must be considered: The noise levels in the test suite must be controlled, and the patient should be positioned so that he cannot watch the movements of the audiologist while the test is being performed.

TEST INTERPRETATIONS (PURE-TONE AUDIOMETRY)

Actual performance of the hearing tests is only one portion of audiologic assessment. The audiologist then interprets audiometric relationships between air conduction and bone conduction by the amount of air–bone gap evidenced in the final test results. These results aid the physician in his final medical determination of the type and extent of hearing loss. The following classification is basic; the reader is referred to Chapter 3, Ear Examination, for more detail.

Conductive Hearing Loss

Attenuation of sound caused by a problem in the outer and/or middle ear results in reduced sensitivity to tones received by air conduction. However, if the inner ear is not impaired, bone-conduction results will be within the normal range of response. An audiogram with reduced air-conduction levels (at least 15 dB poorer than bone-conduction levels) and essentially normal bone-conduction levels is said to represent a conductive hearing loss (Fig. 6–1).

Sensorineural Hearing Loss

Attenuation of sound produced in some portion of the sensorineural mechanism (such as the inner ear) results in reduced thresholds for air conduction (AC). However, it will usually also cause an

FIG. 6–1. Relationship between air conduction and bone conduction for a conductive hearing loss. ●—●, AC, unmasked, RE; [—[, BC, masked, RE.

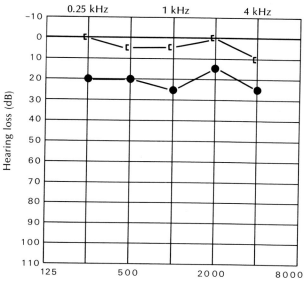

equal reduction in bone-conduction (BC) thresholds. After allowing for individual intra-test variability, we can state that when AC = BC ± 10 dB, the audiogram is reported to represent a sensorineural hearing loss (Fig. 6–2).

Mixed Hearing Loss

As stated, attenuation of sound in some portion of the sensorineural mechanism results in reduced thresholds for bone conduction and air conduction. When there is also a concurrent lesion in the external auditory canal and/or the middle ear, there will be an additional attenuation in thresholds for air conduction. When air-conduction and bone-conduction levels are reduced from normal, and the reduction for air conduction is greater than that for bone conduction, the audiogram is said to represent a mixed hearing loss (Fig. 6–3).

FACTORS INFLUENCING ACCURATE AUDITORY ASSESSMENT

It is certainly important for test procedures to be performed properly for maximum diagnostic utilization. Many factors contribute to accurate threshold determination aside from proper adherence to psychophysical methods. These variables can be classified under four major headings: 1) mechanical; 2) physiologic; 3) procedural; and 4) psychological.

MECHANICAL FACTORS

Equipment Calibration

A regularly and properly calibrated audiometer should provide signals at given intensity levels with some dependability. However, some very significant differences in thresholds may be related to relatively unrecognized mechanical problems associated with the equipment. An audiometer should be calibrated to American National Standards Institute (ANSI) 1969 standards (2) with a sound-level meter at least four times a year, and preferably monthly. In addition to equipment calibration, "real ear" calibration should be done weekly to assure that

1. There are no clicks when the interrupter switch is depressed
2. The hearing attenuator dial appears accurate and linear
3. The frequencies do not sound distorted in pitch characteristics
4. The plug-jacks are in the proper places and are completely connected
5. The earphones appear to be delivering pure

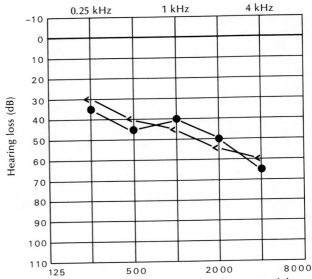

FIG. 6–2. Relationship between air conduction and bone conduction for a sensorineural hearing loss. ●—●, AC, unmasked, RE; <—<, BC, unmasked, RE.

FIG. 6–3. Relationship between air conduction and bone conduction for a mixed hearing loss. ●—●, AC, unmasked, RE; [—[, BC, masked, RE.

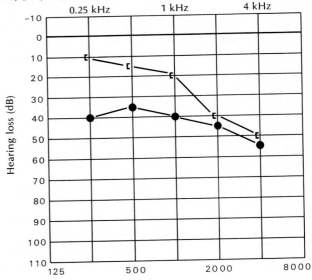

tones of equal loudness to both phones at each frequency

6. The bone-conduction vibrator is performing properly

A quick daily check of the professional's own hearing can grossly estimate the accuracy of threshold measurements in addition to regular weekly and monthly equipment calibration.

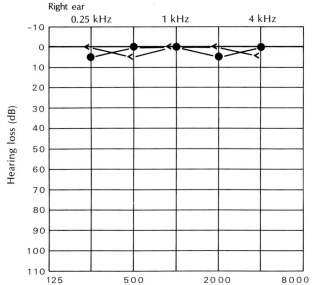
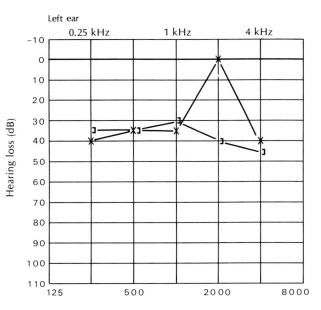

FIG. 6–4. Unexpected "good" hearing by left-ear, AC at 2000 Hz, as a result of equipment "cross-talk." **At left,** ●—●, AC, unmasked, RE; <—<, BC, unmasked, RE. **At right,** x—x, AC, unmasked, LE;]—], BC, masked, LE.

Equipment and the Test Environment

The testing environment must be noise-controlled. The ideal arrangement is a sound-proofed test suite (such as an anechoic chamber), but the cost is generally prohibitive for routine use. Most facilities with two-room test suites either install sound-treated rooms or the new prefabricated test suites. Single-room testing is another alternative. Regardless of the setup utilized, standards have been established for the maximum allowable sound-pressure levels (SPL) for background noise for testing at zero hearing-threshold-level settings of audiometers calibrated to ANSI 1969 values (13):

Octave Band (Hz) 125 250 500 750 1000
1500 2000 3000 4000 6000 8000
SPL allowable (dB) 40 40 40 40 40 42
47 52 57 62 67

Equipment—Earphones

Since the purpose of the earphones is to deliver signals to the patient for threshold determination, it is important that they be well cared for and appropriately used. The headband should hold the cushions snugly against the pinna with the microphone diaphragm directly in front of the opening to the external auditory canal. Problems can arise when the headband pressure is so great that excessive pressure is exerted against the pinna by the earphone. Collapse of the soft cartilaginous portion of the external auditory canal can occur as a result of this pressure by the standard audiometer earphone. The greater the pressure, the greater the likelihood that a false air–bone gap will be observed. (This will be discussed more fully under Physiologic Factors.)

Air Radiation of the Bone Conduction Signal

A mechanical characteristic of the bone vibrator that frequently causes false air–bone gaps at 4 kHz is referred to as **air radiation** of the bone-conduction signal. If the bone vibrator radiates sounds to such a degree that they are picked up by air conduction through the external auditory canal, bone conduction may appear at least 5 dB better than expected, judging from the previously determined air-conduction thresholds. The examiner should be aware of this phenomenon so that when an air–bone gap exists at 4 kHz (after checking for collapsed canal with no air conduction change), air radiation should be suspected.

Equipment—Cross-Talk

Leakage of a pure-tone signal from the test ear to the nontest ear is termed **cross-talk.** It can occur on any audiometer (regardless of manufacturer or age of equipment). Of course, when masking is used, this leakage cannot occur. However, during unmasked portions of the test, leakage can be a significant problem. It is usually easily recognized because of the sudden "improvement" in hearing threshold (in the previously determined poorer ear) at one or two frequencies (Fig. 6–4). Because this leaked signal is generally of a fixed intensity (somewhere between 15 and 20 dB hearing level) the patient will continue to respond at the softest levels on the hearing threshold level dial because the signal is being heard at a level above threshold in the better ear, the nontest ear. The use of a soft masking noise of approximately 40 dB hearing level is normally sufficient to rule out cross-talk

when this unusual configuration suggests its probable presence.

Equipment—Bone-Conduction Vibrator

Placement of the bone-conduction vibrator on the optimum point of the mastoid process can affect threshold measurements as much as 20 dB (Fig. 6–5). Often, when bone conduction thresholds fail to be as good as air conduction levels, poor mastoid placement is the answer. However, it is possible for bone conduction to be slightly depressed in relation to air conduction thresholds (contrary to audiometric mythology), as a result of changes in the inertial and osseotympanic bone-conduction modes produced by abnormal conditions of the ears (15). Moreover, when tuning-fork tests have suggested a conductive hearing loss but pure-tone tests have failed to definitely confirm this, poor placement of the bone-conduction vibrator may be the cause. An audiometric Weber test can quickly identify the reliability of the pure-tone measures, and repeat testing with movement of the vibrator may be necessary. Bone-conduction testing, of course, must be conducted in a very quiet setting. It is apparent that removing the earphones will expose the patient to environmental noises, and unless a significant hearing loss exists, these noises will interfere with the individual's ability to respond to true organic threshold levels for bone conduction.

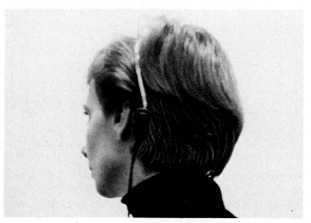

FIG. 6–5. Placement of BC vibrator on mastoid process.

FIG. 6–6. Air conduction and bone conduction thresholds, left ear **(right),** appearing as "shadow curves" from right ear **(left)** resulting from interaural attenuation. **At right, x—x,** AC, unmasked, LE; **>—>,** BC, unmasked, LE; □—□, AC, masked, LE;]—], BC, masked, LE; **diagonal arrows,** no response at maximum output; **SRT,** 50 dB, unmasked; SRT, no response at maximum output, masked. **At left, •—•,** AC, unmasked, RE; **<—<,** BC, unmasked, RE; SRT, 5 dB.

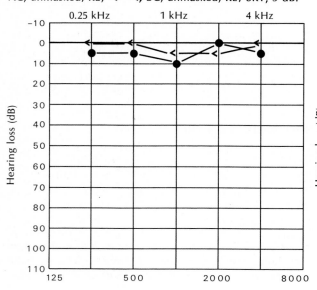

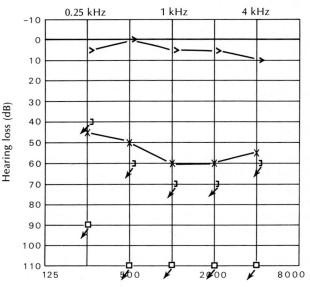

PHYSIOLOGICAL FACTORS

Interaural Attenuation

When a difference in auditory sensitivity exists between the two ears, audiometric results may be inaccurate. Air-conduction and/or bone conduction stimuli, when presented to the poorer ear, stimulate the cochlea of the better hearing ear at certain critical levels. The reduction in energy of the stimuli traveling across the head (from the better ear to the poorer ear) is called **interaural attenuation.** The responses obtained as a result of this phenomenon are referred to as **shadow curves** or **cross hearing** thresholds (Fig. 6–6).

Investigators have attempted to discover the amount of interaural attenuation that exists as a function of frequency for both air-conduction and bone-conduction stimuli. The most current figures (20) for the range of cross-hearing by air conduction are:

Hz:	250	500	1000	2000	4000	8000
dB:	35–70	45–75	45–75	40–80	40–80	40–80

The amount of interaural attenuation for bone conduction stimuli was believed to be 10 dB. However, current investigations (20) have suggested that the interaural attenuation for bone conduction is generally insignificant, and negative values have even been reported (*i.e.,* bone-conduction thresholds obtained from the mastoid process of the anacusic ear are actually better than those obtained from the mastoid process of the hearing ear).

The clinical implications of this phenomenon are as follows:

1. When a difference of 40 dB exists between the bone-conduction threshold of one ear and the air-conduction threshold of the other ear, masking *must* be employed to rule out the interaural attenuation factor (see Ch. 6, section on masking).
2. The range of cross-hearing implies that as large a difference as 85 dB between ears can exist as a result of interaural attenuation, not necessarily true organic hearing thresholds.

Occlusion Effect

The subjective impression of increased loudness of a bone-conducted tone when the pinna is tightly covered (occluded) with an earphone is termed **occlusion effect.** This phenomenon is discussed, in terms of occurrence and diagnostic significance, in Chapter 8, Conductive Loss and Sensorineural Test Batteries, section on Conductive Loss Test Battery.

Tactile Bone Conduction

Patients who demonstrate an air-conduction hearing loss that is severe to profound in degree may exhibit bone conduction thresholds @ 250–1000 Hz near maximum levels. These reflect a vibratory (tactile) response rather than an auditory response to tonal stimuli (17). When these bone-conduction responses are plotted, they may appear on the audiogram to indicate a mixed hearing loss, falsely suggesting potential surgical intervention to deal with a conductive lesion component (Fig. 6–7). One way to audiometrically confirm or refute the suggestion of a mixed hearing loss is to perform acoustic impedance measurements.

Collapsed Canal Effect

Excessive earphone pressure on the pinna can cause the soft cartilaginous portion of the external auditory canal to "collapse," thus preventing complete transmission of air-conducted sound throughout the auditory system. This collapsed canal effect, first described by Scott Reger (11), is known as the **Reger effect.** An artificial conductive hearing loss is found predominantly in the high frequencies, but it also has been observed to extend throughout the frequency range (Fig. 6–8). Tuning-fork tests and an audiometric Weber test should already have alerted the examiner to the possibility of a false air–bone gap.

To eliminate this false air–bone gap, experience has demonstrated that the most consistently effective procedure is to hold a single earphone (separated from the headset) near the pinna but not against it. Air-conduction threshold measurements are then repeated at the frequencies exhibiting the air–bone gap (Fig. 6–9). Routine testing with the earphones held away from the pinna should be avoided, since the patient is then exposed to noises that may interfere with threshold measurements.

In clinical practice, it is our suspicion that this external auditory canal collapse may account for many undefined conductive hearing losses. Routine administration of the audiometric Weber test and acoustic impedance measurements will assist in determining the validity of the pure-tone findings and will clarify the need for repeated testing by some alternative method to the standard placement of the headset and earphones.

Test Environment

Aside from the mechanical factors involved in the test environment, there are some physiological factors that can affect threshold accuracy. The

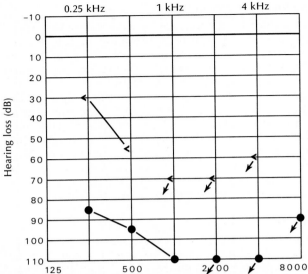

FIG. 6–7. Bone conduction thresholds that appear to indicate a low-frequency conductive hearing loss but are probably only a reflection of vibrotactile response. ●—●, AC, unmasked, RE; <—<, BC, unmasked, RE; **arrows,** no response at maximum output.

FIG. 6–8. Appearance of apparent air-bone gap in high frequencies due to collapsed canal effect (Reger effect). ●—●, AC, unmasked, RE; <—<, BC, unmasked, RE; [—[, BC, masked, RE.

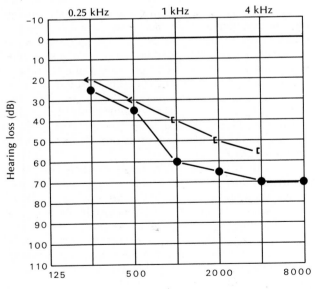

FIG. 6–9. Same ear as in Figure 6–8. Note change in air-conduction thresholds when earphone is held away from ear. ●—●, AC, unmasked, RE; <—<, AC, unmasked, RE.

temperature in the test suites is very important. Excessive heat or poor ventilation can create discomfort for the patient and may even cause drowsiness. The critical listening skills necessary for accurate pure-tone threshold determination may therefore be affected by physical discomfort.

Another factor is the amount of visual distraction in the rooms. Some facilities attempt to make the test suites appear less sterile by painting murals on the walls or filling the room with assorted decorations. The major drawback, especially with regard to pediatric testing, is that such accouterments can be distracting and may actually interfere with the patient's ability to attend to the required task (*i.e.,* listening to pure tone at threshold).

Central Masking

When a masking noise is introduced into the non-test ear, a small shift (averaging 5 dB) in the pure tone threshold may be noted (22). This demonstration of slightly poorer hearing is believed to be caused by efferent inhibition and is referred to as **central masking** (Fig. 6–10). It does not create a significant enough elevation in auditory threshold to create concern, but it should be recognized as the major cause of a 5 dB shift in pure-tone threshold with the introduction of masking noise in the non-test ear.

PROCEDURAL FACTORS

Test Technique

The techniques appropriate for obtaining the most valid and reliable threshold measurements for

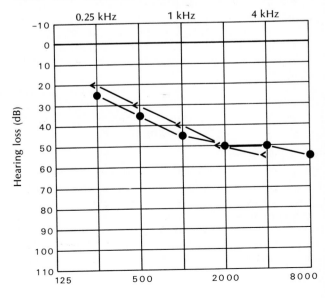

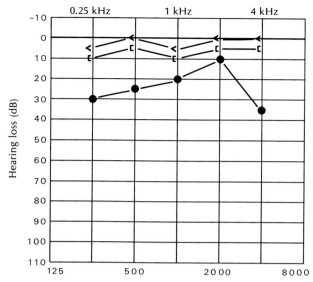

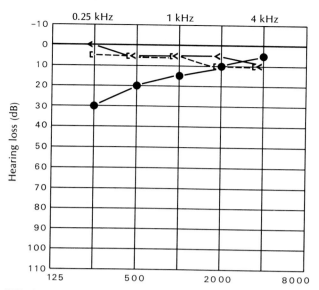

FIG. 6–10. Shift in masked bone conduction hearing thresholds due to central masking effect. ●—●, AC, unmasked, RE; <—<, BC, unmasked, RE; [—[, BC, masked, RE.

FIG. 6–11. Demonstration of need for masking for bone conduction. (Masking noise introduced into nontest ear, at 250–1000 Hz, due to presence of air-bone gap at those frequencies.) ●—●, AC, unmasked, RE; <—<, BC, unmasked, RE; [—[, BC, masked, RE.

FIG. 6–12. Demonstration of need for masking for air conduction. Masking noise introduced into right ear while AC thresholds were retested at all frequencies in left ear because of a 40-dB difference. **At right, x—x,** AC, unmasked, LE; □—□, AC, masked, LE. **At left,** ●—●, AC, unmasked, RE; <—<, BC, unmasked, RE.

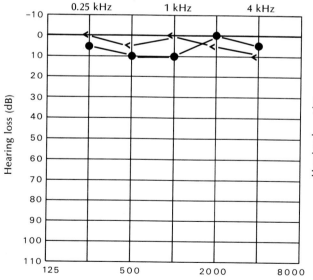

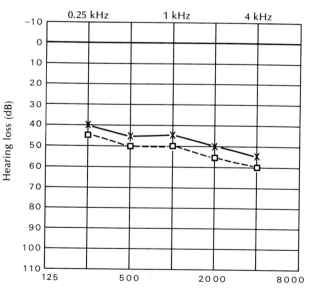

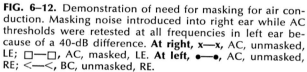

pure-tone and speech signals are well-documented (4). For pure-tone testing, this clinic uses the Psychophysical Method of Limits for exploration of hearing threshold, employing a modification of the Hughson–Westlake technique (4). Hearing threshold level is determined by presenting stimuli in both a descending mode (preparatory phase) and ascending mode (exploratory phase) and shifting from one mode to the other and back again. This procedure is termed **crossing threshold** and serves to determine the level of the stimulus to which a response can be elicited 50% of the time.

The duration of the stimuli can also affect the hearing threshold level (8). When tonal presentation is prolonged, the ear will adapt (*i.e.,* the tone will gradually attenuate) as a result of changes in the auditory system. Adaptation will be less discernible if the stimulus is changing, and especially if the tone is of an on and off nature. The clinical implication of the effect of adaptation of the auditory system is that when a pure-tone test is being performed, the tone should not be left on continuously for a period of time greater than 1 or 2 sec.

Some flexibility in test technique is required, however, when considering the needs of patients with special concerns. One may need to modify signaling techniques or instruction techniques for patients with physical handicaps, developmental delays, low-level language skills, autism, total deafness, age-related problems, etc. If the suggested procedures are followed routinely, utilizing consistency in technique and adhering to psychophysical principles, validity and reliability of the majority of test results can be anticipated.

Masking

Another procedural variable that can significantly affect test results is the appropriate use of masking. Masking involves the introduction of noise into the nontest ear to aid in elimination of inaccurate threshold levels that result from cross-hearing or interaural attenuation. Various types of noises can be used, differentiated by their frequency spectrum and/or band-width characteristics. The only type of noise that should be employed for masking pure tones, is narrow-band white noise (*i.e.,* noise that has been filtered to contain only a restricted band of noise around a central frequency).

Two basic rules should be adhered to in deciding when masking is necessary:

1. Masking is needed for bone conduction whenever there is an air–bone gap in the test ear. Thus one need only look at the results in the one ear in question when deciding whether to mask bone conduction (Fig. 6–11).

2. Masking is needed for air conduction whenever the bone conduction of one ear is 40 dB (or more) better than the air conduction of the opposite ear. Thus, the results for *both* ears are required when deciding whether to mask for air conduction (Fig. 6–12).

Audiometric Weber Test

The audiometric Weber test should be employed whenever there is an inconsistency between tuning-fork test results and audiometric findings. It follows the same principles established for the tuning-fork Weber test (*i.e.,* lateralization will occur either to the ear with the greatest cochlear reserve or to the ear with the largest conductive component, or the sound will register in midline in symmetrical losses). The test differs from the tuning-fork Weber test in that the tonal stimulus is presented via the bone-conduction vibrator to the forehead of the patient, rather than by the stem of the tuning fork. The patient task is the same: to indicate in which ear the stimulus is perceived.

Instruction Technique

The type of instruction technique employed can have an effect on thresholds obtained. The phrasing used is not so critical a factor as is certainty that the concepts involved in the task are understood. Patients differ greatly in terms of age, motivation, intelligence, ability and/or willingness to perform the task. Therefore, it is essential that the patient clearly understand the required task.

In addition, it is necessary that the examiner be flexible enough to adjust the instruction technique for the patient who presents special concerns. Patients, for example, may be 1) conversant only in a foreign language, 2) lacking in language skills, 3) suffering from impaired hearing, 4) developmentally delayed or 5) physically handicapped.

The two most common inaccurate responses that occur are the false-positive (responding when no tone is presented) and false-negative (failing to indicate that the tone has been heard when in fact it has). The examiner must be aware when these situations are occurring and remind the patient of his or her responsibility in the task, without which accurate threshold determination is dubious.

PSYCHOLOGICAL FACTORS

The Patient

As previously mentioned, the patient must take responsibility for the task of attending to tones at threshold. Pure-tone tests are a subjective measure because the patient's responses are voluntary. Confounding results can occur if the patient is unwilling or unable to respond at his true organic threshold level. A patient's inability to attend may be due to the feeling that pure tones are relatively uninteresting to listen to. The task is further complicated by having to listen at extremely soft levels. Some patients, however, are unwilling to respond at threshold, on either a conscious or subconscious basis (see section on Functional [Nonorganic] Hearing Loss which deals with this subject).

The Examiner

There are several reasons why an examiner can affect test results. The most obvious is the lack of necessary skills, due to poor training or lack of experience, to perform the task with the required accuracy. This type of tester error is most evident in evaluation of the pediatric population, the difficult-to-test population, the patients with unilateral hearing loss, and those with functional hearing loss.

Another cause of inaccurate test results involves the "preparatory set" of the examiner. Sometimes the audiologist may observe a patient during the pretest situation and inaccurately estimate the patient's auditory capabilities. These impressions may carry over to the test situation and cause the audiologist to pursue an inaccurate approach. The audiologist should recognize the possibility that initial casual observations may have been incorrect and only an objective, critical test approach will result in accurate threshold determination.

TEST INTERPRETATION (SPEECH AUDIOMETRY)

Speech Reception Threshold

The speech reception threshold (SRT) is the softest hearing threshold level at which a person can repeat correctly approximately 50% of highly familiar two-syllable words (spondees). The SRT is an estimate of the minimum level of conversation to which the person can be expected to respond. It provides a check on the validity of the pure-tone tests, since it should agree with an average of the two best pure-tone thresholds on the audiogram (±5 dB). While it is not a test of discrimination, it does provide gross information about a patient's ability to recognize and respond appropriately to speech.

Speech Awareness Level

The speech awareness (SA) level is a gross means of validating the pure-tone air-conduction thresholds. It is utilized only when a patient lacks the language capability and/or hearing capacity to recognize and repeat familiar words. It is most frequently used with pediatric patients.

The speech awareness level is the softest hearing threshold level at which the patient indicates "hearing" more than half of the stimuli presented (such as vowels and/or diphthongs). The SA level is usually in agreement (±5 dB) with the best threshold at any one frequency on the audiogram.

Speech Discrimination Score

Speech discrimination tests are supra-threshold measures. Speech discrimination is usually measured by presenting monosyllabic word lists, consisting of phonetically balanced words, which the patient is asked to repeat. The percentage of correct responses is referred to as the **speech discrimination score** (SDS).

The speech discrimination word lists are helpful in assisting the physician in determining the anatomic site of lesion in the auditory system (see Ch. 8, Conductive Loss and Sensorineural Test Batteries). They also serve as estimators of conversational ability. They can be used in evaluating hearing-aid performance. Prediction of speech discrimination ability from other audiometric data alone is poor, particularly when sensorineural hearing loss is present. Table 6–1 interprets the effect of various categories of speech discrimination.

Special Central Auditory Nervous System Speech Tests

Special speech tests comprise a portion of the sensorineural hearing loss test battery. For further information and diagnostic implications, see Chapter 8, Conductive Loss and Sensorineural Test Batteries.

FACTORS AFFECTING RELIABILITY OF SPEECH MEASURES

Speech Reception Thresholds

Most of the factors influencing the establishment of pure-tone thresholds are applicable to the measurement of speech reception thresholds (SRT). Therefore, the special considerations discussed here are those peculiar to the establishment of the SRT.

WORD LISTS. Lists of bisyllabic words referred to as spondee words were first developed at the Psycho-Acoustic Laboratories at Harvard (9). These originally lengthy word lists have been shortened to allow for greater flexibility and ease

TABLE 6-1. Speech Discrimination Classifications

Speech discrimination score (%)	Nature of problem
100–88	**No significant problem** This individual should be able clearly to understand speech at normal conversational levels, or when speech is presented @ a level loud enough to compensate for reduction in auditory sensitivity. Amplification, if indicated, usually is employed with great satisfaction.
86–70	**Mild to moderate difficulty** This person will encounter frequent situations in which he misses "parts" of messages. Degree of handicap will depend largely on social and vocational life styles. Amplification is usually employed with satisfaction.
68–50	**Moderate to marked difficulty** This individual will encounter many situations in which difficulty in understanding conversation will be significant. Addition of speech reading can be very beneficial. Amplification is successful only after training in listening skills.
⩽ 48	**Extreme difficulty** This person has difficulty in following most conversation. To function in employment and social life, one must be willing and able to take advantage of every auditory, visual, linguistic, and emotional clue available. Successful communication will depend heavily on this type of behavior. Hearing aid may be of some benefit, particularly if its limitations are understood by the individual.

of administration. The 27 spondee words that clinical practice and research have indicated are the most reliable because they are the most homogeneous in familiarity, intelligibility, and intensity (6) are as follows:

Iceberg	Daybreak
Airplane	Schoolboy
Armchair	Oatmeal
Playground	Whitewash
Woodwork	Farewell
Hardware	Stairway
Cowboy	Toothbrush
Birthday	Drawbridge
Greyhound	Doormat
Eardrum	Inkwell
Sunset	Mushroom
Northwest	Mousetrap
Sidewalk	Padlock
Railroad	

METHOD OF PRESENTATION. It evidently does not matter whether words are presented in decreasing steps of 2 dB or 5 dB (5). However, there is a significant lack of validity if the test is presented without familiarizing the patient with the words (21).

LIVE VOICE VERSUS RECORDED MATERIALS. Disc-recorded versions of any speech-test materials are unreliable because of the poor durability of discs and player needles. Tape-recorded versions are the most reliable and the most commonly used forms. In addition, many facilities are equipped with single-room test suites, which necessitate the use of recorded speech materials. Some patients (i.e., the foreign-speaking, aged, pediatric, etc.) may

require the greater flexibility of live-voice testing. However, live-voice testing does require a two-room test suite.

Whatever materials are used to obtain the SRT (e.g., live voice, recorded, etc.) testing for the SDS must be performed in a similar manner, to ensure consistency in presentation (12).

NEED FOR MASKING. The following strict rule should be followed when testing with speech materials for both SRT and SDS: Whenever speech materials must be presented to a test ear at levels of 50 dB (or more) greater than the bone conduction of the opposite ear, masking should be used in the nontest ear (Fig. 6–13).

Speech Discrimination Score

WORD LISTS. The monosyllabic word lists used to measure speech discrimination were first developed at the Psycho-Acoustic Laboratory at Harvard (PB-50 word lists) (9). Later, after recognizing that many of the words were archaic and unnecessarily difficult, the Central Institute for the Deaf (CID) in St. Louis devised the W-22 word lists (using the same criteria of familiarity and phonetic balance.) Since then, many different word lists for measurement of discrimination of speech have appeared.

The word lists used today in most clinics in the United States are the CID W-22 lists. They consist, however, of extremely simple words, and the tests often fail to distinguish those patients with significant discrimination problems because of the simplicity. Clinical experience suggests that the most reliable word lists for assessment of speech discrimination ability lie somewhere between the

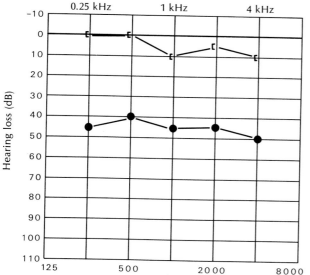
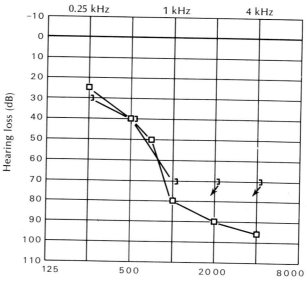

FIG. 6–13. Need for masking in testing with speech materials. **At right,** □—□, AC, masked, LE;]—], BC, masked, LE; **arrows,** no response at maximum output. SRT, unmasked, 45 dB; masked, 45 dB; SDS at 85 dB, unmasked 90%, masked 48%. **At left,** ●—●, AC, unmasked, RE; [—[, BC, masked, RE; SRT, 40 dB; SDS at 80 dB, 100%.

oversimplified W-22 lists and the archaic PB-50 words. Our ranking of the currently available word lists, in order of their increasing difficulty and their ability to differentiate among sensorineural pathologies is: 1) W-22; 2) CNC (or CVC), which represents consonant–vowel nucleus–consonant word lists developed by Peterson and Lehiste; 3) NU-6 word lists developed at Northwestern University; and 4) PB-50.

METHOD OF PRESENTATION. It is important that a carrier phrase be used to present the words, and it may be either of these: "You will say _____" or "Say the word _____." Clinical research has suggested that the carrier phrase is particularly important when live-voice presentation is used (12).

LIVE VOICE VERSUS RECORDED MATERIALS. Highest reliability is obtained using tape-recorded versions of the word lists. Tape-recorded versions should be used to assure intertest consistency of results, particularly when the personnel have limited training or in clinics where multiple personnel with different voices are employed. There are, however, two procedural drawbacks to the tape method: 1) The patient has limited verbal contact with the mechanical tester; thus the word presentations cannot be timed for the patient's response variabilities, nor can the "tape" tester continually ad-

monish the patient to attend or "guess". 2) Tape-recorded presentation is significantly slower than that of live-voice methods.

However, live-voice testing lacks adequate monitoring of control of the word presentation. Also the use of a variety of voices can affect the reliability of this measure (12).

Pediatric Considerations

SPEECH RECEPTION THRESHOLDS. Many of the two-syllable words used to obtain SRT with young children can easily be made up into picture cards. As with familiar objects, the child is not required to repeat words, but merely point to the picture that is named. Because of the effect of the pictures (or objects) being continually visible and limited in number ("closed set") to those most familiar to the young child, the SRT obtained in this manner is often 5–10 dB better than would be predicted from the audiogram. The following list consists of 15 familiar two-syllable words found to be especially successful when testing children:

Pancake	Oatmeal
Birthday	Toothbrush
Sidewalk	Popcorn
Hotdog	Backyard
Baseball	Milkman
Cowboy	Outside
Playground	Icecream
Airplane	

Objects used should be easily recognizable, and most familiar to the child.

SPEECH DISCRIMINATION. Children 6 years old and under often lack the necessary language sophistication and/or familiarity with the words used in the standard adult word lists. Specially constructed word lists (Kindergarten PB word lists—or PBK-50's) are available for children (15).

Another technique for speech discrimination with children utilizes matched word pairs with acoustically minimal phonemic differences. Word cards representing the words are placed on the table and the child is requested to select the appropriate card (when named). This is another example of the "closed set" approach utilizing a very limited number of stimuli, and, as such, it can be expected that the discrimination score will probably suggest somewhat better discrimination ability than that seen in the child's daily functioning. In addition, it is obvious that the child must be able to deal with a multiplicity of items in order to perform this task.

The older child with severe (or profound) hearing impairment may not develop sufficient language sophistication to recognize the words contained in the PBK word lists. Of course, if the words are not familiar, then factors other than discrimination are going to complicate the test results. The Manchester Juvenile (MJ) word lists (7) are useful with children having this severe (or profound) degree of hearing loss.

The Foreign-Speaking Patient

Materials have been developed in several languages (*e.g.*, Spanish, French, etc.) for determining the SRT and SDS. If the examiner is comfortable using these word lists, essentially accurate SRT and SDS can be determined.

However, in our experience, the examiner should avoid using a foreign language unless his use of its accents and idioms is sophisticated. Many foreign patients are only confused by a person attempting to speak their language and using words that sound unfamiliar because of the presentation.

Many foreign-speaking persons can adequately repeat selected English spondees (with prior training). Because of the limited "closed set" used, the results will be somewhat better than would be predicted. Foreign-speaking persons can also repeat W-22 word lists adequately, to obtain a satisfactory *estimate* of discrimination for single words. We do not ask the hesitant patient to attempt this procedure, because of obvious reticence and concern.

Whenever a nonstandardized procedure is employed, the test results must state that fact.

THE BASIC AUDITORY ASSESSMENT BATTERY FOR INFANTS AND CHILDREN

BIRTH TO 24 MONTHS

Parents can expect an infant to begin to be interested in voices, indulge in vocal play with the mother, and in general, to be responsive to the auditory world by no later than 8 months of age. If some or all of these activities fail to develop, a parent will begin to ask questions about the baby's hearing.

These first questions are scattered among any and all professionals who come into contact with the family. A common approach to alleviating this concern is to see if the baby hears the calling of his name, the snap of fingers, or the sound of a noisemaker (such as a bell). Most normally developing infants will promptly and satisfactorily respond to these gross tests.

However, it is imperative to remember that such sounds are complex, with wide frequency range, many overtones, and undetermined intensity. The parent may momentarily be relieved of anxiety by a supposed response to such tests, even though they do not provide adequate information as to the presence or absence of a hearing loss, or its possible configuration.

In our experience, the mother who raises the question of a possible hearing problem in her infant (especially in his first year of life) is most often accurate in her concern. Nevertheless, it is often another 12 months in the infant's life before the next question is heard: "Why isn't he talking?"

When the question is posed about what can be done to assess the infant's hearing level, parents are often *incorrectly* told that a child of this age cannot have accurate hearing testing.

This invalid information tends to delay further appropriate habilitative and rehabilitative procedures. The effect of this delay results in early sensory deprivation. This deprivation, whether caused by conductive hearing loss (*e.g.*, that due to secretory otitis media) or sensorineural hearing loss ranging from mild to profound in degree, is a major factor in limited or delayed language capabilities.

Optimal language and speech development appears to require: 1) exposure to appropriate language stimulation; 2) an efficient sensory input system; 3) an intact auditory feedback mechanism. If a breakdown occurs anywhere along this system, language and speech development may be hindered. The first 36 months of life are considered to be the most critical for language and speech development (18). The concept of critical periods for language acquisition suggests to us that only by applying the proper training procedures during this time can the child's optimum language potential be fulfilled.

Early detection is also essential for appropriate otologic intervention. Prompt medical and/or surgical treatment of some hearing problems (secretory otitis media, mastoiditis, congenital anomalies, etc.) may either completely ameliorate the problem or substantially reduce its deleterious effects.

There are certain behavioral milestones, which if not achieved, necessitate immediate referral for formal otologic and audiologic assessment. Therefore, referral is indicated in the following circumstances:

1. The infant does not localize toward the sound source (or does not show any positive awareness to sound) by 5–6 months of age.
2. Babbling stops (most often noted around 18 months of age) and no specific intelligible words replace it.
3. The infant has not said his first word by 18 months.
4. Jargon persists and is not replaced by actual attempts at speech.
5. Ongoing speech attempts cease or fail to progress at any time.
6. By age 3 years, the child is not using at least two-word combinations.

The case history is one means for discovering which milestones were achieved and at what age. Every audiologic evaluation (following medical examination) should include not only appropriate testing techniques for determination of threshold, but an interview session with the parent or guardian of the infant to

1. Determine developmental history
2. Describe the communication handicap and its effect on the infant and his environment
3. Establish a hypothesis for the definition and management of the hearing loss
4. Establish a basis for counseling regarding fundamental communicative and educational management of the infant.

The newborn nursery would appear to be the prime locale for identification of hearing loss at the earliest possible stage of life, allowing for appropriate intervention almost at the moment of birth. However, neonatal hearing screening has not been enthusiastically endorsed by most investigators, although considerable research has been conducted (18). Some of the problems are the following:

1. The auditory signal required must be at a level sufficiently intense to cause a gross motor reflex. This intensity fails to identify any but the most severe losses. Those infants with mild, moderate, and even some with severe losses will usually not be recognized. Thus, the number of infants identified as having any hearing loss will be small.
2. The sleep state must be light enough to allow for an observable response. The deep sleep of many infants interferes with most procedures.
3. The pass/fail system, under the current methodology, cannot definitively relieve the parent of anxiety, but it should not create undue concern about the presence of a hearing loss in the infant.
4. Cooperation from the parents has been poor when they have been asked to return for further evaluation following notification of their infant's "failing" a newborn hearing-screening test. Thus, the investment in personnel, training, and equipment has not proved to be entirely worthwhile.

The question of neonatal hearing screening has not been dismissed as an identification technique. The Joint Committee on Infant Hearing Screening (1) has recommended it as a research need. One can hope that present and future research will lead to the creation of more reliable techniques and equipment, perhaps utilizing such units as the "Cribogram" (18), or electroacoustic impedance (see Ch. 7, Acoustic Impedance Tests).

Rather than neonatal hearing-screening of all infants, the Joint Committee on Infant Hearing Screening has recommended the mass use of a modified high-risk register:

Supplementary Statement, Joint Committee on Infant Hearing Screening

I. The criterion for identifying a newborn at AT RISK for hearing impairment is the presence of one or more of the following:
   A. History of hereditary childhood hearing impairment.
   B. Rubella or other non-bacterial intrauterine fetal infection (*e.g.*, cytomegalovirus infections, herpes infection).
   C. Defects of ear, nose, or throat. Malformed, low-set or absent pinnae; cleft lip or palate (including submucosal cleft); any residual abnormality of the otorhinolaryngeal system.
   D. Birthweight less than 1500 grams.
   E. Bilirubin level greater than 20 mg/100 ml serum.
II. Infants falling in this category should be referred for an in-depth audiological evaluation of hearing during their first two months of life and, even if

hearing appears to be normal, should receive regular hearing evaluations thereafter at office or well-baby clinics. Regular evaluation is important since familial hearing impairment is not necessarily present at birth but may develop at an uncertain period of time later.

The infants who seem to meet any one of the criteria are identified as being at high risk, and then should be tested individually for possible hearing loss during the first 2 months of life, and subsequently receive a complete hearing evaluation at regular intervals.

A high-risk register, to be effective, should identify a disease that is 14 times more prevalent in the register than in the general population. The modified high-risk register should identify a disease that is 35 times more prevalent in the register than in the general population (18).

Despite present pessimism regarding the screening of newborns, early detection is still possible. In our opinion, valid and reliable in depth audiological evaluations of individual infants (from birth on) can be performed by well-qualified professionals in acoustically controlled environments.

Behavioral and objective approaches can be used for assessing the audition of infants. Behavioral techniques require some degree of participation or cooperation. Objective techniques appraise hearing acuity without active participation and/or cooperation of the patient.

BEHAVIORAL EVALUATION OF THE INFANT

The techniques employed for audiometric assessment of infants have been disputed by experts in many varied fields, despite long years of clinical use. The need for proximity of assessment centers and for immediacy of test results have encouraged inadequately trained personnel to take responsibility for evaluating these infants.

The skilled professional, after supervised experience with infants, can make valid and reliable assessments of behavioral changes in response to auditory stimuli. Judgment of these subtle behavioral changes is a difficult task, which should not be attempted by an inadequately trained examiner who lacks thorough knowledge of normal developmental behavior, typical auditory behavior, or principles of psychoacoustics. Audiologists with only adult experience will require special training in pediatric testing before assuming such evaluation responsibility.

Behavioral evaluation of auditory capability may err in the direction of either a greater or lesser hearing loss than actually exists. Errors can be

avoided by taking the factors of test procedure and interpretation into consideration.

All these factors apply to hearing testing in children of all ages. They are particularly important in infant testing.

TEST PROCEDURAL DETAILS

Calibration of Equipment

It is imperative that sound-field calibration be consistent with the standard which has proved to be reliable and valid as compared to monaural ear-phone testing. We have found in our clinic that sound-field calibration references are best set at levels essentially equivalent to earphone levels of calibration for the normal adult ear (ANSI, 1969). Of course, auditory assessment of infants is best performed in a two-room, noise-controlled test suite (Fig. 6–14).

Preconceived Attitudes of the Examiner (Preparatory Set)

The examiner must have adequate experience to determine whether reliable hearing thresholds have been obtained, and should be comfortable with the most difficult to test infant. If a reliable hearing test is achieved, parents will more confidently follow the recommendations of a professional who exhibits ease in dealing with the child.

The Audiological Assistants

In many clinics the parent functions as a second observer with the child, while the audiologist presents stimuli from the second room. This may create a problem in that the parent is forced into a role that creates emotional separation from the child and denies the child the comfort supplied by the natural parent-child relationship. In addition, direct parental involvement (in the assistant status) often leads to interference with observational procedures, which may confound test results. This is understandable, since parents enter the test situation with anxiety and concern, which often clouds their ability to be objective.

The most consistently effective procedure is to have a nonfamily member work directly with the child, as the assistant to the audiologist. The assistant should be objective and sufficiently experienced to be able to signal the audiologist (in the control room) when a stimulus should be presented, to assist the audiologist in determining whether an observable behavioral change has occurred in response to the stimulus. The trained observer with the infant must be quiet in approach, warm in manner, and loving in response.

Appropriate Assessment Technique

The type of play activity employed should be limited to whatever would adequately engage the interest of the infant, without demanding skills or interests of which he may not be capable. The 12-month-old would not play attentively with a form board, and a 6-month-old

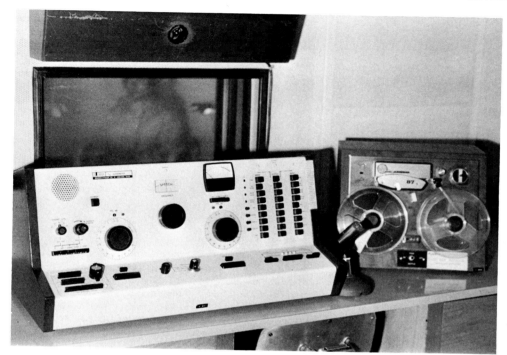

FIG. 6–14. Two-room test suite and audiometer in foreground and patient in background.

FIG. 6–15. A. Infant in high chair is distracted with toys by the audiologist. **B.** Infant localizes to the speaker when stimulus is heard. This behavior is reinforced by the moving toy.

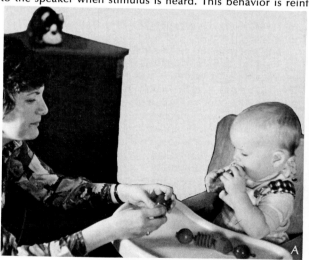

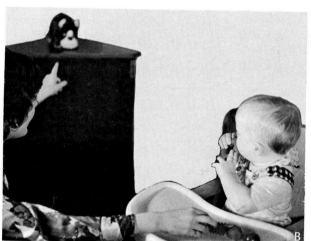

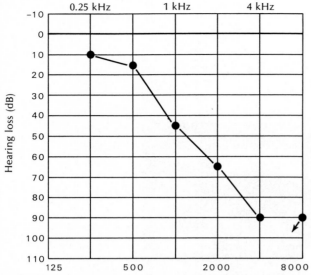

FIG. 6–16. Demonstration of how speech awareness most closely represents best AC thresholds. Therefore, if only speech testing were conducted, the erroneous determination of normal hearing may have been made. ●—●, AC, unmasked, RE; **arrow,** no response at maximum output; speech awareness, 20 dB.

FIG. 6–17. Sound-field AC audiogram on 18-month-old patient. Note slightly better response to speech stimulus than to tonal stimuli. **S—S,** sound field, AC (warble tone), better ear; speech awareness, 15 dB.

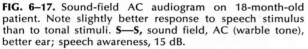

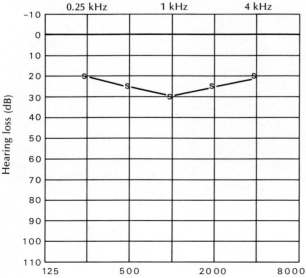

would not be expected to stack cubes. In addition, one would not expect a 3-month-old to turn his head directly to a sound source. Such behavior is more appropriate for the 4- to 7-month-old.

The infant should be allowed to engage in an activity that pleases him, whether it be passive or active. Quiet play or light sleep are the best states for hearing testing.

While conditioned orientation reflex (COR) audiometry or visual reinforcement (VR) audiometry may be successful with the infant as young as 6 months of age, one would not expect it to succeed until the child is functioning at the 12-month level. The COR or VR audiometry is usually applicable and enjoyable until the 30-month level. At 30 months, interest in visually reinforcing toys wanes rapidly.

Types of Stimuli Used

The most interesting and reliable auditory stimuli for infants have been found to be (in rank order): 1) speech; 2) noise bands; 3) music; and 4) environmental sounds (10). These stimuli are complex sounds and give the tester gross information as to hearing capability. They can be presented in the sound field, and the child's behavior at consistent levels of presentation will be noted (Fig. 6–15). The results will reflect only the status of the better hearing ear. They will not reveal the configuration of a hearing loss. Unless further testing is performed, one might erroneously assume that a hearing loss of no more than mild degree exists when there may actually be a hearing loss of greater degree at *some* frequencies. The level of awareness for complex sounds may represent response to only one frequency of a total spectrum (Fig. 6–16).

It is not unusual, when testing infants, to obtain responses to speech that are 5–10 dB better than responses to tonal stimuli. Gross responses will reveal the level of sound at which the infant will show a signal awareness to the parent's voice, and to environmental sounds. Experience suggests these results are related to the infant's greater interest in the complex, broadspectrum, and more meaningful association of speech (Fig. 6–17).

Therefore, it is imperative to attempt to elicit awareness responses to pure-tone stimuli (warble tones) to as many discrete frequencies as possible in the sound field. These stimuli can also be presented monaurally through earphones, to assist in determining significant differences between right and left ears (Fig. 6–18).

Bone conduction testing can also be attempted in the infant (Fig. 6–19). Even while he is sucking a bottle in his mother's arms, it is possible to monitor his behavior, and levels of awareness to auditory signals can be measured. When sound-field air-conduction and monaural bone-conduction tests reveal the existence of an air–bone gap, otologic review for a possible middle ear lesion is essential.

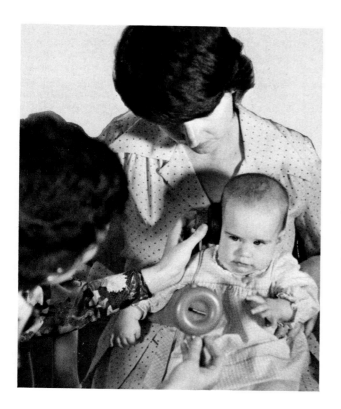

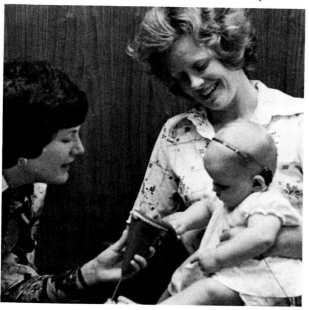

FIG. 6–19. Infant wearing BC vibrator on mastoid process.

FIG. 6–18. Earphone being held to the ear of an infant for monaural evaluation.

FIG. 6–20. Infant's response to stimuli presented via an earphone held next to right ear.

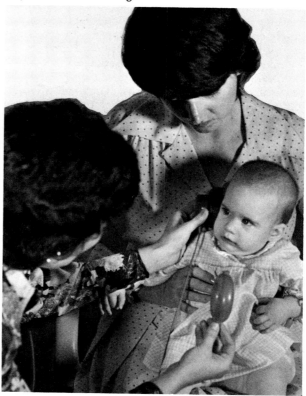

TEST INTERPRETATION

Typical Infant Behavioral Response

The audiologic evaluation of an infant involves not only assessment of peripheral hearing levels, but also recognition of deviant developmental behavior patterns (*i.e.*, those not consistent with a child's chronological age). Atypical developmental behavior calls for pediatric neurologic assessment.

Facial grimaces and brow raising are valid indicators of auditory behavior. The 3-month-old passively resting in an infant's seat or in his mother's lap will demonstrate one of several behaviors, such as eye widening, body startle, etc. (Fig. 6–20). The 6-month-old may initiate or cease activity upon hearing a stimulus.

Application of Appropriate Hearing Standards for the Infant's Developmental Level

Auditory responses follow predictable maturational patterns in the first year of life. Table 6–2 presents data relating to norms for responses to auditory stimuli.

When testing infants, one must remember to apply only the standards appropriate for the child's *developmental* level. As the child progresses developmentally, he continues to increase his ability to attend to less intense sounds, up to a developmental age of 12–15 months. Thus, a 12-month-old infant who has been developmentally assessed as functioning at the 6-month age level will be expected to respond to speech stimuli at 21–40 dB (for pure-tone and speech stimuli). When the same child reaches the developmental level of 12 months, hearing testing reflects his ability to respond differentially to fainter sounds.

THE YOUNG CHILD (2–6 YEARS)

BEHAVIORAL EVALUATION

In the young child's behavioral evaluation, the primary factors previously discussed under Behavioral Evaluation of the Infant are equally important (*e.g.*, calibration of equipment, audiological assistant, etc.). In addition, some procedural problems are specific to the young child.

TEST PROCEDURAL ARRANGEMENT

Appropriate Assessment Technique

Determination of the appropriate test technique for the 3-year-old child will depend on many factors (*e.g.*, social maturity, physical condition, and developmental level). While visual reinforcement (VR) or conditioned orientation response (COR) audiometry is usually successful in children from 12 to 30 months, the orientation response generally habituates rapidly in children over 30 months. Many socially mature 2-year-olds are *able to learn to play the audiometry "game"* and perform reliably, but we recommend VR audiometry as the initial choice for the child from 24–30 months of age.

Sound-Field Technique

All hearing test procedures should proceed from the *most comfortable* and the *least threatening* to those requiring the most conscious cooperation. Therefore, it is best to begin testing with sound-field presentation of speech and tonal stimuli (utilizing either a VR or "play" audiometry technique), and then proceed to bone-conduction testing. Even if the child is resistant to wearing earphones, significant information is obtained, and a negative attitude is averted when testing proceeds in this fashion. Since sound-field air-conduction thresholds and unmasked bone-conduction thresholds relate only to the better-hearing ear, monaural testing should be done as soon as possible.

An example of procedural error is that of a 2-year-old child whose sound-field audiogram suggests a hearing loss of no more than 25–30 dB (Fig. 6–21). Classically, a child of this age with a mild hearing loss has been allowed to wait until the first school experience (kindergarten) to determine his classroom function before any habilitative intervention is offered. Many professionals have operated under the mistaken assumption that a hearing loss of mild degree will have few or no consequences in communicative ability.

This same child may later be found by his kindergarten teacher to have a deviant articulation pattern and distractable auditory behavior, and it is only at this time that he is referred for further testing. Monaural tests then explained the reason for the teacher's report and results revealed a significant bilateral hearing loss (Fig. 6–22).

This case clearly exemplifies the drawbacks in sound-field testing alone. The unusual audiometric configuration of each ear, which would be significant

TABLE 6-2. Auditory Response in the First Year of Life

Age	Speech	White noise	Warbled pure tones
6 wk–4 mo	47 dB (SD* = 2 dB)† 30–45 dB§	45 dB§	70 dB (SD = 10 dB) PTA‡† 500 Hz = 48 dB§ 4000 Hz = 75 dB§
4–7 mo	21 dB (SD = 7 dB)†		51 dB (SD = 9 dB) PTA†
7–9 mo	15 dB (SD = 7 dB)† 15–30 dB§	30 dB§	45 dB (SD = 15 dB) PTA† 500 Hz = 33 dB§ 4000 Hz = 60 dB§
9–13 mo	8 dB (SD = 7 dB)†		38 dB (SD = 8 dB) PTA†

*SD, standard deviation of the mean.
†(Northern JL, Downs MP: Hearing in Children. Baltimore, Williams & Wilkins, 1974)
‡PTA, pure tone average for 500, 1000, and 2000 Hz.
§(Hoversten GH , Moncur JP: J Speech Hear Res 12: Dec, 1969)

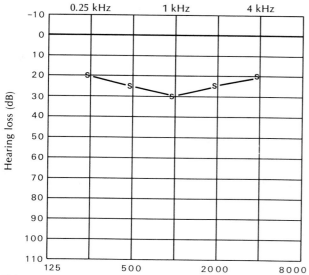

FIG. 6–21. Audiogram obtained when a patient was 2 years of age. Results suggest hearing loss of mild degree. **S—S,** sound field, AC (warble tone), better ear; speech awareness, 25 dB.

for communication purposes, is not revealed until monaural earphone testing is performed. Reliance on sound-field results alone can lead to delay in instituting habilitative measures.

Mastoid-Bone-Conduction Technique

The sound-field testing should be followed by mastoid-bone-conduction testing without masking. Comparison between air conduction and bone conduction, while not revealing which is the better ear, can indicate the presence of an air–bone gap. Such gaps on sound-field and mastoid-bone-conduction have usually been confirmed by later monaural testing with masking.

Play-Audiometry Technique

The youngest patient age at which the audiologist can hope to achieve a complete audiogram by play audiometry is 24 months. This complete test must include monaural air and bone conduction and monaural spondee thresholds (SRT).

Training for the play audiometry "game" is begun in the sound-field (Fig. 6–23). Stacking or shape-sorting toys, varying in complexity, can be employed for play audiometry (Fig. 6–24). They should be geared to the motor and visual capabilities of the child. They should be enjoyable enough to maintain interest throughout the test session, but not sufficiently complex to be totally engrossing.

When the audiologist is certain that the child understands the task, earphones are introduced and monaural testing is conducted (Fig. 6–25). Although earphone testing is accepted at 24 months, not every child can be expected to respond to play audiometry until 36 months of age. The play audiometry technique requires socialization skills not usually present until 3 years of age.

Those behavioral traits seen in the 2- to 6-year-old

FIG. 6–22. Individual monaural test results on same patient shown in Figure 6–21 at 5 years of age. **At left,** ●—●, AC, unmasked, RE; <—<, BC, unmasked, RE; [—[, BC, masked, RE; **arrow,** no response at maximum output; SRT, 25 dB. **At right, x—x,** AC, unmasked, LE; >—>, BC, unmasked, LE;]—], BC, masked, LE; SRT, 25 dB.

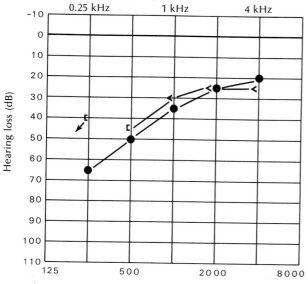

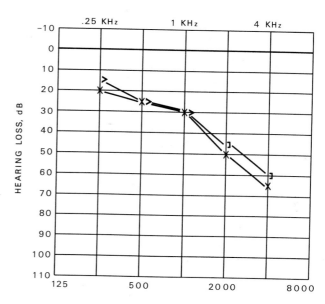

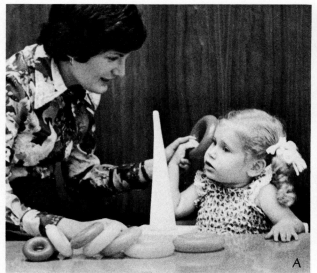
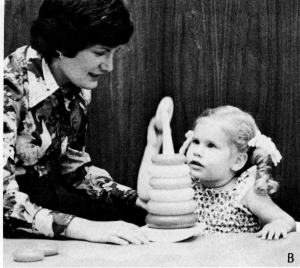

FIG. 6–23. A. Child being trained in sound-field for play audiometry holds toy ring near her ear while waiting for the stimulus. **B.** After the stimulus is heard, the child places the ring on the stick.

FIG. 6–24. Examples of stacking and shape-sorting toys available for play audiometry procedure.

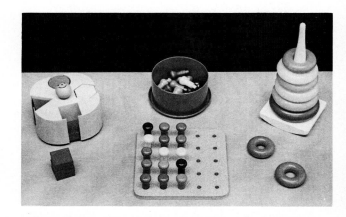

FIG. 6–25. A. Child is being trained for play audiometry while wearing earphones. Initially she held the toy to her ear while waiting for the stimulus. **B.** She acknowledges that the stimulus is perceived by placing the toy in appropriate slot.

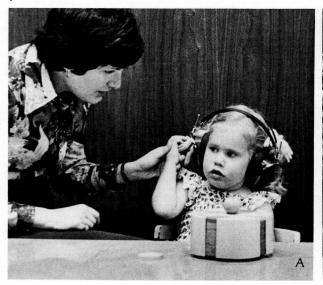
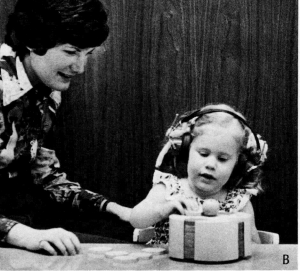

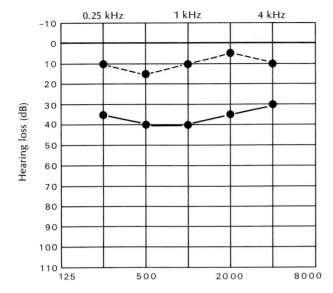

FIG. 6–26. First AC threshold was poor (●—●, AC, unmasked, RE). A test for SRT (10 dB after first test) pointed to better hearing. Second AC threshold (●- - - -●, AC, unmasked, RE) showed agreement with SRT level. Repetition of testing may be indicated.

basis for referral for language and speech therapy. To determine whether a child's linguistic skills are appropriate for his chronological age and/or developmental level, one must have a thorough knowledge of normal language development, much too detailed to discuss here (14). Only then can the audiologist state whether the behavior observed appears to be deviant or appropriate.

In addition, the audiologist should be familiar with a set of norms for speech sound acquisition. The Poole List (19) suggests the outside limits for phoneme acquisition, serving as a guide for determining deviant articulation (Table 6–3).

If the child cannot produce these sounds appropriately by the suggested chronological age then he should be referred for a language and speech evaluation, after a hearing loss or developmental problem has been diagnosed or ruled out.

SPECIAL CONCERNS

The Child With Ongoing Medical Problems

Children with recurrent upper respiratory infections, severe allergies, and comparable disorders present special problems. When an acute condition is present, hearing thresholds may fluctuate, not only in the normal-hearing child but also in the hard-of-hearing child. Normal hearing may decrease to a mild or moderate hearing loss. Mild or moderate hearing loss may decrease to severe hearing loss. Severe hearing loss may decrease to profound hearing loss. Such fluctuations can seriously impede educational and social development. The otologist and audiologist should confer to plan short-term educational and social objectives. If the middle-ear problem will be of relatively long duration, temporary amplification may be necessary. Whether a hearing aid is recommended or

that might interfere with accurate threshold measurement, can be managed by a person trained to work with this age level. With proper behavioral management, threshold responses obtained should be no more than 5–10 dB poorer than actual thresholds, and this notation should be on the audiogram.

Standard adult test techniques are not recommended with children under 6 years of age. Hearing testing should be as enjoyable as possible for a child. Listening to repetitive tones is boring for anyone. The introduction of toys makes the task more enticing, and does not require any more time.

Testing is begun with speech stimuli. Speech is a more interesting and meaningful stimulus than pure tones, and will produce responses closer to threshold. Beginning a hearing test with tonal stimuli and then proceeding to speech stimuli, usually produces dramatically different results (Fig. 6–26).

In specific clinical situations, speech testing is delayed until later in the session. These special situations relate to patients with cleft palate, cerebral palsy, stuttering, reported language delay, deviant articulation patterns, and to the reportedly nonverbal child. In all these cases, language and speech have been areas of great concern for the family as well as the child, and thus, speech testing should not initiate the evaluation procedures.

TEST INTERPRETATION

Indirect Assessment of Linguistic Capabilities

During the evaluation process, the audiologist should make some statement of the linguistic capabilities of the child being evaluated, whether or not he is hearing-impaired. This does not constitute a formal assessment, but it does provide a

TABLE 6-3. Phoneme Acquisition

Chronological age (yr)	Sounds that should have been acquired
3.5	p, b, m, h, w
4.5	t, d, n, k, g, n, j
5.5	f
6.5	ʒ, v, ʃ, l, ʒ
7.5	s, z, θ, hw, r, dʒ

(Poole I: Elementary Eng Rev 11:159–161, 1934)

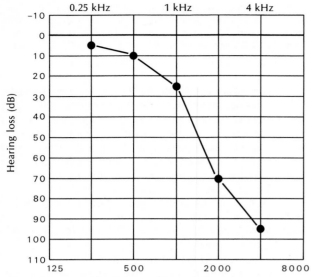

FIG. 6–27. Normal hearing in low frequencies and a high-frequency hearing loss, moderate to severe in degree. The SRT level (10 dB) reflects low frequency hearing; however, SDS (68% at 40 dB) is poor. ●—●, AC, unmasked, RE.

not, the school certainly should be notified so that the teacher can plan modified teaching strategies to allow for decreased response during class sessions.

During ongoing medical treatment, it may also be necessary to refer the child for speech and language evaluation and possible therapy. A child with delayed language and speech development will not spontaneously improve "overnight," following medical treatment, and return to normal hearing. The speech pathologist should evaluate the child and assess receptive and expressive language and speech capabilities. The child can be compared to others of his age and judgments made as to whether he is stimulable and ready for therapy. The speech therapist will also counsel the parents regarding appropriate timing for language and speech therapy.

The Child With a High-Frequency Hearing Loss

The most commonly missed hearing loss is the sharply sloping high-frequency hearing loss, with one or more low frequencies in the range of near-normal hearing or mild hearing loss (Fig. 6–27). These children will be aware of voices and many environmental sounds at a normal intensity level. *Awareness*, however, should not be misinterpreted as *comprehension* of language and speech, which may be severely impaired. This dichotomy is very difficult to explain to parents and teachers who must deal with such a child.

The Overtested Child

A common problem is the child who is consistently being tested, either in the home, at clinics, or at professional agencies. Those who work with children realize how difficult it is to maintain a child's interest in any activity that has been repeated too often, such as "testing" hearing.

Parents with concern about a child's hearing may attempt gross testing at home by banging pots and pans and clapping hands, etc., hoping for a response, however fleeting. Other parents may shop around from one professional clinic to another, often with the unspoken hopefulness that one of them will deny their fears and will claim that the child has normal hearing. This child then comes to an assessment situation overtested and very quickly tires of most activities that can be devised. He also may require sounds that are "louder" than his true threshold before a response can be evoked. In such a case, rehabilitative recommendations and hearing-aid decisions may be founded upon a mistaken impression of hearing poorer than actually exists.

Parents who drift from agency to agency, in addition to overexposing the children to auditory testing, push themselves into blocked situations. Such parents are unable to follow the suggestions of any one of these agencies because they tend to focus on the inconsistencies rather than the commonalities which have been the judgments of the multiple consultants. This self-inflicted parental dilemma will require great patience and tact in the final recommendation.

THE DIFFICULT-TO-TEST CHILD

The child who proves to be difficult to test may be 1) profoundly deaf, 2) developmentally disabled, 3) centrally disordered (sometimes called aphasic), 4) emotionally disturbed (sometimes called autistic), 5) deaf-blind, or a combination of any or all of these disorders. The child who exhibits one or more of these possible disorders needs immediate referral to an experienced pediatric audiologist, even if travel is necessary. Ideally, this audiologist will be part of a diagnostic team, specializing in differential diagnosis. When an unrecognized hearing loss coexists with any of these other diagnoses, the burdens that the *primary* disorder places on the child are significantly complicated by the added disadvantage of the unrecognized and uncorrected hearing impairment.

In addition to previously mentioned concerns, a child may exhibit problems in auditory processing, or may be inattentive, and/or may be auditorily distractible. Hearing testing is indicated for children who exhibit these auditory behavior patterns, to rule out the possibility of peripheral hearing loss. When audiologic evaluation reveals a decrease in thresholds from normal, this loss will interfere with development of communication abilities, regardless of other handicapping problems.

Tangible Reinforcement Operant Conditioning Audiometry (TROCA)

This special behavioral test technique for the difficult-to-test child uses positive reinforcement (such as candy or small toys) to reward appropriate responses to auditory stimuli. The positive reinforcement is withheld for inappropriate responses (*i.e.*, when no sound has been presented). Research has not yet clarified whether continuous reinforcement (*i.e.*, every positive response rewarded) or fixed ratio scheduling (*i.e.*, rewards given for specific number of positive responses) will be the best conditioning method. The test technique is not necessary as a routine, but it is an excellent backup technique with children who do not respond well to traditional reinforcement of social approval.

It may be necessary to modify test procedures to allow for decreased mental or physical function, and/or erratic behavior. However, before these techniques can be appropriately altered, it is imperative that the responsible audiologist have extensive experience with infants and children whose development and behavior are within normal ranges for chronologic ages.

Tests must be structured to allow the child's responses to be judged in relation to **developmental age.** Thus, an 18-month-old child who has been determined as functioning at the 9-month level, must be evaluated as a 9-month-old child, in terms of the kinds of behavioral changes that can be viewed as his levels of response to auditory stimuli. In addition to procedural modifications, speed, accuracy, and flexibility are required to assess hearing levels of "difficult-to-test" children.

THE CHILD WHO IS PROFOUNDLY DEAF

The profoundly deaf child may have so little residual hearing that it is not possible to elicit a response with sounds sufficiently loud to attribute responsiveness to auditory stimuli—*i.e.*, the maximum intensities provided by audiometric equipment may not be sufficient to produce auditory recognition. Such a child may be erroneously considered "autistic" or severely emotionally disturbed.

The child whose hearing loss is of profound degree, however, may respond to a bone conduction vibrator (placed on the hand, fingers, etc.) at near-maximum levels and may even be conditioned to respond to the vibrator if it is placed on the mastoid process, when stimuli are presented at near maximum levels for 250 and 500 Hz. If he then fails to respond to auditory stimulation via earphone or sound-field speaker, he can be assumed to have a hearing loss of severe to profound degree.

THE CHILD WHO IS DEVELOPMENTALLY DISABLED (MENTALLY RETARDED)

These children tend to function at the same developmental level (*i.e.*, are uniform) in all areas of behavior and performance. They are easy to evaluate for auditory acuity, unless hearing evaluation has been delayed for so long that they have developed social mannerisms or other behavioral patterns that might interfere with their ability to cooperate. As a rule, when mental retardation (or developmental disability) is the only handicap, reliable and consistent auditory thresholds can be obtained with modification of techniques to allow for the child's developmental level.

Mentally retarded children may also be congenitally hearing-impaired, perhaps even to the degree of profound hearing loss. They may also be "autistic," and may present a complexity of problems. Discovery of one causal factor does not rule out the possibility of additional handicaps.

THE CHILD WITH A CENTRAL DISORDER ("APHASIC")

Although most children with central language learning disorders exhibit hearing threshold responses within normal limits, it is now known that aphasia and hearing loss can be concomitant disorders. Therefore, when the presumptive diagnosis is a central learning disorder (or severe language delay), the presence of a peripheral hearing impairment must still be ruled out as well.

THE CHILD WHO IS EMOTIONALLY DISTURBED ("AUTISTIC")

The child who is severely emotionally disturbed (autistic) may also be deaf. But a child who does not respond to maximal audiometric stimuli may *only* be profoundly deaf. Many youngsters have hearing losses exceeding those levels now measurable with standard audiometers. The concomitant diagnoses of severe emotional disorder and profound deafness require the multidisciplinary approaches of neurology, psychiatry, pediatrics, psychology, as well as otology and audiology.

It is not the failure to respond to auditory signals that should create suspicion of severe emotional disorder; rather it is lack of affect, failure to make eye contact, and total lack of response to 1) visual, 2) tactile, and 3) auditory stimuli. If a child fails to respond to these three sensory stimuli during an auditory assessment, one must suspect a severe emotional disorder. The child whose primary disorder is in the peripheral hearing mechanism *will* respond to visual and tactile stimuli but will fail to respond to auditory stimulation.

THE CHILD WHO IS DEAF-BLIND

A child with both a visual problem and an auditory disorder is generally labeled as **deaf-blind,** although there may still be usable vision and hearing may also be adequately rendered useful with amplification. These children respond to auditory testing in a very individualistic manner, unique to each child and probably affected by the degree of severity of either of the disorders, as well as the previous exposure to auditory stimulation. It is usually necessary to perform gross tests of hearing (*i.e.,* using noisemakers), to observe the types of behavioral changes that occur in response to sound. Then, when formal audiometric assessment begins, it becomes possible to differentiate true responses to auditory stimuli from random behavioral changes.

Auditory assessment of the deaf-blind child is facilitated when the visual problem is adjusted first. Subsequently, when hearing testing is performed, the child is better able to orient to the visual reinforcement following auditory stimulation, and more accurate estimations of auditory threshold can be made.

The child who is deaf-blind may have concomitant central, emotional, or developmental disorders, which must be diagnosed so that special habilitative measures can be taken.

REFERENCES

1. American Academy of Ophthalmology and Otolaryngology, American Academy of Pediatrics, American Speech and Hearing Association, Joint Committee on Infant Hearing Screening, Dallas, 1970

2. American National Standards Institute, New York, 1969

3. American Speech and Hearing Association, Directory for 1976, Code of Ethics

4. Carhart R, Jerger J: Preferred method for clinical determination of pure-tone threshold. J Speech Hear Dis 24:330–345, 1959

5. Chaiklin J, Ventry I: Spondee threshold measurement: a comparison of 2 and 5 dB methods. J Speech Hear Dis 29:47–59, 1964

6. Curry ET, Cox BP: The relative intelligibility of spondees. J Aud Res 6:419–424, 1966

7. Dale D: Applied Audiology for Children. New York, C Thomas, 1970

8. Hallpike C, Hood J: Some recent work on auditory adaptation and its relationship to the loudness recruitment phenomenon. J Acoust Soc Am 23:270–274, 1951

9. Hirsch I, Davis H, Silverman S et al.: Development of materials for speech audiometry. J Speech Hear Dis 17:321–337, 1952

10. Hoversten G, Moncur J: Stimuli and intensity factors in testing infants. J Speech Hear Res 12:687–702, 1961

11. Kelley N, Reger S: The effect of binaural occlusion of the external auditory meati on the sensitivity of the normal ear for bone conducted sound. J Exp Psych 21:211–217, 1937

12. Kruel EJ, Bell D, Nixon J: Factors affecting speech discrimination test difficulty. J Speech Hear Res 12:281–287, 1969

13. Martin F: Introduction to Audiology. Englewood Cliffs, NJ, Prentice-Hall, 1975

14. Menyuk P: The Development of Speech. Bobbs-Merrill Studies in Communicative Disorders, 1972

15. Naunton R: Measurement of hearing by bone conduction. In Jerger J: Modern Developments in Audiology, 1st ed. New York: Academic Press, 1963

16. Newby H: Audiology, 3rd ed. New York, Appleton-Century-Crofts, 1972

17. Nober EH: Pseudoauditory bone conduction thresholds. J Speech Dis 29:469–476, 1964

18. Northern J, Downs M: Hearing in Children. Baltimore, Williams & Wilkins, 1974

19. Poole I: Genetic development of articulation of consonant sounds in speech. Elementary English Review 11:159–161, 1934

20. Snyder J: Interaural attenuation characteristics in audiometry. Laryngoscope 83:1847–1854, 1973

21. Tillman TW, Jerger JF: Some factors affecting the spondee threshold in normal hearing subjects. J Speech Hear Res 2:141–146, 1959

22. Wegel R, Lane G: The auditory masking of one pure tone by another and its probable relation to the dynamics of the inner ear. Physiol Rev 23:266–285, 1924

FUNCTIONAL HEARING LOSS

Functional hearing loss may be defined as audiometric evidence of hearing impairment where, in fact, no organic basis exists. Nonorganic hearing handicaps range from classic hysterical and psychogenic deafness to conscious, purposeful malingering.

Motivation for manifesting this condition varies, depending upon the age of the patient and history as reported. For example, adults are often motivated by the idea of potential monetary benefit (*i.e.*, the profit motive), whereas children rarely prevaricate for financial gain. Their motivations are usually more serious, involving emotional disturbances, and range from mild to severe in degree. Emotional disorders do not apply solely to the pediatric population; indeed, many adults give false data pointing to hearing loss, a manifestation of serious personal emotional problems.

Regardless of motive, it is the task of the audiologist to discover the existence of a functional hearing loss and to assume the responsibility for determining true audiometric threshold. There are classic behavioral clues in audiometric detection of functional hearing loss.

DISTINCTIVE BEHAVIORAL CLUES TO NONORGANIC HEARING LOSS

1. Inconsistency between air-conduction thresholds and speech-reception thresholds suggests functional hearing loss. Patients generally give more accurate responses to speech tests than to pure tones, unaware of the direct correlation between the two test measures. Speech-reception thresholds should agree within ±5 dB of the best two-frequency average of pure-tone thresholds in the speech frequencies (Fig. 6–28).
2. The lack of a shadow-curve for air or bone conduction in unilateral hearing loss is indicative of nonorganic hearing impairment. If the patient has one normal ear and an organically based hearing loss in the other ear (40–60 dB or poorer), there will be responses to PT on the poorer ear that "shadow" the air-conduction responses on the better ear, before the introduction of masking in the better ear (Fig. 6–29). In addition, the mastoid bone conduction results on the poorer ear should be within 10 dB of those obtained from the better ear. Many patients attempting to feign partial or total unilateral hearing loss are unaware of these natural phenomena, and in their willingness to convince everyone of their sincerity, do not respond to any stimuli presented to the poorer ear. This is a dead giveaway.
3. One should always suspect the possibility of functional hearing loss in legal cases from which a patient may hope to derive significant monetary benefits on the basis of a professed hearing loss.

"INCONSISTENT BEHAVIOR" CLUES TO FUNCTIONAL HEARING LOSS

1. Patients may demonstrate a conversational ability that is not consistent with reported hearing difficulty (*i.e.*, the patient has no trouble understanding directions presented while wearing earphones or when the examiner gives directions at soft conversational levels). When the audiologist later confronts the patient with this inconsistency in behavior, the patient may claim exceptional speechreading ability. (This is not to deny the possibility that a patient with a sudden hearing loss may rely on an innate speechreading ability.)
2. A patient may feign a unilateral hearing loss and exaggerate the use of his "good" ear or claim to be straining to use all residual hearing.
3. A patient may demonstrate normal inflection,

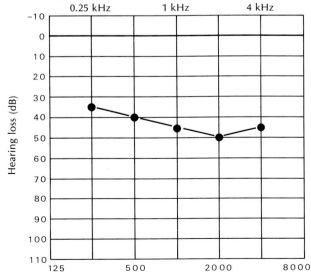

FIG. 6–28. Lack of agreement; SRT (15 dB) versus pure tone average.

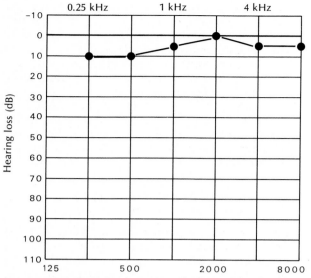

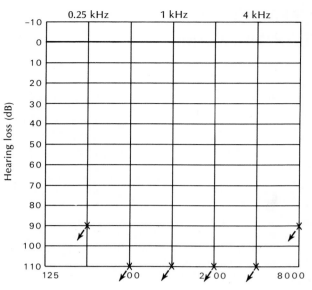

FIG. 6–29. Patient did not respond at all to left ear signals. The response of one with total organic left ear anacusis to unmasked pure-tone stimuli would have been within the range of normal attenuation. **At left,** ●—●, AC, unmasked, RE; SRT, 5 dB. **At right,** x—x, AC, unmasked, LE; **arrows,** no response at maximum output.

FIG. 6–30. Lack of retest reliability. ●—●, AC, unmasked, RE (first test, SRT, 40 dB); ●- - - - -●, AC, unmasked, RE (second test, 5 days later, SRT, 35 dB). Note difference in SRT.

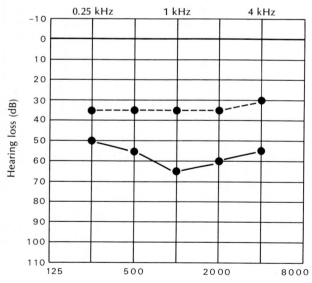

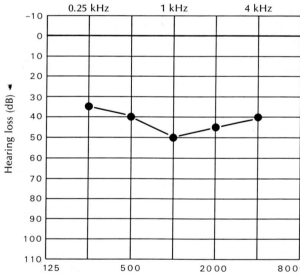

FIG. 6–31. "Saucer" type audiogram. ●—●, AC, unmasked, RE.

voice quality, and articulation ability while claiming a profound bilateral hearing loss. If the auditory feedback mechanism is truly faulty (*e.g.,* due to an organically based hearing loss of long duration), a breakdown in encoding and/or decoding generally occurs, and one would not expect such a patient to have well-modulated voice quality and good articulation.

4. The lack of confirming medical evidence is sometimes cause for suspicion, especially in the presence of other behavioral inconsistencies.

5. Test-retest reliability exceeding 15 dB may be suspect. This is noted with some reservation, bearing in mind the patient with fluctuating thresholds due to secretory otitis media, perilymph fistula, eustachian tube dysfunction, Meniere's syndrome, etc. (Fig. 6–30).

6. A typical audiometric finding is the "saucer" or flat audiogram, which may range from 40 dB to 60 dB (Fig. 6–31). This is based on the assumption that the subject, in trying to establish a reference intensity, responds following equal-loudness contours (usually at his level of "listening" at comfortable loudness).

7. Inappropriate use of a hearing aid can be another alerting clue. For example, a patient's reporting great success with a mild-gain aid, while claiming a profound hearing loss, is cause for suspicion. Also, lack of familiarity with the function of the aid, with battery life, etc., are other clues to watch for.

8. Another common behavioral indication is a half-word response to spondees. Again, a qualification must be stated, because many patients displaying no evidence of nonorganic hearing loss repeat only half the spondee at or near speech reception thresholds.

Demonstration of any or a combination of the foregoing behavior patterns should tend to arouse suspicion (27). Once suspicion is aroused, confirmation becomes the next goal in the evaluation process.

TEST PROCEDURES FOR ASSESSMENT OF FUNCTIONAL HEARING LOSS

Acoustic Impedance Measurement

In our clinic, acoustic impedance measurement is routinely employed as part of the diagnostic test battery on all patients (see Ch. 7, Acoustic Impedance Tests), but it has a special usefulness in determining nonorganic hearing loss. It is often administered at the beginning of the test session in such cases, with the explanation that this test automatically records the patient's response to sounds, for the supposed accurate assessment of the hearing threshold level. This is often sufficient to "cure" an alleged hearing loss. If this ruse does not work, at least the presence of positive acoustic reflexes bilaterally (at levels within the normal range) will rule out a profound unilateral or bilateral hearing loss.

Attempts have been made to employ acoustic reflex thresholds (SPAR) for predicting hearing threshold levels (26). It is our opinion that aural reflex threshold levels (an objective measure), should be used in addition to behavioral or conditioned audiometry (psychophysical measures) to predict hearing thresholds. A test with a 30% error rate is too gross a measure for professional acceptability as a viable technique for determining hearing threshold levels.

The Stenger Test

The Stenger test is an effective classic technique for discovering a nonorganic unilateral hearing loss. It is based upon the assumption that if a tone is simultaneously presented to both ears, it is perceived by the ear in which the tone has greatest intensity. The Stenger test is equally effective if performed as a speech or pure-tone test. It would take a person of great sophistication to cheat on this test.

A pure-tone is presented to the "better" ear at a 10-dB sensation level. A pure tone (same frequency) is presented to the "poorer" ear with increasing intensity (slowly ascending from 0 dB in 5-dB steps). The patient is instructed to continue responding as long as he hears a tone. The patient with a unilateral organic hearing loss will continue to respond to the tone, hearing it in the good ear every time. The patient falsely claiming a unilateral hearing loss will tend to cease responding when the tone becomes louder in the supposed "poor" ear or continue to keep his finger up, despite elimination of the tone in the reportedly "better" ear.

Békésy Test

A type V Békésy tracing (see Ch. 8, Conductive Loss and Sensorineural Test Batteries) is usually found in functional hearing loss. The premise is that the continuous tone is subjectively perceived as being louder than the pulsed tone, and when the patient attempts to respond to tones at equal-loudness levels, he traces the continuous tone at softer intensity levels than for the pure tones. A qualifying statement must be made here, since occasional patients with no functional component or overlay may display a type V pattern. The caution must also be observed that failure to trace a type V pattern does not rule out functionality.

Psychogalvanic Skin Response

The psychogalvanic skin response or electrodermal response audiometry is an objective procedure for evaluating the hearing of the difficult-to-test patient or for determining functionality.

This test is a conditioning technique, which

couples a pure-tone stimulus and an electric shock (via electrodes placed on the fingertips and wrist) for elicitation of an autonomic change in the sweat glands of the skin of the patient. Responses are analyzed from the results indicated on the recorder.

The use of electric shock as a conditioning technique is effective with adults. (For discussion of its use in the pediatric population see section on Objective Audiometry.)

Doerfler–Stewart Test

A patient with a nonorganic hearing loss (or with some functional overlay) establishes and maintains elevated pure-tone and speech thresholds by means of establishing some reference level for responding to the stimuli presented. The Doerfler–Stewart test attempts to disrupt this reference level with the addition of a complex masking noise superimposed upon the primary speech stimulus at various intensity levels.

Its usefulness as a test of functionality is as part of a battery, but it can be employed as a screening test. When positive results are achieved, further investigation is warranted. The Doerfler–Stewart test does not adequately differentiate subjects with a nonorganic hearing loss from those with no functional problem and is a less efficient technique than psychogalvanic skin response audiometry, the relationship between pure-tone average and speech-reception threshold or the pure tone test-retest relationship (23).

Delayed Auditory Feedback

This test is designed to approximate true organic thresholds by introducing a time-delayed message (via earphones) to the patient, while he reads a passage aloud. The secondary (delayed) message, when presented at 20–40 dB above actual hearing level, has been reported to create marked changes in reading rate, fluency, and voice quality and intensity in many subjects (29).

The problem with this procedure is that many patients are minimally affected by the delayed auditory feedback and are able to maintain a consistent reading rate, despite the delay time or intensity of the secondary stimulus. An additional problem concerns the time of the delayed message from the better ear to the supposedly "poorer" ear, where a minimum requirement must be met for maximum reliable interpretation.

The test has been employed at this clinic with good validity. It is especially valuable in confirming functionality, where use of other procedures produce positive results. It is less useful in dubious cases of functionality.

A modification of the delayed auditory feedback employs key-tapping as a motor task of functionality (24, 25). Instead of observing reading-rate changes, rhythmic performance disruption (as a result of delayed feedback) is noted. Further investigation (28) indicated that it was possible to obtain a more accurate estimate of true hearing level than with the original delayed auditory feedback technique. One drawback to this procedure is that some patients get tactile-kinesthetic reinforcement from the tapping, which helps maintain their rhythm pattern and allows them to beat the test.

SUMMARY

The detection of a functional (or nonorganic) hearing loss may appear to be an exciting pursuit. However, the audiologist's concern cannot be limited merely to determining the presence of a functional hearing loss or component. Ideally, the optimal environment in which to see these patients is one in which an otologist and audiologist have direct access to psychological services on the same premises. While the adult feigning a hearing loss may have the direct motivation of monetary gain, we must certainly be concerned about the emotional implications involving the child who presents the same problem.

The need for psychological referral must be individually determined. There are degrees of emotional involvement in this type of patient, as there are in any nonorganic complaint. The audiologist may choose to determine that inconsistencies exist which suggest a nonorganic hearing loss and then may or may not attempt to obtain a more consistent audiogram revealing the essentially normal hearing. However, a casual dismissal of the case after these evaluations can be of significant disservice to the child or adult. Why did he feign hearing loss? How difficult was it to encourage true responses? What was his response to the announcement that he did indeed have essentially normal hearing? These and many other such questions require time and professional skills that the average otologist or audiologist cannot offer.

In the case of the adult seeking monetary compensation, it is the responsibility of the professionals evaluating the patient to discuss the inconsistencies in the test results and explain that they will have to be reported in any summaries requested. This generally has the effect of causing the patient to ask for another chance to perform the hearing test. Many suggestions can be made that will allow the patient to have an "out" and then be able to respond at normal levels for adult thresholds. Among the most successful has been the following: "You have been so worried about your hearing that you are afraid to respond unless you are absolutely certain." Telling the patient to rest and come back in a week to 10 days usually has the effect of relieving him of the anxiety of having to perform again on the same day and affords him the opportunity to save face on the return visit. Many patients then come back telling us that the rest "helped them tremendously." On that second visit we rarely have any problem in obtaining a reliable, consistent audiogram that more closely represents the patient's true hearing levels.

FUNCTIONAL (NON-ORGANIC) HEARING LOSS

23. Chaiklin J, Ventry I: Functional hearing loss. In Jerger J (ed): Modern Developments in Audiology. New York, Academic Press, 1963, pp 76–125
24. Chase R, Harvey S, Standfast S, Rapin I, Sutton S: Comparison of the effects of delayed auditory feedback on speech and key tapping. Science 129:903–904, 1959
25. Chase R, Sutton S, First D: Bibliography: delayed auditory feedback. J Speech Hear Res 2:193–200, 1959
26. Jerger J, Burney P, Mauldin L, Crump B: Predicting hearing loss from the acoustic reflex. J Speech Hear Dis 39:1, 1974
27. Kinstler DB: Functional hearing loss. In Travis L (ed): Handbook of Speech Pathology and Audiology. New York, Appleton Century Crofts, pp 375–398, 1971
28. Ruhm H, Cooper W Jr: Low sensation level effects of pure-tone delayed auditory feedback. J Speech Hear Res 5:185–193, 1962
29. Tiffany W, Hanley C: Delayed auditory feedback as a test for auditory malingering. Science 115:59–60, 1952

OBJECTIVE AUDIOMETRY

Audiometry is based on subjective responses to a variety of auditory signals. Objective audiometry includes a number of techniques designed to elicit clinical information independent of subjectivity.

With the exception of tympanometry (see section 1, Audiologic Assessment in this chapter) and behavioral response techniques for neonatal auditory tests, objective audiometry is based upon electrical response measurements.

Electrodermal measurements of changes in skin resistance have been applied to audiometric testing by conditioning techniques to provide objective responses in special cases.

The historic demonstration of the cochlear microphonic by Wever and Bray (53) in animals (the Wever–Bray effect) was followed by major developments in auditory nerve physiology. Recording of cochlear potentials in humans was reported by Perlman and Case (41), Ruben and colleagues (45), and others (34, 36, 44, 46, 48, 54).

Electrophysiological measurements of the auditory system have been made possible by developments in computer averaging techniques. Berry and co-workers (30) have reviewed such salient aspects as electrocochleography, evoked brain-stem responses, and evoked cortical responses. These are graphically demonstrated in Figure 6–32.

The development of computer signal averaging made possible the detection of very low voltage potentials, and improvement of signal/noise ratio. An early use of this approach was in cortical evoked response audiometry. Early experiments in recording cochlear microphonic measurements from the round window membrane, by Ruben and associates (45), were followed by the development of clinical electrocochleography by Sohmer and Feinmesser (49) and Portmann, Aran, and LeBert (42, 43).

More recently the very early potentials following repetitive click stimuli have been studied by Jewett and Williston (37) and Lev and Sohmer (38). Thus, detection of subcortical and brain-stem responses has become possible.

ELECTRODERMAL PSYCHOGALVANIC SKIN RESISTANCE AUDIOMETRY

Electrodermal or psychogalvanic skin resistance audiometry was developed as an attempt to achieve objectivity in responses from patients otherwise difficult to examine by conventional audiometric tests.

Skin resistance audiometry is based on the objective recording of a conditioned reflex response through a conditioned reflex arc. The objectivity is not a function of direct electrical sequelae from the cochlea or CNS auditory pathway following acoustic stimulation via the external auditory canal. Thus, while the skin resistance technique might well be defined as nonsubjective, it is not truly objective audiometry.

The electrical resistance of the skin varies di-

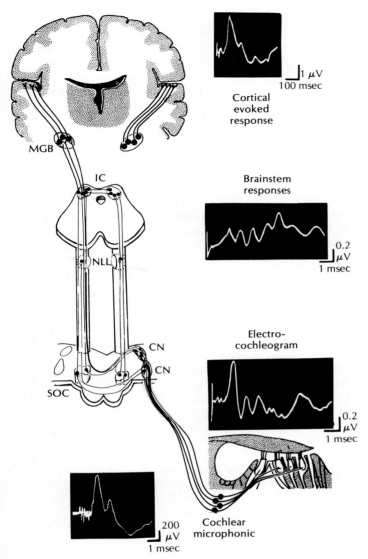

Cortical evoked response

1 μV
100 msec

Brainstem responses

0.2 μV
1 msec

Electro-cochleogram

0.2 μV
1 msec

200 μV
1 msec

Cochlear microphonic

FIG. 6–32. Electrocochleogram shows a large N_1 potential followed by a lower amplitude N_2 response. Brain-stem recording shows an initial eighth nerve action potential followed by the first 10-msec recording following a click stimulus. Cortical evoked response is a later electrical phenomenon, within 500 msec following click stimulus. **CN,** cochlear nucleus; **SOC,** superior olivary complex; **NLL,** nucleus of lateral lemniscus; **IC,** inferior colliculus; **MGB,** medial geniculate body. (Berry H, Briant T, Winchester B: J Otolaryngol 5:3–11, 1976)

rectly with various emotional and physiological changes occurring within the body. The measurement of electrical resistance in ohms is determined by measuring the passage of a minute DC current between two skin electrodes. The conductivity between the electrodes varies with skin resistance as modified by sweat beneath the electrodes, which changes conductivity. The production of sweat beneath the electrodes is moderated by autonomic responses to a variety of stimuli, such as electrical shock, emotional stimuli, and sounds of varying pitch and intensity.

A DC amplifier and a 5-mamp ink recording ammeter is used. A Wheatstone bridge indicates small fluctuations in current flow, usually 2–20 μamp, which is adequate upon amplification to deflect the ink writer for recording and study.

A standard pure-tone audiometer and electrical shocking device complete the equipment setup (Fig. 6–33).

A conditioned reflex is set up after conditioning with a pure tone, followed within 4 or 5 sec by a shock stimulus. The electrical shock stimulus is discontinued when a conditioned response to the sound stimulus has been achieved. A drop in skin resistance occurs between the electrodes as a result of autonomic stimulation and sweat secretion. The skin resistance drop occurs within 1.5–2 sec after the sound stimulus. The intensity of the sound is gradually diminished until threshold is reached. At threshold intensities, usually no change in skin resistance occurs after sound stimulus. The entire sound spectrum is then explored. Details of equipment and testing techniques were described by Goodhill, Rehman, and Brockman (36).

In a study of 150 patients (mostly children), useful audiometric information was obtained in many children who could not respond accurately to ordinary pediatric subjective audiometric tests.

A moderately stable recording base line is found in the normal child and adult. Upon tone stimulation after conditioning, a latent period of approximately 2 sec occurs; this is followed by a sharp drop in skin resistance, as indicated by pen deflection. The pen then returns rapidly to the base line and remains inactive until the following tone stimulus. Some correlation seems to exist between the degree of deflection of the pen and the intensity of the tone stimulus. This ratio of pen deflection to tone stimulus intensity usually makes it possible to approach threshold rapidly.

Incomplete and variable records, due to fatigue, emotional disturbances, or lack of maturation, were obtained in some infants less than 20 months of .age. However, excellent correlations between psychogalvanic skin resistance (electro-audiogram) and standard audiometry were found in many children with cochlear hearing loss of congenital type (Figs. 6–34, 6–35, 6–36).

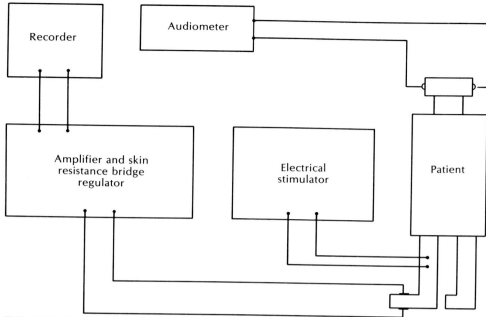

FIG. 6–33. Standard pure-tone audiometer and electrical shocking device.

FIG. 6–34. Congenital, hereditary cochlear hearing loss in 3-year-old child. Test response to condition and sound stimuli good. Occasional marked changes in polarity. Autonomic activity increased as test progressed. Close correlation with pure-tone audiogram. ●—●, pure tone AC, RE; ▲- - - -▲, electroaudiogram. (ASA, 1954)

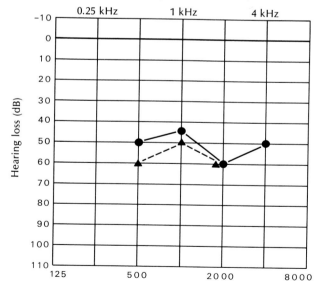

Difficulty in obtaining reliable tests was encountered in brain-damaged children, in which electrical stimulation does not always elicit a response despite considerably greater intensity of stimulation. The latent period is variable, as is the degree of response. The diffuse nature of the response cannot be relied upon, and often a conditioned reflex cannot be obtained. In some instances, when the conditioned reflex is established, it is of a transitory nature, so that constant reinforcement is required.

The responses in brain-damaged children exhibit several characteristic curves that are readily identifiable. The peaks are sharper, of shorter duration, and usually in the form of a crescendo type of response. Continuous short bursts of activity during the ascending and descending portions of the response, and volley effects, are present. This phase is of fairly short duration and then passes into either a hyperactive or refractory stage.

In addition to the role of psychogalvanic skin resistance audiometry as a paraobjective test of hearing, significant neurophysiological information can emerge from the test. The base line in the normal patient is maintained at a moderately stable level, whereas the base line in the patient with neurologic disease shows constant drift and produces a spiked appearance. The base-line drift in these patients must be corrected at

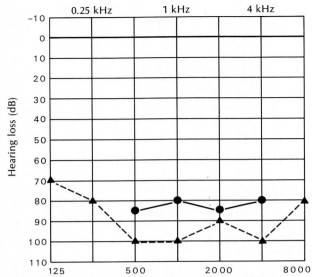

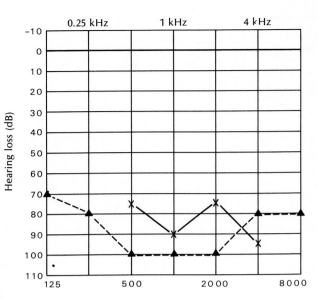

FIG. 6–35. Congenital bilateral Rh-kernicterus cochlear nucleus hearing loss (otologic diagnosis). Very low degree of autonomic activity, of short duration, sharp peaking, and little evidence of volley effect. Close correlation with pure-tone audiogram noted. **At right, x—x,** pure tone AC, LE; **▲ - - - ▲,** electroaudiogram. **At left, ●—●,** pure tone AC, RE; **▲ - - - ▲,** electroaudiogram.

FIG. 6–36. Nonorganic hearing loss in 4-year-old child. Fluctuating type of autonomic responses superimposed on major responses were present. Responses were considerably exaggerated for some frequencies and intensities. Subjective pure-tone audiogram could not be obtained by conventional audiometry. Following psychotherapy, normal hearing on play audiometry and excellent speech were demonstrated. **At right, x—x,** pure tone AC, LE; **▲ - - - ▲,** electroaudiogram. **At left, ●—●,** pure tone AC, RE; **▲ - - - ▲,** electroaudiogram. (ASA, 1954)

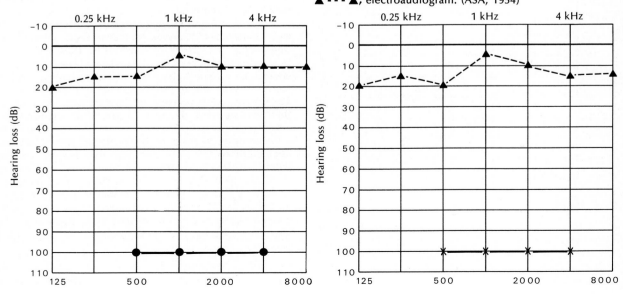

frequent intervals. The drift in base line is in the direction of an increase in skin resistance. Latent periods ranging from several seconds to almost 45 sec were noted in several. The character of these responses is also different—*i.e.*, a slow, steady drop occurs rather than the rapid, sharp drop seen in the normal individual. Various other changes are seen, such as reversal of polarity and abnormally large decreases as well as increases in skin resistance.

The emergence of evoked response audiometry, electrocochleography, and brain-stem audiometry has displaced psychogalvanic skin resistance audiometry use in most clinics. However, it may continue to have a significant place in the future, as one of a group of nonsubjective tests available for diagnosis of problem cases.

EVOKED RESPONSE (CORTICAL) AUDIOMETRY

Evoked response audiometry, or cortical audiometry, is a useful diagnostic tool, especially in infant testing. A number of unanswered questions remain, however, relative to reliability or validity.

Lowell, Lowell, and Goodhill (39) studied 129 infants with a median age of 12 months, in whom hearing loss was suspected. They were then retested at 6-month intervals until they were old enough to be tested by play-type audiometric procedures.

EQUIPMENT

Silver disc electrodes (Grass) were taped on the vertex (active), referred to each mastoid (reference), with a high midfrontal ground (32). Two channels were recorded simultaneously, linking the vertex electrode to the right mastoid and the vertex electrode to the left mastoid. The two mastoids were not linked together to form a single reference. The output from the electrical activity generated went to two Tektronix 122 preamplifiers in tandem with a frequency response setting of 2–250 Hz. The infant's electroencephalogram was recorded on a 4-channel, FM tape recorder (Electro-Medi-Dyne) and analyzed by computer (Mnemotron Computer of Average Transients, Model 400). An X-Y plotter (Houston Instrument Model 200) was utilized to read out the resultant wave-forms.

PROCEDURES

The test was conducted by making 60 presentations of each stimulus during each run. The auditory stimulus consisted of a 500-Hz tone burst of 300 msec duration with a 10-msec rise and delay. The tone bursts were generated by an oscillator (Hewlett-Packard) passed through an amplifier (Scott) and an electronic switch and interval timer (Grason Stadler). The interstimulus rate was every 5 sec. The infants were either held on their mothers' laps or placed in an infant seat 2 feet from and directly in front of the room speaker. Testing was done with a speaker (Altec) or TDH-39 earphones mounted in MX/41 cushions. An attempt was made to gain information at both 500 Hz and 2000 Hz. Observations were made of the child's motor behavior, and testing was curtailed for brief periods when the child was overactive or fussy.

TESTING SEQUENCE

Initial presentation of the 500-Hz tone burst was begun at 50 dB hearing level and increased in 10-dB steps until an auditory evoked response was noted. Two presentations of each intensity level were included in each session. If a response was noted at 40 dB, subsequent stimulus presentations were decreased in 10-dB steps until the response disappeared and then increased in 10-dB increments until the pattern reappeared. The final decision as to the response threshold was determined only after all records for a session had been read out and latency of the predominant peaks was measured.

THRESHOLD RESPONSE

A threshold response was defined as the lowest intensity level at which at least one of four responses (two runs at each intensity level were obtained from the vertex to right mastoid and from the vertex to the left mastoid) conformed to the latency pattern of the responses at higher intensity levels. There were two presentations of 60 stimuli at each intensity level.

Each child was scheduled for two initial tests, a week apart. All families were contacted at 6-month intervals regarding a follow-up appointment for either a retest of evoked response audiometry or a play-type audiogram when the children exhibited signs of sufficient maturity.

LATENCY CHARACTERISTICS

Data were collected on the first prominent negative (N) and positive (P) waves, which are labeled as N_1 and P_2 components. Latencies for both right and left electroencephalogram channels and all intensities were pooled. The mean latency of N_1 was 192 msec, and the mean P_2 latency was 281 msec.

STUDY CONCLUSIONS

In this study group of children with clinical diagnosis of sensorineural hearing loss, the major etiologic factor was rubella; heredity, Rh incompatibility, and birth injuries were other etiologic factors. Conclusions from this study were as fol-

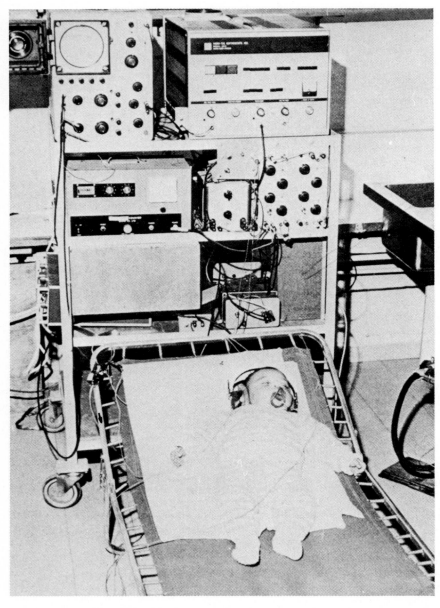

FIG. 6–37. Infant during a test. At rear, mobile cart with all the stimulus and response equipment. There is no Faraday cage or sound-proof room. The cart can be brought to any part of the hospital. (Sohmer H, Feinmesser M: Arch Oto-Rhino-Laryngol (Berlin) 206: 91–102, 1974)

lows: 1) Young children can be tested by evoked response audiometry without requiring sleep or sedation. 2) Correlations between evoked response audiometry testing and behavioral audiograms indicate good agreement. The 12-month tests correlated 0.93 with 500-Hz behavioral results.

ELECTROCOCHLEOGRAPHY

The need for more accurate auditory testing in infants and young children was responsible for the increased interest in human recordings of cochlear action potentials. In 1967 Sohmer and Feinmesser (49) pioneered in this work. In both animal and human studies, they proposed the use of noninvasive techniques with earlobe and scalp electrodes. In 1968 Portmann, Aran, and LeBert (43) advocated the use of invasive transtympanic-membrane surgical techniques for recordings from the cochlear promontory. In addition to the ear lobe and the middle-ear promontory techniques, a third approach has been advocated by Elberling (33) and Montandon and co-workers

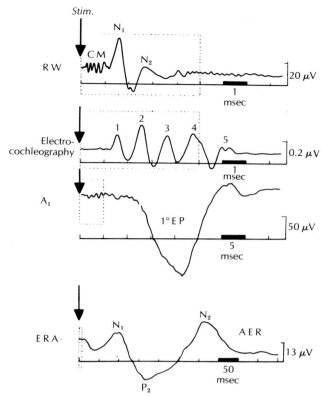

FIG. 6–38. Electrical responses of the auditory system, showing time relations between them. An electrode on or near the round window **(RW)** of the cochlea records cochlear microphonic potential **(CM)** and compound cochlear action potential **(N₁).** Ear lobe—scalp electrodes record five waves (electrocochleography). An electrode on primary auditory cortex **(A₁; cat,** computer average transients) records primary evoked potential (1° EP). Scalp electrode records, much later, the averaged auditory evoked response **(AER)** used in evoked response audiometry **(ERA).** (Sohmer H, Feinmesser M: Arch Oto-Rhino-Laryngol (Berlin) 206: 91–102, 1974)

(40), in which electrodes are placed in the external auditory canal.

Sohmer and Feinmesser (49) have compared the findings of nontraumatic ear lobe and scalp electrocochleography in a number of patients with unusual problems, including brain damage, mental retardation and retrocochlear hearing loss. Their technique is particularly useful in infants (Fig. 6–37). It does not require either a soundproof room or an electrically shielded room. The time relationships between various electrical responses of the auditory system are shown in Figure 6–38. A dramatic example of the value of this

kind of study is demonstrated in a patient with an acoustic neurinoma (Fig. 6–39).

These investigators have also reported the use of both cochlear and cortical audiometry in the same subject (50). Their comparisons of stimulus generation and response in the cochlear and cortical recordings are of great diagnostic significance (Figs. 6–40 to 6–43).

Elberling (33) studied the action potentials along the cochlear partition as recorded from the external auditory canal. Comparisons were made from human adult ears in both high-frequency and low-frequency hearing loss lesions (Fig. 6–44). He concludes that it is possible to examine the entire auditory nerve spectrum as a function of intensity in analysis of response distribution along the cochlear partition, as recorded from the human external auditory canal.

Simmons (47) compares three commonly used recording sites to obtain computer averaged N₁ responses from human subjects to click stimuli. The three recording sites were 1) dermal electrode; 2) subdermal electrode, both in the external auditory canal; and 3) a transtympanic electrode on the cochlear promontory. His studies show that the promontory electrodes were consistently more sensitive and yielded cleaner N₁ wave forms than did the other two sites. In considering the clinical use of N₁ averaging, he concluded that the advantages of the transtympanic method outweighed the risks (Fig. 6–45).

Montandon and colleagues (40) advocate the clinical feasibility of ear canal recordings in patients with various types of otologic problems, including unusual conductive hearing losses with no air–bone gap, and in cases with high frequency "notch" type hearing loss due to acoustic trauma.

M. Portmann has recently summarized a 10 year experience in over 2000 electrocochleography tests. They were carried out on 1.5% of all adults and 12% of children studied audiometrically. He reported a pediatric age distribution of 59% under age three, 10% between ages three and five, and 25% in children older than five years. Electrocochleogram (ECochG) findings appeared to be valuable in masking problems (phantom curves and congenital atresias) in very young children or in behavior problems. In 6% of cases, ECochG findings were considered indispensible because standard audiometry was impossible, i.e., in psychotic or autistic children, in cerebral palsy with severe motor disabilities or in children with associated defects, such as the deaf blind (41a).

BRAIN STEM AUDIOMETRY

Human brain-stem audiometry makes it possible to record electrical activity generated along the auditory pathway in its course from the cochlea to the cortex, using surface electrodes. The use of such "far-field" recording requires computer averaging of generated potentials, at a distance, out of the background electrical noise. According to Starr (52), 1000- to 2000-click trials presented 10/sec are required to resolve brain stem-components. He states: "It is possible to define a series of seven deflections in the first ten milliseconds following click signals. Their amplitudes are in the nanovolt range. Both the latency and amplitude of the components vary in an orderly manner with a signal intensity and can be detected to click signals close to threshold intensity."

An analysis of wave forms indicates a major degree of spatial auditory pathway localization. Thus, lesions can be localized from areas as far apart as the eighth nerve and the inferior colliculus.

In this respect, brain-stem audiometry offers a significant diagnostic advantage.

FIG. 6–39. Audiogram and electrocochleographic and evoked responses from 45-year-old subject with acoustic neurinoma. All responses on left side are normal while on right side there are no behavioral responses (audiogram) or evoked responses. However, the first electrocochleographic wave representing the compound cochlear action potential is present. This, too, contributes to the diagnosis of a retrocochlear lesion. (Sohmer H, Feinmesser M: Arch Oto-Rhino-Laryngol (Berlin) 206:91–102, 1974)

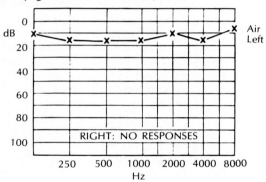

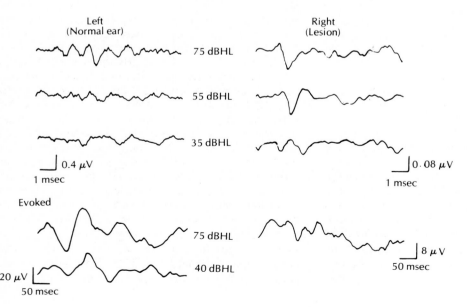

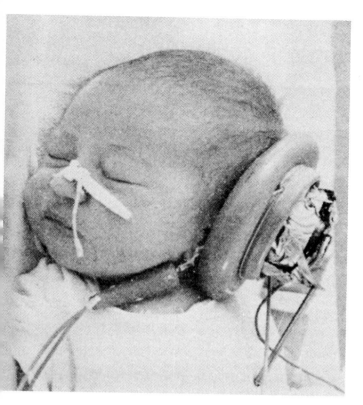

FIG. 6–40. An infant during recording. A clip electrode has been attached to the ear lobe and a disk electrode to the nose. The scalp vertex electrode is hidden from view. The earphone is seen applied to the left ear. (Lieberman A, Sohmer H, Szabo G: Developmental Med & Child Neurology 15(1):8–13, 1973)

FIG. 6–41. Block diagram showing stimulus-generating and response-recording systems. (Lieberman A, Sohmer H, Szabo G: Developmental Med Child Neurology 15(1):8–13, 1973)

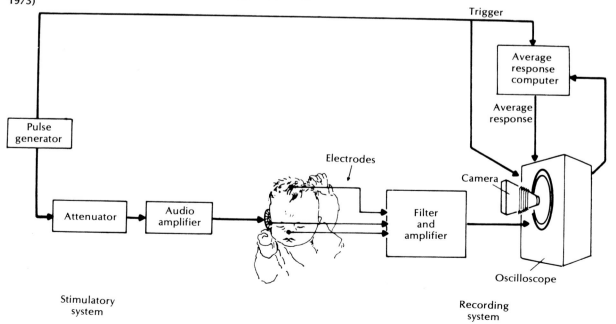

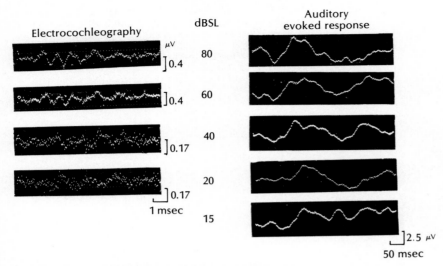

FIG. 6–42. Electrocochleographic and evoked response recordings in an awake, unsedated adult. Note that the first, third and fourth electrocochleographic waves are clearly present even in response to sound stimuli. 20 dB above the subjective threshold of this subject. (Sohmer H, Pratt H, Feinmesser M: Revue de Laryngologie 95, No 7–8, 1974)

FIG. 6–43. Electrocochleographic recordings in a two-year-old child sedated with trichloryl. Note at 0 dB HL, the presence of the first and fourth waves on the left and the fourth wave on the right. (Sohmer H, Pratt H, Feinmesser M: Revue de Laryngologie 95, No 7–8, 1974)

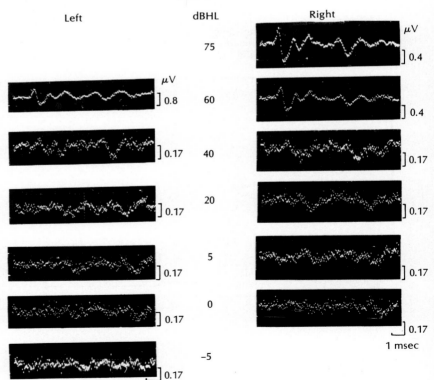

FIG. 6–44. Audiograms **(at top)** and whole nerve AP recordings **(at bottom)** in patients with severe cochlear hearing loss. Latencies of the different frequency bands are indicated in the recordings. **Left.** Patient with high-frequency hearing loss. **Right.** Patient with low-frequency hearing loss. **SPL,** sound pressure level. (Elberling C: Scand Audiol 3:13–19, 1974)

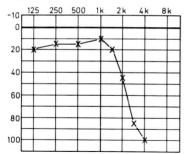

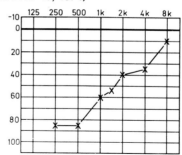

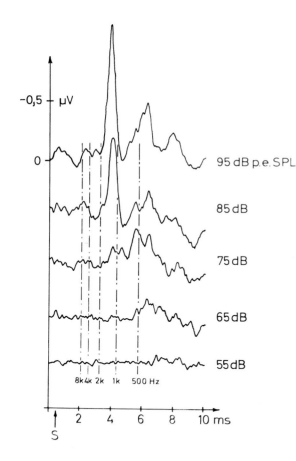

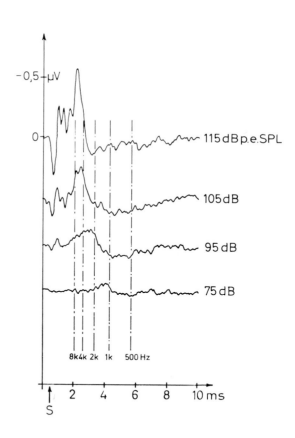

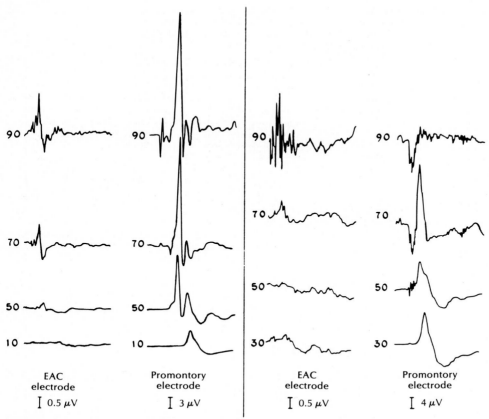

FIG. 6–45. Examples of ear canal and promontory N_1 averaged recordings. Set at **left** is the most sensitive EAC recording obtained in Simmons' study—a threshold of 10 dB (re: normal average perceptual threshold). Set at **right** is more typical. Promontory records are from same subjects but were obtained at different times. The numbers at left of each tracing indicate click stimulus intensity. Length of each tracing is 10 msec. (Simmons FB: Laryngoscope 85:1564–1581, 1975)

CONCLUSIONS

Evoked response audiometry techniques are necessary only in a small number of problem cases, such as infants and children with uncertain diagnoses. Electrical masking of small evoked responses is produced by movement artifacts and muscle action potentials. Such masking can be lessened by testing in sleep, under sedation, or under general anesthesia. In a recent review of various evoked response audiometric techniques, Davis summarizes some of the problems as follows:

For electric response audiometry of young children who require sedation, an indicator is desired that is more reliable than the slow vertex potential. There are four leading candidates: 1) The electrocochleogram (ECochG) is very reliable with a transtympanic electrode on the promontory, but this is a surgical procedure and requires a general anesthetic. 2) The early midbrain responses give similar information with external electrodes, but they are complex and low in voltage. 3) The muscle reflexes (sonomotor responses) are a crude indicator with high and variable thresholds and are not suited to precise audiometry. 4) The "middle" responses, perhaps cortical in origin, are good candidates, but they have not yet been adequately validated in the clinic. For the midbrain responses, and particularly for the ECochG, close synchronization of nerve impulses is essential. This requires a compromise with selectivity of frequency. High tone audiometry by electrocochleography and midbrain responses is satisfactory, but limitations are increasingly severe below 2 kHz, where each sound wave is a separate acoustic stimulus. Low-frequency tones stimulate the basal turn of the cochlea at relatively low sensation levels. This makes assessment of the apical portion of the cochlea very difficult, even with the midbrain "frequency-following response" (F.F.R).

In summary, a number of nonsubjective auditory test procedures have emerged from recent neurophysiological and otoaudiologic research efforts. Long-range evaluative studies will clarify the comparative values of psychogalvanic skin resistance audiometry, evoked response audiometry, electrocochleography, and brain stem audiometry, and other auditory electrophysiological techniques.

OBJECTIVE AUDIOMETRY

30. Berry H, Briant T, Winchester B: Electro-physiologic assessment of the lower portion of the auditory pathway in the human subject. J Otolaryngol 5:3–11, 1976

31. Davis H: Brainstem and other responses in electric response audiometry. Ann Otol Rhinol Laryngol 85:3–14, 1973

32. Davis H, Zerlin S: Acoustic relations of the human vertex potential. J Acoust Soc Am 39:101–116, 1966

33. Elberling C: Action potentials along the cochlear partition recorded from the ear canal in man. Scand Audiol 3:13–19, 1974

34. Elberling C, Salomon G: Cochlear microphonics recorded from the ear canal in man. Acta Otolaryngol (Stockh) 75:489–495, 1973

35. Gavilan C, Sanjuan J: Microphonic potential picked up from the human tympanic membrane. Ann Otol Rhinol Laryngol 73:101–109, 1964

36. Goodhill V, Rehman I, Brockman S: Objective skin resistance audiometry. Ann Otol Rhinol Laryngol 63:22–39, 1954

37. Jewett DL, Williston JS: Auditory evoked far fields averaged from the scalp of humans. Brain 94:681–696, 1971

38. Lev A, Sohmer H: Sources of averaged neural responses recorded in animal and human subjects during cochlear audiometry (electrocochleogram). Arch Klin Exp Ohr-Nas, Keilk Heilk 201:79–90, 1972

39. Lowell MO, Lowell BL, Goodhill V: Evoked response audiometry with infants: a longitudinal study. Audiol Hear Educ 1:32–37, 1975

40. Montandon PB, Megill ND, Peake WT et al.: Recording auditory nerve potentials as an office procedure. Ann Otol Rhinol Laryngol 84:2–10, 1975

41. Perlman HB, Case TJ: Electric phenomena of the cochlea in man. Arch Otolaryngol 34:710–718, 1941

41a. Portmann M: Electrocochleography. J Laryngol 91:665–677, 1977

42. Portmann M, Aran JM, LeBert G: Electrocochleogramme humain en dehors de toute intervention chirurgicale. Acta Otolaryngol (Stockh) 65:105–114, 1968

43. Portmann M, LeBert G, Aran JM: Potentiels cochleaires obtenus chez l'homme en dehors de toute

intervention chirurgicale. Note preliminaire. Rev Laryngol Otol Rhinol (Bord) 88:11, 1967

44. Ruben RJ: Cochlear potentials as a diagnostic test in deafness. In Graham AB (ed): Sensorineural Hearing Processes and Disorders. Boston, Little, Brown, 1967, pp 313–337

45. Ruben RJ, Knickerbocker GG, Sekula J et al.: Cochlear microphonics in man. Laryngoscope 69:665–671, 1959

46. Salomon G, Elberling C: Cochlear nerve potentials recorded from the ear canal in man. Acta Otolaryngol (Stockh) 71:319–325, 1971

47. Simmons PB: Human auditory nerve responses: a comparison of three commonly used recording sites. Laryngoscope 85:1564–1581, 1975

48. Simmons FB, Beatty DL: The significance of round window recorded cochlear potentials in hearing. Ann Otol Rhinol Laryngol 71:767–800, 1962

49. Sohmer H, Feinmesser M: Cochlear action potentials recorded from the external ear in man. Ann Otol Rhinol Laryngol 76:427–435, 1967

50. Sohmer H, Feinmesser M: Cochlear and cortical audiometry, conveniently recorded in the same subject. Isr J Med Sci 6:219–223, 1970

51. Sohmer H, Feinmesser M: Electrocochleography in clinical audiological diagnosis. Arch Otol Rhinol Laryngol 206:91–102, 1974

52. Starr A: Brain stem audiometry. West J Med 131–132, 1975

53. Wever EC, Bray CW: Auditory nerve impulses. Science 71:215, 1930

54. Yoshie N, Yamaura K: Cochlear microphonic responses to pure tones in man recorded by a nonsurgical method. Acta Otolaryngol (Stockh) [Suppl] 252:37–69, 1969

SUGGESTED READING

OBJECTIVE AUDIOMETRY

Beagley HA, Hutton JNT, Hayes R: Clinical electrocochleography. A review of 106 cases. J Laryngol 88:993–1000, 1974

Berlin C: New developments in evaluating central auditory mechanisms. Trans Am Otol Soc 168–176, 1976

Crowley DE, Davis H, Beagley HA: Survey of the clinical use of electrocochleography. Ann Otol Rhinol Laryngol 84:297–305, 1975

Davis H: Principles of electric response audiometry. Ann Otol Rhinol Laryngol [Suppl] 28:85: 1976

Davis H, Hersch SK: The audiometric utility of brain stem responses to low frequency sounds. Int Audiol 15:181–195, 1976

Douek E, Clarke GP: A single average crossed acoustic response. J Laryngol 90:1027–1032, 1976

Elberling C: Transitions in cochlear action potentials recorded from the ear canal in man. Scand Audiol 2:151–159, 1973

Galambos R: Electrophysiological measurement of human auditory function. In Tower DB (ed): Human Communication and Its Disorders, vol 3. New York, Raven Press, 1975

Hecox K, Squires N, Galambos R: Brainstem auditory evoked responses in man. I. Effect of stimulus rise—fall time and duration. J Acoust Soc Am 60:1187–1192, 1976

Hooper RE: Electrocochleography. Surg Forum 23: 1972

Leiberman A, Sohmer H, Szabo G: Cochlear audiometry (electrocochleography) during the neonatal period. Dev Med Child Neurol 15:8–13, 1973

Madsen PB, Pay GW: ERA without tears. Hearing Instruments 27(8):16–17, 1976

Mokotoff B, Schulman-Galambos C, Galambos R: Brain stem auditory evoked responses in children. Arch Otolaryngol 103:38–43, 1977

Montandon PB, Shepard NT, Peake WT et al.: Auditory nerve potentials from ear canals of patients with otologic problems. Ann Otol Rhinol Laryngol 84: 164–173, 1975

Moore EJ, Devgan DK: Questions and answers about electrocochleography (ECOG) and brain-stem evoked responses (BER). Audiol Hear Educ 59:42, 1976

Moore EJ: Recording the electrocochleographic (ECochG) response in humans: a reply to AC Coates [J Acoust Soc Am 56:708–711, 1974]. J Acoust Soc Am 59:1504–1505, 1976

Naunton RF, Zerlin S: Basis and some diagnostic implications of electrocochleography. Laryngoscope 86:475–482, 1976

Olson WO, Noffsinger D: Masking level differences for cochlear and brain stem lesions. Trans Am Otol Soc 82:155–160, 1976

Russ FM, Simmons FB: Five years of experience with electric response audiometry. J Speech Hear Res 17:184–193, 1974

Simmons FB: Electrocochleography. Ann Otol Rhinol Laryngol 83:312–313, 1974

Sohmer H, Feinmesser M, Lez A et al.: Routine use of cochlear audiometry in infants with uncertain diagnoses. Ann Otol Rhinol Laryngol 81:72–75, 1972

Sohmer H, Feinmesser M: Routine use of electrocochleography (cochlear audiometry) on human subjects. Audiology 12:167–173, 1973

Sohmer H, Feinmesser M, Szabo G: Electrocochleographic (auditory nerve and brain stem auditory nuclei) responses to sound stimuli in patients with brain damage. Electroencephalogr Clin Neurophysiol 34:761, 1973

ACOUSTIC IMPEDANCE TESTS

MARSHA R. SIMONS

The acoustic impedance technique provides an objective measurement relating to the function of the peripheral auditory mechanism. An electro-acoustic impedance bridge is used to 1) measure tympanic membrane mobility; 2) determine middle ear pressure; 3) identify eustachian tube function; 4) evaluate the continuity and compliance of the ossicular chain; 5) identify abnormal reflex decay; and 6) aid in identifying the presence of functional hearing loss.

This technique has the advantage of providing significant information without requiring direct patient response. Only passive participation is required. This is of critical importance in the evaluation of multi-handicapped children and other patients who do not respond consistently to conventional subjective hearing tests.

The acoustic impedance test battery includes measures of acoustic impedance (static compliance), tympanometry, and acoustic reflex threshold measurements. Although each portion of the test battery can provide significant information, their diagnostic capabilities are strengthened when results from all three procedures are viewed as a total evaluation.

DEFINITION OF ACOUSTIC IMPEDANCE

The term impedance may be defined as the immobility or resistance offered by a given system to the flow of energy. **Acoustic impedance** is the opposition or hindrance rendered to the passage of sound. Acoustic impedance measurement is expressed in acoustic ohms. **Acoustic compliance** is the reciprocal of acoustic impedance. It describes the mobility or springiness of the middle ear system and refers to the ease of sound transmission through the middle ear. Acoustic compliance is measured in equivalent cubic centimeters of volume.

Another term in use is **acoustic admittance** (7), which (like compliance) defines the ease of energy flow through or into a system. The unit of measurement is the millimho.

Clinically, electroacoustic impedance measurements may be classified as either static or dynamic.

The term static is intended to connote that measurement which is made in the resting state, while the term dynamic implies measurement of how function varies with changes in relative variables. Thus, compliance measured at the resting state will be called static compliance of the middle ear . . . and compliance measured under conditions of varying air pressures in the external canal would be a dynamic measure (11).

In the middle-ear mechanical system, it is the interrelationship between three factors—mass (inertial component), friction (resistive component), and stiffness (elastic component)—that produce the total complex of mechanical impedance at the lateral surface of the tympanic membrane. In the middle ear, mass consists of the three ossicles; friction is caused by the resistance supplied by the muscles and ligaments that dissipate energy within the transmission system. However, these two elements contribute very little influence to the impedance of the middle ear. The third element, stiffness, plays the most prominent role in middle ear impedance. The stiffness component is generated at the footplate of the stapes. Here a large resistive component must be overcome to cause displacement of the ossicular chain, which, in turn, causes displacement of the cochlear fluids and basilar membrane. Therefore, the *impedance of the middle ear system is stiffness-dominated.*

The relationship between these three elements can change when high-frequency probe tones are utilized. Most electroacoustic impedance bridges employ a 220-Hz probe tone, which lies well below the resonance frequency of the middle ear (about 2000 Hz). Above 600 Hz, deviations in the measurements begin to be observed. These deviations are due to the changes in elasticity and mass of the tympanic membrane and ossicles that are caused by the resonance phenomena. No additional diagnostic information of clinical significance appears to be obtained with higher probe-tone frequencies (1). For clinical applicability, a 220-Hz probe tone provides sufficient diagnostic information.

BASIC ACOUSTIC PREMISE

The measurement of acoustic impedance is based upon the principle that sound pressure level (SPL) is a function of closed-cavity volume. That is, for a specified probe tone of a determined intensity and frequency, the SPL will decrease as cavity size increases. If the difference between the intensity of the sound going into the external auditory canal and that reflected back from the tympanic membrane is measured, some inferences can be made regarding stiffness (or compliance) of the middle-ear system.

The cavity volume is altered with concomitant variations in SPL, when pressure changes are made in the external auditory meatus. The pressure and tone are introduced via the probe tip on the headset, which is hermetically inserted into the ear canal. The probe tip actually has three openings: 1) the pressure manometer; 2) a 220-Hz probe tone; and 3) a pickup microphone that receives sound waves reflected off the tympanic membrane.

An earphone is placed on the contralateral ear (Fig. 7–1), through which tones of varying frequency and intensity are presented (in addition to white noise and narrow bands of noise). A schematic view of the electroacoustic impedance bridge as it functions when the probe tip is sealed in the ear canal is presented in Figure 7–2.

Total impedance will be affected by the middle ear lesion that exists closest to the tympanic membrane. Since the lateral ossicle of the ossicular chain, the malleus, is actually part of the tympanic membrane, the malleal condition or the condition of any other portion of the ossicular chain will affect acoustic impedance measurements obtained at the tympanic membrane. This may present a diagnostic problem if two middle-ear lesions coexist, or if these is tympanic membrane disease (*e.g.*, perforation). One observes the lesion closest to the tympanic membrane.

A normal tympanic membrane and middle ear offer relatively low acoustic impedance, implying that appreciable energy is absorbed and transmitted through the middle ear. If a tympanic membrane is thickened or the middle ear contains fluid, the impedance will be increased, less energy will be absorbed, and transmission capabilities will be diminished. In general, if the impedance is higher than normal (*e.g.*, in stapes fixation), one may expect a decrease in the flexibility or compliance of the ossicular chain, an increase in its mass, and an increase in the friction or resistance during ossicular movement. Conversely, ossicular chain discontinuity would be expected to decrease acoustic impedance measurements at the tympanic membrane, since mass and friction (or resistance) would be decreased and compliance would be increased.

ACOUSTIC IMPEDANCE OR STATIC COMPLIANCE

The terms **acoustic impedance** and **static compliance** are usually interchanged and are the inverse of each other. However, it should be remembered that they do not truly measure the same conditions. To determine the acoustic impedance or the static compliance of the middle ear, two equivalent volume measures are taken with the tympanic membrane in two different states of compliance (**C1** and **C2**). The scales and formulas utilized determine total acoustic impedance (or static compliance) of the middle ear.

The initial volume measurement (C1) is made when the tympanic membrane is stiffened by a known air pressure (+200 mm H_2O), where the maximum possible sound is reflected back from the tympanic membrane. After determining the volume (in cubic centimeters) or impedance (in acoustic ohms) at maximum stiffness, the second volume measurement (C2), which is really an equivalent volume measurement, is made with the tympanic membrane at its most compliant state (*i.e.*, when air pressure in the middle ear is equivalent to that in the external auditory canal). Maximum compliance is determined by reducing the pressure from +200 mm and recording the pressure where the balance meter needle just begins to show an increase in impedance. It is here that the maximum amount of sound will be absorbed, thus allowing air pressure to exert no effect on the movement of the tympanic membrane.

These two measures have minimal significance individually because they include the volume of the external auditory canal. By subtracting the two volume measurements (C2 − C1) the "contamination factor" of the external auditory canal can be canceled out, and the resulting difference equals the static compliance of the middle ear.

FIG. 7–1. A. Acoustic impedance headset with probe inserted into right ear and earphone over left ear. **B.** Examiner performing acoustic impedance evaluation.

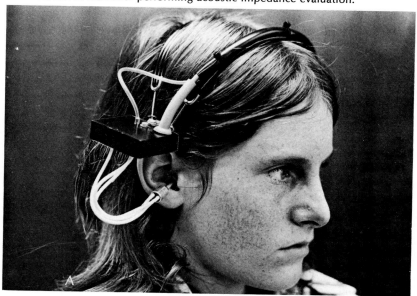

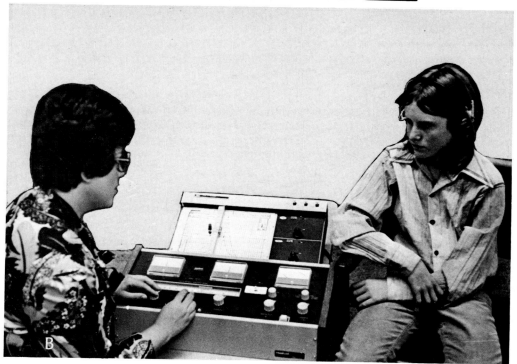

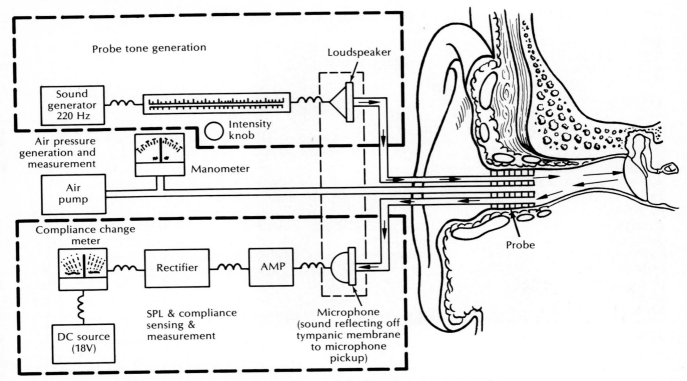

FIG. 7–2. Schematic view of the major functional parts of the impedance measurement system. **SPL,** sound pressure level.

This measurement can be obtained in acoustic ohms by reading the numbers on the "acoustic ohms scale" rather than the "cc scale," and performing the necessary computations (18).

CLINICAL APPLICATIONS OF STATIC COMPLIANCE

Range of Static Compliance

Static compliance contributes meager information to otologic and audiologic diagnosis, compared to the other portions of the impedance battery. This is primarily due to overlapping values of static compliance for various otologic lesions within the normal middle ear mechanism. In addition, middle-ear compliance is influenced by sex, age, and the condition of the tympanic membrane and middle ear. The most significant clinical use is in differentiating between ossicular chain fixation and ossicular chain discontinuity. For clinical utilization, static compliance should be considered abnormally low when the values are smaller than 0.8 cc and abnormally high when they are greater than 2.5 cc. Likewise, acoustic impedance should be considered abnormally low when the values

are smaller than 850 ohms and abnormally high when the values exceed 2750 acoustic ohms.

Diagnosis of disorders that is based solely on compliance or total impedance values is at best tenuous and should be made with *extreme* caution.

Physical Volume Test

Another use for static compliance is identification of tympanic membrane performations. In the presence of a tympanic membrane perforation or a patent ventilating tube (also referred to as the pressure-equalization tube), the probe tone circulates sound throughout the middle-ear space (not just the external auditory canal). Therefore, the volume measured will be quite large, often greater than 3–5 cc. This is compared to normal average findings of 0.06–1.8 cc (1.1 being average) for volume (25). If the ventilating tube is blocked, the volume will more closely resemble "average" volume.

The physical volume test can also be used to evaluate a middle-ear lesion in the presence of a tympanic membrane perforation. Prior to appearance of a middle-ear lesion, values of 4–5 cc will be measured on the physical volume test. If periodic rechecks indicate reduced test values, there would be indications of active growth of a middle-ear space-occupying lesion.

TYMPANOMETRY

TYMPANOMETRY PRINCIPLES AND TECHNIQUES

Tympanometry is a technique that assesses the mobility or compliance of the tympanic membrane during variations of air pressure in a hermetically sealed canal. Various "pressure-compliance" functions or tracings are obtained (tympanograms) each revealing a particular characteristic of the conductive portion of the peripheral auditory system. For diagnostic purposes (and in conjunction with routine pure-tone audiometry, otologic examination, and acoustic reflex measures), tympanometry can provide valuable information for identification of 1) tympanic membrane mobility; 2) middle-ear pressure; 3) tympanic membrane perforations; 4) patency of the pressure equalization tubes; and 5) eustachian tube function. Thus, stated differently, tympanometry comprises the methods and techniques for measuring, recording, and evaluating changes in acoustic impedance using systematic changes in air pressures.

The procedure for obtaining a tympanogram consists of introducing a specified positive pressure into the external auditory canal (usually equivalent to +200 mm H_2O) and subsequently decreasing the pressure to approximately −200 mm H_2O. As the pressure is varied, a certain range of movement will be observed graphically if the tympanic membrane is normal. The shape of the curve that is observed resembles a tepee. The notch, or the highest point of the curve, represents the point of maximum compliance of the tympanic membrane where air pressure in the middle ear equals the air pressure in the external auditory canal. This notch represents a decrease in the sound pressure level of the probe tone present in the sealed external canal. At the same point the patient experiences an increase in the loudness of the probe tone.

In cases with intact tympanic membranes and adequate eustachian tube function, maximum compliance will be shown on the tympanogram at atmospheric pressure (0 mm H_2O) or within approximately 100 mm of atmospheric pressure (Fig. 7–3). When the tympanic membrane is intact but the eustachian tube is functioning poorly, maximum compliance will be observed at negative air pressure values exceeding −100 mm H_2O. Although opinions vary concerning the normal range for maximum compliance, in our experience, pressures greater than ±100 mm H_2O are abnormal. Cases (especially pediatric) in which tympanometry consistently reveals maximum compliance outside the range of normal should be considered at risk for developing secretory otitis media (even without otoscopic visualization of fluid), and the patients should return for periodic otologic and acoustic impedance evaluations. The accuracy of tympanometric measurements of middle-ear pressure within 15 mm H_2O of actual pressure has been demonstrated (6).

The range of movement charted for a tympanogram, as stated previously, is from +200 mm H_2O to −200 mm H_2O (although the negative range can be extended to −600 mm H_2O). A tympanometric interpretation of mobility (or stiffness) can be estimated by comparing observed tympanic membrane movement to "normal" membrane movement within this established range. The otologist can also make statements regarding tympanic membrane mobility based on pneumatic otoscopy; however, the pressure range is considerably larger for the latter procedure (*i.e.*, pressure in excess of ±700 mm H_2O). Therefore, when tympanometry fails to demonstrate membrane mobility (within the established limits), this same conclusion may not be confirmed by pneumatic otoscopy because of the pressure differences employed to assess mobility.

Five basic tympanographic patterns have been assigned alphabetical classifications (10, 17). We prefer to employ operational definitions of these five tympanographic patterns, rather than the alphabetical classifications.

Normal Tympanogram

The normal tympanogram (type A) shows a well-defined maximum compliance at an air-pressure differential of 0 mm H_2O. This curve is most often seen in patients with normal hearing or with "pure" sensorineural hearing loss. In contrast, a normal tympanogram may also be observed in cases of stapes fixation (see Ch. 19, Otosclerosis). The fixed stapes of moderately advanced otosclerosis has a minimal effect on tympanic membrane mobility and varying changes in air pressure. Therefore, the resulting tympanogram for otosclerosis is either normal or shows a somewhat shallow notch, indicating a slight decrease in compliance.

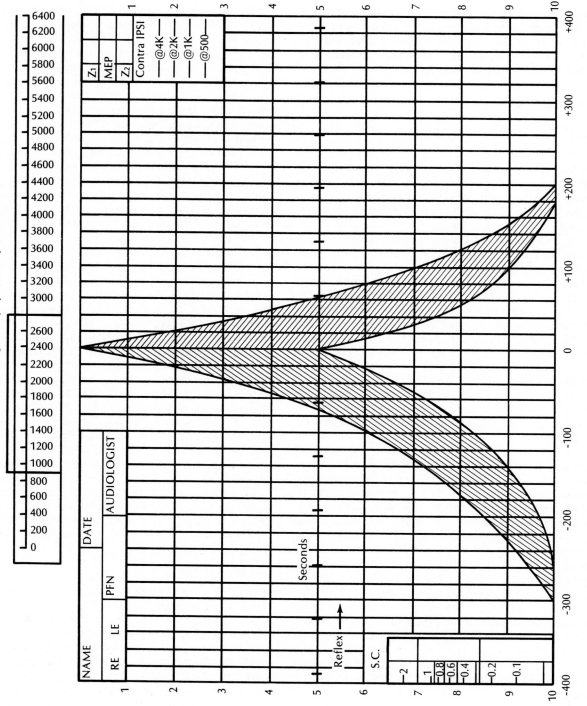

FIG. 7-3. Form for recording acoustic impedance results. Normal range for tympanometry is illustrated.

Therefore, when 1) otoscopic examination reveals a normal tympanic membrane, 2) a conductive hearing loss is present by audiometry, 3) the acoustic reflex is absent, and 4) an essentially normal tympanogram is obtained, these findings point to moderate stapedial fixation (Fig. 7–4).

Restricted Tympanogram

In advanced cases of otosclerosis, lateral fixation of the ossicular chain, tympanic membrane fibrosis, and middle ear tympanosclerosis, the restricted tympanogram (type As) is most often seen. This pressure-compliance function is characterized by normal middle ear pressure and limited compliance relative to normal mobility (Fig. 7–5).

Hypermobile Tympanogram

Large changes in relative compliance and small changes in air pressure will produce a hypermobile tympanogram (type Ad). It is noted in ossicular chain discontinuity or in partial atrophy of the tympanic membrane (large neomembrane). The tympanogram demonstrates a high, open notch, or one with undulations, depending upon the probe-tone frequency used. The significance of this curve is its representation of an extremely flaccid tympanic membrane (Fig. 7–6).

Flat Tympanogram

A flat (type B) tympanogram is characterized by little or no change in middle ear compliance when air pressure is varied in the external auditory canal. No well-defined maximum compliance is observed at any measureable air pressure. This curve is most commonly seen in secretory otitis media with adhesions. It is also noted in patients with: 1) tympanic membrane perforations; 2) congenital middle ear malformations; 3) patent tympanic ventilatory tubes; 4) total occlusion of the external auditory canal by epithelium, cerumen, or foreign body (Fig. 7–7).

Retracted Tympanogram

A well-defined compliance maximum occurring at negative pressures greater than −100 mm H_2O is seen in the retracted tympanogram (type C). This curve may or may not be related to the presence of middle-ear fluid (Fig. 7–8). This differs from the flat tympanogram in terms of tympanic membrane mobility. Persistence of an intact but retracted membrane suggests poor eustachian tube function.

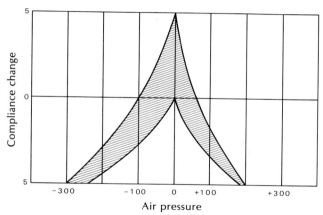

FIG. 7–4. Normal range for tympanometry, type A **(shaded area),** as represented on standard reporting form.

FIG. 7–5. Restricted tympanogram, type As **(shaded area).**

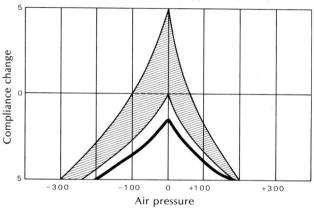

FIG. 7–6. Hypermobile tympanogram, type Ad **(shaded area).**

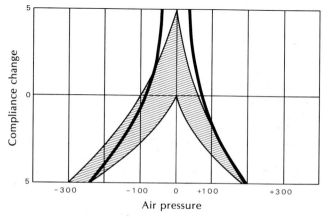

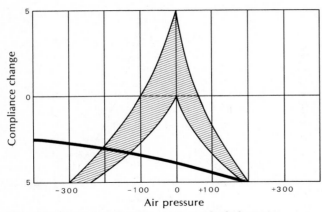

FIG. 7–7. Flat tympanogram, type B **(shaded area).**

FIG. 7–8. Retracted tympanogram, type C **(shaded area).**

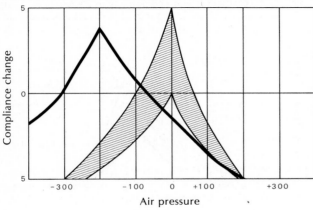

CLINICAL APPLICATIONS OF TYMPANOMETRY

Eustachian Tube Function

Acoustic impedance evaluation may also include assessment of eustachian tube function. Various clinical techniques have been designed for determination of eustachian tube physiology. The measurements can be made either when the tympanic membrane is intact or when there is a perforation in the membrane.

When the tympanic membrane is intact, tubal function can be assessed during tympanometry, by noting the middle-ear pressure at maximum compliance. If middle-ear pressure lies within the range of ± 100 mm H_2O, normal eustachian tube function can indirectly be assumed. Another procedure involves obtaining middle-ear pressure at maximum compliance and then immediately re-evaluating the pressure at maximum compliance after the **Toynbee swallow** (*i.e.*, while holding the nose and swallowing with the jaw closed). There should be an increase in negative pressure after the Toynbee swallow technique if the eustachian tube is functioning normally.

Tubal function testing can also be performed in most patients with tympanic membrane perforations. The testing techniques are included as part of the preoperative examination battery (together with audiometry, otomicroscopy, and x-ray).

Initially, positive pressure is introduced until the eustachian tube spontaneously opens (usually between 280 and 350 mm H_2O). In many cases of tympanic membrane perforation, it is possible to obtain a hermetic seal and create the necessary positive or negative pressure in the external auditory canal since the eustachian tube is normally closed. The patient is instructed not to swallow or in any way open the eustachian tube until requested. If the tube does not open when as much as +400 mm H_2O is introduced, it is indicative of poor tubal function. (The initial addition of positive pressure may also help to clear mucus or other matter that may be partially obstructing the eustachian tube.)

Another means for assessing eustachian tube function in patients with tympanic membrane perforation is to reduce the pressure in the external auditory canal and middle ear to −200 mm H_2O. The patient then attempts to open the eustachian tube, thereby causing equalization of the air pressure between the middle ear and nasopharynx, by swallowing, yawning, etc. It has been suggested that four to six swallows (mouth closed) should be enough to reduce the pressure back to between −50 mm H_2O and 0 mm H_2O (8, 25). Eustachian tube function has been quantified as follows:

Good Eustachian Tube Function. Patient can reduce air pressure to −100 mm H_2O or better.

Fair Tube Function. Patient can reduce air pressure between −200 and −100 mm H_2O.

Poor Tube Function. Patient is unable to reduce pressure with four swallows (25).

The Patulous (Hyperpatent) Eustachian Tube

The major complaint of patients with hyperpatent eustachian tubes is autophony and hearing their own breathing. During tympanometry, the tympanic membrane moves inward, upon inspiration, with mouth closed (increase in compliance) and moves outward upon expiration (decrease in compliance). Movement of the tympanic membrane is diminished with open-mouth breathing and is stilled when breathing momentarily ceases. Large excursions with nasal breathing can be observed at maximum compliance on the impedance bridge and recorded.

Middle-Ear Lesions

Tympanometry is of particular value when a middle-ear or conductive lesion exists with no audiometric evidence of hearing loss, especially in secretory otitis media when no meniscus line or air bubble is visualized on otoscopy.

Postoperative Evaluation of the Middle Ear

Tympanometry can be used to provide objective data on middle-ear function recovery in various surgical procedures. Tympanometry can also help to clarify reasons for postoperative hearing loss following an otherwise technically successful stapedectomy or tympanoplasty.

Tympanometry as a Screening Device

The use of tympanometry as a screening device for detection of middle-ear pathology will be elaborated upon in the section Acoustic Impedance Measurements as a Screening Technique.

THE ACOUSTIC REFLEX

BASIC MECHANISM OF ACOUSTIC REFLEX

The third portion of the acoustic impedance test battery is the acoustic reflex test. The term **acoustic reflex** refers to the contraction of the stapedial muscle in response to stimulation by sound of sufficient intensity. In the individual with normal hearing, the acoustic reflex will be observed following pure tone signals presented between 70–100 dB hearing level (median value, 82.2 dB), and approximately 65 dB hearing level with white noise as a stimulus (9, 19).

The acoustic reflex is determined by monitoring changes in acoustic impedance measurements in response to a loud sound introduced into either ear. The stapedius muscle will contract bilaterally, regardless of which ear is stimulated. Contraction of the stapedius muscle moves the ossicular chain, and thus causes tympanic membrane stiffening, thereby increasing middle ear mechanism impedance. Sound transmitted to the cochlea is attenuated about 10 dB.

The reflex in the ear under evaluation will respond in a manner that is dependent upon the nature of the lesion. If significant impairment exists in the afferent portion of the reflex arc to the pons, stapedial contraction will either be al-

tered or absent. The ear under evaluation, in this case, is the acoustically stimulated ear, and not the probe ear. However, when information is desired regarding ossicular chain integrity or seventh nerve function (the efferent portion of the reflex arc), the probe ear is the ear under evaluation (16). The level at which the acoustic reflex is elicited is recorded on the stimulus ear, although it is observed in the ear with the probe.

The acoustic reflex may be absent (when the contralateral ear is the stimulus ear) when there is 1) a conductive lesion in the probe ear, which prevents ossicular mobility (ipsilateral ear); 2) a loss greater than 80 dB in the stimulus ear (contralateral); 3) damage to the eighth nerve in the stimulus ear (contralateral); 4) paralysis of the seventh nerve (suprastapedial) in the probe ear (ipsilateral); or 5) an absent stapedius muscle in the probe ear (ipsilateral).

The typical impedance results corresponding to different types of disorders are given in Table 7–1.

CLINICAL APPLICATIONS OF ACOUSTIC REFLEX THRESHOLDS

UNILATERAL HEARING LOSS AND ACOUSTIC REFLEX THRESHOLDS

The acoustic reflex is of special diagnostic significance in the identification of unilateral hearing losses, where the accuracy of masking for bone conduction may be questionable. Most often, when the unilateral conductive loss exceeds 30 dB, absent acoustic reflexes occur bilaterally (Fig. 7–9). In other types of unilateral hearing loss, however, the acoustic reflex is generally not absent bilaterally (Fig. 7–10).

The ear with unilateral sensorineural hearing loss will usually show positive acoustic reflexes bilaterally, provided the sensorineural loss does not exceed 80 dB (in the stimulus ear) (Fig. 7–10). If the sensorineural hearing loss is less than 60 dB, there is a 90% chance of eliciting a positive acoustic reflex (Fig. 7–11). As the degree of sensorineural involvement increases, the likelihood of observing a positive reflex decreases. There is a 50% chance of eliciting a positive reflex (when threshold in the stimulus ear is at 85 dB hearing level) and only a 5–10% chance when threshold is at 100 dB hearing level (15).

A unilateral sensorineural anacusic ear, with a contralateral normal ear, will reveal absence of acoustic reflex when the anacusic ear is the stimulus ear and a positive acoustic reflex when the normal ear is the stimulus ear (Fig. 7–12).

TABLE 7-1. Typical Impedance Findings for Common Clinical Diagnosis

Clinical diagnosis	Tympanometry	Tympanogram	Contralateral acoustic reflex	Total acoustic impedance
Bilateral normal hearing	Normal	(tympanogram)	Present	Normal range
Bilateral SNHL (mild to moderate)	Normal	(tympanogram)	Present	Normal range
Unilateral SNHL (mild to moderate)	Normal	(tympanogram)	Present	Normal range
Bilateral SNHL (severe)	Normal	(tympanogram)	Absent	Normal range
Otosclerosis	Normal or restricted	(tympanogram)	Absent	Normal range or high
Lateral ossicular fixation (fixed malleus, incus)	Restricted	(tympanogram)	Absent	High range
Stapedial crural discontinuity	Hypermobile	(tympanogram)	Present	Low range
Lateral ossicular discontinuity (incus necrosis)	Hypermobile	(tympanogram)	Absent	Low range
Otitis media—secretory, serous (SOM)	Retracted	(tympanogram)	Present at elevated levels or absent	High range
Secretory (glue)	Flat or retracted	(tympanogram)	Absent	High range
Adhesive	Flat or retracted	(tympanogram)	Absent	High range
TM perforation or patent PEV tube	Rapid pressure leak or flat	(tympanogram)	CNT* or absent	CNT* or high range
Impacted cerumen	Flat	(tympanogram)	Present or absent	CNT*
Congenital anomalies	Varies depending upon pathology		May be present or absent	Varies, depending upon pathology
Eustachian tube occlusion	Variable—generally retracted	(tympanogram)	Present at elevated levels or absent	Low range or normal range
Eustachian tube hyperpatent	Hypermobile	(tympanogram)	Present	Generally low range; may vary with respiration

*CNT = could not test.

FIG. 7–9. Typical contralateral acoustic reflex findings in unilateral conductive hearing loss ≧ 30 dB. **Shaded area,** reflex absent from monitor (probe) ear. **Clear area,** reflex present in monitor ear.

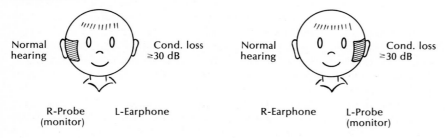

Normal hearing — Cond. loss ≥30 dB
R-Probe (monitor)   L-Earphone

Normal hearing — Cond. loss ≥30 dB
R-Earphone   L-Probe (monitor)

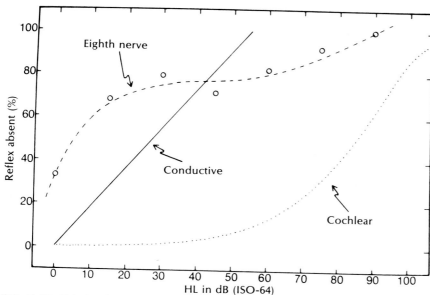

FIG. 7–10. Relation between degree of hearing loss and likelihood of reflex absence in conductive, cochlear, and eighth nerve lesions. ISO–64 = International Standards Organization, 1964. (Jerger J *et al.*: Arch Otolaryngol 99:409–413, 1974)

FIG. 7–11. Typical contralateral acoustic reflex findings with unilateral SNHL < 60 dB. **Shaded area,** reflex absent from monitor (probe) ear; **clear area,** reflex present in monitor ear.

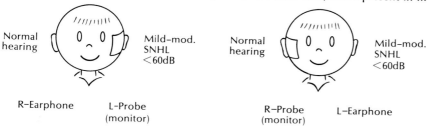

FIG. 7–12. Typical contralateral acoustic reflex findings in unilateral SNHL > 80 dB. **Shaded area,** reflex absent from monitor ear; **clear area,** reflex present in monitor ear.

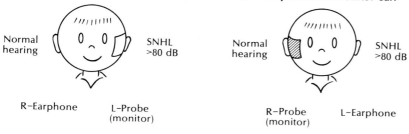

CONDUCTIVE HEARING LOSS AND THE ACOUSTIC REFLEX THRESHOLD

In bilateral conductive hearing loss, the acoustic reflex will be absent bilaterally, since the presence of a lesion in each ear prevents the probe ear from responding to compliance change when the contralateral ear is acoustically stimulated. The presence of an air–bone gap (probe ear) as small as 5 dB is sufficient to obscure the acoustic reflex 50% of the time (12). The acoustic reflex test is a sensitive indicator of most conductive lesions (Fig. 7–13).

THE ACOUSTIC REFLEX AND ABNORMAL LOUDNESS GROWTH

The acoustic reflex has further diagnostic significance as an indicator of cochlear disorders. In sensorineural hearing loss, the presence of an acoustic reflex may be demonstrated at a sensation level less than 60 dB above the auditory pure-tone threshold. This relationship has been attributed to the phenomenon of abnormal loudness growth (usually referred to as recruitment). Regardless of such speculation, it is adequate to consider the lesions as cochlear in location.

THE DIFFERENTIAL LOUDNESS SUMMATION TEST (DLST) OR TEST OF SENSITIVITY FOR PREDICTING ACOUSTIC REFLEX (SPAR)

A recent procedure was reported for calculation of air conduction threshold levels from stapedial reflex measurements (21). A follow-up study was conducted (13) in an attempt to predict the degree of sensorineural hearing loss through the relationship between acoustic reflex thresholds for pure tones and broad-band noise. In the normal ear, the acoustic reflex for broad-band white noise is elicited at a level about 25 dB softer than for

FIG. 7–13. Absence of reflex findings as functions of air-bone gaps in 154 patients with unilateral conductive hearing losses. **Triangle,** sound in good ear; **circle,** sound in bad ear. (Jerger J et al.: Arch Otolaryngol 99:409–413, 1974)

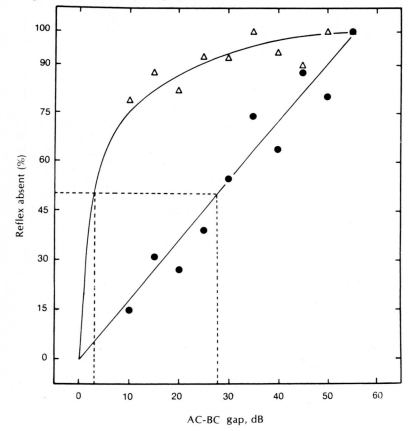

pure tones within the band. It is known that in an ear with sensorineural hearing loss, this difference will be diminished.

In addition to prediction of degree of loss, it is believed that audiometric configuration (or slope) can be predicted by comparing low-pass and high-pass noise bands. It was found that the prediction (predicting audiometric levels from these acoustic reflex threshold relationships) was seriously incorrect in 4% of the cases, moderately incorrect in 36%, and insignificantly different from actual findings in 60% of the patients tested.

If it is assumed that loudness is mediated at the level of the cortex and is a psychophysical correlate requiring subjective interpretation by the patient, then the premise that hearing loss may be predicted on the basis of acoustic reflex thresholds should be viewed as a research problem. Before it is utilized as a routine clinical procedure, the SPAR test requires further clinical research.

ACOUSTIC REFLEX AND EIGHTH NERVE DISORDERS

A number of recent studies have appeared on the use of the acoustic reflex in helping to identify retrocochlear lesions (2, 14). Patients with surgically confirmed retrocochlear lesions either had 1) absent acoustic reflexes, 2) elevated acoustic reflex thresholds, or 3) abnormal reflex decay (all findings in stimulus ear). The criteria established for the presence of *abnormal* reflex decay are 1) presentation of stimulus in the contralateral ear at 10 dB sensation level (in regard to acoustic reflex threshold) at 500 and 1000 Hz; and 2) diminution of amplitude of the reflex by half its original size within 10 sec of tonal stimulation (Fig. 7–14).

When acoustic reflex findings for these patients are compared to conventional tests for site-of-lesion determination (*e.g.,* Bekesy tracings, tone decay results, and performance-intensity function

for phonetically balanced [PB] words), acoustic reflex findings are more diagnostically sensitive. In addition, it is hypothesized that the relative incidences of the various acoustic reflex findings accompanying acoustic tumors will be closely related to the stage at which the tumor is detected (*i.e.,* more significant findings with further progression of the disease).

It should be remembered that measurement of acoustic reflex thresholds at 4 kHz and reflex decay at 2 kHz and 4 kHz does not reveal clinically significant information (24).

ACOUSTIC REFLEX AND SEVENTH NERVE LESIONS

If the acoustic reflex is present (by contralateral stimulation) in the presence of facial paralysis, with no accompanying hearing loss, the site of lesion is probably suprastapedial.

Regular monitoring of the acoustic reflex is a valuable technique in the management of VII nerve paralysis (see Ch. 28, Seventh Nerve Diagnostic Techniques).

IPSILATERAL ACOUSTIC REFLEX MEASUREMENTS

Ipsilateral reflex testing is currently under investigation. The **ipsilateral** technique is the presentation of the stimulus via the probe ear rather than the contralateral ear. For example, if one is trying to assess seventh nerve function in the stimulus ear and there is a conductive hearing loss in the probe ear, the reflex would be obscured by contralateral stimulation. Use of ipsilateral stimulation bypasses the conductive mechanism and the crossed acoustic pathways and allows one to assess ipsilateral afferent and efferent pathways (Fig. 7–15).

Another important diagnostic value of ipsilateral reflex testing is identification of patients with

FIG. 7–14. A. Ten-second stimulation with no evidence of decay. **B.** Ten-second stimulation with half-life decay of acoustic reflex.

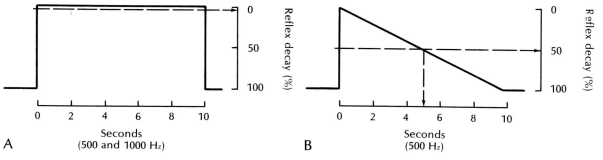

A — Seconds (500 and 1000 Hz)

B — Seconds (500 Hz)

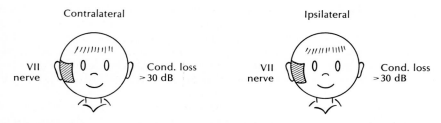

Contralateral   Ipsilateral

VII   Cond. loss   VII   Cond. loss
nerve   > 30 dB   nerve   > 30 dB

R-Probe (monitor)   L-Earphone (stimulus) R-Probe (stimulus)   L-Earphone

FIG. 7–15. Contralateral versus ipsilateral stimuli in patient with VII nerve lesion right ear, and conductive hearing loss > 30 dB left ear. With contralateral stimuli alone, failure to elicit an acoustic reflex could have reflected only the conductive hearing loss in left ear. However, absence of acoustic reflex with ipsilateral stimulation in right ear indicates tonotopic right VII nerve lesion site. **Shaded area,** reflex absent; **clear area,** reflex present.

FIG. 7–16. Ipsilateral versus contralateral stimulation in patient with left brain-stem lesion. **Shaded area,** reflex absent; **clear area,** reflex present.

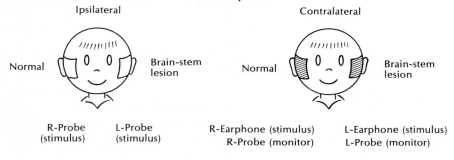

Ipsilateral   Contralateral

Normal   Brain-stem   Normal   Brain-stem
                       lesion   lesion

R-Probe   L-Probe   R-Earphone (stimulus)   L-Earphone (stimulus)
(stimulus)   (stimulus)   R-Probe (monitor)   L-Probe (monitor)

brain-stem lesions. If the stimulated ear is ipsilateral to the lesion, the reflex may be obscured with contralateral stimulation. This occurs because brain-stem lesions usually interrupt the crossed acoustic pathways, thus obscuring contralaterally measured reflexes. In contrast, ipsilateral stimulation will demonstrate the presence of the acoustic reflex (Fig. 7–16). Further studies of these observations will expedite neuro-audiologic diagnosis.

The comparative use of contralateral versus ipsilateral stimulation in oto-audiological diagnosis is presented in Table 7–2.

PEDIATRIC IMPEDANCE EVALUATION

Impedance has become an important diagnostic tool in the auditory assessment of children. It provides valid information about the peripheral auditory mechanism without requiring any active co-operation by the patient. There is virtually no difficulty in obtaining a hermetic seal, and most children will cooperate, once they understand that the procedure is not painful. The children who tend to be the most resistant are those with multiple handicaps or those who have had an unpleasant experience in a medical environment. The two most common difficulties encountered in obtaining impedance information in the pediatric population are the following:

1. Vocalization (*e.g.,* crying, talking), which causes a spontaneous contraction of the stapedius muscle, randomly alters tympanic membrane compliance, rendering impedance measurements impossible.
2. Extraneous movements of the subject, which also create compliance changes, confound test results.

It then becomes the task of the audiologist to attempt, frequently but briefly, to distract and

TABLE 7-2. Contrast Between Contralateral and Ipsilateral Acoustic Reflex Findings for Various Clinical Diagnoses

Clinical diagnosis		Contralateral stimulation		Ipsilateral stimulation	
Right ear	Left ear	Stim. RE	Stim. LE	Stim. RE	Stim. LE
Normal	Normal	+	+	+	+
SNHL with thresholds better than 85 dB hearing level	Normal	+	+	+	+
Profound SNHL with 85 dB or poorer hearing level	Normal	−	+	−	+
Bilateral SNHL with thresholds of 85 dB or poorer		−	−	−	−
Conductive hearing loss 30 dB or poorer	Normal	−	−	−	+
Bilateral conductive hearing loss with thresholds of 30 dB or poorer		−	−	−	−
VII nerve lesion	Normal	+	−	−	+
VIII nerve lesion	Normal	−	+	−	+
Low brain-stem lesion*	Normal	−	+	+	+
High brain-stem lesion†		−	−	+	+
Cortical (temporal) lesion		+	+	+	+

*Lesion in the area between the medial superior olivary complex and inferior colliculus.

†Lesion in the area between the inferior colliculus and the cortex.

Plus sign, present.

Minus sign, absent.

interest the child while the test is being performed. Several successful distraction techniques (23) have been reported by a number of authorities. Despite these pitfalls, the results of acoustic impedance evaluation are quite reliable and relatively simple to obtain.

ACOUSTIC IMPEDANCE MEASUREMENTS AS A SCREENING TECHNIQUE

The goal of hearing-screening programs, as defined by the National Conference on Identification Audiometry, is to "locate children who have even minimal hearing problems so they can be referred for medical treatment of active ear pathology discovered to be present, so that remedial educational procedures can be instituted at the earliest possible date. . . ." (22). Present pure-tone screening techniques will be effective in identifying children with moderate to severe hearing loss. However, since active middle-ear disease can exist without significant hearing loss, pure-tone audiometry alone fails to identify substantial populations of pediatric secretory otitis media.

The most common cause of hearing disorders in young school-age children is secretory otitis media. In one study (4), 50% of subjects (408 ears) with this disorder would have passed a 25 dB screening level, the level set by the American National Standards Institute in 1969. In another study (5), the average hearing loss discovered in secretory otitis media was 14 dB, and less than 50% of middle-ear disorders were detected by pure-tone screening methods. A child having a 15-dB hearing loss resulting from continuous middle-ear problems may be delayed in language skills, as compared to the child with normal hearing and without middle-ear problems (3). In classes for children with severely delayed language development, a significant incidence of previous middle-ear infections has been reported among the children. In addition, untreated middle-ear disease can lead to permanent hearing loss or can be life-threatening.

Acoustic impedance testing is an effective screening measure because it is objective, has a high accuracy in detecting middle-ear fluid, and is not affected by background noise. Reports have shown a 93% overall agreement between impedance screening and otoscopy (20).

Clinical use of acoustic impedance measurements must be considered along with the general diagnostic approach (medical history, physical examination, radiography, and audiometry). No single portion of the impedance test battery is sufficient for definitive conclusion. The total impedance test battery should be used for maximum diagnostic interpretation of the acoustic impedance test results.

REFERENCES

1. Alberti PW, Jerger J: Probe tone frequency and the diagnostic value of tympanometry. Arch Otolaryngol 99:206–210, 1974

2. Anderson H, Barr B, Wedenberg E: Early diagnosis of eighth nerve tumors by acoustic reflex tests. Acta Otolaryngol (Stockh) [Suppl] 263:232, 1970

3. Brooks D: Impedance measurements in screening for auditory disorders in children. Hearing instruments 36:20–21, 1974

4. Cohen D, Sade J: Hearing on secretory otitis media. Can J Otolaryngol 1:27, 1972

5. Eagles E: Selected findings from the Pittsburgh study. Trans Am Acad Ophthalmol Otolarngol 76:343, 1972

6. Elichar I, Sando I, Northern J: Measurements of middle ear pressure in guinea pigs. Arch Otolaryngol 99:172–176, 1974

7. Feldman A, Wilbur L: Acoustic Impedance and Admittance—Measurement of Middle Ear Function. Baltimore, Williams & Wilkins, 1976

8. Holmquist J: Eustachian tube function in diseased ears—assessment and clinical application. Eye, Ear, Nose, Throat Monthly 52:398–403, 1973

9. Jepson O: Middle ear muscle reflexes in man. In Jerger J (ed): Modern Developments in Audiology. New York, Academic Press, 1963

10. Jerger J: Clinical experience with impedance audiometry. Arch Otolaryngol 92:311–324, 1970.

11. Jerger J: Suggested nomenclature for impedance audiometry. Arch Otolaryngol 96:1–3, 1972

12. Jerger J, Anthony L, Jerger S et al.: Studies in impedance audiometry. III. Middle ear disorders. Arch Otolaryngol 99:165–171, 1974

13. Jerger J, Burney P, Maulden L et al.: Predicting hearing loss from the acoustic reflex. J Speech Hear Dis 39:11–22, 1974

14. Jerger J, Harford E, Clemis J et al.: The acoustic reflex in eighth nerve disorders. Arch Otolaryngol 99:409–413, 1974

15. Jerger J, Jerger S, Maulden L: Studies in impedance audiometry. I. Normal and S–N ears. Arch Otolaryngol 96:513–523, 1972

16. Klockhoff I: Middle ear muscle reflexes in man: a clinical experimental study with special reference to diagnostic problems in hearing impairments. Acta Otolaryngol (Stockh) [Suppl] 164: 1961

17. Liden G, Pederson JL, BJorkman G: Tympanometry. Arch Otolaryngol 92:248–254, 1970

18. Lilly DJ: Acoustic impedance at the tympanic membrane. In Katz J (ed): Handbook of Clinical Audiology. Baltimore, Williams & Wilkins, 1972

19. McCandless G, Thomas GK: Impedance audiometry as a screening procedure for middle ear disease. Trans Am Acad Ophthalmol Otolaryngol 78:98–102, 1974

20. Metz O: Threshold of reflex contraction of muscles of the middle ear in recruitment of loudness. Acta Otolaryngol (Stockh) 55:636–643, 1952

21. National Conference on Identification Audiometry. Baltimore, MD, 1966

22. Niemeyer W, Sesterhenn G: Calculating the hearing thresholds from the stapedius reflex thresholds for different sound stimuli. J Audiol Commun 11:84, 1972

23. Northern J, Downs M: Hearing in Children. Baltimore, Williams & Wilkins, 1974

24. Olsen W: Acoustic reflex and reflex decay. Arch Otolaryngol 101:622–625, 1975

25. Rock I: Practical otologic applications and considerations in impedance audiometry. Impedance Newsletter, American Electromedics, Vol 3, Dec 1974

There are a number of diagnostic tests that are helpful in the determination of the site of lesion in auditory disorders. One group of tests comprises the conductive loss battery, utilized to measure cochlear reserve in presumptive conductive hearing loss. A second group, referred to as the sensorineural battery, helps to differentiate between conductive, cochlear, retrocochlear, and central auditory nervous system lesions. The tests may also confirm or refute normal audiometric findings in the presence of abnormal symptoms.

The discussion of these tests will be limited to their applicability to the adult population, as there are two basic problems inherent in applying these tests to the pediatric population:

1. The duration of attention span required to complete these tests exceeds that expected of the typical young child.
2. Children (as a group) find the necessary sophisticated judgments difficult to make—*e.g.*, determining "equal" loudness levels (as in the loudness-balancing test); deciding when a tone is no longer present (as in the tone-decay test); determining barely audible from barely inaudible (as in the Bekesy test); making finite figure-ground distinctions (as in the SISI test); and others.

Although claims have been made that these tests can be used routinely with young children, our experience with a large pediatric practice has shown that only a limited number of youngsters can accurately perform the necessary tasks without requiring numerous clinic visits and extensive professional time.

Although problems exist in employing these special test batteries for diagnostic evaluation of young children, they *should* be attempted when deemed necessary. However, they should not be considered as routine diagnostic procedures in the pediatric population.

Acoustic impedance measurement is the one procedure applicable both to adults and children, since no active patient participation is involved in obtaining meaningful diagnostic information.

We strongly recommend that acoustic impedance measurements be part of the basic audiometric test battery performed on each patient (adult or child). (For the diagnostic implications of the impedance test, see Chapter 7, Acoustic Impedance Tests.)

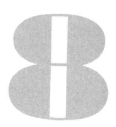

CONDUCTIVE LOSS AND SENSORINEURAL TEST BATTERIES

H. PATRICIA HEFFERNAN, MARSHA R. SIMONS

CONDUCTIVE-LOSS-TEST BATTERY

The majority of patients with conductive hearing loss are adequately identified by conventional mastoid bone conduction (MBC) tests. However, some patients exhibit small audiometric air–bone gaps in the low frequencies (usually 250 and 500 Hz) and/or negative Rinne tuning-fork results, which may be the only diagnostic clues pointing to a conductive disorder, such as in incus necrosis, or ossicular fixation (see Ch. 5, Hearing Loss and Deafness). In these cases the conductive component (tested by MBC) can be obscured. For example, in otosclerosis, MBC can be depressed in the high frequencies because of the relative perilymph immobility caused by stapedial fixation, known as the **Carhart notch** (4). After operation, as the perilymph is "mobilized," the notch disappears. In lateral ossicular chain fixation (malleal and/or incudal), an even greater depression across the frequency range can occur in MBC.

In certain middle-ear disorders, bone conduction thresholds obtained by frontal bone conduction (FBC) and by sensorineural acuity level (SAL) test may be less depressed than MBC responses; in certain middle-ear lesions, as much as a 20-dB average difference may exist between FBC and MBC results (6) (Fig. 8–1).

The advantage of FBC measurements is that they tend to maximize the air–bone gap and enable a more accurate determination of the presence of a conductive component. However, tonal perception for FBC requires greater intensity of presentation than for MBC, because more energy is required at the forehead than at the mastoid. The vibrator used for the frontal bone has the same intensity limitations as the vibrator used for mastoid bone. Therefore, the use of FBC will be limited to cases where bone conduction thresholds are of moderate degree or better.

The conductive loss test battery consists of four tests of cochlear reserve so that the degree of conductive loss can be quantified precisely.

BONE CONDUCTION

Bone conduction is a method of measuring the intensity of auditory signals conducted to the cochlea through the cranial bones. There are two ways of determining bone conduction thresholds: frontal bone and mastoid bone placement.

Frontal Bone Conduction

Pure tones are conducted through a bone conduction vibrator placed on the center of the forehead (Fig. 8–2). A narrow-band masking signal is introduced into the nontest ear, via an insert receiver or standard earphone, for determination of frontal bone conduction thresholds (Fig. 8–3).

Mastoid Bone Conduction

Pure tones are conducted through a bone conduction vibrator placed on the mastoid process (Fig. 8–4). A narrow-band masking signal is introduced (as necessary) into the nontest ear via an insert receiver or standard earphone for determination of MBC thresholds in the unmasked ear (Fig. 8–5).

SENSORINEURAL ACUITY LEVEL (SAL)

The SAL test can be used to determine the degree of cochlear reserve in patients with mixed losses, in whom the amount of air conduction shift (with the introduction of masking via the forehead) is purported to reveal the true cochlear reserve.

Pure tones are presented through nonoccluding (Pederson) earphones (Fig. 8–6). Air conduction thresholds for each ear are recorded without noise and then with the introduction of a narrow-band masking signal (0.5 volt) via a bone conduction vibrator placed in the center of the forehead. The resulting difference in threshold (contrasting masked and unmasked re-

FIG. 8–2. Placement of bone vibrator for FBC testing.

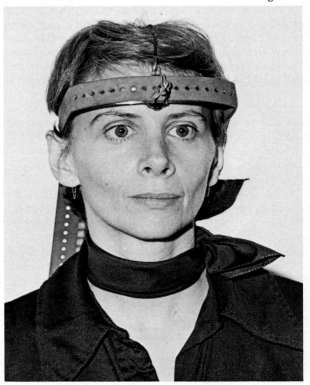

FIG. 8–1. Demonstration of how FBC and SAL reveal a greater air–bone gap than MBC alone. ●—●, AC, unmasked, RE; **solid triangles,** MBC; **x- - - - -x,** sensorineural acuity level; **open triangles,** FBC.

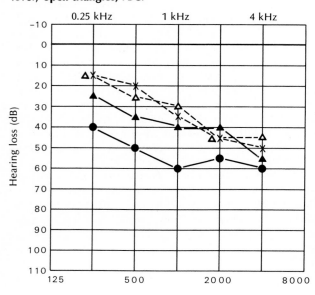

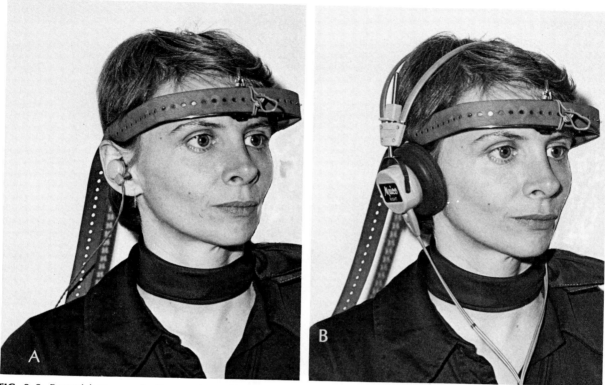

FIG. 8–3. Frontal bone conduction testing with introduction of masking using either an insert receiver (**A**) or an earphone (**B**).

FIG. 8–4. Placement of bone vibrator for MBC testing.

FIG. 8–5. Mastoid bone conduction testing with introduction of masking via earphone.

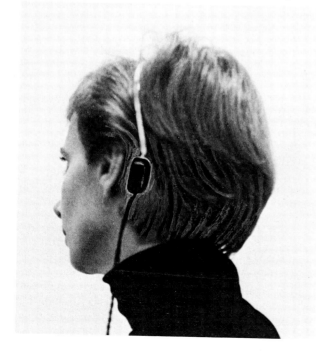

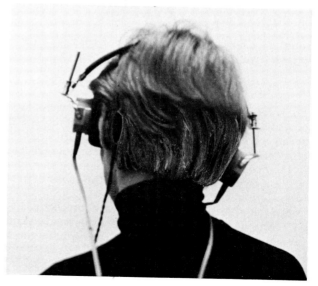

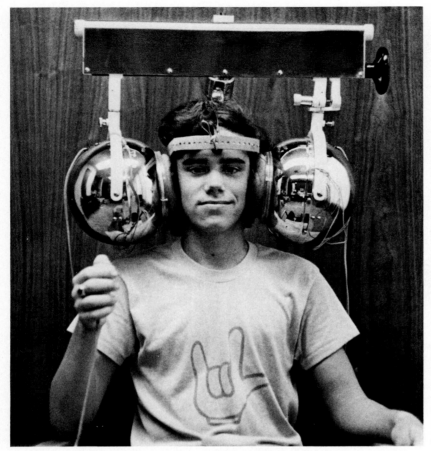

FIG. 8–6. Patient wearing Pederson earphones for SAL testing.

sults) should represent the amount of cochlear reserve at each frequency tested (28).

OCCLUSION EFFECT

The **occlusion effect** is a procedure whereby FBC or MBC is measured by occluding the nontest ear by an air conduction earphone. This can create a temporary, moderate degree of air conduction loss in the occluded ear, with a corresponding increase in bone conduction response (*i.e.*, the tones appear to be amplified and therefore thresholds obtained are better than those obtained without occlusion) (7). The degree of occlusion effect depends upon the volume of air trapped under the earphone and can be explained in part, by changes in osseotympanic conduction. The occlusion effect is present in patients with normal hearing or with sensorineural hearing loss at frequencies 1000 Hz and below.

Testing is performed in the usual manner, by MBC. An earphone is then placed on the test ear, and bone conduction thresholds are measured again, with the ear canal occluded by the earphone. The results of threshold measurements for the two conditions are compared for differences.

Patients with conductive hearing loss are believed to have a "built-in" occlusion effect (*i.e.*, the middle-ear lesion itself mimics the degree of air conduction loss created by the occluding earphone). Bone conduction responses, therefore, should not improve with the introduction of an occluding earphone. When test results reveal a failure of bone conduction thresholds to improve with use of an occluding earphone, the results are consistent with a conductive hearing loss.

Bone conduction results obtained with occlusion of the external ear are referred to as **absolute** and those obtained without external ear occlusion are referred to as **relative.** The presence or absence of this occlusion effect assists in differentiating between middle ear and cochlear sites of lesion.

ACOUSTIC IMPEDANCE MEASUREMENTS

Measurement of acoustic impedance is an objective test to aid in determining the integrity of the middle-ear mechanical system (see Ch. 7, Acoustic Impedance Tests).

Mastoid bone conduction (MBC), FBC, and SAL (in addition to tests for occlusion effect and acoustic impedance measurements) provide several measures of cochlear reserve and/or indications of the integrity of the middle-ear mechanical system, for maximum diagnostic utilization. Each test yields useful supplementary diagnostic information, but individual tests should not be considered a substitute for the complete battery.

With rapid advances in middle-ear surgery, it is increasingly necessary to investigate even a relatively small air–bone gap.

THE SENSORINEURAL HEARING LOSS TEST BATTERY

Pure tone test results reveal gross information about the peripheral hearing mechanism. Findings may show essentially normal hearing or even reduced acuity. It is imperative, where the symptomatology suggests the need, to employ additional test procedures to elicit a more definitive picture of the total auditory system.

The following tests comprise the sensorineural hearing loss test battery, and are designed to aid in more accurately determining the site of lesion.

STANDARD BEKESY AUDIOMETRY

The Bekesy audiometric procedure is utilized diagnostically as a portion of the sensorineural hearing loss test battery. Two tracings are made for each ear, and responses are automatically recorded for pulsed and continuous tones, either at fixed frequencies or continuously variable (sweep) frequencies (Fig. 8–7). The patterns traced are categorized (or classified) numerically, each type of tracing suggesting different sites-of-lesion. Bekesy audiometry may also be employed to detect the presence of functional hearing loss.

The diagnostic significance of Bekesy audiometry (15) is based on the relationship between the pulsed and continuous tracings. Patterns traced are believed to measure the amount of adaptation

in the auditory system, with the more peripheral lesion having the greatest effect on test results, where two or more sites-of-lesion may coexist.

The patient, wearing earphones, holds an interrupter switch throughout the procedure. When the continuous or pulsed stimulus is heard, the switch is depressed. Conversely, when the signal is not heard, the switch is released. The machine automatically traces the responses on a recording chart. The method of instruction can affect the relationship between the continuous and pulsed tracings (12).

The relationships between tracings can be categorized into five types (15):

Type I

The continuous and pulsed tracings interweave. Both excursions may be about 10 dB in width. The type I pattern is characteristic of normal hearing, conductive hearing loss, or mild sensorineural hearing loss (Fig. 8–8).

Type II

The continuous tracing interweaves with the pulsed tracing at some frequencies, but tends to separate at frequencies of 500 Hz and above, and parallel the pulsed tracing (by sweep frequency tracing).

It is not unusual, however, to note separation between continuous and pulsed tracings throughout all frequencies (by fixed frequency tracings). The separation should not exceed 20 dB. In addition, the amplitude of continuous tracing may become quite narrow (3–5 dB in width). The presence of reduced excursion amplitude has been considered either an indirect measure of recruitment or, perhaps more likely, a sign of rapid adaptation (9, 10, 24). The type II pattern is characteristic of a cochlear site-of-lesion. However, in some patients with normal hearing a type II pattern will be noted (Fig. 8–9).

Type III

This pattern is dramatically different from types I and II. Here, the continuous tracing falls below the pulsed tracing, but instead of following a parallel course, as in the type II pattern, it continues to separate precipitously, usually to the upper intensity limits of the Bekesy audiometer. The separation may occur at almost any point in the frequency range.

The type III pattern is usually characteristic of a retrocochlear site-of-lesion (*i.e.,* an internal auditory meatus lesion, such as eighth nerve tumor) and calls for repeated testing at regular intervals (Fig. 8–10).

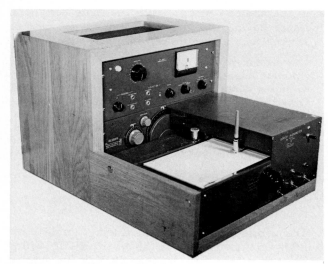

FIG. 8–7. Bekesy E-800 audiometer.

FIG. 8–8. Form for automatically recording Bekesy tracing, showing type I sweep tracing, in which pulsed **(black)** and continuous **(gray)** tracings interweave, found with normal hearing or mild hearing loss.

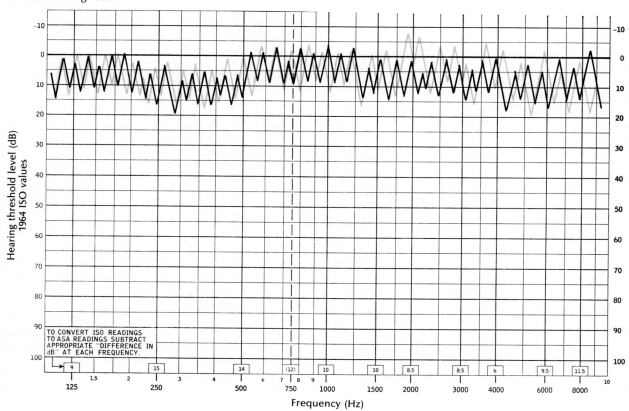

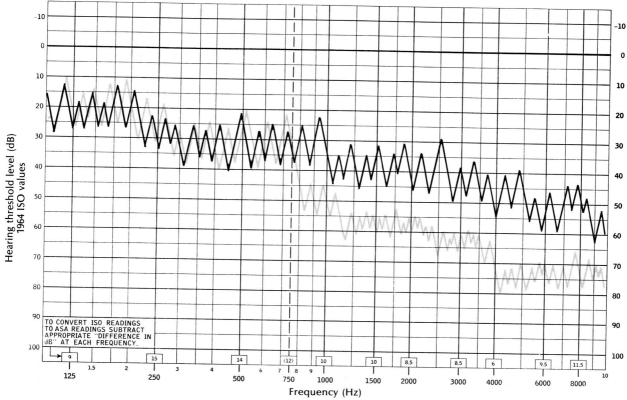

FIG. 8–9. Type II sweep Bekesy tracing, in which separation of the pulsed **(black)** and continuous **(gray)** patterns usually denotes a cochlear lesion.

Type IV

The continuous tracing falls below and runs parallel to the pulsed tracing, as in the type II pattern. However, unlike the type II pattern, the separation between continuous and pulsed is greater than 25 dB (11). An interesting characteristic of the type IV pattern (found in sweep frequency tracings) is that the two tracings may interweave in the mid or high frequencies.

The type IV pattern has been found in patients with Meniere's syndrome. However, it will frequently be found in many other types of sensorineural hearing loss (Fig. 8–11).

Type V

This pattern differs significantly from the others in that the continuous tracing demonstrates better hearing level responses than the pulsed tracing.

The type V pattern is usually found in nonorganic hearing losses (Fig. 8–12).

While classification of the basis of types is convenient, the patterns must be clinically interpreted with caution. It should be kept in mind that an acoustic tumor may generate patterns other than type III, depending upon the size, site, and stage of development of the lesion (20). However, Bekesy audiometry is a useful tool when utilized as part of a total battery determining the sites-of-lesion of auditory disorders.

FORWARD-BACKWARD BEKESY AUDIOMETRY

The forward-backward discrepancy, a variation of the traditional Bekesy technique, compares forward-sweeping continuous tracings (running from low to high frequencies) with backward-sweeping continuous tracings (i.e., running from high to low frequencies). The site-of-lesion determination is based upon the amount of difference between these two continuous tracings.

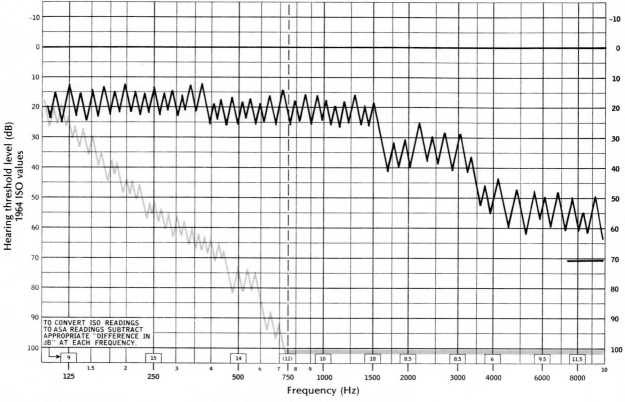

FIG. 8–10. Type III sweep Bekesy tracing, usually indicative of a retrocochlear lesion.

In our clinical experience, this procedure reveals no additional diagnostically significant results. It is based on the premise that if a discrepancy between the two continuous tracings is recorded, it is characteristic of a retrocochlear site-of-lesion (18). It was also shown to have potential diagnostic significance in identifying patients with functional hearing loss. However, the presence of a diagnostically significant discrepancy does not occur in all types of retrocochlear disorders or functional hearing losses.

BEKESY COMFORTABLE LOUDNESS AUDIOMETRY

The premise of Bekesy comfortable loudness is that a suprathreshold tracing procedure would be a more sensitive indicator of retrocochlear disorders. It was proposed (17) that the initial signs of retrocochlear lesions tend to be cochlear in characteristic, and that eighth nerve signs first are visualized at relatively intense suprathreshold levels. Further progression of the lesion may reveal retrocochlear signs at less intense threshold levels. Again, the use of conventional Bekesy types is avoided. Rather the relationship between the continuous and pulsed tracings is compared, when the stimuli are presented within the range of comfortable loudness.

This variation of the traditional Bekesy technique is not a universally employed procedure and has not been utilized routinely at our clinic. This test is difficult to administer because, at this time, the instruction technique has not yet been standardized (e.g., what is comfortable loudness? How does one determine it?).

THE TONE DECAY TEST

The Owens tone decay test (23), the technique employed at this clinic, attempts to quantify the rapidity of decay with increasing intensity and to classify the patterns of this decay into types corresponding to different sites-of-lesion. Interpretation is based upon an analysis of the patterns of response to continuous stimuli (Table 8–1).

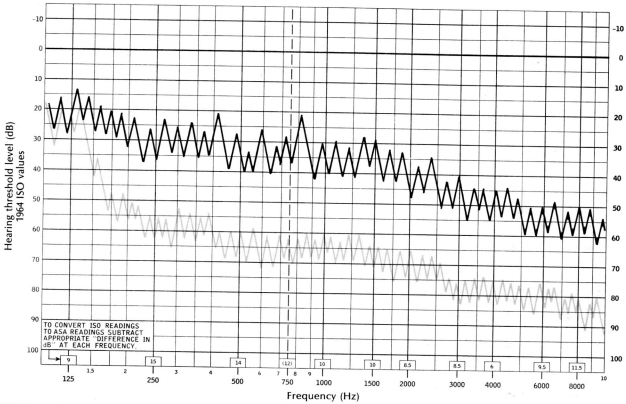

FIG. 8–11. Type IV sweep Bekesy tracing, associated with Meniere's syndrome or other sensorineural hearing loss.

FIG. 8–12. Type V sweep Bekesy tracing, usually found in nonorganic hearing loss.

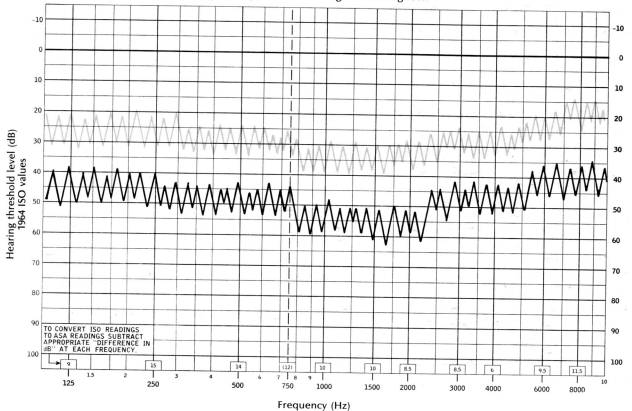

TABLE 8-1. Classification of Tone Decay Patterns

Level above threshold (dB)	I*	II†					III‡
		A	B	C	D	E	
5	60	25	7	12	15	5	14
10		60	34	26	23	14	16
15			60	40	30	18	12
20				60	39	21	14

*Type I, normal or conductive.
†Type II, cochlear.
‡Type III, retrocochlear.
(Owens E: J Speech Hear Disord 29:14–22, 1964)

The purpose of the test is to determine the presence of abnormal threshold tone decay (*i.e.,* an audible tone or sound may become inaudible within a short period of time). This phenomenon is most characteristic in retrocochlear lesions, although it may be present in cochlear disorders.

After the threshold for an individual frequency is established, the patient is instructed to raise one hand for as long as the tonal signal is audible. The method of instruction is important, since the patient may be experiencing several types of perceptual phenomena (8). Four possible levels of presentation are offered at each of the frequencies 500–4000 Hz (5-dB, 10-dB, 15-dB, and 20-dB sensation levels), discontinuing presentation when a response is sustained for 60 sec. The patterns of a response are recorded and categorized as described in the foregoing sections (Fig. 8–13).

SHORT INCREMENT SENSITIVITY INDEX

The short increment sensitivity index (SISI) test is administered, at this clinic, as a screening device, presented at an intensity level (70 dB sound pressure level or greater) sufficient to determine whether small intensity changes can be perceived (manifested as a high or low SISI score). If a high sensitivity is achieved (70–100%), it is believed to reflect a normal phenomenon, characteristic of normal hearing or a peripheral hearing disorder. If a low sensitivity is achieved (0–65%), this finding is considered diagnostically significant as being indicative of a retrocochlear site-of-lesion.

The patient listens, under earphones, to a continuous tone of at least 1-min duration. The patient is instructed to push a signal button (or raise one hand) whenever an increase in loudness is perceived. Responses to the 1-dB increment of intensity change are recorded for 20 presentations, and the percentage of positive responses to these changes is calculated on a basis of 5% per correct response (Fig. 8–14).

The SISI test cannot be considered as a measure of recruitment, nor will it differentiate cochlear from conductive impairment or normal hearing, as originally intended (19), if the intensity level of the cochlea is taken into account (25, 26, 29). Once this factor is allowed for, only a low SISI score (0–65%) at a sufficiently high intensity level of presentation, is indicative of a positive response and diagnostically significant in differentiating between peripheral and retrocochlear disorders. When the SISI is administered at 75 dB SPL to a group of patients with surgically confirmed acoustic neurinomas, the affected ear is incapable of sensitivity to small intensity change (27).

LOUDNESS-BALANCING PROCEDURES

Loudness-balancing techniques are a useful portion of the cochlear battery, to assist in identification of the site-of-lesion of auditory disorders. The alternate binaural loudness balance (ABLB) technique was designed to measure the presence of loudness recruitment, a phenomenon believed characteristic of sensorineural hearing loss (5). However, the presence of subjective loudness recruitment does not absolutely rule out the possibility of other than cochlear sites-of-lesion.

Tones of the same frequency are presented alternately to each ear. Presentation levels to the "better ear" are fixed (as applicable) at sensation levels of 20 dB, 40 dB, and 60 dB in relation to the hearing threshold levels at each frequency. Presentation levels to the "poorer ear" are not fixed but are varied until the patient indicates that the tonal signals appear to be equally loud bilaterally.

Loudness-balance results are generally plotted on a laddergram. This laddergram gives a schematic representation of loudness judgments, and the subsequent interpretation generally falls into four categories:

1. No recruitment . The lines remain parallel (±10 dB) on the laddergram, representing the points where equal sensation levels produce the judgment of equal loudness, (*i.e.,* loudness growth is proportionate bilaterally) (Fig. 8–15).
2. Partial recruitment. There is some converging of the lines on the laddergram, representing the points where the judgment of equal loudness is reached at decreased sensation levels for the poorer ear (*i.e.,* the growth of loudness

FIG. 8–13. Form for recording tone decay test findings.

Name: ______________________ Date: ________________ Age: ___

Audiometer ____________________ Audiologist: ____________________

Tone decay

H. L.	500 R	500 L	1000 R	1000 L	2000 R	2000 L	4000 R	4000 L
0								
5								
10								
15	T							
20	60							
25			T		T			
30			40		25			
35			60		52			
40					60			
45								
50							T	
55							18	
60							32	
65							44	
70							50	
75								
80								
85								
90								
95								
100								
105								

COMMENTS:

FIG. 8–14. Form for recording of SISI findings.

SISI

Name ____________________ Age ______ Sex ______ Date ________ Tester ______________ Diagnosis ________________

Freq.	Ear	Threshold / Level of present	1	2	3	4	5	6	7	8	9	10	11	12	13	14	15	16	17	18	19	20	No. Corr.	% CORR.
1000 Hz	R	40dB / 70dB	√	√	√				√		√	√	√	√	√			√	√		√	√	13	65%
1000 Hz	L	50dB / 70dB	√	√	√		√	√	√	√	√		√	√	√	√	√	√	√	√	√		17	85%

in the poorer ear is more rapid than in the good ear but never reaches equal intensity levels (Fig. 8–16).

3. Complete recruitment. The lines completely converge on the laddergram representing points where the judgment of loudness occurs at equal intensity levels bilaterally (±10 dB) (*i.e.*, the growth of loudness in the poorer ear is disproportionately greater than that in the better ear (Fig. 8–17).

4. Hyperrecruitment. The lines converge in an oblique manner on the laddergram, representing the points where the judgment of equal loudness in the good ear exceeds the intensity level of the poorer ear (*i.e.*, the growth of loudness is so rapid in the poorer ear that it is disproportionate to that in the better ear to a greater degree than with complete recruitment (Fig. 8–18). The determination of hyperrecruitment does not appear to provide any more additional diagnostic information than the interpretation of complete recruitment on patients seen at this clinic.

There are three major pitfalls inherent in this procedure:

1. Patients may report the presence of diplacusis (*i.e.*, tones of the same frequency presented to both ears appear to be different in pitch and/or tonal quality). Although this may be a complicating factor in loudness matching, most patients with diplacusis can perform the desired task.

2. Sophisticated judgments are required (*i.e.*, "equal" loudness determinations are difficult). However, only a small percentage of adult patients seen at this clinic have been unable to perform the task.

3. The potential benefit of this procedure is minimized by the limits to the population for whom this test is applicable. The patient must have a) one ear with hearing no poorer than 20 dB; b) a difference between ears of no less than 20 dB and no more than 55 dB; and c) have one frequency within the normal range (for monaural loudness balance procedure (MLB).

Attempts have been made to correlate the presence of loudness recruitment with 1) decrease in excursion width of the continuous Bekesy tracings, 2) high SISI scores (70–100%); 3) presence of acoustic reflex thresholds at sensation levels less than 60 dB and 4) limited tolerance for auditory stimuli. However, the *only* test measure that provides direct information to which we can apply the term recruitment is the ABLB or the less frequently performed MLB test.

SIMULTANEOUS BINAURAL MEDIAN PLANE LOCALIZATION

The simultaneous binaural median plane localization (SBMPL) test is simple and quick to administer as part of the sensorineural hearing loss battery and can be employed as a screening technique.

Tones of the same frequency are presented simultaneously to both ears. The intensity is kept constant in one ear and varied in the second ear. The patient points to the location on the head where the stimulus appears to be heard.

The SBMPL test, a variation of the loudness balancing technique, involves a judgment in the form of a median-plane localization rather than the equation of equal loudness. The hypothesis is that with integrity of the afferent pathway through some (as yet undetermined) critical subcortical center, a patient would be able to localize sound at the midline, when tones are presented simultaneously to both ears, at relatively equal sensation levels. It is particularly useful in cases in which there is no significant peripheral hearing impairment. The inability to medially localize the signals has been associated with the presence of a central disorder affecting the afferent pathway (14).

One problem noted concerns patients with diplacusis, who are unable to localize medially, reporting that the tones appeared to have different pitch and/or tonal quality characteristics, even at subjectively equal loudness levels.

PERFORMANCE INTENSITY FUNCTION

The performance intensity function (also called the articulation function curve) for phonetically balanced (PB) words was studied in this clinic as a routine part of a differential diagnostic test battery. The results obtained failed *routinely* to assist in differentiating cochlear from retrocochlear lesions, since in some sensorineural hearing losses (especially Meniere's syndrome and presbycusis), the results were similar to those obtained with patients with retrocochlear losses at high intensity presentation levels. This technique merits further investigation and study for inclusion as a routine part of a diagnostic battery.

The use of discrimination scores, as a diagnostic technique for site-of-lesion testing, has been examined (13). It was presumed that with in-

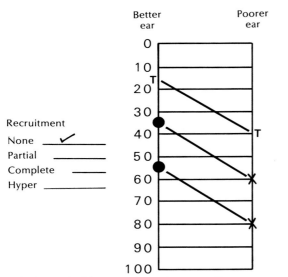

FIG. 8–15. Laddergram form for recording responses on ABLB test. This recording represents no recruitment. **T,** threshold; **solid circle,** right ear, **X,** left ear.

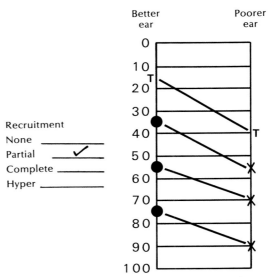

FIG. 8–16. Laddergram, representing partial recruitment. **T,** threshold; **solid circle,** right ear; **X,** left ear.

FIG. 8–17. Laddergram representing complete recruitment. **T,** threshold; **solid circle,** right ear; **X,** left ear.

FIG. 8–18. Laddergram representing hyperrecruitment. **T,** threshold; **solid circle,** right ear; **X,** left ear.

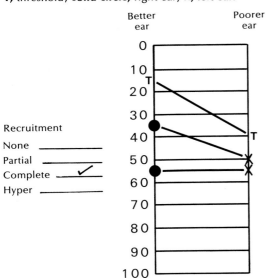

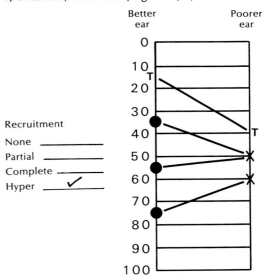

creasing intensity levels of presentation for PB word lists, discrimination scores would become poorer for patients with severe cochlear losses. More recently, this decrease in discrimination has been associated with retrocochlear lesions. It is theorized that with eighth nerve lesions, as compared to cochlear disorders, a more significant decrease in discrimination ability for PB words would occur (16).

SPECIAL CENTRAL AUDITORY NERVOUS SYSTEM SPEECH TESTS

The next set of tests to be discussed as part of the sensorineural hearing loss battery concern the identification of central auditory nervous system (CANS) lesions. The central auditory area in the brain consists of the primary auditory reception centers of the cerebral cortex, which includes the superior temporal gyrus bilaterally, especially the middle and posterior portions.

The need for diagnostic tests aimed at discovering patients with unilateral lesions of the CANS has gained interest, mainly because patients with these lesions may respond to pure tone thresholds within the normal range. Pure tones (which are based on simple frequency and intensity manipulation) are not sensitive enough as diagnostic indicators of the site-of-lesion, because of the redundancy of the signals. As lesions progress closer to the cerebral cortex, redundancy is enhanced by the multiple crossings and interactions in the auditory tract. One of the few diagnostically significant audiologic clues is the reduced ability to discriminate speech on the ear contralateral to the lesion, especially when the task is complicated by the addition of a distortion element.

Therefore, speech stimuli are deliberately distorted, on the assumption that by making the words less understandable, (*i.e.*, reducing their redundancy), heavier demands are placed upon the integrating and synthesizing function of the auditory cortex. Under these stressful conditions, the patient with cortical damage will demonstrate an inability to perform correctly the desired speech task, thus revealing the presence of cortical damage.

There are many varieties of CANS speech tests currently in use, involving different modes of presentation of speech materials. The speech stimuli are distorted in different ways (frequency distortion, time compression, faint presentation, interrupted speech). Regardless of the type of filtering process, they have been found to be sensitive indicators of temporal lobe lesions. Three of the most frequently used tests for CANS lesions are filtered speech tests, dichotic speech tests, and the staggered spondee word (SSW) test.

FILTERED SPEECH TESTS

Filtered (or distorted) speech may be defined as speech that has been altered in a way to increase difficulty in understanding, by eliminating portions of the frequency spectrum.

When distorted speech tests are administered to patients with temporal lobe tumors (3), it has been noted that 1) the ability to discriminate low-pass filtered speech is reduced in the ear contralateral to the lesion; 2) this impairment of discrimination ability in the contralateral ear may improve after surgical removal of the affected area; 3) the ability to discriminate low-pass filtered speech may also improve in the ipsilateral ear after surgery.

The need for these specialized test procedures (as stated previously) arises from the problem that with lesions occurring higher in the central nervous system than the cochlear nuclei, there is no apparent decrease in hearing acuity for pure-tone stimuli. Therefore, the development of more sensitive measures for detection of central auditory disorders have been necessary. More research is needed to standardize these suggested filtered speech tests, to make them more clinically applicable and sensitive enough to identify the locus of lesions within the CANS.

DICHOTIC SPEECH TESTS

Dichotic stimulation concerns the simultaneous presentation of two different messages (usually words or syllables) to each ear. In subjects with normal hearing, the right ear generally outperforms the left ear when speech is the stimulus. However, when two different stimuli (the dichotic mode) are employed, the left ear generally outperforms the right ear. When a temporal lobe lesion exists, the ear contralateral to the lesion gives poorer results than the ipsilateral ear on dichotic speech tests (1, 2).

The theoretical assumption is that while both hemispheres have the capability to extract auditory parameters of a speech signal, the dominant hemisphere may be specialized for the extraction of linguistic features from those parameters. The speech transmission process is believed to go from the right to the left hemisphere and does not work in reverse. If the right hemisphere is disconnected (*e.g.*, by a cerebral lesion) from the dominant left hemisphere, messages essential to the interpretation of speech are not transmitted to the left side. This can result in the patient's being unable to identify and classify the speech material presented.

Whether one hemisphere is dominant and one subordinate is not as important as understanding that each hemisphere appears to have individual, distinctive functions that enable a broad spectrum of activities to be conducted. The left hemisphere appears to be involved in a wide range of linguistic activities, such as conceptualization, perceptual integration of temporal events, etc. Similarly, the right hemisphere appears to exhibit dominance for some diverse motor and perceptual activities.

As yet no complete definition of these distinctive functions of the two hemispheres has been established. Much experimental study is necessary, but the procedure has great potential as a viable test of central auditory disorders.

STAGGERED SPONDEE WORD TEST

The SSW test is another measure of CANS dysfunction. It is a dichotic procedure—*i.e.*, different signals are presented to each ear and the subject is expected to repeat both messages (21, 22). The SSW test differs from other dichotic speech tests in terms of the type of stimuli used—*i.e.*, spondee words rather than monosyllabic words. The purpose of using words with greater redundancy and ease of understanding is that the test is more applicable to a broad spectrum of patients, regardless of age, education, intelligence; and it aids in reducing contamination caused by the possible presence of peripheral hearing disorders. In addition, the test procedure requires little sophistication or training on the part of the patient.

In terms of test interpretation, as with other tests of the CANS, moderately and severely reduced SSW performance is related to dysfunction in the contralateral hemisphere. Sex, intelligence, socioeconomic status do not appear to be confounding variables in interpretation of the SSW. One exception to this exists in terms of a laterality effect, generally favoring the right ear. The SSW might be sensitive to central changes in the audition of the elderly population in this regard. Therefore, in patients 60 years or older, it becomes hard to distinguish whether CANS change is caused by a centrally located auditory lesion or is merely a result of typical central changes occurring with the aging process. Also, this technique has not been shown to be effective for children under 11 years of age.

The unilaterally filtered speech test, patterned after the procedures established by Bocca and coworkers (3) probably does not require the integrity of the same centers as those tests based on separation of binaurally competing messages. In addition, tests that use words that have familiar speech material, containing considerable redundancy, are less likely to be affected by peripheral hearing loss than are those that make use of distorted monosyllabic words.

A battery of central tests might sample the integrity of different auditory areas and thereby provide more specific localization of the brain dysfunction.

REFERENCES

1. Berlin C, Lowe SS: Temporal and dichotic factors in central auditory testing. In Katz (ed): Handbook of Clinical Audiology. Baltimore, Williams and Wilkins, 1972
2. Berlin C, Lowe–Bell S, Janetta P, Kline D: Central auditory deficits after temporal lobectomy. Arch Otolaryngol 96:4–10, 1972
3. Bocca E, Calearo C, Cassinari V: A new method for testing hearing in temporal lobe tumors, preliminary report. Acta Otolaryngol 44:219–221, 1954
4. Carhart R: Effects of stapes fixation on bone conduction response. Otosclerosis. Boston, Little, Brown, 1962, pp 175–197
5. Fowler EP: A method for early detection of otosclerosis. Arch Otolaryngol 24:731–741, 1936
6. Goodhill V, Dirks D, Malmquist C: Bone conduction thresholds: relationship of frontal and mastoid measurements in conductive hypacusis. Arch Otolaryngol 91:250–256, 1970
7. Goldstein D, Hayes C: The occlusion effect in bone conduction hearing. J Speech Hear Res 8:137–148, 1965
8. Green D: Threshold tone decay. In Katz J (ed): Handbook of Clinical Audiology. Baltimore, Williams and Wilkins, Ch 13, 1972
9. Harbert R, Young I: Clinical application of hearing tests. Arch Otolaryngol 76:55–67, 1962
10. Harbert R, Young I: Threshold auditory adaptation. J Aud Res 2:229–246, 1962
11. Hughes RL: Current audiometric practices. Voice 16:82–87, 1967
12. Hughes RL: Bekesy audiometry. In Katz J (ed): Handbook of Clinical Audiology. Baltimore, Williams and Wilkins, Ch 12, 1972
13. Huizing HC, Reyntjes JA: Recruitment and speech discrimination loss. Laryngoscope 62:521–527, 1952
14. Jerger J: Observations of auditory behaviors in lesions of the central auditory pathways. Arch Otolaryngol 71:797–805, 1960
15. Jerger J: Hearing tests in otologic diagnosis. ASHA 4:139–145, 1962

16. Jerger J, Jerger S: Diagnostic significance of PB word functions. Arch Otolaryngol 93:573–580, 1971

17. Jerger J, Jerger S: Diagnostic value of bekesy comfortable loudness (BCL) Tracings. Arch Otolaryngol 99:351–360, 1974

18. Jerger J, Jerger S, Mauldin L: The foreward-backward discrepancy in bekesy audiometry. Arch Otolaryngol 96:400–406, 1972

19. Jerger J, Shedd J, Harford E: On the detection of extremely small changes in sound intensity. Arch Otolaryngol 69:200–211, 1959

20. Jerger J, Waller J: Some observations on masking and on the progression of auditory signs in acoustic neurinomas. J Speech Hear Dis 27:140–143, 1962

21. Katz J: The use of staggered spondaic words for assessing the integrity of the central auditory nervous system. J Aud Res 2:327–337, 1962

22. Katz J: The SSW test—an interim report. J Speech Hear Dis 33:132–146, 1963

23. Owens E: Tone decay in eighth nerve and cochlear lesions. J Speech Hear Dis 29:14–22, 1964

24. Suzuki T, Kubota K: Normal width in tracing on bekesy audiogram. J Aud Res 6:91–96, 1966

25. Swisher LP: Response to intensity change in cochlear pathology. Laryngoscope 76:1706–1713, 1966

26. Swisher LP, Stephens MM, Doehring DG: The effects of hearing level and normal variability of sensitivity to intensity change. J Aud Res 6:249–259, 1966

27. Thompson G: A modified SISI technique for selected case with suspected acoustic neuroma. J Speech Hear Dis 28:299–302, 1963

28. Tillman TW: Clinical applicability of the SAL test. Arch Otolaryngol 78:20–32, 1963

29. Young I, Harbert R: Significance of the SISI test. J Aud Res 7:303–311, 1967

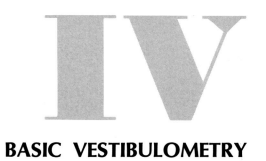

IV

BASIC VESTIBULOMETRY

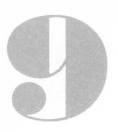

EQUILIBRIUM AND DIZZINESS

VERTIGO, THE VESTIBULE, AND THE VESTIBULAR SYSTEM

Equilibrium, spatial orientation, and proprioception are vital biologic functions involving interactions between complex peripheral and CNS structures. These functions involve more than the vestibular system alone.

The term **vestibular system** was derived from the labyrinthine "vestibule." The **vestibule** is the largest cubic component of the bony labyrinth. Within the vestibule, which is filled with perilymph, are suspended delicately interconnected viscera containing endolymph. These endolymphatic viscera include primarily the utricle and saccule, the utricle connecting with the semicircular canal system and the saccule connecting with the cochlear duct system. The total continuous system is a vestibulocochlear organ that behaves as one complex sensory organ. The cochlear system is, more or less, a "silent partner" in "vestibular" function; the vestibular system is organized to deal with information-processing relating to acceleration (angular and nonangular) as well as to static displacement. The vestibular system, peripherally, is a statokinetic system. Because of the role played by the utriculosaccular–semicircular canal end organ system, it has become common usage to link disorders of equilibrium, spatial orientation, and proprioception with the vestibule. However, the lesions causing the symptoms may not be specifically vestibular—*i.e.*, relating to the vestibule in the inner ear. The symptoms may be due to lesions anywhere in the entire afferent and efferent peripheral and central vestibular system, with interactions between the end organ and a number of CNS structures.

Since the discovery by Flourens more than a century ago that an experimental fistula in the horizontal canal of a pigeon caused head movements in the horizontal plane, much research has been directed to the vestibular labyrinth. Head movements and eye movements (nystagmus) have been studied extensively. Ewald, in 1892, proposed three vestibular laws. The first Ewald law states that eyes and head move in the direction of endolymph flow, in the plane of the canal stimulated. The second Ewald law states that endolymph flow toward the ampulla in the lateral semicircular canal (ampullipetal) produces a greater stimulus than flow away from the ampulla (ampullifugal). The third Ewald law relates to the superior and posterior canals (which have a common crus), in which the ampullifugal stimulus is greater.

The directional aspect of ampullar stimulation is related to cellular polarization and directional aspects of the arrangements of the kinocilium relative to the other hair-cell stereocilia. The cilia are polarized for directional effects. Similar ciliary specialization exists in saccular and utricular maculas.

The vestibular system is organized to deal with information-processing relating to acceleration, (angular and nonangular) as well as to static displacement. Peripherally, it is a statokinetic system.

Normal equilibrium is the state of harmonious symmetry between the right and left vestibular systems as they function to maintain the proper relationships between the person and the environment. The vestibular systems are complex, involving 1) the right and left peripheral vestibular labyrinths, each with three semicircular canals and utriculosaccular organs; 2) the lower CNS vestibular pathways; and 3) the higher integrative CNS vestibular pathways involving cerebellar and/or cerebral functions.

The vestibular end organs in the semicircular canals, utricle, and saccule function dynamically in three ways: 1) At rest, they are constantly discharging resting signal patterns from cristas and maculas to the CNS vestibular system. 2) When stimulated, the semicircular canal cristas respond to radial accelerations. 3) The maculas of the utricle and saccule respond to linear displacement patterns.

There is an intricate partnership between the right and left vestibular systems. In response to motion, the two systems (right and left) are stimulated in different quantitative patterns. These differences in afferent signals are processed by the

CNS vestibular system. In response to radial (angular) acceleration, semicircular canal stimulation produces nystagmus. In response to linear displacement, utriculosaccular stimulation produces ocular counterrolling.

Nystagmus is a response to head motion involving angular acceleration that causes an unequal endolymphatic concentration on one side of the semicircular canal cupulas. This displacement creates an afferent signal resulting in nystagmus, an alternating involuntary movement in both eyes, characterized by a slow movement (slow component) to one side, with a corrective fast return movement to the other side (quick component).

The direction of nystagmus may be horizontal, vertical, diagonal, or rotary. Nystagmus may be manifest or occult: manifest if observable with the naked eye, in ordinary light, and occult if observable only under magnification with +20 lenses to abolish fixation or recorded by electronystagmography in the dark with abolition of ocular fixation.

Ocular counterrolling is a response to otoconial displacement with afferent vestibular impulses from each macula, relating to gravity induced changes. Ocular roles in spatial orientation involve retinal postural reflexes, integrated with labyrinthine impulses. Both labyrinthine and ocular mechanisms are further modified by the muscle spindles and specialized nerve endings of the proprioceptive system.

The orientating role of the vestibular labyrinths is linked to a unified coordinating mechanism consisting of both labyrinths, their vestibular nerves, ganglia, nuclei, central ocular pathways, the spinal cord, cerebellum, medial longitudinal fasciculus (bundle—MLF), red nucleus, thalamus, hypothalamus, and cerebellar cortex.

The role of the MLF is most important, since its fibers connect the vestibular pathways with eye muscle nuclei, oculomotor and trochlear nerves in the midbrain, and abducens nerve in the pons. The MLF also relates the vestibular pathway to the functions of other cranial nerves and to the anterior horn cells of the spinal cord which supply extremity muscles.

In clinical physiology, ocular nystagmus is the major response to be considered as the sequel of crista ampullaris stimulation following angular acceleration. The quick (compensatory) component is used by convention to describe direction of nystagmus. Deflection of cilia responsible for nystagmus also occurs in response to the thermosiphon effect of caloric stimulation. Ear canal irrigation with water significantly cooler or warmer than body temperature will create thermosiphon currents adequate to stimulate vestibular receptors and produce nystagmus.

Cool or warm air currents can produce the same response. Electronystagmography is the clinical method for quantitative studies of nystagmus patterns (see Ch. 10, Examination of the Dizzy Patient).

Galvanic neck stimulation can also be used clinically for similar response patterns, in addition to nystagmus studies. Body sway and deviations in step pattern are other post-vestibular-stimulation phenomena useful in clinical diagnostic procedures.

Utricular macular responses to linear acceleration produces counterrolling of the eyes, although nystagmus patterns have also been observed under some conditions.

THE TERMS DIZZINESS, VERTIGO, DYSEQUILIBRIUM, AND MOTION SICKNESS

Dizziness is one of the most common symptoms in medicine. Dizziness and vertigo are not necessarily synonymous. Terms such as "giddiness," "motion sickness," "imbalance," "wooziness," "faintness," and "passing out" are frequently loosely equated with equilibrium disorders. Thus, the word **dizziness** may be used to describe cortical or visual disorientations, altered states of consciousness, and limb incoordinations in addition to equilibrium disorders.

Two specific terms will be used to describe these disorders: 1) vertigo, and 2) dysequilibrium.

1. Vertigo. The term **vertigo** will be used specifically to describe symptoms of the vestibular (equilibrium) system. This includes peripheral labyrinthine, retrolabyrinthine, and/or CNS vestibular system disorders.
2. Dysequilibrium. The term **dysequilibrium** will be used to describe symptoms of spatial disorientations not caused by either peripheral (labyrinthine or retrolabyrinthine) or CNS vestibular system disorders. It also describes ataxia (CNS limb incoordinations) as a form of dysequilibrium, which must be differentiated from vertigo.

A misunderstanding of the differences between vertigo and dysequilibrium is responsible for much confusion in diagnosis, and for much inappropriate drug and surgical therapy for the "dizzy

TABLE 9-1. "Dizziness": Differentiation Between Vertigo and Dysequilibrium

	Vertigo	Dysequilibrium
Symptoms	True sensations of disturbed motion	Illusions of spatial disorientation or incoordination
Findings	Nystagmus	No nystagmus
Causes	Peripheral (labyrinthine or retrolabyrinthine) or CNS vestibular system disorders	Systemic disorders or nonvestibular CNS disease

patient." Table 9–1 presents the basic differences in symptoms, findings, and causes between vertigo and dysequilibrium.

True motion sickness is a complex syndrome related to the vestibular, proprioceptive, and visual systems. It is a maladaptation syndrome related to various types of motion. Thus it is a form of vertigo, with superimposed symptoms of pallor, cold sweating, nausea, and vomiting. It differs from dysequilibrium in that it does involve peripheral and central vestibular pathways.

VERTIGO

VERTIGO AND NYSTAGMUS

VERTIGO—THE SYMPTOM

Vertigo is the symptom denoting specific *illusions of motion,* related either to a sensation of turning or to a sensation of falling. It results from an asymmetrical neuronal firing pattern between the right and left vestibular systems. Vertigo may be "objective," in which the patients feels that the environment is turning or falling, or it may be "subjective," in which the patient feels that he or she is turning or falling. Combinations of both may occur. Sensations of abrupt turning may be directional, either to the right or left, and may be horizontal or rotary in pattern. They may also be described as vertical illusions of motion, related to a feeling of falling, as one would experience in a rapidly descending elevator or airplane.

NYSTAGMUS—THE FINDING

Nystagmus, the objective finding that accompanies vertigo, is related to head motion involving angular acceleration that causes an unequal endolymphatic concentration on one side of the cupulas of the semicircular canals. This displacement produces an afferent signal that results in nystagmus.

Nystagmus is usually an alternating involuntary movement of both eyes. It is characterized by a slow movement (slow component) to one side with a corrective fast return movement to the other side (quick component). By convention, nystagmus is identified by the direction of the quick component. Thus, a nystagmus to the left means a nystagmus which has a slow movement to the right and a quick corrective component to the left. The quick component actually represents the CNS corrective reflex. Although the slow component is the true index of cupular labyrinthine response, the quick component is more easily noted and quantified.

The direction of nystagmus may be horizontal, vertical, diagonal, or rotary. When describing the direction of rotary nystagmus, the horizontal component of the rotary nystagmus is utilized. Nystagmus, the objective component of vertigo, is the basis for nystagmography.

McCabe (1) defines vestibular nystagmus as a repetitive attempt to retain the field of last gaze by a conjugate movement of the eyes and a rapid reflex return of the eyeballs across the midline in compensation.

Nystagmus may be manifest or occult. Manifest nystagmus can be observed with the naked eye, in ordinary light. Occult nystagmus is that which can be observed either under magnification using +20 Frenzel lenses to abolish fixation, or that recorded by electronystagmography in the dark with abolition of ocular fixation.

CAUSES OF VERTIGO AND NYSTAGMUS

Vertigo and nystagmus can be produced either by peripheral (labyrinthine) or by central (CNS) disorders of the vestibular system and occasionally by combined lesions (Fig. 9–1).

Peripheral vertigo and nystagmus can originate from the semicircular canals and probably from the utricle and saccule of the labyrinth. They may originate from extralabyrinthine pathways, *i.e.,* the vestibular neurons and ganglia (Scarpa's ganglion), and from central afferent vestibular nerves in the internal auditory canal and meatus.

FIG. 9–1. Peripheral and central pathways for vertigo and nystagmus.

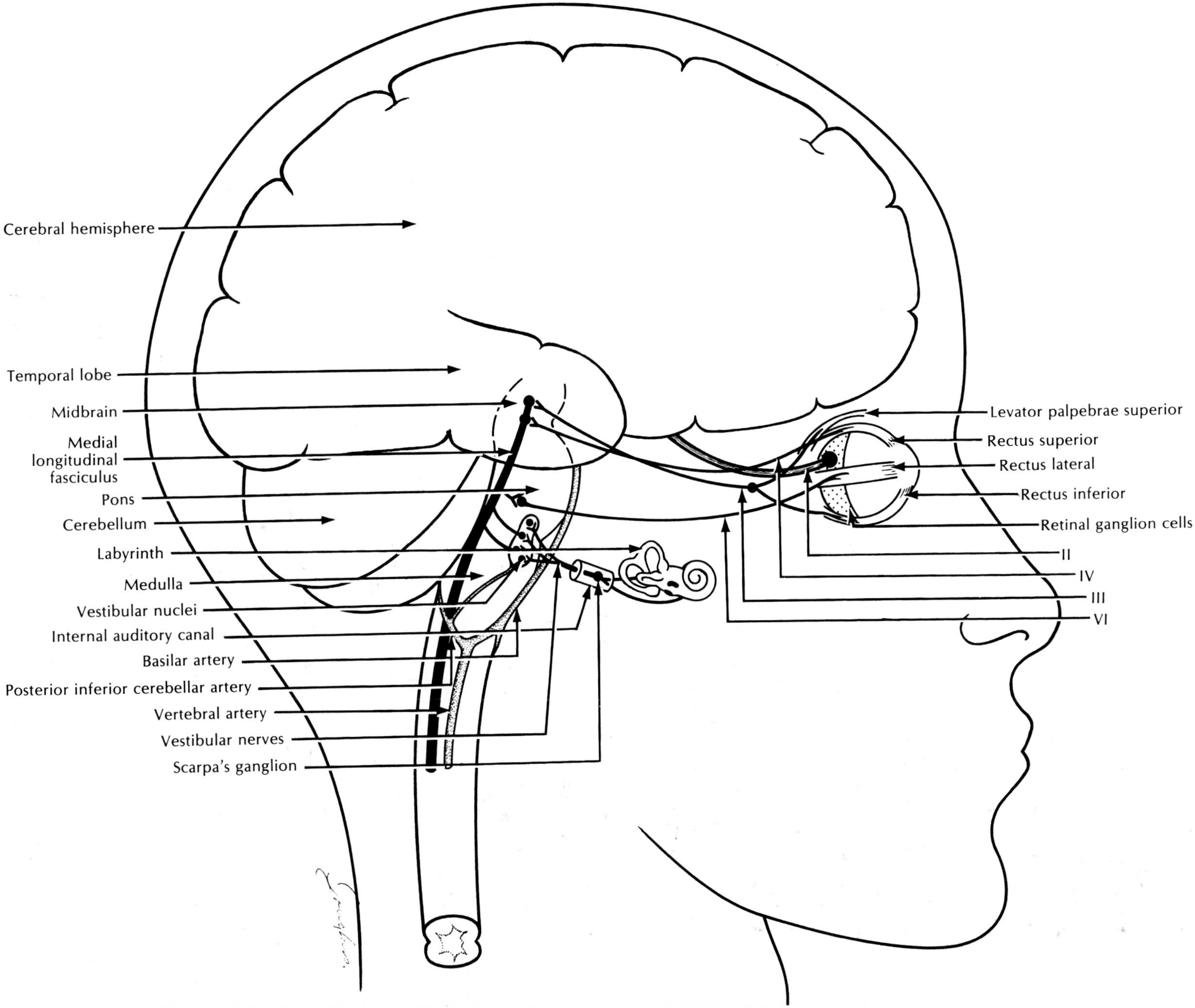

Levator palpebrae superior
Rectus superior
Rectus lateral
Rectus inferior
Retinal ganglion cells
II
IV
III
VI

Cerebral hemisphere
Temporal lobe
Midbrain
Medial longitudinal fasciculus
Pons
Cerebellum
Labyrinth
Medulla
Vestibular nuclei
Internal auditory canal
Basilar artery
Posterior inferior cerebellar artery
Vertebral artery
Vestibular nerves
Scarpa's ganglion

Central vertigo and nystagmus may be caused by a tumor in the temporal lobe (transverse gyrus of Heschl), by cerebral arteriosclerosis, and by lesions of the midbrain, pons, cerebellum, and brain stem. Lesions of the posterior inferior cerebellar artery will involve vestibular nuclei and their connections to the medial longitudinal fasciculus. Peripheral and central pathways can interact.

Peripheral vertigo is usually due to an assymmetry in neural firing patterns from labyrinthine sense organs or from their afferent nerve fibers. Labyrinthitis, Meniere's disease, and labyrinth fistulas are examples of common causes of peripheral vertigo. The symptoms of vertigo may be accompanied by symptoms of nausea, vomiting, and generalized malaise.

Peripheral vestibular or labyrinthine system vertigo is due either to intralabyrinthine or extralabyrinthine causes. Both intralabyrinthine and extralabyrinthine lesions may involve either 1) cochlear and vestibular sense organs (cochleovestibular), or 2) vestibular sense organs alone.

Cochleovestibular Disorders

These disorders will usually produce auditory symptoms and findings (hearing loss and tinnitus), as well as vestibular symptoms and findings (vertigo and nystagmus). Cochleovestibular lesions occur either in the labyrinth, the internal auditory canal and the internal auditory meatus or in the cerebellopontine angle.

Vestibular Disorders

These disorders will produce only vertigo and nystagmus, and can occur in the labyrinth, the internal auditory canal and internal auditory meatus, or in the cerebellopontine angle.

Because the seventh nerve (facial nerve) accompanies the eighth nerve (auditory-vestibular nerve) throughout its internal auditory canal course from the temporal bone petrosa through the internal auditory meatus to the cerebellopontine angle, seventh nerve symptoms and findings may accompany either intralabyrinthine or extralabyrinthine lesions.

The following outline presents the types of lesions which may occur in the peripheral vestibular system:

I. Cochleovestibular disorders (hearing loss and tinnitus, vertigo and nystagmus).
   A. Intralabyrinthine
      1. Meniere's disease
      2. Otosclerosis and sequelae of otosclerosis surgery
      3. Otomastoiditis with complications including labyrinthitis and labyrinthine fistula
      4. Hereditary or acquired congenital or delayed cochleovestibular syndromes
      5. Trauma of middle and inner ears
      6. Osteodystrophies
      7. Viropathies
      8. Syphilis
      9. Ototoxic drugs
      10. Tumors
   B. Extralabyrinthine (internal auditory meatus and cerebellopontine angle)
      1. Intracanalicular tumors and anomalies
      2. Cerebellopontine angle tumors and anomalies of blood vessels
      3. Herpes zoster oticus
II. Vestibular diseases (vertigo and nystagmus only)
   A. Intralabyrinthine
      1. Motion sickness, congenital vestibular end organ asymmetry, associated with sensory maladaptation
      2. Benign paroxysmal positional vertigo, otolithic vertigo
   B. Extralabyrinthine (retrolabyrinthine)
      1. "Toxic" vestibular neuronitis
      2. Viral vestibular neuronitis

CENTRAL NERVOUS SYSTEM VERTIGO AND NYSTAGMUS

Central nervous system vertigo and nystagmus come from lesions in the four vestibular nuclei in the brain stem, or from midbrain, cerebellum, and higher CNS vestibular pathway lesions.

Both vascular lesions and nonvascular lesions in the CNS will produce vertigo, nystagmus, occasionally hearing loss, and occasionally tinnitus.

The types of lesions that may produce CNS vertigo and nystagmus are listed:

I. Vascular lesions
   A. Subclavian and other "steal" syndromes
   B. Cervical spondylosis
   C. Intermittent vertebral-basilar insufficiency
   D. Vertebral-basilar "migraine"
   E. Posterior inferior cerebellar artery syndromes
   F. Anterior inferior cerebellar artery syndromes
   G. Internal auditory vestibular branch syndromes
II. Degenerative, neoplastic, or traumatic lesions
   A. Multiple sclerosis
   B. Vertiginous epilepsy (tornado)
   C. Cerebellar lesions (degeneration and tumors)
   D. Head injury

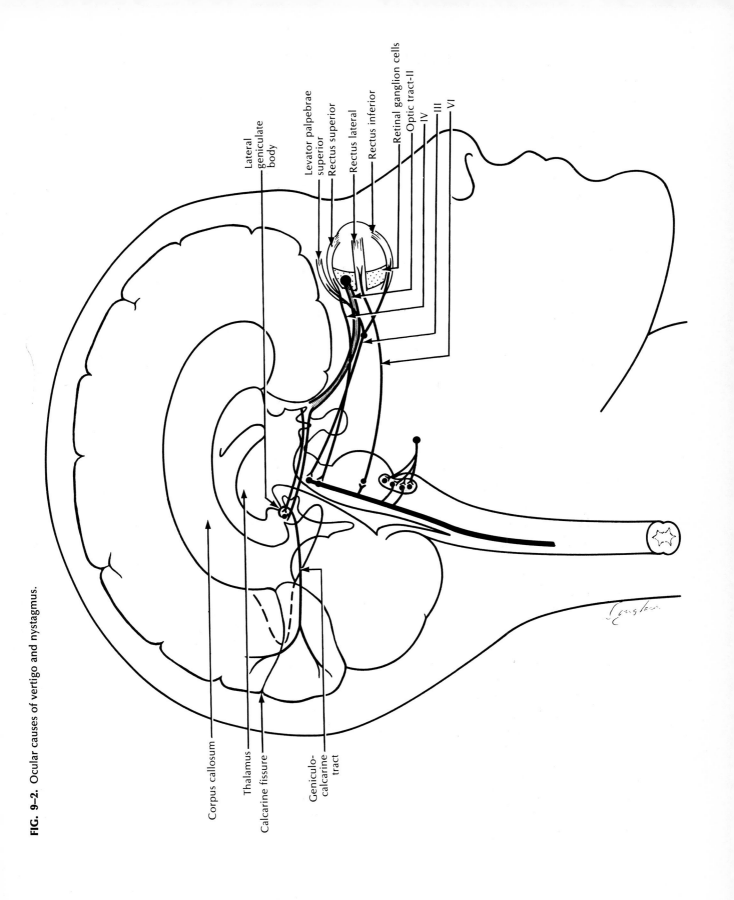

FIG. 9–2. Ocular causes of vertigo and nystagmus.

Lateral geniculate body

Levator palpebrae superior
Rectus superior
Rectus lateral
Rectus inferior
Retinal ganglion cells
Optic tract-II
III
IV
VI

Corpus callosum

Thalamus

Calcarine fissure

Geniculo-calcarine tract

FIG. 9–3. Vagal symptoms of respiratory rate changes, cardiac arrhythmia, nausea and vomiting, which can accompany vertigo.

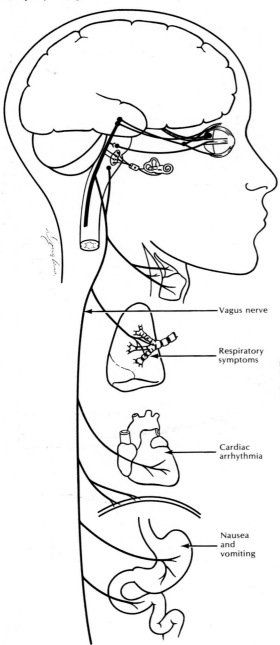

Vagus nerve

Respiratory symptoms

Cardiac arrhythmia

Nausea and vomiting

NEUROANATOMIC INTERRELATIONSHIPS IN VERTIGO AND NYSTAGMUS

Vertigo and nystagmus are also potential sequelae of any one of a number of neuroanatomic relationships involving the ears, the eyes, the CNS, the cardiovascular system, and the abdominal viscera.

A person normally oriented in space (2) is one in whom there is a harmonious integration of the afferent impulses *from each ear*—from labyrinthine semicircular canal cristas (angular rotary acceleration sensations), from labyrinthine otolithic maculas (gravity change-induced linear sensations), and *from each eye* (retinal postural reflexes). In addition to integration of right and left labyrinthine and ocular impulses, orientation in space is also modified by the muscle spindles and specialized nerve endings of the proprioceptive system (bones, muscles, and joints of the neck, trunk, and extremities).

A complete analysis of vertigo and nystagmus must also take into consideration the unified, coordinating mechanism, which consists of both labyrinths, the vestibular nerves, their ganglia and nuclei, ocular pathways, the spinal cord, cerebellum, medial longitudinal fasciculus (bundle), red nucleus, thalamus, hypothalamus, and the cerebral cortex.

The fibers of the medial longitudinal fasciculus (MLF) connect the vestibular pathway with eye muscle nuclei (oculomotor and trochlear nerves in the midbrain, abducens nerve in the pons). The MLF also relates the vestibular pathway with the spinal accessory nerve, and the anterior horn cells of the spinal cord supplying extremity muscles.

Nystagmus may result from MLF connections in lesions of the medulla, pons, or midbrain. Where past-pointing and the tendency to fall in a specific direction are present, the vestibulospinal tract has probably lost its normal regulatory control of anterior horn cells in the spinal cord.

Ocular lesions may participate through the MLF in vestibular symptoms. The relationships between the optic nerve and the vestibular nuclei are shown in Figure 9–2 in the neural arcs of the ocular vertigo and nystagmus pathway. Axons from the ganglion cells of the retina travel through optic nerve, optic chiasm, and the optic tract, which terminates in the lateral geniculate body. The geniculocalcarine pathway reaches the calcarine fissure of the occipital lobe and has intimate relationships with the nuclei of the oculomotor and trochlear nerves and the midbrain colliculus region. Synapses with the MLF make possible connections with brain-stem vestibular ganglia. A number of visual conditions have been implicated in episodic vertigo, probably because of dissociation of impulses coming from the retina, the eye muscle nuclei, and the vestibular apparatus.

Nausea and vomiting frequently accompany vestibular symptoms, either of peripheral or central origin. The vestibular nuclei have neuronal connections through the MLF to the visceral motor nucleus of the tenth (vagus) nerve and to the reticular activating system. In Figure 9–3 these vestibular, MLF, and tenth nerve relationships are illustrated with special reference to vagal connections with respiratory, cardiac, and gastric reflexes. Therefore, a patient with acute vertigo may present with irregular cardiac action, respiratory and gastrointestinal disturbances (especially nausea and frequently vomiting).

Motion sickness is a classic example of a vestibular syndrome complicated by interactions with cortical, ocular, and medial longitudinal fasciculus CNS pathways (see Ch. 27, Central Nervous System Vertigo and Motion Sickness).

REFERENCES

1. McCabe BF: Vestibular physiology: its clinical application in understanding the vertiginous patient. In Paparella M, Shumrick D (eds): Otolaryngology, Vol 1. Philadelphia, WB Saunders, pp 318–328, 1973
2. Spector B: Neuroanatomic mechanisms underlying vertigo and nausea. Bull N Engl Med Ctr 10:145–154, 1948

10

EXAMINATION OF THE DIZZY PATIENT

VICTOR GOODHILL
IRWIN HARRIS

VERTIGO OR DYSEQUILIBRIUM?

Since the patient with the complaint of "dizziness" may or may not have true vertigo, the first diagnostic task is to differentiate between the possibilities of vertigo and dysequilibrium. **Vertigo** is a disorder originating either in the peripheral or central vestibular system. **Dysequilibrium** may be the result of any one of a number of ataxic or systemic conditions. In the differential diagnostic approach, the first step is a special "dizziness" history. This is followed by a basic medical examination and a basic otologic examination. This preliminary study of the dizzy patient will frequently result in the diagnosis of dysequilibrium and a detailed vestibular electronystagmographic study will not be necessary.

SPECIAL HISTORY ON DIZZINESS

The challenge of the patient who says, "I am dizzy," involves a major problem in differential diagnosis. The history is the single most important diagnostic tool; it must be sufficiently detailed to elicit specific differences between the symptoms of vertigo and dysequilibrium. A systematic approach is essential. While it may be done informally, a written questionnaire is recommended. The following six sets of questions have been found extremely important in elucidating the problem.

However, before the patient is asked to respond to the six sets of questions, one basic question is asked by the examiner: "Please tell me what happens when you get dizzy? What happens to you? You may answer this question in any way, except that you may not use the words 'dizzy' or 'dizziness.' Use any other words you please." After the patient has described the subjective pattern of the "dizziness," a Dizziness Questionnaire is useful, either in oral or written form.

DIZZINESS QUESTIONNAIRE

This questionnaire deals with six approaches to dizziness: chronology; general pattern; hearing loss, tinnitus, or ear disease; ocular problems; CNS-ataxia problems; and dysequilibrium.

Chronology
1. When did your dizziness start?
2. Is your dizziness constant?
3. If your dizziness comes in attacks, how often?
4. Give dates (approximate) of most recent attacks.
5. How long does an attack last?
6. What kind of "warning" do you have before an attack?
7. Are you free of dizziness between attacks?
8. Does your dizziness start when you awaken in the morning?
9. Do you get airsick or seasick?
10. Do you get carsick, especially in the back seat?
11. Did your dizziness come on after a severe flu?
12. Did your dizziness follow a recent airplane trip?
13. Did your dizziness follow swimming or diving or physical exertion?

General Pattern
1. When you have an attack, do you feel as if you are falling?
   To the right _____ To the left _____
   Forward _____ Backward _____
2. Do you have nausea during an attack? Vomiting?
3. What position provokes an attack?
4. What do you think brings on an attack?
5. When you are dizzy, must you support yourself when you are standing?
6. Do you have a sensation of objects spinning or turning around you?
7. Do you have a sensation that you are turning or spinning inside?
8. Do you have "loss of balance" when walking?
9. Do you know anything that will stop your dizziness? Or make it feel better? Or make it worse?
10. Do you feel better if you sit or lie down when

you become dizzy?

11. Has there been any dizziness in any member of your family?

Hearing Loss, Tinnitus, or Ear Disease

1. Do you have a draining ear?
2. Have you ever had any kind of ear surgery?
3. Do you have a feeling of stuffiness in your ears when you have a dizzy spell?
4. Does your hearing seem to change at times?
5. Do you have any buzzing, ringing, or hissing in either ear?
6. Do you have any increase in ringing or buzzing before a dizzy attack; or after a dizzy attack?
7. Do you have a hearing loss in either ear?
8. Do you have earaches?

Ocular Problems

1. Do you ever have double vision?
2. Do you have trouble walking in the dark?
3. Do you have periods of blurred vision?
4. Do you ever have spots before your eyes?
5. Did you get new glasses recently?

CNS-Ataxia Problems

1. Do you ever have numbness of the face, arms, or legs?
2. Do you have a weakness in your arms or legs?
3. Do you have a feeling of clumsiness in your arms or legs?
4. Do you drop books or dishes unintentionally?
5. Do you have difficulty in speaking?
6. Is it hard for you to get words out, even though you know what you want to say?
7. Do you have difficulty with swallowing?
8. Do you ever have any tingling around your mouth?
9. Have you ever had a head injury? Were you unconscious?

Dysequilibrium

1. When you feel dizzy, are you lightheaded?
2. When you are dizzy, do you have a swimming sensation in the head?
3. When you are dizzy, do you feel as if you are going to black out?
4. When you are dizzy, do you lose consciousness?
5. When you are dizzy, do you also have a headache?
6. When you are dizzy, do you have a feeling of pressure in the head?
7. Do you feel faint when you are dizzy?
8. Do you get dizzy after overwork or exertion?
9. Do you get dizzy when you are hungry?
10. Do you have dizziness related to your menstrual cycle?
11. Do you use the "pill" (oral contraceptive)?

12. Do you get upset easily and cry easily?
13. Have you been under great emotional stress?
14. Do you smoke?
15. Do you drink alcohol?
16. What medications are you taking?
17. Do you have high blood pressure? Low blood pressure?
18. Are you anemic?
19. Are you on thyroid medication?
20. Do you feel dizzy when you turn over in bed, or when you first get up out of bed?

GENERAL MEDICAL EXAMINATION OF THE DIZZY PATIENT

A patient who complains of dizziness requires a careful general medical examination. It may seem simplistic to state that no patient complaining of dizziness should be approached primarily as an otologic, ophthalmologic, or neurologic problem. However, such approaches are frequently used, with mistaken diagnosis. A careful medical history and the special Dizziness Questionnaire should precede the basic medical examination.

Special concern should be given to the presence or absence of manifest nystagmus or ataxia, or otoscopic or tuning-fork test abnormalities, along with fundamental laboratory studies including urine, blood, chest x-rays, electrocardiogram, and other indicated procedures.

Thus, in the very first history and in the basic medical examination, positive findings may be discovered to attribute the dizziness to dysequilibrium caused by any one of a number of medical conditions.

The primary medical history, special dizziness history, and the general medical examination may reveal no manifest, spontaneous, or postural nystagmus or ataxia. Systemic abnormalities, however, may be disclosed that will point to the probability of dysequilibrium (pseudovertigo).

DYSEQUILIBRIUM (PSEUDOVERTIGO)

"Dizziness" may or may not be due to vertigo. It occasionally is due to ataxia, but in most instances it can be described by the general term, dysequilibrium (pseudovertigo).

Nonvestibular conditions frequently produce subjective symptoms of spatial disorientation. These symptoms may be accompanied by a number of findings, but no nystagmus can be detected and no disturbances of vestibular function can be elicited on vestibular examination.

Patients with such dizziness may describe feelings of disturbances of equilibrium or states of altered consciousness. Thus, patients may use the word "dizziness" to convey the feelings of blacking out, fainting, sinking, instability, drunkenness, light-headedness, inability to concentrate, floating in space, or visual confusion.

The term dysequilibrium includes a host of nonspecific illusions of orientation characterized by vagueness, lack of directionality, and by unclear time-linked relationships.

Dysequilibrium is usually constitutional in etiology. It may be related to cerebral oxygenation, blood pressure changes, or to various metabolic disorders. It may be due to drugs, visual disturbances, or to emotional disturbances.

No significant auditory or vestibular symptoms are associated with dysequilibrium. There is no spontaneous or positional nystagmus; caloric responses are usually normal on electronystagmographic vestibular examination, and auditory tests are usually normal. There are only occasional signs of ataxia in certain patients.

Dysequilibrium can result from a number of constitutional or CNS (nonvestibular) conditions.

POSTURAL HYPOTENSION

Hypotensive states may produce dysequilibrium. These are patients in whom significant transitory decreases in blood pressure may resemble vasovagal syncope and indicate a delayed cardiovascular system response to positional changes.

True orthostatic hypotension, a disease of the autonomic nervous system, is usually secondary to CNS or endocrine disease.

A number of hypotensive drugs used in hypertension may produce symptoms similar to orthostatic hypotension, especially in patients with varying degrees of carotid sinus hyperirritability.

Vertigo and nystagmus are rare in postural hypotension. The vague symptoms of "swimming," "giddy," "partial blackout," and "woozy" are the complaints of most of these patients. The diagnosis is suggested by the history, and symptoms may be elicited during examination by having the patient quickly change from supine to sitting to standing. The patient may manifest unsteadiness but no nystagmus. It is possible to measure significant changes in blood pressure upon such positional changes.

HYPERVENTILATION

Hyperventilation symptoms have been variously estimated as occurring in 10–27% of the population. Hyperventilation episodes are involuntary, and the patient is not aware of hyperventilating. The CO_2 reduction with subsequent changes in blood pH may constrict brain arterioles, reducing cerebral blood flow significantly. The reduced oxygen saturation of cerebral tissue produces slowing of brain waves and may give rise to the symptoms of imbalance and possibly ataxia, but rarely true vertigo. Emotional and metabolic factors may be etiologic.

Hyperventilation may occur quite commonly in young girls and has even been reported in "epidemics." Group patterns of hyperventilation have also been reported in military recruits.

Diagnosis of hyperventilation syndrome with dysequilibrium is easily made by having the patient breathe vigorously with the mouth open for several minutes. No vertigo or nystagmus will result, but the patient will usually complain of feeling giddy, lightheaded, distant, and occasionally true syncope may result.

Psychogenic functional causes undoubtedly play significant roles in the hyperventilation syndrome.

ARTERIOSCLEROSIS

Arteriosclerosis with symmetrical changes involving the carotid and vertebral systems rarely produces true episodic vertigo. In the majority of such patients dizziness is most commonly due to dysequilibrium. The transient ischemia attack is a frequent cause of dysequilibrium. It can produce vertigo and nystagmus if the lesion is specifically unilateral in relation to lower CNS vestibular pathway lesions.

HYPERTENSION

The hypertensive patient with pulsating tinnitus and headache may complain of dizziness. This is usually dysequilibrium unaccompanied by nystagmus or vestibular abnormalities as determined by electronystagmography.

HEMATOLOGIC DISORDERS

A number of hematologic disorders will affect cerebral blood flow and thus produce dizziness symptoms comparable to both postural hypotension and hyperventilation. Anemia, polycythemia, leukemia, microglobulinemia, and many other hematologic lesions may be characterized by periodic episodes of dysequilibrium. It is possible for hematologic disorders to produce true vertigo and nystagmus when there is asymmetric peripheral labyrinthine involvement. Leukemia, myeloma, and other hematologic lesions may specifically involve one or both labyrinths, with resultant true vertigo in addition to dysequilibrium.

METABOLIC DISORDERS

Dizziness may be a dysequilibrium related to menstrual cycles and/or hormonal drugs, including hormonal contraceptives.

Some women, both users and nonusers of oral contraceptives have described symptoms of "giddiness" in the immediate premenstrual period. Since ovarian hormones are known to have the capacity occasionally to produce edema, and since some cases of premenstrual tension have been explained as the result of cerebral edema, it has been postulated that a similar mechanism might be involved in the production of giddiness—dysequilibrium in women using oral contraceptives. A study was conducted (8) in an attempt to localize the equilibrium complaint to either the vertigo or dysequilibrium states. A search was made for positional and/or spontaneous nystagmus, and responses to calorization were studied. No significant consistent findings of spontaneous or positional nystagmus could be observed. Neither was there any true abnormality on caloric studies using electronystagmography. It was therefore concluded that the dizziness associated with hormonal conditions and that associated with hormonal contraceptives was a type of dysequilibrium and not true vertigo.

ATAXIA

The term ataxia is defined as *spatial incoordination* of the extremities. One example of ataxia is the gait disturbance in neurosyphilitic tabes dorsalis. Another example is the gait disturbance that may occur in darkness and is produced by bilateral peripheral vestibular paralysis resulting from streptomycin or other ototoxic drugs.

Subjective spatial extremity incoordination is accompanied by objective ataxia on various neurologic tests, *e.g.*, finger to nose adiodochokinesia.

Chronic ataxia is usually a CNS disease. However, an acute ataxic staggering can follow the same stimuli that produce vertigo and nystagmus of peripheral or central vestibular system origin.

THE DIZZY PATIENT—DIAGNOSTIC APPROACH

1. The symptom dizziness may be due to vertigo or to dysequilibrium.

2. Vertigo is the symptom of a peripheral or CNS vestibular disorder and is accompanied by manifest or occult nystagmus. Complex peripheral and CNS pathways may be involved in vertigo.
3. Dysequilibrium is a nonvestibular symptom of spatial disorientation. It is not accompanied by nystagmus.
4. The diagnostic approach to the dizzy patient requires both general medical and otologic considerations.
5. A number of constitutional or nonvestibular CNS conditions may produce dysequilibrium.
6. Since the dizzy patient may have either a general medical problem causing dysequilibrium or an otologic or neurootologic problem causing vertigo, the primary diagnostic approach must involve a systemic medical survey to rule out the various conditions that are responsible for dysequilibrium.
7. Such a medical study may uncover a definitive systemic explanation for the dizziness which is dysequilibrium rather than vertigo.
8. If the dizziness problem is not clearly systemic dysequilibrium a neurootologic study is necessary. This involves the detailed methodical dizziness history *and* a neurootologic examination.

The first approach to the dizzy patient is the management of any obvious medical problems discovered. With such management, the symptom of dizziness may disappear. If general medical examination does not suggest dysequilibrium, an otologic evaluation is indicated. The initial medical examination may reveal adiadochokinesia, or ataxic gait, or other neurologic abnormalities suggestive of ataxia, in which case, a neurologic evaluation is also indicated.

BASIC OTOLOGIC EXAMINATION OF THE DIZZY PATIENT

The basic ENT examination is described in Chapter 2. The basic otologic examination of the dizzy patient includes basic ENT, audiometric, radiologic, vestibular, and screening neurologic examinations. Such an approach will result in a specific diagnosis without further special studies.

BASIC ENT EXAMINATION

The otologic examination is preceded by an examination of the nose, paranasal sinuses, pharynx, oral structures, and larynx. The neck is examined for masses and auscultated for bruits. The maxillas and mandible are palpated. A preliminary examination for ocular paralysis or manifest spontaneous nystagmus is made.

Examination of the postauricular area, auricle, external auditory canal, and tympanic membrane is made. Adequate visualization of the external auditory canal and tympanic membrane may require preliminary careful removal of cerumen and epithelial debris. Material from a discharging ear should be examined by appropriate smears and cultures.

Examination of the tympanic membrane includes a careful search for perforations, granulomas, or tumors, and should involve an examination of tympanic membrane mobility by pneumatic otoscopy and by observation of mobility following Valsalva inflation, and politzerization. In the presence of a perforation, careful pneumatic compression may elicit a possible fistula response in terms of nystagmus or atypical nystagmoid eye deviations. A positive fistula test may or may not be accompanied by a sensation of sudden dizziness and nausea. Occasionally, a positive fistula test with nystagmus or ocular deviation may occur with an intact tympanic membrane (12).

BASIC AUDIOLOGIC STUDY

Careful measurement of hearing function begins with Rinne and Weber tuning-fork tests with 128-, 256-, and 512-Hz forks. The standard audiogram (pure tone, air conduction, bone conduction, speech reception threshold, and speech discrimination studies with appropriate masking) is followed if necessary by the special differential sensorineural diagnostic auditory test battery, and in some cases by the conductive loss test battery (see Ch. 6, Audiologic Assessment, Functional Hearing Loss, and Objective Audiometry).

BASIC RADIOLOGIC STUDY

The minimal radiographs required for an otologic examination are plain Schuller views of the mastoids and Stenver view of the petrous pyramid—the internal auditory canal and the meatus. Additional radiographs may be indicated (see Ch. 4, Otoradiology), including transorbital views, polytomographic studies, CAT scan or contrast studies if suggested by otoaudiologic and/or vestibular findings.

In cases where there is a question of contributory rhinologic disease, a plain Waters' view sinus film is indicated. Occasionally, other sinus views and skull films may be necessary.

THE BASIC VESTIBULAR STUDY

The semicircular canal system, arranged in pairs bilaterally at 90° planes, allows one pair of canals for each three-dimensional plane. Movement of the contained endolymph stimulates the crista and its ampulla: 1) Rotation of a patient in a chair will produce sensory stimuli because of fluid motion with resultant series of reflexes; 2) calorization by irrigation of an ear canal with cold water or warm water will produce a thermosiphon effect and result in a reflex response because of stimulation of the crista.

Two basic reflex arcs are associated with semicircular canal stimulation, the vestibulospinal arc and the vestibuloocular arc. Both are useful in clinical studies of the vestibular system.

The vestibulospinal reflex pattern is tested in the Romberg, walking, and past-pointing tests. The vestibuloocular reflex is tested in ocular nystagmus studies.

Nystagmus, an alternating involuntary movement of both eyes, is most frequently horizontal and is characterized by a slow movement to one side with a corrective fast movement to the other side. By convention, nystagmus is identified by the direction of the quick component. Thus, a nystagmus to the left means a nystagmus that has a slow component to the right and a quick corrective movement to the left. The quick component represents the CNS corrective reflex. The slow movement is the true index of cupular response from the labyrinth, but the quick component, the corrective component, is more easily noted and quantified.

The rapid eye movements that occur as the gaze is shifted to "place" visual objects into the macular part of the visual field, are known as saccades. Saccadic movement is very fast. Alcohol and some drugs can reduce saccadic velocity markedly (19).

Direction of nystagmus is usually horizontal, but can be vertical, diagonal, or rotary. When describing the direction of rotary nystagmus the horizontal component of the rotary nystagmus is utilized. Nystagmus intensity is usually described as being of first, second or third degree.

The utriculosaccular system, responding to gravity changes upon the otoliths and their maculas, is more difficult to assess clinically. Although true nystagmus appears to be evoked by horizontal or vertical stimulation, it is slower and more difficult to interpret. Counter rolling of the eyes is a proven method of measuring the gravity receptor otolith system, but its recording techniques and interpretation facets have not yet been fully developed for clinical use.

Nystagmus is not a normal phenomenon. It can occur in a number of vestibular lesions, either as spontaneous nystagmus or an evoked reaction. Postural nystagmus is evoked by changing positions of the head. Nystagmus can also be evoked by rotation or calorization.

Thus, examination of the vestibular system involves, first, detection of spontaneous nystagmus, then positional nystagmus. Evoked nystagmus studies following rotation and calorization stimuli complete the vestibular study.

The basic vestibular study does not require elaborate equipment. Electronystagmography is useful, but it is not always essential. It is frequently possible to get adequate diagnostic information by ordinary visual examination for manifest (spontaneous and positional) and evoked nystagmus. The use of +20 diopter Frenzel lenses will eliminate eye reflex inhibition by gaze fixation.

Spontaneous Nystagmus

The Romberg and past-pointing tests precede a search for spontaneous nystagmus. The patient, sitting erect, may show evidence of spontaneous nystagmus of first, second, or third degree. Gaze nystagmus may be noted on lateral gaze command.

Positional Nystagmus

Positional testing is performed with patient lying on a couch in a number of positions.

Spontaneous horizontal nystagmus is usually of peripheral origin (labyrinthine or vestibular disease). Spontaneous vertical, rotary, or diagonal nystagmus is usually of CNS origin. Positional-direction-changing nystagmus without apparent vertigo is highly suggestive of a CNS lesion. Extremely active spontaneous nystagmus without vertigo indicates a CNS lesion.

Evoked Caloric Nystagmus

The classic approach to examination of the thermosiphon effect of the semicircular canal system was through the ice-water caloric study, a method of mass or suprathreshold stimulation now reserved for special problems. The limited use of only cold stimulation gives only one set of response parameters to the examiner, frequently obscuring proper diagnosis.

The development of the Hallpike bithermal caloric test technique is a very important advance over the ice-water caloric test. Not only is the bithermal test more comfortable for the patient, but it is much more sensitive, allowing the examiner to make comparisons of various responses to quan-
titatively determine *right or left labyrinthine preponderance* (usually a sign of peripheral vestibular disease) or *directional preponderance* (considered to be a sign of CNS disease, but still debated).

The Hallpike bithermal caloric test is performed by having the patient lie on a couch with head elevated on a pillow at 30°. Comparisons between right and left ear responses and between warm (44° C) and cold (30° C) calorization responses make possible such definitive findings as those of a hyporeactive (canal paresis) labyrinth, a nonreactive ("dead") labyrinth, or directional nystagmus preponderance.

Evoked Rotation Nystagmus

Sinusoidal rotation in a chair or torsion swing will evoke nystagmus (usually horizontal). Absence of nystagmus points to bilaterally nonresponsive vestibular systems, which may be due to labyrinthine or CNS lesions.

It is possible for adequate diagnostic information to be obtained by such noninstrumental studies of nystagmus, preceded or followed by an otoneurologic survey. However, in many cases, more precise and detailed approaches to the patient with vertigo are necessary. Vestibular electronystagmographic study is then indicated.

THE OTONEUROLOGIC EXAMINATION

The otoneurologic examination includes a systemic, cranial nerve, and CNS survey. Comparative right and left blood pressures are examined for detection of possible "steal" syndromes. This is followed by auscultation of the skull (supraorbital regions, temporal squamae, and mastoid processes) and neck for evidence of bruits.

Since CNS causes of vertigo are frequently accompanied by cranial nerve involvements other than the eighth nerve, methodical cranial nerve survey is necessary.

Otoneurologic Examination
(Check List)

Blood pressure
    Right arm
    Left arm
Auscultation for bruits
    Over eyes
    Mastoids
    Temporal squamae
    Neck
Cranial nerves
      I Nerve: olfactory nerve
        Smell—check whether patient, with eyes
          closed, can identify smells of

        Coffee
        Tobacco
        Cloves
        Mint
   II Nerve: optic nerve
        Spontaneous nystagmus—degree
        Pupillary responses
           Light reflex
           Consensual reflex
           Accommodation
        Fundoscopic examination
  III, IV, and VI Nerves: oculumotor, trochlear, and
     abducens nerves)
        Eye motion
        Conjugate motion
    V Nerve: trigeminal nerve
        Open mouth against resistance
        Corneal reflex
        Facial sensation
  VII Nerve: facial nerve
        Facial motion
        Taste
   IX Nerve: Glossopharyngeal nerve
        Palatal and pharyngeal reflex
        Position of soft palate
    X Nerve: Vagus nerve
        Vocal cord examination
        Motion of soft palate
        Sensation of skin of external auditory canal
   XI Nerve: Accessory nerve
        Forced motion for head turn
        Shoulder shrug
  XII Nerve: Hypoglossal nerve
        Motion of tongue

Cerebellar function
    Finger-to-nose test
    Adiodochokinesia
    Walking forward and backward
    Romberg test
    Tandem studies
    Deep tendon reflexes

VESTIBULOMETRY BY MEANS OF ELECTRONYSTAGMOGRAPHY

Although valuable and frequently diagnostic vestibular information can be obtained without instrumentation, a number of diagnostic advantages make electronystagmographic (ENG) examination preferable.

For example, although the Hallpike bithermal caloric test can be performed and give useful information without recording techniques, it is far more valuable to be able to examine and measure an ENG record and thus quantify test findings. The measurement of nystagmus amplitudes, latencies, and duration can be accomplished by ENG recording of nystagmus beats and nystagmus patterns.

Various methods are used to compute the characteristics of vestibular responses to caloric stimulation. Vestibulometry gives information regarding specific amplitudes of slow and quick components, dysrhythmia, and other graphic aspects of the response pattern. Information from vestibulometry as an analogue to audiometry has expedited otologic differential diagnoses.

The problem of ocular fixation can cause confusion in non-ENG studies of nystagmus patterns, although it is possible to reduce ocular fixation by the use of +20-diopter glasses. In electronystagmographic vestibular examinations carried out in a darkened room, abolition of ocular fixation is possible, and responses with both eyes either closed or open can be obtained. Both responses are useful diagnostically.

THE ELECTRONYSTAGMOGRAPHIC TEST TECHNIQUE

Electrical recording of the displacement of the cornea–retina potential on movement of the eye is the basis for current clinical electrical graphic recordings of nystagmus. It provides a permanent, objective record that can be carefully measured and evaluated. It is more sensitive than visual observation and can record nystagmus behind closed or open eyes in a darkened room (removing the suppressive effect of visual fixation). A one-channel recording of horizontal nystagmus is commonly used clinically, but two-channel recordings for both horizontal and vertical nystagmus are used now increasingly in many clinics. Four channels may be used to record horizontal, vertical, and two diagonal channels. In our clinic the four-channel method has been in use for several years as a clinical investigative tool. The vertical and diagonal channels may prove to have additional diagnostic value in the future (Figs. 10–1, 10–2).

Clement and Goodhill (3) have reported the use of such four-channel ENG recordings in animal experiments. It was possible to record induced nystagmus as a response to parallel-swing linear acceleration, probably generated by the otolith system.

In our clinic, nystagmus is recorded on the Beckman Dynograph, model R. This recorder has microvolt sensitivity up to 1 mv and a high-frequency cutoff at 26 Hz. An AC coupler is used with a time constant of 5 sec. Skin electrodes made of silver and silver chloride are employed. Electrolyte paste makes the only contact between skin and the electrode.

Testing is performed in a semidark room. The patient is tested with eyes closed, thus eliminating

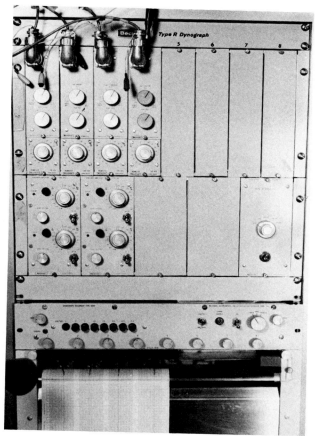

FIG. 10–1. Four-channel recorder for electronystagmography (ENG).

FIG. 10–2. Four-channel ENG tracing.

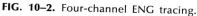

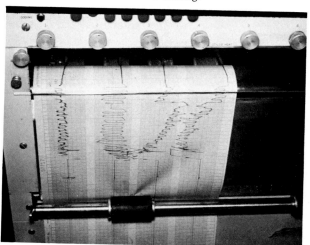

light and fixation, factors known to inhibit nystagmus. The patient is asked to count backwards during the test to maintain an "alert" state, a factor that facilitates the appearance of an existent nystagmus. The speed of the slow component of the nystagmus at its culmination is chosen as the representative criterion of its intensity.

Pretest Instructions

Prior to examination, the patient is given a set of instructions explaining the ENG procedure and directing the patient not to wear makeup and to avoid alcohol and certain medications, *i.e.*, sedatives, tranquilizers or antivertigo drugs, for at least 48 hours prior to the examination. Figure 10–3 shows suppression of nystagmus by drowsiness. Drowsiness produced by such drugs can suppress nystagmus needle excursions through cortical (central) mediation of the reflex arc.

The Electronystagmographic Examination

PREPARATION OF THE PATIENT AND CALIBRATION. The skin around the eyes is cleansed, removing all makeup and surface oils. Electrodes are attached firmly to the skin close to the eyes. A ground electrode is attached to the forehead (Fig. 10–4). A lack of good skin–electrode contact may result in poor recording. Within a minute or two, the electrode paste has set, and calibration of eye movements may be performed and recorded. A calibration board with alternately flickering lights is used to calibrate eye movements (20° of eye movement per 20 mm movement of the needle on the electronystagmogram). This calibration is performed for each channel, to compare accurately the amplitude between channels (Fig. 10–5). Horizontal calibration is performed, followed by similar vertical and optional diagonal calibration.

The patient is placed on a comfortable couch or table in the supine position with head elevated 30° and is asked to look back and forth on command between two lights set 20° apart. The excursion for horizonal nystagmus is 10° to the right of center and 10° to the left of center. If the patient has an artificial eye, only the one seeing eye is used, with all electrodes placed around that eye. Calibration patterns of eye movements are observed for deviations from the normal. Such a deviation is significant in what has been described as "calibration overshoot," which is frequently a sign of cerebellar disease (an ocular form of past-pointing).

Blinking should not be confused with nystagmus. Blinking patterns can easily be detected and differentiated from nystagmic beats by their shape (Fig. 10–6).

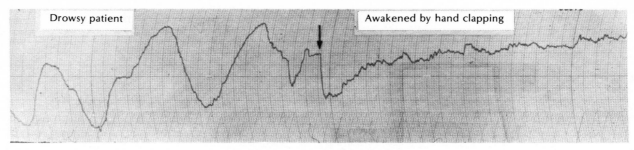

Drowsy patient | Awakened by hand clapping

FIG. 10–3. An ENG tracing of drowsy patient awakened by hand-clapping.

FIG. 10–4. Electrodes attached. Calibration underway.

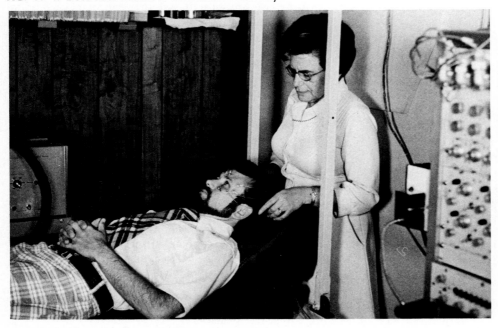

FIG. 10–5. At top, horizontal calibration. **At bottom,** vertical calibration. (The same board can be used for diagonal calibration.)

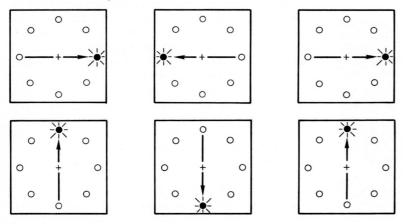

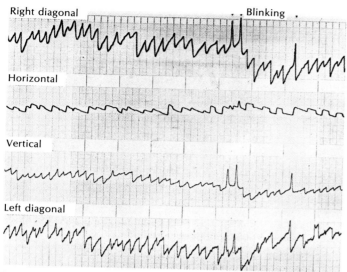

FIG. 10–6. Blinking pattern, contrasted with nystagmus beats. Blinking is noted most clearly in vertical and in diagonal channels.

SPONTANEOUS NYSTAGMUS. Spontaneous nystagmus, if present, may be recorded with the patient in the straight, erect sitting position. Measurements are obtained with eyes open and eyes closed. Each position for either spontaneous or positional nystagmus testing is maintained for at least 90 sec. Since voluntary suppression can result in nystagmus modification, the patient is asked to perform a mental exercise such as counting backward which requires concentration. Such instruction will usually eliminate voluntary nystagmus suppression. If either spontaneous (Figs. 10–7, 10–8) or positional nystagmus persists (unlimited duration), it usually is considered pathologic.

GAZE NYSTAGMUS AND POSITIONAL NYSTAGMUS. The gaze test is performed at the beginning of positional testing, while the patient is supine, with the head elevated 30°. The patient is asked to gaze alternately at lights, 15 sec per light, which are 20° to the right and 20° to the left of a midline. Gaze nystagmus in either direction is considered abnormal.

Positional testing (Figs. 10–9, 10–10) is performed in the following positions: supine, eyes open, eyes closed; right lateral, eyes open and eyes closed; left lateral, prone, hanging head, sitting with head turned to the right, and sitting with head turned to the left.

CALORIZATION—HALLPIKE BITHERMAL CALORIC TEST. The purpose of the bithermal test is to compare warm and cold stimulation parameters for each ear. Conventionally, the ears are irrigated first with water at 30°C and then with water at 44°C (Figs. 10–11, 10–12). These temperatures have been shown to elicit maximal response without undue discomfort. The pattern of each is observed insofar as 1) *duration* is concerned. Since the range of normal may be from 50 sec to 5 min, care must be taken in interpreting results. More precise information is obtained with reference to 2) *amplitude.* Cold stimuli produce contralateral nystagmus; warm stimuli produce ipsilateral nystagmus.

In a normal labyrinth, cold irrigation (30°C) on the left results in a contralateral nystagmus (quick component to the right—right-beating nystagmus). Cold irrigation (30°C) on the right will result in a quick component nystagmus to the left—left-beating nystagmus. Warm irrigation (44°C) on the left results in a left-beating nystagmus, and warm irrigation (44°C) on the right results in a right-beating nystagmus.

HALLPIKE PREPONDERANCE FORMULA. Horizontal eye movement calibration is rechecked prior to each irrigation. During this test, the patient is once again in the supine position with head elevated 30° so that the horizonal semicircular canal is in a horizontal plane. At least four 30-sec caloric irrigations (approximately 250 cc each) are performed. Each ear is irrigated at intervals of 10 min, beginning with water of 30°C and then at

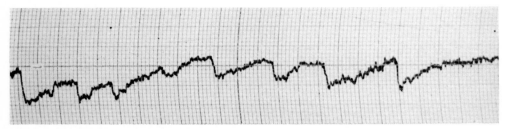

FIG. 10–7. Spontaneous nystagmus to left.

FIG. 10–8. Spontaneous nystagmus to right.

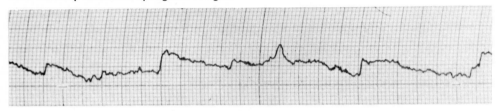

FIG. 10–9. Only three electrodes were used in this patient for the two-channel ENG recording. **A, B, C,** and **D.** Various positions used to elicit spontaneous nystagmus.

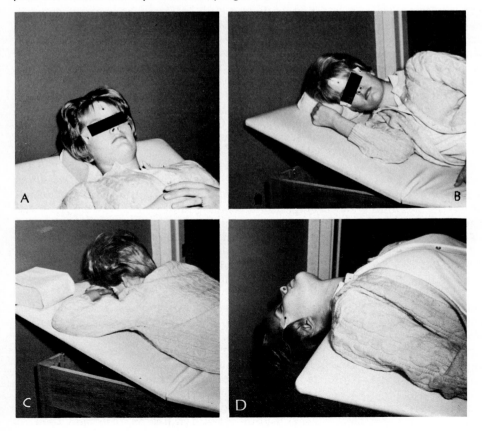

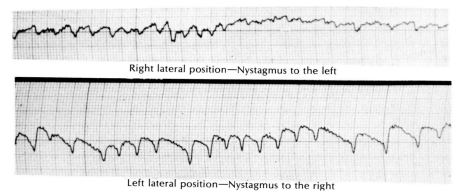

Right lateral position—Nystagmus to the left

Left lateral position—Nystagmus to the right

FIG. 10–10. ENG tracings of positional nystagmus, right and left.

FIG. 10–11. Controlled thermal irrigator for Hallpike bithermal caloric test.

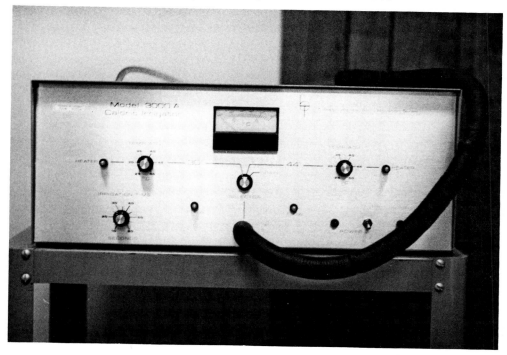

44°C (7° below and above normal body temperature). The patient should rest for at least 8 min between irrigations.

When any one caloric response is greatly skewed (high or low), it is repeated. To avoid voluntary inhibition of nystagmus, the patient is asked to perform mental concentration activity (backward counting) immediately following each irrigation, while the nystagmus is being recorded.

Maximum response is usually observed between 30 and 60 sec following irrigation. Sixty seconds following irrigation, the patient is asked to open the eyes, and nystagmus suppression is observed: Such suppression is considered normal, and absence of suppression is considered pathologic.

To objectively measure calorization results, the maximum speed of the slow phase following each irrigation is measured. Degrees of nystagmus, of

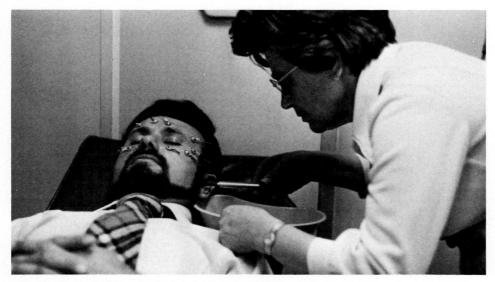

FIG. 10–12. Technique of caloric irrigation for Hallpike test.

FIG. 10–13. Hallpike caloric stimulation diagram. **A.** Normal response. **B.** Left canal paresis = right labyrinthine preponderance. **C.** Right directional preponderance (CNS?)

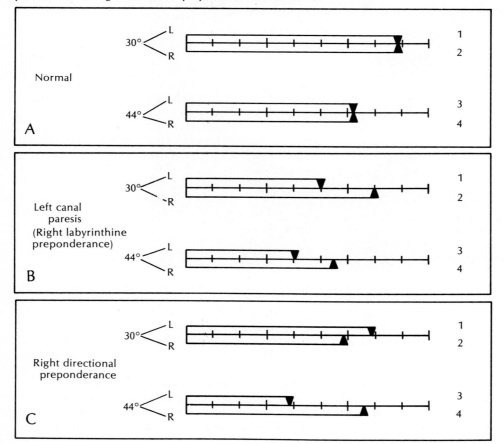

both the right and left ear, and right and left beating directions are computed.

The standard formula used to express labyrinthine preponderance (*LP*) or directional preponderance (*DP*) with the speed of the slow component of the nystagmus in degrees per second is as follows:

1. Left cold: nystagmus to the right
2. Right cold: nystagmus to the left
3. Left warm: nystagmus to the left
4. Right warm: nystagmus to the right

$$LP = (1 + 3) - (2 + 4)/(1 + 2 + 3 + 4) \times 100\%$$

$$DP = (1 + 4) - (2 + 3)/(1 + 2 + 3 + 4) \times 100\%$$

The *LP* (difference between ears) is considered significant when it is 14–30% or greater, and the *DP* is considered significant when it is 18–30% or greater.

The preponderance diagram affords a visual representation of caloric responses (Fig. 10–13).

In labyrinthine preponderance, the conventional *implication is that the ear contralateral to the preponderant ear* is pathologic. Thus, a left labyrinthine preponderance of 40% implies that the vestibular response of the right labyrinth is depressed or hypoactive (also termed **canal paresis**). There are differing opinions concerning this interpretation. Not infrequently, the preponderant ear will demonstrate audiologic findings pointing to ipsilateral disease rather than contralateral disease. Can a preponderant vestibular response point to vestibular hyperactivity or vestibular *recruitment* (increased sensation response to stimulation)? This question is still unanswered.

The significance of directional preponderance relative to CNS disease is still debated.

Positional nystagmus recorded before calorization may have an effect on observed nystagmus during calorization. In such a case, ice-water stimulation (of at least 0°C) is used to verify the activity of the tested labyrinth. Ice water is also used when there is no response to the standard 7° temperature changes. A 15-sec irrigation is performed. If there is a resulting nystagmus beating to the expected or contralateral direction in the supine position, the patient is maneuvered into the prone position, in which the nystagmus is expected to reverse direction if it has originated in the labyrinth stimulated calorically. This is a currently debated concept, but it is an important diagnostic dilemma that requires solution.

Positional nystagmus may be a normal finding if it appears in three or four head positions in low amplitudes. It becomes an abnormal finding if it occurs in most of the test positions and if the speed is great (high amplitude). Positional nystagmus that occurs in a few positions at low amplitudes is not of pathologic significance. However, unexplained positional nystagmus calls for repeated vestibular studies for clarification.

Positional alcoholic nystagmus (PAN) has been known for many decades. It is a temporary finding, with many variables. Total vestibular system responses to alcohol ingestion are still under study.

DRY CALORIZATION. Dry calorization may be performed by using a finger cot to confine the irrigation. When a patient has a tympanic membrane perforation, an open mastoid cavity, or any other otologic condition in which caloric irrigation would be medically contraindicated, finger cots are placed in both ears and a 40-sec irrigation is performed using cold temperatures of 25°C and warm temperatures of 49°C (Fig. 10–14). Equipment is now also available to substitute warm and cool air in place of water for caloric stimulation (Figs. 10–15, 10–16). The finger cot technique is simple, reliable, and inexpensive (7).

SINUSOIDAL ROTATION TEST. The sinusoidal rotation test has supplanted the traditional Barany rotation tests in our clinic. Following calorization, after the patient has rested at least 10 min, a rotational test is administered in the form of sinusoidal stimulation. The patient is turned to the left and the right in sinusoidal fashion while sitting in a rotating chair (Fig. 10–17), with eyes closed, facing straight ahead. The movement results in the stimulation of both the labyrinths at the same time. Differences between the left and right beating nystagmus are computed by measuring the number of beats to each direction (Figs. 10–18, 10–19).

OPTOKINETIC TEST. The patient is placed before a screen illuminated by an optokinetic drum that projects images normally producing optic stimulation. Striped patterns are moved to the left and then to the right. Slow and fast speeds are used in each direction. Asymmetry and differences in intensity of nystagmus between directions is considered abnormal and indicative of a CNS site of lesion.

Electrodes are removed following the optokinetic test, and the clinician calculates and records the ENG studies. These findings are then correlated with other examination results concern-

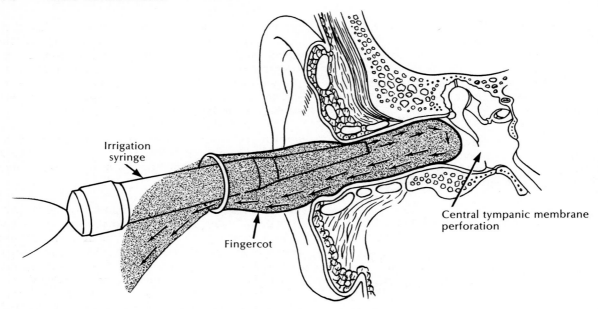

FIG. 10–14. Diagrammatic drawing of dry calorization method using fingercot to protect a diseased ear from direct irrigation.

FIG. 10–15. Poor nystagmus was evoked in **B** because of thermal insulation, but there was close correlation between **A** and **C** when temperature was increased by 5°.

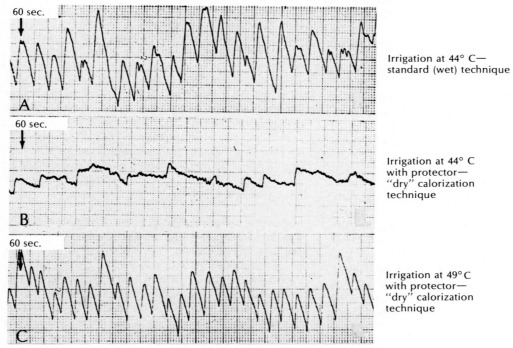

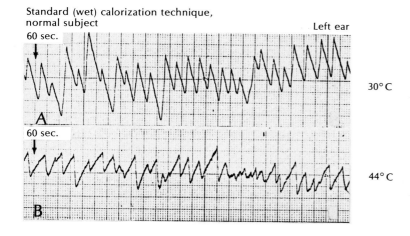

Standard (wet) calorization technique,
normal subject

Left ear

60 sec.

30° C

A

60 sec.

44° C

B

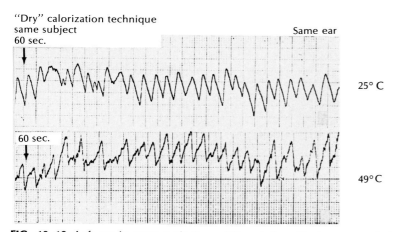

"Dry" calorization technique
same subject

Same ear

60 sec.

25° C

60 sec.

49°C

FIG. 10–16. Left ear in same patient on different days illustrates correlation between standard wet calorization and dry calorization technique.

ing the site and nature of the lesion, for the purpose of determining, quantifying, and comparing data for test-retest purposes.

COMPARISON OF OPTOKINETIC, COMMAND, AND FOLLOWING RESPONSES. Significant indications of CNS disease can be obtained by comparing responses to the optokinetic images, to eye-movement command, and to following a moving finger or pencil of light in the ENG examination.

Dix (5) pointed out the diagnostic importance of such observations. In Figure 10–20 the normal relationships are demonstrated. In Figure 10–21, in a patient with basal ganglion disease, dramatic differences may be noted. The responses to commands to shift the gaze are slow and irregular, the optokinetic responses show gross abnormalities, and when the optokinetic drum is reversed from left to right the eyes deviate to the right.

An obvious objective of the optokinetic examination is to differentiate between vertigo of peripheral origin and that of central origin. However, localization of the site of vestibular disease is not always simple. Morisette *et al.* made a comparative study of 15 normals, 10 patients with unilateral labyrinthectomy, and 8 patients with neurologically confirmed brain-stem lesions (11). They found a pattern of decreasing eye response to increasing drum speed to be characteristic of brain-stem lesions. Stare optokinetic nystagmus was not much affected by a peripheral vestibular lesion even as severe as complete unilateral labyrinthectomy.

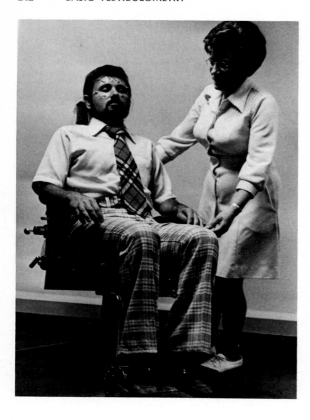

FIG. 10–17. Sinusoidal rotation test.

FIG. 10–18. Nystagmoid responses to sinusoidal rotation.

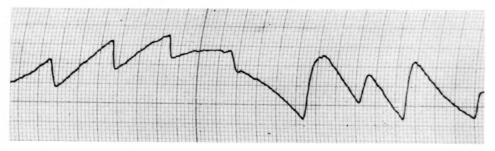

GALVANIC VESTIBULAR STIMULATION. The passage of a direct current stimulus between the two mastoid regions produces several vestibular responses. Varying reports of significance of galvanic testing have appeared from time to time. Weiss and Tole (18) report studies pointing to the necessity for intact vestibular nerve for measurement of galvanic effects. They believe that quantifiable galvanic techniques for vestibular testing will be developed.

Coats (2) reported that galvanic body sway responses have lower thresholds than nystagmic responses. He reports that because of this low threshold, body sway response can be elicited painlessly with monoauricular and monopolar stimulation. It is believed that such studies will expedite differential diagnosis between vestibular and retrovestibular lesions.

AGE AND VESTIBULAR FUNCTION

Vestibular studies can be performed on infants and young children, and are extremely important in a number of differential diagnostic problems.

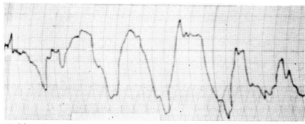

Calibration

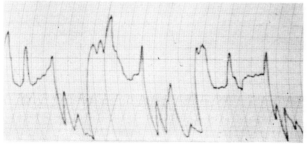

Sinusoidal rotation responses

FIG. 10–19. Calibration and sinusoidal rotation responses in an 18-month-old child.

FIG. 10–20. Command, following, and optokinetic responses in a normal subject. **Arrows,** drum reversal. (Dix MR: Proc Roy Soc Med 64:857–860, 1971)

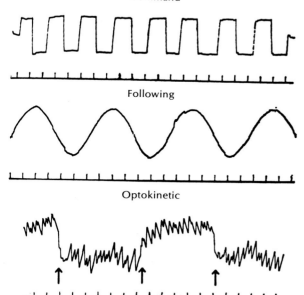

Command

Following

Optokinetic

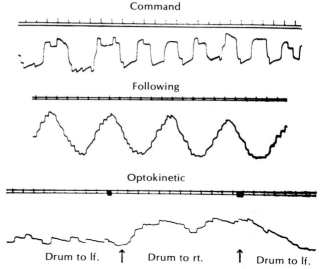

Command

Following

Optokinetic

Drum to lf.   ↑   Drum to rt.   ↑   Drum to lf.

FIG. 10–21. Command, following, and optokinetic responses in a patient with basal ganglion disease. (Dix MR: Proc Roy Soc Med 64:857–860, 1971)

There is a definite correlation between birth weight and maturation of vestibular responses as an index of CNS maturation (6).

Vestibular studies may be performed on infants and young children by the simple sinusoidal rotation test (Fig. 10–22). The child is seated on the mother's lap during the rotation test, which may be performed either with or without electronystagmographic registration. Nystagmus will be elicited in most children. Preterm babies and term babies will differ in vestibular responsiveness. However, at the age of 6 months, most infants may show fairly normal responses to vestibular stimulation, either by sinusoidal rotation or in response to calorization.

In adults there are some differences between younger and older individuals. In young people a nystagmus with small frequency and large amplitude is usually found. In older people the nystagmus will show a higher frequency and a smaller amplitude.

SPECIAL AND UNUSUAL ELECTRONYSTAGMOGRAPHIC FINDINGS

OCULAR DYSMETRIA

In addition to conventional electronystagmographic studies, both pendulum tracking and individual eye testing, with the other eye covered, will be of significant diagnostic value. Severe ocular dysmetria is characterized by a change in the normal sine wave in pendulum tracking to a very erratic curve.

THE TULLIO PHENOMENON

Ever since the experiments of Tullio (17), who showed in the pigeon that the ampulla of a semicircular canal can be excited by an acoustic stimulus, attempts at studying auditory-vestibular relationships have been made. A sonoocular test has been worked out that is based upon ENG response to acoustic signals. (15). This can be very helpful in diagnosing labyrinthine fistula and in certain congenital labyrinthine disorders. The technique requires ENG with eyes closed and acoustic stimulation with pulsed tones of varying frequencies.

MULTIPHASIC SLOW COMPONENT IN INTRACRANIAL DISEASE

Torok (16) described qualitative factors in vestibular nystagmus that are of help in differential diagnosis. A normal monophasic slow component in the standard ENG may be replaced by a multiphasic slow component in space-occupying intracranial lesions (Fig. 10–23).

VESTIBULAR "DECRUITMENT"—FATIGUE

Vestibular fatigue is a central phenomenon. It can be detected on the ENG when a very minimal stimulus evokes a greater response than a strong stimulus.

COMMAND ELECTRONYSTAGMOGRAPHIC TEST ABNORMALITIES IN CERTAIN DISEASE STATES

In a study of 33 cases, Dix (5) described clinical features common to ataxic patients who had either Huntington's chorea, progressive supranuclear palsy, familial ataxia, and vascular lesions. All of these CNS lesions manifested unsteadiness of gait, deranged speech, and abnormal eye movements. Comparisons of command, following, and optokinetic responses showed significant changes in all three patterns.

VECTOR ELECTRONYSTAGMOGRAPHY

A four-channel approach to ENG has been under study in our clinic. The addition of two diagonal channels to the horizontal and vertical channel may create the possibilities of a vector type of

FIG. 10–22. Sinusoidal rotation test on a child. **A.** Electrodes attached to face. **B.** Child seated on lap of adult in rotating chair.

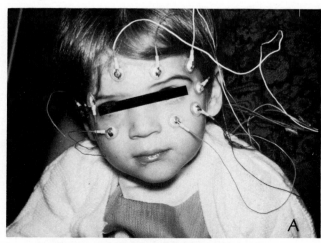

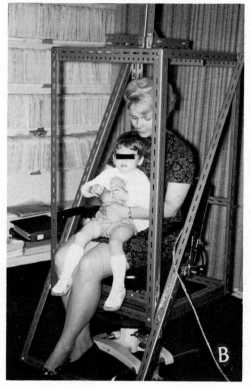

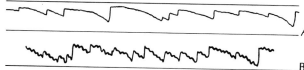

FIG. 10–23. A. Smooth deflection ENG pattern, monophasic response to caloric stimulation in a normal subject. **B.** Multiphasic slow component of caloric ENG response in subject with intracranial lesion. (Adapted from Torok N: Qualitative evaluation of vestibular nystagmus. Fifth International Congress of Oto Rhino Laryngo Broncho Oesophagology. Amsterdam: Koninklijke Van Gorcum & Co, 1953)

FIG. 10–24. Mechanical stimulation **(arrow)** of utricle before labyrinthectomy is followed by a short latency period and then by short duration nystagmus in all channels but the horizontal.

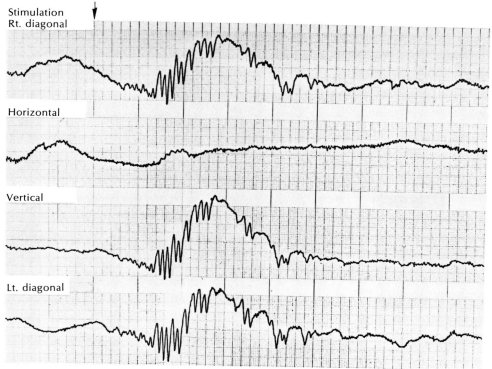

response integration analysis technique. Although the horizontal channel is the main vector in calorization responses in most subjects, it is possible to show significant differences between the four channels in a number of conditions. For example, in labyrinthectomy, peroperative stimulation of the utricle produces major responses in vertical and diagonal channels, but the horizontal channel response is barely noticeable (Fig. 10–24).

CLINICAL SIGNIFICANCE OF SPONTANEOUS AND POSITIONAL NYSTAGMUS

A classification of positional nystagmus proposed by Nylen (13) and modified by Aschan (1) consists of three types.

Type I (PN I) is direction-changing. As the head position is changed, the nystagmus direction changes. Onset is immediate and it is persistent.

It has been attributed to posterior fossa lesions. Type II (PN II) is direction-fixed, with varying etiologies. Type III (PN III) is transitory, fatigable, direction-changing in character, and is accompanied by postural vertigo. It has been known as **benign positional vertigo,** and usually recovers spontaneously.

Dayal and colleagues (4), in a study of 302 patients with peripheral, brain stem, and cerebellar lesions, concluded that the term benign paroxysmal nystagmus should be discontinued, since it is not always benign and can occur in CNS lesions.

Harrison and Ozsahinoglu (9) reported that "categoric classification of the type of positional vertigo into benign and central forms does not appear to be justified. . . ."

BILATERAL "DEAD" LABYRINTHS

Bilateral labyrinthine areflexia (14) (labyrinths nonresponsive to caloric or rotational stimulation) is seen in a number of conditions—*e.g.*, congenital deafness, ototoxicity, post meningitis, etc. However, it is important to note that vestibular nonresponse can be due to habituation. Hood (10) describes a number of vestibular habituation patterns, such as those encountered in skaters, ballet dancers, and in certain psychiatric disorders.

SUMMARY

A precise examination of the dizzy patient is possible by utilization of a methodical series of neuro-otologic tests. The electronystagmographic (ENG) approach facilitates quantitative and qualitative examination of the vestibular system.

Specific lesions producing vertigo and nystagmus and their management are described under peripheral causes and central causes (see Ch. 26, Peripheral Vertigo, Labyrinthitis, and Meniere's Disease; and Ch. 27, Central Nervous System Vertigo and Motion Sickness).

REFERENCES

1. Aschan G, Bergstedt M, Stahle J: Nystagmography —Recording of nystagmus in clinical neurootological examination. Acta Otolaryngol [Suppl] (Stockh) 46:129, 1956
2. Coats AC: Galvanic body sway in normals and patients with VIII nerve lesions. Adv Otorhinolaryngol 19:857–860, 1971
3. Clement PAR, Goodhill V: Four channel electronystagmographic (ENG) studies of eye movements induced by linear accelerations. ORL 37:193–208, 1975
4. Dayal VS, Tarantino L, Farkashidy J et al.: Spontaneous and positional nystagmus: a reassessment of clinical significance. Laryngoscope 84:2033–2043, 1974
5. Dix MR: Disorders of balance: a recent clinical neuro-otological study. Proc R Soc Med 64:857–860, 1971
6. Eviatar L, Eviatar A, Naray I: Maturation of neurovestibular responses in infants. Dev Med Child Neurol 16:435–446, 1974
7. Eviatar A, Goodhill V: A dry calorization method for vestibular function. Laryngoscope 78:1746–1755, 1968
8. Eviatar A, Goodhill V: Dizziness as related to menstrual cycles and hormonal contraceptives. Arch Otolaryngol 90:301–306, 1969
9. Harrison MS, Ozsahinoglu C: Positional vertigo. Arch Otolaryngol 101:675–678, 1975
10. Hood JD: The clinical significance of vestibular habituation. Adv Otorhinolaryngol 17:149–157, 1970
11. Morisette Y, Abel SM, Barber HO: Optokinetic nystagmus in otoneurodiagnosis. Can J Otolaryngol 3:348–362, 1974
12. Nadol JB: Positive fistula sign with an intact tympanic membrane. Clinical report of three cases and histopathological description of vestibulofibrosis as the probable cause. Arch Otolaryngol 100:273–278, 1974
13. Nylen CO: Positional nystagmus. A review and future prospects. J Laryngol 64:295–318, 1950
14. Secretan JP: Labyrinthine areflexia. ORL 36:141–149, 1974
15. Stephens SDG, Ballam HM: The sono-ocular test. J Laryngol 88:1049–1059, 1974
16. Torok N: Qualitative Evaluation of Vestibular Nystagmus. Fifth International Congress of Oto Rhino Laryngo Broncho Oesophagology. Amsterdam, Koninklijke Van Gorcum & Co, 1953
17. Tullio P: Das Ohr und Die Enstehung Der Sprache und Schrift. Berlin-Vienna, Urban & Schwartzengerg, 1929
18. Weiss AD, Tole JR: Effect of galvanic vestibular stimulation on rotation testing. Adv Otorhinolaryngol 19:311–317, 1973
19. Wilkinson IMS: The influence of drugs and alcohol upon human eye movement. Proc R Soc Med 69:479–480, 1976

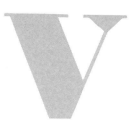

BASIC OTOLARYNGOLOGIC
RELATIONSHIPS

HEAD AND NECK LESIONS RELATED TO EAR PROBLEMS

SPECIFIC RELATIONSHIPS BETWEEN NOSE AND THROAT AND EAR PROBLEMS

OTITIS MEDIA AND OTOMASTOIDITIS

Tonsil and Adenoid Problems

Acute otitis media and its potential sequelae, secretory otitis media and chronic otomastoiditis are intimately related to nose and throat problems. The relationship involves normal aerial continuity between nose and throat and middle ear via the eustachian tube, which must adequately oxygenate and pressurize the middle ear. Nose-and-throat mucosal diseases are transmitted cytologically through eustachian tube mucosa as well as through vascular and lymphatic channels from the nasopharynx to the middle ear and the temporal-bone cell system.

In infants and children, the central adenoid mass, the palatine tonsils, and the associated lymphoid areas in Rosenmueller's fossas play major roles in initiation and continuance of acute otomastoiditis, secretory otitis media, and their complications. It is impossible to treat otitis media in children (and in many adults) without considering concomitant diseases of the adenoid and tonsil area.

Immunologic deficits, nasal allergy, and tonsil and adenoid disease all appear to play etiologic roles in pediatric otitis. The role of tonsil and adenoid infections is occasionally ignored because of undue stress upon allergy. Conversely, allergy frequently goes unrecognized as an etiologic factor, and the tonsil and adenoid infection is incorrectly assumed to be the basic cause of sustained, or recurrent episodes of secretory otitis media.

In the child acute otitis media that apparently subsides (in terms of fever, pain, and bulging, inflamed tympanic membrane) may still remain an unresolved infection, with the middle ear completely or partly filled with exudate. In this situation, the tonsil and adenoid problem may be primary. Such children may not complain of sore throat, and therefore inspection of the pharynx and nasopharynx may be casual and inadequate. Bacterial cultures from the throat may have been omitted. Antibiotic therapy may have been administered empirically without regard to such cultures and antibiograms. The antibiotic treatment may have been administered in inadequate dosage and for an insufficient length of time.

A major cause of persistent secretory otitis media is neglect of underlying episodic tonsil-adenoid reinfections.

Tonsillectomy and adenoidectomy is not a panacea in the management of secretory otitis media, but in many cases it is the key to successful treatment (see Ch. 15, Secretory Otitis Media).

Nasal Septal Problems

Nasal septum fractures may go unnoticed because of lack of external deformity, especially in children. *Nevertheless, a child may have a markedly obstructive septal defect due to birth or postnatal injury.* A septal deflection may produce either unilateral or bilateral blockade of the ostium with secondary sinusitis, which may be ipsilateral or contralateral to the deflection.

Nasal Mucosal Problems

Allergy may be a major cause of otitis media. The pale swollen mucosa of intermittent allergic edema is easily recognized. Smears for eosonophils will be helpful diagnostically. Eosinophilia on complete blood counts will frequently be present. Allergic nasal polyps become significant in persistent secretory otitis media.

Sinusitis

Unrecognized paranasal sinus disease may be etiologic in otitis media. An apparently quiescent maxillary sinusitis (occasionally ethmoiditis or sphenoiditis) with or without symptoms of localizing pain, pressure, or discharge may remain the primary cause for lack of resolution of secretory otitis media.

Multiple Etiology

In recurrent pediatric acute or secretory otitis media, multiple etiologic factors may consist of infected tonsils and adenoids, ipsilateral, contralateral, or bilateral sinusitis, nasal allergy and immunoglobulin deficiencies. Some children will require patient reevaluations of nose, throat, and sinus problems along with long-term management of food and inhalant allergies, and other immunologic deficiencies.

TYMPANOPLASTIC SURGERY

Reconstructive tympanoplastic surgery in otomastoiditis will include repair of the tympanic membrane and various ossicular lesions or defects. Surgical techniques can be combined in one procedure or may be staged. Reconstruction may be combined with management of such lesions as tympanosclerosis, keratoma (cholesteatoma), ossicular defects, granulomas, polyps, and other middle ear, attic, and mastoid diseases. All such procedures are designed not only for removal of disease, but for the ultimate purpose of improving tubotympanic physiology and hearing. Fundamental to any surgical procedure of this type is the assumption that eventually there will be effective eustachian tube function to deal with ventilation of the middle ear and mastoid air-cavity system. Although there are occasional exceptions to this rule—in which a permanent indwelling myringostomy (middle ear ventilation) tube may take the place of a nonfunctioning eustachian tube—in the majority of instances, the effectiveness of the otosurgical procedure depends upon the satisfactory role of the eustachian tube mucosa and its muscles in modulating intratympanic air pressures. Such pressure dynamics are of extreme importance in tympanolabyrinthine function. The integrity of a normal tubotympanic air space maintained by the normal cycle of spontaneous tubotympanic ventilatory functions has relevance not only to tympanic membrane and ossicular system function but also to labyrinthine window function (the oval window stapedial footplate, and the round window membrane).

The eustachian tube role is dependent upon nose and throat physiology. Thus, the otologist involved in major reconstructive surgery must consider nose and throat relationships both before and after operation. Preoperative assessment of the nose, paranasal sinus, nasal mucosa, and nasopharyngeal status is crucial to the predictability of tympanoplastic results.

A number of eustachian tube manometric and other function measurement methods, including tympanometry, are in use. Dye studies have been used to assess tubal functional visually. Radiopaque dyes are also under study to assess eustachian tube and middle ear functions adequately.

STAPES SURGERY

Nose and throat relationships are important in the preoperative and postoperative aspects of otosclerosis surgery. Examination of the nose and throat prior to stapes surgery is necessary to rule out significant acute or chronic infections, severe allergic problems, or other lesions. Adequate eustachian tube function is essential for ventilation of the middle ear in stapedectomy as in other microsurgical otologic procedures.

The timing of stapes surgery in a patient with chronic allergic rhinitis should be considered relative to seasonal hay fever episodes.

The allergic patient whose poststapedectomy hearing gain has not come up to expectation, may have a blocked eustachian tube primarily due to allergic eustachian tube edema. Unrecognized food or inhalant allergy may be a cause. Prompt elimination of offending foods, attention to environmental and epidermal (fur, animal dander, etc.) inhalants, accompanied by oral decongestant use, and gentle Politzer inflation may improve the hearing level by 20–25 dB. Lack of recognition of a nasal problem may cause the poststapedectomy hearing level to be depressed. Before revision surgery is considered, attention should be directed to nose, sinus, and nasopharyngeal mucosa for a possible explanation.

NOSE AND THROAT INFECTION AND ROUTINE ANTIBIOTIC PROPHYLAXIS BEFORE AND AFTER EAR SURGERY

Varying opinions continue in the debates regarding prophylactic antibiotic therapy in so-called "elective clean surgery."

Surgery of the middle ear cannot be unequivocally considered clean surgery. This is obvious in chronic otomastoiditis but not in stapes surgery. The middle ear and eustachian tube are analogous to a paranasal sinus and a sinus ostium. Undetected or unrecognized presence of low-grade nasopharyngeal infection may well prove to be a problem in healing in the middle ear or in postoperative ear infections. The eustachian tube mucosa represents an "escalator," transmitting potentially pathogenic organisms from the nasopharynx to the tympanic mucosa and possibly into the vestibule, following removal of the footplate. For this reason we advise preoperative and postoperative broad-spectrum prophylactic antibiotic therapy for all ear surgery, including stapes surgery. We advise our patients to see their general physicians after ear surgery whenever there is onset of a true upper respiratory infection (common cold), with sore throat and fever. Following a throat culture, appropriate prophylactic antibiotic therapy should be immediately started. Patients who have had successful stapedectomies or tympanoplastic surgical procedures may have ear complications following untreated upper respiratory infections. The middle ear is in contact with a potentially contaminated area—namely, the nasopharynx. Reports of immediate or delayed serious infections (labyrinthitis and meningitis) have appeared in the literature in patients who have not received such prophylactic antibiotic therapy.

THE PEDIATRIC TONSIL AND ADENOID DILEMMA

The role of chronic or recurrent tonsillitis and/or adenoiditis is very important in otitis and mastoiditis, especially in children. Much controversy continues regarding such relationships.

The complex interrelationship between nose-and-throat disease and ear disease should not be considered in a simplistic fashion.

Routine tonsillectomy and adenoidectomy was not advised by competent otorhinolaryngologists in the past and is not in the present. Before advising tonsil and adenoid surgery in the management of ear disease, careful consideration should be given to other etiologic possibilities, including classic nasal allergy, special immunologic deficiency states, congenital anomalies, active sinusitis, and hypometabolic problems.

However, chronic or recurrent tonsillitis or adenoiditis is an important cause of either primary or secondary eustachian tube disease. The superior tonsillar pole may play just as important a role in tubal obstruction or in tubal infection as lateral adenoid tissue, or the lymphoid follicles in Rosenmuellers fossas.

The decisions for tonsil and adenoid surgery require experience, individualization, and above all, an accurate history of tonsil and adenoid infections, preferably observed by the physician responsible for the otologic management. Where indicated, properly performed tonsillectomy and adenoidectomy may be the most important single treatment in a resistant or recurrent otitis media problem. Proper technique is important. It includes meticulous removal of lymphoid tissue, with careful preservation of the mucosal and muscular surfaces. This is especially necessary in adenoidectomy. "Blind" adenoidectomy, without

elevation and direct visualization of central and lateral nasopharyngeal regions, is frequently inadequate and may be harmful. Nasopharyngeal scars produced by pharyngeal muscle damage may result in permanent tubal dysfunction. Proper adenoid removal requires monitoring by mirror examination to visualize the nasopharynx during surgery before and after removal of the lymphoid tissue. Such visualization takes less than a minute, and will yield significant information to permit anatomically accurate adenoidectomy (whether primary or secondary).

RELATIONSHIPS BETWEEN HEAD AND NECK CONDITIONS AND EAR PROBLEMS

SALIVARY GLANDS

The parotid and submaxillary salivary glands can produce a number of ear symptoms. Calculi in either parotid or submaxillary ducts, with ductal obstruction, can produce otalgia or ear fullness.

Parotid gland mixed tumors may first be recognized because of otalgia or ear fullness.

Congenital branchial cleft fistulas may involve external auditory canal and/or middle ear tracts contiguous with parotid glands.

CAROTID ARTERY–JUGULAR VEIN LESIONS

Pulsating tinnitus, subjective and/or objective (bruits), can be due to a number of lesions of the external or internal carotid artery or of the external or internal jugular vein. Occlusions, arteriovenous aneurysms, carotid body tumors, and jugular vein chemodectomas can produce a number of ear symptoms, including pain and discomfort, in addition to bruits and pulsating tinnitus.

CERVICAL SPINE LESIONS

Cervical osteophytes, osteoarthritis, and trauma (whiplash) can produce episodic or constant otalgia.

REFERRED OTALGIA

Ear pain is not always due to ear disease. Ear pain accompanied by a tender auricle is usually due to some form of external otitis. Ear pain without a tender auricle is a common symptom of acute otitis media or acute exacerbation of chronic otitis media.

Otalgias, however, may also be due to pain referred from remote areas, such as the teeth, larynx, hypopharynx, styloid process, or the parotid gland. Otalgia is frequently due to cervical plexus pain referral and can be associated with cervical arthritis or other orthopedic neck problems. It is very commonly due to temporomandibular joint syndromes of various types, as already mentioned.

Otalgia is occasionally associated with intracranial tumors, including acoustic neurinomas and meningiomas. Otalgia can also be referred from any one of a number of cranial nerves, including neuralgia of the fifth, seventh, ninth, and tenth nerves.

Carcinoma of the tongue, hypopharynx, upper esophagus, or larynx may be first manifested by otalgia. Cranial nerve neuralgias (fifth and ninth nerves) can produce otalgia. A throbbing otalgia may be related to ischemic cardiac episodes.

TEMPOROMANDIBULAR JOINT LESIONS

Temporomandibular joint fractures, osteoarthritis, neoplasms, and the temporomandibular joint syndrome (Costen's syndrome) produce a number of ear symptoms. Although management of temporomandibular joint problems is not usually within the clinical responsibility of the otologist, it is frequently the otologist who will discover such a problem.

A number of otologic symptoms are definitely attributable to temporomandibular joint disorders. A patient with ear pain or pain radiating from the ear to the throat or with a feeling of stuffiness or fullness in the ear, may have no evidence of otologic disease. The cause of such an ear complaint may remain an unsolved mystery unless a few simple tests are made with reference to temporomandibular joint dysfunction. It cannot be assumed that a patient who has been recently examined by a dentist does not have a temporomandibular joint dysfunction. There are many conflicting conceptions regarding such problems among general dentists and dental specialists who tend to focus their attention on the teeth alone. Some dentists are unaware of borderline temporomandibular joint problems, the only symptoms of which may be otologic.

Four different types of pathologic condyle positions in the fossa with the teeth in centric occlusion have been described by Gerber (2) and by de Boever (1). They include upward displacement with compression of the disc, downward displacement, medial displacement, and dorsal displacement.

These may be diagnosed by palpation and by simple temporomandibular joint radiographs.

Temporomandibular joint dysfunction with referred pain may affect the adolescent undergoing orthodontic treatment, the young or middle-age adult with missing molar teeth and particularly the senior citizen with dentures.

A common complaint is pain anterior to the auricle or in the ear canal in a patient in whom there are no significant external or middle ear findings to explain the pain. Likewise, there may be no significant pharyngeal, laryngeal, or neck lesions to explain the pain. The evidence of missing unilateral upper or lower molar teeth may indicate a direction for further studies. Significant diagnostic information may be obtained by comparative temporomandibular joint palpation in open and closed positions, looking for localized pain or tenderness and/or a cracking sensation on movement. An additional informative diagnostic or therapeutic test is that of placing a small pad of gauze or a wrapped tongue blade between the molar teeth and having the patient bite down. This temporary change of bite will frequently change the symptoms. Most commonly, the patient's major complaint of pain, stuffiness, or fullness in the ear will be completely or partly alleviated. Occasionally the reverse may be true, with the original symptom greatly exaggerated by this temporary change in the bite dimensions. Palpation of the joints (Fig. 11–1) laterally and intraorally will frequently elicit marked differ-

FIG. 11–1. Temporomandibular joint palpation.

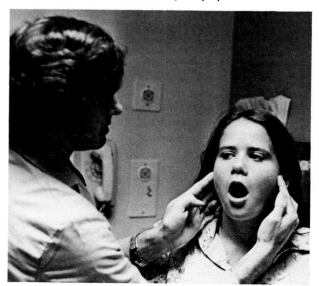

ences in sensitivity between the right and left temporomandibular joint areas. Digital palpation of joint motion through the external auditory canal may be informative. X-ray films of the temporomandibular joint areas in open and closed positions are frequently diagnostic.

The functional aspects of temporomandibular joint problems are very important. One of the major causes other than missing molar teeth or other mechanical irregularities is that of nocturnal grinding of teeth (bruxism) due to emotional factors of which the patient may be unaware. A simple device to test this hypothesis is the trial use of a bite block, a plastic splint, which can be made very simply by any dentist. The patient wears the splint for several weeks as a clinical test (see special communication by David Marcus, D.D.S., later in this chapter).

Significant symptomatic relief is obtained by most patients within 10 days by three simple measures: 1) the application of moist heat to the affected area to relieve spasm and encourage circulation; 2) a soft diet to put the joint at rest; and 3) a muscle relaxant-analgesic.

After careful examination, reassurance that there is no evidence of serious ear or mastoid disease is of great value to the patient, for this is usually the reason for seeking otologic consultation. Referral to the dental temporomandibular joint specialist is required when symptoms persist.

In general, the majority of patients with such symptoms who do not have serious diseases such as tumors, advanced arthritis, or fractures, etc., can be helped by careful bite corrections without the need for major surgery.

Abnormalities of the temporomandibular joint are great "masqueraders" of ear disorders, and muscle spasms in the joint area may produce a number of ear symptoms that will clear up following correction of the temporomandibular joint problem.

A number of unsubstantiated reports purport to show relationships between temporomandibular joint dysfunctions and various types of hearing losses. No definitive evidence of hearing loss can be attributed to such joint dysfunctions. Realignments or surgery, while very effective for the relief of pain, have no demonstrable effects on either hearing loss or tinnitus.

DENTAL CAUSES OF EAR SYMPTOMS (3)

Ear symptoms are encountered by the dentist frequently. Dental causes of such symptoms and their management are discussed in the following communication by David Marcus, DDS.

Dental symptoms which come to the attention of the otologist for care fall into the following broad areas:

1. Otalgia, unilaterally and bilaterally, radiating generally from the ear areas to the mandibular molar, occipital, and parietal areas of the head externally and internally. Pain may be constant or intermittent and may or may not be aggravated by the movements of mastication.
2. Stiffness and decreased temporomandibular joint mobility unilaterally and bilaterally are often present. Many patients often complain of increased symptoms upon awakening, especially after deep sleep. Jaw opening is sometimes restricted to varying degrees.
3. Ear noises, such as clicking, popping, or ringing, both unilaterally and bilaterally may occur intermittently or constantly for varying time periods.
4. Pain in and around the teeth and mouth may occur upon mastication.
5. Periodontal lesions ranging from simple bleeding to advanced bone loss with attendant suppuration and loss of teeth.

All these symptoms may derive from a variety of causes—physical trauma such as yawning; biting hard substances; or actual blows in the mandibular or maxillary areas, or anywhere in the head and neck area. A careful history should be taken as to the possibilities of physical trauma, recently or remotely incurred, including dental operations of varying types, oral surgery, reconstructive dental operations, possible changes in occlusion due to dental procedures, or general wear and tear of the masticatory apparatus.

These conditions are often transitory and are many times amenable to relaxants of various types. Here, time, and a soft diet will often produce favorable results.

It is the presence of intractable symptoms for long periods of time that presents problems requiring a different approach to therapy. When no specific pathologic reasons can be found for the continued presence of symptoms, direction should then be given to the possibility that these symptoms are of dental origins, resulting from either poor occlusion or functional problems.

If dental occlusion defects are corrected but symptoms persist, attention should then be directed to the possibility that these symptoms are the result of clenching and grinding the teeth, especially during sleep, and possibly during work,

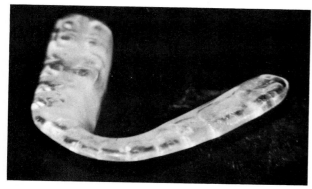

FIG. 11–2. Bite plate covering the occlusal and incisal surfaces, and extending lingually to just beyond the linguogingival borders.

FIG. 11–3. Bite plate in position, mouth open.

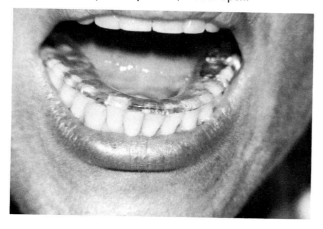

FIG. 11–4. Bite plate in position, mouth closed.

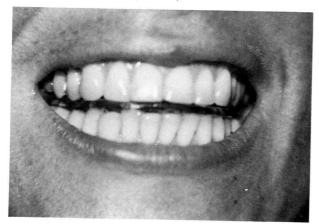

when work demands great concentration, as in writers, performers, artists, stenographers, etc.

In my experience, the symptoms in most patients, regardless of physical or pathologic conditions present, will be improved or will disappear by the use of a simple splint, worn by the patient primarily during sleep. The patient's dentist should construct a mandibular arch bite plate made of clear soft impact plastic approximately 1 mm in thickness, covering the occlusal and incisal surfaces, and extending lingually to just beyond the linguogingival borders (Fig. 11–2). The splint should be very flat, should offer absolutely no resistance to lateral or protrusive movements and should be corrected to the basic centric position (Fig. 11–3).

It goes without saying that an attempt to correct basic problems of occlusion is necessary, but every effort should be made to postpone prolonged dental reconstruction until acute symptoms are eased or disappear by the use of the bite-plate splint.

The splint or bite plate (Fig. 11–4) acts as a shock absorber between the hard surfaces of the upper and lower teeth and reduces trauma to the underlying osseous and soft tissues within the mouth and thus eases the tension in the musculature in and around the mandibular, maxillary, and temporomandibular joint areas.

Not only should this bite plate be worn during sleep, but it should also be worn during the day when very acute symptoms are present. The period of time necessary for the usage of the splint will depend primarily on the length of time that the underlying subacute conscious or unconscious emotional status factors result in clenching or grinding of teeth.

REFERENCES

1. De Boever J: Temporomandibular joint—function and dysfunction. Oral Sci Rev 2:100–117, 1973
2. Gerber A: Kiefergelenk und Zahnokklusion. Dtsche Zahnaerztl Z 26:119, 1971
3. Marcus D: Personal communication

12

BASIC OTOSURGICAL PROCEDURES

In microsurgery for otologic lesions, a number of basic incisions and surgical procedures are employed. They are briefly described in this introductory chapter for reference purposes.

INCISIONS

Four basic types of surgical incisions are in use. They include intra-auricular, endomeatal, endaural, and postauricular incisions. In each, a number of subtypes are available for special purposes.

INTRA-AURICULAR INCISIONS

Intra-auricular incisions are used for excision of auricular tumors and for incision and drainage of auricular abscesses. The tragus is approached surgically to obtain autogenous cartilage and/or perichondrium for reconstructive uses, especially in tympanoplasty. A number of auricular incisions are used for auriculoplasty, a plastic surgical procedure.

ENDOMEATAL (TRANSCANAL) INCISIONS

A number of otosurgical incisions are performed through an endomeatal (ear speculum) approach. These transcanal incisions are the most common incisions used in otosurgical practice.

External Auditory Canal Incisions

Incisions of the cartilaginous-bony margin of the external auditory canal may be posterior, anterior, superior, or inferior. Occasionally they are combined. Removal of osteophytes (osteomas) and other bony and soft tissue lesions of the external canal is possible through such incisions.

The incision is preceded by local anesthetic block with 1.5% xylocaine with 1:200,000 epinephrine. If necessary, in special cases, this may be supplemented by general anesthesia. A 30-gauge needle is used through an oval or round ear speculum. The surgical microscope is used for illumination and magnification.

Wherever possible, the incision is made on the posterior wall of the external auditory canal, since additional access to the lesion may be obtained by removal of lateral mastoid cortical bone. Microsurgical angulated instruments are used for incision and tissue elevation. The incision is made through skin and periosteum to bone, and the flap is elevated medially, as required, and replaced at the completion of the procedure. The incision usually requires no sutures, the margins being approximated and held in place by packing (Fig. 12–1).

Posterosuperior Flap (Omega Incision— Posterior Tympanotomy)

This is the most common incision used in approaching posterior middle-ear lesions. It is used in stapedectomy, ossiculoplasty, myringoplasty, incudomalleal fixation, transfenestral labyrinthectomy, and in the removal of many intratympanic tumors.

The posterosuperior flap is made through a speculum following a circumferential xylocaine-epinephrine block in the external canal. The subcutaneously injected solution is massaged with a moist cotton applicator to create diffusion and extension of the solution to the fibrous annulus area of the tympanic membrane. A superior curved incision starts above the malleal short process and extends laterally to the cartilaginous–bony junction. An inferior curved incision starts posteriorly to the posterior annulus, slightly below the level of the malleal umbo. The incisions meet posterolaterally, extending through skin and periosteum to bone. (Fig. 12–2). The flap is then elevated down to the fibrous annulus.

The annular margin is carefully enucleated from the bony annulus, and the posterior middle ear exposed. Annular bone is removed with curets or the surgical drill to gain additional exposure. Care is necessary to avoid trauma to the chorda tympani nerve (Fig. 12–3).

Myringotomy Incision

This is the most common ear operation. It is a temporary incision through the tympanic membrane and is made either through the posteroinferior or anteroinferior quadrant in radial fiber direction (Fig. 12–4).

Myringostomy

Myringostomy is a semi-permanent myringotomy accomplished by insertion of a middle ear ventila-

FIG. 12–1. Lateral endomeatal incision.

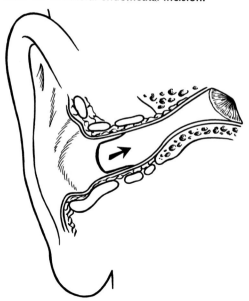

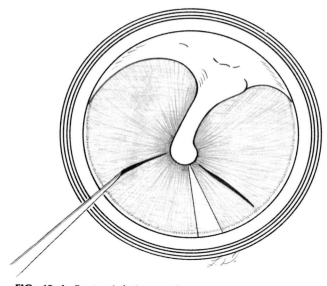

FIG. 12–4. Posteroinferior and anteroinferior quadrant myringotomy incisions.

FIG. 12–5. Middle ear ventilation tube through postero-inferior myringostomy incision.

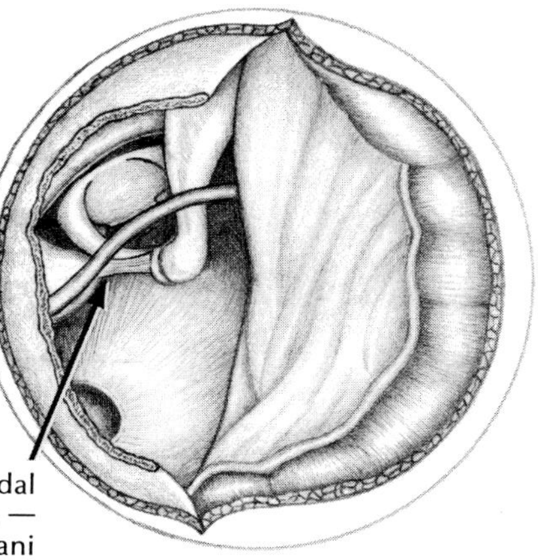

FIG. 12–2. Posterior omega incision.

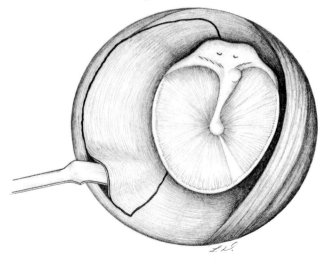

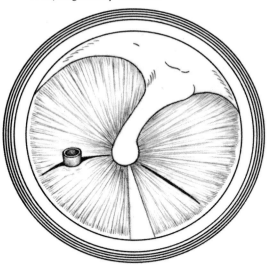

Pyramidal
recess —
sinus tympani
region

FIG. 12–3. Posterior tympanotomy following removal of marginal posterosuperior canal wall bone.

tion tube through a posteroinferior quadrant or anterioinferior quadrant myringotomy (Figs. 12–5, 12–6).

Double Myringotomy and/or Myringostomy

Occasionally two incisions (postero- and anteroinferior) are made (for drainage) through the tympanic membrane. One allows air to enter while fluid is withdrawn through the other by a suction tip (Fig. 12–7).

ENDAURAL INCISIONS

Standard Endaural Incision

This is a transauricular intercartilaginous or "auricle sectioning" incision created anterior to the conchal cartilage and extending superiorly anterior to the spina helicis. The auricle is thus sectioned diagonally. The tragus is retracted anteriorly and the auricle posteriorly. Elevation of subcutaneous tissue and superficial auricular muscles exposes the temporalis fascia, temporalis muscle, and the periosteum of the lateral surface of the temporal bone. Additional periosteal incision and further retraction posteriorly and/or anteriorly exposes the lateral mastoid cortex widely (Figs. 12–8, 12–9).

Extended Endaural Incision

The standard endaural incision is extended posterosuperiorly over the squama, curving into the postauricular cleft. This allows auricular retraction in a posteroinferior direction (Fig. 12–10).

POSTAURICULAR INCISIONS

Several types of postauricular incisions are in use, most of them optional, in place of the endaural incision. The postauricular incision is usually preferred for pediatric mastoid surgery to prevent postoperative canal stenosis.

The Standard Postauricular Incision

The standard postauricular incision is created in the postauricular fold crease. The auricle is reflected anteriorly. Access to the external canal requires either concurrent use of an endomeatal

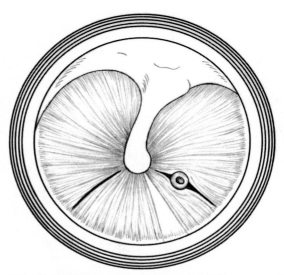

FIG. 12–6. "Collar button" type of middle ear ventilation tube through anteroinferior myringostomy incision.

FIG. 12–7. Suction applied to lips of myringostomy incision in removal of middle ear fluid.

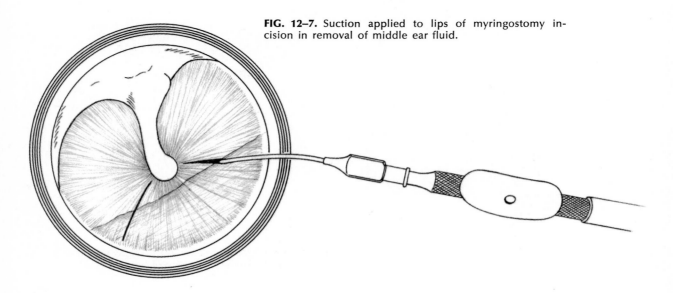

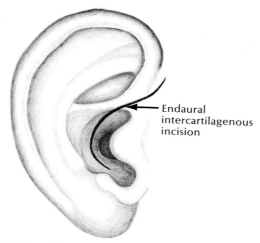

FIG. 12–8. Endaural incision.

FIG. 12–9. Endaural retractors with mastoid bone exposure.

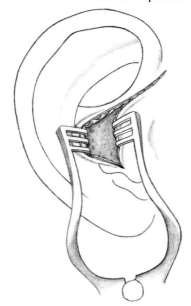

FIG. 12–10. Extended endaural incision.

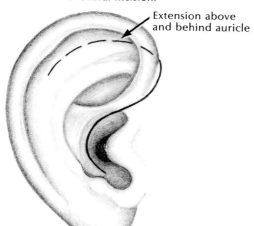

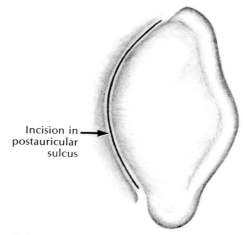

FIG. 12–11. Postauricular incision.

FIG. 12–12. Postauricular retractor with mastoid bone exposure.

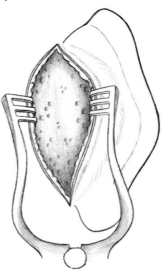

FIG. 12–13. Linear posterior incision in infant to avoid region of superficial infantile stylomastoid foramen for VII nerve.

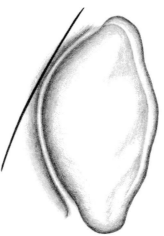

incision or transsection of the posterior canal wall skin (Figs. 12–11, 12–12).

The Retrofold Postauricular Incision

The retrofold postauricular incision is used in infants to avoid possible injury to the seventh nerve at the stylomastoid foramen, which is more superficial in the infant's temporal bone (Fig. 12–13).

SURGICAL PROCEDURES

TYMPANOLYSIS

The posterior omega incision is used for tympanolysis in the posterior middle-ear compartment, a procedure for sectioning scar tissue bands that limit the mobility of the ossicular chain or that of an ossiculoplastic restoration.

STAPEDIOLYSIS, STAPEDECTOMY, AND FENESTRATION

These operations are for the surgical treatment of otosclerosis, and related diseases involving the stapes and oval window and are described in detail in Chapter 19, Otosclerosis.

MASTOIDECTOMY

The basic term **mastoidectomy** refers to the surgical exposure and removal of mastoid air cells. An endaural or postauricular incision may be used for any of the following types of mastoidectomy.

Simple Mastoidectomy

A limited exenteration of the primary cellular system of the mastoid process is involved in simple mastoidectomy, omitting exploration of the tympanic cavity, the epitympanum, or of other significant cell groups. This limited procedure provides inadequate information and inadequate removal of disease and is virtually obsolete today. It has been replaced by the atticomastoidectomy.

Atticomastoidectomy

The basic complete mastoid operation is the atticomastoidectomy, which includes exploration of the entire "attic" or epitympanum, in addition to the major mastoid air cell groups. The procedure is usually done through an endaural or postauricular incision, and permits visualization and management of lesions of any portion of the mastoid cellular system, in addition to lesions involving the epitympanum, the body and short process of the incus, the head and neck of the malleus, and

the incudomalleal joint. It also allows access to the entire horizontal portion of the facial nerve, including the geniculate ganglion. This operation frequently includes an exploratory posterior tympanotomy. To accomplish the latter, it is often sufficient to separate the skin of the membranous canal from the bony canal down to the annulus tympanicus, and to enucleate the latter, reflecting the posterior canal wall skin anteriorly. It may or may not be necessary to remove annular bone for visualization (Fig 12–14).

Radical Mastoidectomy

The radical mastoidectomy is the classic operation, involving atticomastoidectomy plus removal of the posterior bony canal wall, the tympanic membrane. the malleus, and the incus, leaving only the stapes or the stapedial footplate. In the classic radical operation, no attempt is made to save either the bony or the fibrous annulus. The removal of the posterior bony canal wall converts the exenterated mastoid cellular area and the external auditory canal into a single cavity, a "stoma" in direct communication with the external auditory meatus. The cavity, also called the mastoid "bowl" or open "mastoidostomy" can be examined and treated directly through the external auditory meatus (Fig. 12–15).

Modified Radical Mastoidectomy

The term **modified radical mastoidectomy** is applied to a group of operations in which only a portion of the posterior bony canal wall is removed, with creation of a permanent mastoidostomy cavity, but in which the tympanic membrane and the ossicles are not removed. The modified radical

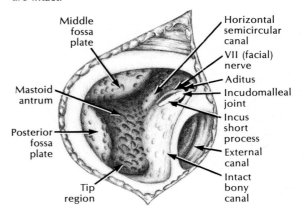

FIG. 12–14. Complete atticomastoidectomy, so called "simple" mastoidectomy. Ossicles and posterior bony canal are intact.

Middle fossa plate

Mastoid antrum

Posterior fossa plate

Tip region

Horizontal semicircular canal

VII (facial) nerve

Aditus

Incudomalleal joint

Incus short process

External canal

Intact bony canal

mastoid operation has been largely replaced by newer mastoid-tympanoplastic techniques.

TYMPANOPLASTY

Tympanoplasty is the reconstruction of the tympanic-membrane–ossicle transformer mechanism by the grafting of autogenous or homogenous tissues, which are used to repair or to reconstruct tympanic-membrane–ossicular defects. Tympanoplastic operations are frequently carried out in conjunction with mastoid operations of one type or another. Such procedures are designated **mastoidectomy-tympanoplasty.**

Basic principles of tympanic physiology are utilized in the planning of tympanoplastic operations. Wullstein (13) contributed a useful classification of five types of tympanoplasty based upon the progression of problems encountered in tympanic defects. At the present time (with developments in ossiculoplasty) a modification of the types I, II, III, IV, and V classification is used.

Type I Tympanoplasty

Basic tympanoplasty is the reconstruction of all or part of the tympanic membrane and is the primary goal in tympanoplasty. Closure can be accomplished by Gelfilm (induction-regeneration) of a tympanic membrane defect in the presence of an intact, normally mobile ossicular chain, and an otherwise healthy middle ear. The term **myringoplasty** may be reserved to describe the closure of a small central tympanic membrane perforation which does not involve either the ossicular chain or the tympanic annulus, and is confined to not more than one quadrant of the membrane. Larger defects, with or without involvement of the ossicular chain and bony and fibrous annulus should be described as type I tympanoplasty (Fig. 12–16A).

Type II Tympanoplasty-Ossiculoplasty

A type II procedure includes a type I tympanic membrane repair (tympanoplasty) and ossiculoplasty. **Ossiculoplasty** is a surgical reconstruction of the middle-ear ossicular system to connect with a functioning tympanic membrane or a tympanoplastic substitute. Because of the unique characteristics of the incudomalleal joint (within the epitympanum), the original three-ossicle arrangement is not reconstructed or replaced with allografts to reproduce a normal malleus, incus, and stapes chain. Instead, a bypass is usually created surgically. If the tympanic membrane is normal, ossiculoplasty alone is performed.

The most common defect requiring ossiculo-

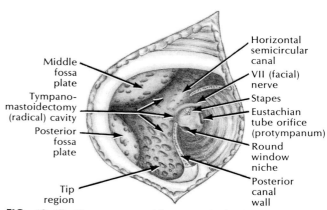

FIG. 12–15. Tympanomastoidectomy (radical mastoidectomy). Malleus, incus, and posterior canal bone have been removed. A common cavity includes external canal, middle ear, and mastoid antrum and periantral cells.

plasty is loss of all or part of the incus. In most instances this requires restoration of contact between the stapes and the malleus, which is usually mobile. The stapes arch may or may not be present. Thus, two basic types of ossiculoplasty can be performed: 1) lateral ossiculoplasty (with intact stapes arch); and 2) medial ossiculoplasty (with absent stapes arch).

LATERAL OSSICULOPLASTY (INTACT STAPES ARCH). This reconstruction involves acoustic reconnection between malleus and capitulum of the stapes, usually accomplished by the insertion of a sculptured ossicular bone autograft or allograft between the two. Reconstruction of such a defect requires the presence of an intact malleal manubrium, head, and neck. In addition, the malleal ligaments and tensor tympani tendon should be intact and mobile (Fig. 12–16B).

EXTENDED OSSICULOPLASTY (ABSENT STAPES ARCH). This operation is the ossiculoplastic reconstruction of a defect between the malleal manubrium and the oval window (healthy, mobile oval window neomembrane or normal stapedial footplate). A sculptured ossicular bone graft is inserted to bridge the gap (Fig. 12–16C).

Type III Tympanoplasty

MYRINGOSTAPEDIOPEXY. In a shallow middle-ear condition with a hypermobile malleal manubrium, it may be advisable to avoid an ossiculoplasty. Instead, the tympanic membrane or the reconstruction of it is rotated to a more medial position so that the retroumbo or umbo region of the tympanic

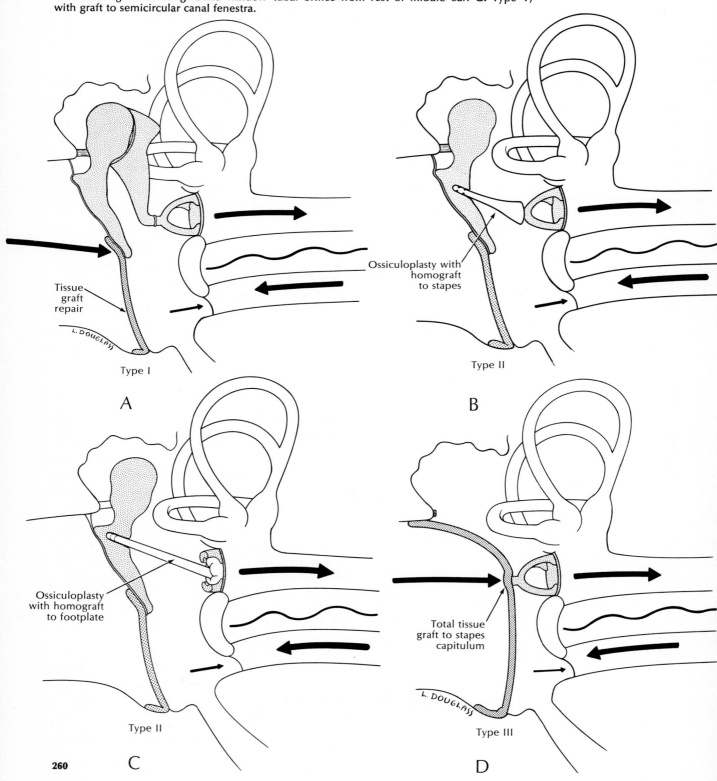

FIG. 12–16. Five types of tympanoplasty. **A.** Type I repair of tympanic membrane (TM) defect. **B.** Type II combined TM repair with homograft to stapes capitulum. **C.** Type II, with homograft to footplate. **D.** Type III, with tissue graft directly to stapes (myringostapediopexy). **E.** Type III, with conjoint cartilage-tissue T graft to footplate. **F.** Type IV cavum minor type, with tissue graft isolating round window–tubal orifice from rest of middle ear. **G.** Type V, with graft to semicircular canal fenestra.

Tissue graft repair

Type I

A

Ossiculoplasty with homograft to stapes

Type II

B

Ossiculoplasty with homograft to footplate

Type II

C

Total tissue graft to stapes capitulum

Type III

D

L. DOUGLASS

FIG. 12–16 (*continued*)

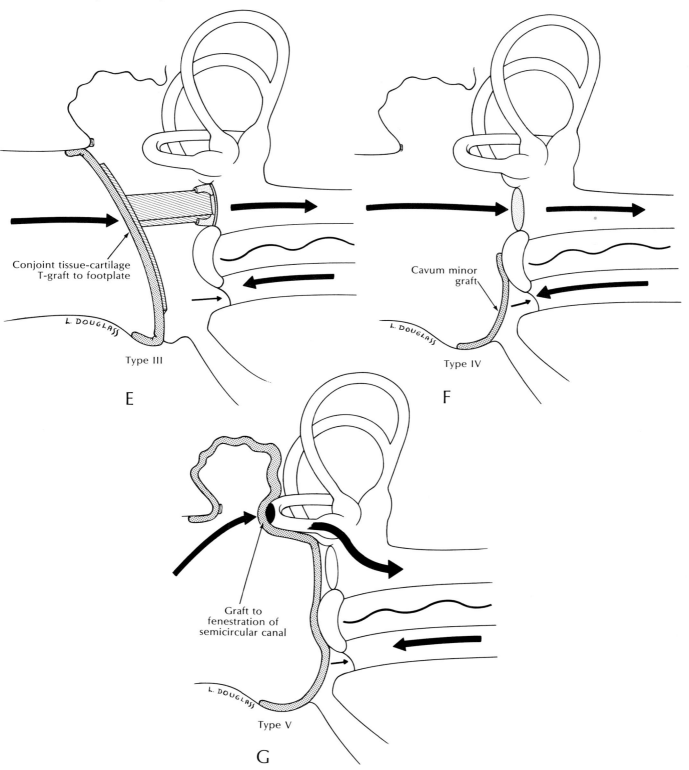

Conjoint tissue-cartilage
T-graft to footplate

L. DOUGLASS

Type III

E

Cavum minor
graft

L. DOUGLASS

Type IV

F

Graft to
fenestration of
semicircular canal

L. DOUGLASS

Type V

G

membrane effectively contacts the mobile sta-pedial capitulum. This direct tympanic mem-brane-to-stapes linkage is a type III tympanoplasty (myringostapediopexy) (Fig. 12–16D).

In this procedure, acoustic energy from the tympanic membrane is transferred directly to the stapedial arch. Sound-pressure transformation can be restored partially because there is still an adequate *area dif-ference* between the tympanic membrane or neo-mem-brane and the stapedial footplate. The only thing that is lost is the lever action of the malleus and the incus, which is not a crucial factor in the transformer func-tion of the middle ear mechanism.

"T CARTILAGE-PERICHONDRIUM" TYMPANOPLASTY. In instances of total absence of the tympanic membrane, malleus, incus, and stapedial arch, it is possible under favorable middle ear and eusta-chian tube mucosal circumstances to reconstruct the entire sound-transformer system. A composite autogenous graft is fashioned from tragal carti-lage and its attached, partially separated peri-chondrium (Fig. 12–16E).

Type IV Tympanoplasty—Cavum Minor Operation

In instances in which there has been a loss of stapedial capitulum and crura, but in which the footplate is still mobile, a cavum minor (small-cavity) operation may yield sufficient sound pro-tection to the round window membrane to re-store the sound-pressure difference between the two windows.

This "baffle" operation, in which the round window is protected or shielded from sound, is usually produced by rotation of a mucosal graft inferiorly from the promontory over the round window niche and cover-ing this mucosal graft with a fairly thick, connective tissue graft in continuity with the anterior tympanic fibrous annulus. This creates a small middle ear, which provides continuity of air space between the tympanic eustachian orifice and the round window. The oval-window region and the mobile footplate or neofoot-plate membrane in that window are exteriorized to air-borne sound (Fig. 12–16F). The round window baffle effect will frequently permit restoration of thres-holds from 60 dB to the 30 dB level. The obvious loss of the transformer action of the middle ear still exists, but this improvement in hearing may be significantly helpful in certain cases.

Type V Tympanoplasty—Semicircular Canal Fenestration

If the oval window footplate area is fixed by an obliterative lesion, hearing may still be partially restored by the dual procedure of a round window baffle type IV cavum minor procedure and fenes-

tration of the horizontal semicircular canal (Fig. 12–16G).

The new semicircular canal fenestra provides a portal of entry for air-borne sound into the scala vestibuli perilymph space. The sound protection of the round window via the baffle effect may yield a hearing gain of approximately 30 dB in some cases (similar to that of the type IV tympanoplasty).

Type IV cavum minor and type V fenestration proce-dures are not used very frequently, but they do have a place in tympanoplastic surgery. They provide the potential of significant gains in hearing, which may range up to the 25- to 30-dB level, particularly in the 2000 Hz frequency range. Such a level of gain con-stitutes a significant hearing improvement in an other-wise inoperable conductive lesion of major magnitude.

EVALUATION OF OTOSURGICAL HEARING RESULTS

In otosurgical procedures performed primarily for eradication of infections, tumors, or other con-ditions that threaten the lives or well-being of patients, maintenance or improvement in hearing is, of course, desirable, but hearing may have to be compromised to prevent serious sequelae to other vital structures.

In many otosurgical procedures, however, the primary goal is restoration or improvement in hearing. In such conditions, it is desirable to have quantitative guidelines to evaluate and compare various otosurgical techniques. Simple decibel gain measurements are useful but are physio-logically inadequate for evaluation of surgical ef-ficacy. Achievement of a set improvement goal—*i.e.,* the attainment of a 25-dB or 20-dB level—is desirable, but by itself, it does not offer a quanti-tative method of comparing different techniques.

The only useful method of evaluating otosur-gical techniques relating to hearing restoration in middle ear surgery must take into consideration the relative "closure" of the air–bone gap. This principle for evaluation can be used in individual cases and in groups of cases by measuring the degree of closure of the air–bone gap, expressed as a percentage: The **percentage closure** of the **air-bone** gap is the only valid quantitative approach in evaluating hearing results in middle-ear surgery. The formula for calculating the percentage is as follows:

Preop. AC minus Postop. AC/Preop. AC minus Preop. BC *or* AC gain/air-bone gap = % improvement

This is illustrated in Figure 12–17. These measurements are predicated on improvement in the speech reception threshold (SRT), and it is assumed, of course, that the postoperative speech discrimination score (SDS) remains unchanged, an indication of good cochlear function preservation.

SURGICAL AUDIOMETRY

In the early development of stapedolysis (mobilization) surgery, we devised a method of surgical audiometry that was very useful in mobilization surgery. Although it was possible to judge visual and tactile factors, elements of unpredictability and unreliability were present. Surgical audiometry, as originally designed to titrate manipulations in mobilization techniques, is still used and recommended in the performance of various types of stapedectomy (12) as well as in ossiculoplasty, tympanoplasty, and in related conditions under local anesthesia.

The possibility for determining hearing status during surgery was realized a long time ago. Blake (1) described operative hearing tests on two patients during stapedectomy, by using the Politzer acoumeter, tuning forks, and the Galton whistle. Holmgren (10) described a technique of operative audiometry, and Nilsson (11) described such a technique during fenestration surgery. Surgical audiometry and a nomograph guide in stapes mobilization surgery have been described (8). Audiometry can be performed in the ordinary operating room, provided ambient noise is cut down to a minimum. The patient uses a push button for response signaling, and is instructed in the response technique. An air-conduction receiver, enclosed in a sterile sleeve

(Fig. 12–18), is held in place over the speculum within the external auditory canal (Fig. 12–19), and threshold determinations are made for three test frequencies: 500 Hz, 1000 Hz, and 2000 Hz.

An averaged response threshold is used. The Fletcher formula for conversion of pure-tone thresholds to an equivalent speech-reception threshold (SRT) consists of selecting the two "best" thresholds (highest levels) at 500 Hz, 1000 Hz, or 2000 Hz, and averaging these two values. This gives an equivalent SRT (Fig. 12–20) or single "figure of merit" for evaluating each surgical step. An example is illustrated in stapes surgery, by measurement of **threshold shifts** following surgical steps. Hearing is tested at four specific steps in a middle-ear reconstructive surgical procedure, if the preoperative status of the tympanic membrane was intact.

TEST 1, MIDDLE EAR CLOSED. This test is performed following the completion of the flap elevation, with enucleation of the tympanic fibrous annulus from the tympanic sulcus, so that the middle ear has been opened and then temporarily closed again with the skin–periosteal–tympanic–membrane flap approximated to the original incision.

TEST 2, MIDDLE EAR OPEN. The second test is made after the middle ear has been reopened. This step will be used for comparison with critical step 3.

TEST 3, COMPLETION OF SURGICAL RECONSTRUCTION, MIDDLE EAR STILL OPEN. Test 3 is performed upon completion of the procedure and is compared with test 2 for evidence of threshold shift. Significant improvement depends on several factors, as monitored by a nomograph. The gain in decibels is determined by a ratio, as determined below.

TEST 4, MIDDLE EAR CLOSED. This final test is performed when the posterior-skin–tympanic-membrane flap is replaced as in step 1. Test 4 obviously will differ from the threshold determination to be made after the operation in a sound-treated room, when healing has occurred.

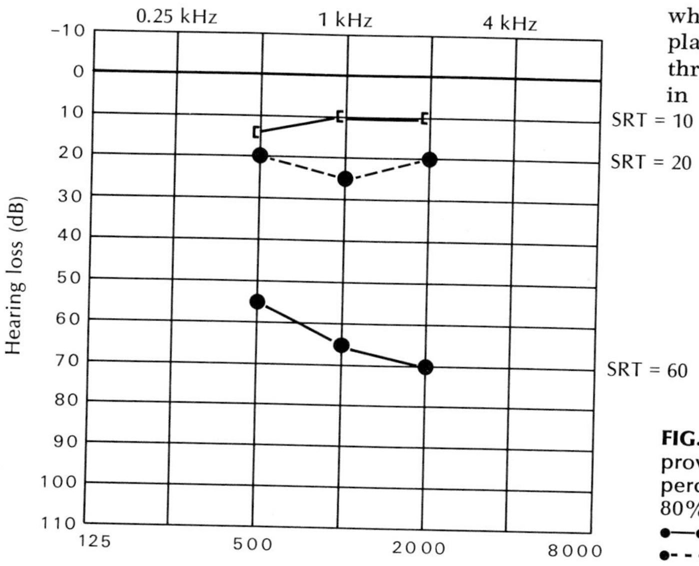

FIG. 12–17. Audiograms before and after surgery to improve hearing. The formula is applied to determine the percentage of improvement: 60 − 20/60 − 10 = 40/50 = 80% improvement (80% closure of the air–bone gap). ●—●, AC before operation; [—[, BC before operation; ●- - -●, AC after operation.

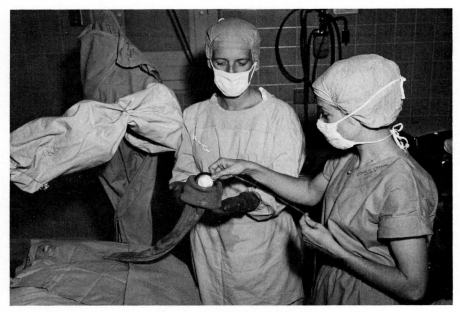

FIG. 12–18. Air-conduction receiver placed in sterile sleeve.

FIG. 12–19. Surgical audiometry in process. Speculum remains in canal under draped receiver. The anterior surgical position is used.

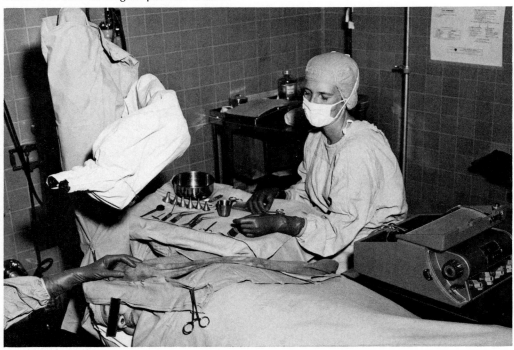

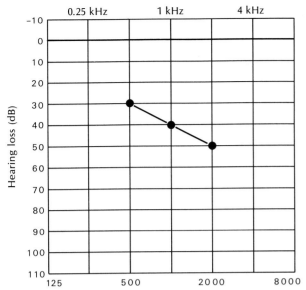

FIG. 12–20. Using the figures of this three-frequency audiogram, the "best" two levels are selected (30 dB at 500 Hz and 40 dB at 1000 Hz) and used in the following formula: $(30 + 40)/2 = 70/2 = 35$ dB, SRT.

ANALYSIS OF THE FOUR TESTS. Test 1 usually measures well below preoperative air conduction, because of the presence of edema. Test 2, with the middle ear open, is lower. Test 3 in successful cases shows an SRT gain. The final test should show a further gain.

The Nomograph

A surgical audiometric nomograph is used, with a Fletcher equivalent SRT for BC, preoperative AC, and for each of the four surgical audiometric AC steps. The SRT values are then plotted to indicate predictively the desirable objectives for thresholds of steps 3 and 4. The ordinates (vertical axis) of the graph are in dB ratios with respect to the normal audiometric zero level. The abscissa (horizontal axis) divisions are made arbitrarily equal to the ordinate, representing the four tests in surgical audiometry. The preoperative BC (SRT) level is drawn as a dashed horizontal (abscissa) line at its ordinate dB level, establishing the idealized surgical objective of success.

The SRT values are plotted at six positions, as used to indicate (1) the preoperative AC level, the four (2, 3, 4, 5) surgical audiometric tests and finally (6) the actual postoperative AC (SRT) level to be charted two weeks following surgery.

The crucial step in the surgery is at test 3, where a completed reconstruction is apparently satisfactory. A predictive formula is used to judge the physiologic adequacy of the surgical procedure, as determined by change in the air–bone gap, which differs from case to case. Thus, an air-bone gap of 20 dB, in a case with a preoperative 20 dB BC level and a 40 dB AC level poses a decision different from the one with a 50 dB

air–bone gap in a case with a preoperative 15 dB BC level and a 65 AC level. Both of these examples occur in otosclerosis and in other lesions.

The nomographic technique (Fig. 12–21), as originally devised for stapes surgery, has been described in detail in several publications (2–9).

SUMMARY

Microsurgery has been largely pioneered in otology. Many refinements in technique have been added since the 1940's. In addition to the basic otosurgical procedures described in this chapter, many additional special techniques involving seventh nerve, eighth nerve, and otoneurosurgical procedures are dealt with in chapters devoted to specific areas.

Audiologic advances have kept pace with otosurgical innovations, and thus preoperative and postoperative audiologic guidelines play major roles in otosurgical decision-making and in operative and postoperative evaluations.

REFERENCES

1. Blake CJ: Operation for removal of the stapes without ether. Boston Med J 127:551, 1892
2. Goodhill V: Transincudal stapedolysis for stapes mobilization in otosclerotic deafness (under audiometric control). Laryngoscope 65:693–710, 1955
3. Goodhill V: Surgical audiometry in stapedolysis (stapes mobilization). Arch Otolaryngol 62:504–508, 1955
4. Goodhill V: Present status of stapedolysis (stapes mobilization). Laryngoscope 66:333–381, 1956
5. Goodhill V: Stapedolysis (stapes mobilization) and the nomograph technic. J Speech Hear Res 1:179–190, 1958
6. Goodhill V: Evaluation of stapes mobilization results and surgical audiometry. Arch Otolaryngol 71:246–247, 1960
7. Goodhill V: Stapes Surgery for Otosclerosis. New York, Paul B Hoeber, 1961, pp 86–110
8. Goodhill V, Holcomb A: The surgical audiometric nomograph in stapedolysis (stapes mobilization). Arch Otolaryngol 63:399–410, 1956
9. Goodhill V, Holcomb A: A study of 500 stapes mobilizations. Laryngoscope 67:615–642, 1957
10. Holmgren G: In Kopetzky (ed): Surgery of the Ear, 2nd edition. New York, Thas Nelson and Sons, 1947, p 399
11. Nilsson G: The immediate improvement of hearing following fenestration operation. Acta Otolaryngologica 39:329, 1951; [Suppl] 98:1, 1952
12. Sooy FA: Personal communication
13. Wullstein H: Theory and practice of tympanoplasty. Laryngoscope 66:1076–1093, 1956

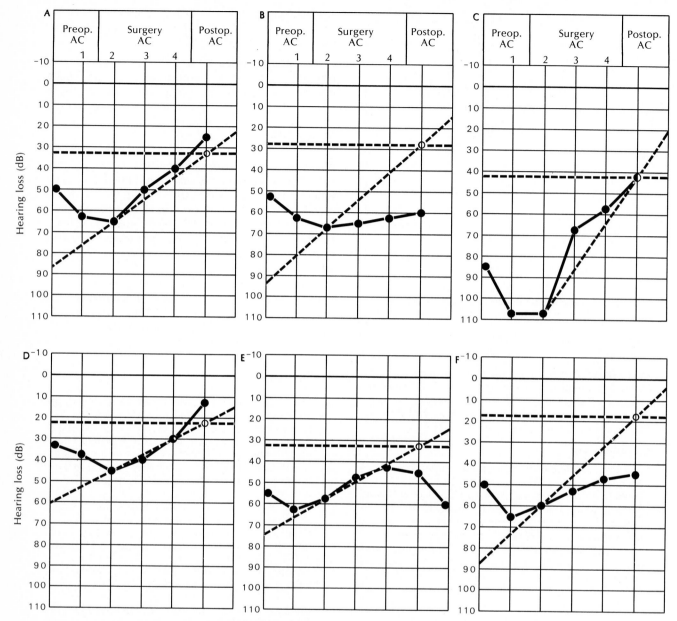

FIG. 12–21. A. In a successful case, the preoperative tests and postoperative AC levels lie to the left of the predictive line. **B.** In an unsuccessful case the threshold in test 4 is practically identical with that of test 1. The 2-week postoperative AC level is below the preoperative AC level. **C** and **D.** These cases are both successful, although it will be apparent that they differ widely in air–bone gap. **E.** In this case (stapedolysis) there is evidence of good mobilization but early reankylosis. **F.** This case is an example of a small gain in air conduction as a result of partial stapedolysis. The gain was only partial, and the operation was not successful.

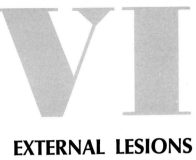

EXTERNAL LESIONS

13

EXTERNAL EAR DISEASES

Lesions of the auricle (pinna) and external ear canal may include any skin, cartilage, or bone disease. Relationships of the external ear to the middle ear, mastoid, scalp, skull, neck, parotid, and to the temporomandibular joint regions create many differential diagnostic problems and require a number of therapeutic approaches.

Congenital, acquired, and traumatic external ear diseases can also produce secondary lesions in eighth nerve (auditory and vestibular) and in seventh nerve systems.

Thus, external ear diseases involve far more complexities than simplistic considerations under "external otitis."

EXAMINATION OF THE EXTERNAL EAR

Proper examination of the auricle, external auditory meatus and external auditory canal requires the use of an electric headlight and a binocular magnifying loupe in addition to the ordinary electric otoscope (see Ch. 3, Ear Examination). The surgical binocular microscope is ideal but not essential. The patient's head must be immobilized by use of a headrest or use of an examining table. Sterile speculums, suction tips, fine cotton-wrapped metal applicators, and blunt metal cerumen spoon curets are needed for removal of dequamated epithelium, cerumen, and/or foreign bodies from the canal. The electric otoscope is useful, but it should usually be preceded by bimanual examination with headlight, magnifying loupe, and cleansing of the external auditory meatus and canal. Many diagnostic errors are due to premature otoscope examination prior to inspection and debridement with binocular vision and magnification.

Examination of the inflamed and infected external ear may be painful. A normal ear canal is moderately sensitive to instrumentation. The rapid introduction of an otoscope with a metal speculum may produce extreme discomfort even in a normal external auditory canal.

It is helpful to "desensitize" the ear by a conditioning maneuver prior to use of the speculum or any instrument. A simple gentle touch upon the auricle and external auditory meatus with a cotton-tipped applicator will prepare the patient for examination of the external meatus and canal. Such preliminary "warning palpation" is extremely helpful and takes but a second.

A frequent error in otoscopy is that of hiding a lesion with the speculum of the otoscope. A small meatal or canal lesion will be missed if the examiner places the speculum on the lesion without prior examination of the auricle and the external auditory meatus and canal with no instrument. Posterosuperior elevation of the auricle with anterior digital retraction of the tragus will frequently disclose a lesion otherwise blocked from view by insertion of a speculum (Fig. 13–1). An infected sebaceous cyst, a tumor, a foreign body, or an abrasion will be hidden and may well be missed by immediate use of a speculum.

After examination of the external auditory meatus, a speculum with the largest possible diameter is selected for adequate visualization of the cartilaginous external auditory canal.

Unilateral auricular external meatal or canal hypesthesia may be noted. Unilateral hypesthesia has been reported in several lesions, including acoustic neurinoma. However, it has also been noted in Meniere's disease. The diagnostic significance of unilateral hypesthesia remains unclear (2).

Hyperesthesia is found in temporomandibular joint problems as well as in cervical plexus neuritis.

MALFORMATIONS OF THE AURICLE, EXTERNAL AUDITORY MEATUS, AND EXTERNAL AUDITORY CANAL

CONGENITAL AURICULAR APLASIA

Total auricular aplasia is not common. When it occurs, it is most usually associated with defects of the external auditory meatus and canal. Occasionally, there may be a normal but small external meatus and canal. Very commonly, associated malformations of the tympanic membrane and middle ear accompany auricular and external meatal and canal malformations. A number of congenital syndromes with combined malforma-

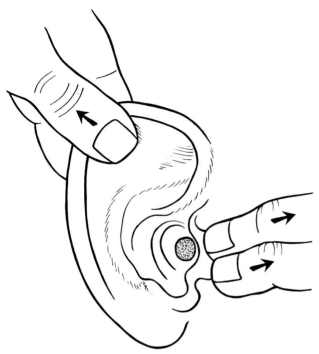

FIG. 13–1. Preliminary external ear digital examination without speculum.

tions of the ear and other structures are discussed in Chapter 32, Hereditary Congenital Ear Syndromes.

Auricular aplasia may be unilateral or bilateral. No urgent surgery is indicated in infancy. If it is unilateral and the contralateral ear is entirely normal with normal hearing, there is no need for haste in therapeutic management, since no significant communication deficit exists. Language and speech development will be acquired in normal fashion, if there are no associated congenital lesions. There is no urgency in considering the cosmetic aspect of the absent or malformed auricle or surgical reconstruction of the involved external auditory meatus and canal or middle ear.

The problems of auricular aplasia, the "lop" ear, the prominent auricle, and other malformations, and the pros and cons of reconstructive auriculoplasty surgical techniques and uses of auricular prostheses are discussed in Chapter 32.

The problems of combined auricular, external meatal and canal, and middle ear malformations require collaborative otosurgical and plastic surgical approaches. In general, the surgical reconstructions of combined ear malformations should be staged, with primary attention directed to tympanoplastic procedures for external meatal and external canal atresia and middle ear and ossicular reconstruction. Auriculoplasty or auricular prosthetic corrections can then be instituted following correction of the hearing defects.

CONCHAL BLOCKADE (PHYSIOLOGICAL EFFECT OF MALFORMATION OF CONCHA)

A "collapsed," anteriorly displaced conchal fold and cartilage may be responsible for blockade of the external auditory meatus, producing fluctuating conductive hearing loss (Reger effect). The abnormally forward-lying conchal cartilage may make contact with the posteromedial surface of the tragus. The condition is usually bilateral and some patients with this condition learn that they can hear better if the auricle is pulled backwards and upwards, pulling the conchal fold away from the tragal contact area. Such conchal malformation may produce only intermittent ear blockade and hearing loss, particularly when there is additional obstruction by cerumen, moisture, or the swelling of external otitis.

The audiometric characteristics of the Reger effect are variable and are demonstrated in Chapter 6, Audiologic Assessment, Functional Hearing Loss, and Objective Audiometry.

The diagnosis of conchal blockade is frequently missed because of the primary use of the otoscope alone, without prior examination of the auricle and tragus region with binocular vision, an examination that should be performed *without the use of a speculum.* The primary conventional use of an otoscope speculum simply pushes the conchal cartilage out of the way and is responsible for many missed diagnoses of this lesion (Fig. 13–2).

Patients with conchal blockade will require frequent removal of cerumen. The frequency of removal is not due to the amount of cerumen but to the fact that the very narrow cartilaginous external auditory meatus is open only when there is no cerumen in the meatal area. If simple cerumen removal accomplishes relief, no further treatment is necessary.

However, if the problem is not solved by cerumen removal and there is chronic annoyance because of hearing fluctuations requiring frequent physical elevation of the auricle by the patient, the only solution is a surgical canal-plasty, involving subtotal removal of the anterior conchal cartilage lip.

Surgical Correction of Conchal Blockade

This operation is performed under local or general anesthesia. Following a low endaural incision, the anterior presenting edge of the conchal cartilage is exposed. Skin and perichondrium are elevated to ex-

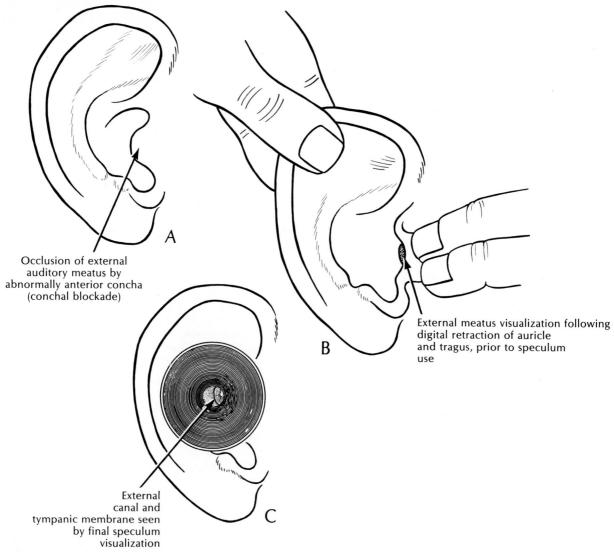

Occlusion of external
auditory meatus by
abnormally anterior concha
(conchal blockade)

External meatus visualization following
digital retraction of auricle
and tragus, prior to speculum
use

External
canal and
tympanic membrane seen
by final speculum
visualization

FIG. 13–2. Conchal collapse with Reger effect. **A.** Occlusion of external auditory meatus by abnormally anterior concha (conchal blockade). **B.** External meatus visualization following auricular and tragal digital retraction prior to speculum use. **C.** External canal and tympanic membrane seen by final speculum visualization.

pose conchal cartilage. A partial semilunar resection of obstructive anterior conchal cartilage lip is carried out along with removal of excess skin and primary closure of the incision (Fig. 13–3). In some cases, removal of additional superior conchal skin in the meatal portion of the endaural incision is necessary to facilitate the canal-plasty. In some cases it advisable to use an indwelling arterial Dacron tube (1×2 cm) to maintain patency during the 2-week healing period. The tube is sutured to the upper wound margins and remains in the external auditory meatus and canal until the incision is completely healed.

PREAURICULAR BRANCHIAL CLEFT FISTULAS

Preauricular congenital fistulas are quite common and are usually bilateral. A tiny dimple anterior to the helix is usually the external opening of a branchial cleft cyst. Its tract may be single or racemose, of variable length and direction. Uninfected preauricular cysts are minor cosmetic problems and usually require no treatment. There may be secondary infection due to skin bacteria and to manipulation by the patient. An infected pre-auricular cyst (Fig. 13–4) may respond to con-

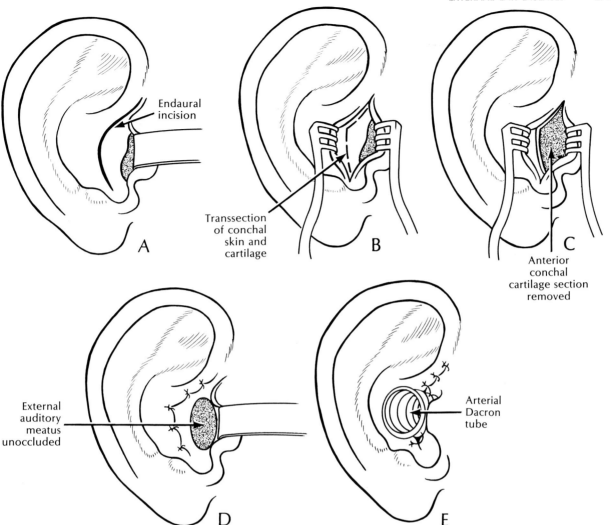

FIG. 13–3. Surgical correction of conchal collapse.

servative treatment consisting of hot compresses and appropriate antibiotic therapy, following cultures and sensitivity tests of secretions from the cyst opening. Frequent recurrences of infections in such preauricular cysts call for excision.

Excision of a preauricular congenital fistula may involve extensive dissection, since the tract can extend into the ear canal, into the parotid gland, the pharynx, the tonsillar fossa, or into the retrosubmandibular area of the neck. Excision of a preauricular congenital fistula should not be undertaken as a minor procedure. An extensive tract may be intimately related to branches of the facial nerve and to major vessels of the neck. Many congenital preauricular cysts have long complex tracts that may be multiple and noncommunicating. Incomplete excision will cause frequent major recurrences with more difficult second-stage excisions because of scarring and obliteration of normal landmarks (Fig. 13–5).

DISEASES OF THE AURICLE AND PERIAURICULAR REGION

POSTAURICULAR LESIONS

Acute postauricular swelling may be encountered in acute mastoiditis, especially in children. Either periostitis or a postauricular abscess due to cortical bone necrosis will produce a tender soft-tissue swelling with obliteration of the postauricular sulcus and forward displacement of the auricle (see Ch. 14, Acute Otitis Media and Mastoiditis).

A thin linear scar in the postauricular sulcus may be evidence of a childhood mastoidectomy, of which the patient may have been unaware. This finding may solve a diagnostic problem in a patient with a conductive hearing loss, an intact tympanic membrane, and no obvious cause. In mastoidectomy during infancy, the incus may

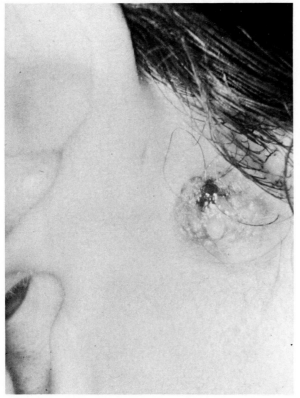

FIG. 13–4. One small uninfected dimple is at the margin of the helix; a larger, congenital, preauricular fistula anteriorly is infected.

FIG. 13–5. Congenital preauricular fistulas. **A.** A simple "dimple" pit, which is superficial. **B.** An example of possible major racemose extensions into pharynx and neck.

have been dislocated or removed, producing a total conductive hearing loss. The only obvious sign may be a tiny previously unrecognized postauricular sulcus scar.

A very deep postauricular scar (Fig. 13–6) may be found in older patients who had mastoid surgery in the decades prior to the 1940's. Postauricular mastoidectomy techniques in that period frequently resulted in deep scars because of superficial wound closure methods, which resulted in acquired external canal atresia in addition to the postauricular deformation.

A postauricular fistula into the mastoid is usually the result of an unhealed postauricular mastoidectomy wound (Fig. 13–7), occasionally accompanied by recurrent keratoma (cholesteatoma), tympanosclerosis, or granulomatous otomastoiditis. A postauricular fistula may be accompanied by intermittent or constant purulent drainage (Fig. 13–8). Revision mastoidectomy is usually indicated in such cases, either as a stage or as a concomitant of a postauricular fistula repair (see Ch. 17, Otomastoiditis Surgery—Mastoidectomy and Tympanoplasty). Postauricular eczema and dermatitis may accompany a number of scalp dermatologic lesions.

Postauricular tumors in children and adults range from relatively benign lesions, such as histiocytic granuloma to highly malignant lesions such as rhabdomyosarcoma (see Ch. 22, Temporal Bone Tumors).

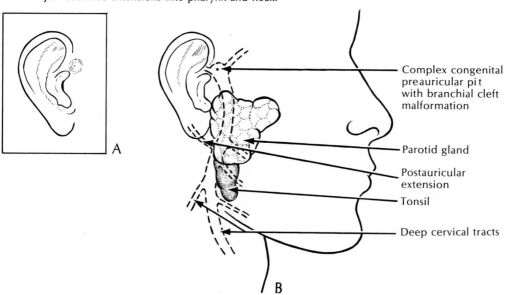

A

Complex congenital preauricular pit with branchial cleft malformation

Parotid gland

Postauricular extension

Tonsil

Deep cervical tracts

B

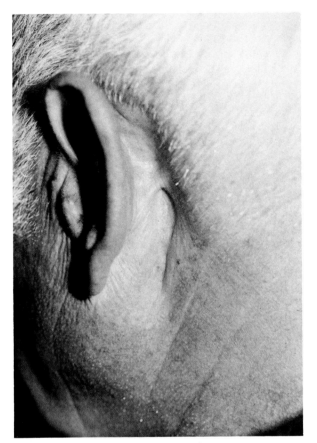

FIG. 13–6. Deep postauricular mastoidectomy scar.

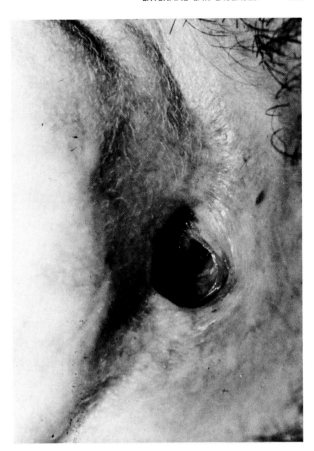

FIG. 13–7. Postauricular dry fistula due to old unhealed postauricular mastoidectomy incision.

PREAURICULAR LESIONS

Acute tender preauricular swelling extending to the zygomatic process of the temporal bone or to the zygoma itself may accompany acute mastoiditis. This is usually due to extension of epitympanic infection into zygomatic cells, which may break through into the squamous temporal bone area (see Ch. 14, Acute Otitis Media and Mastoiditis).

A preauricular scar may be the result of previous endaural ear surgery or a face lift operation. Such scars occasionally become infected, but usually respond to conservative measures without surgery.

LESIONS OF THE AURICLE

Dermatologic Lesions

Auricular dermatologic lesions may include all common skin diseases which appear in the auricle as well as in the scalp. Treatment, in general, is based upon dermatologic therapy of the scalp lesions.

Tumors of the Auricle

Tumors of the auricle are frequent, and include basal-cell carcinoma, squamous-cell carcinoma, malignant melanoma, and rhabdomyosarcoma (especially in children), as well as many benign tumors. Treatment is based on the nature of the lesion and usually requires excision and postexcision radiation therapy in some cases (see Ch. 22, Temporal Bone Tumors).

Auricular Inflammatory Lesions—Chondritis, Perichondritis

An acutely swollen, tender auricle, especially the concha and tragus, can accompany acute external otitis. Acute auricular tenderness serves as an important differential diagnostic sign between acute external otitis and acute otitis media. The latter is rarely accompanied by tenderness in the auricle. However, it is possible for acute external

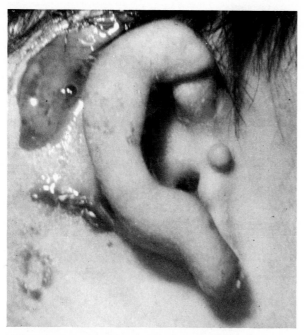

FIG. 13–8. Draining granuloma from recurrent postauricular mastoid fistula. Note preauricular "tag."

otitis to be accompanied by a major conductive hearing loss similar to that noted in otitis media because of occlusion of the external auditory canal. It is also possible for a patient to have coexisting external otitis and otitis media, especially in gram-negative infections such as *Pseudomonas*. Tenderness of the auricle is usually an indication of infection in meatal and canal wall skin rather than in the otomastoid area. Mastoid x-rays, cultures, and serial audiologic studies are necessary for differential diagnosis.

Auricular perichondritis and chondritis may follow frostbite, burns, and trauma (see Ch. 24, Traumatic Diseases of the Ear and Temporal Bone). Recent popularization of acupuncture therapy is responsible for many cases of chondritis.

The "cauliflower" ear of the boxer is due to repeated multiple contusions, hemorrhages, and fibrotic lesions with secondary chondritis. Treatment involves incision and drainage of acute suppurative infections, combined with appropriate antibiotic therapy. Reconstructive plastic procedures may be necessary for major auricular deformities.

Infections following ear piercing are not uncommon, especially since most ear piercing is not performed by physicians. Infections of the lobe usually respond to simple cleansing, warm soaks, and appropriate antibiotic therapy. It is also possible for viral hepatitis to follow ear piercing (4).

Infections may follow inflammatory reactions to the earring metal. Nickel, used in gold earrings, predisposes to allergic reactions. Use of 14-carat gold, stainless steel, or platinum is advisable.

Relapsing Generalized Polychondritis

Generalized relapsing polychondritis is a serious mesodermal disease of obscure nature. Perichondritis of the auricle may be associated with generalized polychondritis, and may also be accompanied by cochlear hearing loss of varying degrees and severity. The relationship of degenerative labyrinthine lesions and the polychondritis is unclear at the present time. The presence of a tender swollen auricle in a patient who has an inner ear hearing loss should call for a careful general medical examination with study of other cartilaginous areas, including ribs, trachea, etc. Steroid and antibiotic therapies have been used. The lesion is still a diagnostic and therapeutic dilemma: It appears to be an autoimmune problem with a common molecular target (6).

LESIONS OF THE EXTERNAL AUDITORY MEATUS AND EXTERNAL AUDITORY CANAL

"EAR WAX"—HYPERCERUMINOSIS

The Problem of Ear Wax

The most common ear lesion encountered in the practice of medicine is "ear wax," and the most common ear procedure in medical practice is ear wax removal. Although it is very frequently performed, removal may be inadequate and/or traumatic. Primary reasons for failure in cerumen removal are poor visualization and instrumentation.

There are great variations in the amount and frequency of cerumen production and in diversities of lipid chemical cerumen types. There are people who are definitely categorized as "wax formers." Such cerumen formation may recur rapidly. Symptoms are ear stuffiness, itching, and hearing loss. Symptomatology will depend not only on the type and rate of accumulation, but also on the anatomic aspects of the ear canal. A narrow, tortuous cartilaginous bony canal junction will be responsible for frequent cerumen impactions, which may contact the tympanic membrane. Impactions may produce discomfort or severe otalgia, especially if water enters the canal and increases the mass of the cerumen impaction. Secondary external otitis is commonly a sequel of cerumen impaction.

Patients should be cautioned not to attempt self-removal of cerumen with the use of cotton applicators, hairpins, or other devices. Such attempts are followed frequently by increased impaction and secondary infections. In general, the use of cotton-tipped applicators in the ears should be discouraged. Patients are told to leave their ears alone and not to attempt to be "too neat" about cleansing ears following showers and baths. It is perfectly adequate and safe to dry the ear with the end of a towel.

Removal of Ear Wax

A headlight and binocular loupe magnification are essential (see Ch. 3, Ear Examination). The electric otoscope is inadequate, and its primary use in wax removal is discouraged. Cerumen may be removed by irrigation, by blunt ear curet, by alligator or "cup" forceps, by suction, or by a combination of all methods. The otoscope can be used for final examination, including pneumatic otoscopy.

Cerumen diagnoses in new patients may be incorrect. An accumulation of cerumen may surround an unsuspected tumor, keratoma, granulomatous polyp, or foreign body.

Before cerumen removal in a new patient, a careful history is essential and may reveal information regarding 1) tympanic membrane perforation, 2) previous ear surgery, or 3) previous acute otitis media or chronic otomastoiditis. Mastoid x-rays (Schuller view) may show evidence of childhood or acquired mastoiditis, or a surgical defect. Cerumen irrigation in a patient whose tympanic membrane has not been previously seen should be avoided.

Removal of cerumen in a new patient is best done with the use of suction (Fig. 13–9) and the GENTLE use of both "naked" and cotton-wrapped cerumen curets (Fig. 13–10). In a "new" patient a primary cerumen irrigation before tympanic membrane visualization may be unwise. Cerumen and/or water may be forced through an unknown perforation into the middle ear, with potentially serious sequelae.

In "old" patients who are known to the physician as "wax formers," it is possible to expedite wax removal by careful syringing, using water at body temperature with a metal ear syringe (Fig. 13–11), or through a compressed-air washbottle system (Fig. 13–12).

The ear canal and tympanic membrane must be examined following ear wax removal. If irrigating solution has been used, any remaining in the canal should be gently wiped out with cotton-wrapped metal applicators. The water may be suctioned or blown out with the use of compressed air pressure. It is essential that the tympanic membrane and the anterior sulcus of the external auditory canal be visualized following cerumen removal.

A number of annoying yet "minor" external auditory canal problems other than cerumen require management. Epithelial collections due to desquamation and debris collections due to unusually dense hair growth in the cartilaginous external auditory meatus and canal require ear hygiene. Frequently, irrigation and simple curettage are ineffective. The use of H_2O_2 on applicators, applied liberally prior to removal, will usually loosen debris and allow more effective irrigation or curettage. Periodic instillation by the patient of 5–10 drops of 1% boric acid in 70% ethyl alcohol (at body temperature) twice daily will frequently give relief and result in less frequent debris accumulations in the external canal.

The itching ear compounded by scratching frequently results in epithelial slough, and a thin, sterile serous otorrhea. Gentle insufflation of boric acid powder (1%) will coat the desquamated area and allow prompt healing. Similarly, the use of boric acid in a lanolin-petrolatum base is helpful for dryness and its resulting itching.

FOREIGN BODIES IN THE EXTERNAL AUDITORY CANAL

In addition to epithelial debris and cerumen, foreign bodies may be present in the external auditory canal. Patients—adults or children—frequently push absorbent cotton, crumpled toilet paper, crumpled tissue, toothpicks, matches, and many other foreign bodies into the external auditory canal. An unimpacted foreign body is best removed with a blunt curet under direct vision, with loupe and headlight visualization (Fig. 13–13). A foreign body may remain in the canal for many years, as an undiagnosed and unrecognized cause of conductive hearing loss.

Foreign bodies in the external canal are potentially serious, and when impacted at the junction of the cartilaginous and bony external canal, safe removal is impossible without anesthesia, particularly in a child (Fig. 13–14). Foreign bodies may be inadvertently pushed through the tympanic membrane into the middle ear, with serious sequelae (Fig. 13–15), such as ossicular chain disruption with tympanic membrane perforation, secondary otitis media, facial paralysis, and labyrinth damage by penetration ruptures

FIG. 13–9. **A** and **B.** Suction removal of cerumen.

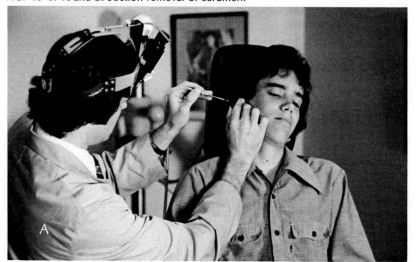

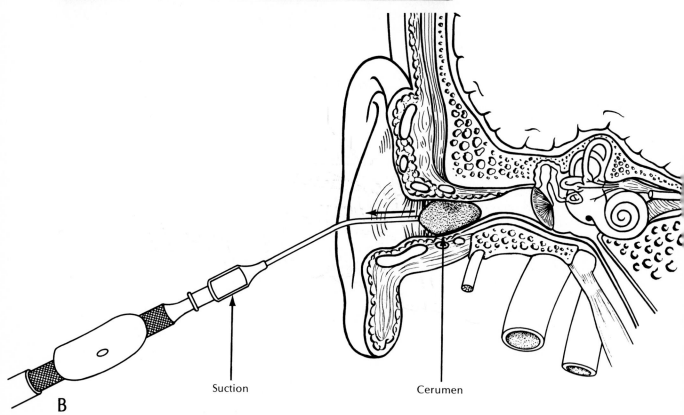

Suction   Cerumen

FIG. 13–10. A. Cerumen removal with blunt curet under direct vision with headlight and magnifying loupe. **B.** Cerumen removal with blunt curet.

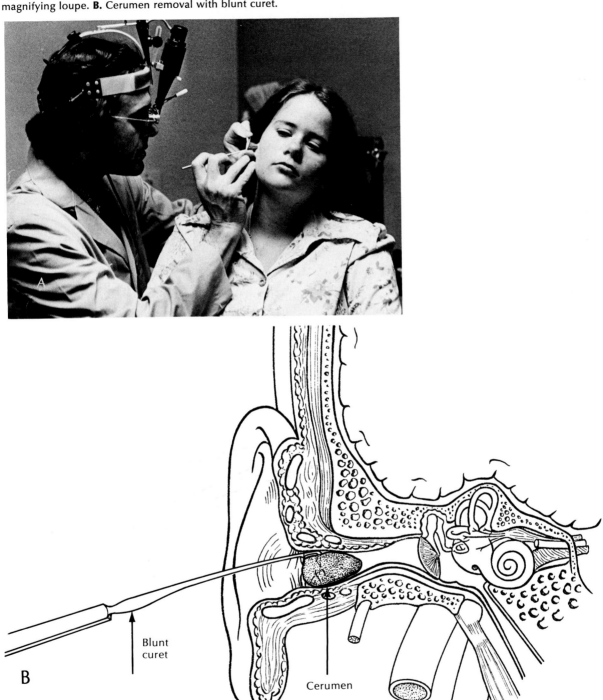

Blunt
curet

Cerumen

B

FIG. 13–11. A. Cerumen irrigation with cerumen syringe. **B.** Cerumen syringe in use.

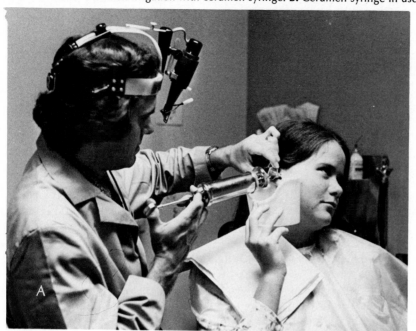

A

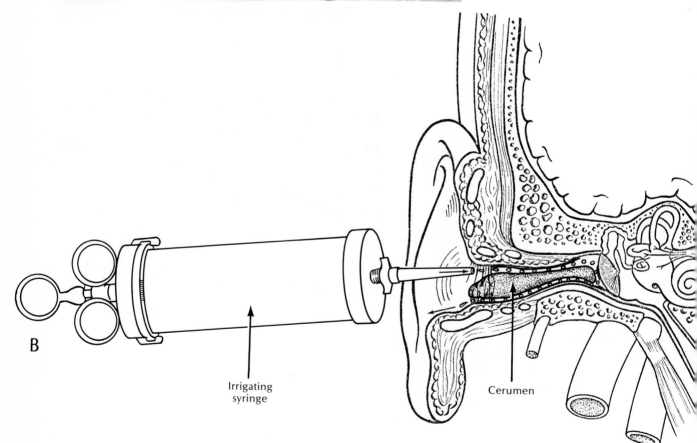

B

Irrigating
syringe

Cerumen

FIG. 13–12. A. Cerumen irrigation with compressed air irrigation—bottle system. **B.** Irrigation bottle for cerumen removal.

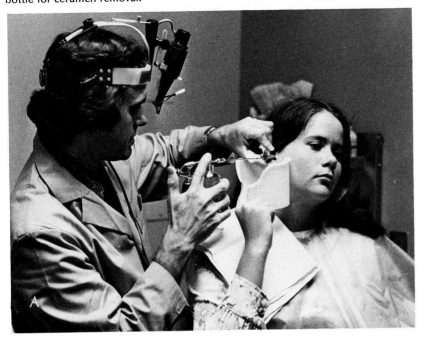

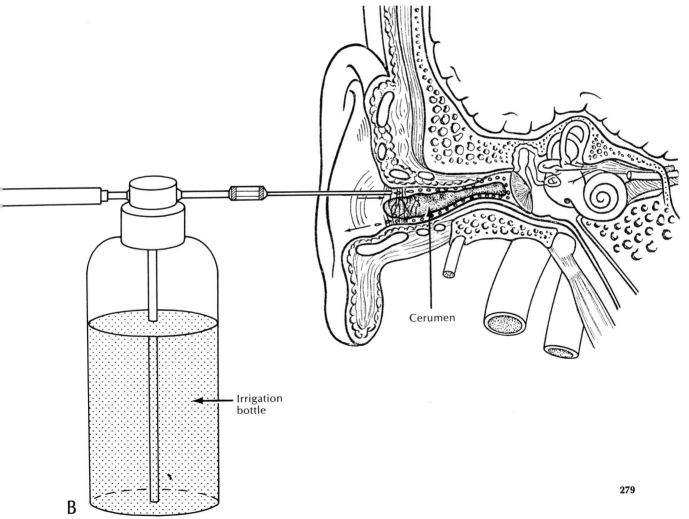

Cerumen

Irrigation
bottle

through the round window membrane or the oval window.

When a fixed foreign body is encountered, outpatient attempts at removal should cease. The patient should be hospitalized following x-ray and audiometric studies. Examination and removal should be an operating room procedure with adequate general anesthesia and the use of the surgical microscope. In some cases, endaural or postauricular incision may be necessary for adequate visualization and instrumentation (Fig. 13–16).

DERMATOLOGIC LESIONS OF THE EXTERNAL AUDITORY MEATUS AND CANAL

Seborrheic Dermatitis

Seborrheic dermatitis affects the ear as part of scalp involvement. (See Color Fig. 3.) The erythematous, greasy eruption with itching is frequently followed by scratching and secondary neurodermatitis. Factitial bacterial infections frequently follow neurodermatitis. Thus, acute external otitis may be the sequel of seborrheic dermatitis, followed by neurodermatitis and self-inflicted secondary bacterial or fungus infections. The treatment of auricular seborrheic dermatitis is basically dermatologic, with special attention to the treatment of the underlying scalp lesions. Frequently, appropriate dermatologic treatment of the scalp lesion will be followed by spontaneous resolution of the external auditory canal lesion.

Allergic Dermatitis

A number of contact substances may produce atopic contact dermatitis due to specific hypersensitivities. Patients may be allergic to plastic or metal in eyeglasses and earrings, to perfumes, shaving cream, hair dyes and cosmetics.

Asteatosis—the Dry Ear

An important cause of the itching ear is the dry external auditory canal lacking cerumen, with inadequate sebaceous lubricating secretion. There appears to be a racial etiology in asteatosis, with a higher incidence in Orientals, American Indians, and Eskimos. It may be associated with other skin problems in older people. Such deficiency of normal "lubrication" of the external auditory canal will usually respond to the use of a simple boric acid lanolin-petrolatum base ointment, preferably applied by the patient at bedtime once or twice weekly with a clean finger and not with a cotton applicator. In general, the use of cotton applicators for ear cleansing or ear medication should

be discouraged. The severe itching phases will usually respond to short courses of steroid cream applications (twice daily for 7 days).

ACUTE INFECTIOUS DISEASES OF THE EXTERNAL EAR CANAL

A number of diseases can cause acute external otitis. Such lesions can be of viral, mycotic, or bacterial origin.

Viral External Otitis

Herpes simplex of the auricle or external canal resembles herpes on the face or elsewhere in the body. Local treatment is confined to the use of a mild lanolin-boric acid ointment applied several times daily. If the herpetic lesion is in the external auditory canal, the ointment is applied on a 0.25-in. gauze trailer left in the canal and changed at least once daily. Response is reasonably rapid and recurrences are relatively infrequent.

Viral bullous myringitis involving the outer tympanic membrane layer can spread laterally beyond the tympanic sulcus into the bony external canal. (See Color Fig. 5.) Topical use of warm, simple, nonantibiotic glycerol preparations will give some relief. The bullas will usually rupture spontaneously. Occasionally, surgical incision of a bulla will be necessary to relieve pressure and pain. Gentian violet may be beneficial for local treatment. It should be applied on a very fine applicator gently to the ruptured bullous area. The canal should be kept closed with sterile cotton changed twice daily. In the event secondary bacterial infection of the middle ear or external auditory canal occurs, it should be treated with appropriate antibiotic medication as a specific bacterial acute otitis media or bacterial canal infection.

The Ramsay Hunt syndrome is a serious herpes zoster viral disease of the geniculate ganglion, which should not be confused with herpes simplex of the external auditory canal or auricle. The lesion is accompanied primarily by facial nerve paralysis and occasionally by labyrinthine involvement due to cochlear and vestibular eighth nerve involvement.

Specific treatment for the Ramsay Hunt syndrome does not exist at the present time. Secondary bacterial infection is not common. The primary problem involves compression of the geniculate ganglion, which may respond to steroid therapy or require facial nerve decompression (see Ch. 30, Seventh Nerve Lesions and Injuries).

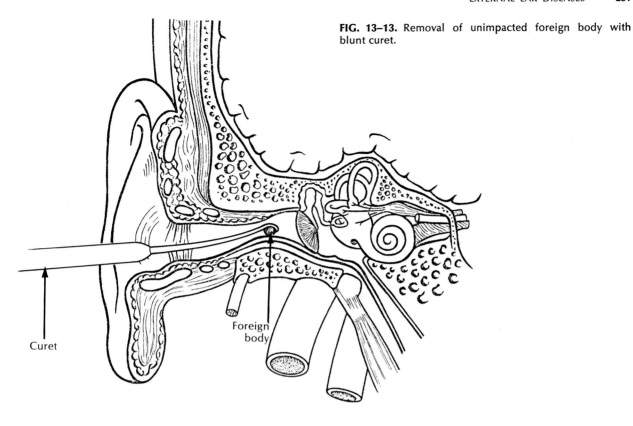

FIG. 13–13. Removal of unimpacted foreign body with blunt curet.

Curet

Foreign
body

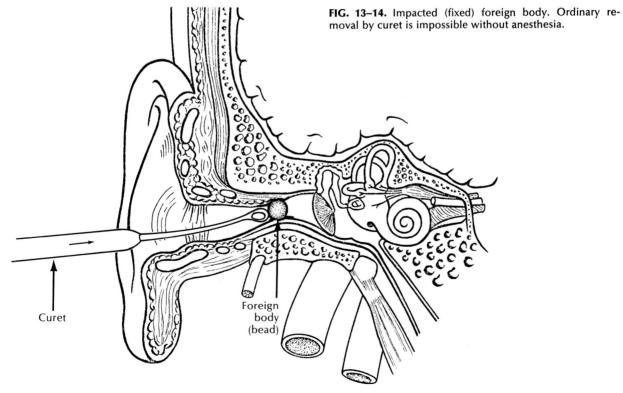

FIG. 13–14. Impacted (fixed) foreign body. Ordinary removal by curet is impossible without anesthesia.

Curet

Foreign
body
(bead)

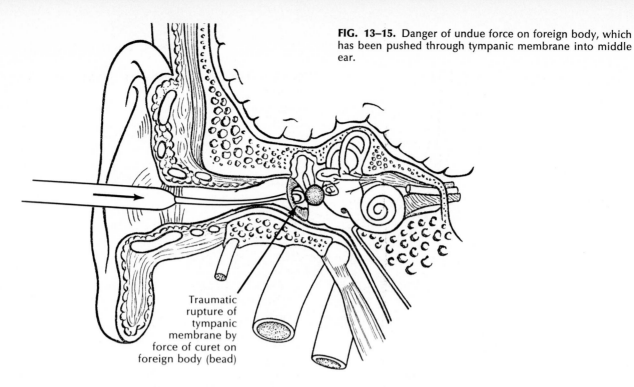

FIG. 13–15. Danger of undue force on foreign body, which has been pushed through tympanic membrane into middle ear.

Traumatic rupture of tympanic membrane by force of curet on foreign body (bead)

FIG. 13–16. Endaural surgical approach for external canal impacted foreign body (bead) removal. **A.** Endaural incision. **B.** Skin flap elevated by extension of incision. **C.** Posterior canal wall bone removal. **D.** Atraumatic removal of foreign body. **E.** Flap replaced.

Endaural Incision   Incision extended   Bone removed

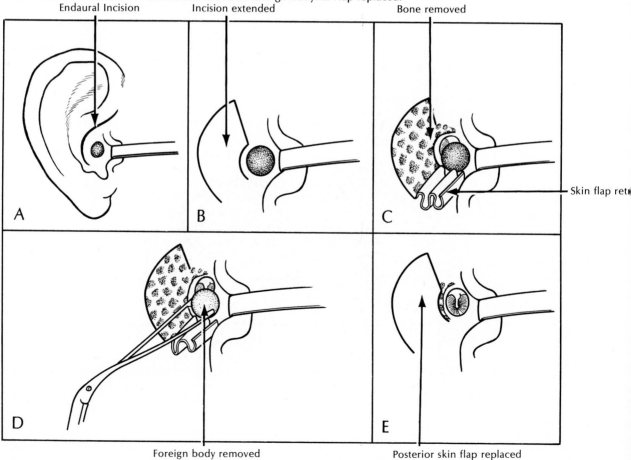

Skin flap ret▶

Foreign body removed   Posterior skin flap replaced

Mycotic External Otitis—Otomycosis

True otomycosis is characterized by gross yeast or fungus infections that can be seen otoscopically. (See Color Fig. 4.) The specificity of the infection can be confirmed by microscopic studies.

There is a characteristic otoscopic appearance to most fungus infections of the external auditory canal. The lesions may appear as a "forest" of "trees," which may vary in color from white to black, including many variations. Very frequently the skin under the fungus area, particularly if it is in the bony canal, will have been eroded, and the mycotic lesion will actually be in contact with bare bone. Fungous diseases are more common in tropical or subtropical climates. Among the fungi responsible have been members of the following groups: Aspergillaceae, Mucoraceae, yeast-like fungi, dermatophytes, and a number of miscellaneous fungal groups. The characteristic beginning of a true mycotic infection is that of itching in the ear. Very frequently the itching will be rapidly followed by pain. If the fungal mass is large, there may well be complaints of "blockage," fullness in the ear, and conductive hearing loss.

Removal of overlying cerumen by gentle suction and curettage, under binocular headlight loupe or examining microscope visualization, and the preparation of smears for examination under the microscope will usually reveal the presence of mycelia spores, and other cells.

As the disease progresses, pain may become intense. The patient may be unable to chew, there may be hearing loss and tinnitus, and the external auditory canal will be entirely occluded by marked cellulitis that can extend into auricular perichondrium and skin. Edema and lymphadenopathy in the periauricular and subauricular regions will be accompanied by enlargement of the anterior and posterior cervical lymph nodes.

The treatment of otomycosis consists primarily of thorough and complete removal of the fungal masses with the use of suction and careful cleansing with sterile, fine cotton-tipped applicators under direct vision. Irrigation is occasionally advisable in the removal of such fungal masses from the external auditory canal. Local antimycotic therapy is usually very effective. A number of agents are useful. Most of them are rather nonspecific with reference to fungal identification and specificity. Classic treatments of fungal infections in the past have included a number of topical drugs that were extremely effective but usually very painful. These include 90% ethyl alcohol, 1% thymol in 90% alcohol, and ether. The recent introduction of a number of antifungal drugs has made it possible to treat most of these infections without the need for use of painful drugs. The new drugs, in ointment or suspension form, include tolnaftate, nystatin-iodochlorhydroxyquin, etc. They are applied on a sterile 0.25-in. gauze wick saturated with the medication under direct vision with a fine forceps. The entire involved area of the external auditory canal is covered by the medicated gauze, which is changed daily.

Such treatment is usually followed by prompt recovery.

In *Aspergillus niger* infections, the skin of the osseous meatus and tympanic membrane is covered with a moist gray membrane with numerous black spots. The membrane may be suctioned or gently removed by irrigation. After the removal of the fungal membrane, the skin appears desquamated, red, and swollen. Occasional perforations of the tympanic membrane are present. The infection may respond to treatment with antifungal drugs only to reappear with renewed vigor at intervals of weeks or months. Long-term observations are advisable.

Bacterial External Otitis

The pathologic findings in both acute and chronic external otitis will vary according to etiology and duration. However, the essential findings are those of marked edema, inflammation, miliary abscess formation, hyperkeratosis, infiltrates surrounding sebaceous and apocrine glands, and vascular congestion (Fig. 13–17).

In temperate climates the most common type of bacterial external otitis is that due to gram-positive organisms, most commonly staphylococci. However, *Pseudomonas* organisms are noted with increasing frequency. Such an external otitis may take the form of furunculosis, which occurs as an isolated lesion, or more commonly, it will take the form of diffuse external otitis. Occasionally, both furunculosis and diffuse external otitis may coexist.

The first symptom is usually pain, and in most instances it is possible to get a history of a predisposing cause, such as the use of cotton-tipped applicators by the patient for an itching ear, swimming, or some other irritating event, such as shampooing the hair. Pain is variable although it may be very severe in some patients. Occlusion of the external auditory canal can be accompanied by tinnitus, fullness, and hearing loss.

Examination will reveal external auditory meatus and canal redness and edema, which can involve conchal, tragal, and auricular cartilages.

Very frequently the canal will be closed tightly so that it may be impossible to insert even an infant's speculum into it. Secretions from the area should be cultured. Gram-negative and/or gram-positive organisms may be encountered.

Dr. Ben H. Senturia (5), with vast experience in the management of acute diffuse bacterial external otitis, recently summarized a new study with the following conclusions:

1) Ears with mild acute diffuse external otitis consistently showed *Pseudomonas* organisms, which should respond to simple "Coly-mycin" or "polymyxin B" preparations. The contralateral, uninfected ear showed only *Staphylococcus* epidermidis. Response to treatment of the mild infection was very good.

2) The moderate and severe grades of infection showed a broad flora of exogenous organisms which, in addition to *Pseudomonas*, included *Proteus mirabilis,*

Klebsiella pneumoniae and beta hemolytic streptococci. Such infections required broad coverage antibiotic ear drops and frequently needed supplementary systemic therapy. In order to provide proper therapy for these grades of ear infection, cultures should be obtained routinely prior to institution of therapy.

3) Clear evidence for the use of a corticosteroid incorporated in the otic drops is not available in this study, but clinical experience with these patients strongly suggested its use. Where there was secondary eczematization of the auricle and periauricular areas, a steroid cream was very effective.

4) These studies clearly demonstrated that spontaneous subsidence of symptoms and disappearance of exogenous organisms does not occur during the hot, humid weather; that early and effective treatment is important for the prompt control of acute diffuse external otitis.

5) Sensitivity tests did not support the routine use

FIG. 13–17. A. Normal epidermis in cartilaginous external canal. **B.** External otitis. Note hyperkeratosis, fluid in stratum corneum, abscess infiltrates, edema, acanthosis, and elongated rete pegs.

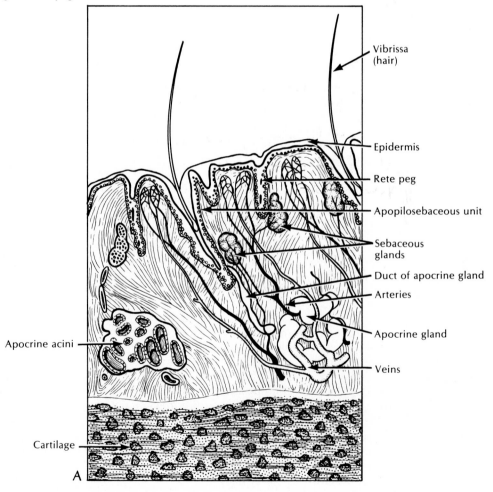

Vibrissa (hair)

Epidermis

Rete peg

Apopilosebaceous unit

Sebaceous glands

Duct of apocrine gland

Arteries

Apocrine gland

Veins

Apocrine acini

Cartilage

A

FIG. 13–17 B (*continued*)

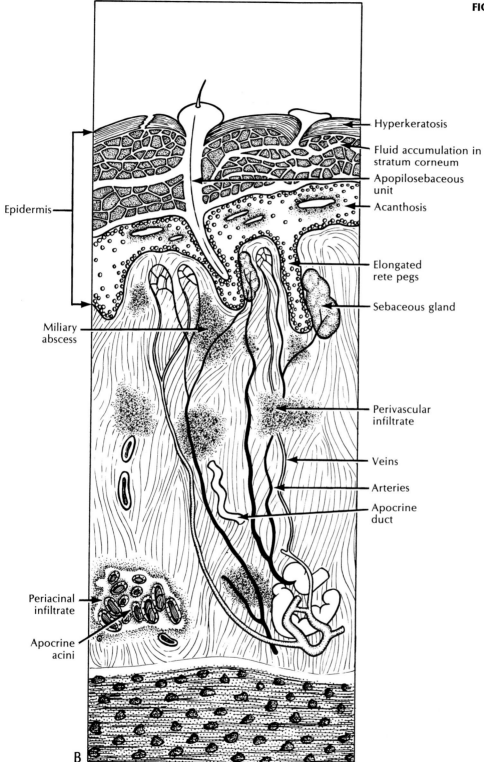

Hyperkeratosis

Fluid accumulation in stratum corneum

Apopilosebaceous unit

Acanthosis

Epidermis

Elongated rete pegs

Sebaceous gland

Miliary abscess

Perivascular infiltrate

Veins

Arteries

Apocrine duct

Periacinal infiltrate

Apocrine acini

B

of oral tetracyclines for the treatment of moderate and severe cases, although there appeared to be some good clinical responses in the severe grade of infection. Fortunately, oral systemic therapy is available for most of the exogenous organisms except *Pseudomonas*. When necessary in severe infections, because of poor response to local therapy, hospitalization for intramuscular and/or intravenous therapy with gentamicin and carbenicillin may be indicated.

6) It appeared that the mild form of acute diffuse external otitis can be treated effectively by an antibiotic-steroid combination ear drop preparation. However, the moderate and severe forms required the used of an antibiotic-steroid combination in a vehicle impregnated in a cotton or gauze pack inserted into the ear canal which will reduce the inflammatory edema of the skin. When the edema had subsided sufficiently, the ear drop combination was substituted successfully.

7) In order to effectively treat all forms of external otitis, further careful studies need to be performed on otic preparations, including ear drops containing single and multiple antibiotics, antibiotic-steroid combinations, antibiotics in cream and ointment vehicles and antibiotic-steroid combinations in other vehicles.

In addition to local therapy and systemic antibacterial therapy, adequate pain medication is always necessary. It is also advisable for the patient to limit physical activity, since it is not unusual for external otitis to spread into the middle ear, producing acute otitis media, or to spread to the periauricular area with cellulitis extending into the check, over the parotid region, down into the neck, and into the scalp.

In most cases, rapid resolution will follow combined local and systemic therapy. Inflammatory edema usually subsides within a few days, with relief of pain and obstruction.

Furunculosis may occasionally accompany acute diffuse external otitis and may require incision and drainage if there is a definitely pointing abscess. Such an abscess may drain spontaneously. In general, it is wise to avoid incision and drainage unless there is definitive evidence of localization. Conservative therapy of furunculosis will usually be followed by rapid therapeutic response. Warm compresses, using either warm saline or aluminum sulfate solution, are effective. Following resolution of the furunculosis, local therapy previously described for the external auditory canal is continued until total resolution of the external otitis.

Swimmer's Ear

External otitis (acute or chronic) related to swimming is very frequently encountered in tropical or subtropical climates. The more common types of swimmer's external otitis are due to either gram-negative organisms such as *Pseudomonas* or to fungal or yeast infections.

Swimming *per se* may not be etiologic in this type of external otitis. The real cause may be related to excessive attempts at ear cleansing following swimming. It frequently occurs as a result of a combination of temperature and humidity factors and absence of a protecting sebaceous lipid cover by normal ear gland secretions. The symptoms may be identical to those seen in acute gram-positive external otitis, although furunculosis is less common in gram-negative infections.

Local therapy is of greater value than systemic therapy in these infections although one should not hesitate to use systemic therapy with appropriate antibiotic drugs after culture and sensitivity tests have been performed. The primary treatment locally is that of meticulous cleansing, using suction and dry sterile applicators followed by insertion of gauze trailers medicated with one of the specific antibacterial drugs for gram-negative organisms. Among these effective drugs are chloramphenicol (Chloromycetin) and colistin sulfate (Coly-Mycin). Frequently acetic acid alone may be a useful treatment for gram-negative organisms. Simple vinegar as a common external otitis medication was very effectively used in the pre-antibiotic era. A nonaqueous solution of acetic acid in a propylene glycol vehicle is useful as prophylactic therapy in areas known to be endemic for swimmer's external otitis (3).

The secondary spread of either gram-positive or gram-negative organisms into auricular perichondrium and/or into the middle ear is not rare. External otitis with gram-negative organisms can be particularly dangerous in elderly diabetic patients. A serious temporal bone disease has recently been identified and termed "malignant external otitis."

MALIGNANT EXTERNAL OTITIS (FULMINATING OTITIS, MASTOIDITIS)

The term **malignant external otitis** is a useful description of a very serious disease that may start as a gram-negative external otitis infection which then spreads to the middle ear, causing otitis media and mastoiditis, with further intracranial and hematogenous spread. It is difficult to ascertain the primary cause of the lesion in many patients. Most commonly it occurs in elderly diabetics with varying degrees of vascular disease. The term "malignant external otitis" may give the erroneous impression that it is only an external otitis. The more profound bony and potentially intracranial aspect of this infection is discussed under the heading of Fulminating Otitis—Mastoiditis, Diabetic (see Ch. 16, Chronic Otomastoiditis—Diagnosis and Management).

SUBACUTE AND CHRONIC EXTERNAL OTITIS

Subacute and chronic forms of external otitis of bacterial or mycotic origin are not as common as the acute forms. In most instances, such infections are secondary to a dermatitis complicated by factitious infections. The "itching ear" is a common problem in dermatoses. It becomes an infected ear by virtue of the "scratching finger" or by the vigorous rubbing of the ear canal with a cotton-tipped applicator. Skin is removed by such trauma, and secondary infections are created.

Secondary External Otitis

Careful differential diagnosis must be based on an awareness of other sources of infection. Most important is the unrecognized existence of chronic otitis-mastoiditis with otorrhea. Secondary external otitis may be the first sign of a previously undiagnosed microperforation or marginal annular perforation of the tympanic membrane.

Careful otologic investigation is necessary in all chronic, subacute, or intermittent cases of infectious external otitis. This should include pneumatic otoscopy with magnification and radiographic and audiologic examinations.

In addition to unrecognized otomastoiditis, malformations, external keratoma, and early tumors (ceruminoma, carcinoma) may be the underlying causes of secondary infectious external otitis.

Primary Subacute, Chronic, or Intermittent Infectious External Otitis

Only after the possibility has been ruled out that the external otitis is secondary to some other primary problem should the management be based upon the consideration of a primary problem in the external auditory canal.

Chronic external otitis is usually due to deep infections of the meatal skin, involving subepithelial areas and usually in hair follicles, or in apocrine or cerumen glands.

Symptoms may alternate between itching and pain. Otorrhea may be scant or copious. Microbiologic studies by smear and culture are necessary for proper identification of organisms.

Treatment is usually based on careful cleansing of debris, preferably with suction, and followed by local medication. Specific antibiotic preparations may be used either in solutions or emulsions, or in the form of ointments. In the case of liquid preparations, techniques are similar to those described for acute external otitis. Attention to penicillin allergy and other sensitization must be given before local agents are selected.

Patients should be discouraged from cleansing or self medication with cotton applicators. Superinfections, secondary dermatitis and bleeding may follow any such self-treatment. Careful use of appropriate ear drop instillation or the use of a powder blower for powder insufflations may be advisable.

A number of commercial otic preparations are widely advertised and used. Most contain neomycin and hydrocortisone, and in addition some contain other ingredients such as colistin sulfate, polymyxin B, acetic acid, or other ingredients. Neomycin is potentially ototoxic. Care should be taken to prevent neomycin from entering the middle ear, with possible labyrinth penetration through the oval window or round window.

In general, true external otitis is of cartilaginous canal and meatal origin and is not due to bony canal (medial) lesions. Thus, local medication should be directed to the lateral two-thirds of the external auditory canal. Gauze trailers saturated with appropriate medications and carefully placed under direct vision by the physician are far more effective therapeutically than ear drops used by the patient, although the ear drops may be used to resaturate the gauze trailer every few hours. Trailers are usually removed in 24–36 hours.

Empirically, it has been found that many stubborn external canal bacterial infections will respond to certain dyes if they are resistant to antibiotics. Among these dyes are scarlet red and gentian violet in ointments that may be topically applied directly or applied by the use of a gauze trailer.

ACQUIRED CANAL ATRESIA

A relatively uncommon sequel of external otitis is that of acquired fibrotic atresia of the external otitis. It occasionally may be associated with chronic otitis—mastoiditis.

The presenting finding is that of a closed or an almost closed external meatus (Fig. 13–18). There may or may not be some degree of inflammatory change accompanying the edema and fibrosis in the meatal skin, but all that can be visualized is a tiny pinpoint opening, or the external auditory canal may be completely closed.

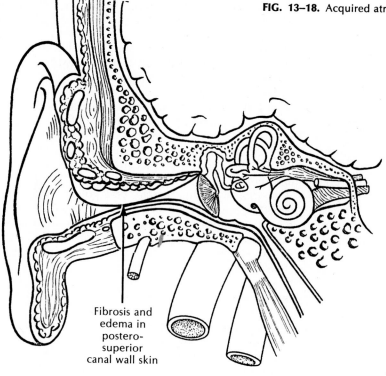

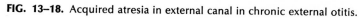

FIG. 13–18. Acquired atresia in external canal in chronic external otitis.

Fibrosis and edema in postero-superior canal wall skin

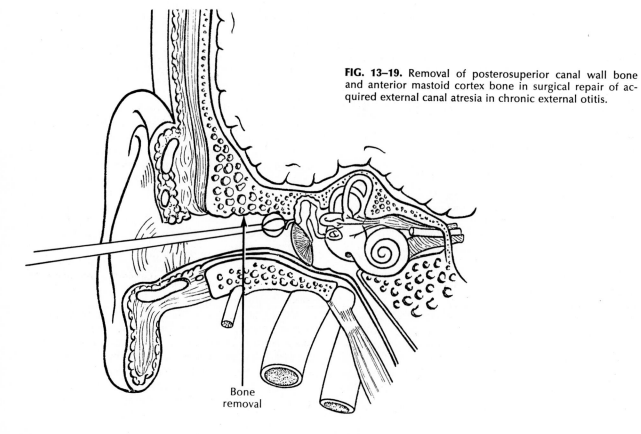

FIG. 13–19. Removal of posterosuperior canal wall bone and anterior mastoid cortex bone in surgical repair of acquired external canal atresia in chronic external otitis.

Bone removal

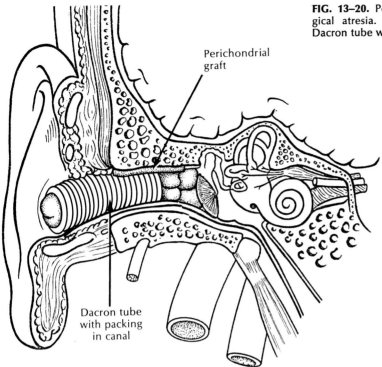

Perichondrial graft

Dacron tube with packing in canal

FIG. 13–20. Postoperative packing following repair of surgical atresia. Surgically enlarged canal contains arterial Dacron tube with packing.

Occasionally, local treatment of such a long-standing chronic inflammatory external otitis with secondary atresia is successful. It involves precise microbiologic diagnosis obtained by scrapings and cultures. Frequent reinsertions of medicated trailers may be followed by a reduction of the edema. In many patients, however, all attempts at such local treatment fail, and the treatment is surgical excision of the atretic region and surgical reconstruction of the external auditory canal.

Surgical Atresia Repair in Chronic External Otitis

The surgical procedure is best performed under local anesthetic block, but general anesthesia may be used. It is assumed that preoperative radiographic and audiologic studies have been carried out and have shown a normal mastoid and a conductive hearing loss. If there are additional findings (either audiologic, vestibular, or radiographic) surgical intervention more extensive than that of atresia correction may be necessary.

An endaural incision is made, with exposure of posterior canal wall skin. The entire anterior canal wall skin area should remain untouched. The skin of the posterior canal wall is elevated medially, accompanied by removal of subcutaneous tissue down to and including the periosteum of the anterior mastoid cortex (the posterior canal wall bone) region.

It may or may not be possible to carry the dissection down to the tympanic membrane in one stage. Anterior mastoid cortex (posterior external auditory canal wall) bone removal is necessary to create an enlarged canal. A significant amount of anterior mastoid cortical bone is removed (Fig. 13–19), preferably using diamond burrs with careful bone removal and irrigation, under surgical microscopic control.

It is also necessary to plan removal of obviously thickened and irreversibly hypertrophic skin and subcutaneous tissue from the posterior canal wall region. Removal of the periosteitic tissue and accompanying hyperostotic bone, which is secondary to the long-standing chronic inflammatory process, is necessary.

The only way to create a new canal is to obtain space at the expense of anterior cortical (posterior canal) bone. Usually it is possible to do this without opening into the mastoid cell system. Microscopically controlled bone removal is carried out in an elliptical fashion to create a generous meatal diameter. When the bony annulus region is reached medially, the dissection stops. The retention of the anterior canal wall skin, even though it is thick and boggy and obviously obstructive, is extremely important. It is quite common for such thickened anterior canal skin to decrease dramatically in thickness in the healing period. A perichondrial graft is obtained from the tragus (see Ch. 17, Otomastoiditis Surgery—Mastoidectomy and Tympanoplasty).

The perichondrial graft is sutured laterally to the posterior aspect of the endaural incision, and is kept in place very effectively by the use of an arterial Dacron tube of proper size, which is placed in contact with the intact anterior canal wall skin and posteriorly with the perichondrial graft (Fig. 13–20). The arterial Dacron graft is filled with antibiotic–steroid-saturated gauze, and the tube is sutured to the superior margins of the endaural incision so that it remains in place for at least 2–3 weeks. Prophylactic broad-spectrum oral antibacterial medication is advisable. The Dacron tube may be removed as an office procedure. At that time the perichondrial graft is epithelialized, and the generously enlarged canal allows good visualization of at least the posterior half of the tympanic membrane. The anterior canal wall skin may still remain edematous for many months before the chronic inflammatory changes subside. It is rarely necessary to do further surgical removal of anterior canal wall skin and subcutaneous tissue. It may be advisable to use a stent after the operation to prevent recurrent atretic adhesions, in some cases (1).

THE ITCHING EAR

This common problem is challenging diagnostically and therapeutically.

Causes of itching ear may be of ear or other origin. The management of an itching ear has been discussed earlier under Asteatosis—the Dry Ear, in the section on Lesions of the External Auditory Meatus and External Auditory Canal.

FIG. 13–21. Keratoma (cholesteatoma) of external bony canal has been removed. Note large bony defect in posterior canal bone (**on left**). The tympanic membrane annulus and tympanic membrane are **at right**.

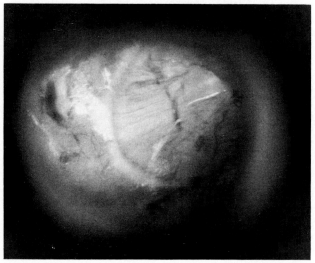

EAR CAUSES

1. Skin allergy to hair dyes, perfumes, hair sprays, eye glass metal, and jewelry
2. Low-grade mycotic or bacterial infection
3. Asteatosis—senile absence of lubricating oils even if cerumen is present

OTHER CAUSES

1. Nasal allergy to foods, pollens, or epidermals (The "ear itch" is usually not due to a lesion in the external auditory canal but to an allergic nasopharyngeal or "throat itch" which is referred to the ear.)
2. Temporomandibular joint problems (Very frequently these problems will be manifested by itching in the ear, in addition to pain and soreness.)

TUMORS OF THE AURICLE AND EXTERNAL AUDITORY CANAL

For discussion of temporal bone tumors, see Chapter 21, Temporal Bone Granulomas and Dystrophies, and Chapter 22, Temporal Bone Tumors.

BENIGN TUMORS

Common Benign Skin Tumors

Most common benign skin neoplasms may occur in the skin of the auricle and in the cartilaginous external auditory canal, including lipomas, sebacious cysts, and others. Treatment follows the usual principles of excision if the tumor is space-occupying or shows signs of growth or secondary infection.

Keratoma (Cholesteatoma) of the External Auditory Canal

Keratoma (epithelial or epidermoid cholesteatoma) is a relatively common tumor, usually of inflammatory origin, in the middle ear (chronic otomastoiditis). (See Color Fig. 12.) It is relatively rare for keratoma to occur as a primary mass in the external canal. When it does, it produces progressive widening of the bony canal, usually in a painless fashion. Areas of typical keratinaceous epithelium are found usually lateral to the bony annulus and in most instances lateral to the tympanic membrane (Fig. 13–21). Large excavations may occur in the inferior bony external canal, reaching down almost to the region of the jugular bulb. Similar erosions may occur anteriorly, posteriorly, and superiorly, resulting in a rather dramatic skeletinization of the peri-annular regions of the canal. Rarely, such an external canal keratoma will involve the mastoid and the middle ear. Usually, complete removal can be accomplished microsurgically via an endo-meatal or endaural approach. The cause of kera-toma in the external canal is unknown, but it is probably related to epithelial metaplastic changes in the canal wall.

MALIGNANT TUMORS OF SKIN AND SUBCUTANEOUS TISSUES

Among the various malignant tumors of skin that can occur in the external canal are common epi-thelial neoplasms, including squamous-cell car-cinoma. Special types of tumors, however, also occur in the external auditory meatus and canal, the most common of which is ceruminoma (see Ch. 22, Temporal Bone Tumors).

MIXED TUMORS OF THE SALIVARY GLAND

"Mixed tumors" of parotid and submaxillary gland types may occur in the preauricular region, involv-ing the auditory meatus and canal secondarily.

BENIGN TUMORS OF BONE: OSTEOPHYTES, OSTEOMAS, EXOSTOSES

Partial or complete narrowing of the bony external canal as a result of bony growths is common. These growths are variously described as osteomas or osteophytes (see Ch. 22, Temporal Bone Tumors).

MALIGNANT BONY TUMORS

In infants and children, malignant bony tumors are encountered in the sarcoma group. Thus rhab-domyosarcoma may manifest itself in early child-hood as a progressively enlarging, deforming, bony-ear-canal mass, removal of which has usually been unsatisfactory and the prognosis for which is usually poor. Recent developments, however, are encouraging (see Ch. 22).

RADIONECROSIS OF TEMPORAL BONE

Radiation therapy to lesions involving the peri-auricular or postauricular area (*e.g.,* basal cell carcinoma, etc.) may cause radionecrosis of the temporal bone at any time following therapy. The very first manifestation of temporal bone radio-necrosis can occur in bony external auditory canal. It will be manifested by a discharging and usually painless lesion due to bone necrosis and secondary infection. External canal skin is missing, and the bare bone is necrotic, frequently sloughing out in pieces. Discharge is intermittent and occasionally accompanied by slight bleeding. Topical treatment is of value in the mild cases. Gentian violet and scarlet red ointment are quite efficacious in clear-ing up low-grade secondary infections and in stopping the discharge.

When the radionecrosis extends into the mas-toid cells, there is usually secondary mastoiditis. The mastoiditis then frequently results in purulent otomastoiditis, accompanied in most cases by spontaneous tympanic membrane perforations and middle ear otorrhea. In such cases, surgical mastoid exenteration of necrotic areas is indicated. Repeated surgical debridement may be necessary as new necrotic areas appear. It is possible to perform limited mastoid bone removal if the middle ear has been spared (see Ch. 17, Otomas-toiditis Surgery—Mastoidectomy and Tympano-plasty).

REFERENCES

1. Beales PH: Atresia of the external auditory meatus. Arch Otolaryngol 100:209–211, 1974
2. Eviatar A, Goodhill V: Hypesthesia of the external auditory canal. Diagnostic significance. Arch Oto-laryngol 87:65–67, 1968
3. Garrity JD, Halliday TC, Glassman JM: Prevention of swimmers ear by simple prophylactic regimen. Curr Ther Res 16:437–441, 1974
4. Lazar P: Answer to question "Viral hepatitis pre-vention in ear piercing." JAMA 233:1316, 1975
5. Senturia BH: External otitis acute, diffuse evalu-ation of therapy. Ann Otol Rhinol Laryngol [Suppl] (82)8:22, 23, 1973
6. Swain R, Stroud M: Relapsing polychondritis. Laryngoscope 82:891–898, 1972

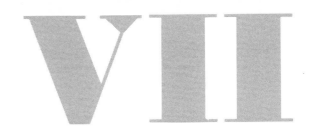

VII

OTOMASTOIDITIS

14

ACUTE OTITIS MEDIA AND MASTOIDITIS

OTOMASTOIDITIS

TUBOTYMPANITIS-OTITIS-MASTOIDITIS CONTINUUM

Acute otitis media and its frequent sequel, acute mastoiditis, are common diseases related to upper respiratory infection. Since the eustachian tube is analogous to a sinus ostium, infections of the nose and nasopharynx are directly transmissible to the middle ear in the same manner as such infections spread to the paranasal sinuses. In addition to infections, other conditions (allergic, metabolic) can comparably involve the middle ear. Foreign material (water, inhaled particles, regurgitated esophageal contents, etc.) can enter the middle ear via the eustachian tube. Last, but not least, barometric pressure changes, which cause positive and negative pressure variations in the contained air of the middle ear and mastoid cell system (Fig. 14–1), also are etiologic factors.

All these factors, separately or in combination, constitute common considerations in the pathologic continuum of tubotympanitis, otitis media, mastoiditis, and their complications.

EUSTACHIAN TUBE ROLE IN ACUTE OTITIS MEDIA

The eustachian tube orifice, in the lateral nasopharynx, and the middle ear mastoid air-cell system may be considered as an analogue of a paranasal sinus. The crucial difference between a paranasal sinus and the middle ear mastoid cell system relates to the contents of the latter. The

acoustic-vestibular (eighth nerve) system, the middle-ear–mastoid course of the seventh nerve, and major intracranial boundaries are located within the air-filled middle-ear–mastoid system.

Because of paranasal and parapharyngeal anatomicophysiological contiguity, the eustachian tube and its mucosal lining participate in every pathologic process affecting the nose, paranasal sinuses, and pharynx. Thus, tubotympanitis, on an infectious, allergic, metabolic, or mechanically obstructive basis, accompanies almost all nose and throat lesions.

ACUTE TUBOTYMPANITIS

The mucosa of the pharyngeal end of the eustachian tube is part of the mucociliary system of the middle ear. Tubal closure by mucosal edema, negative intratympanic pressure, lymphatic and vascular nasopharyngeal lesions, and direct extension of infection from the pharynx predispose to tubotympanitis, an extremely common disease. It accompanies every "common cold," every episode of allergic rhinitis, and is related to every lesion of the nasopharynx.

Tubotympanitis is an inflammatory lesion of the tubotympanum. This includes the entire eustachian tube and the protympanum. The latter is the funnel-shaped junction of the medial aperture of the bony eustachian tube and the anterosuperior middle ear.

Tubotympanitis, as an extension of nasopharyngitis, is the first step in the continuum of temporal bone infections. The second step is otitis media. Tubotympanitis and otitis media blend almost imperceptibly into the third and final entity of mastoiditis.

ACUTE OTITIS MEDIA

Acute otitis media, as an extension of acute tubotympanitis, may be a transitory condition that subsides spontaneously with subsidence of tubotympanitis. Persistent acute otitis media leads to secretory otitis media or to acute mastoiditis. Secretory otitis media is the common subacute-chronic middle ear lesion (see Ch. 15, Secretory Otitis Media). In virulent infections, acute otitis media leads directly to acute otomastoiditis without an interim episode of secretory otitis media.

ACUTE OTOMASTOIDITIS

Pneumatic relations of the middle ear with the mastoid air-cell system are complex. The most

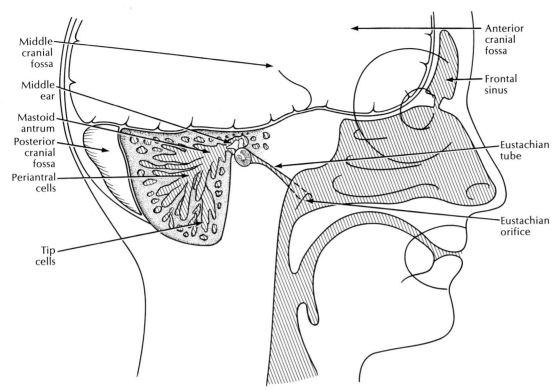

FIG. 14–1. The air-filled mucosa-lined continuum extends from nasal and oral cavities through the eustachian tube into middle ear, mastoid antrum, and total temporal bone cellular system.

direct route is through the aditus ad antrum, an expansion of the posterior epitympanum connecting with cell groups in the mastoid process, the squama, and the petrosa. All are described clinically as *mastoid air cells.* Infection in any part of this air-cell system is termed mastoiditis. Acute otitis media and acute mastoiditis constitute the clinical lesion known as acute otomastoiditis.

CHRONIC OTOMASTOIDITIS

Acute otomastoiditis and secretory otitis media are the most common antecedents of chronic otomastoiditis, which is a mucosal-osseous lesion. Two basic subtypes of chronic otomastoiditis can occur. Type A lesions are potentially reversible pathologically and include granulomatous, purulent, and fibrotic processes. Type B lesions are irreversible with two prototypes—keratoma (cholesteatoma) and tympanosclerosis.

SEQUENTIAL PATTERNS OF THE TUBOTYMPANITIS-OTOMASTOIDITIS CONTINUUM

Acute tubotympanitis and acute otomastoiditis that do not respond to therapy lead to complications. Many chronological patterns and pathologic variations create a mosaic of inflammatory lesions of middle-ear–mastoid mucosa, bone, and air spaces.

An example of a potential sequential continuum is listed below, not necessarily in the exact order, and not necessarily involving every lesion. Both acute and chronic patterns with exacerbations can occur.

1. Acute and Subacute Patterns
    A. Transitory tubotympanitis (mild mucositis, negative pressure, no middle ear fluid)
    B. Acute tubotympanitis (mucositis, negative pressure, clear serous or serosanguineous middle ear fluid)

C. Acute purulent otitis media (tubotympanic mucositis, negative pressure, seropus, pus)

D. Subacute or chronic secretory otitis media (tubotympanic mucositis, tubal blockade, sustained negative pressure, seromucoid fluid—"glue" ear)

E. Acute otomastoiditis (tympanomastoid mucositis plus osteitis, mucopurulent middle ear and mastoid exudate)

F. Acute otomastoiditis with complications (labyrinthitis, lateral sinus thrombophlebitis, meningitis, etc.)

2. Chronic—Type A

A. Chronic otomastoiditis with tympanic fibrosis, (healed osteitis, no middle ear fluid, middle ear and mastoid fibrosis, tympanic membrane perforations

B. Chronic purulent otomastoiditis (otomastoiditis, mucosal polyposis, granulomatosis, osteitis, ossicular necrosis, purulent exudate, tympanic membrane perforation)

3. Chronic—Type B

A. Chronic purulent otomastoiditis with tympanosclerosis (otomastoiditis, osteitis, mucositis, tympanosclerosis, ossicular necrosis, and/or fixation, mucopurulent middle ear exudate, tympanic membrane perforation)

B. Chronic purulent otomastoiditis with keratoma (cholesteatoma), (otomastoiditis, osteitis, granulomatosis, polyposis, ossicular necrosis, keratoma in middle ear, mastoid, or both, and tympanic membrane perforation)

C. Chronic purulent otomastoiditis with tympanosclerosis and keratoma (cholesteatoma)

D. Chronic purulent otomastoiditis with keratoma (cholesteatoma), and/or tympanosclerosis, and complications (cranial nerve, meningitis, sigmoid sinus thrombophlebitis, brain abscess) (Fig 14–2).

ACUTE OTITIS MEDIA AND OTOMASTOIDITIS

ACUTE OTITIS MEDIA

ETIOLOGY

Acute otitis media, a complication of the "common cold," probably accompanies every viral and/or bacterial upper respiratory infection. The nasal, paranasal, and pharyngeal mucositis spreads to involve eustachian tube and middle ear mucosa, as a tubotympanitis. In most cases of this type, the otitis is transitory and subsides without significant symptoms or findings.

The primary cause of acute otitis media is more commonly a viral upper respiratory infection with tubotympanitis as a secondary bacterial superinfection, although primary bacterial infection is frequent. Common etiologic organisms are the *Pneumococcus* group, the *Haemophilus influenzae* group, and *Staphylococcus aureus*, beta-hemolytic streptococcus, *Escherichia coli*, *Pseudomonas aeruginosa*, and other gram-negative bacilli. In infants and young children, *H. influenzae*, frequently nontypable, is very common. In older children and adults, *Diplococcus pneumoniae* is a more frequent cause. Quasiepidemic episodes of acute otitis media occur in given communities following epidemics of viral or bacterial upper respiratory infection. In addition to these viral and bacterial miniepidemics, seasonal allergic acute otitis media miniepidemics may occur. In the schools, the periodic influxes of many young children with impaired immunologic responses to upper respiratory infections frequently lead to such miniepidemics. Swimming in congested swimming pools during summer months is another cause of increased incidence of acute otitis media. Air travel during miniepidemics of upper respiratory infection is associated with a high incidence of aerootitis media.

Acute otitis media may be unilateral or bilateral, depending upon anatomic, nasal, and nasopharyngeal factors. Viral ("pure viral") otitis is less common than the bacterial type and is related to epidemics of viral upper respiratory infection. The clinical manifestations are those of bullous myringitis, accompanied by serosanguineous middle ear effusions and frequent extensions of the myringitis to medial external auditory canal skin.

PATHOLOGY

Acute otitis media starts as an inflammatory mucositis of the eustachian tube, protympanum, middle ear, and tympanic membrane. Leukocytic and lymphocytic infiltrates accompany the mucosal edema. Periostitis occurs in the promontory of the tympanic cavity and in ossicular periosteum. Eustachian tube function virtually stops because of blockade from tubal mucositis and ciliary paralysis. The middle ear cavity becomes filled with serous, hemorrhagic, or purulent exudate, and the tympanic membrane becomes thickened by inflammatory edema, frequently rupturing spon-

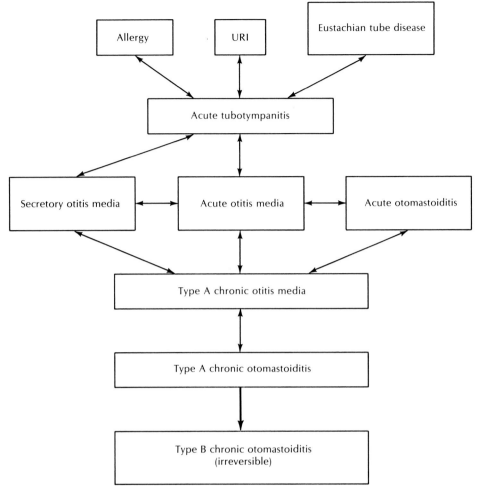

FIG. 14–2. Patterns of progression of otitis media and otomastoiditis.

taneously because of increased pressure in the middle ear.

In cases primarily of viral origin, the major lesion frequently is in the tympanic membrane itself. All three tympanic membrane layers undergo rapid inflammatory edema, with bullous blebs, especially in the external epithelial layer of the membrane. This viral lesion, myringitis, can be limited to the tympanic membrane or can spread to the remainder of the middle ear. Secondary bacterial invasion is frequent in primary viral myringitis.

HISTORY AND SYMPTOMS

The onset of ear symptoms, primarily otalgia, can occur within hours of upper respiratory infection onset or may be delayed days or weeks. Nasal and

ear stuffiness and hearing loss may precede or follow otalgia, which can vary from a slight "earache" to an excruciating pain, spreading to the temporal area and rarely relieved completely by analgesics.

FINDINGS

NOSE AND NASOPHARYNX EXAMINATION

Examination of the nose usually reveals vascular congestion, edema, crusting, and purulent discharge, especially, but not exclusively, on the ipsilateral side. The nasopharynx mucosa is red and edematous with mucopurulent discharge, or a very dry exudate with crusts will be present. The uvula is frequently edematous. Pathogenic bacteria are usually cultured both from nose and naso-pharynx. Sinusitis frequently is a concomitant finding.

EXTERNAL EAR EXAMINATION

Examination of the auricle and periauricular region usually reveals no abnormalities. There is rarely redness, swelling, or tenderness in the auricle or in the cartilaginous canal. Manipulation of the auricle rarely causes discomfort, in sharp contrast to the findings in external otitis. However, in acute viral myringitis or in viral acute otitis media with secondary pneumococcal, beta-hemolytic streptococcal, or other bacterial infections, the tympanic membrane swelling may spread to involve the tissues of the external auditory canal with edema, erythema, and auricular pain and tenderness.

OTOSCOPY

The diagnosis of acute otitis media is usually made on otoscopic examination. Adequate oto-scopic visualization requires careful cleansing of external ear canal, with removal of cerumen and epithelial debris prior to tympanic membrane visualization (see Ch. 13, External Ear Diseases). The external auditory canal may contain seropus because of spontaneous rupture of the tympanic membrane.

Classic otoscopic findings in acute otitis media include marked vascularization of the entire tympanic membrane, frequently spreading beyond the tympanic annulus to the skin of the external auditory canal. Normal sharp annular tympanic membrane margins are blurred. In early acute otitis media, the two primary bony landmarks, the malleal *short process* and the *umbo* are visible, although they might be distorted by intense arteriolar and venous engorgement. (See Color Fig. 6.) As the infection proceeds from mucositis to marked submucosal edema and progressive closure of the eustachian tube, rapid middle ear exudation occurs. The exudate changes from serous to serosanguineous to seropurulent and finally to the purulent stage rapidly. Early blurring of the malleal short process, due to epitympanic mucositis, is followed by edema and bulging of the pars flaccida (Shrapnell's membrane).

With the progression of mesotympanum involvement, loculations of tympanic exudate occur because of rapid friable fibrosis. Swelling of the tympanic membrane will be anterior, posterior, or posterosuperior (Fig. 14–3). These differences are due to preexisting tympanic fibrosis from previous episodes of acute otitis media. Finally, total blurring of all tympanic membrane landmarks occurs (Fig. 14–4), including the umbo and short process. Additional spread of edema to the tympanic annulus can blur the boundaries between the tympanic membrane and the external auditory canal, so that no definitive tympanic membrane landmarks are recognizable (Fig. 14–5).

HEARING TESTS

The degree of conductive hearing loss will depend upon the amount and viscosity of middle ear exudate, middle ear fibrosis, and tympanic membrane edema. Thus, conductive hearing loss may vary from 5–10 dB to 40–50 dB, with primary involvement of low frequencies, occasionally high frequencies. The hearing loss may be combined conductive and cochlear if there is labyrinthine extension, but it is relatively rare (Fig. 14–6).

FEVER

Fever of varying degrees is usually present, depending upon the immunologic responses and bacterial specificity; it can be masked by analgesics or antibiotics.

LABORATORY TESTS

Mastoid radiographs (Schuller) will reveal haziness in periantral cells or in the entire mastoid, even in early acute otitis media. Certainly this finding by itself does not warrant consideration of mastoid surgery. Complete blood counts will usually show leukocytosis, with predominant polymorphonuclear responses. In allergic patients there may be additional eosinophilia. Urine examination is usually normal. Bacteriologic studies of nasal, nasopharyngeal, and ear exudate are discussed in detail under Management.

COURSE OF ACUTE OTITIS MEDIA

Acute otitis media frequently progresses rapidly to spontaneous tympanic membrane rupture and otorrhea, which may be serous, serosanguineous, seropurulent, or purulent. (See Color Fig. 9.) If pain, fullness, and hearing loss are not relieved by spontaneous otorrhea, either intratympanic purulent loculation has occurred, or there is marked severity of the infectious process, or both. Acute otitis media is potentially a serious disease

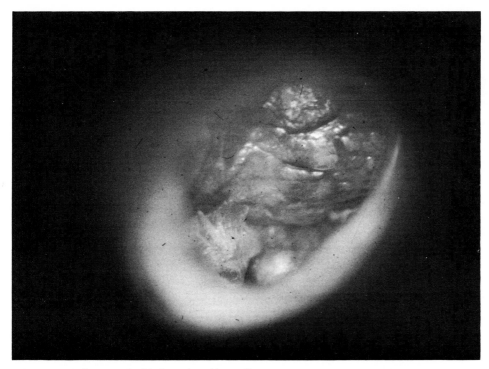

FIG. 14–3. Bullous myringitis in early otitis media.

FIG. 14–4. Acute seropurulent otitis media.

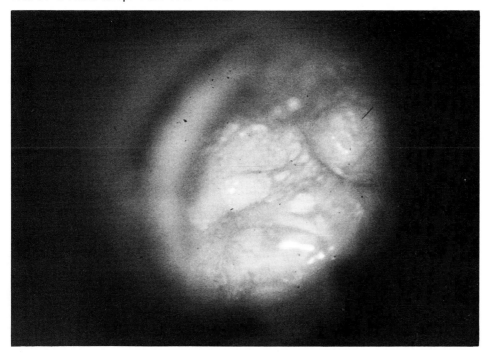

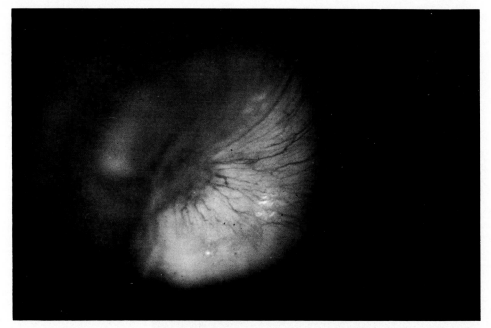

FIG. 14–5. Acute purulent bulging otitis media.

FIG. 14–6. Types of hearing loss in acute otitis media. **A.** Mild conductive loss, seen in most cases. ●—●, AC, unmasked, RE; [—[, BC, masked, RE; SRT, 25 dB; SDS, 98%. **B.** More advanced conductive hearing loss with sloping high frequency AC and BC curves, accompanied by lower SDS percentage, suggestive of a superimposed acute cochlear lesion. ●—●, AC, unmasked, RE; [—[, BC, masked, RE; SRT, 40 dB; SDS, 76%.

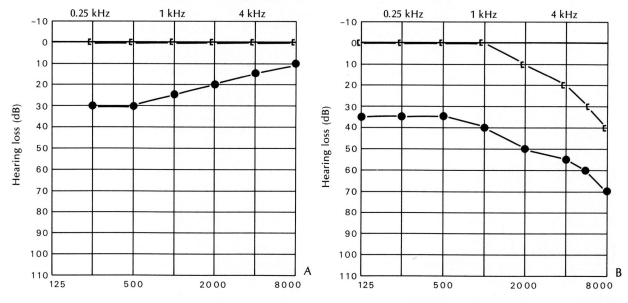

and deserves serious attention. Acute complications range through mastoiditis, labyrinthitis, to intracranial complications, including meningitis and brain abscess. Chronic complications include perforations, keratoma (cholesteatoma), tympanosclerosis, ossicular necrosis, as well as labyrinthitis and chronic intracranial complications.

MANAGEMENT

MEDICAL TREATMENT

The general treatment is that of any potentially serious viral or bacterial invasive disease. Bedrest, fluids, light diet, and avoidance of irritants (smoking) are important. Nasal decongestion is necessary, and includes oral Phenylpropanolamine HCl, 25 mg, and tripelennamine, 25 mg, or comparable decongestants and antihistaminics every 4 hours, accompanied by the use of intranasal warm oxymetazoline hydrochloride nasal spray or comparable nasal decongestants.

The management of acute otitis media and acute otomastoiditis was revolutionized with the introduction of sulfonamide chemotherapy in the late 1930's. Resolution either without surgery or with less drastic surgery became possible in a significant number of cases. However, a more dramatic shift to effective medical therapy came with the introduction of antibiotic therapy. The discovery of penicillin was rapidly followed by introduction of its use in acute and subacute mastoiditis by Macbeth (2). With his historic report of a series of 50 cases treated by closure of wounds and perfusion with penicillin, a new era in the management of acute otitis media and acute otomastoiditis started.

Definitive antibiotic therapy should be based on specificity, as determined by bacteriologic cultures and antibiotic sensitivity tests. However, immediate antibiotic therapy is entirely empiric, followed by a revised antibiotic program based upon ear culture after spontaneous otorrhea or myringotomy and/or nasopharyngeal cultures. Since *Diplococcus pneumoniae* infections are the most common in children and adults, ampicillin is the antibiotic of choice for immediate treatment. If there is no history of penicillin allergy, empirical ampicillin therapy should be started as soon as the diagnosis is made and continued for 10 days, pending a possible change of antibiotic upon completion of antibiograms from ear cultures and nasopharyngeal cultures. In conflicting ear and nasopharynx cultures, primary consideration is given to ear cultures.

Amoxicillin (Larotid) may have advantages over ampicillin, in terms of better absorption. Penicillin G or V is usually effective in older children and adults. In patients allergic to penicillin, erythromycin should be used. It can be effectively combined with sulfonamides in younger penicillin-sensitive children. If medical antibiotic therapy is followed by prompt resolution of all symptoms with return to normal otoscopic findings (intact normal tympanic membrane) and restoration of hearing to normal, only follow-up care is needed.

SURGERY—MYRINGOTOMY

Although antibiotic therapy is essential, there is danger in reliance on antibiotic therapy alone. The increasing worldwide incidence of secretory otitis media (see Ch. 15, Secretory Otitis Media) is largely due to reliance only upon antibiotic therapy in the treatment of acute otitis media. In the preantibiotic era, the treatment of choice for the disorder was prompt myringotomy. In the present antibiotic era, myringotomy has almost been forgotten, an amnesia responsible for a marked increase in chronic "lurking," "latent" complications of acute otitis media, primarily secretory otitis media.

Myringotomy in mild acute otitis media is elective if there is no prompt resolution of the acute process with medical management, including bedrest, nasal decongestion, and appropriate antibiotic therapy. However, when the otitis is rapidly progressive, with a red, bulging tympanic membrane, severe otalgia, and fever, the ideal treatment is *immediate myringotomy accompanied by medical antibiotic therapy*. Indications for myringotomy in purulent middle ear abscess loculations are the same as the indications for incision and drainage of pus in any closed cavity or viscus. Pus under pressure in a contained space will work its way out. The most common "way out" in acute otitis media is through the tympanic membrane to the external auditory canal; less commonly it is into mastoid cells. Less frequently, the way out is into and through the labyrinthine windows, the perineurium of the facial nerve, or into the subarachnoid space through epitympanic fissures. Thus, mastoiditis, labyrinthitis, facial paralysis, meningitis, and sequelae can follow "simple" acute otitis media.

In infants and very young children there is usually no need for anesthetic for myringotomy.

With good illumination, magnification, and adequate restraint of the child, a skillful rapid myringotomy can be performed in a few seconds. In older children and in adults, appropriate general anesthesia, preferably under hospital conditions, is advisable. An endomeatal xylocaine-epinephrine block is occasionally adequate for analgesia. Recent introduction of iontophoresis may also prove helpful in anesthesia.

Use of the conventional otoscope is not the best approach to myringotomy. The ideal equipment consists of an electric headlight, a binocular magnifying loupe (see Ch. 3, Ear Examination), appropriate speculums, sterile suction, and a *sharp* myringotomy knife. A surgical microscope provides excellent magnification and illumination, but is not essential.

Prior careful cleansing of the external auditory canal without production of bleeding should precede the myringotomy. This involves gentle removal of cerumen and epithelial debris, preferably with a fine suction tip and sterile, cotton-wrapped, fine metal applicators. The patient should be lying comfortably on an examining table. Myringotomy done with the patient sitting up is usually an unpleasant and sometimes dangerous procedure. It is necessary to have adequate assistance to keep the patient's head completely immobilized so that there is no unexpected movement that might significantly endanger the procedure.

Bimanual technique is recommended, in which the speculum is held in one hand and the myringotomy knife in the other. The ideal location of the myringotomy incision should be based upon the location of the major tympanic membrane lesion. The primary swelling may be either anterior or posterior. The incision should be approximately 2.5–4 mm in length and in the direction of the inferior radial fibers (see Ch. 13, External Ear Diseases).

It is advisable to send the myringotomy knife with its purulent material to the laboratory in a sterile tube for culture and sensitivity tests. The external auditory canal is kept lightly closed with sterile cotton, which should be changed every few hours as long as otorrhea continues. The external canal should not be irrigated. Suction may be used by the physician, with a sterile suction tip as necessary in examination. Antibiotic therapy should be continued until there is complete resolution, with subsidence of pain, fever, exudate, and hearing loss. It is usually advisable to continue such full antibiotic therapy for at least 10 days, assuming a rapid favorable clinical response.

FOLLOW-UP CARE

Acute otitis media that responds rapidly to medical therapy alone or to combined medical therapy and myringotomy requires careful follow-up and long-range observation. Care must be taken to detect an unresolved secretory otitis media, which can occur as a sequel of acute otitis.

In the present antibiotic era, there has been a drastic diminution in incidence of serious complications, particularly acute coalescent mastoiditis. However, antibiotic therapy may be responsible for the masking of such symptoms as pain, fever, and hearing loss in many patients. One of the cardinal signs of incomplete resolution is the persistence of hearing loss with minimal or no otoscopic evidence of persistent middle ear exudate.

Acute otitis media represents not only a cavity infection but involves a cavity containing a delicate and complex sense organ. The function of this sense organ must be evaluated in assessing progression or resolution of the disease. Visual reliance upon otoscopic findings is inadequate in the judgment of adequate treatment for acute otitis media. Attention primarily to hearing function and, to a lesser extent, to equilibrium is essential in management. Ideally, audiometric examinations should be started early in the course of acute otitis media to establish a base line for judging the adequacy of treatment. There are no valid alternatives to audiometry. Tuning-fork tests can be of great assistance but cannot be relied upon entirely. The reversal of a negative Rinne to a positive Rinne is helpful but no more reliable than changes in responses to whispered or spoken voice tests. If tuning-fork tests are used for a crude guide, the ideal fork should be the 128- or 256-Hz cycle fork. Higher frequency forks will occasionally give wrong information regarding changes in conductive hearing loss.

The most common sequel of inadequately treated acute otitis media is persistent painless middle ear fluid which is serous, mucoid, or a mixture. Lack of recognition of such subacute middle ear fluid leads to chronicity and to later complications of secretory otitis media, acute otitis media, and mastoiditis. The mistaken impression that myringotomy is virtually an obsolete procedure in acute otitis media is indeed unfortunate. There is no real debate of "myringotomy versus antibiotics." (See Color Fig. 8.) Treatment should be based upon the sound principles of control of infection, and drainage of pus from and ventilation of the middle ear. One cannot assume spontaneous complete resolution in every case, regardless of therapy. The subsidence of pain, fever, stuffiness, and subjective hearing loss are inadequate assurances that the infection has cleared. A low-grade tubotympanitis can persist for several weeks or months. The patient with acute otitis media, in whom all acute symptoms have subsided, should be reexamined by otoscopy and audiometric tests 3–4 weeks following apparent subsidence of the acute infection. Normal otoscopic and audiometric findings should precede discharge of the patient.

In addition, attention should also be directed to the nasopharyngeal, nasal, and sinus areas. A persistent nasopharyngitis, maxillary or ethmoid sinusitis, can remain as a focus for possible reinfection of the same middle ear or the contralateral middle ear weeks or months later. The middle ear cannot be considered an isolated separate chamber. It is a contiguous mucosal partner of the nose and the nasopharynx. Its mucociliary "ramp" remains a source of viral/bacterial communication from nose, sinuses, and nasopharynx to the most remote mastoid or petrous apical cell in the temporal bone system.

COMPLICATIONS

The most common complication of acute otitis media is secretory otitis media (see Ch. 15, Secretory Otitis Media). A less common complication is a persistent tympanic membrane perforation, which may require tympanoplastic reconstruction. A relatively uncommon complication of acute otitis media in this antibiotic era is *acute mastoiditis*. Because it is now uncommon, greater vigilance is necessary to detect its presence. A rare complication is fulminating pneumococcic meningitis without apparent acute mastoiditis. This problem, and other intracranial complications, is discussed in Chapter 18, Complications of Otomastoiditis.

ACUTE MASTOIDITIS

ETIOLOGY

Acute suppurative mastoiditis has not completely vanished in the antibiotic era. It is more common in infants and children but also occurs sporadically in the adult population, especially following epidemics of upper respiratory tract viral infections. Resistant secondary bacterial organisms are often the offending etiologic agents, especially when antibiotic therapy has been used without myringotomy in the treatment of early acute otitis media. Bacterial organisms encountered after a viral infection are *Diplococcus pneumoniae*, *Haemophilus influenzae*, *Staphylococcus aureus hemolyticus*, beta-hemolytic *Streptococcus*, *Pseudomonas* and other gram-negative bacteria.

PATHOLOGY

Acute otitis media is usually accompanied by transitory acute mucosal mastoiditis, which is potentially a prelude to acute osteitic mastoiditis. The nasopharyngeal mucositis, tubotympanitis, and middle ear mucositis, accompanied by ciliary paralysis, extends to the mucosa of the aditus ad antrum with rapid osteitis. Mucositis and osteitis from *aditus ad antrum mastoideum* spreads throughout the diploetic spaces, marrow spaces, and into the small, medium, and large cell groups of the entire mastoid process. There may be involvement of squama, petrous apex, and perilabyrinthine cell groups. In addition, extension occurs to hypotympanic, peritubal, digastric, and into retrosinus cell groups.

In most patients with acute mastoiditis, rapid recovery follows adequate treatment of the primary acute otitis media with minor persistent changes in either the mucous membrane or the intercellular septums of the mastoid air-cell system.

However, in some instances, because of problems of bacteriologic drug resistance or of specific immunity deficiency, unusual nasopharyngeal-sinus problems, or coexistent systemic diseases, acute mastoiditis will not respond to treatment of acute otitis media and becomes a persistent and spreading lesion. It is characterized by increased mucosal edema and cell partition necrosis. Polypoid blockage may occur in the aditus ad antrum, the major air connection between the middle ear and the mastoid. The mucositis is followed by periostitis and osteitis, and pus formation. Mastoid air cells, normally containing only air and lined with flat endothelial cells, become filled with pus as inflammatory changes produce marked edema of the lining membrane.

The term "coalescent" mastoiditis accurately describes the pathologic process as seen grossly at surgery. The previous normal cell boundaries disappear in many areas and the result is a coalescence of cellular areas filled with hyperplastic mucosa and pus. Microscopically diffuse osteo-clasia is also seen (1).

HISTORY

With the development of periostitis and osteitis, mastoid symptoms begin to occur. In some cases, such extensions into mastoid cellular areas may be "masked" and asymptomatic, but in most instances the spread is accompanied by pain and tenderness, in the retroauricular, supraauricular, and infraauricular regions. With the pain and tenderness, fever and leukocytosis may increase. In most cases there will be an accompanying increased conductive hearing loss. Headache and general malaise are usually present.

FINDINGS

Otoscopic findings will show changes from those noted at the onset of acute otitis media. There will be obliteration of the view of the malleal short process. The superior tympanic membrane and the superior external auditory canal wall area will present a blurred undemarcated appearance. There will be "sagging" of the posterosuperior wall of the external auditory canal, with narrowing of the medial canal lumen. Otorrhea may be absent or present. If present, it will be serous, seropurulent, or mucopurulent. It can be pulsatile (in rhythm with the patient's pulse) as a result of transmitted middle ear fluid pressure. The perforation (spontaneous or postmyringotomy) is usually obscured because of intense edema of the tympanic membrane and external auditory canal.

The appearance of mastoid symptoms calls for repeated radiographic studies. Mastoid radiographs (Schuller view) are diagnostic in most cases. Previous mild haziness (during acute otitis media) in the mastoid air cells, is now followed by evidence of trabecular breakdown. The petrous apex cells should also be studied radiographically (Stenver view) (Fig. 14–7).

Audiologic tests usually show an increased conductive hearing loss. There may also be bone conduction depressions, producing a "mixed loss." Such bone conduction hearing loss is usually of a "mechanical" type and is not usually due to cochlear involvement. Patterns are similar to those in acute otitis media (Fig. 14–6).

In fulminating acute mastoiditis, however, the patient may have true cochlear hearing loss due to oval window and round window extensions. In such cases, speech discrimination scores will drop, an indication of true cochlear labyrinthitis.

Vertigo is uncommon, but if it occurs, and if accompanied by manifest spontaneous nystagmus, it may be assumed that labyrinthitis is present, as a result of retrograde vascular spread or direct spread through fistulization of the otic capsule, either in the vestibule or in the semicircular canal system region.

COURSE

Acute mastoiditis appears as a concomitant of acute otitis media in cases of unusual bacterial virulence or unusually poor immunologic response in a debilitated individual (diabetic adult) or in infants. Such acute mastoiditis may respond (along with the acute otitis media) to prompt myringotomy, intensive antibiotic therapy, and general supportive measures, including hospitalization.

Acute mastoiditis which follows onset of acute otitis media by several days or a week can subside with increased or changed antibiotic therapy if there is adequate middle ear drainage. In some cases, however, there is no response to such therapy and mastoid surgery must be considered. If adequate middle ear drainage and appropriate antibiotic therapy are not followed by rapid disappearance of pain, tenderness, systemic findings, and improvement in hearing, mastoid surgery should be considered.

INDICATIONS FOR MASTOID SURGERY IN ACUTE OTOMASTOIDITIS

The following signs indicate the advisability of mastoid surgery:

1. Definite radiographic changes in the mastoid, including increasing cloudiness of cell contents and beginning destruction of bony cell walls, typical of coalescent mastoiditis
2. Persistence or increase of conductive hearing loss
3. Persistent fever
4. Sagging of the posterosuperior wall of the external auditory canal
5. Edema of Shrapnell's membrane and obliteration of malleal tympanic membrane landmarks, especially the short (lateral) process
6. General systemic malaise
7. Persistent leukocytosis

It is not necessary that all of the above indications be present. Surgical judgment will indicate appropriate time for surgical intervention.

The surgical procedure of choice in acute or

FIG. 14–7. A. Normal right mastoid in a 6.5-year-old child. Hazy cells and cellular break-down in left mastoid. **B.** Normal right petrous apex. Marked density of small left petrous apex cells with indistinct cell walls.

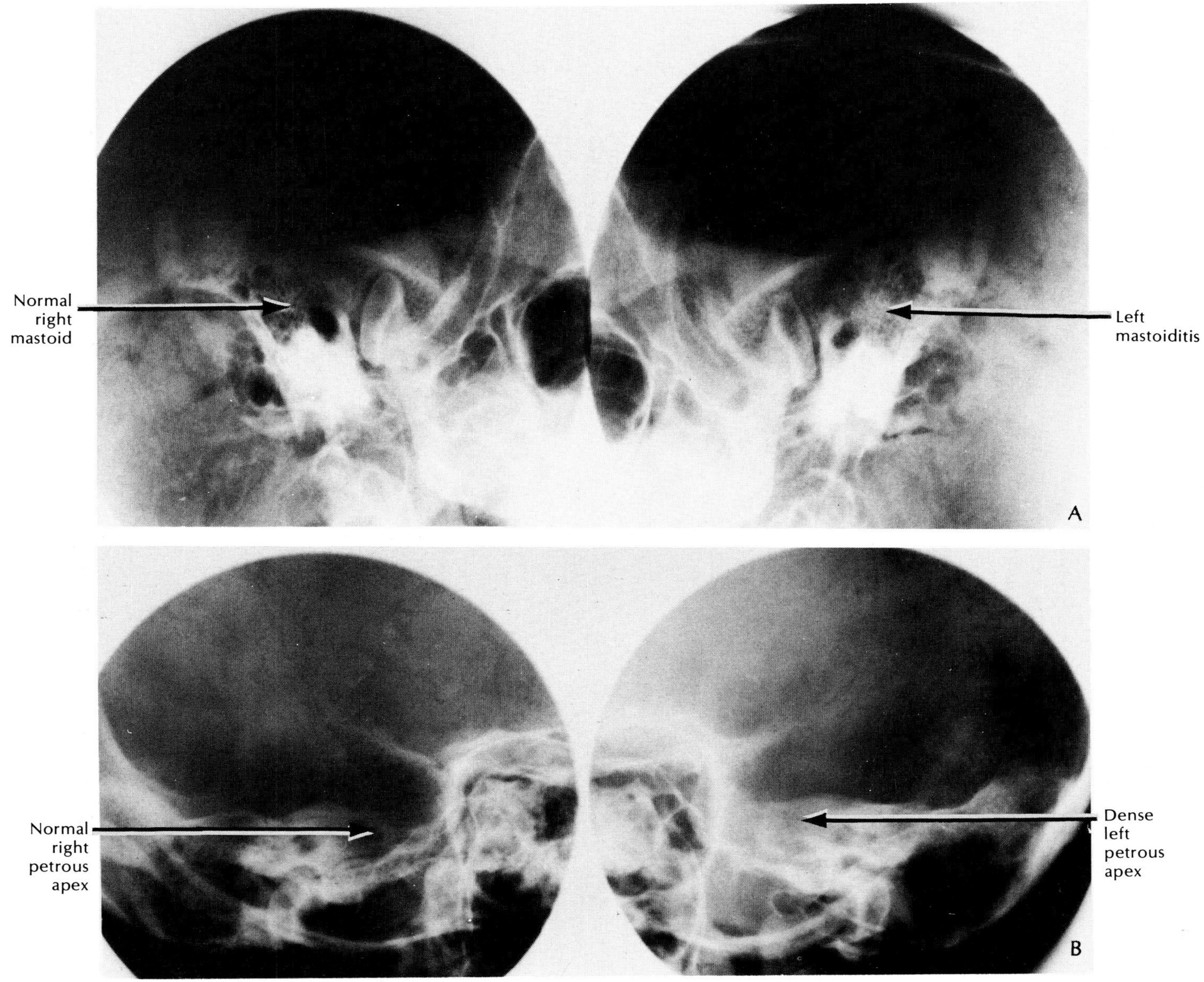

subacute coalescent mastoiditis is atticomastoid-ectomy. Prolonged undue reliance upon antibiotic therapy alone in persistent acute mastoiditis may lead to complications that can involve the labyrinth, facial nerve, the sigmoid sinus, or the intracranial cavity. Even if these complications do not occur, persistent subacute mastoiditis will lead to chronicity, *i.e.*, to chronic otitis media and chronic otomastoiditis.

When there are indications for mastoid surgery in acute mastoiditis, surgical intervention should be carried out regardless of age or general condition of the patient. Appropriate general supportive therapy with the collaboration of the pediatrician or internist is necessary.

The usual surgical procedure for an acute mastoiditis is atticomastoidectomy. Only rarely is radical mastoidectomy or tympanoplasty advisable in acute mastoiditis.

MASTOIDECTOMY TECHNIQUE IN ACUTE OTOMASTOIDITIS

The basic operation, atticomastoidectomy, is performed either through a postauricular or endaural incision. The purpose is removal of infected mastoid cell mucosa and bony cell walls, and restoration of tubotympanic-mastoid pneumatic continuity.

The operation starts with removal of the lateral mastoid cortex and mastoid antrum cell group. The procedure must include identification of the mastoid antrum and visualization of the posterior epitympanum. The posterior bony canal wall is identified but not disturbed; neither is the canal wall skin, tympanic membrane annulus, mesotympanum, hypotympanum, or anterior epitympanum. The ossicular chain is not disturbed. The short process of the incus must be identified, as must the horizontal semicircular canal, and the seventh nerve posterior genu. Failure to identify these structures is an indication that the antrum (the primary mastoid cell) has not been opened.

Koerner's septum is a bony bridge between the lateral antrum wall and lateral cell tracts. If present, it obscures the approach to the mastoid antrum. Removal of the Koerner's septum is essential to gain adequate access to the mastoid antrum and its periantral area. Many failures of mastoid surgery in either acute or chronic mastoiditis are due to failure to recognize a Koerner's septum, which will frequently resemble the medial aspect of the antrum. Familiarity with these pneumatic variations is essential in mastoid surgery.

Radical mastoidectomy is necessary in acute mastoiditis if there is evidence of irreversible type B disease, such as keratoma (cholesteatoma), necrotizing tympanosclerosis, or clinical evidence of intracranial complications.

Following exenteration of infected periantral cell groups, the incision is closed loosely. The mastoid cavity is not packed. A soft silicone rubber drainage tube is placed in the antrum and sewn to the incision (either postauricular or endaural). The drain is allowed to remain *in situ* for 5–10 days to make sure there is adequate egress for secretions and that ventilation will be insured until eustachian tube aeration function returns.

Postoperative mastoid care includes maintenance of antibiotic therapy with periodic reexaminations for antibiotic bacteriologic specificity to make sure that appropriate antibiotic coverage is being maintained. Antibiotic therapy should be continued until there is no drainage from the middle ear or mastoid cavity and until the incision is healed and the patient is asymptomatic.

Follow-up audiologic studies are always necessary. Lack of clearing of conductive hearing loss is an indication of continued mucositis or ossicular disease. The tympanic membrane and its perforation must be observed with the otoscope to detect persistence of infection that will lead to chronic otomastoiditis with all its sequelae. The patient should be rechecked at monthly intervals for a period of 6 months following subsidence of acute otomastoiditis and should be discharged only when there is a healed tympanic membrane, return of hearing to normal, and resolution of all symptoms.

REFERENCES

1. Friedmann I: Pathology of the Ear. Oxford, Blackwell Scientific Publications, 1974
2. Macbeth RG: A series of 50 cases of acute and subacute mastoiditis treated by closure of wound and perfusion with penicillin. J Laryngol Otol 60:16–23, 1945

15

SECRETORY OTITIS MEDIA

VICTOR GOODHILL
SEYMOUR J. BROCKMAN

Tubotympanitis due to upper respiratory infection or to allergy frequently subsides completely. If it persists because of infection, it progresses to acute otitis media. If its persistence is due to allergy, it usually progresses to secretory otitis media. Acute otitis media either subsides completely or progresses rapidly to acute otomastoiditis in many cases. However, acute otitis media frequently does not subside but progresses to a subacute–chronic phase. This phase persists as a "steady state" or "détente" condition, *e.g.*, secretory otitis media, also known as subacute middle ear effusion, unresolved otitis media, nonsuppurative otitis media, chronic middle ear effusion, otitis media with effusion, hydropic otitis media, the "glue ear," and serous otitis. Thus, secretory otitis media can develop without previous infection, as in allergic tubotympanitis, or it can develop as a sequel to acute otitis media.

This painless lesion is characterized by middle ear fluid, an intact tympanic membrane, and a fluctuating or stable conductive hearing loss; it is a stage in the continuum of otitis–mastoiditis (see Fig. 14–2). At times it may be an active bacterial infection, but usually the middle ear fluid is sterile. Negative intratympanic pressures and abnormal cytologic changes are characteristic of secretory otitis media.

Although secretory otitis media was recognized in the preantibiotic era, its incidence has greatly increased in the antibiotic era. Etiologic factors include undue reliance on antibiotic therapy, chronic respiratory allergy, changing bacterial biology, and omission of indicated surgical drainage by myringotomy. Secretory otitis media is frequently but not always reversible; it usually precedes chronic otomastoiditis and destructive middle ear lesions.

Secretory otitis media that follows acute otitis media can progress to a clear middle ear transudate or to an exudate that may last days or weeks as a subacute form of the secretory condition. Although a sequel of viral-bacterial acute otitis media, secretory otitis is usually a sterile lesion. In the chronic form, it becomes the viscous glue ear. Secretory otitis media can remain as a limited middle ear lesion for months or years but frequently also involves mastoid cells. Both type A and type B chronic otomastoiditis can follow secretory otitis media. Type A forms include granulomatosis, polyposis, and tympanic fibrosis, and may be accompanied by ossicular lesions. Type B forms include tympanosclerosis, keratoma (cholesteatoma), and their complications. Both type A and type B lesions can produce ossicular necroses.

Sterile secretory otitis media may follow negative intratympanic pressure without infection, as commonly seen following barotrauma or allergic tubotympanitis. It can follow eustachian tube obstruction by hypertrophic adenoid tissue or by nasopharyngeal tumor.

Secretory otitis media has been known for more than a century but continues to elude diagnosis because it is asymptomatic in many patients. It rarely causes discomfort or pain and may produce only a conductive hearing loss. If it is unilateral in a child, it may elude recognition. Otoscopic recognition may be difficult, and the condition may remain undiagnosed for months or years. It is frequently difficult to differentiate a slightly scarred tympanic membrane from that in secretory otitis media with hidden serous, seromucoid, or mucopurulent middle ear fluid.

Infectious secretory otitis media is frequently the antibiotic era version of the acute purulent otomastoiditis before the advent of antibiotics. Before the use of sulfonamides and penicillin, acute otitis media was frequently and rapidly followed by acute mastoiditis with fever, pain, mastoid-cell and cortex necrosis, and postauricular swelling. Although such acute mastoiditis still occurs, it is rare, and has been displaced by secretory otitis media as the primary sequel to acute otitis media.

Allergic secretory otitis may occur as a primary lesion in some cases. Age is an important factor in pediatric cases, the vast majority occurring within the first 7–8 years of life. In addition to age, sex seems to play a role in the predominance of male children over female children in secretory otitis media statistics.

Combined infectious-allergic secretory otitis cases are very common, especially in children. Management for infection alone or allergy alone in such cases will usually fail.

ETIOLOGY

The acute viral and/or bacterial causes of acute otitis media are also primary in the etiology of secretory otitis media. However, allergy and a number of other predisposing factors are also involved in the development of secretory otitis.

Predisposing congenital anatomic factors include septal deviations, congenital anomalies of the nasopharynx, tubal and tympanic anomalies, and abnormalities (clefts) of the hard and soft palate, all of which contribute to poor tubal ventilation and predispose to recurrent acute and chronic tubotympanic malfunctions. The prime congenital example is the patient with cleft palate. Choanal atresia (unilateral or bilateral) is not a rare cause.

Predisposing acquired nasopharynx factors include adenoid lymphoid hyperplasia, chronic infectious adenoiditis, postoperative recurrence of adenoid tissue, scarring or diseased lymphoid tissue masses in Rosenmüller's fossas, poor lymphatic drainage in the lateral nasopharynx, and polypoid degeneration of posterior turbinate tips. Benign and malignant nasopharyngeal tumors may also produce swelling and blockade of one or both eustachian tube orifices.

Chronic paranasal sinusitis with postnasal discharge and secondary nasopharyngitis is a frequent cause of intermittent tubal obstruction with impaired tubotympanic ventilation.

Chronic allergic rhinitis is a major factor in many cases of secretory otitis media. Both allergy and infection (viral and bacterial) produce similar physiologic and cytologic sequelae in the eustachian tube and middle ear. Infectious and allergic primary etiologies may vary with geography and climate. In tropical or subtropical areas, perennial inhalant allergies may be responsible for the serous and seromucoid varieties of secretory otitis.

In temperate and cold climates, seropurulent and mucopurulent complications occur more frequently.

ACUTE HYPERSENSITIVITY AND IMMUNOCHEMICAL FACTORS

The role of allergy in secretory otitis media has been disputed for decades. In a recent study (2), an incidence of allergy in 25–30% of patients with secretory otitis was found. However, the immunohistologic and immunochemical studies did not implicate the middle ear mucosa as an allergic shock organ. It was concluded that nasal and nasopharyngeal allergenic roles were primary.

However, in a study on middle ear immunochemistry (3), data suggested that there is a distinct secretory immune system in the middle ear with significance relating to infections in that area.

In another immunologic study (10) higher levels of IgA, IgG, and lysozyme were found in the effusions than in corresponding serums, indicating local production. The mucoid types contained higher levels of immunoglobulins and lysozymes than the serous types of effusions. Bacteria were identified in 77% of smears and in 52% of cultures. The study showed that immunoglobulin production slowly reaches maturity at about 8 years of age. This finding points to the significant role of maturation of the local immune system as well as the enzyme defense system. The high incidence of secretory otitis media in children under 7–8 years of age is probably related to those immunologic factors, at least in part.

EUSTACHIAN TUBE FACTORS

The role of the eustachian tube in secretory otitis media has always been recognized as very important. A recent study (4) described the "floppy" nature of the eustachian tubes in young children as easily collapsible. At about age 8 the tube becomes stiff enough to function properly.

IATROGENIC FACTORS

Iatrogenic factors are significant in secretory otitis media because of undue reliance upon antibiotic therapy alone in the treatment of acute otitis media. Neglect of myringotomy and neglect of predisposing factors contribute to apparent frequently "recurrent" acute otitis media. It is a great temptation to ignore myringotomy when a patient "responds promptly" to antibiotics. What is meant by "respond promptly"? It usually means relief of pain and fever and apparent return of the tympanic membrane to "normal," without *accurate audiometric confirmation of normal hearing.* Many patients appear for otologic examination months or years after acute otitis media complaining only of hearing loss. If the patient is a child and the secretory otitis media is unilateral, the hearing loss may go unnoticed indefinitely. It is unfortunately necessary, therefore, to include iatrogenic factors among predisposing causes.

Secretory otitis media that follows acute otitis is usually self-limited and spontaneously reversible when tubal function returns to normal. The persistent phase usually occurs as a result of tubal obstruction and subsequent irreversible tubotympanic mucosal changes.

PATHOLOGY

The histopathology of secretory otitis media involves changes in the middle ear mucosa or in that of many cell groups within the complex tubotympanic continuum. In a recent report on the earliest stage of secretory otitis media, as observed in a 3-month-old infant, Tos (15) and Bak-Pedersen (1) studied the entire mucosa. Inflammatory changes begin with lymphocytic infiltrates and dilatation and increases in numbers of blood vessels, mucosal hyperplasia followed by metaplasia into pseudostratified ciliated epithelium, increase in goblet-cell density, and formation of mucous glands. It is the mucous accumulation from goblet cells that characterizes the disease clinically.

Sade and Eliezer (13) describe the histopathology of secretory otitis media as related to a defective role within the normal mucociliary middle-ear system. Mucosal stem cells can differentiate into mucous cells, ciliated cells, and keratin-producing cells. Abnormal numbers of mucus-producing cells are formed in the presence of inflammation. The normal ciliated columnar (pseudostratified) epithelium changes, in secretory otitis media, to a hypertrophied epithelium with enlarged mucous glands staining PAS-positive.

Sade (14) further demonstrated that keratinizing stratified squamous epithelium may form as a pathogenic differentiation from mucous cell groups in secretory otitis.

Lim and Birck (8) showed the electron microscopic differences between mucoid secretory otitis media and serous otitis media. The most distinctive features of the mucoid type were described as 1) a prominent thickened connective tissue layer (lamina propria), and 2) a proliferated mucosal epithelium with numerous secretory cells. There were also many glandular and cystic structures lined with secretory cells.

The serous (seromucoid) type was characterized by tissue edema and round-cell infiltrations, consisting mainly of lymphocytes, monocytes, and plasma cells. The pure serous type lacks mucus-secreting elements, in contrast to the mucoid type, in which abundant mucus-secreting elements predominate. The epithelial cells of both serous and mucoid types were formed by cuboidal and simple squamous cells, although occasionally they can be formed by large, tall, columnar secretory cells.

This study also revealed the pleomorphism of secretory otitis media and the possibility that the condition might change to cholesterol granuloma, a phase that has been frequently noted clinically. The histologic features described that relate to cholesterol granuloma include large numbers of lipoid cytoplasmic inclusions in addition to secretory granules in the epithelial cells. Cholesterin crystals were found embedded in the tissues, surrounded by numerous foreign body giant cells. Crystalline structures were found in both ciliated and secretory cells.

Other mucosal histochemical studies (12) show acid phosphatase, lactate dehydrogenase, and malate dehydrogenase as strong precipitates in middle-ear epithelium. Periodic acid-Schiff–positive mucus (neutral mucopolysaccharide evidence) appeared in the epithelium and in the free mucus, but it was definitely the lesser product of secretory glands when compared with acid mucopolysaccharides.

HISTORY AND SYMPTOMS

A history of preceding acute otitis media is helpful in the diagnosis, but it may be forgotten by the patient. The symptoms in most patients are vague. In children, there may be no symptoms at all, the hearing loss being noticed first by a parent or teacher. In adults, there is a greater awareness of blockade and fullness in the involved ear or in that side of the head. There may be constant or pulsating tinnitus which is usually "visceral" (see Ch. 42, Tinnitus) as a result of masking of ambient noise by the conductive hearing loss. The hearing loss may be subjectively exaggerated if the lesion is unilateral, since the contrast will produce greater awareness. Diplacusis or "double hearing" (a subjective awareness of different pitch sensations in response to the same stimulating tone frequency, either from a tuning fork or an audiometer) may occur. Diplacusis is not uncommon and the adult patient may mention it. Pain is rarely present, either in children or adults. Dizziness is a rare symptom. Deep ear "itching" may be an adult's complaint but is relatively uncommon in children.

FINDINGS

The diagnosis of secretory otitis media depends upon a high index of suspicion, and involves special attention to the findings in ear, nose, and throat examination, in audiologic tests, in radiography, and in middle-ear aspiration. All diagnostic steps should involve attention to *subtle changes.*

The nose and throat findings in secretory otitis are rarely dramatic. Primary attention is directed to otoscopic examination, but nose and throat findings are critically important.

OTOSCOPIC EXAMINATION

Otoscopic diagnosis in secretory otitis media is a challenge because the tympanic membrane may appear deceptively normal. Otoscopic examination must be done under both *manifest* and *evoked* conditions.

In *manifest otoscopy* (at rest), the tympanic membrane may be normal or retracted or slightly bulging, depending upon previous scarring, thickening, and proportions of air to fluid in the middle ear. There may be a clear-cut fluid level with meniscus line and air bubble (Fig. 15–1) or an opalescent sheen, which may range in color from yellow to brown to dark blue and even to blue-black in some cases, as a result of mucosal hemorrhage (idiopathic hemotympanum). (See Color Figs. 6 and 7.)

In *evoked otoscopy*, delicate middle-ear pressure changes are produced to mobilize contained tym-

FIG. 15–1. Intratympanic fluid in secretory otitis media.

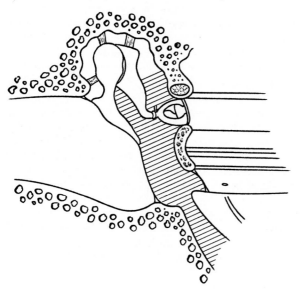

panic fluid. The pneumatic otoscope is used to induce slow, pneumatic, positive compressions and negative rarefactions. Similar changes can be induced by tubotympanic pressure changes via Valsalva inflation, politzeration, or tubal catheterization and inflation. These evoked pressure changes can be noted by otoscopy or by auscultation (see Ch. 3, Ear Examination).

On otoscopic pneumatic compression-rarefaction of the tympanic membrane, fluid level changes or air bubble movements or tympanic membrane immobilization may be noted. Characteristic "clickings" and "gurgles" may be heard. Another dynamic otoscopic technique is that produced by gravity. The patient's head is moved up and down or rocked to and fro while the ear is under otoscopic observation. The fluid level in the middle ear may become apparent by changes on positional movement.

NOSE AND THROAT EXAMINATION

Nasal examination is directed to deformities of the nasal dorsum, nasal bones, cartilaginous areas, and the tip. Nasal obstruction of significant degree can be completely missed if examination consists only of an intranasal survey using a nasal speculum. The speculum insertion may obscure a physiologically obstructive soft-tissue tip lesion involving nasal alae. External examination with digital elevation of the nasal tip is important. Conventional examination with a headlight or head mirror and an intranasal speculum then follows. Septal irregularities and changes in inferior and middle turbinates are noted. In most instances it is advisable to examine the nose before and after the use of a nasal decongestant, which will permit more complete examination of the posterior choanal region, the middle meatus, and the middle turbinate areas. Polyps, adhesions, spurs of the septum, collections of mucopus, and accumulations of crusts may not be noticed until after nasal decongestion. It is also possible to see the superior nasopharynx transnasally, but this does not constitute a total examination of the nasopharynx.

Paranasal sinus disease may be etiologic in some cases of secretory otitis media. Diseases of the maxillary, ethmoid, and sphenoid sinuses can cause persistent or recurrent tubotympanic disorders. Sinuses should be examined by palpation for tenderness, for obvious external deformities, and by transillumination. The latter is valuable for screening but does not always suffice. Radiographic examination is necessary for definitive evaluation of the sinuses. Additional studies may require cytologic smears and cultures of nasal secretions. Diagnostic aspiration of sinuses may be necessary in some cases.

In anterior transnasal examination, it is frequently possible to see the upper nasopharynx, and the search may be assisted by having the patient swallow or phonate the letter "K." This will also reveal soft palate mobility problems and occasional obstructive polyps or tumors, or obstructive adenoid tissue.

Indirect peroral mirror nasopharyngeal examination is necessary for the lower half of the nasopharynx. Such an examination is possible even in many children and will yield important information regarding nasopharyngeal lesions, particularly with reference to adenoid tissue, cysts, tumors, and antrochoanal polyps.

In some cases, mirror nasopharyngeal examination is either impossible or inadequate. The transnasal use of a nasopharyngoscope after adequate local anesthesia of nasal mucosa is extremely helpful and can be carried out in most adults and some children with little or no discomfort. Nasopharyngoscopy may reveal an unexpected cause of secretory otitis media, such as nasopharyngeal fibroma, chordoma, or malignant tumor.

The Berci-Ward-Hopkins peroral nasopharyngoscope (16) furnishes brilliant illumination in a large-field view of the nasopharynx. The instrument is introduced through the mouth with no need for anesthesia. The instrument can then be rotated for detailed examination of the lateral pharynx, the epiglottis, and larynx.

Digital examination of the nasopharynx was used by otolaryngologists for many decades. It is a crude, gross, and relatively traumatic method of examining the nasopharynx, and is no longer in common use. When nasopharyngeal examination is necessary in a child, definitive observations can be made only under general anesthesia with mirror examination, while the soft palate is elevated with a palate retractor. Whenever transnasal and mirror nasopharyngeal examinations have been unsatisfactory, there is no choice but to recommend intraoral intubation for general anesthesia, allowing the use of a palate retractor and mirror for adequate direct peroral visualization of the nasopharynx.

Lateral radiography of the nasopharynx is very helpful in evaluating adenoid tissue in some cases and may make it unnecessary to resort to major examination procedures for an accurate nasopharyngeal diagnosis.

AUDIOLOGIC TESTS

Tuning-Fork Tests

Tuning-fork tests do not displace careful audiometric examinations. However, they are useful as ancillary diagnostic tools. Comparative tuning-fork tests of air conduction may show "loudness" differences or time duration differences between the right and left ears. Occasionally, diplacusis (different pitch responses to same fork between right and left) may be noted.

In advanced unilateral secretory otitis media, a negative Rinne response is found. The upper incisor Weber test will be "referred" to the involved ear, or in bilateral secretory otitis, to the poorer hearing ear. However, in cases with slight or moderate hearing loss, the Rinne responses may be positive (air conduction/bone conduction) with 512-Hz and 256-Hz forks, and negative (bone conduction/air conduction) with the 128-Hz fork.

Tuning-fork tests are helpful in home or hospital examinations as a prelude or follow-up to audiometry.

Audiometric Tests

Audiometric assessment is essential in every case of secretory otitis media. Continual fluctuations in air conduction thresholds are not uncommon, depending upon intermittent tubal ventilation efficiency, which is rarely total and fixed. A frequently observed behavioral manifestation of this disability is the presence of many false positive responses to air conduction pure-tone stimuli.

The presence of an air–bone gap, predominantly occurring in the low frequencies (250-1 kHz) is a typical audiometric finding. However, secretory otitis media can exist *without* any audiometric evidence of an air–bone gap. The study by Eagles, Wishik and Doerfler (5) revealed that the average hearing loss of preschool-age children with secretory otitis media was 15 dB, an amount previously considered insignificant for acquisition of language and speech. In fact, children with a "hearing loss" of less than 20 dB would not even be discovered on a routine audiometric screening test; yet they may have active middle-ear disorders.

The air–bone gap associated with secretory otitis media may vary from 0–50 dB, but generally appears in the 15–30 dB range (Fig. 15–2). The configuration of the audiometric findings cannot be predicted. There has been considerable interest evidenced in the use of limited-frequency hearing tests to identify children with secretory otitis media (Fig. 15–3). Some clinicians recommend testing at 250 and 500 Hz, while others are in favor of testing at 2000 and 4000 Hz. Yet many children in need of medical attention for secretory otitis media have been found to have hearing losses at some specific frequencies only (Fig. 15–4). Table 15–1 shows the relationships between hearing losses occurring in the first few years of life and effects on language development. This table is applicable to patients with hearing loss, regardless of the conductive/sensorineural components.

The child with chronic secretory otitis media may also have depressed bone conduction responses, usually at 2000 and 4000 Hz. Typically, the decreased bone conduction thresholds average 15–20 dB below normal (Fig. 15–5). After treatment, the bone conduction levels usually return to normal thresholds (Fig. 15–5).

Early identification and treatment of secretory otitis media is obviously important medically, but is also serious because of education retardation resulting from undetected hearing losses during the early years of life. The child with unrecognized or inadequately treated secretory otitis media with lack of awareness of a moderate hearing loss, will have a sensory deprivation during the optimal time for the development of language. These children have been shown to be significantly delayed in all language skills requiring the receiving or processing of auditory stimuli or the production of verbal responses. It cannot be assumed that the resultant dysfunction can easily be overcome. This is true, even for the patient with mild hearing loss occurring at various intervals during infancy and early childhood (7, 9).

The child with mild–moderate congenital sensorineural hearing loss and superimposed secretory otitis media becomes severely handicapped. Such children must be carefully followed by otologic examinations and audiologic studies (Fig. 15–6).

The impedance test (especially the tympanometry portion), has been particularly useful in identifying secretory otitis media (see Ch. 7, Acoustic Impedance Tests) (11).

RADIOGRAPHIC EXAMINATION

In patients with suspected or evident chronic secretory otitis media, the mastoids and maxillary sinuses should be radiographed. In the mastoid

FIG. 15–2. A. Preoperative audiometric test. Note air–bone gap accompanied by a sloping high-frequency BC curve. A 4000-Hz notch is accompanied by depressed right BC response at 4000 Hz. Postoperative test. Note return of hearing virtually to normal. It is especially important to note the dramatic restoration of hearing in the high frequencies, especially at 4000 Hz. ●—●, AC, unmasked, RE, preoperative test; [—[, BC, masked, RE, preoperative test; ●- - -●, AC, unmasked, RE, postoperative test. **B.** Preoperative audiometric test. There is virtually no air–bone gap. There is a 1000-Hz AC notch and a 4000-Hz AC notch. Postoperative test. As in the right ear, hearing virtually returns to normal. There is a dramatic restoration of hearing at 4000 Hz. **x—x,** AC, unmasked, LE, preoperative test;]—], BC, masked, LE, preoperative test; **x- - -x,** AC, unmasked, LE, postoperative test.

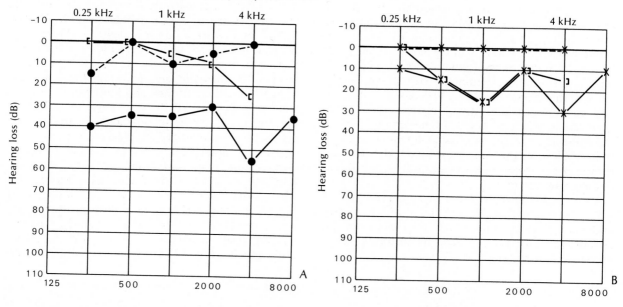

FIG. 15–3. A. Note AC hearing levels in both ears at 250 Hz and 4000 Hz. This child with bilateral secretory otitis media would have passed a low-high frequency screening test. ●–●, AC, unmasked, RE; [—[, BC, masked, RE; **x—x,** AC unmasked, LE;]—], BC, masked, LE; SRT, RE, 10 dB; SRT, LE, 10 dB. **B.** The small right air–bone gap due to secretory otitis media would have been missed on all conventional screening tests. ●–●, AC, unmasked, RE; [—[, BC, masked RE; SRT, 5 dB; **x—x,** AC, unmasked, LE; SRT, dB.

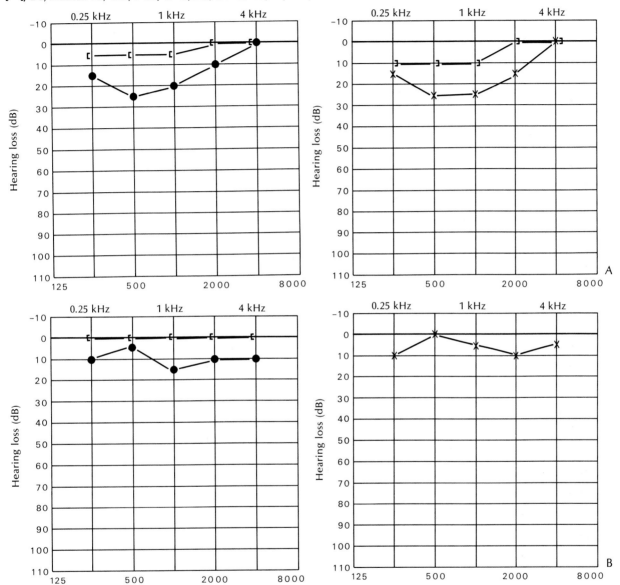

FIG. 15–4. A. It is possible for secretory otitis media to exist with no air–bone gap in the high frequencies at all. In this instance, the child would have passed a limited high-frequency test. ●—●, AC, unmasked, RE; [—[, BC, masked, RE; x—x, AC, unmasked, LE;]—], BC masked, LE; SRT for both ears was zero. **B.** This child with bilateral secretory otitis media would have passed a low frequency screening test.

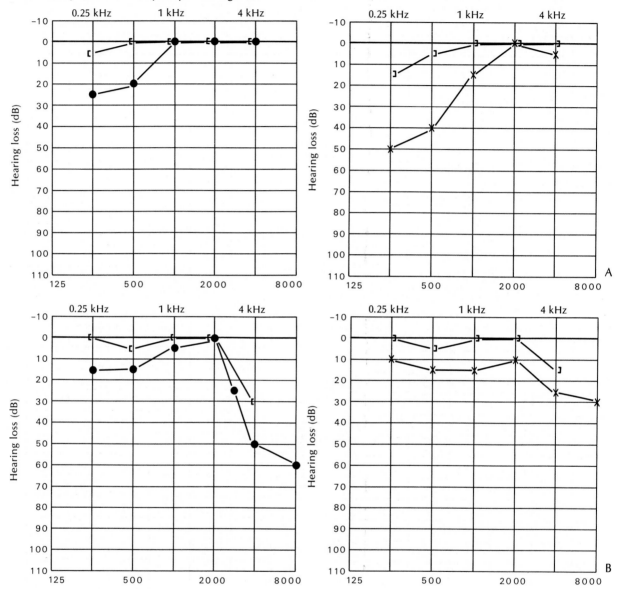

TABLE 15-1. Handicapping Effects of Hearing Loss

Hearing level (dB)*	Description	Condition	Sounds heard without amplification	Degree of handicap (if not treated in first year of life)	Probable needs
0–15	Normal range	Serous otitis, perforation, monomeric membrane, tympanosclerosis	All speech sounds	None	None
15–25	Slight hearing loss	Serous otitis, perforation, monomeric membrane, sensorineural loss, tympanosclerosis	Vowel sounds heard clearly; may miss unvoiced consonant sounds	Mild auditory dysfunction in language learning	Consideration of need for hearing aid; lipreading; auditory training; speech therapy, preferential seating
25–40	Mild hearing loss	Serous otitis, perforation, tympanosclerosis, monomeric membrane sensorineural loss	Hears only some louder-voiced speech sounds	Auditory learning dysfunction, mild language retardation, mild speech problems, inattention	Hearing aid, lipreading auditory training, speech therapy
40–65	Moderate hearing loss	Chronic otitis, middle ear anomaly, sensorineural loss	Misses most speech sounds at normal conversational level	Speech problems, language retardation, learning dysfunction, inattention	All the above, plus consideration of special classroom situation
65–95	Severe hearing loss	Sensorineural or mixed loss due to sensorineural loss plus middle ear disease	Hears no speech sounds of normal conversation	Severe speech problems, language retardation, learning dysfunction, inattention	All the above, plus probable assignment to special classes
≥95	Profound hearing loss	Sensorineural or mixed loss	Hears no speech or other sounds	Severe speech problems, language retardation learning dysfunction, inattention	All the above; plus probable assignment to special classes

*Average hearing, 500–2000 Hz (ANSI).
(Adapted from Marion Downs: In Northern J (ed): Hearing Disorders. Boston, Little Brown, 1976)

FIG. 15–5. Before operation there was a marked air–bone gap in each ear, accompanied by both AC and BC losses at 2000 Hz and 4000 Hz. **At left,** ●—●, AC, unmasked, RE; [—[, BC masked, RE; **At right,** x—x, AC, unmasked, LE;]—], BC, masked, LE. After operation, hearing returned to normal in both ears. It is especially noteworthy that hearing is normal at 4000 Hz in each ear, indicating that the 2000 Hz and 4000 Hz dips were purely conductive and not cochlear. **At left,** ●- - -●, AC, unmasked, RE; <- - -<, BC, unmasked, RE; **At right,** x- - -x, AC, unmasked, LE; >- - ->, BC, unmasked, LE.

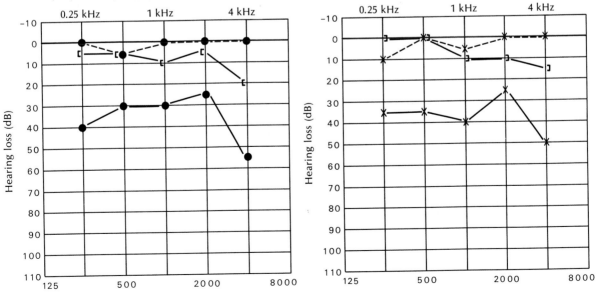

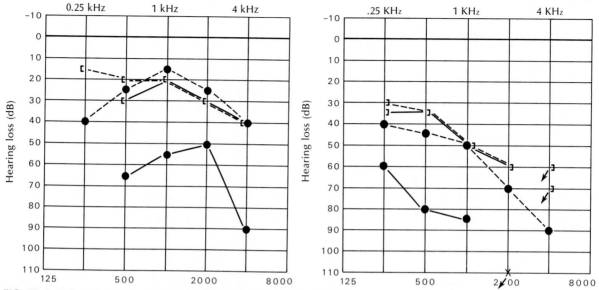

FIG. 15–6. Before operation there was a bilateral mixed loss with asymmetric air–bone gaps. ●—●, AC, unmasked RE; [—[, BC masked, RE; SRT, 45 dB. After operation, there was a significant closure of both air–bone gaps with a persistent asymmetrical cochlear loss. This example of secretory otitis media superimposed upon cochlear hearing loss is extremely significant since children with congenital cochlear hearing losses are just as susceptible to secretory otitis media as children with no previous hearing loss. ●- - -●, AC, unmasked RE; [- - -[, BC, masked SRT, 20 dB.

FIG. 15–7. A 15-year-old patient with right chronic secretory otomastoiditis. Right mastoid is less well pneumatized, with haziness in all cell groups **(arrow, RE)**. Left mastoid is well developed and normally aerated **(arrow, LE)**.

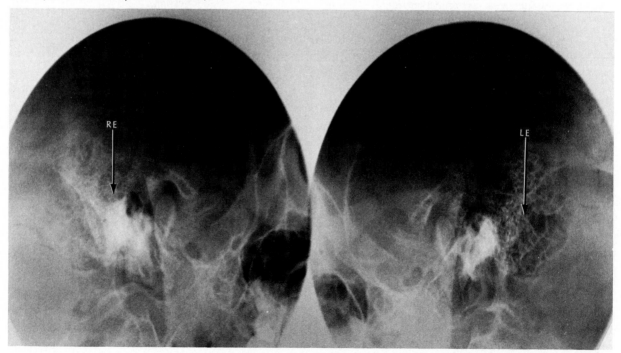

(Schuller's view), cellular air spaces are hazy and there is trabecular halisteresis seen as a "fuzziness" of cell walls, in cases of long duration. The petrous apex (Stenver's view) may also show air-cell haziness (Fig. 15–7).

Maxillary radiograms (Water's view) of the sinuses will often reveal ipsilateral (occasionally bilateral or contralateral) mucosal edema or polyposis. The sinus lumen is cloudy (Fig. 15–8). In chronic allergy, bilateral mucosal edema is present, not only in the maxillary sinuses, but also in the ethmoid, frontal, and sphenoid sinuses.

In patients with long-standing secretory otitis media that has been unresponsive to medical therapy, surgical drainage, and middle-ear ventilation tube aeration, in whom hearing losses of 30 dB or greater are present, the possibility of unrecognized ossicular necrosis, keratoma, and other otomastoiditis complications must be considered. In such patients, additional diagnostic assistance will be obtained from polytomographic radiographs. Routine polytomography is not necessary in the majority of secretory otitis media lesions.

MIDDLE EAR DIAGNOSTIC
ASPIRATION (TYMPANOCENTESIS)

In recurrent cases or those of long duration, tympanic membrane edema and scarring will prevent definitive diagnosis by manifest, induced, or gravity otoscopy. In questionable cases, diagnostic aspiration through the tympanic membrane (tympanocentesis) may be indicated, through each inferior tympanic membrane quadrant. Usually no anesthesia is necessary in adults. Local endomeatal lidocaine (Xylocaine) or iontophoresis block may be necessary. Contents are aspirated into a sterile tube for cytologic and bacteriologic studies. Frequently, the culture is reported negative for bacteria. In some cases, eosinophilia can be demonstrated on stained smear. The primary indication for transtympanic aspiration is to answer the question: is there fluid in the middle ear?

In children, diagnostic aspiration usually requires general anesthesia as a hospital procedure and is performed in conjunction with some other definitive surgical procedures, *i.e.*, tonsillectomy and adenoidectomy, adenoidectomy revision, direct nasopharyngoscopy, maxillary sinus irrigation, or any combination of these procedures. Only occasionally does the condition arise in children when diagnostic aspiration *per se* justifies general anesthesia.

DIFFERENTIAL DIAGNOSIS

Many conditions resemble secretory otitis media. This does not refer to such obvious differential diagnostic problems as otosclerosis, or pseudo-otosclerosis, in which the primary similarity is audiometric conductive hearing loss. In the differential diagnosis of secretory otitis, one must consider cases of conductive hearing loss with an intact tympanic membrane but abnormal otoscopic findings in the membrane and the middle ear. Among these conditions are congenital vascular middle ear anomalies, otomastoiditis, tumors, sequelae of trauma, and other lesions.

CONGENITAL VASCULAR ANOMALIES
OF THE MIDDLE EAR

Intratympanic Jugular Bulb

The jugular bulb usually does not project above the floor of the hypotympanum. In congenital anomalies it is possible for the jugular bulb, either covered or uncovered by bone, to be present in the hypo- or mesotympanum. This will usually create a discoloration behind the tympanic membrane. If the bulb is not pressing against the tympanic membrane, there will be no bulging but only discoloration (bluish or reddish sheen), which may mimic the color of the fluid in secretory otitis media. If the tympanic membrane is bulging, the bulb will simulate middle ear tumor. Inadvertent myringotomy in such cases can result in serious jugular bulb hemorrhage.

Aberrant Tympanic Internal Carotid Artery

Another anomaly is the presence of the internal carotid artery in the mesotympanum. Like the anomalous jugular bulb, it may simulate secretory otitis media. The artery's presence may not displace the tympanic membrane but simply produce opacity similar to that of middle ear fluid. There may be no hearing loss in the case of an anomalous internal carotid artery in the middle ear unless deformations of the ossicular chain occur. Inadvertent myringotomy incision may produce dangerous carotid arterial hemorrhage.

Persistent Obturator Artery

The obturator artery, which is present in fetal life and usually disappears after birth, is a large vessel that occupies the entire space of the obturator foramen in the stapes arch. A persistent large obturator artery can also produce discolora-

FIG. 15–8. Bilateral secretory otomastoiditis in a 5-year-old child. Note concomitant left maxillary sinusitis. **A.** Bilateral poorly developed mastoids, with haziness and indistinct bony cellular outlines **(arrows). B.** Left maxillary sinus (Waters view) is opaque **(arrow)** as result of advanced mucositis and fluid. Right is normal.

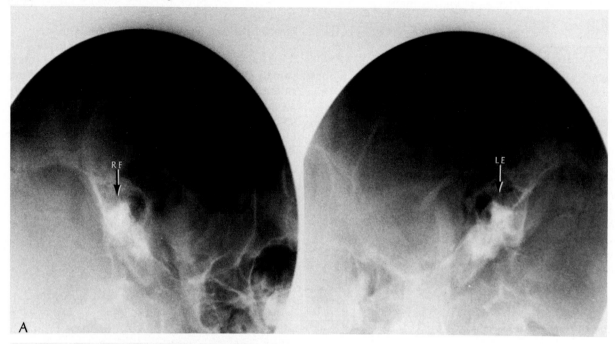

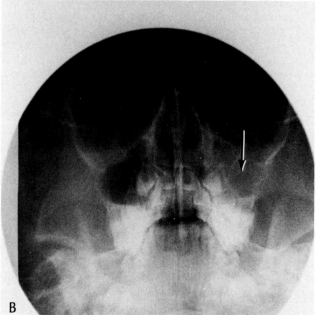

tion and an opaque but intact tympanic membrane and may be accompanied by conductive hearing loss. Inadvertent myringotomy may produce significant arterial hemorrhage.

Intratympanic Arteriovenous Aneurysm

An intratympanic arteriovenous aneurysm involving the internal carotid artery and/or the jugular bulb may be present behind an intact tympanic membrane, producing changes in texture and color that resemble those seen in secretory otitis media. Inadvertent incision of such an aneurysm results in severe hemorrhage.

OTOMASTOIDITIS WITH INTRATYMPANIC MASSES

Cholesterol Granuloma

Cholesterol granuloma may well be a sequel of secretory otitis media. It may be a concomitant of chronic otomastoiditis accompanied by middle-ear fluid and middle-ear granuloma behind an intact tympanic membrane. Although it may be a late sequel of secretory otitis media, it requires mastoid surgery and illustrates the need for mastoid radiographs in every patient with suspected secretory otitis.

Tympanic Keratoma (Cholesteatoma)

Quiescent or "lurking, latent" keratoma (cholesteatoma) (6) frequently occurs behind an intact tympanic membrane with no history of previous otomastoiditis. This is especially common in children. Usually radiographic abnormalities and conductive hearing loss are present. Myringotomy incision will rarely yield fluid. However, squamous (keratomatous) epithelial tissue will be found, identifiable as keratin on a stained smear.

Tympanosclerosis

Tympanosclerosis may follow secretory otitis media but can present as a different sequel to acute otitis media. The tympanic membrane, in most cases, is thickened, with white-gray tympanosclerotic plaques. Secretory otitis may be found concurrently with previously healed tympanosclerosis. Mastoid radiographic findings are usually helpful in differential diagnosis. Myringotomy will usually yield no fluid but may yield a thick mucoid fluid. There will be resistance to the incision because of the calcific nature of the thickened tympanic membrane and the blocking tympanosclerotic intratympanic masses.

POSTTRAUMATIC INTRATYMPANIC CEREBROSPINAL FLUID

Intratympanic clear fluid may not be serum or transudate in a suspected case of secretory otitis media but cerebrospinal fluid coming from a recent or old, known or unknown, tympanic tegmen skull fracture with cerebrospinal fluid filling the middle ear (see Ch. 24, Traumatic Diseases of the Ear and Temporal Bone). Upon myringotomy in such a case, a brisk and usually pulsating flow of clear fluid will appear and will not readily stop. It will rapidly refill on aspiration. Chemical studies for glucose and protein, tomographic, radiographic studies, and tympanoepitympanic surgical exploration will be necessary to rule out a tegmental skull fracture. In some cases, an accompanying meningoencephalocele may protrude through a tegmen fracture, along with the presence of cerebrospinal fluid.

TYMPANIC PERILYMPH

Middle ear perilymph may resemble secretory otitis media fluid. Such perilymph collections are not common. They occur occasionally following poststapedectomy oval window fistulas. The hearing loss may be purely conductive and thus mimic that in secretory otitis, but more commonly the hearing loss is mixed conductive and cochlear. Such perilymph collections may also occur following traumatic labyrinthine fractures and may simulate cerebrospinal fluid in the middle ear, as well as the fluid in secretory otitis media (Fig. 15-9).

TUMORS

Nasopharyngeal Tumors

Benign tumors of the nasopharynx usually produce tubal obstruction with secondary secretory otitis media. An example is nasopharyngeal fibroma or chordoma. The secretory otitis may be unilateral or bilateral. This problem underscores the great need for careful study of the nasopharynx in every case of secretory otitis media.

Malignant carcinomas of the nasopharynx may be first manifested by secretory otitis. This is common in adults with transitional-cell carcinoma (lymphoepithelioma). The first complaint may be a conductive hearing loss. Otoscopic examination will frequently reveal yellow or amber intratympanic fluid comparable to that seen in secretory otitis. Myringotomy and insertion of middle-ear

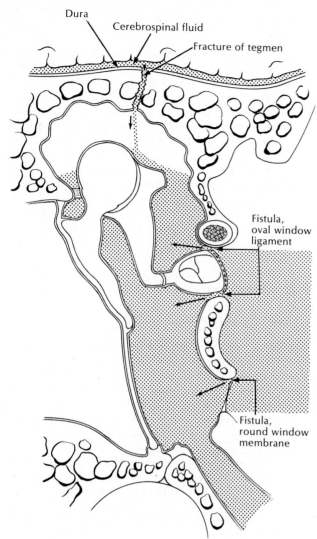

FIG. 15–9. Middle-ear fluid due to either cerebrospinal fluid from a tegmen bony defect (as in skull fracture) or to perilymph fistulas in oval or round windows.

ventilation tubes in such a case, without careful and repeated nasopharyngeal examinations, may result in a missed carcinoma diagnosis. Nasopharyngeal lymphomas will produce similar tubal obstruction with secondary secretory otitis.

Middle Ear Tumors

Benign tumors of the middle ear may simulate secretory otitis media. The most common differential diagnostic problem is that concerning the chemodectoma group. Tympanic glomus tumors, prior to causing the tympanic membrane to bulge, will produce simple color changes and opacity which will mimic secretory otitis. Inadvertent myringotomy in such a case may be followed by hemorrhage. Small glomus tumors in the middle ear may elude diagnosis, and conventional mastoid radiographs may indicate a normal state. For this reason, in obscure cases, the middle ear should be examined via exploratory tympanotomy, even when polytomographic temporal-bone radiographs are apparently normal.

Choristoma, an uncommon anomalous intratympanic salivary gland pseudotumor secretes saliva into the middle ear, creating a condition that simulates secretory otitis. It usually is accompanied by ossicular necrosis and conductive hearing loss. Myringotomy will yield saliva. Definitive treatment requires removal by middle ear and mastoid surgery.

Carcinoma may occur in the middle ear with or without involvement of the external auditory canal. Primary carcinoma of the middle ear can occur behind an intact tympanic membrane, with opacity and conductive hearing loss simulating that in secretory otitis. The tumor will be recognized on tympanotomy for middle-ear exploration (see Ch. 22, Temporal Bone Tumors).

Intracranial Tumors

Meningioma may involve the temporal bone. The en-plaque variety frequently is accompanied by fibrous dysplasia with epitympanic and middle-ear fluid, producing secretory otitis media. If middle-ear exploration yields fluid and tympanic fibrosis is present, primary meningioma should be considered.

Meningoencephalocele in the middle ear simulates secretory otitis, with cerebrospinal fluid in the middle ear appearing as a clear secretion. The only presenting complaint may be mild or moderate conductive hearing loss. Myringotomy is followed by persistent fluid flow. Such unusual fluid seepage calls for exploratory tympanotomy, and appropriate polytomographic radiographic studies. Further transmastoid exploration may be necessary to identify the transtegmen tumor.

Mastoid Tumors

Tumors of the mastoid may be primary, with secondary middle-ear findings. Carcinoid tumor of the mastoid may present as secretory otitis media with a conductive hearing loss. Carcinoid tumors are not highly malignant and usually respond favorably to surgical excision and postoperative radiation. Sarcomas of the mastoid and histiocytic granuloma tumors rarely produce fluid in the middle ear.

POSTRADIATION TEMPORAL BONE NECROSIS

Patients who have received radiation therapy for various head and neck tumors, such as basal-cell carcinoma (auricular or postauricular), may develop delayed postradiation temporal bone necrosis. This may manifest itself first by middle-ear fluid prior to the actual appearance of necrotic bone lesions. The fluid is a result of reactive osteitis and middle-ear mucositis. Radiographic studies and surgical exploration, in addition to careful history, will result in definitive diagnosis.

OSTEODYSTROPHIES AND MESODERMAL DYSPLASIAS OF THE TEMPORAL BONE

Benign mesodermal dysplasias may produce secretory otitis media. This group includes monostotic fibrous dysplasias, eosinophilic granuloma, and other forms of histiocytosis X and Paget's disease.

These lesions involve both middle-ear and mastoid air-cell mucosa and occasionally produce middle-ear fluid. Mastoid, skull, and long-bone radiographs followed by diagnostic surgical exploration, are diagnostic (see Ch. 21, Temporal Bone Granulomas and Dystrophies).

MANAGEMENT PRINCIPLES IN SECRETORY OTITIS MEDIA

Acute otitis media requires not only proper antibiotic therapy, but also prompt surgical drainage through myringotomy in many cases. Antibiotic therapy alone is frequently inadequate in acute otitis media. Secretory otitis media is usually a sequel to acute otitis media and will be diagnosed only if there is a high index of suspicion.

The management of secretory otitis is based on two principles: 1) elimination of the underlying cause or causes, and 2) the removal of fluid and the ventilation of the middle ear, regardless of cause. Persistent fluid and lack of middle-ear ventilation, regardless of cause, frequently lead to a number of serious sequelae, including tympanic fibrosis, middle-ear mucosal dysplasia, ossicular necrosis, irreversible atelectatic and monomeric changes in the tympanic membrane, and all the sequelae of chronic otomastoiditis.

Careful study of tympanic and paratympanic areas, including nasopharynx and mastoid, must be included in the management plan. Nasal, sinus, nasopharyngeal, allergenic, metabolic, immunologic, and other factors must be carefully evaluated in each case.

In some cases, institution of adequate nasal ventilation, restoration of tubotympanic function, and the use of appropriate antibiotic, antihistaminic, decongestive, and antiallergic measures may be sufficient to produce spontaneous resolution of secretory otitis media.

In pediatric secretory otitis, throat cultures, nasal and nasopharyngeal examination, and sinus and mastoid radiographs are essential in management. In adult secretory otitis, in addition to the same considerations involved in pediatric cases, special attention is directed to possible nasopharyngeal neoplasms.

SPECIAL MANAGEMENT OF PEDIATRIC SECRETORY OTITIS MEDIA

BASIC PEDIATRIC SECRETORY OTITIS MEDIA PROBLEMS

Secretory otitis media is primarily a pediatric problem, although adult cases are not rare. Two factors play roles in this pediatric predominance: 1) the tonsil-adenoid factor, and 2) respiratory allergy. Pediatric immunologic problems are linked to both.

Debates regarding tonsil-and-adenoid and allergy roles have dominated ear, nose, and throat and pediatric journals for decades. The debates continue. There are no simple solutions to these complex problems. An awareness of both factors, thorough examinations, and clinical judgment derived from pediatric-ENT experience will expedite management of pediatric secretory otitis media problems. Thorough evaluation must be based upon otologic, audiologic, and radiologic studies (initial and serial), combined with thorough pediatric-immunologic evaluations. There are no panaceas in the management of pediatric secretory otitis.

Secretory otitis media may appear to respond to one treatment, only to recur and require other therapy. What is required in the management of pediatric secretory otitis is an awareness of the complexity of the upper respiratory system and its relationships to the tubotympanic mastoid cellular system. In addition, constant attention must be directed to the auditory-vestibular system, which is in intimate contiguity with the tympanomastoid cellular system.

EXAMINATION

The child with secretory otitis media requires three basic examinations: 1) ENT examination; 2) audiologic tests; and 3) radiographs of mastoids and sinuses. No responsible judgment can be made without these three examinations, which should follow a careful chronologic history.

TONSIL-AND-ADENOID INFECTIONS AND SINUSITIS IN SECRETORY OTITIS MEDIA

This combination plays an etiologic role in a large percentage of pediatric cases of secretory otitis media. When there is a history of repeated febrile acute otitis media attacks, accompanied or preceded by tonsillitis, cervical adenitis, and purulent rhinosinusitis, wise management will include tonsillectomy and adenoidectomy, irrigation of involved maxillary sinuses (depending upon radiographic findings), myringotomy with aspiration and ventilatory intubation of the middle ear in the involved ear or ears. In many cases bilateral secretory otitis media is present.

The surgery should be preceded and followed as a joint responsibility of the pediatrician and the otolaryngologist. Follow-up joint care should be long-range, including periodic audiologic studies, otoscopy, and radiographs. Recurrences are frequent. Decisions regarding swimming and other activities require joint management.

TONSIL-AND-ADENOID INFECTIONS, SINUSITIS, AND ALLERGY

When allergy is present, in addition to recurrent tonsillitis, adenoiditis, and sinusitis, the therapeutic problem increases in complexity. In addition to the management outlined in the foregoing paragraphs, special consideration of allergy is necessary.

ALLERGY IN SECRETORY OTITIS MEDIA

Allergy can be the primary or sole cause of secretory otitis media in some children. In some cases it may be the underlying factor with secondary infection superimposed. Allergy and chronic infection can coexist as etiologic factors producing tubal malfunction, ciliary hypofunction, and development of permanent or semipermanent changes in mucosal cytology in the middle ear, such as large increases in goblet-cell populations. Both transudates and exudates with varying proportions of mucus, serum proteins, and other components may be present because of the mixed etiologic pattern.

In some patients simple attention to elimination of common allergenic foods, such as milk, wheat,

eggs, chocolate, shellfish, and nuts, may be sufficient to eliminate a major ingestant allergic cause. In other patients additional allergic measures are necessary, including attention to house dust, animal dander, pollens, and other inhalants. In some patients and in certain specific geographic areas, pollen factors may play dominant roles and specific hyposensitization may be essential before treatment of secretory otitis becomes effective. In addition to dietary elimination and specific inhalant hyposensitization, the intermittent use of antihistaminic and decongestant drugs may be helpful. The use of such drugs should not be prolonged unduly, since they may produce excessive mucosal dryness. The use of tripelennamine (25 mg) and thenylpropanolamine HCl (25 mg) taken together two to three times a day is beneficial in many patients. Such therapy may be alternated with liquefying agents, such as potassium iodide solution or hydriodic acid during "dry" phases.

In stubborn allergic cases, which are resistant to conventional approaches in the management of allergy, corticosteroid therapy in short-term courses is effective. Steroid therapy, administered with great care, in correct dosage, and for limited fixed periods of time, can be extremely helpful in the management of nonresponsive secretory otitis media. It should not replace attention to adenoid tissue problems, paranasal sinus disease factors, and other infectious aspects of secretory otitis. Such steroid therapeutic regimens may be repeated several times a year if necessary to deal with exacerbations of secretory otitis. Obviously, attention to possible complications of corticosteroid therapy is necessary. Joint pediatric-otologic management is preferred.

ANTIBIOTIC AND SULFONAMIDE THERAPY IN SECRETORY OTITIS MEDIA

Penicillin in one form or another is the primary antibiotic therapy used in dealing with bacterial aspects of secretory otitis media. Since middle-ear cultures in secretory otitis are frequently sterile, reliance on repeated nasopharynx cultures and sensitivity tests may be required for antibiogram guidance. Erythromycin and cephalexin monohydrate are indicated in some cases. Attention to possible antibiotic allergy must be considered in all cases. Tetracycline should be avoided in children under the age of 8 years because of danger of dental staining.

The empiric use of triple sulfa drugs has been a helpful adjunct in a small percentage of cases of secretory otitis media that recurs in spite of adequate attention to T&A problems, sinusitis, and allergy, and use of conventional antibiotics. In occasional pediatric cases of secretory otitis shown to be resistant to other therapeutic programs, favorable responses have been noted following long-range daily sulfonamide therapy. Microorganisms sensitive to sulfonamides are those that must synthesize their own folic acid (pteroylglutamic acid). Sulfonamides "compete" with these bacteria for the utilization of paraaminobenzoic acid, essential for manufacture of pteroylglutamic acid.

Such sulfonamide therapy may be necessary for months, or even years, in an occasional child. Careful attention to urine, blood, and general systemic effects is necessary. Dosages are maintained at 500–1000 mg daily. As in all pediatric cases of secretory otitis media, joint pediatric-otologic consultations are advisable.

SURGICAL MANAGEMENT OF PEDIATRIC SECRETORY OTITIS MEDIA

When conservative treatment—*i.e.*, management of predisposing causes and medical therapy—fails, surgical management is necessary. Surgical management basically consists of myringotomy with aspiration of middle-ear fluid and ventilatory intubation of the middle ear.

Surgical drainage and ventilation may be necessary prior to, concomitant with, or following medical therapy. There is no simple, clear-cut formula. Experience and judgment will determine proper timing and combination of medical and surgical therapy.

In general, myringotomy, aspiration, and ventilatory intubation of the middle ear are carried out simultaneously with tonsillectomy, adenoidectomy, and/or maxillary sinus irrigation procedures, as deemed necessary in each case. Variations on this theme will be dictated by specific findings. General anesthesia is used.

The myringotomy and ventilatory intubation of the middle ear may be single or double, *i.e.*, in anteroinferior and posteroinferior quadrants of the tympanic membrane (Fig. 15–10), depending upon the nature of the middle-ear fluid. In "serous" secretory otitis media, posteroinferior and anteroinferior quadrant incisions and ventilatory tubes are necessary (Fig. 15–11). Fluid is suctioned alternately from each incision, and specimens are sent for laboratory study. Either one or both inferior quadrant incisions may be intubated.

Many tube types are in use for ventilating the middle ear. In thin serous secretory otitis, simple tubes for short-term use are adequate (Fig. 15–12). In glue ear otitis, some type of long-term tube is desirable, such as the "collar button" tube, made of silicone, Teflon, or metal (Figs. 15–13, 15–14, 15–15).

Special techniques are necessary in cases of secretory otitis with complications, such as tympanic fibrosis or atelectasis.

SECRETORY OTITIS MEDIA WITH TYMPANIC FIBROSIS

Progressive intratympanic fibrosis is a frequent sequel to secretory otitis and occurs in several forms as a result of irreversible mucosal changes. Compartments usually result in pseudocystic intratympanic "pockets" of middle-ear fluid.

Simple myringotomy and intubation will not suffice in most cases of this type, but a trial of the procedure may be advisable. If there is no resolution of the secretory otitis, it will be necessary to follow with a definitive tympanolysis procedure. A tympanotomy is performed and fibrous bands in the middle ear are carefully sectioned.

SECRETORY OTITIS MEDIA WITH ATELECTASIS OF THE TYMPANIC MEMBRANE

Recurrent chronic secretory otitis media that is untreated may result in atelectasis of the tympanic membrane with atrophy of the middle (fibrous) layer. The tympanic membrane consists of two types of cells (lateral epithelium and medial mucosa) and is an exceedingly thin so-called monomeric membrane, which frequently becomes adherent to the incus, to the incudostapedial joint, or to the middle-ear promontory. This is a common finding in patients with cleft palate but occurs in many other cases also. Myringostomy is possible and requires delicate use of suction to pull the monomeric tympanic membrane portion laterally, prior to the myringostomy procedure. A collar-button ventilatory tube is inserted into the anteroinferior quadrant (preferably), and the redundant monomeric membrane is elevated from the middle-ear adhesions. The collar-button tube becomes a space retainer in addition to its role as a ventilatory tube for the middle ear. (See Color Fig. 8.)

Such careful myringotomy and intubation may be followed by reestablishment of an improved

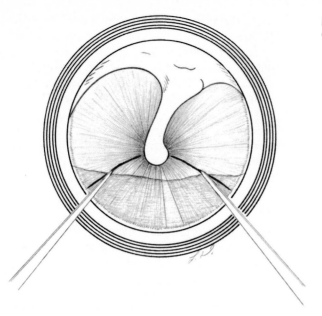

FIG. 15–10. Double myringostomy incisions in inferior quadrants.

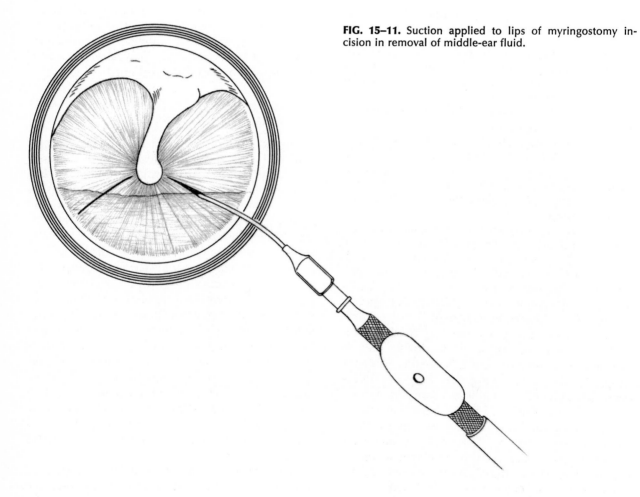

FIG. 15–11. Suction applied to lips of myringostomy incision in removal of middle-ear fluid.

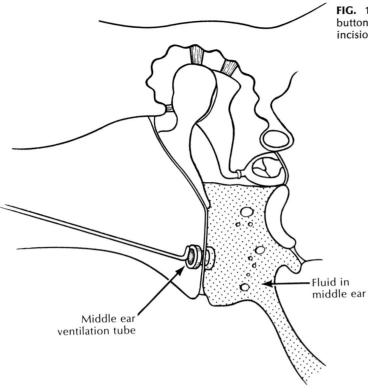

FIG. 15–12. Insertion of middle-ear ventilation collar-button tube through tympanic membrane myringostomy incision for fluid drainage and middle-ear ventilation.

Fluid in
middle ear

Middle ear
ventilation tube

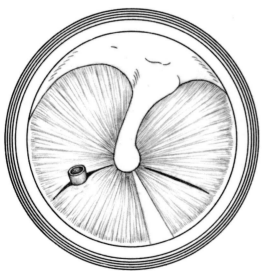

FIG. 15–13. Middle-ear ventilation tube inserted through posteroinferior myringostomy incision.

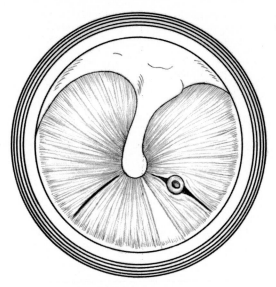

FIG. 15–14. Collar-button type middle-ear ventilation tube through anteroinferior myringostomy incision.

FIG. 15–15. Secretory otitis media with collar-button middle-ear ventilation tube.

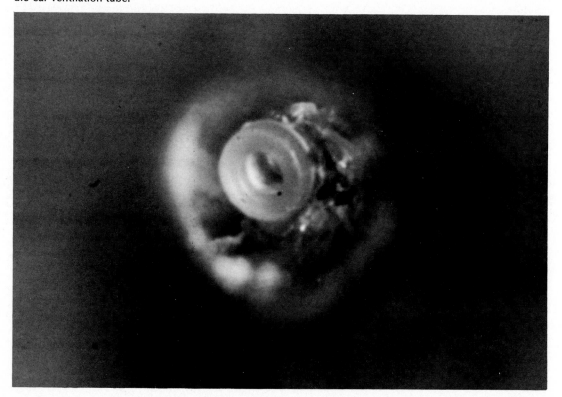

middle-ear air space. It may be necessary to leave the tube in position for months or years. Lack of response will require definitive tympanoplastic reconstruction.

SECRETORY OTITIS MEDIA WITH MASTOIDITIS

Secretory otitis media may be the presenting finding in several forms of mastoiditis, especially in cholesterol granuloma of the mastoid. Mastoid radiographs will be diagnostic in most cases and treatment will require mastoid surgery. Simple myringotomy and ventilatory intubation of the middle ear will usually be inadequate (see Ch. 16, Chronic Otomastoiditis—Diagnosis and Management).

SECRETORY OTITIS MEDIA IN PATIENTS WITH CLEFT PALATE

Cleft palate malfunctions usually involve peritubal muscles and lymphoid tissue. Secretory otitis media is present in almost every patient with cleft palate.

Primary management principles for the secretory otitis remain unchanged, except for variable approaches to tonsil and adenoid management. In general, routine T&A is not recommended in most cases of cleft palate. Some advocate tonsillectomy and lateral adenoidectomy with retention of central adenoid. Others are either more conservative or more radical.

The management of the middle-ear problem, *per se,* is the same as in the child with a normal palate. Early diagnosis, proper medical therapy, and long-duration ventilatory intubation of the middle ear is recommended in most cases of cleft palate.

MANAGEMENT OF SECRETORY OTITIS MEDIA IN ADULTS

BASIC FACTORS IN SECRETORY OTITIS MEDIA IN ADULTS

There are significant differences between adult and pediatric cases of secretory otitis. These may be summarized as follows:

1. More intensive and long-range search is necessary in the adult for predisposing factors listed in the section on etiology earlier in this chapter.

In particular, this relates to tumors of the nasopharynx and middle ear.
2. More detailed radiographic studies of the mastoid may be necessary to rule out undetected mastoid lesions.
3. Tonsil and adenoid problems are less common, but cannot be disregarded, as persistent infected adenoid masses do occur in even middle-aged adults.
4. Sinusitis is just as common a predisposing factor as in pediatric secretory otitis.
5. Tympanic fibrosis is more common in adult patients with secretory otitis media.

SURGICAL TECHNIQUES IN ADULTS WITH SECRETORY OTITIS MEDIA

In adult cases, simultaneous attention is directed to the diagnosis of predisposing factors and to fluid aspiration from the middle ear.

The first approach is tympanocentesis, as described previously. Myringostomy is the next procedure; in adults it can be performed in the office. This technique has also been described previously, but it should be modified as follows.

Myringotomy

Single or double radial fiber myringotomy, involving an incision in one or both inferior quadrants is performed. This is followed by suction to the lips of the incision. Such suction is frequently expedited if, first, Valsalva inflation, politzerization, or eustachian tube catheterization gently forces hypotympanic or protympanic middle-ear fluid into the mesotympanum, from where it may be more readily aspirated.

If aspiration reveals thin fluid and ready emptying of the middle ear, no further measures are indicated unless the fluid reforms. If aspiration reveals a thick, gluelike fluid, myringotomy is necessary with insertion of tubes for ventilation and drainage of the middle ear. One tube is usually used, but it may be advisable to use two tubes in some cases, one in each inferior quadrant incision, so that if one becomes plugged, the other will still be effective in maintaining aeration, ventilation, and possible drainage. Collar-button drainage tubes made from Supramid, Silastic, Teflon, or stainless steel are designed to prevent premature extrusion. Polyethylene tubes (size PE 90) may be used in some cases, in which long-term intubation is not necessary.

In chronic cases of secretory otitis with thick

gluey fluid, tubes may require replacement, preceded by suction, several times before resolution and recovery occur. Tympanic atelectasis may develop, requiring special management as described under Special Management of Pediatric Secretory Otitis Media.

Tympanic fibrosis is more common in adult secretory otitis and may be the result of repetitive previous episodes of the disorder in childhood. In such cases, repetitive myringotomy and ventilatory intubation of the middle ear is ineffective. A definitive tympanolysis through an endomeatal incision will be necessary to lyse tympanic fibrous compartments. Intubation will then be more effective.

The posterior tympanotomy through an endomeatal omega incision reveals pockets of fibrous tissue. It will be necessary to lyse these fibrous partitions to obtain adequate aeration and drainage. Tympanolysis requires meticulous, gentle, and careful dissection of scar-tissue bands between the ossicles, between the ossicular chain and the tympanic membrane, and between the ossicular chain and the promontory. Frequently, a peri-stapedial fibrous tent will entrap a collection of fluid. Similar scar tissue bands must be removed from the round window niche and occasionally from the anterior tympanic compartment, where they block eustachian tube ventilation. A ventilatory tube is then inserted into the middle ear through an anteroinferior quadrant radial fiber incision.

FIG. 15–16. Large mastoid drainage and ventilation tube in place in sutured endaural incision following atticomastoidectomy for persistent secretory otomastoiditis.

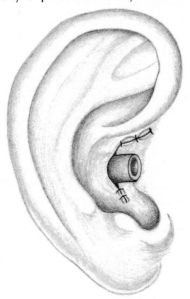

Persistent secretory otitis media may be secondary rather than primary. This is especially the case in subacute chronic polypoid seromucoid mastoiditis. Limited middle-ear surgery will be ineffective. Definitive mastoid surgery will be necessary.

When clinical and radiographic findings reveal definite changes in the mastoid, an atticomastoidectomy will usually reveal pockets of cystic fibrous tissue with fluid collections, frequently of the glue type, in which the exudate is very sticky and difficult to remove by suction. It is necessary to do a thorough mastoidectomy, following anatomic cell tracts in methodical fashion to create a well-aerated mastoid bowl without disturbing the incus or the incudomalleal joint and without removal of the posterior canal wall. Prolonged drainage is usually advisable (Fig. 15–16). In addition to one or two ventilatory tubes in the middle ear, a large inert ventilation tube (Silastic or Teflon) is left in place within the mastoid antrum to emerge either through the endaural or postauricular incision. During the period of such drainage and ventilation (2–4 weeks) broad-spectrum antibiotic coverage is maintained, along with indicated treatment of the nasopharynx, nose and nasal sinuses, and antiallergic measures, as necessary. Prompt recognition of chronic secretory otitis media and polypoid mastoiditis and the surgical elimination of mastoid and middle-ear lesions will frequently prevent late changes and the need for such procedures as tympanoplasty.

COMPLICATIONS OF SECRETORY OTITIS MEDIA

Major complications of secretory otitis media are due to progression from simple tubotympanic mucositis to major irreversible changes in mucosa, periosteum, ossicular chain, and in mastoid bony trabeculae. Tympanosclerosis and keratoma (cholesteatoma) are not uncommon complications of secretory otitis media.

Thus, both type A and type B chronic otomastoiditis are the significant problems requiring management. Diagnostic and therapeutic aspects of these lesions are described in Chapters 16, 17, and 18.

Iatrogenic complications may be due to inadequate or to overzealous treatment. There is danger of paracentesis combined with transcanal inflation in attempts to obtain drainage of the middle ear forcefully through the eustachian tube. Congenital defects may exist in labyrinthine windows, or in the tegmen tympani, which can lead to intracranial complications.

REFERENCES

1. Bak-Pedersen K, Tos M: Density of goblet cells in chronic secretory otitis media: a temporal bone report. Rev Laryngol Otol Rhinol 94:27–34, 1973

2. Bernstein J, Reisman R: The role of acute hypersensitivity in secretory Otitis Media. Am Acad Ophthal Otolaryngol 78:ORL 120–127, 1974

3. Bernstein J, Tomasi T, Ogra P: The immunochemistry of middle ear effusions. Arch Otolaryngol 99:320–326, 1974

4. Bluestone C, Beery Q, Andrus W: Mechanics of eustachian tube as it influences susceptibility to and persistance of middle ear effusions in children. Ann Otol Rhinol Laryngol [Suppl] 83 (11):27–34, 1974

5. Eagles EL, Wishik SM, Doerfler LG: Hearing sensitivity and ear disease in children. A prospective study. Laryngoscope 5: [Suppl] 77:1–274, 1967

6. Goodhill V: The lurking latent cholesteatoma. Ann Otol Rhinol Laryngol 69:1199–1213, 1960

7. Holm VA, Kunze LH: Effect of chronic otitis media on language and speech development. Pediatrics 43:833–839, 1969

8. Lim D, Birck H: Ultrastructural pathology of the middle ear mucosa in serous Otitis Media. Ann Otol Rhinol Laryngol 80:838–853, 1971

9. Ling D, McCoy RH, Levinson EV: The incidence of middle ear disease and its educational implications among Baffin Island Eskimo children. Can J Pub Health Oct, 1969, pp 385–390

10. Liu Y, Lim D, Lang R et al.: Chronic middle ear effusions. Arch Otolaryngol 101:278–286, 1975

11. McCandless GA, Thomas GK: Impedance audiometry as a screening procedure for middle ear disease. Trans Am Acad Ophthalmol Otolaryngol 78:ORL 98–102, 126, 1974

12. Palva T, Palva A: Mucosal histochemistry in secretory otitis. Ann Otol Rhinol Laryngol 84:112–116, 1975

13. Sade J, Eliezer N: Secretory Otitis Media and the nature of the mucociliary system. Acta Otolaryngol (Stockh) 70:351–357, 1970

14. Sade J: The biopathology of secretory Otitis Media. Ann Otol Rhinol Laryngol 83:59–70, 1974

15. Tos M, Bak-Pedersen K: The outset of chronic secretory Otitis Media. Arch Otolaryngol 101:123–128, 1975

16. Ward P, Berci G, Calcaterra T: Advances in endoscopic examination of the respiratory system. Ann Otol Rhinol Laryngol 83:754, 1974

SUGGESTED READING

Lim DJ, Liu YS, Birck H: Secretory lysozyme of the human middle ear mucosa: immunocytochemical localization. Ann Otol Rhinol Laryngol 85:50–66, 1976

Paparella MM, Hiraide F, Oda M et al.: Pathology of sensorineural hearing loss in Otitis Media. Ann Otol Rhinol Laryngol 81:632–647, 1972

Shemada T, Lim DJ: Distribution of ciliated cells in the human middle ear. Ann Otol Rhinol Laryngol 81:203–212, 1972

Terrahe K, Fromme HG, Schulz J: Die Schalleitungskette des Mittelohres bei chronischer epitympanaler Otitis. Eine rasterelektron-mikroskopische untersuchung. Z Laryngol Rhinol Otol 50:548–556, 1971

16

CHRONIC OTOMASTOIDITIS— DIAGNOSIS AND MANAGEMENT

Chronic otomastoiditis is the sequel of untreated or nonresponsive acute otomastoiditis or secretory otitis media and is the final phase of the continuum beginning with tubotympanitis (see Ch. 14, Acute Otitis Media and Mastoiditis).

The continuum of tubotympanitis–otitis–mastoiditis varies greatly in chronology, sequence, and variety of lesions. The "détente" phase of secretory otitis media frequently is a midpoint in the continuum, which finally ends in chronic otomastoiditis.

A tympanic membrane perforation, dry or draining, is characteristic of chronic otomastoiditis. The "chronic draining ear" is a sign of chronic otomastoiditis unless proved otherwise.

Lesion specificity in chronic otomastoiditis involves two pathologic types: type A (potentially reversible), comprising mucositis, osteitis, polyposis, granuloma lesions; and type B (irreversible), comprising epithelial migration and metaplastic mucosal, osteolytic, keratinizing, and osteitic lesions. Significant differences in management characterize these two types.

Location (anatomic) of the lesion (type A or type B) will modify management crucially. The entire pneumatic system or any portion of the temporal bone and its constituent structures may be involved. This includes the tympanic membrane, middle ear, ossicular chain, labyrinth, facial nerve, mastoid cell groups, arteries, veins, and middle and posterior fossa bony plates.

Loss of function almost always involves a conductive hearing loss. Secondary cochlear hearing loss can occur. Vestibular function disturbances will occur with labyrinthitis and fistula.

Laboratory findings, particularly bacteriologic, will modify management approaches in the various combinations of types A and B lesions and their anatomic locations.

These four approaches to care constitute the **4L equation** in evaluating a patient's status.

Medical management is important and may be curative in type A (potentially reversible) cases. In many type A cases and in most type B (irreversible) cases, some type of surgery is necessary.

Surgery for chronic otomastoiditis usually requires some form of mastoidectomy for eradication of infected tissues, and tympanoplasty for reconstruction of the tympanic membrane and middle-ear structures.

Mastoidectomy and tympanoplasty constitute interrelated surgical approaches. Basic surgical planning and technical details in this and following chapters represent otosurgical experiences of my colleagues and me.

ETIOLOGY

Chronic otomastoiditis is usually the result of previous acute otitis media, acute otomastoiditis, or secretory otitis media. Most of the infections are bacterial, although viral infections may precede bacterial involvement.

There are significant bacteriologic differences between acute otitis media and chronic otomastoiditis. A recent study showed both pure and mixed infections, with *Pseudomonas* found in 42.1%, staphylococci in 39.8%, *Proteus* in 23.2%, and *E. coli* in 8.3% of lesions (2). *Pseudomonas aeruginosa* infections were sensitive to colistin, polymixin B and gentamicin, and resistant to penicillin, chloramphenicol (Chloromycetin), and sulfonamides. Staphylococci were sensitive chloramphenicol and other drugs, but 80% resistant to sulfonamides. Proteus was sensitive to gentamicin, neomycin and streptomycin, and resistant to tetracycline, colistin, and polymixin B.

Specific unusual bacterial causes, such as tuberculosis, actinomycosis, and related mycoses, create special management needs. Constitutional problems, *i.e.*, syphilis, diabetes, radiation necrosis, and others may be direct or contributory etiologic factors.

Allergy, which can be primarily etiologic in secretory otitis media (see Ch. 15, Secretory Otitis Media), undoubtedly plays a role in those cases of chronic otomastoiditis that follow chronic secretory otitis media.

PATHOLOGY

A number of diverse pathologic lesions occur in chronic otomastoiditis. In general, two basic types are involved, either of which may be specific to the disorder. Type A lesions, usually primary, are the pathologic sequelae of acute inflammatory lesions within the mesodermal tubotympanomastoid air-mucosa-bone system. Type B lesions are usually secondary sequelae of type A primary lesions. They may be produced by 1) migration of squamous epithelial cells from the tympanic membrane and external auditory canal into the mesodermal eustachian tube-middle ear-mastoid air-cell system; or 2) they may be due to metaplastic middle ear mucosal changes; or 3) may follow type A osteolytic bony changes.

Chronic otomastoiditis lesions frequently represent combined sequelae of both type A and type B as mixed lesions.

Because of differences in bacterial etiology, systemic diseases, reinfections, mucosal metaplasia, and osteitic progression, multiform pathologic combinations frequently coexist.

In spite of these possible complexities, from the standpoint of clinical management it is useful to divide chronic otomastoiditis into the two clinicopathologic types, type A lesions and type B lesions.

Type A lesions are usually nonspecific fibrogranulomatous otomastoid lesions. They include cholesterol granuloma, mastoid-middle ear polyposis, fibrosing lesions that produce tympanic fibrosis and tympanic atelectasis and various forms of osteitis, most commonly involving ossicles. In general, most type A lesions are partially or completely reversible with relatively conservative medical and surgical management.

Type B lesions constitute the two primary chronic forms of chronic otomastoiditis: 1) **Keratoma (cholesteatoma)** can occur in the middle ear and in any portion of the entire mastoid system, and is due to keratinizing changes in type A lesions; occasionally it is a primary lesion. 2) **Tympanosclerosis** is usually due to hyaline collagen changes with chronic irreversible sclerotic lesions, primarily involving the middle ear and epitympanum and, rarely, the total mastoid air-cell system.

SPECIAL PATHOLOGY OF TYPE A LESIONS

Mucosal, mucoendosteal, and periosteal lesions occur as a result of inflammatory changes from the mucosa and mucoendosteum of the tubotympanomastoid air-cell system. These may vary from the cytologic changes of middle ear mucosa, such as seen in secretory otitis media, to major mastoid polyposis and granulomatosis such as occur in cholesterol granuloma. In addition, fibrosing lesions and polypoid lesions result in middle ear tympanic fibrosis, tympanic atelectasis, and aural polyposis. Although mastoid osteitis requiring radical surgical removal is relatively uncommon in type A lesions, osteitis does occur, but it is usually limited and frequently will respond to medical treatment or to conservative surgical procedures. The exception, however, is osteitis of the ossicles, especially the incus, which frequently results in aseptic necrosis requiring ossiculoplasty.

Type A mastoid lesions usually result in thickened edematous mucosa with obliteration of mastoid cell lumens, perivascular fibrosis, and osteitis.

Polypoid granuloma (aural "polyps") represented by hyperplastic mucosa, will frequently fill the mastoid antrum and also occur as extensions into the middle ear and extrude through tympanic membrane perforations into the external auditory canal (Fig. 16–1). Although such polypi occur frequently in type A lesions, they also occur in type B lesions associated with keratoma, tympanosclerosis, or both. (See Color Figs. 10 and 11.)

Cholesterol granuloma appears grossly at surgery as "fatty" and "greasy" tissue filling the mastoid cells. It is not to be confused with keratoma, a type B lesion, although it can coexist in mixed type-A–type-B lesions. Cholesterol granuloma is related to mucosal hemorrhage factors in mastoiditis. Microscopic examination reveals cholesterol deposits and macrophages (Fig. 16–2).

Ossicular lesions (bone destruction) have been demonstrated in 83% of nonkeratoma lesions, i.e., in type A or "simple" chronic otitis media cases (12).

In general, type A pathologic lesions carry the potential of reversibility, even though there may well be histologic evidence of healed osteitis, thickened mucosa, and diminished air space within the mastoid cells. Many type A lesions can respond to medical therapy. Surgery may not be necessary, or if it is, may not require radical tissue removal.

Although type A lesions are usually relatively benign from the standpoint of bacterial infection, there are major exceptions to the rule. It is possible for a type A lesion, i.e., a fibrogranulomatous lesion, to be clinically more serious in its pathologic implications than relatively low-grade irreversible type B lesions of keratoma or tympanosclerosis. Two examples are the type A lesions that occur in tuberculosis and those that occur in elderly patients, mostly diabetic, who are susceptible to gram-negative "malignant external otitis."

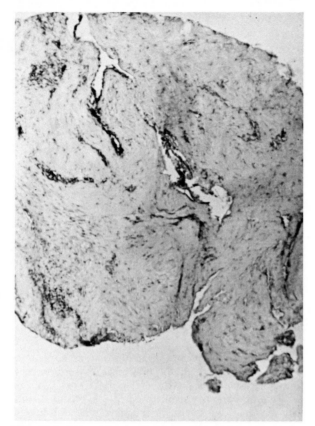

FIG. 16–1. Polypoid granuloma (aural polyp), a type A lesion, with dense fibrous tissue and columnar cells.

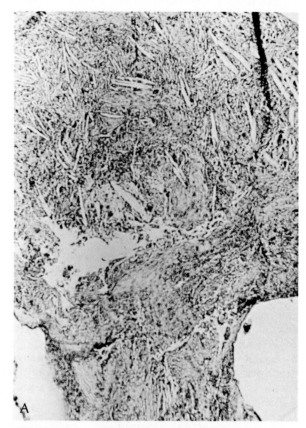

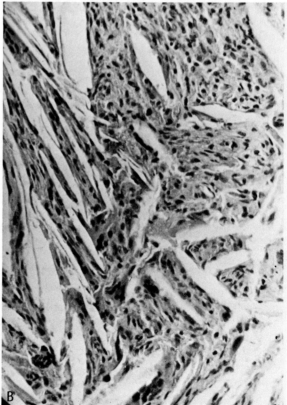

FIG. 16–2. A. Cholesterol granuloma (type A otomastoiditis). Note cholesterol clefts and reactive cellular infiltrate. (Low power.) **B.** Cholesterol granuloma. High-power view of another specimen. Note cholesterol clefts, which are characteristic.

Tuberculous mastoiditis is not common but still occurs in children and in adults, in spite of antibiotic therapy. It occurs generally in pneumatized mastoids, although it may occur in a sclerotic mastoid. Specific tuberculous granulation tissue fills air cells or perivascular spaces. Tubercles containing epithelial cells, lymphocytes, and Langhans giant cells will be noted. Caseation can also occur.

Fulminating diabetic mastoiditis usually starts as "malignant external otitis" of gram-negative bacterial etiology (most commonly *Pseudomonas*) and is a rapidly necrotizing lesion. Acute osteomyelitis and marked vascular changes characterize the special pathology of this type A lesion, which has a high mortality (1).

SPECIAL PATHOLOGY OF TYPE B LESIONS
(KERATOMA, TYMPANOSCLEROSIS)

A type A lesion, mild or severe, will become transformed into a type B lesion if there is squamous epithelial migration from the tympanic membrane or external auditory canal into the middle ear or if mucosal metaplasia in the middle ear results in keratinization or hyalinization.

The keratinizing lesions of keratoma and the hyalinizing lesions of tympanosclerosis are prototypes of type B chronic otomastoiditis. In both forms, bone involvements (mastoid osteitis and ossicular osteolysis) are common. They are irreversible, and usually require more extensive surgery than type A cases for disease removal and for functional hearing and vestibular improvement. As in type A cases, specific bacterial pathogens (especially gram-negative) will influence the course and management of type B lesions.

It is possible for type A and type B lesions to coexist. It is also common for both type B forms (keratoma and tympanosclerosis) to coexist.

Type B cases present the majority of chronic otomastoiditis problems requiring prolonged care and surgical intervention. Even surgical intervention may not be curative and the need for recurrent surgical procedures is not uncommon in type B lesions.

Lesions

The two major type B lesions, keratoma and tympanosclerosis, have several features in common. The histopathologic lesions are irreversible, rarely respond to medical therapy, and result in fixed, nondiminishing, and potentially necrotizing lesions.

Locations

Both keratoma and tympanosclerosis occur in the middle ear. Keratoma frequently invades the entire mastoid. Tympanosclerosis usually involves the middle ear but stops at the aditus, rarely involving the mastoid cellular system. Both produce ossicular necrosis and both can produce labyrinth invasion, seventh nerve paralysis, and intracranial complications.

Loss of Function

Both type B lesions can cause major conductive hearing losses and can produce labyrinthine invasion with additional cochlear hearing losses. Vestibular problems due to labyrinthine fistulas and seventh nerve paralysis occur in a significant number of type B cases.

Laboratory Findings

Most type B lesions are eventually characterized by drug-resistant gram-positive and especially gram-negative infections. Radiologic changes usually are those of sclerosis and necrotizing osteolysis in keratoma; sclerosis, trabecular necrosis and haziness characterize tympanosclerosis. Since many Type B lesions start in early life, poorly pneumatized temporal bones are the rule in both varieties of type B lesions.

SURGICAL PATHOLOGY OF KERATOMA

Keratoma of the temporal bone is the most common cause of persistent otomastoiditis with bone necrosis. (See Color Fig. 12.) It has been called "cholesteatoma" for more than a century. Friedmann states: "Cholesteatoma is a misnomer in that it is neither a tumor nor does it necessarily contain cholesterol" (3).

Keratoma can produce tympanic membrane perforations, necrosis of the malleus, incus, and stapes, mastoid cell-wall destruction in any part of the temporal bone, and can involve the facial nerve, labyrinth, and temporal bone vessels.

One cannot improve upon the description of gross keratoma written by Adam Politzer (10) a century ago:

We often observe the growth of circumscribed tumors which are covered with a glistening mother-of-pearl pellicle, and which are composed of a homogenous mass, or of concentric stratified lamellae. These tumors . . . begin to develop either during the time of suppuration or after the process has run its course.

The lining membrane of the cavities in the temporal bone, enlarged by the growth of the cholesteatoma, presents a tendon-gray, smooth, shining, mother-of-pearl appearance, and is covered with a layer which is *firmly united with the bone,* and resembles the reta Malpighii.*

He then describes the "onion-like stratified cholesteatoma" and how "cholesteatomatous masses *forced their way into the Haversian canals . . .* a condition which explains the obstinate *relapses of cholesteatomata* even *after the operative opening of the middle-ear spaces.*"

Politzer's gross pathology description is still unchallenged almost a century later.

The size of cholesteatoma varies from that of a hemp-seed to that of a walnut and over. Their form is round or oval, or they may correspond to the concavities of the middle ear, or show a very irregular outline in conformity with the cavities in the temporal bone produced by the destruction and absorption of the bony tissue. The surface, which is usually iridescent, is smooth or glandular, with club or nipple-shaped projections. The masses sometimes show on cross section, a stratified, laminated, iridescent structure of various colors, occasionally present the appearance of freshly made cheese.

In describing the lesion as seen by microscopy, he stated: "They consist of large, round or polygonal, often non-nucleated, squamous, epithelial cells, with the addition of granules, giant cells, fat globules, *cholesterine crystals,* and *bacteria.* Caseated exudate or semi-fluid masses of detritus are occasionally found alongside of, and between, the epithelial masses" (11).

Politzer's masterful clinicopathologic descriptions of gross and microscopic lesions are still authoritative. He described the most common secondary cholesteatoma, as well as the rare primary cholesteatoma.

Keratinizing squamous epithelium or a fibrous granulation tissue stroma lines the characteristic structure, which contains laminated keratin (Fig. 16–3). The lesion should not be confused with the nonepithelial aspect of cholesterol granuloma (type A). Although keratomas frequently start in the epitympanum (attic), they can start in the pars tensa. They may be associated with either marginal or central tympanic membrane perforations. They can occur in the external auditory canal with no apparent middle ear or mastoid involvement. (See Color Fig. 15.)

Most keratomas are secondary to squamous epithelial "invasion" or to metaplasia. Primary keratomas as congenital lesions are rare and can

---

* The latter layer is a clear description of what is designated surgically as "matrix" at the present time.

occur in temporal bone, in the central nervous system, and in the skull other than the temporal bone area (see Fig. 22–16). The cerebellopontine angle is the occasional site of a primary keratoma.

An intact keratoma (cholesteatoma) "pearl," as described by Politzer, is usually covered with simple squamous or tall columnar type of epithelium, including both goblet and ciliated cells. This epithelial layer is known as "matrix" clinically. The matrix, which is composed of epidermis, is surrounded by perimatrix composed of the connective tissue layer, the lamina propria of the cholesteatoma. The perimatrix is formed of loose connective tissue containing collagen fibers with fibrocytes. Occasionally the perimatrix is infiltrated with round cells, especially where there is secondary evidence of inflammation.

The matrix epidermis is composed of keratinizing squamous epithelial cells. Within this matrix, keratin, granular, malpighian, and basal layers are clearly demonstrable. Scanning electron microscopic characteristics of a typical pearl-like keratoma are clearly illustrated in Figure 16–4.

Recent research on acid mucopolysaccharide, collagenase, and unresorbed fetal mesenchyme factors may widen our etiopathologic concepts of keratoma.

SURGICAL PATHOLOGY OF TYMPANOSCLEROSIS

It is difficult to improve upon the words of von Tröltsch (13) who, in 1864, described

A pathological process, in which the mucous membrane becomes denser, more rigid and inelastic. These changes impair the vibrating power of the membrana tympani . . . and of . . . the fenestra rotunda, and fenestra ovalis. They finally lead to a complete rigidity, calcareous or osseous degeneration of the membrane surrounding the stapes, ankylosis of the stapes, or of the membrane of the fenestra rotunda.

Tympanosclerosis is frequently due to repair of healing phases of secretory otitis media. It can be a sequel of acute otitis media and acute otomastoiditis with primary features of collagen hyalinization and secondary calcification. (See Color Fig. 13.)

Harris and Weiss (8) described histologic characteristics of tympanosclerosis as follows:

1. Chronic inflammatory process includes granulation tissue, lymphocytes, plasma cells, and histiocytes.
2. There is dense fibrosis with areas of hyalinization (*i.e.,* sclerosis) (Fig. 16–5).
3. There are various stages of secondary bone destruc-

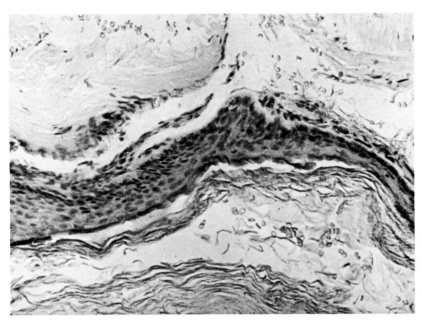

FIG. 16–3. Keratoma (cholesteatoma). Keratinizing squamous epithelium above characteristic layers of laminated keratin.

FIG. 16–4. A. Pearl-like cholesteatoma shows epidermis **(Ep)**, lamina propria **(Lp)**, and mucous membrane **(M).** A large fibrocyte is seen in the lamina propria. (Scanning electron micrograph.) **B.** Matrix **(Ep)** and perimatrix **(Lp).** Mucous membrane **(M)** is covered with typical ciliated as well as secretory cells. **Arrows,** dendritic Langerhans cell. (Scanning electron micrograph.) Insert. Surgical microscopic view of pearl-like cholesteatoma. (Lim D, Saunders W: Ann Otol Rhinol Laryngol 81:2–12, 1972)

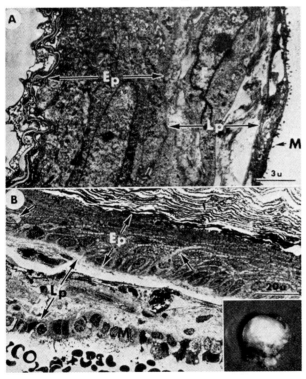

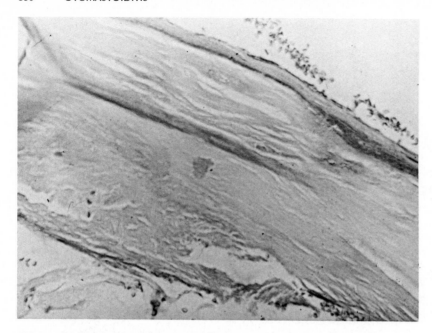

FIG. 16–5. A sheet of tympanosclerosis (fibrosis and hyalinized collagen).

FIG. 16–6. Tympanosclerosis and bone marrow fibrosis—incus necrosis.

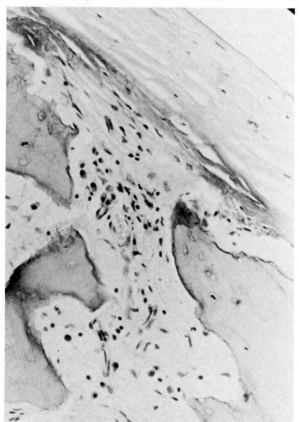

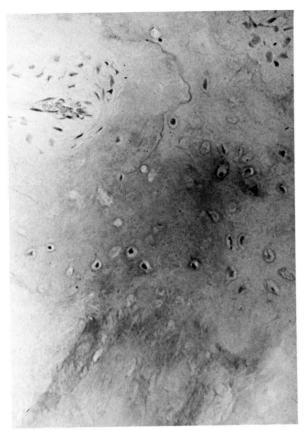

FIG. 16–7. New bone formation in a tympanosclerotic lesion.

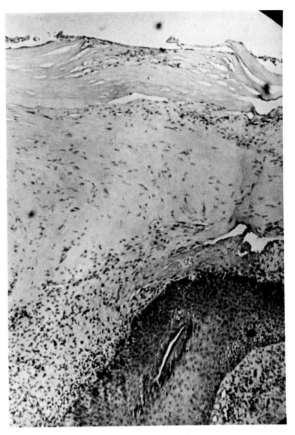

FIG. 16–8. Tympanosclerosis layer covering a keratoma.

tion, intertrabecular fibrosis and new bone formation.

4. Epithelium over the lesion (Figs. 16–6, 16–7) may vary from columnar to keratinizing squamous epithelium. (See Color Fig. 14.) The latter appears to originate by metaplasia from the former and is the source of desquamating keratin, thus forming a keratoma within a tympanosclerotic mass (Fig. 16–8).

5. Some lesions show evidence of hemorrhage and hemosiderin-containing granuloma.

6. Tympanosclerosis has been found as an unsuspected lesion in the presence of acute mastoiditis with and without keratoma.

Clinical tympanosclerosis occurs in two forms: 1) a sclerosing mucositis, which seems to be more superficial and amenable to complete surgical removal; and 2) an apparently invasive embedded osteoclastic mucoperiostitis which defies complete removal (see Ch. 19, Otosclerosis; Figs. 19–27, 19–28, 19–29).

HISTORY AND SYMPTOMS

Otorrhea and hearing loss are the two most common complaints in chronic otomastoiditis. Otalgia is not a common complaint except in acute exacerbations. Vertigo, intermittent and mild, is not a common complaint. It can be a major complaint in the presence of a labyrinthine fistula.

Many patients are more distressed by the otorrhea than by the conductive hearing loss, unless the disease is bilateral. A unilateral conductive hearing loss does not disturb patients as much as persistent malodorous otorrhea.

Many patients relate the onset of chronic otomastoiditis to a childhood episode of acute otitis media, with or without a definitive history of upper respiratory infection. In some, the onset and duration is described vaguely. A history of nonspecific ear treatment is frequently given, with recollection of casual prescriptions of "ear drops" in the majority of cases.

Exacerbations and remissions of otorrhea are common, but hearing loss is relatively stable. Occasional otalgia follows upper respiratory infections or follows accidental water in the ear following bathing or swimming. Surprisingly, some patients with otorrhea histories swim and dive with impunity.

Otorrhea varies in degree, timing, and character of discharge. Some patients are not aware of otorrhea at all. However, upon questioning, a patient will describe that the ear forms much "wax," which requires frequent removal with finger, cotton-tipped applicator, or tissue. This wax usually consists of dried middle-ear secretions, and crusts consisting of epithelial debris, cerumen, and middle-ear mucopus or pus.

FINDINGS

OTOSCOPIC EXAMINATION

Otoscopic findings will vary greatly. If otorrhea is present it may be seen in the external auditory canal. A specimen should be taken for direct smear, bacterial cultures, and an antibiogram. The remaining secretion is gently aspirated with sterile suction tips until the external canal and tympanic membrane landmarks are noted. Ideally, such examination should be performed with a focusing headlight and a binocular magnifying loupe or with the surgical microscope. The external canal should be inspected for dehiscences, fistulas, and crusts, following removal of epithelial debris and cerumen. It is not unusual to discover a posterosuperior bony canal defect due to chronic osteitis and a fistula between the external canal and the mastoid cell system. Simple aspiration of secretions from tympanic membrane perforations or from such a fistula may evoke vertigo. Occasionally, manifest spontaneous nystagmus will follow such suction-manipulation, indicating a probable labyrinthine fistula.

A defect in the pars tensa of the tympanic membrane, or the pars flaccida, or both, is present in most cases, frequently with annular bone erosion. Atelectatic lesions are frequently seen in the pars tensa, more commonly in epitympanic pars flaccida. The external attic wall (scutum) may be partly absent allowing a direct view of keratoma or tympanosclerotic lesions. (See Color Fig. 16.) In some cases, ossicular lesions, granulomas, polypi, crusts, and blood clots, are seen through the otoscope.

A variety of defects occur in the tympanic membrane (Fig. 16–9). The entire membrane may be absent, or appear to be absent, because of atelectatic adherence to the medial tympanic wall. Squamous epithelial invasion may continue from the external auditory canal into the middle ear and fuse with the ossicles or the middle-ear promontory (Figs. 16–10 through 16–15).

The tympanic membrane may be intact, usually edematous, but occasionally relatively normal in appearance. However, translucency is usually absent and mobility is severely impaired on pneumatic otoscopy. Similar impairment of mobility can be noted on tympanometry.

NOSE AND THROAT EXAMINATION

Nose, throat, and neck may be entirely normal on examination. However, in many cases, an assortment of predisposing or contributory lesions will be noted. Infected tonsils and/or adenoid tissues, tonsil "tags," nasal and postnasal crusts, paranasal sinusitis, mucopurulent nasopharyngeal discharge, nasal polyposis, cervical lymphadenopathy, and other manifestations of recurrent upper respiratory diseases may be found. (Benign or malignant cysts and other lesions are occasionally seen in the nasopharynx. They are not common causes of chronic otomastoiditis.)

These pathologic nose and throat findings are important, not only for primary etiologic explanation, but also as factors to be concerned with in recurrences of chronic otomastoiditis. Nose and throat lesions require definitive treatment as an essential component of the general management of chronic otomastoiditis.

AUDIOLOGIC AND VESTIBULAR STUDIES

Standard audiometry in chronic otomastoiditis usually shows a conductive hearing loss, the degree of which is usually related to the severity of the middle-ear lesion. Tympanic membrane defects, ossicular discontinuity, middle-ear fluid, and varying stiffness lesions are additive. Because of physiologic acoustic complexities, however, surprising inconsistencies may be noted between pathologic middle ear and mastoid lesions and audiologic measurements. It is not unusual, in a case of keratoma and incus necrosis, to note a 20-dB speech reception threshold and 100% speech discrimination score. This may be due to the fact that the keratoma itself is acting as a temporary effective transformer mechanism. The patient literally hears with the help of the keratoma. However, in most cases, there is a con-

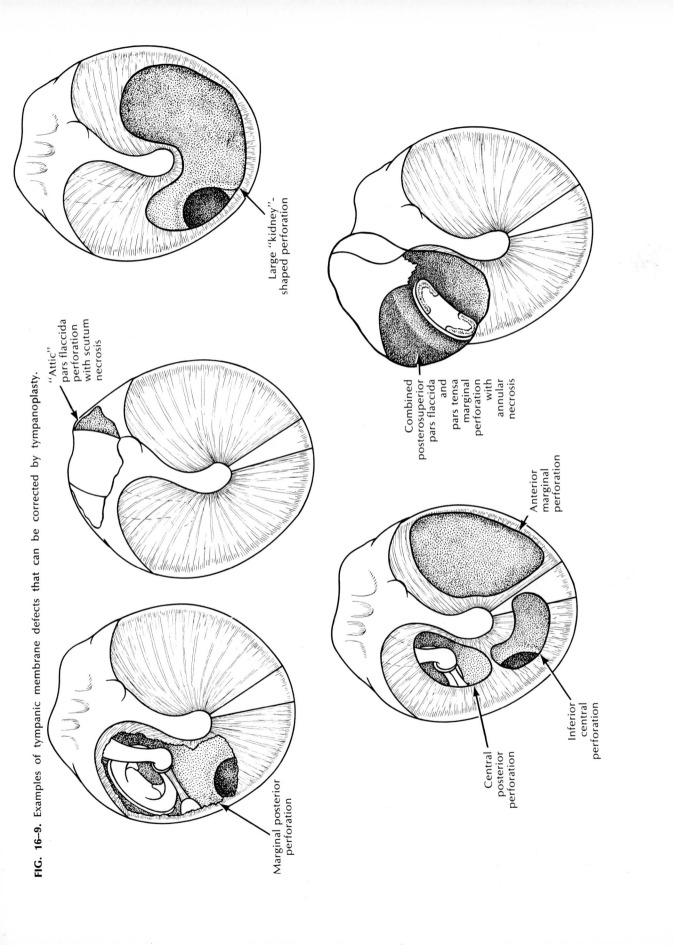

FIG. 16–9. Examples of tympanic membrane defects that can be corrected by tympanoplasty.

Large "kidney"-shaped perforation

Combined posterosuperior pars flaccida and pars tensa marginal perforation with annular necrosis

"Attic" pars flaccida perforation with scutum necrosis

Marginal posterior perforation

Anterior marginal perforation

Central posterior perforation

Inferior central perforation

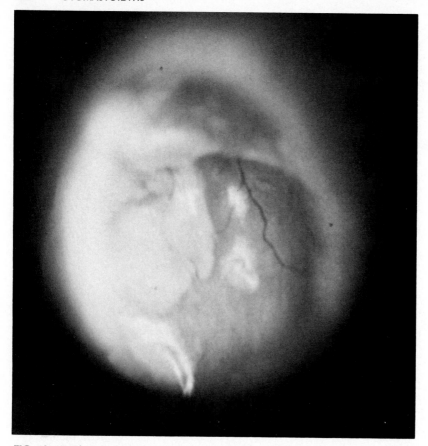

FIG. 16–10. Chronic secretory otitis media with tympanosclerosis.

FIG. 16–11. Large middle ear keratoma projecting into external canal (simulating osteoma).

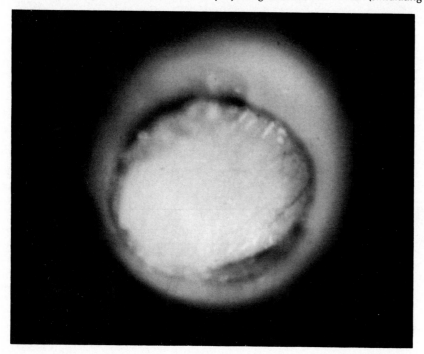

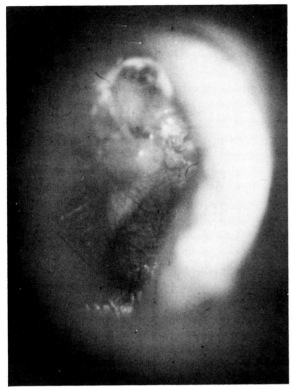

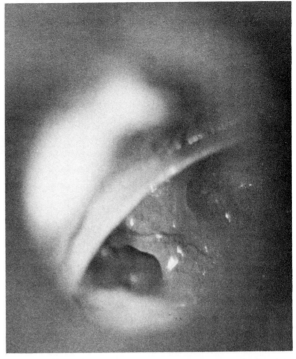

FIG. 16–14. Large central tympanic membrane perforation.

FIG. 16–12. Attic (epitympanic) marginal erosion by keratoma.

FIG. 16–15. Small–medium central, dry perforation.

FIG. 16–13. Tympanosclerosis and large central perforation.

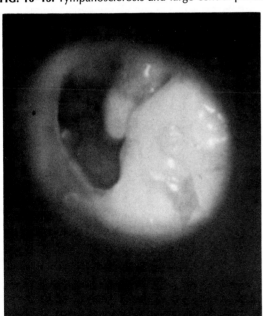

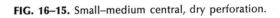

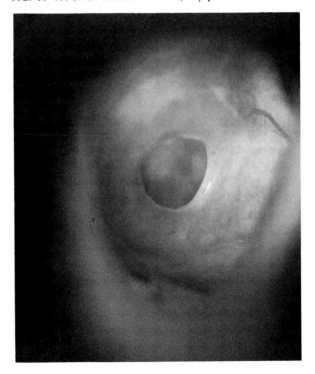

FIG. 16–16. Chronic type A otomastoiditis with onset in early childhood in an 80-year-old man. **A. At left,** cellular development is poor. **At right,** only the antrum can be seen **(arrow).** There are no other cells. **B.** Dense, pneumatized apex on each side **(arrows).**

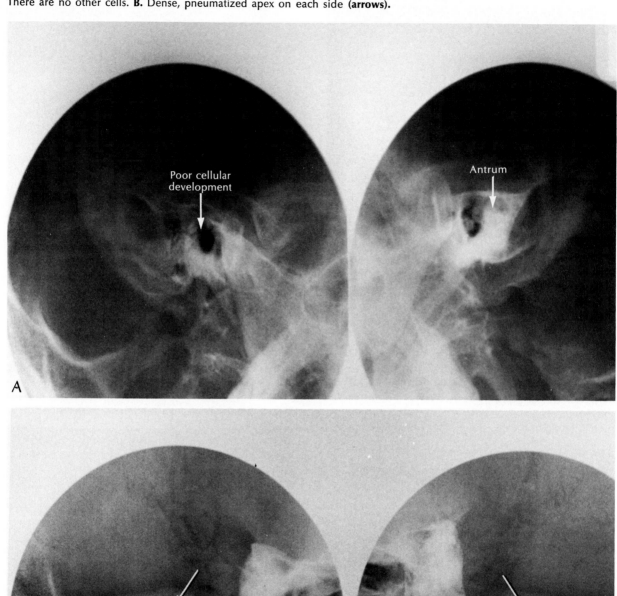

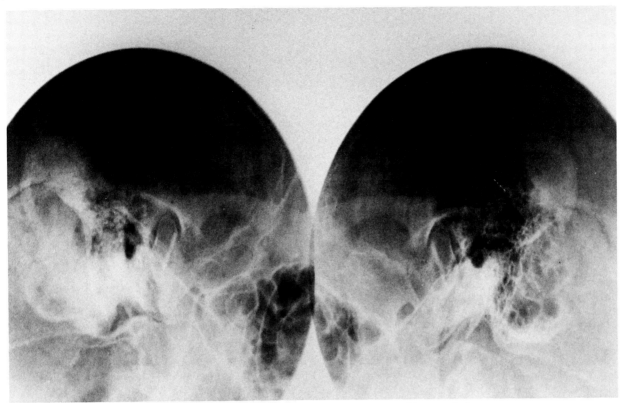

FIG. 16–17. Chronic tympanosclerosis involving right mastoid in a 51-year-old man. Left mastoid **(at right)** is well pneumatized and normal.

sistent relationship between the severity of the lesion and the degree of conductive hearing loss.

In patients with vertigo or neurologic symptoms indicating possible labyrinthine complications, more detailed audiologic studies will be necessary. In such cases, Békésy studies and other components of the differential diagnostic auditory test battery may reveal cochlear or retrocochlear involvement (see Ch. 6, Audiologic Assessment, Functional Hearing Loss, and Objective Audiometry).

Tympanometry is of diagnostic value: Impedance, compliance, and stapedial reflex studies will yield useful diagnostic data in many patients (see section on Acoustic Impedance Measurements, Ch. 7).

Vestibular studies are of great diagnostic value in patients with chronic otomastoiditis and vertigo. In addition to tests for sinusoidal rotation, spontaneous nystagmus and positional nystagmus, dry calorization tests are indicated in such cases to evaluate vestibular function (see Ch. 10, Examination of the Dizzy Patient).

RADIOGRAPHIC EXAMINATION

Radiographs of the mastoid are essential for accurate diagnosis in every case of chronic otomastoiditis. The Schuller view is most informative. The degree of pneumatization is compared with that of the opposite ear to assess duration of the disease. A nonpneumatized or poorly pneumatized mastoid will usually indicate childhood onset of the otomastoiditis (Fig. 16–16). Changes in cell-wall outline and haziness of air spaces (Fig. 16–17) are frequently seen in chronic otomastoiditis. The destructive, punched-out, rounded or oval lesion of keratoma can be seen frequently (Fig. 16–18).

The Stenver view of the petrous pyramid is also essential in assessing possible extension of disease to the apex. Polytomographic information is most

FIG. 16–18. A. Large radiolucent excavation due to keratoma **(arrow at left)** seen on Schuller view. Left mastoid is normal **(arrow at right). B.** Stenver view of same keratoma **(arrow).**

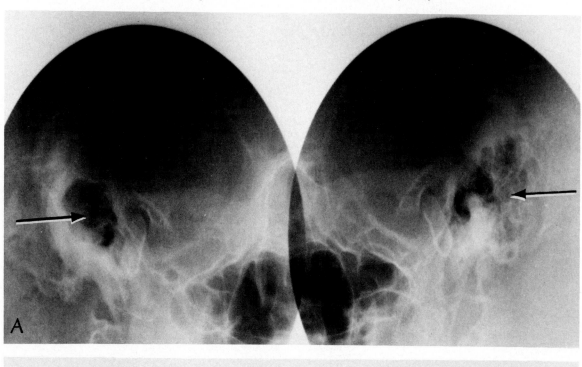

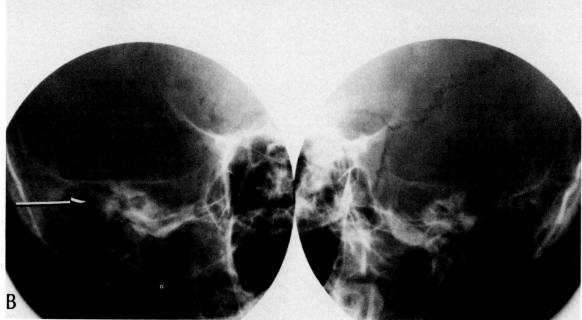

useful but is not essential in the average case of chronic otomastoiditis. In suspected labyrinthine fistula, polytomography may be diagnostic. In some diagnostic special problems, polytome views of the middle ear will be helpful in assessing ossicular status (see Ch. 4, Otoradiology).

CLINICAL LABORATORY FINDINGS

Direct smears for fungi and yeasts, bacterial cultures, and antibiograms are essential in evaluating the otorrhea exudate. The management of the lesion is to a great extent based upon these microbiologic findings.

Gram-negative organism infections (*Pseudomonas aeruginosa, E. coli, Proteus*, etc.) constitute difficult management problems, with higher incidences of complications and recurrences.

Urine and blood examinations are essential to identify possible significant concomitant constitutional diseases such as diabetes. The course of otomastoiditis is greatly influenced by such systemic conditions.

MASKED MASTOIDITIS

Chronic mastoiditis may occur without symptoms following upper respiratory infections. Antibiotic therapy may result in such "masking," but the clinical entity of masked mastoiditis was recognized even in the preantibiotic era.

There may be only a slight conductive hearing loss and/or a feeling of fullness in the ear, accompanied by an intact tympanic membrane, although it is an abnormal membrane with thickening suggestive of intratympanic middle-ear fluid and characterized by loss of normal landmarks. The first sign may be any one of a number of complications, especially meningitis. Most frequently masked mastoiditis is due to a type A lesion.

DIFFERENTIAL DIAGNOSIS

The diagnosis of chronic otomastoiditis is based upon the history of otorrhea, evidence of conductive hearing loss, otoscopic demonstration of tympanic membrane and middle ear lesions, and radiographic evidence of changes in mastoid air-cell system. All these aspects have been described.

In differential diagnosis, problems may arise in cases in which the tympanic membrane is intact but other findings (audiologic and radiologic) are indicative of chronic otomastoiditis. The "intact" tympanic membrane is not always normal. It may be bulging, reddened, atelectatic, and scarred, and normal landmarks may be blurred or missing. In such cases, the differential diagnosis should be based upon a consideration of lesions which may mimic either secretory otitis media or chronic otomastoiditis in which the tympanic membrane appears to be intact. The following differential diagnostic considerations are discussed in detail in other chapters:

Congenital vascular middle ear anomalies
1. Intratympanic jugular bulb
2. Aberrant tympanic internal carotid artery
3. Persistent obturator artery
4. Intratympanic arteriovenous aneurysm

Posttraumatic intratympanic cerebrospinal fluid

Tumors
1. Nasopharyngeal tumors with middle-ear fluid
2. Middle-ear tumors
3. Intracranial tumors with extension to middle ear
4. Mastoid tumors with extension to middle ear

Postradiation temporal bone necrosis

Osteodystrophies and mesodermal dysplasias of the temporal bone

MANAGEMENT OF OTOMASTOIDITIS

BASIC PRINCIPLES

The management of otomastoiditis involves medical therapy alone in some cases, and combined medical-surgical approaches in others. The ultimate goals are 1) removal of the lesion, and 2) retention of function or repair of functional losses.

Management involves considerations of the "4L" equation: lesion (pathology), location (anatomy), loss of function (hearing, vestibular, facial nerve), and laboratory findings (bacteriology, etc.).

Lesion, Types A and B

Differences between type A (potentially reversible) lesions (mucositis, osteitis, polyposis, and granulomatosis) and type B (irreversible) lesions (keratoma, and tympanosclerosis) dictate different managements.

Adequate eradication of a lesion is an obvious

necessity. The term "adequate" eradication is used rather than "total" or "complete." While complete eradication of a lesion is obvious and desirable, it must be remembered that the middle-ear–mastoid complex is part of the total temporal-bone cellular system. It is neither possible nor necessary to achieve an absolute surgical removal of every single cell in the complex tympanomastoid-squamopetrosal air-cell system.

Type A cases may respond to medical therapy alone, but they may also require surgery frequently. Type B cases usually require surgery. In keratoma, total removal of the lesion is necessary unless unacceptable sacrifices of vital structures are encountered. In tympanosclerosis, however, total removal of the lesion may not be possible or desirable.

A number of tympanoplasty methods, now in developmental phases, are based upon the assumption of the possibility of total lesion removal. Routine "intact canal wall" and musculoplastic obliterative procedures are examples of methods based on such assumptions. With such techniques, there may be possible recurrences of hidden lesions. Because total removal is not always possible, preplanned "staging" of surgery may be necessary (6).

Location

The maintenance or reconstitution of anatomic integrity are elements that may challenge those of restoration of function. Thus, repair of a tympanic membrane perforation may be a more important consideration than a hearing gain in some cases; the reverse may be true in others.

Loss of Function

The previous two elements (lesion eradication and anatomic location) have been considered for more than a century. Concern for loss of function (primarily hearing) is the chief motivation for the development of tympanoplasty. The acoustic physiological factors that underlie tympanoplasty are complex. Eustachian tube physiology and tympanic membrane/oval window geometric ratios are elementary considerations in tympanoplastic planning. Finer aspects of tympanolabyrinthine physiology are those involved in mass, stiffness, and elasticity coefficients, as well as in consideration of stapedial and tensor tympani muscle functions. In addition to these middle ear structures, labyrinthine function and seventh nerve function must be included in the loss of function element within the 4L equation.

Laboratory Findings

The fourth element in the 4L equation, laboratory findings, may modify management of the first three elements. A resistant gram-negative organism in a diabetic patient with type A disease may require more radical management, both medical and surgical, than an extensive type B tympanosclerosis lesion in which bacteriologic cultures show mixed gram-positive organisms with an antibiogram indicating favorable responses to all common antibiotics.

THERAPY

With the introduction of tympanoplastic surgical techniques in the 1950s, zealous efforts have been made to deal surgically with most, if not all, type A and type B lesions, regardless of the 4L equation evaluation.

In newly evolving approaches to surgical restoration of hearing function or to avoidance of a mastoidostomy (exteriorized mastoid bowl), some elements in the 4L equation have been ignored. Some lesions are irreversibly advanced and require radical surgical extirpation. In other special problems, merely palliative surgery may lead to preservation of adequate or borderline hearing levels. In some tympanoplastic procedures, primary hearing gains may be short-lived, resulting in poorer hearing eventually. It is possible to damage cochlear, vestibular, or seventh nerve function through overzealous lesion eradication or inappropriate reconstruction procedures.

In consideration of medical versus surgical therapy, we must deal with the definition of **a successful result.** It may not be enough to define success, for example, as a dry ear with a gain in hearing. Neither the dry ear nor the gain in hearing may be long-lasting. A dry ear in which keratoma continues to grow and spread without signs of recognition of a final seriously destructive sequelae in the middle ear and mastoid is not a success. A preliminary gain of hearing from a 50-dB level to a 25-dB level may eventually result in a greater loss accompanied by labyrinthine fistula and vertigo. In the present era of developing tympanoplasty, a fifth element that modifies the 4L equation—*time*—plays a great role in the consideration of management methods in chronic otomastoiditis.

Management of chronic otomastoiditis involves several of the traditional mastoidectomy procedures. However, the introduction of tympanoplasty and ossiculoplasty with modern microsurgical technology has changed previous surgical approaches to chronic otomastoiditis. These surgical techniques and indications are described in detail in Chapter 17, Otomastoiditis Surgery—Mastoidectomy and Tympanoplasty.

SPECIAL MANAGEMENT OF TYPE A LESIONS

BASIC PRINCIPLES

Type A lesions (mucositis, osteitis, polyposis, granulomatosis) are potentially reversible. However, location, loss of function, and laboratory findings may change the management of type A lesions to more formidable proportions approaching or even surpassing some of the clinical problems in type B lesions.

Lesion

The type A lesion may be any one of a number of variations of middle ear and mastoid infections produced by mucositis, osteitis, granulomatosis, and polyposis. These are potentially reversible lesions, with the exception of tympanic membrane perforations and ossicular necrosis.

Location

In general, type A mastoid lesions involve most of the temporal bone cellular area. Type A lesions occur more frequently in well-pneumatized mastoids than do type B lesions. This is probably related to the fact that type B lesions frequently start in infancy or in early childhood, with resulting pneumatization arrest. Scientific disputes exist with reference to theories of the genesis of type B lesions as related to pneumatization. Type A lesions uncommonly cause labyrinthitis or seventh nerve paralysis. Intracranial complications do occur, especially in acute exacerbations of chronic type A lesions. Spontaneous otorrhea through a central tympanic membrane perforation is frequent. Although marginal perforations occur in type A cases, the most common perforation is the central "kidney" type. Although the ossicles, especially the incus, may be involved by mucosal and osteitic change, major ossicular necrosis is not so common as in type B cases. However, incus necrosis does occur frequently as a result of slowly developing periostitis with secondary osteitis and bone atrophy.

Loss of Function

The primary loss of function in type A lesions is a fluctuating conductive hearing loss, usually related to the size of the tympanic membrane perforation, otorrhea, and degree of mucosal edema. Hearing losses usually fluctuate from 20 to 40 dB. Cochlear function is usually intact with speech discrimination scores of 90–100%. Vertigo is rare, since labyrinthitis is uncommon in type A cases. Seventh nerve paralysis is also rare in type A cases because of the infrequent occurrence of necrotizing disease in the bony wall of the facial canal.

Laboratory Findings

Many type A lesions are associated with *Pneumococcus*, *streptococcus*, and *staphylococcus* organisms. However, gram-negative superinfections do occur. In most type A cases, the gram-positive organisms are antibiotic-sensitive. Medical therapy with systemic and local antibiotics is frequently effective, either in cure or in alleviation of the disease process.

MEDICAL MANAGEMENT

Many type A middle ear-mastoid lesions will spontaneously respond to treatment of associated nasal-sinus-nasopharyngeal lesions. An ipsilateral maxillary sinusitis with or without allergy is a common concomitant of type A lesions. Attention to the rhinopharyngeal infection and management of allergic factors frequently results in spontaneous cessation of otorrhea and improvement of hearing.

Medical treatment is indicated in a number of type A conditions. Episodic mucoid or mucopurulent otorrhea occurs in quiescent type A chronic otomastoiditis associated with a central perforation of the tympanic membrane and no radiographic evidence of keratoma, tympanosclerosis, or active granulomatosis. Episodic mucoid otorrhea in such cases is frequently associated with upper respiratory infections. Water introduced into the external auditory canal in bathing or swimming will also cause such intermittent episodes of otorrhea. Suction cleansing under magnification, laboratory studies of exudate, radiographs, and audiologic studies are indicated in all such cases. If the hearing loss is minimal and the patient is elderly, neither mastoidectomy nor tympanoplasty may be indicated. Appropriate local therapy may suffice to achieve a dry ear. Attention to predisposing nasal, sinus, nasopharyngeal and allergy factors is necessary.

The ideal management of a type A dry central perforation is tympanoplastic closure of the perforation. This ideal, however, is neither possible nor advisable in some patients. The risks of graft rejection and possible cochlear complications are not insignificant. Reconstructive procedures even in simple perforations must be undertaken with careful study and consideration of possible consequences. This is especially true when there is hearing in only one ear. Periodic medical therapy will be necessary in many cases and may suffice.

Medical treatment is based on two factors: 1) cleansing, and 2) local and/or systemic medication.

Cleansing involves meticulous removal of epithelial debris, cerumen, and canal exudate, using sterile suction, applicators, blunt curets and micro-alligator forceps with binocular visualization and other instrumentation techniques under magnification. It cannot be done adequately with the use of an otoscope alone.

Local and/or systemic medications are used. Antibiotics play important roles in medical therapy. Local antibiotic therapy should be based on microbiologic studies and antibiograms wherever possible. Insufflation of antibiotic powders into the middle ear under direct vision is effective in a large percentage of patients, with both gram-positive and gram-negative infections. Chloramphenicol (Chloromycetin) powder insufflation is very effective in a broad spectrum of cases. It is used sparingly under direct vision; a gentle, mild insufflation through the perforation to the middle ear mucosa is advisable. Very frequently, one such insufflation of chloramphenicol powder may result in immediate cessation of an otorrhea recurrence. Care must be taken to avoid its use or the use of any other antibiotic in patients with histories of specific drug allergy.

A number of ear drops are commercially available. Many are effective against both gram-positive and gram-negative organisms. Neomycin is an ingredient of many commercial ear-drop preparations and is an effective agent, but it calls for some concern because of its known ototoxicity. When used, it should be used carefully, with every attempt made to prevent pooling of the neomycin in the middle ear, in either the oval window niche or the round window niche. Neomycin-saturated gauze trailers or wicks placed in contact with tympanic membrane perforations are effective and safer than indiscriminate use of such ear drops.

In acute infections with profuse otorrhea, systemic antibiotic treatment is necessary. Broad-spectrum oral antibiotics should be used, as guided by otorrhea antibiogram findings, with special concern for possible allergy and careful frequent observation. Ampicillin, tetracycline, erythromycin, and sulfonamide drugs are frequently effective orally.

In some gram-negative infections, acetic acid ear-drop preparations may be efficacious and should be considered especially in patients with known antibiotic allergies. In acutely ill patients with life-threatening, fulminating gram-negative mastoiditis (e.g., diabetic mastoiditis, malignant external otitis) potentially ototoxic antibiotics may be necessary systemically—i.e., gentamicin, kanamycin, etc.—depending upon bacteriologic and antibiogram findings.

SURGICAL MANAGEMENT

Surgery is not necessary in many type A cases. Where surgery is necessary in type A cases resistant to medical management, an atticomastoidectomy procedure with intact canal wall usually suffices. Exenteration of polypi and granulomas will be necessary and the exploration of the middle ear will usually reveal primarily mucosal edema. If there is incus necrosis, primary or secondary ossiculoplastic reconstruction will be required. Antibiotic therapy is advisable before and after operation. It is also advisable to maintain mastoid drainage through a soft Silastic tube for a period of 10–14 days, with prolongation of antibiotic therapy for 2–4 weeks. Premature cessation of antibiotic therapy may result in a flare-up of what is basically a reversible disease.

The results of surgery are usually quite satisfactory, with frequent improvement in hearing. Perforations may heal spontaneously. If not they may require secondary tympanoplastic procedures of either type I or ossiculoplastic type II varieties.

In chronic type A cases, the atticomastoidectomy may be combined with an appropriate tympanoplastic reconstruction in one stage. Radical mastoidectomy (mastoidostomy) is rarely necessary in type A disease. However, in diabetics or in patients with tuberculous mastoiditis, in debilitated elderly patients with evidence of small-vessel sclerosis, and in patients with drug-resistant bacterial infections, radical mastoidectomy may be the only solution. This is also true in children with evidence of immunologic deficiencies who are prone to recurrent infections with or without upper respiratory preludes. Conservative medical therapy alone is inappropriate in nonresponsive immunologic/bacteriologic problems.

A relatively reversible type A lesion can become a fulminating irreversible lesion with spread to the labyrinth and the intracranial areas. A type A lesion can be modified by location, loss of function, and laboratory findings into an irreversible problem requiring radical surgery and heroic medical measures.

SPECIAL TYPE A PROBLEMS

Several varieties of otomastoiditis occur in which the primary problems are not lesion, location, or loss of function. The primary problems in such cases are related to laboratory findings of threatening microbial–host relationships. Although such fulminating lesions may occur in both type A and type B cases, they occur more often in type A lesions. They are more frequent in conjunction with debilitating diseases. They are encountered in children with various immunologic deficiencies. They occur not infrequently in diabetics. They are produced most frequently by gram-negative (*Pseudomonas, Proteus,* and *E. coli*) infections.

Malignant External Otitis

The lesion termed "malignant external otitis" (1) falls into the category of resistant, fulminating chronic otomastoiditis. The location designation is unusual in that a resistant gram-negative external otitis spreads to the middle ear and mastoid and is frequently fatal. However, malignant external otitis is neither neoplastic nor malignant; it is not cancer, and it is not primarily an external otitis except in terms of primary onset location.

Rapidly progressive nonspecific inflammatory changes occur in the skin, periosteum, and bone of the external auditory canal. Periostitis, osteitis, myringitis, tympanic membrane perforations, mastoiditis, and other lesions occur in varying sequences, including type A chronic otomastoiditis.

The laboratory findings of 1) resistant gram-negative organisms and 2) constitutional disease (*i.e.,* diabetes) and the radiologic changes are diagnostic.

Radiologic changes in fulminating diabetic gram-negative lesions depend upon whether the lesion is primary or secondary. A primary lesion in a previously uninfected mastoid produces air-cell density and trabecular erosion in a well-pneumatized mastoid. A secondary fulminating lesion may represent either a flare-up of a subacute otomastoiditis or a completely new infection in a previously healed otomastoiditis. In such instances, the usual radiologic findings are trabecular changes in undeveloped or moderately developed mastoids.

The management of fulminating otomastoiditis requires intensive combined medical and surgical care. Fatalities do occur in these lesions. Hospitalization and collaboration between infectious disease specialist, diabetes specialist, neurosurgeon, and otologic surgeon are usually necessary. Intensive treatment with potentially ototoxic drugs may be indicated in such life-threatening infections if the lesion does not respond to less toxic agents and to surgical exenteration.

In most instances, the surgical procedure should be an extensive complete radical mastoidectomy with no attempt at reconstruction or tympanoplastic staging. Prolonged antibiotic therapy, both systemically and locally, will be necessary in most cases. Constant collaborative internal medical participation is necessary to deal with accompanying, predisposing, and contributory constitutional problems.

In adult fulminating otomastoiditis, the primary candidate is the elderly diabetic with a *Pseudomonas* infection in the external auditory canal. Thus, even a seemingly minor but resistant *Pseudomonas* external otitis should alert the physician to the possibility of an insidious spread to a smoldering temporal bone infection that will eventually involve not only the external auditory canal and the tympanic membrane, but the entire middle-ear–mastoid cellular system. Early surgery and intensive long-range antibiotic bacteriologic control are necessary to lessen the probability of complications and fatality. Gentamicin and carbenicillin have been the principal antibiotics used in 1976–1977. Recent experiences with metronidazole (Flagyl) in Great Britain have been very encouraging, with demonstrated superior effectiveness—even in nonsurgical control of cases. Early administration seems to be necessary (9).

Fulminating Pediatric Otomastoiditis

In fulminating otomastoiditis in children, the possibility of meningitis and/or other intracranial complications is high. A constant alert must be maintained to detect meningitis, sigmoid sinus thrombophlebitis, and cerebral and cerebellar lesions. Facial-nerve paralysis is not rare in such cases. Immunologic defects are commonly present in fulminating pediatric otomastoiditis. The pediatric immunologist's collaboration in management is essential.

Tuberculosis and Mycoses

Tuberculosis is not a common temporal bone disease at the present time, since tuberculosis, in general, has become a less common pulmonary and constitutional disease. However, tuberculous mastoiditis still does occur both in children and in adults. It is usually an accompaniment of pulmonary tuberculosis, but it may be secondary to gastrointestinal or other nonpulmonary tuberculosis. It is characterized by an indolent course with relatively little pain. The lesions of middle-ear and mastoid tuberculosis are usually type A (granulomatous and frequently polypoid). They may produce irregular or punched-out lesions (as seen on radiographs) which resemble keratoma, but keratoma is uncommon.

In most instances there is a foul otorrhea, and routine bacteriologic studies will show nonspecific mixed organisms. Unless there is a high index of suspicion and acid-fast and other special tuberculosis studies are requested, the diagnosis may be missed. Tympanic membrane perforations may be central, marginal, or combined. There is usually a very thickened margin to the perforation. There is rarely tenderness over the mastoid. There may be accompanying cervical lymphadenopathy. In some instances, the diagnosis is not made until mastoid granuloma tissue is sent for histologic study. Thus the diagnosis may first be uncovered in the pathology laboratory.

The management of tuberculous mastoiditis involves the collaboration of the otologist and the tuberculosis specialist. Special care is required in specific antituberculosis antibiotic therapy because of drug ototoxicity problems. The tuberculous temporal bone lesion may produce labyrinthine complications with cochlear hearing loss and vertigo. Both may be accentuated by drug ototoxicity.

Combined medical antituberculosis treatment and specific otosurgical treatment may be necessary over a long period of time in the patient with tuberculous mastoiditis, in addition to obvious necessary treatment of any other systemic manifestations of the disease. Surgery should be based on eradication of the lesion and exteriorization. Tympanoplasty is rarely advisable as a primary procedure.

Specific mycoses such as actinomycosis and coccidioidomycosis occur in the temporal bone. Their manifestations are comparable to those of tuberculosis. The surgical and medical management is dictated by specific 4L equation findings. The utilization of appropriate antibiotic and other systemic medications will be necessary, along with otosurgical lesion exenteration. It is, in general, inadvisable to attempt tympanoplastic reconstruction of mycotic temporal bone diseases. Tympanoplastic surgery may be possible at some later period following the complete resolution of the temporal bone and constitutional mycotic lesions.

SPECIAL MANAGEMENT OF KERATOMA (CHOLESTEATOMA)

BASIC PRINCIPLES

The management of keratoma is almost always surgical. In rare cases, in which there are constitutional surgical contraindications, temporizing medical management may be the only treatment possible. Ideally, the treatment of keratoma is surgical removal.

The lesion is described in the section on Pathology early in this chapter. In some cases an otoscopic diagnosis is possible immediately. A dry or wet attic keratoma may appear on primary otoscopic examination, extending from the epitympanum (Fig. 16–19) or from the mesotympanum through a marginal or central perforation into the external auditory canal. It may be purely white and glistening in appearance or covered by muco-

FIG. 16–19. Cholesteatoma sac **(Ch)** situated medial to the ossicular chain. Its connecting neck is seen to pass between the incus and malleus, ending in a Shrapnell perforation. Contacts with bone **(arrows).** (Sade J: In McCabe B, Sade J, Abramson M (eds): Cholesteatoma: First International Conference. Birmingham, Aesculapius Publishing Co., 1977, p 216)

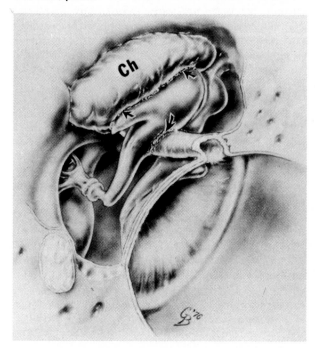

purulent exudate and crusts. Secondary infection may impart a characteristic fetid odor to the otorrhea.

Location

Keratoma may involve any portion or all of the tympanic membrane, including the annulus. Large tympanic membrane defects and scutum defects may be present with exteriorization of a necrotic malleus and incus. Extensions of bone necrosis into the posterior external auditory canal wall may allow visualization of the mastoid cavity through a large fistula between the external canal wall and mastoid. Occasional necrosis may occur in the anterior canal wall, with exposure of the soft tissues in the temporomandibular joint. Radiographs of the mastoids will frequently show smooth erosive lesions characteristic of keratomatous mastoid necrosis.

In addition to the obvious exteriorized keratoma, there are a number of varieties that may be described as "lurking latent cholesteatomas" (4). They may lurk behind dry or moist central perforations, or behind intact tympanic membranes. This type of hidden keratoma may either be primary or secondary.

Keratoma may be accompanied by all the other common varieties of chronic mastoiditis. Thus, keratoma with tympanosclerosis or keratoma with polypoid granulomatosis is not uncommon. In fact, it is possible to see keratoma combined with tympanosclerosis, cholesterol granuloma, and chronic polypoid mastoiditis. A chronic keratoma may first appear clinically with an acute concomitant hemorrhagic mastoiditis. Unsuspected keratoma may be found in an emergency mastoidectomy for a patient with acute mastoiditis with secondary labyrinthitis and/or meningitis.

A special type of keratoma occurs frequently in children, occasionally in adults. It is known as keratosis (cholesteatosis). This may exist in a well-pneumatized mastoid with little change on radiographs to be of diagnostic value. Keratosis may occur as a primary tympanomastoid disease. The etiology is still a controversial issue. The important issue, however, is that cholesteatosis involves a nonloculated type of keratoma, with a different variety of matrix from the more common type in children, and may be a very "silent" process for years or months, with an apparently intact and normal tympanic membrane and frequently without recognizable hearing loss. When it is finally recognized because of an acute flare-up or suppuration that does not respond to medical therapy, surgery will disclose masses of keratoma which can be found in any or every portion of the temporal bone, and frequently the lesion may break through conventional temporal bone boundaries. It is not uncommon for a child with cholesteatosis to have a perforation through the zygoma, or into the temporomandibular joint area, or complete destruction of the posterior fossa dural plate or the middle fossa dural plate or both. (See Color Fig. 15.) Keratosis usually involves necrotization of any or all of the three ossicles. It is not uncommon to find necrosis of most of the malleus, all of the incus, and the stapedial head, neck, and crura. Occasionally even the stapedial footplate will have been replaced by the margin of the invasive cholesteatotic mass. Semicircular canal fistulization is not rare in cholesteatosis.

Loss of Function

Loss of function in keratoma is multifaceted. Hearing loss may vary from minor conductive loss to total sensorineural loss due to labyrinthine destruction. Vertigo due to labyrinth fistula can mimic Meniere's disease and produce electronystagmographic abnormalities which vary from a hyperactive (hyperresponsive) labyrinth to canal paralysis. Seventh nerve paralysis is not rare in keratoma, due to erosion, fistualization, and pressure on the exposed seventh nerve in any portion of it, especially in the posterior genu or in the sinus tympani area.

Laboratory Findings

Laboratory findings in keratoma are frequently diagnostic. Simple Gram stain of lesions from the external auditory canal will show squamous or keratin debris with cholesterol granules. Bacterial infections may be gram-positive, gram-negative, or mixed. Fungi and yeast superinfections are not uncommon. Intracranial complications of keratoma invasion may be manifested by meningeal spinal fluid changes.

Radiologic Findings

Radiologic findings in cholesteatoma most usually occur in a characteristic combination of a non-pneumatized mastoid and periantral sclerosis, and occasionally one may see evidence of radiolucency in some portion of the temporal bone. In some instances radiolucency may not be apparent. Occasionally, as in keratosis in some children, keratoma may occur in a well-pneumatized temporal bone. Usually there is a deficiency in pneumatization. Keratoma usually will start in infancy or early life, but may not be diagnosed until late adult life in some patients.

SURGICAL MANAGEMENT OF KERATOMA (CHOLESTEATOMA)

Adequate surgical removal with conservation of vital structures is the ideal. In some instances of extensive invasion with secondary complications, the surgical procedure may require the removal of ossicles completely incarcerated by keratoma, removal of tympanic membrane remnants, annular bone, scutum, and posterior bony canal wall. In most instances a nonsurgical removal of the posterior bony canal wall has already been performed by the keratoma. The surgeon completes the removal of those remnants that prevent adequate exteriorization of the mastoid bowl.

The options available to the surgeon dealing with keratoma are based entirely upon the extent of the lesion. Although it is possible in many cases to remove the keratoma completely, without removal of posterior bony canal wall or middle ear components, it is not always feasible to successfully remove the keratoma mass and spare such vital structures. Modern temporal bone microsurgery has made possible more conservative procedures, which should be employed whenever possible and wherever the total removal of the lesion is not compromised.

Reconstructive tympanoplastic surgery may be combined with transmastoid removal of the keratoma in many cases. In other cases it is necessary that tympanoplastic procedures be deferred or staged, or omitted.

Thus it is possible to describe a broad spectrum of available surgery for keratoma. The classic radical mastoidectomy is the basic approach, in which the mastoid disease produced by the keratoma is removed, the posterior bony canal wall is removed, the malleus and incus and drum remnants are removed, and in some instances, the stapedial crura are also removed. It is rarely necessary to disturb the stapedial footplate which usually acts as a microbarricade between the middle ear and the scala vestibuli of the labyrinth.

In some cases, however, it is possible to remove a small keratoma through the epitympanic access route, via an endomeatal speculum approach, without disturbing the mastoid process at all.

All procedures must be based upon careful and thorough preoperative radiologic studies, including in many instances, polytomography. These new diagnostic advances, combined with adequate exposure and delicate microsurgical techniques may make possible a host of conservation tympanoplastic procedures without disturbing the integrity of the external auditory canal and without creating an external canal-mastoid communication or bowl—the mastoid bowl or mastoidostomy procedure which results in an exteriorized mastoid cavity and requires permanent postoperative care. In many instances the mastoid bowls will be covered with healthy epithelium and require little or no treatment with no morbidity.

Multilocular keratoma in adults poses a serious challenge both as to preservation of the posterior bony canal wall and to definitive grafting techniques regardless of tissue employed. A conventional autogenous graft tympanoplasty may be apparently successful for a number of years. However, recurrences occur frequently. In view of this fact, it is safer to avoid primary definitive grafting in some cases. An attempt to perform an inductive, deliberate spontaneous tympanoplasty with absorbable gelatin film (Gelfilm) may be made with no compromise of safety (5, 7). The naturally formed regenerative neomembrane is thin and does not tend to block exteriorization of a delayed keratomous recurrence.

Application of primary tympanoplastic reconstruction in cases of pediatric cholesteatosis seems unwise at the present stage of our experience.

Keratoma is a potentially serious disease of the temporal bone and usually calls for surgical removal.

Keratoma may lurk behind dry central tympanic membrane perforations and behind an intact tympanic membrane. It is not a rare disease. It is one of the most common diseases of the temporal bone, and its presence must always be considered until ruled out by appropriate measures.

SPECIAL MANAGEMENT OF TYMPANOSCLEROSIS

Lesion

The lesion of tympanosclerosis occurs in two forms: 1) hyalinization as a healing response to earlier acute otomastoiditis or secretory otitis media and manifested as submucosal sclerosis, and/or 2) osteoclastic mucoperiostitis. Each represents different stages of the same chronic inflammatory disease.

The superficial lesions of submucosal sclerosis are easily and cleanly removed. They leave an intact substructure and invite tympanoplastic repair. The more destructive form, osteoclastic mucoperiostitis, has been noted to have transformed an involved stapes into an amorphous mass of bone, has resulted in cochlear erosion, has destroyed middle ear mucosa and mucoperiosteum and ossicles, and thereby has prevented successful tympanoplastic repair. Tympanosclerosis is more commonly an adult disease, in contrast to keratoma.

If it is not possible to remove all of an embedded lesion, it is likely that epithelial elements may be left behind to progress into keratomatous disease.

The dense hyaline sclerotic tissue may be superficial and subepithelial, or deep and apparently invasive if bone destruction was significant. Calcification and new bone formation may be part of the process. Granulation tissue, as evidence of still active inflammation, may be present. Because of metaplasia of the overlying epithelium, keratoma may accompany tympanosclerosis. Less frequently, as residue of prior hemorrhage, siderogranuloma and cholesterol granuloma may also be present. The lesion may recur after prior eradication.

Location

The location of tympanosclerosis is predominantly in the middle ear, epitympanum, eustachian tube, and aditus ad antrum. It rarely extends into the more posterior part of the mastoid antrum or into the general cellular mastoid architecture.

Loss of Function

Loss of function in tympanosclerosis includes conductive hearing losses of all degrees, frequent secondary cochlear hearing losses, occasional vertigo due to labyrinth capsule erosion, and occasional seventh nerve paralysis due to pressure erosion.

Laboratory Findings

Laboratory findings in tympanosclerosis include radiologic findings of diminished aeration in mastoid cells and nonspecific mixed bacterial flora from middle ear cultures, if otorrhea is present.

Medical treatment is not curative. Local medication will frequently be effective in obtaining a dry ear, intermittently.

Surgery for tympanosclerosis is indicated for removal of granulomatous or suppurative lesions. Tympanoplasty is more frequently successful in the superficial submucosal sclerosis type. The danger of secondary keratoma formation is always present if embedded tympanosclerosis is left *in situ*, but removal over the cochlear promontory, the seventh nerve, and from oval and round window niches may be impossible with safety. Tympanoplastic repair in the presence of embedded osteoclastic tympanosclerosis is usually not recommended. Recurrences of tympanoscle-

rosis are frequent. Thus, exteriorization of such lesions is safer than attempts to close tympanic membrane perforations.

MANAGEMENT OF COMBINED KERATOMA AND TYMPANOSCLEROSIS LESIONS

Location

Tympanosclerosis lesions primarily involve 1) the middle ear, including the protympanum, epitympanum, mesotympanum, and hypotympanum, with replacement of normal tympanic membrane epithelium; and 2) promontory, labyrinth window, and ossicular periosteal and bony lesions, which usually stop at the aditus with only rare mastoid involvement.

Keratoma can be monolocular, multilocular, or diffuse, as in keratosis, and be located anywhere in the temporal bone.

Combined lesions are common in chronic otomastoiditis, with primary keratoma involvement in the mastoid and primary tympanosclerosis involvement in the middle ear.

Loss of Function

Keratoma lesions cause ossicular necrosis, perforations of the tympanic membrane, mastoid bone disease, and erosions of the labyrinth, and seventh nerve, and in general involving any or all temporal bone "viscera." When combined with tympanosclerosis, complex surgical problems are produced, especially in relation to labyrinthine and seventh nerve complications. Hearing losses range from simple to total conductive losses associated with mild to severe cochlear hearing losses. Sclerosing lesions of tympanosclerosis create ossicular fixation more commonly than do the lesions of keratoma, which usually produce ossicular discontinuity. Stapes fixation is more often the contribution of the tympanosclerosis component.

Laboratory Findings

Bacteriologic lesions can be similar in both diseases. Pure or mixed gram-positive or gram-negative infections occur in varying combinations in combined keratoma-tympanosclerosis lesions.

Radiologic findings are characterized by pleomorphism, with predominantly underdeveloped sclerotic mastoid and evidence of halisteresis, hazy cells, and generalized lack of landmark definition. Polytomography may show incus necrosis and/or ossifying incudomalleal lesions.

Management of mixed keratoma and tympanosclerosis lesions is usually surgical and frequently results in complete removal of the keratoma but incomplete removal of the tympanosclerosis because of the different types of lesions produced by each entity. In general, total removal of keratoma is more commonly possible. Removal of tympanosclerosis in osteoclastic forms may be hazardous to the labyrinth, especially in the region of the oval window, round window, and promontory of the cochlea. Erosions of these areas are frequently noted.

In general, it is safer to be more conservative and less radical with tympanosclerosis removal than with keratoma removal.

Ultimate decisions must be based on an awareness of the surgical pathologic differences between these two type B lesions.

REFERENCES

1. Chandler JR: Pathogenesis and treatment of facial paralysis due to malignant external otitis. Ann Otol Rhinol Laryngol 81:648–658, 1972

2. Decher H, Daum L: Zur bakteriologie der chronischen mittelohreiterung und frage der erregeremp-findlischkeit auf antibiotika. Z Laryngol Rhinol Otol 52:583–589, 1973

3. Friedmann I: Pathology of the Ear. London, Blackwell Scientific, 1974

4. Goodhill V: The lurking, latent cholesteatoma. Ann Otol Rhinol Laryngol 69:1199–2013, 1960

5. Goodhill V: Cholesteatoma, mastoiditis, and gelfilm induction tympanoplasty. Trans Pac Coast Otoophthalmol Soc 52:217–242, 1971

6. Goodhill V: Tympanoplasty—Four heterodox techniques. Ann R Coll Surg Engl 59:17–24, 1977

7. Harris I, Barton S, Gussen R et al.: Gelfilm induced neotympanic membrane in tympanoplasty. Laryngoscope 81:1826–1837, 1971

8. Harris I, Weiss L: Tympanosclerosis: superficial and embedded forms. Trans Am Acad Ophthalmol Otolaryngol 66:683–714, 1961

9. Harrison DFN: Personal communication

10. Politzer A: Das cholesteatom des gehörorgans vom anatomischen und klinischen standpunkte. Wien Med Wochenschr 41:8–12, 1891

11. Politzer A: A Text-Book of the Diseases of the Ear for Students and Practitioners, 5th ed. Philadelphia, Lea & Febiger, 1909, pp 453–457

12. Sade J, Berco E: Bone destruction in chronic otitis media. A histopathological study. J Laryngol 88:413–422, 1974

13. Von Tröltsch A: The Diseases of the Ear: Their Diagnosis and Treatment. New York, William Wood and Co, 1864

Surgery for chronic otomastoiditis before 1950 was limited primarily to removal of irreversible lesions of bone and soft tissue from the temporal bone. The two major objectives were 1) safety, by removing lesions liable to cause serious complications, and 2) dry ear, by removing obstructive or necrotizing lesions responsible for chronic or intermittent otorrhea. These two objectives were accomplished primarily by some form of mastoid surgery prior to the modern era of tympanoplastic surgery.

Mastoidectomy applies to any one of several procedures used to remove diseased bone and soft tissues from the mastoid and its contiguous areas.

The most common otosurgical procedures used in chronic otomastoiditis prior to the advent of tympanoplasty were 1) atticomastoidectomy, 2) modified radical mastoidectomy, and 3) radical mastoidectomy. In addition to these three procedures on the mastoid, two other procedures were used in chronic otomastoiditis: 4) tympanic ossiculectomy, and 5) aural polypectomy. All five operations were directed to lesion eradication, not to reconstruction.

The development of tympanoplastic techniques, since 1950, has modified the uses of these five surgical procedures. All five, however, are still in use, either alone or, more usually, combined with tympanoplastic reconstruction.

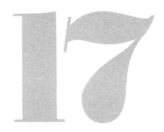

OTOMASTOIDITIS SURGERY— MASTOIDECTOMY AND TYMPANOPLASTY

VICTOR GOODHILL
SEYMOUR J. BROCKMAN
IRWIN HARRIS
JOEL B. SHULMAN
STEPHEN H. COOPER

MASTOIDECTOMY AND RELATED EAR SURGERY

ATTICOMASTOIDECTOMY

Atticomastoidectomy, the primary mastoid operation for acute mastoiditis, also has application in chronic otomastoiditis, especially in certain type A cases (as determined by the 4L equation) (see Ch. 16, Chronic Otomastoiditis—Diagnosis and Management).

A postauricular or endaural incision is used to gain access to the lateral mastoid cortex (see Ch. 12, Basic Otosurgical Procedures). Cortical bone is removed with cutting burrs, irrigation, and suction. Cell groups are identified by their relationships to the major landmarks: middle fossa plate, posterior fossa plate, posterior bony canal wall, aditus, incus short process, horizontal semicircular canal, and the posterior epitympanum. Major differences in pneumatization will dictate degrees of actual bone removal in pneumatic, diploic, and sclerotic mastoids. The middle ear is explored by elevation of posterior canal wall skin and exposure of the middle ear and its contents.

The purpose of atticomastoidectomy is accomplished when mucosal and bony trabecular lesions (usually type A) are removed and grossly normal cells remain, in adequate pneumatic continuity with the epitympanum.

In some cases, as determined by the 4L equation evaluation (Ch. 16), tympanoplastic reconstruction may be performed simultaneously.

The term **simple mastoidectomy** has been used somewhat inaccurately in the past to describe atticomastoidectomy. The connotation of "simple" is misleading as compared with "radical." In many type A lesions, an atticomastoidectomy requires far more extensive and time-consuming bone removal than radical mastoidectomy in some type B lesions. Thus, for example, atticomastoidectomy for extensive cholesterol granulomatosis due to a resistant gram-negative organism, with vascular, mucosal and bony changes in a well-pneumatized mastoid, may require a procedure far more complex than a radical mastoidectomy in a small, contracted, sclerotic mastoid for removal of a quiescent monolocular keratoma.

RADICAL MASTOIDECTOMY AND VARIATIONS

Radical mastoidectomy is an operation in which infected mastoid cell groups are removed, along with the posterior bony canal wall, incus, malleus, and tympanic membrane remnant. The operation is in essence a mastoidectomy, myringectomy, lateral ossiculectomy, and conversion of the mastoid cavity, external auditory canal, epitympanum, and middle ear into one contiguous space. A total exteriorized stoma then remains, consisting of the mastoid cavity–external auditory canal–middle ear cavity. This total cavity, a mastoidostomy, or stoma, or mastoid bowl can be examined after the operation directly through the external auditory meatus.

The classic radical operation was characterized by an attempt at abolition of the eustachian tube orifice by plugging it with various tissues or with foreign materials. In addition, the annular floor of the tympanum was usually drilled down to or below the level of the external auditory canal so that the canal and middle ear floor (hypotympanum) were at the same level. Squamous epithelium was encouraged to migrate into the middle ear to cover the medial tympanic wall completely. The total result was a skin-lined cavity of the entire exenterated mastoid–external auditory canal–middle ear bowl.

Present-day radical mastoidectomy technique avoids such attempts at obliterating the eustachian tube and avoids removal of the bony or fibrous annulus. It is no longer considered desirable to encourage squamous epithelial migration into the middle ear. It is preferable to leave an open eustachian tube and an exposed middle ear mucosa so that the cavity can be inspected carefully. Episodes of mucosal otorrhea can be treated when they occur. Most importantly, such a technique always leaves possible the consideration of a subsequent, carefully timed, secondary tympanoplastic repair. Deliberate closure of the eustachian tube and encouragement of deliberate squamous migration into the middle ear defeats any possibility of subsequent staged tympanoplastic reconstruction.

A number of modified radical mastoidectomy procedures involve various compromises in attempts to preserve some middle ear structures and function. Varying degrees of conservation of the posterior bony canal wall and middle ear structures are employed, ranging from total conservation of the ossicular chain and tympanic membrane to partial ossiculectomies.

OSSICULECTOMY

Transcanal epitympanic ossiculectomy as a specific operation, was used widely, prior to the present era of tympanoplasty. Ossicles were removed either through a tympanic membrane incision or through a tympanic membrane or epitympanic perforation for removal of keratoma and diseased ossicles or part of ossicles. Similar efforts were also made to remove granulomas or tympanosclerotic lesions. These conservative epitympanic ossiculectomy procedures were frequently successful and represented early approaches to modern tympanoplastic surgical concepts.

Such ossiculectomies were successful only in cases in which there was no active mastoid disease. They failed in many instances because of unrecognized active mastoid disease. They also either failed to improve hearing or were responsible for further hearing losses. The primary favorable result was a dry ear, by removal of circumscribed lesions and diseased ossicles. An occasional hearing improvement was fortuitous, due to spontaneous formation of ossicular adhesions.

AURAL POLYPECTOMY

Polyps (polypoid granulomas) resulting from active ossicular necrosis or from chronic otomastoiditis are frequently noted in the external auditory canal, usually accompanying suppuration, either in type A or type B lesions. Aural polypectomy was a common primary office procedure in the past. Polyp "ear snares" and cup forceps were used for removal. In general, primary aural polypectomy has been abandoned as a procedure. A primary aural polypectomy is a blind procedure, since the source of the polypoid growth is usually unknown. Instances of cochlear, vestibular, and seventh nerve damage have been reported following such primary blind procedures.

After an operation, however, granulomatous polyps can be removed occasionally on an outpatient basis (as a secondary polypectomy procedure).

TYMPANOPLASTY

BASIC TYMPANOPLASTY PRINCIPLES

For years it was known that spontaneous closures of tympanic membrane perforations and spontaneous total regeneration of the tympanic membrane with or without hearing improvements could follow either no treatment, medical treatment, or various surgical resection procedures, including mastoidectomy (simple, modified-radical, and radical), ossiculectomy, or aural polypectomy.

With increasing knowledge of physiological acoustics, audiology, plastic surgery, and the stimulating successes of otosclerosis surgery, definitive approaches to reconstructive ear surgery became possible. Zöllner (8) and Wullstein (7) pioneered in the development of tympanoplasty.

These developments made possible a combination of a disease-resection operation (*i.e.*, mastoidectomy) with a reconstructive operation aimed at midde ear function restoration. Thus, the tympanoplasty concept was evolved as an advance over radical mastoidectomy and modified radical mastoidectomy. Many tympanoplastic techniques have emerged in the past 25 years.

The basic Zollner-Wullstein approach was based on modified radical mastoidectomy, in which a mastoidotomy (open mastoid bowl) was created, but it was accompanied by tympanic membrane and middle ear reconstruction.

The Wullstein types I through V tympanoplasty classification is useful conceptually as an introduction to tympanoplastic planning (see Fig. 12–16).

Five tympanic function requisites are necessary for normal hearing or restoration of normal hearing.
1. Patent external canal
2. Normal tympanic membrane
3. Intact continuity of tympanic membrane, ossicular chain (or substitute columella), and mobile footplate (transmission piston)
4. Yielding but shielded round window membrane
5. Tympanic air-space equalization by normal tubal function

Five representative tympanic physiological problems require tympanoplastic solutions.
1. Acoustic reception lesions (tympanic membrane perforations)
2. Acoustic transmission lesions (incus necrosis)
3. Window fixations (oval or round window fixation)
4. Loss of sound pressure difference (defective round window–eustachian tube ventilation).
5. Acoustic "short circuits" (lack of tympanic ossicles, with scar tissue connecting round window niche and oval window niche)

Five classic tympanoplasty procedures may restore function (see Ch. 12).
1. Type I tympanoplasty, basically to repair a tympanic membrane defect
2. Type II tympanoplasty, a neotympanic membrane graft to malleus or incus
3. Type III tympanoplasty, a reconstruction by a neotympanic membrane graft connected directly to the stapes
4. Type IV tympanoplasty (*cavum minor*), a round window baffle procedure with a graft isolating the round window membrane–eustachian tube air space continuum from a mobile oval window footplate
5. Type V tympanoplasty, an adaption of a type IV cavum minor operation combined with horizontal semicircular canal fenestration

OSSICULOPLASTY, INTACT CANAL WALL TECHNIQUES, AND CONTEMPORARY TYMPANOPLASTY

Improvements in microsurgical technology and developments in prosthetic implants and in autograft and homograft ossicle substitutions were responsible for the emergence of ossiculoplastic methods for hearing restoration. These methods were accompanied by conservation of the external auditory canal through retaining the posterior bony canal wall and avoiding an open mastoid cavity (intact canal wall technique). These advances led also to modifications of the original Wullstein five tympanoplastic types.

The present approach to mastoid surgery—tympanoplasty—is based upon a selective decision-making process that takes into consideration the two basic clinical categories of otomastoiditis, type A and type B pathologic lesions and the 4L equation of lesion, location, loss of function, and laboratory findings. The modified Wullstein tympanoplasty procedures may be accompanied or preceded by appropriate mastoid surgery.

The primary problem to be solved in most tympanoplasties is tympanic membrane repair, partial or total. This is accomplished by transplantation of autograft tissues in most cases.

Spontaneous tympanic membrane healing also occurs frequently. There are at least two mechanisms that play major roles in growth and repair of the tympanic membrane: 1) the induction effect of the fibrous annulus, and 2) the special nature of basement-membrane laminas in the middle layer of the tympanic membrane and in the fibrous annulus.

These two factors may be responsible for growth and dedifferentiation characteristics of grafts applied to this area. Indeed, it is possible to expedite spontaneous healing by placing a disc of absorbable gelatin film (Gelfilm) in contact with the fibrous annulus.

Our experiences with such induction phenomena have been crystallized into the deliberate use of absorbable gelatin film instead of tissue in the solution of *some special problems* that contraindicate tissue transplants. Details regarding such "no graft" tympanoplasty techniques are described in the section Special Tympanoplasty Techniques later in this chapter.

Tissues for tympanoplastic repair grafts have included postauricular skin, skin from the wall of the external auditory canal, and a number of mesodermal tissues. At the present writing, meso-

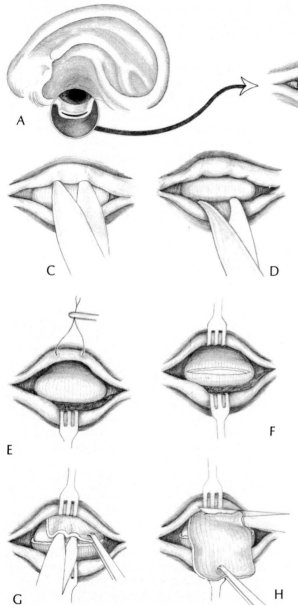

FIG. 17–1. A. Following subcutaneous lidocaine-epinephrine infiltration, linear incision is made over tragal dome. **B.** Exposure of dome of tragal cartilage. **C.** Dissection of subcutaneous tissues from posteromedial (canal) tragal surface. **D.** Dissection of subcutaneous tissue from anterolateral (facial) tragal surface. **E.** Retraction of skin surface with either a rake retractor or a silk traction suture. **F.** Linear incision of perichondrium of tragal dome to expose tragal cartilage. **G.** Dissection of posteromedial (canal) tragal perichondrium from tragal cartilage. **H.** Excision of hemigraft of perichondrium. (Goodhill V: Arch Otolaryngol 85:490, 1967. Copyright 1967, American Medical Association)

dermal tissues have largely displaced skin grafts, and primarily include temporalis fascia, and perichondrium. To a lesser extent, adipose and vein grafts are also used.

For 15 years, surgeons in our group have preferred the use of perichondrium obtained from the tragus. The advantages of perichondrium from the tragus are 1) accessibility in the operative site, 2) availability in adequate amount, 3) useful contour characteristics, and 4) rare rejection.

Tragal perichondrium can be used either from the posteromedial (canal) side or from the anterolateral (facial) side as a hemigraft, or the entire tragal cartilage may be removed and both perichondrial surfaces used in continuity as a total graft. The choice of either hemigraft or total graft is based upon the size of the defect and upon desirable geometry in relation to the defect requiring repair. The tragal dome shape makes possible an anteroposterior graft, which has a concavity and a convexity. These geometric features can be exploited surgically in a number of ways. For this reason, perichondrium has an advantage over shapeless tissues such as temporal fascia.

Perichondrium is obtained from the tragus as follows. Following subcutaneous infiltration of lidocaine (Xylocaine) with epinephrine (1.5% lidocaine with 1:200,000 epinephrine) into the tragal dome, utilizing approximately 1 cc of the anesthetic solution, a linear vertical incision is made with a rounded mini-bladed knife. Dissection of the subcutaneous tissue brings the cartilage dome into clear view, following which either the posterior or anterior surface is exposed, or both surfaces may be dissected if a total graft is necessary (Fig. 17–1).

If a perichondrial hemigraft is desired, a linear incision is carried down to the tragal cartilage. The cut perichondrial surface is gently grasped with a delicate, toothed forceps, and the perichondrium is dissected free from the underlying cartilage with the minibladed knife and a curved fine scissors and removed. Such a hemigraft usually measures about 12 × 14 mm.

If total perichondrial graft is needed, the entire tragal cartilage is removed from the tragal pocket, following superior, caudal, and connecting medial in-

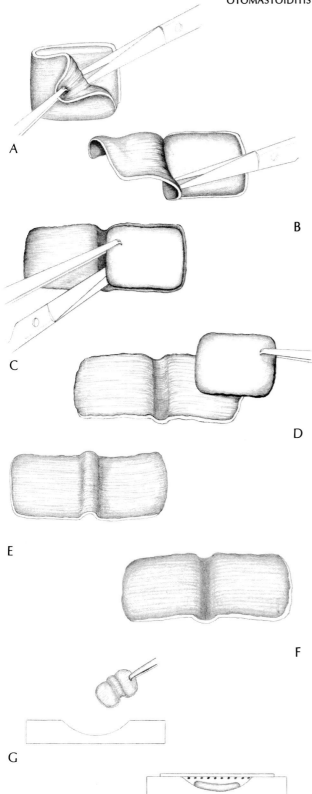

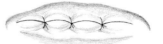

FIG. 17–2. A. Beginning dissection of one surface of perichondrium from tragal cartilage. **B.** Continuation of dissection over tragal dome area proceeding to the other surface. **C.** Completion of dissection in continuity. **D.** Total perichondrial autograft removed from tragal cartilage. **E.** Total perichondrial graft illustrating built-in convexity in region of dome. **F.** Internal view of total perichondrial autograft illustrating built-in concavity. **G.** Shaped total autograft placed in graft plate. **H.** Graft in well of graft plate, covered with moistened glass slide. (Goodhill V: Arch Otolaryngol 85:490, 1967. Copyright 1967, American Medical Association)

FIG. 17–3. Closure of tragal incision with black silk sutures (4-0). (Goodhill V: Arch Otolaryngol 85:490, 1967. Copyright 1967, American Medical Association)

cisions, freeing it from its surrounding soft-tissue attachments superiorly and from its union inferiorly with the cartilaginous isthmus. The perichondrium is then dissected in continuity from both surfaces of the excised lamina tragi cartilage, creating a graft which measures approximately 14 × 25 mm. The graft is placed in the shallow well of a plate made of synthetic plastic material and covered by a moistened glass slide. It is not immersed directly in any solution since there is adequate humidity in the enclosed "well" to prevent excessive drying (Fig. 17–2).

In the event a cartilage columella is necessary, the cartilage of the tragus (lamina tragi) is used, either for the creation of a composite cartilage-perichondrium T graft or for the procurement of a separate cartilage graft to be used in contact with the perichondrial graft as a substitute for the stapes head and crura. In some instances, tragal cartilage is used to create a composite perichondrial-cartilage batten graft when a temporarily stiff tympanic membrane graft is desirable.

If it is necessary to use the entire tragal cartilage, the tragal incision is closed with three black silk 4-0 sutures. No cosmetic deformity results from the removal of the entire tragal cartilage. If, however, it is not necessary to use the cartilage, it is slipped back into the tragal pocket and the incision closed (Fig. 17–3). Such conservation of the tragal cartilage usually results in recreation of another perichondrial covering that occasionally is useful, if necessary, for a secondary procedure.

THE CONTEMPORARY FIVE TYPES OF TYMPANOPLASTY

TYPE I

Type I tympanoplasty is the fundamental tympanic membrane repair procedure. It is indicated in cases with an intact, mobile, ossicular chain and a dry middle ear, free of active mucosal-bony type A disease. Special techniques are used in type B disease—keratoma (cholesteatoma) and tympanosclerosis. Different techniques are used for small to medium perforations and large or marginal perforations of the tympanic membrane. Repairs of small to medium perforations have also been described under the term **myringoplasty.** It is recommended that the term **type I tympanoplasty** be used to describe all tympanic membrane reconstructions in which there is an intact ossicular chain or whenever ossicular reconstruction (ossiculoplasty) will be performed as a second-stage procedure. The term myringoplasty should be limited to relatively small central perforations, which will be described in the following section.

Small to Medium Perforation Repair by Myringoplasty

REGENERATIVE INDUCTIVE MYRINGOPLASTY. Spontaneous regeneration in small central perforations (2–5 mm in diameter) has been recognized as a therapeutic possibility for many decades. The term **patching** has been used to describe this technique, and the procedure was used long before inductive regenerative growth processes were recognized as playing primary roles in such spontaneous healing. Small central perforations that lend themselves to inductive patching may be of traumatic origin or may follow acute, secretory, or chronic otitis media. In general, type I tympanoplasty (myringoplasty) is indicated if the middle ear is dry, if radiographs of the mastoid show no active bone disease, and if a conductive hearing loss no greater than 20–30 dB exists. Inductive (patching) myringoplasty can be done successfully in relatively small perforations. Such techniques are performed as outpatient procedures without anesthesia or with an endomeatal local anesthetic block.

The external auditory canal is thoroughly cleansed. A "cigarette paper" patch of proper size is moistened slightly in 10% AgNO₃, and the patch is gently applied laterally to the perforation so that it overlaps the margin by approximately 2 mm in all directions. A drop of 10% AgNO₃ is then applied gently circumferentially to the paper so that the patch adheres to the margin

of the tympanic membrane. Care is taken not to allow any of the AgNO₃ solution to enter the middle ear. Alternative techniques use other patching substances such as absorbable gelatin film and other stimulating solutions such as trichloroacetic or chromic acid (Fig. 17–4).

The purpose is to create a bridge for epithelial growth across the perforation. Patching procedures can be successful in 70–80% of cases of small tympanic membrane perforations. There is a danger in the use of highly irritating solutions to stimulate patching. Instrumentation must be very careful, and stimulating solutions must not enter the middle ear. Sudden cochlear deafness may follow the use of such solutions.

SURGICAL MYRINGOPLASTY (LATERAL GRAFT TYMPANOPLASTY). Surgical myringoplasty (lateral graft tympanoplasty type I) is used if patching

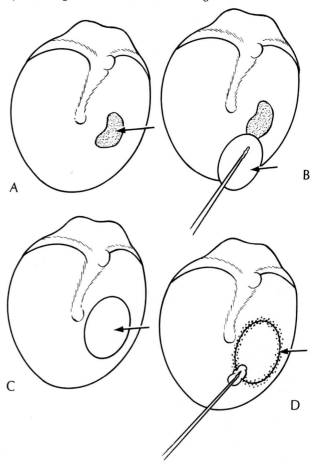

FIG. 17–4. "Inductive" repair of small perforation in dry ear. (Regenerative inductive myringoplasty.) **A. Arrow,** small central perforation. **B. Arrow,** thin paper patch advanced to cover perforation. **C. Arrow,** patch in position. **D. Arrow,** patch margins moistened with 10% Ag No₃.

fails or as an alternative to patching in small to medium perforations. A lateral tissue graft is successful in 90% of cases. The procedure may be done under local or general anesthesia. In adult cases with external auditory canals of large dimensions, a transcanal endomeatal approach is frequently possible. In narrow or angulated external auditory canals and in children, an endaural approach is necessary. Such procedures in adults are done under local anesthesia. In children, combined local and general anesthesia is used.

The entire squamous epithelial layer of pars tensa is removed, using a 1-mm angulated spud curet. The removal is begun circumferentially and approaches the margin of the perforation in a radial fashion. It is thus possible not only to remove the squamous layer *en masse,* but also to simultaneously remove the invaginated squamous margin of the perforation in toto. Care must be taken to be sure that there is no medial keratoma. In some cases an exploratory tympanotomy may be necessary to rule out such a possibility (which would contraindicate this procedure).

A perichondrium graft is obtained from the tragus, adequate in dimension to cover the entire denuded pars tensa to the bony annulus. This graft is set upon a backing of dry, compressed, absorbable gelatin sponge (Gelfoam) and meticulously placed so that it is in good contact with the entire denuded (deepithelialized) surface (Fig. 17–5). The graft is then snugly placed into position by packing with additional gelatin sponge and gauze. Prophylactic broad-spectrum antibiotic therapy administered orally is maintained for 7–10 days.

Repairs of Large Tympanic Membrane Perforations

Type I tympanoplasty (mediolateral graft) is used to repair a large perforation with an intact ossicular chain, or as the first stage of a planned second-stage ossiculoplasty. It should be limited to dry ears, with no radiographic evidence of active mastoid bone disease, a conductive hearing loss no greater than 30–40 dB, and no evidence of eustachian tube closure. Eustachian tube patency can be demonstrated, before operation, by tympanometry or by direct otoscopic visualization following politzerization with nebulized vapor. However, neither test may be completely reliable. Surgical judgment and experience take precedence over most current tests for evaluating eustachian tube function.

The procedure (under local or general anesthesia) commences with a transspeculum examination of the tympanic membrane perforation and the middle ear. When the diameter of the external auditory canal is adequate, the examination and the tympanoplasty are both done by an endomeatal speculum approach. The circumferential surgical approach (described later in

this chapter) to the tympanic membrane and middle ear enables a total area survey. The crucial determinations include 1) visualization of the anterior sulcus of the external auditory canal, 2) epitympanum and sinus tympani exploration, and 3) ossicular chain status. Examination of the two latter areas requires different approaches in anterior and posterior perforations. The term **marginal perforation** has been used to identify perforations that extend to the annulus.

An **anterior perforation** is one that is primarily anterior to the umbo. A **posterior perforation** is primarily posterior to the umbo (see Ch. 16, Chronic Otomastoiditis—Diagnosis and Management). Some posterior perforations are complicated by atelectatic adhesions and annular erosions, usually associated with sinus tympani lesions.

ANTERIOR PERFORATION MEDIOLATERAL GRAFT TECHNIQUE (FIG. 17–6). In an anterior perforation, the procedure consists of the following steps:

FIG. 17–5. Lateral graft type I tympanoplasty. **A. Arrow,** deepithelialized anterior pars tensa. **B. Arrow,** removal of perforation margin. **C. Arrow,** perichondrial graft.

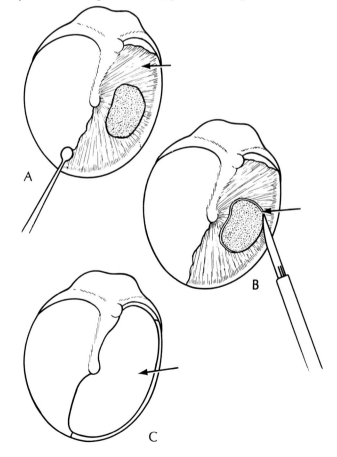

FIG. 17–6. Mediolateral graft tympanoplasty steps.

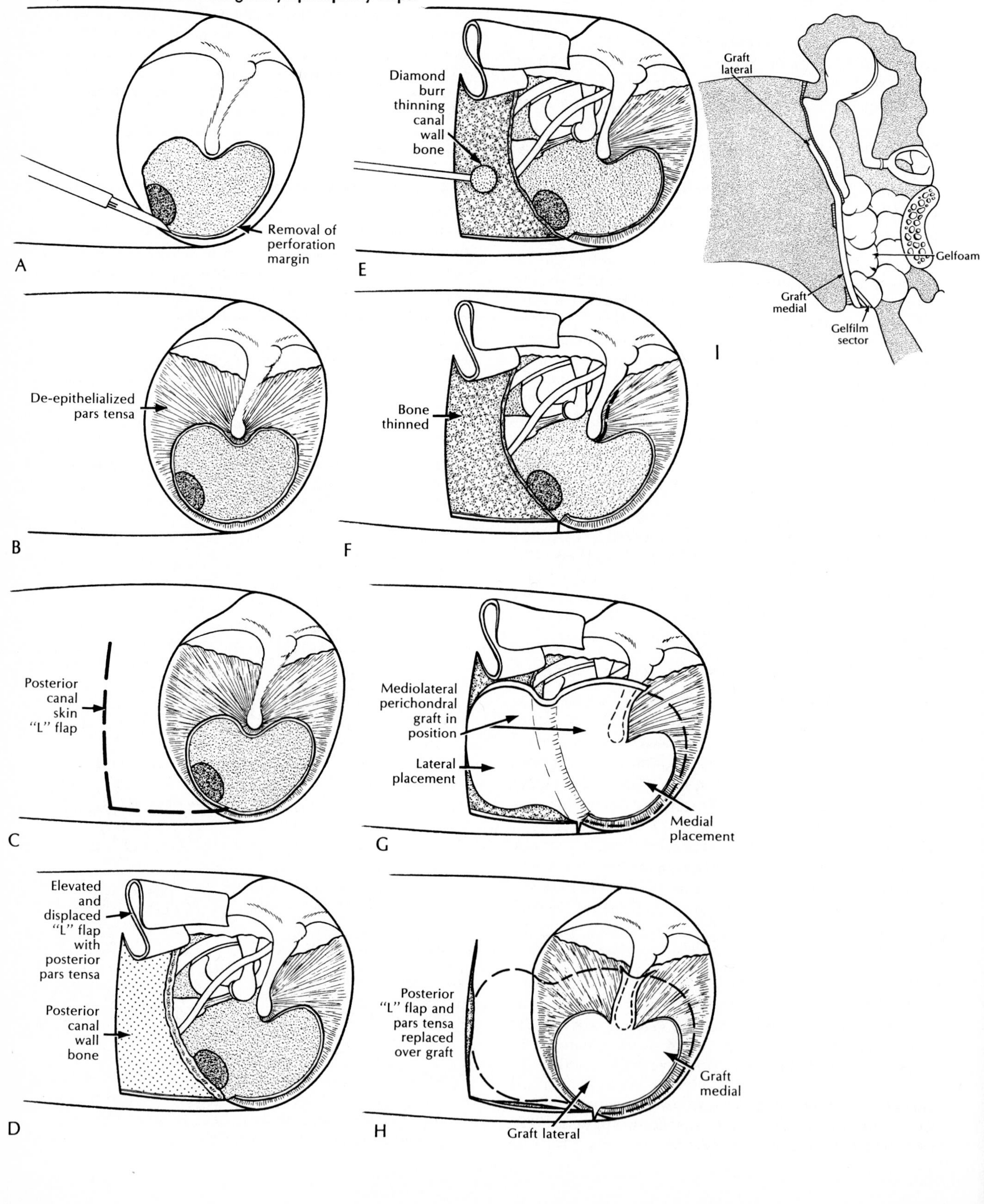

A — Removal of perforation margin

B — De-epithelialized pars tensa

C — Posterior canal skin "L" flap

D — Elevated and displaced "L" flap with posterior pars tensa; Posterior canal wall bone

E — Diamond burr thinning canal wall bone

F — Bone thinned

G — Mediolateral perichondral graft in position; Lateral placement; Medial placement

H — Posterior "L" flap and pars tensa replaced over graft; Graft medial; Graft lateral

I — Graft lateral; Graft medial; Gelfoam; Gelfilm sector

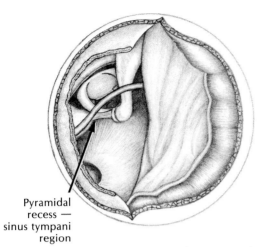

Pyramidal
recess —
sinus tympani
region

FIG. 17–7. Omega flap approach to posterior tympanotomy.

1. Deepithelialization of the pars tensa is carried out, with resection of the entire rim of the tympanic membrane perforation.
2. A posterior omega flap is created, as in stapedectomy.
3. The omega flap is elevated, and removal of an adequate amount of posterior bony annulus is carried out for inspection of the sinus tympani region (suprapyramidal recess and infrapyramidal recess), ossicular chain, and windows (Fig. 17–7).
4. If no significant abnormalities are found, the omega flap is replaced and a limited mediolateral graft is placed.
5. The mesodermal (perichondrial or fascial) graft is placed medially into the anteroinferior middle ear space on a middle ear platform of absorbable gelatin film sectors and absorbable gelatin sponge squares to assure coaptation of the graft to the medial surface of the tympanic membrane remnant, anterior to the region of the anteroinferior perforation margin.
6. A 1.5-mm slit is made vertically anterior to the umbo, through periumbo fibrous tissue. A similar inferior slit is made directly inferior, through the fibrous annulus and the margin of the tympanic membrane perforation to the bony annulus.
7. These two slits serve as exit routes for the graft as it assumes the lateral aspect of a mediolateral graft. The lateral portion of the graft is placed in firm contact with the deepithelialized area surrounding the posterior portion of the tympanic membrane perforation and is firmly packed with absorbable gelatin film and gelatin sponge squares.

POSTERIOR PERFORATION MEDIOLATERAL GRAFT TECHNIQUE. In a posterior central or posterior marginal perforation, the procedure is as follows:

1. Deepithelialization of the inferior two-thirds of the pars tensa remnant is carried out, with resection of entire rim of the tympanic membrane perforation.
2. A superior to inferior incision is made in the posterior canal wall 6–8 mm lateral to the posterior tympanic annulus. It extends from the level of the malleal short process to 1 mm above the floor of the external auditory canal.
3. From the lower end of the lateral incision, a 90° medial cut converts it into an L-shaped incision. The medial cut is made through skin and periosteum but, in addition, also through the fibrous annulus and through the posterior margin of the tympanic membrane perforation, creating a superiorly based posterior canal wall flap.
4. The posterior flap is dissected upward from the posterior canal wall as a superiorly based flap, by elevation of the posterosuperior fibers from the bony sulcus as a continuous skin flap from the annulus to the tympanic membrane; the flap is then tucked into the region of the roof of the external auditory canal temporarily.
5. The posterior canal bony annulus is removed to the extent necessary to obtain adequate visualization of sinus tympani, incus, stapes, and oval and round window niches. Ossicular mobility is checked using round window reflex visualization, which is greatly expedited by the anterior surgical position of the circumferential approach.
6. If such inspection reveals invasive type B disease with mastoid and/or epitympanic extension, a decision is necessary regarding mastoidectomy, ossiculectomy, or other procedures. At this point, a decision may be made not to proceed through the endomeatal-speculum approach. An endaural or postauricular incision is then necessary for adequate exposure of sinus tympani, facial recess, and mastoid cell regions.
7. However, if inspection reveals a normal sinus tympani, epitympanum, ossicular chain and windows, and if there is an adequate access to the external auditory canal, a type I tympanoplasty proceeds as an endomeatal transspeculum procedure.
8. The entire bony posterior canal wall uncovered by the posterior flap is thinned down by diamond burrs approximately 1.5 mm, to widen the external canal slightly in its posterior aspect.
9. Graft placement now proceeds. The anterior portion of the graft is placed on a middle ear (anteroinferior quadrant) bed of absorbable gelatin film and sponge for middle ear support to assure coaptation of the graft to the medial surface of the anteroinferior tympanic membrane remnant.
10. A superior to inferior slit is made in the margin of the tympanic membrane perforation. The slit should be anterior to periumbo connective tissue to

create an exit route for the lateral aspect of the mediolateral graft.

11. The lateral aspect of the mesodermal graft is then placed lateral to the umbo to rest on the umbo and is then draped onto the exposed posterorinferior bony annulus region and brought laterally onto the thinned posterior bony canal wall, avoiding contact with incudostapedial joint. The placement of the graft lateral to the umbo assures an adequate space maintenance to avoid incudo-stapedial joint contact. Coaptation of this graft is also expedited by a bed of absorbable gelatin film sectors and gelatin sponge squares in the postero-inferior middle ear space, sufficient to give the graft adequate medial support for its lateral placement.

12. The posterior canal wall flap is then rolled down to cover the lateral graft placement. In essence, this is not a true mediolateral graft. It is primarily medial since it rests on the posterior bony canal wall and is covered by canal wall skin. However, there is a small exposed *lateral* segment between the slit exits at the inferior margin of the tympanic membrane margin and the covered canal wall portion. This is rapidly epithelialized during the healing period (Fig. 17–8).

TOTAL PARS TENSA PERFORATION. In every chronic perforation, large or small, great care is necessary to examine the entire medial surface of remaining tympanic membrane. *En-plaque* keratoma-squa-mous epithelium without keratoma-cyst formation frequently results from squamous epithelial mi-gration and/or keratinizing metaplasia formation so that virtually the entire pars tensa remnant is keratomatous on its medial surface. Such a kera-toma may extend anteriorly into epitympanum, protympanum, eustachian tube, or superiorly, en-veloping the malleus or incus, or posteriorly, into the aditus ad antrum, or into sinus tympani. In such major extensions, type I tympanoplasty is contraindicated. Management is described in the section on type B lesion management (Ch. 16) and requires consideration of combined mastoid-tympanoplasty-ossiculoplasty, possibly staged.

However, keratoma limited to the tympanic mem-brane is not uncommon, and mastoidectomy-ossiculec-tomy is not necessary (assuming complete exploration for possible extensions has been carried out). There is, therefore, an indication for type I tympanoplasty in keratoma limited to the tympanic membrane. An endo-meatal approach (Fig. 17–9) is appropriate in a large external auditory canal, or an endaural or post-auricular incision may be used. Total excision of keratomatous tympanic membrane is necessary, with special attention to possible retroumbo and retro-manubrial keratoma. Following such excision, a wide open middle ear, with exteriorized manubrium, long

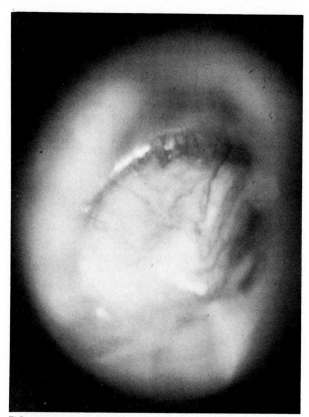

FIG. 17–8. Healed perforation after tympanoplasty.

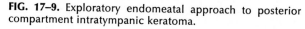

FIG. 17–9. Exploratory endomeatal approach to posterior compartment intratympanic keratoma.

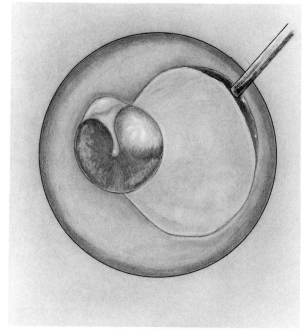

process of incus, incudostapedial joint, and stapes, is in view.

In instances of keratoma surrounding the entire malleal manubrium and/or incus or stapes, attempts at type I tympanoplasty are discontinued. In such extensive keratoma, the possibility of total removal is nil. Ossicular involvement by keratoma is common. In such cases, removal of the ossicles (radical mastoidectomy) is necessary and type I tympanoplasty is impossible. If the posterior canal wall is uninvolved by disease, keratoma removal is carried out with special attention to the sinus tympani area, and it is advisable to defer further reconstruction to a secondary stage, at which time an ossiculoplastic tympanoplasty (type II or type III) will be indicated.

The repair of total absence of the pars tensa is carried out with a large perichondrial graft similar to the procedure described for large posterior defects. The L flap incision previously described is created and the posterior flap elevated superiorly. A mediolateral graft is used. The perichondrial tragal dome concavity is used to good advantage geometrically. The lateral aspect of the perichondrial graft is placed medially after the entire hypomesotympanum area has been completely explored and found to be free of keratoma or adhesive otitis. A bed of absorbable gelatin film and sponge is built up throughout the middle ear, and the perichondrial graft is placed under the anterior bony annulus to fill the entire middle ear cavity anteriorly to the region of the malleal umbo. At the umbo region, the perichondrial graft is brought out of the middle ear laterally and allowed to rest on the malleal manubrium and umbo.

The graft should be so tailored that the posterolateral portion traverses the posterior middle ear, with the perichondrial dome concavity coming into contact with the posterior bony annulus. A new pseudofibrous annulus is, therefore, represented by the perichondrial dome concavity, the rest of the graft having been brought laterally onto the bared bony canal wall. This mediolateral placement should leave adequate space between the graft and the incudostapedial joint.

Following perichondrial graft application onto the thinned posterior bony canal wall, the L flap is rolled down to cover the perichondrial graft. The canal is packed with absorbable gelatin sponge and gauze as previously described.

Type I Tympanoplasty with Mastoidectomy

The discovery of active type A or type B disease (in addition to the tympanic membrane defect) in the sinus tympani does not necessarily rule out a type I tympanoplasty. Polyps, granulomas, limited tympanosclerosis, or limited keratoma without ossicular or epitympanic involvement are indications for mastoid exploration as part of the surgical procedure (see Ch. 12, Basic Otosurgical Procedures).

Exploration of the mastoid requires an additional incision for access. This may be endaural (intercartilaginous) or postauricular. Either incision is satisfactory. In using an endaural incision, there will be no need to modify the canal flap incision previously made. Following the incision, the anterolateral mastoid cortex periosteum is elevated, and classic removal of lateral cortical mastoid bone and cell groups is carried out. Extensions of type A or type B disease from the middle ear into the mastoid are carefully traced in a complete mastoidectomy. If there is no posterior canal wall destruction, a procedure with intact canal wall is usually feasible. However, if there is obvious posterior canal-wall necrosis and/or granulomatous osteitis of type A disease, or if type B (keratoma or tympanosclerosis) disease is present, with involvement of the incus, malleus, and/or stapes, plans for simultaneous tympanoplasty are abandoned. A thorough eradication of the type A or type B lesion is carried out by atticomastoidectomy, or by modified or classic radical mastoidectomy.

If the mastoid exploration reveals only type A disease (*e.g.*, cholesterol granuloma or polypoid granulomatosis), it is perfectly safe to resume the plans for a type I tympanoplasty following the completion of the mastoidectomy procedure as an intact-canal-wall procedure. The identical techniques previously described are carried out.

Postoperative antibiotic coverage and careful postoperative hygiene for the external auditory canal are necessary.

TYPE II (TYMPANOPLASTY–OSSICULOPLASTY)

This designates either a type I tympanoplasty accompanied by ossiculoplasty, or ossiculoplasty independently performed in the presence of an intact tympanic membrane or neotympanic membrane and may be accomplished by repositioning entire or resculptured, homogeneous, preserved ossicles (allografts). Recently, the use of prefabricated allografts has been introduced (5).

The most common lesion requiring ossiculoplasty is an absent or diseased incus. In the presence of a functioning mobile stapes and a mobile malleus, the incus defect can be corrected by replacement with the incus remnant, resculptured as an autograft, or by a precisely prefabricated preserved homograft (allograft) ossicle. (Metal and/or plastic prostheses were originally used to correct such defects, but because of frequent extrusions, such artificial protheses have been largely abandoned.)

If the stapedial crura are absent but the footplate is intact and mobile, a specially sculptured autograft or allograft can be used from the malleus-tympanic membrane complex to the footplate. Two essentials must be present: 1) a mobile, healthy stapedial footplate or footplate substitute (mesodermal autograft), and 2) a mobile malleal manubrium with an intact tensor tympani insertion. The tympanic membrane defect may be repaired simultaneously.

Columellization reconstruction techniques represent the primary aspects of ossiculoplasty. A common technique in use has been that of incus transposition (Fig. 17–10), using either an autogenous or homogeneous total or partially remodeled incus. We found transposition of the entire incus to be an unwieldy procedure with predispositions to postoperative middle-ear adhesions. The mass effect of a total incus transplant is frequently audiologically undesirable. Autogenous tragal cartilage is functionally favorable when used as a "short columella," i.e., from malleus to capitulum. It can be used when the middle ear is shallow. Cartilage loses some stiffness, but this does not significantly interfere with hearing results in the utilization of a short columella. However, it is difficult to sculpt cartilage for precise columellization use.

We now prefer the use of prefabricated allograft ossicular columellae, sculptured in the laboratory, to correct middle-ear defects. The **columella** is the interposed structure between the malleus and either the stapedial capitulum or the footplate. The short columella is interposed between the malleus and the stapedial capitulum. The long columella is interposed between the malleus and footplate or neofootplate membrane.

FIG. 17–10. Autogenous incus remodeling for use in ossiculoplasty.

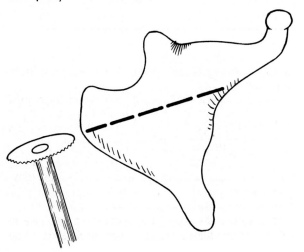

The prefabricated ossicular columella can be locked into a surgically prepared malleal trough laterally (Fig. 17–11). A posterior malleal neck trough is made by careful use of cutting and diamond burrs above the level of the crossover region of the chorda tympani to the malleus. The trough is approximately 1 × 1.5 mm in dimensions.

The prefabricated allograft ossicles are prepared in an approved ear tissue bank, observing tested procedures. A short-saddle columella is used from malleus to stapes and a long-rod columella from malleus to oval window. The short-saddle columella is prefabricated from an allograft malleus. The long-rod columella is prefabricated from an allograft incus. Both the long columella and the short columella may be prepared from either right or left ossicles for use on either side.

The prefabrication is carried out with the use of a large diamond burr. The ossicle may be hand-held or held in a forceps. Since the essential process is that of sculpture, technical dexterity is obviously necessary (Fig. 17–12).

The Short Columella (Saddle)—Malleal Trough to Stapes

A malleus allograft is used. The final shape is an elongated cone with the base (medial end) hollowed out to form a saddle to fit over the capitulum, neck, and stapes tendon. The dimensions vary from 3.5–4.5 mm in overall length. The saddle is approximately 1.50–1.75 mm in diameter. The lateral rod end for attachment to the malleal trough is 0.75–1 mm in diameter, and is scored to provide a slightly rough surface to expedite fibrous tissue anchorage.

The Long Columella (Rod)—Malleal Trough to Oval Window

An incus allograft is used. The final shape is that of a slightly tapered rod.

The length of the rod varies from 5.75–6.5 mm. The lateral end is identical in measurement to that of the saddle, 0.75–1 mm in diameter. The medial end is slightly narrower, 0.65–0.8 mm.

"Bone-Rivet" Columella

In relatively unusual instances to be described later, rivet modifications of both long and short columellae may be necessary, if malleal trough preparation is not feasible. Lateral attachment is secured by deliberate penetration through the perimanubrial region of the pars tensa. This columella has lateral ends comparable in dimensions to those described above, but the columella is capped with a flat head.

Surgical Techniques—Indications and Contraindications

The malleal trough technique is adaptable to most forms of repair problems—i.e., intact tympanic membrane or large or small tympanic membrane perforations in any location (either the pars tensa or the pars flaccida). It is assumed that adequate removal of the lesion has preceded the reconstruction, either as a combined or as a staged procedure. The essential ana-

Chorda tympani

Tensor tympani tendon

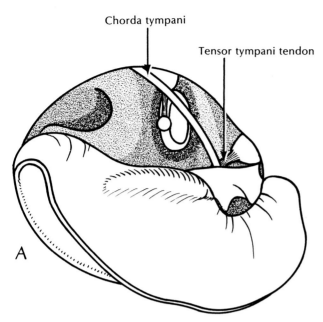

A

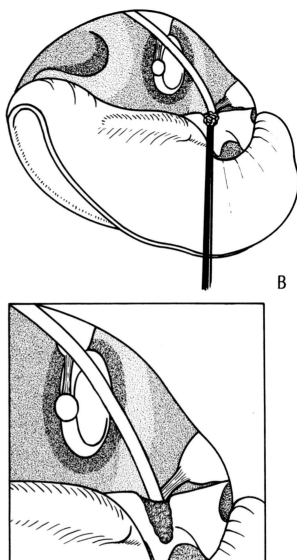

B

C

FIG. 17–11. A. Elevation of canal wall, tympanic membrane, and soft tissue flap. Malleal neck and short process are denuded of periosteum. **B.** Beginning preparation of malleal trough, lateral to level of insertion of tensor tympani tendon, and superior to chorda tympani malleal crossover. **C.** Completed trough in malleal neck and short process (Goodhill V, Westerbergh AM, Davis C: Trans Am Acad Ophthalmol Otolaryngol 78:417–420, 1974)

tomic prerequisite is an intact mobile head, neck, and short process of the malleus, and an intact tensor tympani tendon. It is also desirable, for stabilization purposes, that the anterior epitympanic pouch system (Prussak's pouch and the anterior pouch of von Tröltsch) and anterior ligament and tympanic folds be intact.

An appropriate columella is selected from the sterile collection available after middle ear measurements have been obtained.

The malleal trough having been prepared as previously described, the lateral end of a short or long columella is fitted into the trough (Fig. 17–13, A, B), so that it engages snugly. Minor modifications of trough dimensions are made if necessary to secure snug engagement.

If there is an inadequacy in posterior pars flaccida tissue components, the lateral end of the columella in the trough should be covered by a tragal cartilage-perichondrium graft (Fig. 17–13, C). The cartilage stopple will act as a "cork" over the shaft in the trough. The perichondrium will protect the trough–columella area and is in turn covered laterally by reflection of the remaining components of the posterior pars flaccida, the soft tissues of von Tröltsch's, and Prussak's spaces. If there is a total posterior perforation, the shaft-trough-cartilage-perichondrium area is covered by the

perichondrial graft used to repair the tympanic membrane defect.

When a short (saddle—golf tee) columella is used, the saddle is carefully manipulated into good contact with the stapes (Fig. 17–13 A). With the use of a long (rod) columella, the medial end is placed over the oval window (Fig. 17–13 B). If the footplate is intact, gentle elevation of the mucoperiosteum should be followed by placement of two 1×1 mm perichondrial grafts on the footplate to stabilize and protect the position of the rod in relation to the footplate.

If there is a preexisting fibrous oval window as a result of either surgical repair following removal of the

FIG. 17–12. A. Prefabrication of saddle (short) columella from either right or left malleus. **B.** Prefabrication of rod (long) columella from either right or left incus. **C.** Beginning sculpture prefabrication of golf-tee (short) homograft from malleus. Diamond burr is used. **D.** Saddle concavity produced with diamond burr at base of pyramid-shaped saddle. **E.** Lateral end scored. **F.** Saddle will vary from 3 to 4.5 mm in length. **G.** Diamond burr sculpture to produce rod (long) columella from incus. **H.** Scoring of lateral end. **I.** Completed rod (long) columella measures 5.75 to 6.5 mm. **J.** Specal saddle columella with penetrating cap—"rivet." **K.** Special rod columella with penetrating cap—"rivet." (Goodhill V, Westerbergh AM, Davis C: Trans Am Acad Ophthalmol Otolaryngol 78:417–420, 1974)

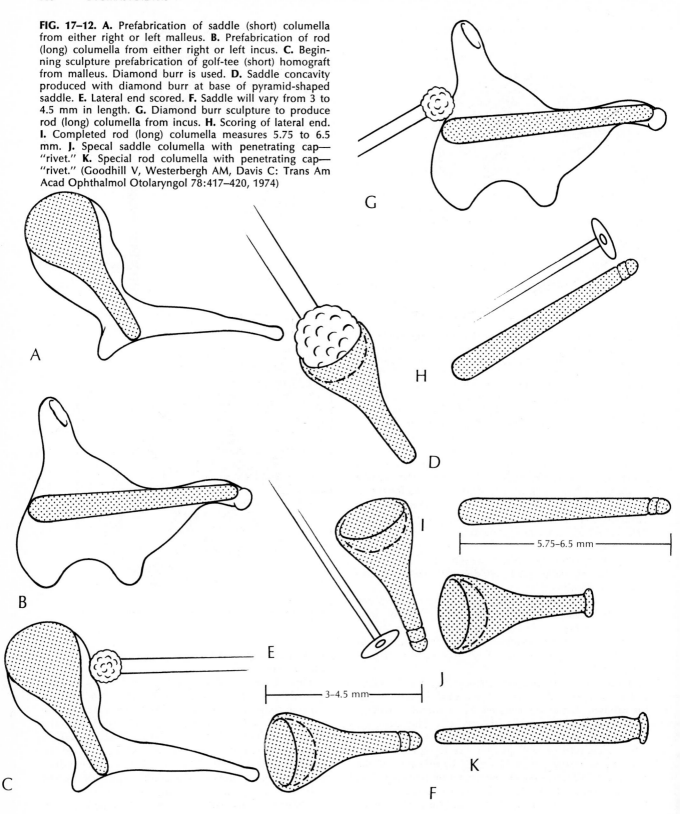

FIG. 17–13. A. Golf-tee columella in position over stapedial capitulum. **B.** Rod columella in position on footplate surrounded by tissue grafts for stabilization. **C.** Cross section of trough columella junction showing closure of trough either by reflected soft tissue posterior flap or by use of cartilage perichondrium "stopple." (Goodhill V, Westerbergh AM, Davis C: Trans Am Acad Ophthalmol Otolaryngol 78:417–420, 1974)

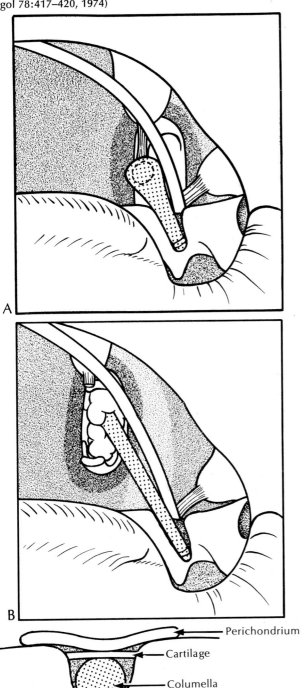

Perichondrium

Cartilage

Columella

Trough

bony footplate, or spontaneous neomembrane regeneration of the oval window, the area must be carefully examined to make sure that the membrane is sufficiently thick to receive the rod without danger of perforation. If it is a thin neomembrane, it should be covered by a concave canoe-shaped fresh perichondrial graft.

Special Problems

The anatomic prerequisite for malleal trough columellae is an intact mobile head, neck, and short process of the malleus, and an intact tensor tympani tendon. If the manubrium has no attachment to these epitympanic structures, or if the malleal head is absent or completely separated from the neck and short process, the trough approach may not be possible.

One alternative is the rivet perimanubrial technique, which utilizes the principle of a projecting columella, the lateral end of which is exterior to the tympanic membrane (Fig. 17–14). Following diamond-burr dermabrasion of the perimanubrial area, a sharp stab incision, 2.5 mm in length, is made through the postmanubrial periosteum and radial fibers above the umbo.

In the long columella application (no stapes arch), the rod is introduced laterally through this stab. It is topped with a flat head to maintain it in contact with the manubrium and to prevent it from slipping. Its medial end is placed as described before.

If the stapes is present, a short columella is introduced from a medial approach, the cap being introduced through the slit. The medial placement of the saddle on the stapes is as previously described. The presenting cap lateral to the tympanic membrane, in either the long or the short columella, is covered by a small perichondrial graft.

Another alternative is the use of a crutch-saddle or a crutch-rod prefabricated columella. The crutch portion is placed laterally, in contiguity with mobile manubrium. Friction forces are used to maintain slight tension between the crutch-manubrium region and the stapes capitulum or between the crutch-manubrium region and the footplate region.

TYPE III TYMPANOPLASTY (MYRINGOSTAPEDIOPEXY)

The basic type III myringostapediopexy of Wullstein is a useful procedure when the stapedial arch is high (long mediolateral dimension) and the tympanic or neotympanic membrane is displaced medially so that the tympanic membrane or the umbo region of the tympanic membrane-manubrium complex can easily contact the stapedial capitulum. If there is adequate lateral projection of the stapedial capitulum, a direct connection between it and the tympanic membrane or membrane substitute may be simpler and more desirable than the placement of an ossicle between them (Fig. 17–15).

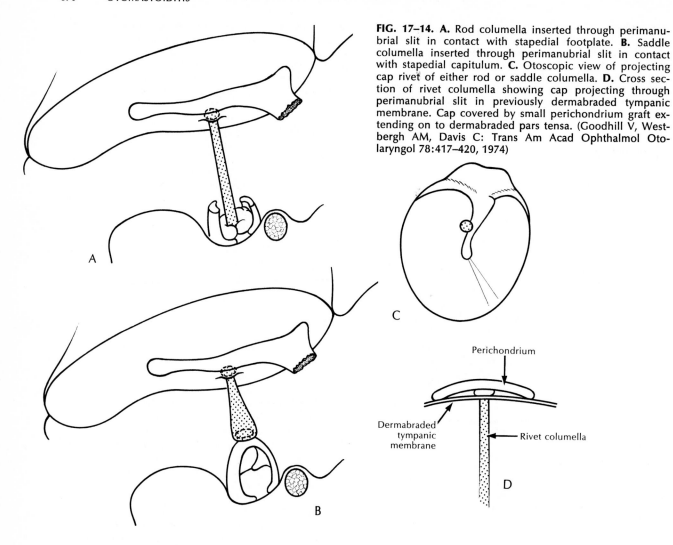

FIG. 17–14. A. Rod columella inserted through perimanubrial slit in contact with stapedial footplate. **B.** Saddle columella inserted through perimanubrial slit in contact with stapedial capitulum. **C.** Otoscopic view of projecting cap rivet of either rod or saddle columella. **D.** Cross section of rivet columella showing cap projecting through perimanubrial slit in previously dermabraded tympanic membrane. Cap covered by small perichondrium graft extending on to dermabraded pars tensa. (Goodhill V, Westbergh AM, Davis C: Trans Am Acad Ophthalmol Otolaryngol 78:417–420, 1974)

In the event that the dimensions of a middle ear space are so narrow that the entire graft has a tendency to adhere medially, not only to the stapedial capitulum but to other medial tympanic surfaces, the graft is tailored primarily from the tragal cartilage so that it includes a circumferential cartilage "batten" for increased stiffness (Fig. 17–16). This cartilage batten will aid in maintaining a lateral position for the graft since the peripheral cartilage segment will be placed in contiguity with the bony annulus. Thus, the medial aspect of the graft covers only the stapedial capitulum and contacts no other surfaces of the medial tympanic wall.

If the stapes arch, incus, malleus, and entire tympanic membrane are absent, tympanoplasty and allograft ossiculopasty, as described, may be considered, with use of a total tympanic membrane-ossicular allograft technique.

An alternative autograft technique involves use of tragal perichondrium and tragal cartilage, used either separately or jointly, as a T cartilage graft.

In the first (separate) procedure, one or two stages may be employed. A perichondrial neotympanic-membrane graft is applied to the annular margins as a lateral graft. A cartilage columella is prepared from the remaining tragal cartilage. It is placed in contact with the crural remnants and footplate medially and the perichondrial graft laterally (Fig. 17–17).

When used as a joint one-stage procedure a composite T columella-perichondrial graft is preferred (Figs. 17–18, 17–19).

TYPE IV TYMPANOPLASTY (CAVUM MINOR)

The type IV (cavum minor) operation is used when the lateral epitympanic wall is missing and there is no possibility for establishment of an epitympanic air space. A graft is placed below the oval window niche to create a sealed air space

FIG. 17–15. Myringostapediopexy. Perichondrial graft used for conventional type III tympanoplasty with convexity placed medially to contact stapedial capitulum. (Goodhill V: Arch Otolaryngol 85:490, 1967. Copyright 1967, American Medical Association)

FIG. 17–16. A. Circumferential cartilage batten still attached to one surface of a total perichondrial autograft. **B.** Composite perichondrial cartilage batten autograft in position lateral to deepitheliated annulus with convexity of graft in contact with stapedial capitulum. (Goodhill V: Arch Otolaryngol 85:490, 1967. Copyright 1967, American Medical Association)

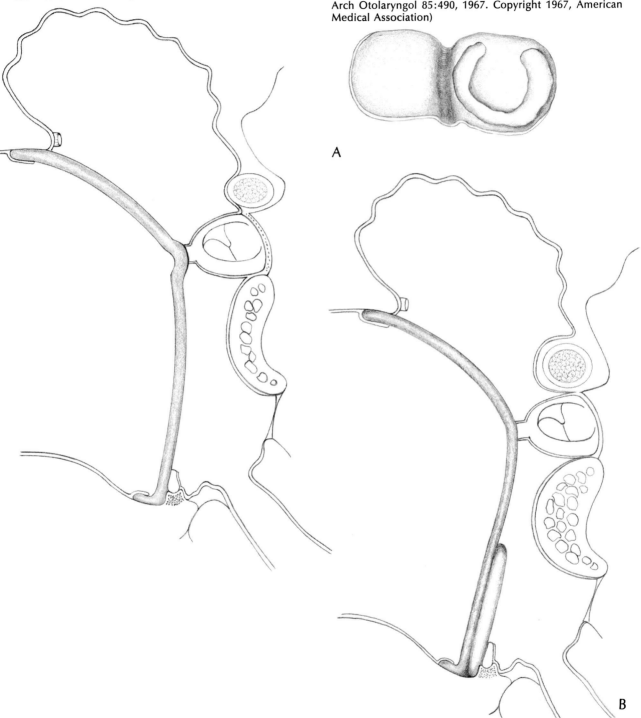

A

B

between the eustachian tube and round window niche. This shielding procedure can result in 20- to 30-dB hearing gains (see Ch. 12, Basic Otosurgical Procedures).

The cavum minor type IV operation is used infrequently. It can only result in a hearing gain comparable to that with the type V tympanoplasty (fenestration operation).

An alternative is a total allograft reconstruction involving the use of preserved tympanic membrane, ossicles, and canal wall bone. Another alternative is creation of an epitympanic wall by an autograft cartilage graft or an allograft bone graft. These procedures are still in experimental phases and are not always successful.

TYPE V TYMPANOPLASTY (SEMICIRCULAR CANAL FENESTRATION)

This approach is possible in cases with a mastoid bowl and no posterior bony canal wall, accompanied by obliterative fixation of the oval window, comparable to that seen in obliterative otosclerosis (see Ch. 19, Otosclerosis). It requires fenestration of the horizontal semicircular canal, with a special epidermal flap and a hemitympanic membrane bridged over the facial nerve to contact a prepared horizontal semicircular canal fenestra (see Fig. 12–16 G). Acoustically there is a loss of aerial ratio transformer function. However, a hearing improvement can result from a shearing force transfer mechanism between the hemitympanic-membrane–skin-flap complex and the fenestra. Moderate degrees of hearing gain that may reach 25–30 dB air conduction speech reception thresholds are primarily attributable to specific improvements in hearing at 2 kHz. In some cases this may mean a gain from a preoperative 60-dB level to a postoperative 35- to 40-dB level, which is significant and valuable if no alternatives are available. Although it may seem less than perfect to the patient, it may allow the use of a less powerful, less inconvenient hearing aid. Under certain circumstances, such unaided hearing may be adequate, depending upon the acoustic environment.

SPECIAL TYMPANOPLASTY TECHNIQUES

STAGING AND INTACT-CANAL-WALL TECHNIQUES

The understandable enthusiasm for intact-canal-wall tympanoplasty techniques is based upon the desirability of avoiding the exteriorized cavity (mastoid bowl—mastoidostomy) of radical mastoidectomy. Although exteriorized mastoid cavities

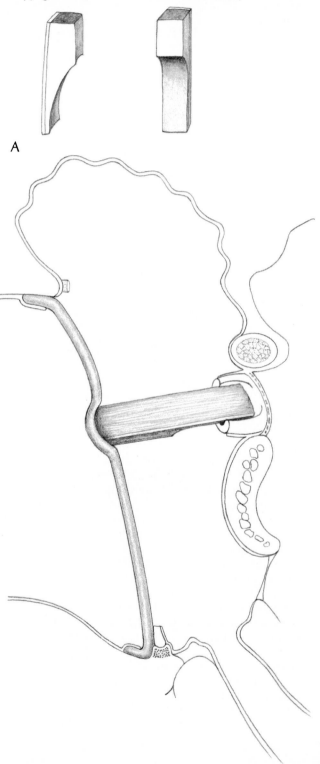

FIG. 17–17. A. Prepared cartilage columella with perichondrial surface still intact on one side. **B.** Conventional cartilage columella in position on stapedial footplate, its lateral extremity in contact with convexity of perichondrial autograft. (Goodhill V: Arch Otolaryngol 85:490, 1967. Copyright 1967, American Medical Association)

A

FIG. 17–18. A. Perichondrium elevated from both surfaces of tragal cartilage. **B.** Tailoring of tragal cartilage to create T cartilage-perichondrial composite graft. **C.** Medial aspect of columella thinned and perichondrium shaped to proper size. **D.** T cartilage-perichondrial graft in place, its medial aspect in contact with mobile stapedial footplate after partial amputation of crura. Note adequate tympanic air space. (Goodhill V: Arch Otolaryngol 85:490, 1967. Copyright 1967, American Medical Association)

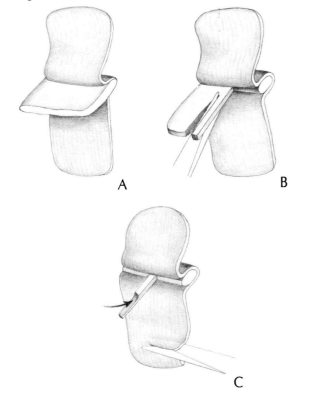
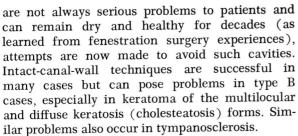

A   B

C

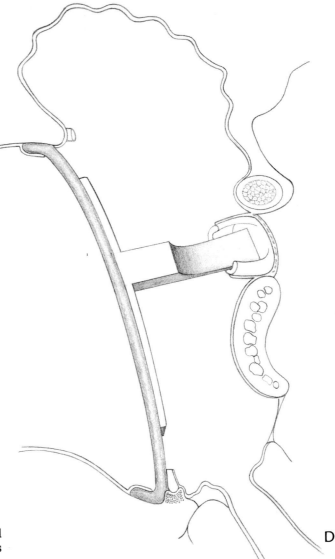

D

are not always serious problems to patients and can remain dry and healthy for decades (as learned from fenestration surgery experiences), attempts are now made to avoid such cavities. Intact-canal-wall techniques are successful in many cases but can pose problems in type B cases, especially in keratoma of the multilocular and diffuse keratosis (cholesteatosis) forms. Similar problems also occur in tympanosclerosis.

Recurrences are not rare in intact-canal-wall procedures for type B lesions and also occur in type A lesions due to resistant organisms. Some surgeons employ only the intact-canal-wall technique and advocate deliberate secondary "prophylactic" operations to inspect the middle ear and mastoid areas. Patients are told that they will require secondary operations in 1 or 2 years, even if they are asymptomatic. The reason for such concern is most commonly attributable to deep keratoma within the sinus tympani area of the posterior middle ear region.

The standard tissue graft (neotympanic membrane) tympanoplastic reconstruction may obscure otoscopic evidence of recurrent keratoma or other lesions.

In attempts to obtain in-depth visualization of the sinus tympani area, a number of procedures have been devised that involve delicate bone dissection in the facial recess area, and extensive intramastoid dissection. In the commonly infantile, densely sclerotic temporal bone encountered in many keratoma cases, the facial recess approach is accompanied by significant surgical risks to the facial nerve and to the horizontal semicircular canal.

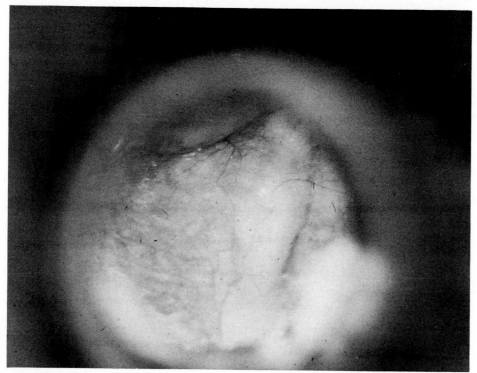

FIG. 17–19. Postoperative cartilage perichondrium T-graft reconstruction of middle ear (with neither ossicles nor drum before operation).

Two alternative techniques have been introduced to minimize the problems in intact-canal-wall operations of 1) unrecognized recurrent keratoma behind a tissue graft, demanding routine staging, and 2) major bone dissections in the facial recess area with risks of seventh-nerve damage and horizontal semicircular canal damage. These two techniques are the induction tympanoplasty using absorbable gelatin film (no graft) and the circumferential tympanomastoid access approach to the sinus tympani area.

REGENERATIVE (INDUCTION) TYMPANOPLASTY
(NO-GRAFT TYMPANOPLASTY)

Spontaneous cicatricial neotympanic membrane healing has been observed frequently during the past century of ear surgery (6, 3). Such neomembrane formation is due to an induction process that probably relates to chemical characteristics in the fibrous tympanic annulus (Fig. 17–20). An inductive signal originates from the cross-linked insoluble structure of fibrous proteins. It is a chemical substance probably related to collagen protein and mucopolysaccharides.

In some cases of advanced type A lesions and in many type B lesions, the lesion, the location, the loss of function, and clinical laboratory findings may indicate a poor prognosis for a tissue graft tympanoplasty. Since it has been observed repeatedly that some tympanic membrane defects heal spontaneously, advantage was taken of this phenomenon to create an alternative to the dilemma of intact-canal-wall retention in some borderline cases. The possibility of creating a safe "bridge" for spontaneous neomembrane formation has been realized in 40–50% of cases by induction using absorbable gelatin film (no-graft tympanoplasty) (1).

Neomembrane formation from the annulus may be enhanced in an inductive manner when the gelatin film and the annulus are in contact (Fig. 17–21). This concept was the basis of the description of the process of "annular induction and basement membrane" formation in inductive tympanoplasty (2).

The absorbable gelatin film (Gelfilm) is sterile and nonantigenic. It is nonporous and, therefore, nonhemostatic. It is approximately 0.075 mm thick and when dry it has the appearance and texture of cellophane. When moistened, it assumes a rubbery consistency and can then be cut to

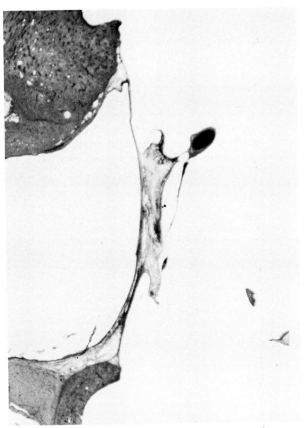

FIG. 17–20. Experimental induction of neotympanic membrane formation by gelatin film in a cat. (Low power)

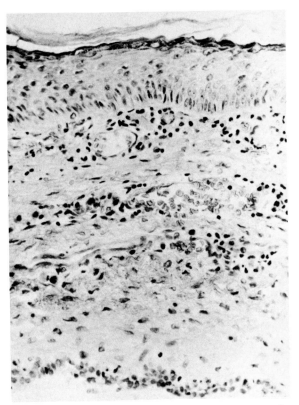

FIG. 17–21. Neotympanic membrane 21 months after placement of a gelatin film disc; appropriate epithelial covering on upper and lower surfaces with well-vascularized fibrous core simulating normal tympanic membrane. (H&E, × 300) (Harris I, Barton S, Gussen R *et al.: Laryngoscope* 81:6–7, 1971)

desired sizes and shapes and fitted to rounded or irregular surfaces. It is most commonly used in the form of circular or oval disks or as sectors prepared from disks.

An assortment of sizes of the disks are quickly and easily obtained by utilizing ear speculums in a biscuit-cutter fashion. The film is placed on a plastic cutting block and various size disks and sectors are quickly prepared, providing the surgeon with a choice of inserts (Fig. 17–22).

After complete removal of middle ear or mastoid lesions, the disk is placed lateral to the fibrous annulus and into contact with healthy ossicles to simulate a type I, II, or III tympanoplastic repair (Fig. 17–23). The skin wall of the external auditory canal is replaced so that it is in coaptation contact with the gelatin film disk or partially covers it laterally. The external auditory canal is then packed with absorbable gelatin foam (Gelfoam) for pressure stabilization of the position of the disk. The outer canal is packed with gauze.

CIRCUMFERENTIAL TYMPANOMASTOID ACCESS TO SINUS TYMPANI

The sinus tympani problem is extensive in type B lesions and plays a major role in recurrences and in elective staging techniques in intact-canal-wall tympanoplasty.

The standard approach, with posterior tympanotomy to the facial recess requires major temporal bone removal through a transmastoid posterior tympanotomy with dissection of the facial recess to visualize the sinus tympani from a posterior to anterior view through the mastoid cavity (4).

This approach to the posterior tympanum and sinus tympani requires the removal of facial recess bone between the vertical segment of the facial nerve and the chorda tympani to create a communication from posterior to anterior—from the mastoid into the middle ear. The bone removal frequently requires exposure of the vertical course of the facial nerve and close to a

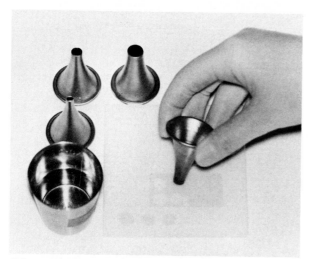

FIG. 17–22. Sheet of gelatin film is dipped in saline and placed on plastic cutting block. Ear speculums are used in a "biscuit cutting" technique to punch out assorted size discs. (Harris I, Barton S, Gussen R et al.: Laryngoscope 81: 6–7, 1971)

"blue line" endosteal view of the horizontal semicircular canal. There are hazards due to variations that depend upon pneumatization, duration, and extent of the disease. Although this posterior tympanotomy-facial-recess approach does bring into view much of the posterior tympanum and sinus tympani, it is impossible, through this approach, to obtain a view of the complete posterorinferior and the posteromedial extensions of the sinus tympani, which may measure anywhere from 1–6 mm. In some instances, it is necessary to uncover the facial nerve and the entire course of the stapedius muscle to see retropyramidal and medial pyramidal aspects of the sinus tympani. Even if such vital structures are uncovered, blind instrumentation is still conceded to be necessary in certain instances.

An alternative approach has been in use for several years. The anteroposterior aspect of a circumferential access approach allows direct view of this critical area. The surgeon standing in front of the patient can look posteriorly to explore the sinus tympani in a posterior, superior, and especially in a medial direction in its relationship to the eminentia pyramidalis and to the vertical segment of the facial nerve. Thus, the difficult and occasionally hazardous posterior tympanotomy-facial recess approach can be entirely avoided in many cases, and the area that is so frustrating in the surgical approach to extensive sinus tympani keratoma (cholesteatoma) can be dealt with by the simple expedient of looking toward the disease instead of trying to look underneath the facial nerve from a posterior approach. In addition, unnecessary bone removal, conducive to adhesions, is avoided.

This "circumnavigation" surgical approach to the temporal bone from a posteroinferior to an anteroinferior position makes possible 270° of visualization (Figs. 17–24 through 17–26).

OBLITERATIVE TECHNIQUES—MUSCULOPLASTY

Another approach to the avoidance of a mastoid bowl or mastoidostomy is to fill the mastoid cavity with viable tissue or nonviable material so that the cavity is no longer a bony hole but has been virtually obliterated by a tissue graft or plastic

FIG. 17–23. Technique using gelatin film: 1) endaural approach; 2) preservation of bony and fibrous annulus; 3) complete lateral deepithelialization; 4) lateral placement of film disc. (Harris I, Barton S, Gussen R et al.: Laryngoscope 81:6–7, 1971)

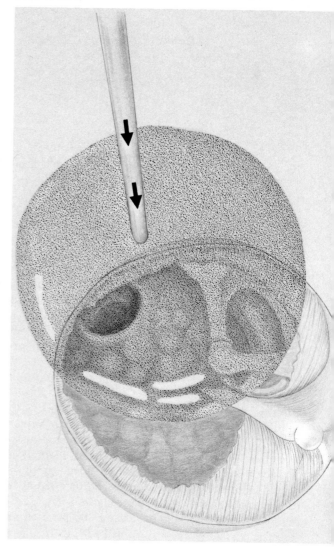

implant. The most common approach to accomplish this purpose is musculoplasty. Enthusiasm for musculoplasty techniques has varied during the past decade. In a combined one-stage mastoidectomy and tympanoplasty, the posterior bony canal wall is removed in most cases. The bony bridge may be narrowed and preserved in other cases. The external auditory canal is recreated "in kind" by a fascial graft using fascia temporalis, and the mastoid cavity is obliterated by a flap of subcutaneous tissue and muscle from the temporal muscle. This is usually a rotation flap rather than a free graft. It is possible to obliterate a cavity successfully by musculoplasty and thus do away with the problem of an open mastoid bowl. However, in our experience, such procedures frequently are followed, several years later, by shrinkage of the muscle and spontaneous reopening of the previously closed mastoid bowl. In other instances, musculoplasty procedures can be followed by such postoperative complications as recurrent deep keratoma or polypoid granulation tissue due to reinfection in the mastoid cells.

SUMMARY

1. In the light of recent surgical advances in mastoid-tympanoplasty and with due consideration to the 4L equations of lesion, location, loss of function, and laboratory findings, the prognosis for most cases of chronic otomastoiditis is very good. However, no one standard technique of mastoid-tympanoplasty can be advocated for the solution of the many diverse problems that occur in the middle ear and mastoid.

2. The planning of a reconstructive tympanoplastic procedure should not compete with, or compromise, the first objective of treatment for the temporal bone disease—namely, adequate eradication of an irreversible lesion.

3. Compulsive attempts to close tympanic membrane perforations to restore hearing or to avoid exteriorizing operations should be avoided in certain specific 4L equation problems. Tympanic reconstruction is not always innocuous to audiovestibular and other functions.

4. In some cases, the wise course of action is adequate exenteration of the lesion and exteriorization, for observation and for local medical therapy. Hearing improvement by means of hearing aid use may be more prudent than tympanoplasty in such cases.

5. With the growth of tympanoplastic experience, more frequent use of deliberate surgical staging will probably be adopted.

FIG. 17–24. Posteroanterior view and anteroposterior view of operating table arrangements. (Goodhill V: Ann Otol Rhinol Laryngol 82:547–553, 1973)

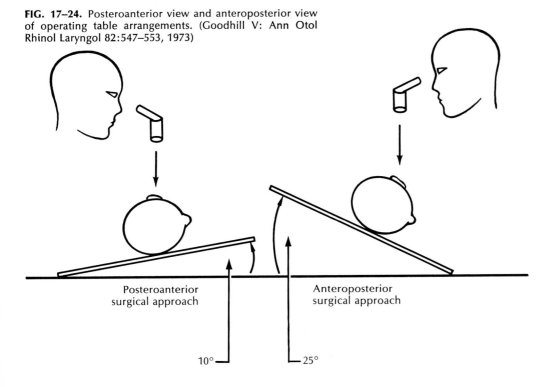

Posteroanterior
surgical approach

Anteroposterior
surgical approach

10°

25°

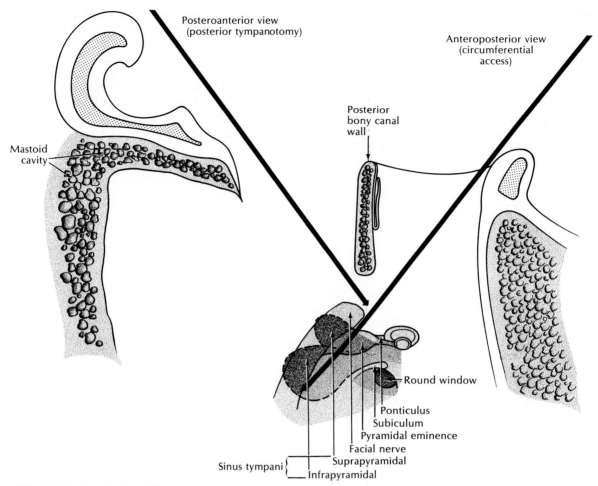

FIG. 17–25. Visualization differences between the posteroanterior and anteroposterior views. (Goodhill V: Ann Otol Rhinol Laryngol 82:547–553, 1973)

FIG. 17–26. Circumferential access approach. (Goodhill V: Ann Otol Rhinol Laryngol 82: 547–553, 1973)

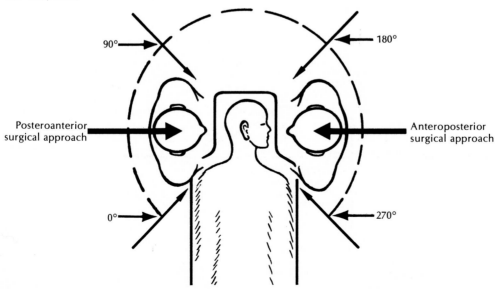

REFERENCES

1. Goodhill V: Deliberate "spontaneous" tympanoplasty. Roles of annular induction and basement membranes. Ann Otol Rhinol Laryngol 75:866–880, 1966
2. Goodhill V: Cholesteatoma, mastoiditis and gelfilm induction tympanoplasty. Trans Pac Coast Oto-ophthalmol Soc 52:217–242, 1971
3. Goodhill V: Circumferential tympano-mastoid access. The sinus tympani area. Ann Otol Rhinol Laryngol 82:547–553, 1973
4. Goodhill V, Westerbergh AM, Davis C: Prefabricated homografts in ossiculoplasty. Trans Am Acad Ophthalmol Otolaryngol 78: ORL 411–422, 1974
5. Harris I, Barton S, Gussen R et al.: Gelfilm induced neotympanic membrane in tympanoplasty. Laryngoscope 81:1826–1837, 1971
6. Politzer A: A Textbook of the Diseases of the Ear for Students and Practitioners, 5th ed. Philadelphia, Lea & Febiger, 1909
7. Wullstein H: Theory and practice of tympanoplasty. Laryngoscope 66:1076–1093, 1956
8. Zöllner F: The principles of plastic surgery of the sound conducting apparatus. J Laryngol Otol 69:637–652, 1955

SUGGESTED READING

Sheehy JL: Surgery of chronic otitis media. In Maloney WH (ed): Otolaryngology, Vol. II. New York, Harper and Row, 1973

18

COMPLICATIONS OF OTOMASTOIDITIS

Complications of otomastoiditis may be encountered in both acute and chronic cases of otomastoiditis. The most dramatic acute otomastoiditis complication is meningitis in an infant or young child. An example of a less severe chronic complication is a slowly developing labyrinthine fistula with episodic vertigo, in the course of chronic otomastoiditis that has been relatively silent for many years, except for intermittent episodes of otorrhea and hearing loss.

Facial nerve paralysis may occur either secondary to the disease itself or secondary to surgery for otomastoiditis.

A fistula may occur in the seventh nerve bony canal, in the oval window niche, the round window niche, in any one of the three semicircular canals, or in any combination of these areas.

Petrous apicitis (petrositis Gradenigo's syndrome) is a complication involving isolated cellular diploetic or sclerotic areas within the petrous apex that are either contiguous with a generalized cellular otomastoiditis or separate and loculated.

Thrombophlebitis of intracranial venous sinuses occurs either in acute or chronic otomastoiditis. Most commonly, there is involvement of the lateral (sigmoid) sinus, with occasional involvement of the jugular bulb and internal jugular vein.

Otogenic (otitic) meningitis occurs in very young infants, less commonly in older children or adults. It may be an acute concomitant of, or sequel to, acute otitis media or chronic otomastoiditis.

Brain abscesses (subdural, intracerebral, cerebellar) may result from contiguous mastoid lesions or as a result of retrograde thrombophlebitic spread from acute or chronic otomastoiditis.

Otitic hydrocephalus (intracranial, otogenic cerebrospinal fluid hypertension) is a relatively uncommon complication due to thrombophlebitis and a defect in arachnoid absorption.

Cerebrospinal otorrhea may result from dural or bony lesions either in otomastoiditis or as a result of external or surgical trauma.

Any combination of these complications may occur. A high degree of suspicion and alertness to intratemporal and extratemporal intracranial complications must accompany the clinical management of otomastoiditis.

FACIAL NERVE (SEVENTH NERVE) PARALYSIS

Bell's palsy, the most common type of facial nerve paralysis, is a disease of either viral or vascular origin, unrelated to otomastoiditis. An apparent Bell's palsy may be a facial paralysis directly related to either diagnosed or unrecognized occult otomastoiditis. Seventh nerve paralysis may occur as a result of otomastoiditis or as the iatrogenic result of surgical management of otomastoiditis.

Facial nerve paralysis in the course of otomastoiditis can be the result of preexisting bony canal dehiscence in the horizontal portion, the posterior genu, or the vertical portion. Such a dehiscence may predispose to direct inflammatory involvement of the seventh nerve perineurium in its intratemporal course during acute otitis media or acute otomastoiditis but more frequently during the course of chronic otomastoiditis.

The onset of seventh nerve paralysis with otomastoiditis calls for immediate careful study for the site of lesion and degree of nerve damage (see Ch. 28, Seventh Nerve Diagnostic Techniques and Ch. 30, Seventh Nerve Lesions and Injuries). In many instances, surgical exposure of the seventh nerve is essential without delay.

Facial nerve paralysis can occur almost simultaneously with the onset of acute otitis media, particularly in an infant or young child, in whom the seventh nerve bony canal is incompletely formed. Such seventh nerve paralysis calls for active surgical intervention (myringotomy), intensive antibiotic therapy, and consideration of early atticomastoidectomy and possible seventh nerve decompression.

Complete seventh nerve paralysis noticed immediately following any surgical procedure for otomastoiditis is an immediate indication for complete surgical exposure of the course of the nerve from geniculate ganglion to stylomastoid foramen. Although postoperative seventh nerve paralysis may be attributable to traumatic edema, and may be a transitory neuropraxia, the paralysis should be considered presumptive evidence of seventh nerve trauma until proved otherwise by immediate reexploration of the mastoid.

If there is anesthesiologic contraindication to prolonging such surgical intervention, seventh nerve exploration should be undertaken as soon as possible in a second-stage operation.

The extent of surgical exposure depends upon individual judgment. It may be adequate to expose the nerve from geniculate ganglion to stylomastoid foramen. Some surgeons prefer to slit the perineurium, and others advise simple exposure and removal of possible penetrating bone fragments.

If reexploration shows actual surgical destruction of a portion of the facial nerve, immediate reconstruction is indicated. This may be accomplished by rerouting and end-to-end anastomosis or by a nerve graft. If rerouting and anastomosis is not possible, an autograft from the greater auricular nerve is taken, interposed between freshened cut ends, sutured superiorly and inferiorly with 6-0 sutures, and covered with absorbable gelatin film (Gelfilm) or polymeric silicone (Silastic) to prevent fibrous tissue ingrowth (see Ch. 30, Seventh Nerve Lesions and Injuries).

LABYRINTH FISTULA—LABYRINTHITIS OSSIFICANS

Labyrinthine fistula is most commonly the sequel of keratoma (cholesteatoma) or tympanosclerosis in type B chronic otomastoiditis although it may occur in type A (granulomatous polypoid) disease. The most common location for such a fistula is in the dome of the horizontal semicircular canal. The fistula may be total, with complete exposure of the perilymphatic space, or subtotal, with bone erosion and only marginal exposure of the perilymphatic space endosteum (1) (Fig. 18–1).

The most common sign of fistula is vertigo accompanied by spontaneous nystagmus, which may be manifest or which may be detected only on electronystagmographic vestibular examination. Dry calorization electronystagmography will usually show a hypoactive response. Occasionally a hyperactive response on the affected side will be demonstrated.

Acute labyrinthine fistula is uncommon during the course of acute otomastoiditis. It may occur with acute fulminating beta *Streptococcus hemolyticus* infections and may accompany other complications, such as seventh nerve paralysis.

In chronic otomastoiditis, a fistula may occur not only in the horizontal semicircular canal but in any of the semicircular canals, depending upon mastoid process pneumatization and upon the lesion, *i.e.*, keratoma (cholesteatoma), tympanosclerosis, or granuloma. A fistula may occur through the oval window following necrosis of the stapedial arch and footplate, or through the bony cochlear wall (1) (Fig. 18–2). This will occur more commonly with a keratoma than with tympanosclerosis or granulomatosis, but it may occur with any otomastoid lesion. With such a fistula there will be a slow, but occasionally rather sudden, hearing loss due to cochlear involvement, with vertigo as a concomitant. Comparable lesions occur occasionally in the round window, with rupture through the round window membrane and fistulization into the scala tympani.

It is possible for a fistula to develop with a delicate monomeric membrane separating the bony lesion from the scala vestibuli perilymph space or scala tympani perilymphatic space.

A horizontal semicircular canal fistula may develop slowly. As long as a shielding membrane remains between the lesion and the perilymph space, the fistula may remain asymptomatic, although vertigo is not infrequent.

The surgical management of fistula requires delicate techniques to remove the necrotizing lesion without opening the perilymph space. It may be accomplished frequently with maintenance of normal cochlear and vestibular function.

A quiet, latent, unsuspected labyrinthine fistula may be encountered during a surgical procedure for otomastoiditis in a patient who has had no vertigo and no change in hearing. Removal of a keratoma lesion or a tympanosclerotic plaque from the region of the horizontal or vertical semicircular canals or the labyrinthine oval window or round window areas requires high magnification and delicate microsurgical technique to prevent penetration into a delicately sealed perilymphatic system.

The management of a surgically encountered fistula requires delicate microsurgical removal of the specific etiologic lesion and closure of the fistulous area in the otic capsule by a tissue graft of either tragal perichondrium or fascia temporalis.

Labyrinthitis ossificans, in contrast to labyrinthine fistula, produces new bone formation. In most cases the lesion starts in the round window region. Suga and Lindsay (5) have described the lesion as occlusion of the round window by new bone and fibrous tissue (Fig. 18–3). A mixed conductive cochlear hearing loss will result from this type of occlusion. The hearing loss, however, may become severe or total with continued ossification.

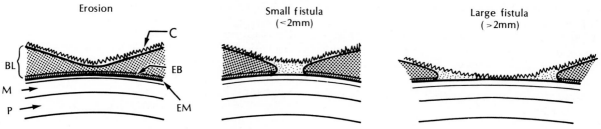

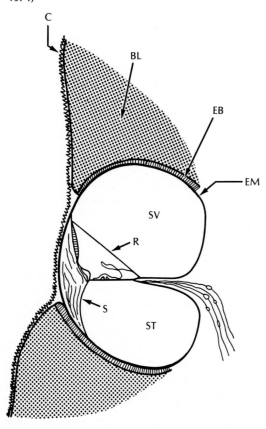

FIG. 18–1. Histologic structures involved in erosion and fistulization of a bony semicircular canal. **BL,** bony labyrinth; **C,** cholesteatoma matrix; **EB,** endosteal bone; **EM,** endosteal membrane; **M,** membranous semicircular canal; **P,** perilymphatic space. (Gacek RR: Ann Otol Rhinol Laryngol [Suppl 10] 83:5, 1974)

FIG. 18–2. Histologic features in cochlear fistula. **BL,** bony labyrinth; **C,** cholesteatoma matrix; **EB,** endosteal bone; **EM,** endosteal membrane; **R,** Reissner's membrane; **S,** spiral ligament; **ST,** scala tympani; **SV,** scala vestibuli. (Gacek RR: Ann Otol Rhinol Laryngol [Suppl 10] 83:5, 1974)

PETROSITIS (PETROUS APEX DISEASE, GRADENIGO'S SYNDROME)

The petrous apex of the temporal bone varies markedly in cellularity from the rest of the temporal bone in some patients. It is not uncommon in an extensively pneumatized temporal bone to find large petrous apical cells comparable to those seen in the mastoid and squamous portions of the temporal bone. However, in moderately pneumatized or mixed pneumatic-diploetic-sclerotic temporal bones, there may be isolated petrous apical cells separated from the rest of the temporal bone pneumatic area by dense sclerotic bone. Because of the heterogeneous nature of petrous apical pneumatization, petrositis occurs relatively sporadically and infrequently in the course of otomastoiditis.

In many instances, a petrosal inflammatory process may be asymptomatic and respond to medical or surgical management of the basic middle ear or mastoid lesion (atticomastoidectomy or radical mastoidectomy). No specific petrosal infection symptoms or signs may be noted.

However, there are cases in which isolated petrosal apical infections may produce loculated areas of bone disease with highly specific symptomatology known as Gradenigo's syndrome or the petrosal apicitis syndrome. Because of the proximity of the apex to Dorello's canal, through which the sixth nerve courses, and because of the proximity of the apex to the trigeminal ganglion, petrosal apical infections are frequently accompanied by intense fifth nerve pain and sixth nerve paralysis, accompanied by intermittent otorrhea, occasionally by fever, leukocytosis, and other signs of acute inflammatory disease.

The onset of sixth nerve paralysis and fifth nerve pain during the course of an otomastoiditis is usually a sign of petrositis.

In the preantibiotic era, petrositis was a very serious complication that did not respond to conventional mastoid exenteration procedures (either simple or radical mastoidectomy) because the apex is frequently separated by sclerotic bone from

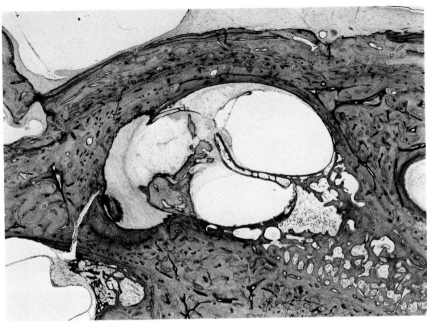

FIG. 18–3. Horizontal section of left cochlea viewed through round window and lower basal turn. Scala tympani at the round window region is filled with fibrous tissue and new bone; round window membrane shows marked fibrous thickening. Degeneration of organ of Corti and spiral ganglion is apparent in lower basal turn. (H&E) (Suga F, Lindsay JR: Ann Otol Rhinol Laryngol 84:37–44, 1975)

the central mastoid pneumatic region. Direct surgical drainage was the only modality available for treatment before antibiotics. A number of surgical procedures were devised to uncap the petrous apex. The Lempert petrous apicectomy involved an anteroinferior route, with the internal carotid artery as chief surgical landmark. The internal carotid artery bony wall is uncapped, and by following the artery to the apex, it is possible to reach the entrapped apical cells and thus drain the abscess.

Petrositis has decreased dramatically in incidence in the antibiotic era. However, petrositis still occurs, and because of antibiotic therapy, its symptomatology and management have undergone changes, making recognition and diagnosis more difficult. Classic symptoms of Gradenigo's syndrome are less common. Polytomographic studies facilitate diagnosis. Surgical approaches may be transmastoid, pericarotid, or via the middle fossa with elevation of the temporal lobe dura.

THROMBOPHLEBITIS—SIGMOID (LATERAL) SINUS AND JUGULAR BULB

Retrograde thrombophlebitis of small vessels occurs in a number of acute middle ear infections.

Similar extensions may occur from mastoid cells, especially from cells posterior to the posterior vertical semicircular canal, in close contiguity with the posterior fossa dural plate. Infections of the hypotympanum may extend through small vessels to the jugular bulb. Thrombophlebitis of the sigmoid lateral venous sinus can occur in both acute and chronic cases of otomastoiditis unresponsive to antibiotics. Persistent fever with or without chills in chronic otomastoiditis, with poor response to adequate mastoid surgery and antibiotic therapy, should point to the possibility of subclinical or occult thrombophlebitis of some portion of the jugular bulb and venous sinus system. Blood cultures are indicated, and should be repeated until diagnosis is clarified.

The classic signs of acute thrombophlebitis of the lateral sinus are sepsis, chills, and fever, accompanied in most instances by a positive blood culture. Tenderness of the jugular vein may be present. Specific diagnosis may be by the manometric Queckenstedt (Toby-Ayer) jugular compression test during spinal puncture. Definitive diagnosis may also be aided by retrograde jugulography, and related special radiographic studies.

The management of lateral sinus thrombophlebitis involves adequate surgical exposure of the lateral sinus. Incision and removal of the thrombus is necessary. The lateral sinus is packed with absorbable gauze superiorly and inferiorly to the thrombus region following posterior fossa dural plate removal. After preliminary ligation of the internal jugular vein, the sinus is incised and the clot evacuated. The absorbable sterile gauze packing absorbs spontaneously. Removal of the major clot reduces the chances of embolization and is usually followed by favorable response to medical therapy, including antibiotics and anticoagulants.

OTOGENIC MENINGITIS

Otogenic meningitis, formerly a very common complication of otomastoiditis, still occurs as a serious complication of otomastoiditis. It has not disappeared into ancient medical history. Deaths still occur as the result of otogenic meningitis. There are differing concepts regarding relationships of concomitant acute otitis media or acute otomastoiditis and meningitis due to *H. influenzae*, *D. pneumoniae*, and *N. meningitidis* infections. Some clinicians consider the two conditions as separate lesions without causal relationships. Clinical response to massive dosage antibiotic therapy alone has been considered evidence of lack of causal correlation. There are cases, however, that are nonresponsive to massive courses of antibiotic therapy, in which improvement follows surgical attention to acute otitis media that may not have been previously recognized. Myringotomy in some cases and mastoidectomy in other cases (accompanied by removal of the middle fossa and posterior fossa plates) are required before the meningitis responds to therapy.

Otologists who treated otogenic meningitis in the preantibiotic era are aware of definitive etiologic relationships insofar as retrograde thrombophlebitic routes to the meninges are concerned. In the preantibiotic era, dramatic therapeutic responses frequently followed the removal of middle and/or posterior fossa dural plates, in addition to atticomastoidectomy. Such surgery should still be considered in infantile (predominantly pneumococcic) meningitis cases that are unresponsive to antibiotic treatment and show otoscopic and radiographic evidence of otomastoiditis.

Obvious evidence of acute otitis media calls for immediate myringotomy. If there is doubt concerning the normality of the tympanum, tympanocentesis is indicated. Tympanocentesis (needle aspiration of the middle ear through the tympanic membrane) and cultured needle contents may reveal clear evidence of middle ear disease (due to *D. pneumococcus, H. influenzae,* or *N. meningitidis*). Mastoid radiographic findings and otoscopic, myringotomy, and/or tympanocentesis findings will guide the surgeon to further necessary otosurgical steps.

Mastoidectomy may be necessary, and should be done as indicated when there is no contraindication to general anesthesia.

In type A cases with osteitis and/or polypoid granulomatosis, an atticomastoidectomy will suffice. It can be performed very rapidly in the infant and young child.

Radical mastoidectomy is indicated in meningitis in a patient with evidence of keratoma or tympanosclerosis (type B chronic otomastoiditis). No attempt at tympanoplasty should be made.

Temporal bone studies in pneumococcal meningitis frequently reveal bilateral purulent labyrinthitis (2, 4). Whether the labyrinthitis is tympanogenic or meningogenic is an academic question. Undue reliance on antibiotic therapy alone in patients with evidence of tympanomastoid disease is unwarranted.

BRAIN ABSCESS

EXTRADURAL ABSCESS

Extradural abscess management is usually considered separately from subdural, intracerebral, or intracerebellar abscess. However, in many cases there may be simultaneous extradural and intracerebral or intracerebellar abscesses (Fig. 18–4).

Both acute and chronic otomastoiditis may be complicated by extradural abscess, usually due to necrotization of the middle fossa or the posterior fossa dural plates, secondary to pressure or secondary to retrograde thrombophlebitic extension from epitympanic or mastoid bone osteitis. An extradural abscess is frequently asymptomatic, and is discovered accidentally at surgery.

INTRACEREBRAL ABSCESS

Subdural abscesses can occur simultaneously or independently of extradural abscesses. Dural softening due to pressure will result in extradural abscess extension through the dura with development of a subdural abscess. In retrograde thrombophlebitic extension, both subdural and intracerebral abscesses may occur, either in the temporal lobe or in the cerebellum. The abscess usually liquefies and encapsulates in several weeks. Symptomatology will depend upon the virulence of the organism, degree of response to

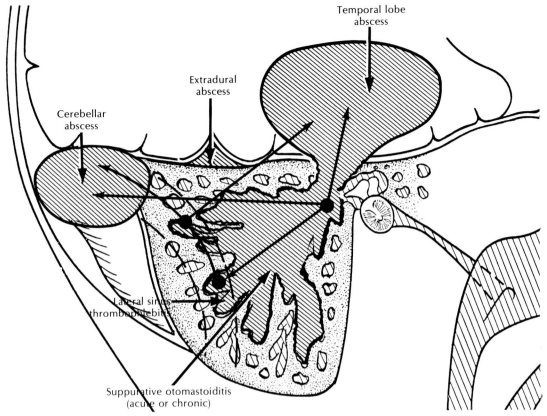

FIG. 18–4. Complications of otomastoiditis with examples of vascular and intracranial spread.

antibiotic therapy, and the localization of the lesion.

Temporal lobe abscess symptoms include vomiting, convulsions, headache, limb weakness, visual hallucinations, and visual field defects. A temporal lobe abscess need not be ipsilateral. It may be contralateral or multiple. The retrograde vascular spread of infection may produce multiple bilateral abscesses from a right or left otomastoiditis, although more commonly the spread will be in contiguity with the mastoid infection.

Cerebellar abscesses produce symptoms with evidence of greater intracranial pressure, including greater intensity of headache, vomiting, and lethargy, in addition to nystagmus and ataxia.

Neurologic symptoms in the course of acute or chronic otomastoiditis call for immediate neurological consultation and neuroradiologic studies. Polytomography and computerized axial tomography (CAT) scanning techniques are frequently diagnostic in localizing and determining the extent of intracerebral as well as extradural abscesses. Cerebral and cerebellar abscesses as complications

of otomastoiditis call for joint otosurgical and neurological management. Diagnostic steps include various combinations of spinal fluid studies, electroencephalography, and cerebral arteriography with subtraction techniques and isotope scanning.

Neurosurgical explorations will be necessary to drain and exteriorize an abscess capsule. Deep lesions may require repeated needle taps or catheter drainage. It may not be possible to remove all of the capsule in some abscesses. The results of neurosurgical management will vary, depending upon location and the degree of brain damage. Neurologic deficits are not uncommon and may include hemiparesis, hemianopsia, and chronic convulsive disorders.

Otosurgical exenteration of the middle ear mastoid lesion may be done simultaneously with the neurosurgical procedure, or as a separate procedure either preceding or following neurosurgical drainage. Precise management methods will be based upon individualization of cases. Joint otosurgical-neurosurgical collaboration is imperative.

OTITIC HYDROCEPHALUS

An unusual intracranial complication, especially in children, is otitic hydrocephalus, which results from sinus thrombosis associated with otomastoiditis. Intracranial venous drainage impairment interferes with the resorptive function of the arachnoid in the superior sagittal sinus. The result is a generalized cerebral swelling, flattening of the gyri, and what might be described as a "general intracranial hypertension." The increased intracranial pressure produces severe papilledema, accompanied by nausea and vomiting.

The primary etiologic factor, otomastoiditis, which may have been undetected, demands prompt surgical attention. Neurosurgical collaboration is necessary and cerebrospinal fluid shunt surgery may be required.

CEREBROSPINAL OTORRHEA

Otorrhea containing cerebrospinal fluid may follow physical or otosurgical trauma. It is not a common complication of chronic otomastoiditis, but it can follow tegmen necrosis in type B lesions. It may be due to temporal bone osteomyelitis, with dural and arachnoid perforation. Congenital tympanomastoid tegmen bony dehiscences may cause such fistulas in type B lesions.

Symptoms of cerebrospinal otorrhea can be elusive. "Watery" unilateral rhinorrhea, or otorrhea, may be observed. Tympanocentesis may yield clear fluid which can be examined for sugar and proteins.

Radiologic studies by polytomography, CAT scans, and dye studies are usually diagnostic.

Surgical repair may be approached otosurgically, neurosurgically, or through a combined approach. Middle fossa exploration combined with otomastoid visualization is frequently helpful. Dural sutures and muscle grafts are usually employed successfully.

SUMMARY

Otogenic complications, which were extremely common in the preantibiotic era, occur much less frequently. This diminished incidence, however, has been accompanied by diagnostic difficulties. Intratemporal bone complications—*i.e.*, seventh nerve paralysis and labyrinthine fistulas—do not pose significant problems because the symptoms are clear-cut.

Intracranial complications, however, can be deceptive symptomatically. Majer (3), who recently reviewed salient diagnostic aspects of otogenic intracranial complications, pointed out the significance of headache, drowsiness, vomiting, speech disturbances, aphasia, ocular paralysis, and choked disk. Subjective "dizziness" without nystagmus and the cerebellar nystagmus of Neumann are important diagnostic features. Acute otomastoiditis more commonly causes meningitis and thrombophlebitis. Chronic otomastoiditis is the primary cause of most brain abcesses.

REFERENCES

1. Gacek RR: The surgical management of labyrinthine fistulae in chronic otitis media with cholesteatoma. Ann Otol Rhinol Laryngol [Suppl 83] 10: 5, 1974
2. Igarashi M, Saito R, Alford B et al.: Temporal bone findings in pneumococal meningitis. Arch Otolaryngol 99:79–84, 1974
3. Majer E: Symptomatology and therapy of otogenic intracranial complications. ORL Digest July, pp 11–15, 1975
4. Schuknecht H, Montandon P: Pathology of the ear in Pneumococcal meningitis. Arch Klin Exp Ohr-Nas-n Kehlk Heilk 195:207–225, 1970
5. Suga F, Lindsay JR: Labyrinthitis ossificans due to chronic otitis media. Ann ORL 84:37–44, 1975

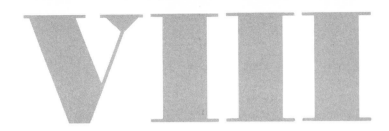

VIII

TYMPANO–OSSICULAR LESIONS

19

OTOSCLEROSIS

Otosclerosis, a common cause of hearing loss, literally means "hardening of the ear" and is an osteodystrophy limited to the temporal bone, primarily affecting the otic capsule of the labyrinth. It usually results in stapes fixation but may also involve the cochlea and other parts of the labyrinth.

Otosclerosis has been described histologically in fetuses and has been observed surgically in very young children as well as in adults of all ages. Characteristically, the onset is usually in early or middle adult life, although it may begin as late as the seventh or eighth decade.

The disease, usually bilateral and symmetrical, is not rare. Histologic otosclerosis was found in 8.3% of temporal bones of white Americans (44). In patients with unilateral clinical otosclerosis, bilateral histologic otosclerosis may be present. The exact incidence of clinical otosclerosis is unknown, but it has been estimated at between 5% and 10% of the white population. It occurs less commonly in blacks and Orientals and shows geographic variability. The disease is more common in women, in a ratio of 2.5:1, and frequently becomes worse during pregnancy and lactation. Some women with otosclerosis show increased incidence of dental caries during pregnancy, although no definitive pattern of calcium-phosphorus abnormality is found in otosclerotic patients. Heredity is a significant factor in otosclerosis, but it is not a constant. Its genetic aspect has been described both as dominant (7) and as recessive autosomal in type.

There are no known systemic effects of otosclerosis. Symptoms are confined to the auditory and vestibular systems. The primary lesion occurs in the otic capsule surrounding the anterior aspect of the oval window niche involving the annular ligament of the stapes footplate and encroaching upon the anterior footplate and anterior crus (Figs. 19–1, 19–2, 19–3). The footplate becomes progressively immobilized with subsequent involvement of posterior crus. In some cases circumferential fixation of the footplate occurs simultaneously. A conductive hearing loss is the usual sequel.

The disease can also involve the vestibular (Fig. 19–4) and cochlear (Fig. 19–5) labyrinths. Vertigo and/or cochlear hearing loss occasionally coexist with stapes fixation. A patient with classic stapedial otosclerosis in one ear occasionally will have a purely cochlear loss in the contralateral ear. "Nerve deafness" (cochlear hearing loss) can be due to otosclerotic involvement of the cochlea, round window niche, and/or internal auditory meatus in some patients.

ETIOLOGY AND PATHOLOGY

Although genetic and basic histologic patterns have been identified in otosclerosis there is no definite agreement as to etiology or precise pathogenesis.

Genetic aspects of otosclerosis were reported recently in a well documented study of 974 otosclerotic individuals carried out in Lithuania by Gapany-Gapanavicius (8). He concluded that otosclerosis is not inherited as a simple autosomal monogenic trait which is purely dominant or recessive. There is autosomal dominant transmission with incomplete penetrance and variable expressivity. Although he found more than twice as many females as males in his patients, he ruled out the hypothesis of sex-linked recessive or dominant inheritance. The female preponderance was attributed to endogenous endocrine factors.

In its earliest stage, the dystrophy is actually an otospongiosis, a softening or "spongiosis" due to increased vascularity and resorption of bone in the otic capsule. This spongy vascular form is most commonly seen when the disease occurs in children or young adults (Fig. 19–6). The more typical form, as seen in the mature adult, is that of sclerosis, which probably represents new bone formation and remodeling (Fig. 19–7). The large vascular spaces in otospongiosis are replaced by dense, mosaic-patterned immature bone with its unusual staining characteristics and architecture. Combinations of both phases are frequently seen in the same specimen. Schuknecht (39) described four classic stages in the pathogenesis and progression of otosclerosis:

FIG. 19–1. Portion of normal stapedial footplate and crus. Note cartilage lining along joint surface at right and along inner ear (vestibule) surface at bottom. (H&E) (Gussen R: The ear. In Coulson W (ed): Surgical Pathology. Philadelphia, JB Lippincott, in press)

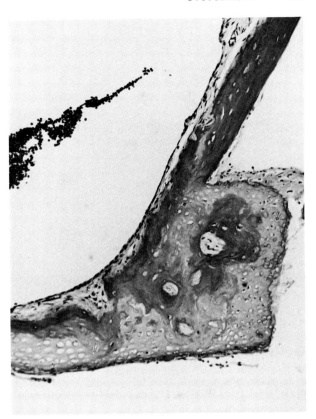

FIG. 19–2. Otosclerosis of oval window and stapedial footplate. (H&E) (Gussen R: J Laryngol 84:1027–1031, 1970)

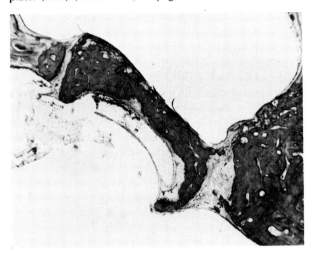

FIG. 19–3. Otosclerosis of oval window, anterosuperiorly, and partially lining facial nerve canal. (H&E, × 14) (Gussen R: Arch Otolaryngol 94:484–487, 1973. Copyright 1973, American Medical Association)

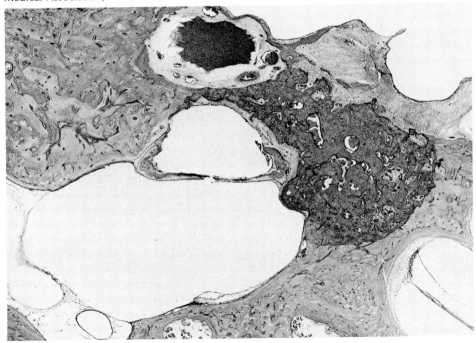

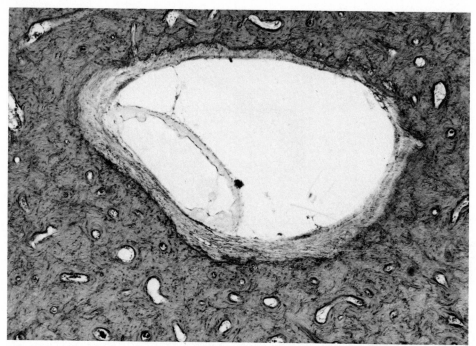

FIG. 19–4. Semicircular canal surrounded by otosclerotic bone. Note widening (uncovering) of collagenous endosteum, with bony surface set farther back. (H&E, × 70) (Gussen R: Arch Otolaryngol 101:438–440, 1975. Copyright 1975, American Medical Association)

FIG. 19–5. Cochlear otosclerosis. Spiral ligament is abnormal. Its fibrils are parallel and close together, with marked loss of "spaces." The eroded otosclerotic bone surface has a thickened collagenous endosteum. (H&E, × 175) (Gussen R: Arch Otolaryngol 101:438–440, 1975. Copyright 1973, American Medical Association)

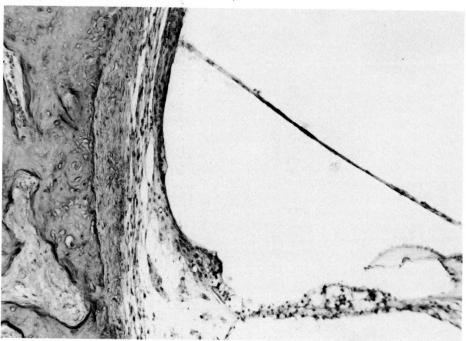

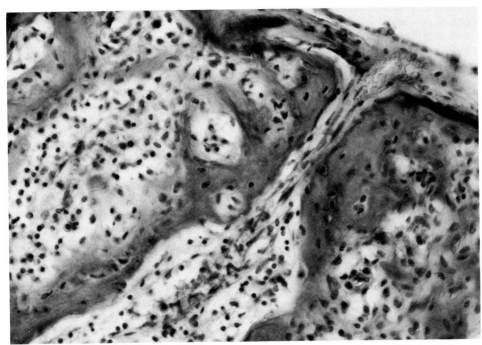

FIG. 19–6. Cellular otosclerosis (otospongiosis). Areas of bone resorption are filled with large numbers of osteoblasts and mononuclear cells, surrounding capillaries. (H&E, × 420) (Gussen R: Arch Otolaryngol 101:438–440, 1975. Copyright 1975, American Medical Association)

FIG. 19–7. Otosclerosis of oval window, anterosuperiorly (postoperative stapediolysis). Tantalum wire removed before processing of specimen. Loose fibrous tissue replaces gelatin sponge material about the wire. Otolithic membrane of the saccule is partially encapsulated. (H&E, × 16) (Gussen R: Arch Otolaryngol 97:484–487, 1973. Copyright 1973, American Medical Association)

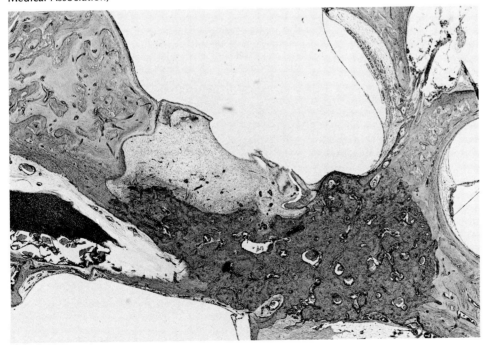

1. Resorptive changes produce destruction of enchondral bone. The resorption is attributed to lysosomal hydrolases. In addition, osteoclasts may absorb calcium by pinocytosis.
2. Immature basophilic bone is produced by mucopolysaccharide osteoid deposits within the fibroblastic collagen.
3. New mature acidophilic laminated bone is laid down.
4. Highly mineralized mosaic bone patterns finally emerge.

The major etiologic theories of otosclerosis deal with the presence of unstable embryonic cartilage rests within the capsule and fissula ante fenestram, the effects of intrinsic and extrinsic mechanical forces on the bone of the otic capsule, and the breakdown and resorption of nonviable bone related to vascular changes.

Any theory of otosclerosis must explain its occurrence in both the labyrinthine capsule and in the stapediovestibular joint, taking into account the prevalence of otosclerosis in the region of the joint.

Bast and Anson described the presence of unstable embryonic cartilage rests which they believed capable of changing into abnormal bone, similar in appearance to otosclerotic bone (2).

Intrinsic mechanical stresses affecting the bone of the otic capsule proper were considered significant by Mayer (30). Sercer and Krmpotic (40) believed that extrinsic mechanical forces increased throughout childhood due to the increasing angulation of the base of the skull, with resultant rotation of the otic capsule, and that these mechanical stresses acted most strongly on the areas of predilection to otosclerosis.

Many investigators related the development of otosclerosis to the blood supply of the bone. Mayer (31, 32) believed that otosclerotic foci developed in areas of decreased blood supply, resulting from vasomotor changes and organic disease of the vessel walls. Wittmaack (47) stated that congestion was the basic cause of changes in the bone. Wolff and Bellucci (48) related the pathogenesis of otosclerosis to increased acidity of the tissue fluids of the perivascular bone, with resultant decalcification and breakdown of the bone. Mendoza and Ruis (34) described nonviable bone in the otic capsule throughout life and related it to the obliteration of large numbers of arteries. Gussen described the changes in the labyrinthine capsule as similar to age changes of bone in general (20). These age changes consist of plugging of the vascular canals of the bone, obliterating the vessels, with loss of osteocytes, and mineralization of the empty lacunas and canaliculi (micropetrosis). Increased plugging of vascular canals and nonviable bone with increasing age (Fig. 19–8) were described by Gussen (21). Greatly increased numbers of vascular canal plugs were found in specimens from persons with severe generalized arteriosclerosis, with more extensive areas of nonviable bone, micropetrosis, and erosions. Gussen believes, therefore, that the breakdown of bone in the otic capsule proper is a result of vascular insufficiency related to changes of the vascular canals and micropetrosis.

Gussen also presented a composite anatomic and functional view of the stapediovestibular joint whereby the fissula ante fenestram and fossula post fenestram are extensions of the joint, by virtue of the direct continuation of the articular cartilage and the insertion of annular ligament fibers deep within the fissula ante fenestram (22). With this interpretation, the new cartilage and/or bone seen occasionally within the fissula ante fenestram can be related to physiologic mechanical loading. She also described the physiologic changes of aging of the articular surfaces of the stapediovestibular joint and showed progression of these changes to degenerative arthritis. With severe degenerative arthritic changes, not only is there erosion of the articular cartilage, but deeper erosion involving the underlying bone of the oval window or footplate may occur. New bone forms as a means of repair and appears to be identical to otosclerotic bone. The prevalence of degenerative arthritis of the joint explains the prevalence of otosclerosis of this region. Gussen (21, 22) therefore, considers that the steps leading to otosclerosis are different in the joint and in the otic capsule proper. The breakdown of bone in the otic capsule is the result of vascular insufficiency related to changes of the vascular canals and micropetrosis, whereas the breakdown of bone in the stapediovestibular joint is the result of severe degenerative arthritis. Such factors as mechanical stress associated with genetic predisposition, hormonal and metabolic factors

FIG. 19–8. Otic capsule, 62-year-old male. Note plugged vascular canal (P) and nonviable, micropetrotic perivascular bone (M) and interstitial bone (M). Partial bone plugs are present (B). Note repolymerizing, cellular bone (R) about normal vascular canals. (H&E, × 16) (Gussen R: Ann Otol Rhinol Laryngol 78:1305–1315, 1969)

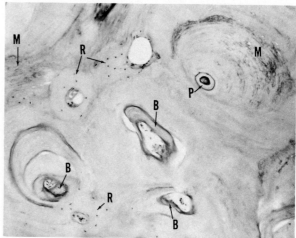

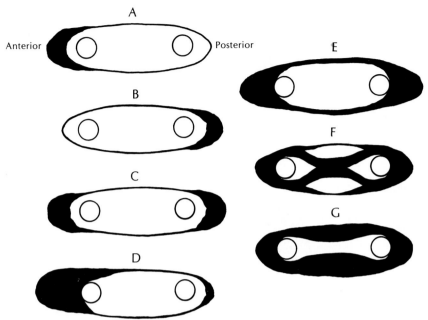

FIG. 19–9. Schematic illustration of typical otosclerotic lesions. **A.** Anterior peribasal lesion. **B.** Posterior peribasal lesion. **C.** Anterior and posterior peribasal lesion. **D.** Anterior peri-crural, posterior peribasal lesion. **E.** Anteroposterior pericrural lesions. **F.** Anteroposterior pericrural lesions connected by transfootplate bar. **G.** Extensive circumferential otosclerosis with small central island.

(such as pregnancy and ochronosis), certain of the osteochondrodystrophies, and irradiation may predispose to degenerative arthritis and, therefore, may predispose to otosclerosis of the stapediovestibular joint. Once erosion of bone occurs in either the joint or the otic capsule, new membrane bone, identical to otosclerotic bone, may form within the eroded areas as a repair mechanism.

In early lesions (regardless of the age of the patient) there is increased vascularity of the mucoperiosteum of the promontory and the peristapedial tissues, as well as that of the stapedial arch itself. This increased vascularization, frequently accompanied by edema, may be responsible for the positive Schwartze sign, a red blush noted on otoscopic examination. The redness seen through the tympanic membrane, if the membrane is not excessively thickened, reflects increased vascularization of the mucoperiosteum of the promontory. This phase of the disease may be described as vascular otospongiosis. Later, repair of the breakdown and resorption of bone by new bone formation produces the final form of otosclerosis.

When the middle ear is exposed surgically, an avascular sclerotic lesion in the oval window involves all or part of the footplate and its annular ligament. Corona-type lesions occur in the peristapedial cochlear promontory area and adjacent to the bony canal of the horizontal portion of the facial nerve. In some cases both vascular and avascular lesions appear in the oval window and promontory areas.

The most significant early physiopathologic sequel is increased mechanical stiffness of the stapedial arch and footplate, resulting in ultimate bony fixation of the stapedial vestibular joint (oval window ligament). Thus, *a fixed stapes is the most common result of otosclerosis.* In some patients, labyrinthine otosclerosis occurs, which may or may not affect hearing and/or vestibular function. These cochlear and vestibular lesions may coexist with the oval window otosclerosis and create complex otoaudiologic findings.

Otosclerotic lesions may occur anteriorly, posteriorly, superiorly, inferiorly, and in varying combinations (Fig. 19–9). Not only may the lesions fix the footplate itself, but they may also create bony fixations between the crura and promontory and between the crura and the seventh nerve bony canal (Fig. 19–10). Otosclerotic extensions may involve the stapedial tendon partially or completely, as well as the articular capsule of the incudostapedial joint. Otosclerotic invasion of the

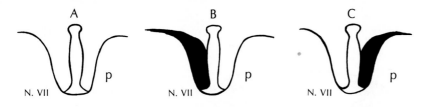

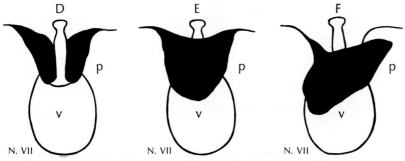

FIG. 19–10. A. Normal stapes. **B.** Superior otosclerotic lesion from bony facial canal with crural fusion. **C.** Inferior lesion fusing crus to promontory. **D.** Superoinferior lesions with complete crural fusion. **E.** Massive oval window niche lesion obliterating medial aspect of crura and footplate, with vestibular extension. **F.** Massive otosclerotic lesion obliterating crura and footplate and extending into cochlear promontory **(P)** and into the vestibule **(V)** extensively. **VII,** seventh nerve bony canal.

FIG. 19–11. Otosclerotic involvement of stapedial footplate. Note cellular membrane bone with closely spaced osteocytes, considerable osteoblastic activity and numerous vascular channels. (H&E) (Gussen R: The ear. In Coulson W (ed): Surgical Pathology. Philadelphia, JB Lippincott, in press)

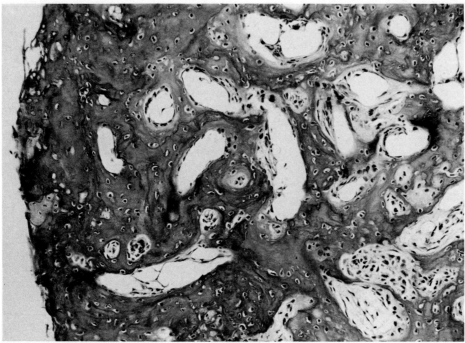

FIG. 19–12. **A.** Moderate oval window lesion. **B.** Extensive oval window lesion with partial round window involvement. **C.** Obliterative oval and round window lesions.

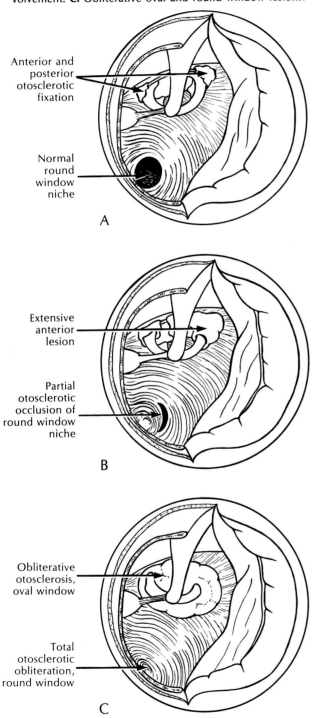

Anterior and posterior otosclerotic fixation

Normal round window niche

A

Extensive anterior lesion

Partial otosclerotic occlusion of round window niche

B

Obliterative otosclerosis, oval window

Total otosclerotic obliteration, round window

C

incus and malleus is rare. Fixation of the incudomalleal articulation may occur as a secondary torsional sequel of otosclerosis. The lateral ossicular chain (incus and malleus) must be examined for mobility at the beginning of a stapedectomy.

The footplate is partially or completely invaded and may be completely replaced by otosclerosis (Fig. 19–11). Extensions of otosclerotic bone may invade the vestibule, narrowing it into a very small channel or obliterating the scala vestibuli completely. Otosclerotic involvement of the round window niche is not rare. In most instances such infiltration is incomplete (Fig. 19–12) and does not interfere with round window membrane function (Fig. 19–13), but in rare cases it may be complete, with total bony replacement of the round window membrane.

Otosclerotic involvement of the cochlea occurs in some temporal bones, along with stapedial otosclerosis. It may occur as an isolated lesion. Otosclerotic involvement of the internal auditory meatus and/or canal has been observed radiologically and pathologically. Its role in otosclerosis sensorineural hearing loss is still debatable.

DIAGNOSIS

The clinical diagnosis of otosclerosis is made on the basis of a conductive hearing loss, an intact mobile tympanic membrane, a functioning eustachian tube, and no x-ray evidence of active mastoid disease. However, such a combination of findings may also occur in nonotosclerotic lesions. The conductive loss may vary audiometrically from 10–100 dB, but it is limited to a range of 10–65 dB in uncomplicated stapedial ankylosis (without cochlear involvement). When the air conduction hearing level exceeds 65 dB, cochlear otosclerosis probably coexists with a fixed stapes. However, a patient may have otosclerosis and another coexisting intratympanic lesion. Thus, it is possible for a patient to have adhesive otitis with otosclerosis, or tympanosclerosis accompanying otosclerosis.

HISTORY AND SYMPTOMS

The primary symptom of otosclerosis is hearing loss, which starts slowly and may not be noticed by the patient for several years. Otosclerosis may start at any time in life, but there are certain ages at which maximum occurrence and more rapid growth are encountered. Otosclerosis has been observed in infants and in children. Successful surgery has been performed on children as young as

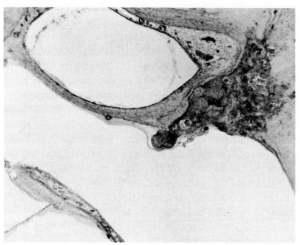

FIG. 19–13. Otosclerosis involving round window, which was direct continuation of nonankylosing otosclerosis of stapediovestibular joint. (Goodhill V: Surgery for otosclerosis: stapedectomy, stapedioplasty, and fenestration. In English GM (ed): Otolaryngology, Volume II. Hagerstown, Harper & Row, 1976, p 5)

4 years of age. Most frequently the disease is encountered between the third and fifth decades. It is more commonly seen in females, frequently starting during or after pregnancy.

The onset of the hearing loss may be very slow. If it is bilaterally symmetrical, the awareness of a hearing loss may escape the attention of both patient and family for some time. However, as the hearing loss level reaches 25–30 dB, it becomes definitely handicapping.

The speech of a patient with otosclerosis becomes soft. Members of the family and associates may become aware of the patient's communication problem before the patient recognizes either the hearing loss or a change in speech amplitude.

The hearing loss itself is usually progressive. The progression may occur in direct linear form or may be plateau-like in character (Fig 19–14). No clear predictions of ultimate thresholds can be made on the basis of serial audiometric studies in patients. The progression in one ear cannot be accurately predicted from the progression in the other ear, although there are frequent examples of symmetrical progression.

The hearing loss, if limited to stapedial involvement, is strictly conductive in the majority of patients. Patients will frequently experience the familiar phenomenon of **paracusis of Willis** (better hearing ability in a noisy environment) if there is no complicating cochlear involvement. It can be very adequately compensated, in most cases, by hearing aid amplification, and patients are able

to tolerate rather wide ranges of amplification. They do not usually exhibit "recruitment of loudness" characteristics and actually enjoy increased loudness, either through a hearing aid or through any simple amplifying system.

Occasionally a patient with otosclerosis may have the impression that the loss of hearing suddenly followed an incident of trauma, an emotional shock, or an acute illness. It is difficult to evaluate the real significance of such apparent causal relationships.

Although otosclerosis is most common as a bilateral lesion, it occurs unilaterally in 15% of cases. When it occurs bilaterally, it is generally symmetric in symptomatology, rate of extension, and degree, but it may be variable. The rate of progression may fluctuate, and an ear that at one time showed greater involvement may be surpassed in hearing loss by the contralateral ear a decade later. If the stapes otosclerotic process is accompanied by cochlear involvement, losses in bone conduction levels as well as deficits in speech discrimination scores will be noted. Occasionally the vestibular labyrinth may be involved, and vertiginous episodes may occur.

Temporary ear pain, usually vague and aching in character, occasionally occurs. Tinnitus is one of the most common and annoying symptoms of otosclerosis. It may be quite varied in its manifestations, being either unilateral or bilateral and roaring, hissing, or pulsating in character. The

FIG. 19–14. Progression of hearing loss in otosclerosis. Steady losses (**solid line**) occur in some patients. In others, the hearing losses occur in plateau forms (**dashed line**), and in many patients both steady and plateau features occur together.

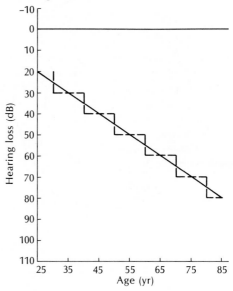

tinnitus may fluctuate greatly in intensity and may be related to metabolic and endocrine disturbances. Thus, tinnitus may have a certain rhythmicity in women with relation to menstrual cycles. Tinnitus is more common in the early stages of otosclerosis and usually disappears as the disease matures.

OTOSCOPIC FINDINGS

Otoscopic examination should include observation of the tympanic membrane at rest, during pneumatic massage, and following tubal insufflation. The Schwartze sign is not a constant finding, except in very early cases. The tympanic membrane and malleus are usually mobile to pneumatic bulb compression and rarefaction.

There are no diagnostic otoscopic findings other than negative ones in otosclerosis. As a matter of fact, the tympanic membrane may be atrophic or thickened, freely mobile or partly fixed, and it may have a transmitted red Schwartze sign from the promontory, or it may have none. Its response to pneumatic massage may be brisk or sluggish, and its response to tubal insufflation may be marked or slight. Some patients with otosclerosis will have had unrelated previous or concomitant otitis media with healed perforations, and varying degrees of tympanic membrane scarring. In general, a tympanic membrane that is *within rather wide limits of normality* is characteristic. However, a high index of suspicion regarding nonotosclerotic conductive hearing loss is especially important in the differential diagnosis of the *unilateral case*.

RHINOPHARYNGEAL EXAMINATION

Examination of the nose, sinuses, and nasopharynx is essential in every case to rule out the possibility of rhinopharyngeal disease for two reasons: 1) The conductive hearing loss may be due to undiagnosed tubotympanitis with secondary otitis media masquerading as otosclerosis. Such a tubotympanitis may be inflammatory or neoplastic. Thus rhinopharyngeal examination is essential in differential diagnosis. 2) An active infection in the rhinopharyngeal area may contribute to poststapedectomy complications.

RADIOGRAPHIC STUDIES

STANDARD PLAIN FILM X-RAYS

Mastoid x-rays (Schuller's view) and internal acoustic meatus x-rays (Stenver's view) are essential in every otologic examination. Otosclerotic involvement of either the oval window or round window niche or of the labyrinth are not usually seen on plain films. They may frequently be seen on polytome radiographs. However, polytomography is not essential in the diagnosis and differential diagnosis of most otosclerosis cases. Polytomography is important, however, in special problems to be discussed.

Schuller and Stenver's x-rays are advisable in all otosclerosis cases for the purpose of differential diagnosis. Such x-rays may reveal unexpected latent lurking keratoma (cholesteatoma), undetected secretory otomastoiditis, erosion of the internal acoustic meatus that is caused by an unsuspected acoustic neurinoma, petrous tip sclerosis, or any one of a number of skull lesions, such as Paget's disease and meningioma, which may produce hearing losses similar to those of otosclerosis. Such possible unexpected pathologic x-ray findings may exist and be unaccompanied by any other clinical findings except a conductive hearing loss. X-rays are therefore absolutely essential in the differential diagnosis of otosclerosis.

POLYTOMOGRAPHY

Polytomography is useful in complex diagnostic problems. Ossicular details regarding malleus, incus, and crura can help in differential diagnosis between otosclerosis and ossicular discontinuity or fixations. The size and topography of oval and round windows can be determined in many cases.

TUNING-FORK TESTS

The Rinne and Weber tests performed with 128-Hz, 256-Hz, and 512-Hz tuning forks will usually (but not always) be suggestively diagnostic in otosclerosis. A negative Rinne response to the low-frequency forks, 128 Hz and 256 Hz, will be found in most patients with early otosclerosis. In patients with coexistent cochlear involvement it may be difficult to demonstrate an air–bone gap by standard audiometric studies, but it may be possible to demonstrate an air–bone gap quite clearly by such negative Rinne responses. This assumes that purely tactile (nonauditory) responses have been ruled out. The dental Weber test (incisor teeth) with 128-Hz, 256-Hz, or 512-Hz forks is confirmatory when it shows lateralization to the affected side in unilateral otosclerosis or to the poorer hearing ear in bilateral otosclerosis.

This discussion of tuning-fork tests is not meant to imply that one may make an accurate diagnosis of otosclerosis by tuning-fork tests alone. Tuning-fork responses may be extremely helpful as screening tests in patients who do not show clearly defined air–bone gaps on conventional audiometry. The recent development of the "conductive loss test battery" and impedance audiometry have clarified many of these borderline problems. As newer audiologic techniques become available, tuning-fork tests are still valuable in otologic diagnosis.

AUDIOMETRIC TESTS

STANDARD AUDIOMETRY

A classic physiopathologic-audiometric pattern of progression occurs in otosclerosis. Although there are exceptions, several stages occur in most patients. Shape and width of the *air–bone gap* are the crucial audiometric findings in otosclerosis.

1. As an early anterior peribasal lesion increases the stiffness of the stapediovestibular joint, hearing decreases progressively for low frequencies, and a "stiffness tilt" is seen in the pure-tone air-conduction audiogram, with a slight air–bone gap (Fig. 19–15).
2. As the lesion further invades the posterior peribasal region, the footplate becomes completely fixed. With increased mass of the otosclerotic footplate, a "mass tilt" occurs in the pure-tone air-conduction audiogram. The high-frequency hearing level also drops (Fig. 19–16), producing an equal loss for all frequencies. The air–bone gap increases (widens).
3. As frictional elements are added to the fixation, the pure-tone air-conduction level continues to drop. Both low frequency and high frequency pure-tone air-conduction levels continue to drop throughout the range. The air–bone gap becomes greater (Fig. 19–17). In a smaller number of patients, superimposition of a cochlear otosclerotic lesion (such as at the basal turn of the cochlea) adds a further high frequency component by bone conduction and air conduction (Fig. 19–18). Speech discrimination scores begin to drop if cochlear involvement increases. However, a high-frequency air and bone conduction loss may be purely mechanical (middle ear) in origin, and not due to a cochlear otosclerotic lesion. In such a case the speech discrimination scores remains high.

Although the air–bone gap is the classic audiologic finding, there are instances when the air–bone gap findings are not clear-cut. A very small air–bone gap, especially in the low frequencies, can be entirely spurious, as a result of tactile bone-conduction responses. However, it may actually be much greater than measured because of some inherent problems of bone-conduction testing. Not only is it necessary to clarify an air–bone gap (conductive versus cochlear problems), but it is necessary to differentiate between otosclerotic and nonotosclerotic conductive lesions.

LOW-FREQUENCY AIR–BONE GAP

A conductive hypacusis (hearing loss) is determined essentially by the difference in hearing levels between air and bone conduction (16) and is traditionally indicated by the negative Rinne response with tuning forks. With the advent of pure-tone audiometry, the air–bone gap became the distinguishing characteristic of conductive hypacusis; thus, the negative Rinne and the air–bone gap are the two diagnostic criteria for conductive losses.

In some cases, one sees a special phenomenon that is observed in the low-frequency region of the auditory spectrum and is best described as **the low-frequency air-bone gap.** This may occur in a continuous (diminishing) form or as a fragmentary isolated form. It may be associated with negative 128 and 256 Hz Rinne responses and with unexpectedly high speech discrimination scores. It may be a fixed (manifest) observation, or it may appear slowly (evolving) over a period of months or years.

Some time ago, we noted that the first sign of beginning reankylosis in stapes surgery was frequently a reversal of the positive Rinne at 250 Hz to a negative Rinne, even though the 500 Hz and the 1000 Hz forks remained Rinne-positive and even though there was still a closure of the audiometric air–bone gap. As the reankylosis progressed, the 500 Hz and later the 1000 Hz Rinne responses became negative, also. This was accompanied by return of the air–bone gap. This phenomenon was then confirmed by reverse observations in successful stapedectomy—namely, that the change from negative to positive Rinne could be noted in the first few postoperative weeks as a function that occurred last in the low-tone forks.

It began to appear that the most sensitive index of stiffness in the ossicular chain was mirrored by the low-frequency air–bone gap, especially as noted in tuning fork Rinne tests. Every effort was made to alert patients to the problem of confusing tactile perception with acoustic perception when low-frequency fork tests were made. With our increasing awareness of this low-frequency air–bone gap sensitivity, forks of 128 Hz and 64 Hz were brought into use. Most of these fork observations were then verified by audiometric replication of low-frequency air–bone gaps.

Of greatest significance is that group of otosclerotic patients in whom the audiologic evidence demonstrates a purely sensorineural lesion. Not only may scrutiny

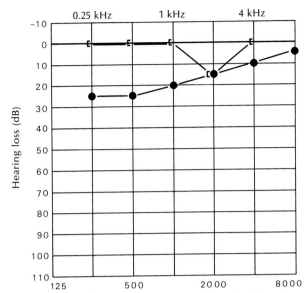

FIG. 19–15. Stiffness tilt in early otosclerosis. Note low-frequency air conduction tilt with little change elsewhere. Note 2-kHz bone conduction dip, attributable to Carhart notch. ●—●, AC, unmasked, RE; [—[, BC, masked, RE.

FIG. 19–16. Mass tilt added to stiffness tilt seen in preceding figure. ●—●, AC, unmasked, RE; [—[, BC, masked, RE.

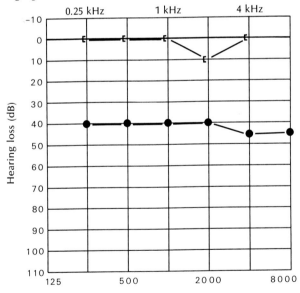

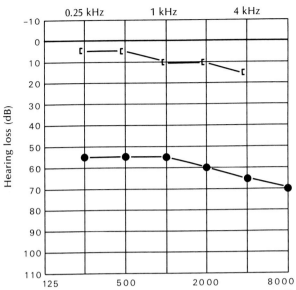

FIG. 19–17. Frictional component adds high-frequency tilt to both air conduction and bone conduction levels. ●—●, AC, unmasked, RE; [—[, BC, masked, RE; **SRT,** 55; **SDS,** 100%.

FIG. 19–18. Cochlear involvement superimposed on stiffness, mass, and frictional tilts adds high-frequency air and bone conduction losses to the previous levels. Speech discrimination score **(SDS)** has dropped to 68%. ●—●, AC, unmasked, RE; [—[, BC, masked, RE; **SRT,** 60 dB.

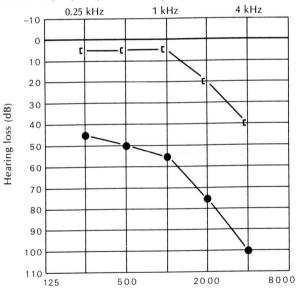

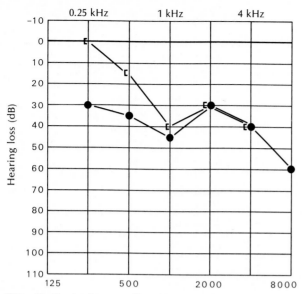

FIG. 19–19. Audiogram illustrating diminishing air–bone gap. •—•, AC, unmasked, RE; [—[, BC, masked, RE.

FIG. 19–20. Audiogram showing only fragmentary evidence of an air–bone gap. •—•, AC, unmasked, RE; [—[, BC, masked, RE; **arrows,** no response at maximum output.

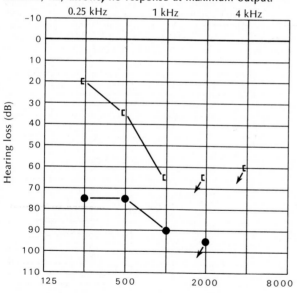

of the low-frequency air–bone gap enable us to detect a conductive component in what is really a combined lesion, but occasionally we find also that the apparent basic sensorineural lesion is not real. This has been repeatedly observed by otologists in stapes cases in which postoperative air conduction levels have reached normal thresholds in spite of major preoperative bone conduction level depressions (in excess of Carhart notch reversals).

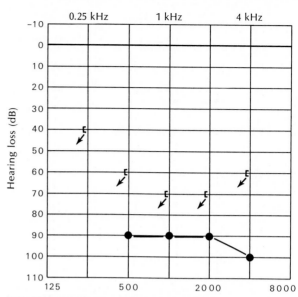

FIG. 19–21. Audiogram illustrating case with no measureable bone conduction although the patient had negative Rinnes in the low frequencies. •—•, AC, unmasked, RE; [—[, BC, masked, RE; **arrows,** no response at maximum output.

The Manifest Group

DIMINISHING AIR–BONE GAP. This term is applied to cases in which the bone conduction curve meets the air conduction curve at 1000 or 2000 Hz or at lower frequencies and then either remains superimposed upon it or crosses over, continuing on its downward slope (Fig. 19–19).

FRAGMENTARY AIR–BONE GAP. This term is applied to the case in which the bone conduction curve is present in the low-frequency area only, usually not higher than 750 Hz, and then vanishes completely. It never reaches the air conduction curve at any point. In some cases, there may be bone conduction responses at only one frequency (Fig. 19–20).

NEGATIVE RINNE WITH NO MEASURABLE BONE CONDUCTION. This term applies to those cases that show definite negative Rinne responses yet have no measurable bone conduction (Fig. 19–21).

The Evolving Group

This group of cases is characterized by the initial absence of any air–bone gap audiometrically and demonstration of positive Rinne responses even with the 128 and 256 Hz forks. With the passage of time, usually years, telltale signs of an air–bone gap in the low-frequency area begin to appear. The first sign may well be a shift of the previously central Weber response, done at the upper incisor teeth, to the poorer ear. The second sign may be the gradual Rinne con-

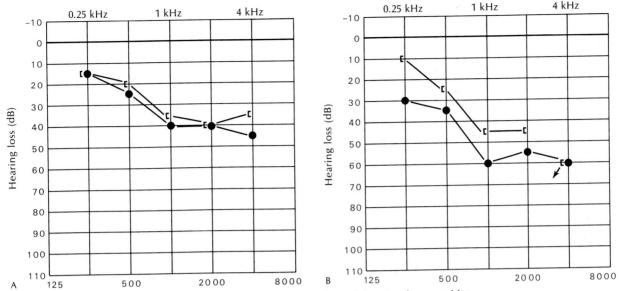

FIG. 19–22. A. Initial audiogram showing an apparent sensorineural hearing loss, positive Rinne responses, and a high SDS. ●—●, AC, unmasked, RE; [—[, BC masked, RE; SDS, 98%. **B.** Three years later, the audiogram reveals a drop in AC and the evolving diminishing air–bone gap. Negative Rinne response at 256 Hz. The SDS (98%) remained unusually high. ●—●, AC, unmasked, RE; [—[, BC, masked, RE; **arrow,** no response at maximum output.

version from positive to negative with first changes in the 128 and 256 Hz forks. The third sign is the development of an air–bone gap at 250 Hz and then at 500 Hz audiometrically. This shift may follow either an air-conduction drop or occasionally an apparent bone conduction "improvement"! Occasionally, it is possible to predict such a chronologic transformation. As an example, we can consider the patient with a fairly typical bilaterally symmetric sensorineural or "perceptive" curve with no air–bone gap or even with a bone conduction curve substantially depressed below the air-conduction curve. The only finding that might lead to a prediction of developing otosclerosis would be the unusually good speech discrimination score—e.g., a 98% SDS in a case with a 45 dB "perceptive" loss. If the hearing in one ear begins to decrease unilaterally, it may then be possible to elicit a Weber shift from central to the poorer side. This may eventually be followed by a change in the Rinne (Fig. 19–22).

FRONTAL BONE-CONDUCTION THRESHOLDS

Clinical bone conduction measurements have traditionally been performed with the vibrator located on the mastoid process. As early as the 1930's, however, Bekesy (3) and Barany (1) suggested that this position on the skull may be one of the least favorable for clinical testing. The frontal bone has received the most attention as an alternate site and was the subject of comparative investigations begun in our laboratory in 1967. Detailed results of the preliminary study of 60 cases with diverse middle-ear problems were published

by Dirks and Malmquist (5). To summarize briefly, the main conclusions of the study were that mastoid and frontal bone conduction thresholds both are influenced by middle ear lesions, but for certain types of lesions, thresholds obtained at the frontal bone are less depressed than those at the mastoid process, because of mechanical artifacts. For the 60 subjects tested, the average difference between measurements at the two sites was 5 dB when reported in terms of hearing level. In some cases, however, thresholds at the frontal bone were reduced as much as 20 dB from comparative thresholds at the mastoid. Of the 60 subjects, 38 were subsequently operated on, and details of the middle ear impairment were obtained. The following findings were of interest. In 7 of the 38 subjects, the frontal bone–mastoid differences exceeded those observed in normal listeners, and surgery revealed that the patients had either malleus fixation or ossicular discontinuity due to incus necrosis or absence of the incus. In 17 cases with stapes fixation due to otosclerosis, no differences were found between frontal-bone and mastoid results. The range of frontal bone–mastoid differences was the same for the stapes fixation group as for listeners with normal hearing. It was suggested that the large frontal bone–mastoid differences observed in the aforementioned seven cases could be identified in clinical settings and that the comparison of frontal and mastoid bone conduction results might be of potential significance for differential diagnosis of some middle ear impairments.

On the basis of our experiences with the low-frequency air–bone gap previously discussed, we felt that it was increasingly important to discover even the relatively small air–bone gap and have thus encouraged the use of the frontal bone as an additional site for performing routine clinical bone-conduction measurements. Our observations suggest that these measurements can provide additional important information in the differential diagnosis of middle ear lesions (15); however, we emphasize that testing at the frontal bone alone, exclusive of other measurements of sensorineural acuity, is not always sufficient for confirmation of a conductive component and certainly not for detailed differential diagnosis of middle ear lesions.

Recent developments in sensorineural acuity level tests (SAL) in frontal bone-conduction measurement techniques and in acoustic impedance studies have been incorporated into the conductive loss test battery. These new methods can clarify many differential diagnostic problems.

THE CONDUCTIVE LOSS TEST BATTERY

Frontal Bone-Conduction and Sensorineural Acuity Level (SAL) Measurements

Routine mastoid bone conduction measurements have now been expanded to include the SAL battery. Thus, a more precise comparison may be made of mastoid, frontal, and air-conduction thresholds. Air conduction is tested first in quiet and repeated with the addition of narrow-band masking noise presented at the forehead. The amount of threshold shift can then be compared to that obtained in the normal ear. In a conductive loss, as might be expected, the shift more closely approximates the normal shift, and the SAL thresholds may reveal a greater difference between air and bone conduction than those recorded at the mastoid. The greater the sensori-

neural involvement, the less difference between air-conduction and bone conduction levels in quiet and in noise (see Ch. 6, Audiologic Assessment, Functional Hearing Loss, and Objective Audiometry).

Acoustic Impedance

Acoustic impedance of the middle ear is a term used to describe the opposition afforded by the middle ear to the passage of sound. It is determined by measuring the amplitude of the incident and reflected sound waves in response to a pure tone of fixed frequency. It is measured in units termed *acoustic ohms*. To differentiate between the normal middle ear, otosclerosis, lateral fixation, or ossicular discontinuity, three indexes are used.

THE ACOUSTIC REFLEX. This is the acoustic reflex of the stapedius muscle. In the normal ear one would expect a positive acoustic reflex—that is, a bilateral contraction of the stapedius muscle would be reflected on the acoustic bridge (see Ch. 6). In otosclerosis there will be no (negative) acoustic reflex.

TYMPANOMETRY. Tympanometry is a graphic representation of tympanic membrane mobility. Since the normal tympanic membrane is not hindered by fixation of any sort, characteristic ear drum movements are recorded (Fig. 19–23). In otosclerosis the tympanometry findings may be normal in an early case but will show restricted tympanic membrane mobility in more advanced cases.

TOTAL IMPEDANCE. When there is no mechanical block in the middle ear, there is no sound absorp-

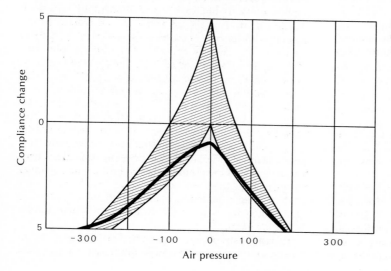

FIG. 19–23. Note otosclerotic restricted mobility curve. Air pressure, cross-hatching, normal range; solid line, otosclerosis, stapes fixation.

tion or reflection. The normal range of total impedance is 900–2800 acoustic ohms. In otosclerosis the total impedance is usually high (2400–4800 acoustic ohms).

DIFFERENTIAL DIAGNOSIS— PSEUDO-OTOSCLEROSIS

The diagnosis of otosclerosis is usually made on the basis of a conductive hearing loss, an intact and mobile tympanic membrane, patent eustachian tube, negative Rinne test, and a significant audiometric air–bone gap. *But such a patient may not have otosclerosis.* **Pseudo-otosclerosis** is a term used to describe a number of diseases that mimic otosclerosis.

Under the differential diagnosis of otosclerosis, we need not include such other middle ear diseases as tympanic perforations with or without otorrhea, tympanic polyposis, and other lesions with obvious signs of active tympanic disease. The cases that mimic otosclerosis and thus warrant the term pseudo-otosclerosis (10) are characterized by an intact tympanic membrane and a significant conductive hearing loss. The vast majority of these cases are unilateral. Although unilateral otosclerosis does occur, the possibility of pseudo-otosclerosis is greater in unilateral cases.

Four groups of lesions are included in pseudo-otosclerosis: 1) middle ear lesions; 2) incus and malleus lesions; 3) nonotosclerotic stapes lesions; and 4) congenital anomalies of ossicles and labyrinth windows.

MIDDLE EAR LESIONS

Secretory Otitis Media

Secretory otitis media is an important cause of conductive hearing loss, which may persist for years as a stable, painless hearing loss, unaccompanied by tinnitus or vertigo. The tympanic membrane may be slightly thickened (Fig. 19–24), and definitive fluid may or may not be seen on otoscopy. Conductive hearing losses will resemble those in otosclerosis. Haziness or density on on Schuller's x-ray views of the mastoid will be diagnostic (see Ch. 15, Secretory Otitis Media).

Middle Ear Fibrosis and Granulomatosis

Granulomatous otitis media can mimic otosclerosis on otoscopic examination and be accompanied by conductive hearing losses varying from 25–60 dB (Fig. 19–25). Mastoid x-ray findings should differentiate this condition from otosclerosis (see Ch. 16, Chronic Otomastoiditis—Diagnosis and

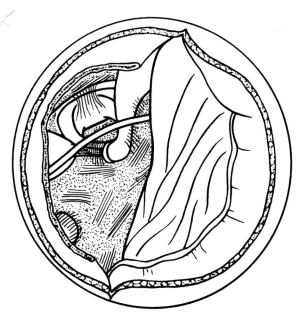

FIG. 19–24. Chronic secretory otitis media—fluid and fibrosis.

FIG. 19–25. Granulomatous otitis.

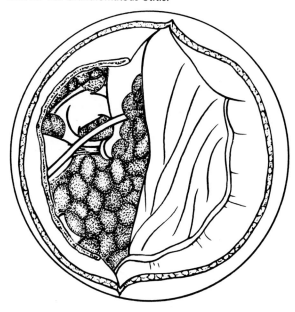

Management). Middle ear fibrosis produces findings (Fig. 19–26) similar to those of granulomatous otitis media.

Tympanosclerosis

Tympanosclerosis, a variant of chronic otitis media, can produce stapes fixation or total os-

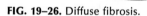

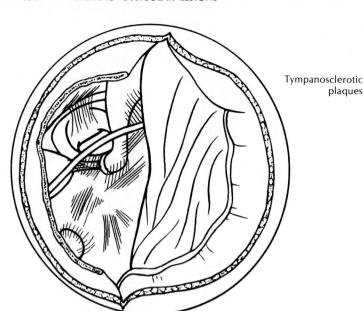

FIG. 19–26. Diffuse fibrosis.

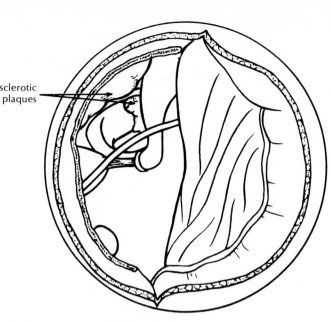

Tympanosclerotic plaques

FIG. 19–27. Tympanosclerosis. Note tympanosclerotic lesion confined to crura and footplate of stapes.

sicular fixation (30- to 60-dB conductive hearing loss).

Tympanosclerosis may occur in the middle ear with minor tympanic membrane abnormalities and thus mimic otosclerosis (Figs. 19–27, 19–28, 19–29).

FIG. 19–28. Tympanosclerosis, diffuse. Note tympanosclerotic lesions on the incus, on the stapes, and on diffuse areas of the otic capsule.

Primary Keratoma

Primary or congenital keratoma can lurk behind an intact tympanic membrane and mimic otosclerosis with a painless and unilateral conductive hearing loss varying from 15–60 dB (Fig. 19–30).

Cerebrospinal Fluid or Perilymph in the Middle Ear

A patient with unilateral conductive hearing loss of long duration, normal tympanic membrane, and an audiometric pattern typical of early otosclerosis, may have a middle ear filled with fluid detectable only on tympanotomy. The fluid is clear and refills on aspiration. Careful exploration to determine its origin is essential. The fluid may be cerebrospinal fluid from an unsuspected fracture of the epitympanic tegmen tympani due to a previous head injury (see Ch. 24, Traumatic Diseases of the Ear and Temporal Bone). The fluid may be perilymph from a fracture or dislocation

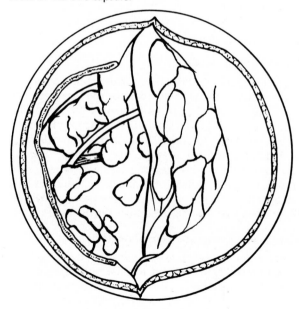

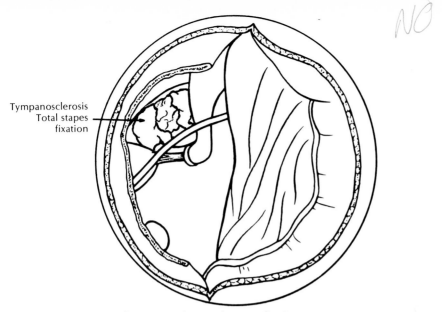

Tympanosclerosis
Total stapes
fixation

FIG. 19–29. Tympanosclerosis causing total stapes fixation.

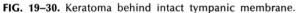

FIG. 19–30. Keratoma behind intact tympanic membrane.

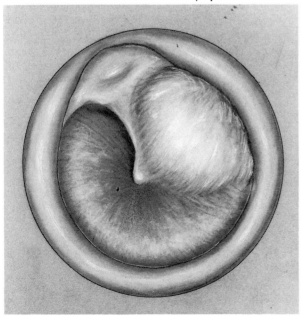

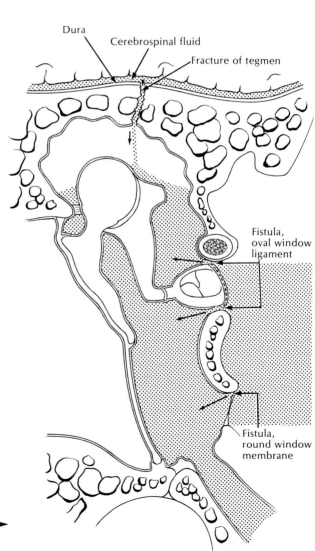

Dura

Cerebrospinal fluid

Fracture of tegmen

Fistula,
oval window
ligament

Fistula,
round window
membrane

FIG. 19–31. Middle ear fluid (either cerebrospinal fluid or ▶ perilymph), which can mimic clinical findings of otosclerosis.

of the stapes, with perilymph leaking from the scala vestibuli. The fluid also could be perilymph leaking from the scala tympani through an unsuspected rupture of the round window membrane (Fig. 19–31) (see Ch. 37, Sudden Hearing Loss Syndrome).

Special diagnostic studies and a second-stage surgical procedure will usually be necessary to deal appropriately with this type of pseudo-otosclerosis.

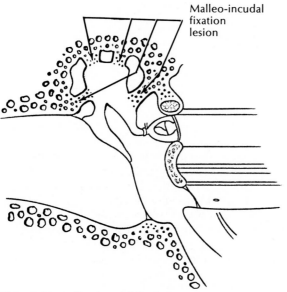

Malleo-incudal fixation lesion

FIG. 19–32. Malleo-incudal fixation.

FIG. 19–33. Fusion of the incus with annulus. Note bony union between long process of incus and annulus.

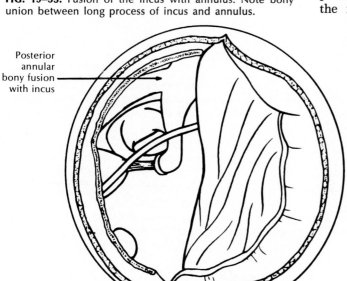

Posterior annular bony fusion with incus

INCUS AND MALLEUS LESIONS

Lateral Ossicular Fixation

The incus and/or malleus can become partially or completely fixed, producing a variety and a continuum of conductive hearing losses.

PANOSSICULAR ARTHRITIC FIXATION. A true osteoarthritis may involve the entire ossicular chain with not only a fixed stapes but also a fixed incudomalleal joint and a fixed incudostapedial joint. Such a case may be clinically indistinguishable from otosclerosis before operation. However, it is usually unilateral, and tympanometry may be helpful in differential diagnosis. The stapedius reflex will be negative, and total impedance will be high.

THE FIXED MALLEUS-INCUS SYNDROME. The fixed malleus-incus syndrome is a special category of nonotosclerotic (pseudootosclerosis) lateral fixation involving either stiffness or fixation of the malleus alone, of the incus alone, or of both malleus and incus without involvement of the stapes (Fig. 19–32). This lesion is a classic example of pseudo-otosclerosis and frequently is not recognized before operation. Stapedius reflex will be negative and total impedance very high (see Ch. 20, Lateral Ossicular Fixation).

This lesion is very often missed during stapes surgery. The surgeon who makes the diagnosis of otosclerosis on the basis of the usual criteria, with a predetermined plan to remove the stapes completely, may do so without testing the mobility of the incus and malleus. An excellent technical

NO

FIG. 19–34. Tympanometry curves in ossicular discontinuity, otosclerosis, and ossicular fixation (lateral).

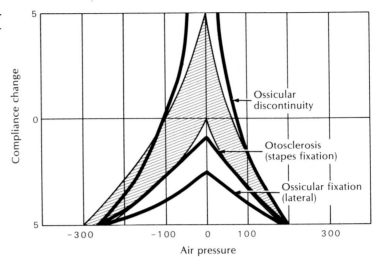

FIG. 19–35. Incus appears to be normal before palpation.

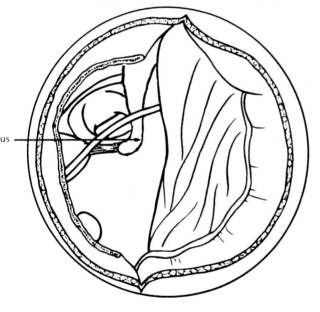

stapedectomy may be accomplished with good placement of the stapes substitute and good closure of the oval window, *but with no improvement in hearing.* Such instances of so-called stapes surgery failures are usually due to lack of recognition of a fixed malleus and incus. The conductive hearing loss and otoscopic findings may be exactly the same as those of otosclerosis. Conductive loss battery and impedance studies will frequently avert such a mistaken diagnosis and mistaken surgical procedure, but the primary safeguard is palpation of the malleus and incus before proceeding with definitive stapedectomy during the surgical procedure.

INCUS–ANNULUS FUSION. In tympanic fibrosis of long duration, eventual osteogenic activity may produce bony fusion in several areas. Occasionally this is characterized by an attachment of the incus to the bony annulus, which produces a secondary type of lateral ossicular fixation (Fig. 19–33). Findings are similar to those in the fixed malleus-incus syndrome. Management is based on ossiculoplasty principles (see Ch. 17, Otomastoiditis Surgery—Mastoidectomy and Tympanoplasty).

Discontinuity of the Incus

Tympanometry is important diagnostically in the following three incudal problems. The reflex is negative, but there is abnormal tympanic membrane compliance, and a low impedance system is usually found (Fig. 19–34) (see Ch. 6, Audiologic Assessment, Functional Hearing Loss, and Objective Audiometry).

INCUDAL LONG PROCESS ATROPHY AND NECROSIS. In contrast to the problem of fixation of the incus, it is possible for a major conductive hearing loss (pseudo-otosclerosis) to result from fibrous atrophy of the long process of the incus in which the periosteum remains intact but there is no bony continuity (Figs. 19–35, 19–36, 19–37). Such an atrophic incus is no longer capable of transmitting acoustic energy because of loss of stiffness. This condition of apparent incudal continuity because of the intact periosteum produces a surgical diagnostic trap. Palpation of the incus quickly reveals the bony discontinuity.

Actual necrosis of the long-process bone is easily recognized. There is a gap between an incudal long-process stump and the stapedial

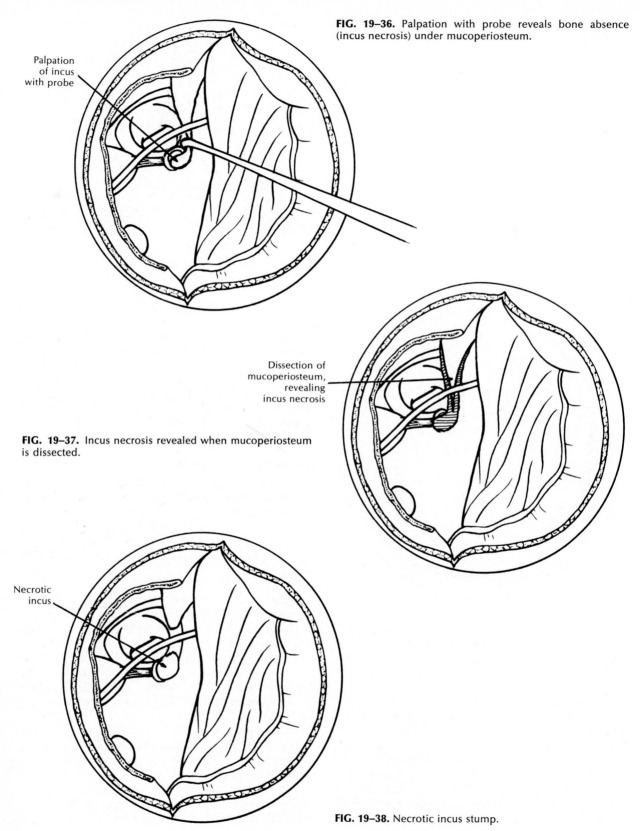

Palpation
of incus
with probe

FIG. 19–36. Palpation with probe reveals bone absence (incus necrosis) under mucoperiosteum.

Dissection of
mucoperiosteum,
revealing
incus necrosis

FIG. 19–37. Incus necrosis revealed when mucoperiosteum is dissected.

Necrotic
incus

FIG. 19–38. Necrotic incus stump.

FIG. 19–39. Discontinuity between incus and stapes due to lenticular process necrosis.

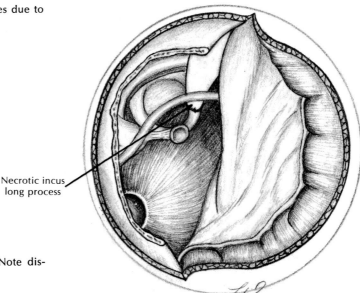

Necrotic incus
long process

FIG. 19–40. Traumatic dislocation of the incus. Note discontinuity between dislocated incus and stapes.

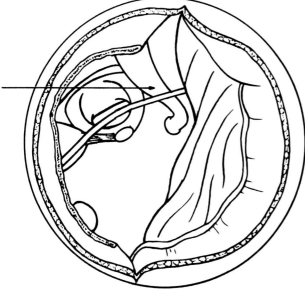

ncus
ated

The treatment of lenticular process necrosis is essentially similar to that of incus atrophy— namely, that of ossiculoplasty. However, in occasional cases, in which the lenticular process defect is less than 1 mm, it may be possible to restore excellent continuity through the use of a tragal cartilage disk, wedged between the long process and stapes capitulum.

TRAUMATIC DISLOCATION OR ABSENCE OF INCUS. One should suspect pseudootosclerosis in the patient with presumptive otosclerosis who gives a history of an infantile mastoidectomy and in whom there is a small postauricular scar. Not infrequently such a patient has a perfectly mobile stapes, with the conductive loss attributal to a traumatically dislocated incus at the time of the infant mastoid operation (Fig. 19–40). The incus may have been dislocated into the mastoid antrum or the epitympanum, or it may have atrophied so that it will not be found anywhere. Not too infrequently, such a condition may occur bilaterally; the patient will know of a bilateral conductive hearing loss since childhood with no history of ear suppuration in adult life. The tympanic membrane is intact and there may be a well-pneumatized mastoid on the affected side or sides.

The treatment of the case of absent incus is best carried out by ossiculoplasty, through the use of a prefabricated homograft, which is anchored to a trough drilled in the region of the malleal neck. The medial saddle of the homograft is placed in contact with the mobile stapedial capitulum.

capitulum. Incus necrosis and/or atrophy is usually due to chronic otitis media but occasionally may be due to an anomalous developmental condition. Surgical repair requires ossiculoplasty (Fig. 19–38) (see Ch. 17, Otomastoiditis Surgery —Mastoidectomy and Tympanoplasty).

INCUDAL LENTICULAR PROCESS NECROSIS. A common cause of conductive hearing loss is necrosis of the lenticular process of the incus (Fig. 19–39). This is frequently seen during mastoidectomy and tympanoplastic surgery but may also occur behind an intact, apparently normal tympanic membrane. In such cases it may definitely mimic otosclerosis.

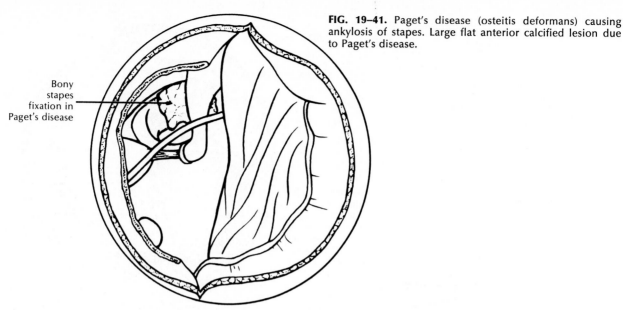

Bony
stapes
fixation in
Paget's disease

FIG. 19–41. Paget's disease (osteitis deformans) causing ankylosis of stapes. Large flat anterior calcified lesion due to Paget's disease.

NONOTOSCLEROTIC LESIONS OF THE STAPES

Paget's Disease

Paget's disease, a deforming progressive bone disease with primary involvement of the skull and long bones (Fig. 19–41) also involves the temporal bone, in which ankylosis of the stapes may occur. This disease, also known as osteitis deformans, can mimic otosclerosis very closely. Petrous apex and otic capsule involvement may also produce sensorineural hypacusis (cochlear hearing loss).

Paget's disease involvement of the stapes can be differentiated from otosclerosis at surgery by the absence of true otosclerosis coronae in the promontory or anywhere surrounding the footplate. The fixation is usually in the region of the stapedial footplate ligament, but hypertrophic deformations are also seen in the stapedial crura. A successful stapedectomy is possible in many patients with Paget's disease stapedial fixation. The oval window should be sealed with a tissue graft, such as perichondrium.

Osteogenesis Imperfecta (Van der Hoeve's Syndrome)

Osteogenesis imperfecta also known as fragilitas ossium, osteopsathyrosis, periosteal dysplasia, Lobstein's disease, Eddowes' syndrome, is a systemic disease characterized by the occurrence of multiple fractures with poor healing, not only in the long bones but in the calvarium. Although true otosclerosis may coexist in a rather high incidence, this is more commonly a pseudootosclerosis, a conductive hypacusis caused by some other middle

FIG. 19–42. Crural necrosis in osteogenesis imperfecta.

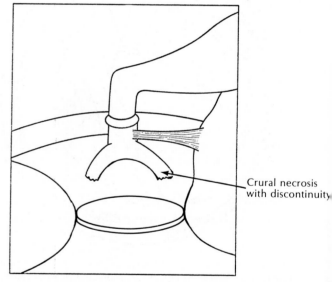

Crural necrosis
with discontinuity

ear lesion, especially crural and incudal necrosis and atrophy (Figs. 19–42, 19–43).

Tympanometry can be most helpful in such cases. If the primary lesion is crural necrosis, an abnormal tympanic membrane compliance will be demonstrated with a positive stapedial reflex.

The diagnosis of van der Hoeve's syndrome is based upon a history of multiple fractures, and the findings of blue sclerae, and conductive hearing loss. The treatment of the hearing loss in osteogenesis imperfecta depends upon the lesions in

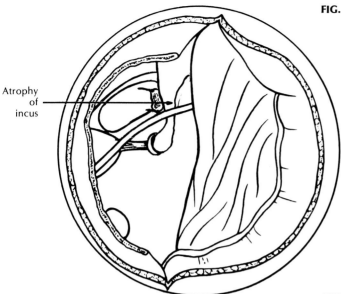

FIG. 19–43. Atrophic incus in osteogenesis imperfecta.

Atrophy
of
incus

FIG. 19–44. Footplate arthritis. Circumferential lesion involving entire annular ligament without otosclerosis.

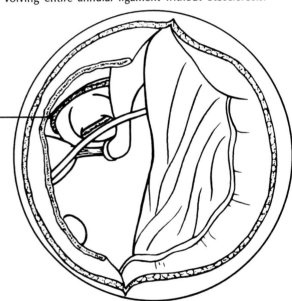

Annular
osteoarthritis
of stapes

the ossicular chain. It may be necessary in some cases to do a staged procedure involving an ossiculoplasty at the first stage and a stapedectomy at the second stage.

Tympanosclerosis of the Stapes

Tympanosclerosis, a hyalinized collagen process, is probably a healing variant of chronic otitis media (see Ch. 16, Chronic Otomastoiditis—Diagnosis and Management), but it may not always represent a subsiding process; it may have invasive properties. The lesion may invade the labyrinthine capsule and destroy the stapedial crura and footplate. Tympanosclerosis can occur behind an intact tympanic membrane, producing marked conductive hypacusis, thus mimicking otosclerosis.

A fairly classic stapedectomy procedure may be possible in stapedial tympanosclerosis, but great care must be taken in footplate removal to avoid damage to the cochlea. Tympanosclerotic plaques frequently are markedly erosive, with extensive invasion of the cochlear promontory and bone of the otic capsule.

Degenerative Footplate Arthritis

Arthritic degeneration of the peristapedial annular ligament may accompany tympanic fibrosis (Fig. 19-44). It may occur alone and mimic otosclerosis by ossification of the annular ligament. In the latter case, there is no visible typical otosclerotic corona, but the fixation is circumferential and quite diffuse.

Stapedectomy may be performed in footplate arthritis. In most instances the results are equivalent to those seen in true otosclerosis.

Crural Atrophy

Chronic latent otitis media may produce complete crural necrosis in an apparently normal middle ear, simulating otosclerosis. If crural atrophy is the only lesion, it can be predicted before operation by abnormal tympanic membrane compliance on tympanometry and a positive stapedial reflex. If crural necrosis is encountered, the stapedial reflex will be absent. The lesion may or may not be combined with other ossicular lesions. The footplate is usually mobile and intact. If the incus is normal, any type of prosthetic stapedectomy restoration may be employed, such as the use of a tantalum ribbon prosthesis or a stainless steel "wire" between the long process of the incus and the mobile stapedial footplate.

Peristapedial Fibrous Tent

A peristapedial fibrous tent may be the only sequel of a previous chronic secretory otitis media that has subsided, either spontaneously or as a result of treatment. The stapes may be partly or completely fixed by a dense fibrous tent without any involvement of the rest of the middle ear or the incus or malleus. Preoperative tympanometry may show an absent or a reversal reflex and normal tympanic membrane compliance.

Careful dissection of the fibrous tent may be possible, with restoration of mobility of the stapedial footplate. Stapedectomy may be necessary. A reconstruction employing a tissue graft such as perichondrium and the use of a metal prosthesis is usually quite successful in restoration of hearing function.

CONGENITAL ANOMALIES OF OSSICLES AND LABYRINTH WINDOWS

Several tympanic anomalies producing conductive defects are indistinguishable from otosclerosis prior to operation. These include 1) absent incus

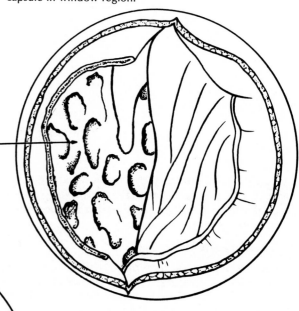

FIG. 19–46. Prototype of congenital malformation of otic capsule in window region.

Congenital lack of oval and round windows

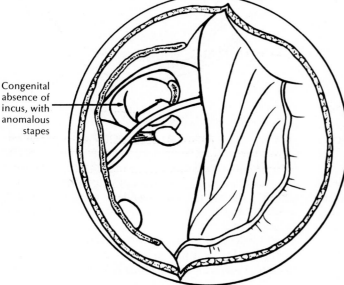

FIG. 19–45. Congenital anomaly. No incus, and abnormal stapes represented by a posterior crus with a lenticular process and a short stub of an anterior crus.

Congenital absence of incus, with anomalous stapes

and abnormal stapes (Fig. 19–45); absent incus and stapes with ill-defined promontory window area (Fig. 19–46); and 3) congenital stapes fixation, occasionally accompanied by abnormal patency of the cochlear aqueduct or abnormally wide medial vestibular foramina.

A persistent stapedial artery may be present. This embryonically large artery may occupy the entire obturator foramen space of the stapes and fixes the stapes partially or completely. Occasionally secondary osteoarthritic fixation of the stapes accompanies a long-standing congenitally persistent stapedial artery.

Surgical stapedectomy techniques in such anomalous cases are technically extremely difficult. These are high-risk stapedectomy cases from the point of view of possible cochlear damage and facial nerve injury.

MEDICAL MANAGEMENT

Medical treatments for otosclerosis have been proposed from time to time. Siebenmann recommended phosphorous therapy (43); Gray advised the use of thyroxine (17); and a number of other medical modalities appear in the older otologic literature. No significant reports of hearing improvement ever appeared.

Following a study of reversal of experimental halisteresis in rats, Guggenheim and co-workers (19) proposed a program of dicalcium phosphate for the medical therapy of otosclerosis, especially for use in pregnant women with otosclerosis and rapidly advancing hearing loss during pregnancy. Although no significant long-range studies followed these original experiments and clinical studies, a good deal of clinical evidence was accumulated to indicate that dicalcium phosphate therapy with vitamins seems to play a role in slowing the rapid progression of otosclerosis (especially the cochlear phase) in some pregnant women. When such calcium therapy was employed, a significant decrease in the indications for therapeutic abortions was noted in women with otosclerosis. Since fenestration surgery for otosclerosis came into wide use at that time, this calcium program was discontinued. There may be a place for reconsidering such a therapeutic approach in otosclerosis in women of child-bearing age, and possibly in all young patients (under 20). The basic concept was an attempt to convert the active process of otospongiosis to a quiescent otosclerotic state, thus producing some degree of limitation to the extent of the otic capsular disease.

In 1952, in a pilot study of the use of cortisone therapy in otosclerosis, no significant hearing improvements were reported by Goodhill (9).

Shambaugh and Scott (42) reported the use of sodium fluoride for arrest of otosclerosis, especially in cochlear otosclerosis. Shambaugh and colleagues (41) advised a dosage of 20 mg of enteric-coated sodium fluoride taken twice a day, equaling 40 mg per day. They recommended, in addition, 0.5 g calcium gluconate twice daily and one multivitamin tablet containing 400 units of Vitamin D daily. This program was advised for 2 years. The investigators recommended that if there were further sensorineural loss, continued positive Schwartze sign, or polytomographic evidence of continued or increased activity of the focus, the sodium fluoride be increased to 60 mg daily. They also advised a maintenance dose of 15–20 mg daily, once definite stabilization of the process occurred.

In a November 1976 Medical Letter report (33) dealing with fluoride therapy in osteoporosis, it was pointed out that fluorosis can occur after long-term ingestion of fluoride in amounts over 20 mg per day. The report concluded as follows: "Medical Letter consultants recommended that fluoride intake from all sources be limited to no more than 10 mg per day."

In a June 1977 editorial, "Sodium Fluoride and Cochlear Otospongiosis,"* Donaldson pointed out that the Food and Drug Administration does not recognize any sodium fluoride preparation that provides "a fluoride ion concentration greater than 1 mg per tablet or capsule as safe and effective for any use."

Sodium fluoride for the treatment of otospongiosis has not been approved. Donaldson states: "Before sodium fluoride can be approved by the FDA for the treatment of cochlear otospongiosis, substantial evidence of safety and effectiveness must be presented to the agency and evaluated by it. As yet, the agency has not received such evidence."

It appears, therefore, that more data are necessary to validate the use of sodium fluoride in the medical management of cochlear otosclerosis. At the present time (1977) there is no final answer on definitive medical therapy or medical preventive therapy in the management of otosclerosis.

SURGICAL MANAGEMENT

HISTORY

The first attempt to deal surgically with otosclerosis was a direct surgical approach to the stapes. In 1878 Kessel (after experiments with Mach in 1870) first "mobilized" the fixed stapes (27). Miot in 1891 reported results from more than 200 cases of stapes mobilization with many surgical successes (35). Other investigators also performed some stapes operations. Because of controversial reports, however, stapes surgery was abandoned at the beginning of the twentieth century.

The second attempt to deal surgically with oto-

* Donaldson JA: Sodium fluoride and cochlear otospongiosis. Arch Otolaryngol 103:313, 1977

sclerosis was through fenestration of the labyrinth. Passow (37) in 1897 had fenestrated the cochlear promontory. Floderus (6) in 1899 suggested fenestration of the horizontal semicircular canal. Fenestration surgery was further developed by Jenkins (26) in 1913, Holmgren (25) in 1923, and Sourdille (45) in 1930. Lempert utilized the endaural approach and developed a practical one-stage technique in 1938 (28, 29). His version of the semicircular canal fenestration really started the present era of surgery for deafness.

In December 1952 Rosen (38) reintroduced the operation of Miot in stapes surgery, with a number of modifications. Rosen's work in mobilization surgery established stapes surgery as the primary management for otosclerosis. Mobilization was followed by techniques involving removal of the footplate. Thus, *stapedectomy* became the basic approach for the treatment of otosclerosis. The fenestration operation became a secondary procedure and is used relatively infrequently at the present time.

STAPES SURGERY

The most common surgical procedure for otosclerosis is some type of stapes surgery. In special situations stapediolysis (mobilization) without removal of any part of the stapes may be indicated. Although fenestration of the labyrinth (the Lempert operation) is used rarely at the present time, a number of patients who have had previous fenestration operations still require postoperative care. Special aspects of postfenestration stapes surgery and other aspects relating to fenestration patients are discussed later in this chapter.

CANDIDATE SELECTION FOR STAPES SURGERY

The average patient with otosclerosis and a bone conduction level of 0–20 dB in the speech range and an air conduction level of 35–65 dB is a candidate for stapes surgery.

In general, stapes surgery is indicated for the patient with otosclerosis, regardless of age, who has an air–bone gap of at least 15 dB (particularly in the lower frequencies) and a speech discrimination score of 60% or better, and who has no anatomic or general medical contraindications to exploratory tympanotomy under local anesthesia.

The new tools of tympanometry and impedance audiometry and the overall conductive loss battery make preoperative assessment of otosclerosis more precise. The presence of an occlusion effect would point to possible diagnostic error or incomplete fixation. A positive stapedius reflex would point to some form of pseudootosclerosis. An open-end tympanogram would point to ossicular discontinuity. An air–bone gap may not be present with conventional mastoid bone conduction measurement, but can frequently be detected by frontal bone studies of bone conduction and SAL.

For the average case the upper limit for air conduction threshold would be approximately 80–85 dB. At higher loss levels a greater air–bone gap would be desirable. For example, a 25-dB air–bone gap at 65 dB, a 35-dB air–bone gap at 75 dB, and a 40-dB level gap at 85 dB. The criteria can be expanded for advanced otosclerosis. Thus, a patient with a bone conduction level even as low as 40–45 dB and an air conduction level of 95–100 dB may be considered a candidate for stapes surgery. Evidence of adequate cochlear reserve, as measured by speech discrimination scores, is necessary. The ultimate aim is *restoration of available cochlear function,* even though this may not always carry with it *the possibility of unaided hearing.* These are guidelines, and the experienced otologist will make exceptions as necessary. Such exceptions can include patients with a past history of clear-cut otosclerosis with very poor speech discrimination scores or no speech discrimination response and air conduction levels at the limit of the audiometer output, provided that a conductive-loss battery shows a measurable air–bone gap by frontal bone conduction and sensorineural acuity level studies, and impedance studies demonstrate an absent stapedius reflex, absent occlusion effect, and appropriate tympanogram (see Ch. 6, Audiologic Assessment, Functional Hearing Loss, and Objective Audiometry).

Patients with losses in the 90- to 100-dB range and no *measurable* cochlear reserve on speech discrimination scores may still be candidates for stapes surgery if the history pointing to otosclerosis is clear-cut, particularly from the points of view of progression, classic audiometric findings in the opposite (usually) better ear, and history of previous favorable response to hearing-aid amplification. In such extremely advanced cases, stapes surgery may indeed be very valuable for the possibility of restoring hearing only for the purpose of hearing aid use in an ear which was previously totally useless.

PREOPERATIVE MANAGEMENT

The probability and definition of surgical success are carefully explained to the patient and the alternative of hearing-aid use is discussed. In most cases, patients have already been using hearing aids without great satisfaction, prior to requesting surgery.

It is advisable to obtain pertinent general medical information prior to stapes surgery. This includes cardiocirculatory status, drug and other allergies, possible psychiatric problems, possible special preanesthesia and presurgery advice from the general physician (*e.g.*, patients on anticoagulant therapy), and possible contraindications to the use of routine local anesthetic drugs.

SURGICAL TECHNIQUE

The adequately sedated patient is brought to the operating room and moved to an operating table capable of lateral tilting of 20–25° in addition to normal head and foot area mobility.

The binocular surgical dissecting microscope is virtually universally used and in most clinics the surgeon stands or sits behind the patient's head in the posterior position. Straight oculars are customarily employed.

A stockinet cap (Fig. 19–47) with an opening for the auricle is placed on the patient's head. An ad-

ditional adhesive dressing protects the surgical field from hair. Opinions vary as to the efficacy of so-called orthopedic preparation of external canal skin. Strong drugs and excessively vigorous scrubbing of this area may be more harmful than prophylactically useful. A clear plastic drape is allowed to adhere to the prepared field. The patient receives oxygen at 0.6 liter/min through nasal tubing. A self-retaining speculum holder is useful.

My colleagues and I prefer an anterior or frontal position and use inclined oculars. This approach is based on purely anatomic grounds. The post-tympanic compartment is more conveniently visualized by this approach in our experience. It requires tilting the patient toward the surgeon approximately 20–25° (Figs. 19–48 through 19–51).

Local Anesthesia

Local anesthesia is preferred by most American otologic surgeons although basal and general anesthesia are in wide use in other parts of the world. In the use of general anesthesia, it is wise to add local anesthesia also, to obtain better control of bleeding.

FIG. 19–47. Head dressing for ear and mastoid surgery.

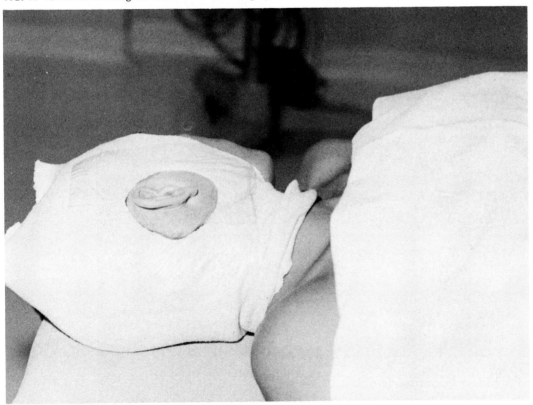

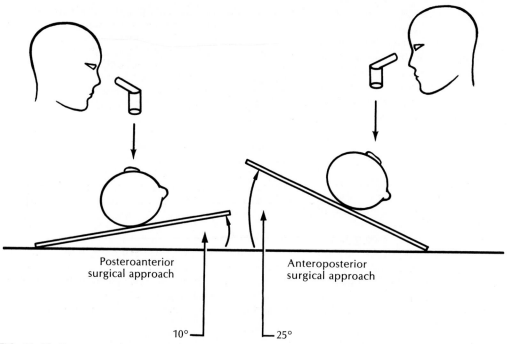

Posteroanterior
surgical approach

Anteroposterior
surgical approach

10°

25°

FIG. 19–48. Posteroanterior view and anteroposterior view of operating table arrangements.

FIG. 19–49. Operating table tilted 20–25° toward surgeon for the anteroposterior approach.

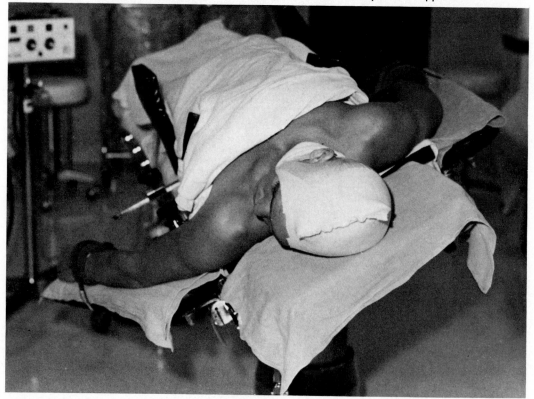

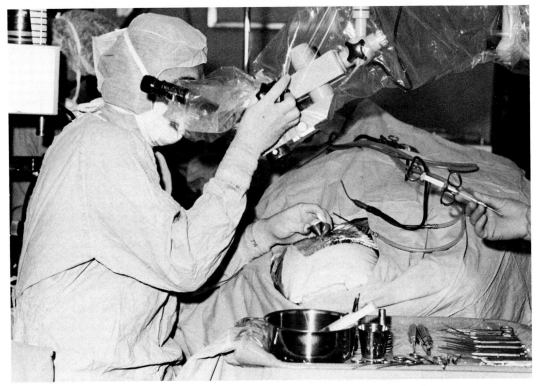

FIG. 19–50. Patient tilted. Surgeon sits in front (anterior) for better visualization of posterior tympanic compartment.

FIG. 19–51. Patient tilted 10% posteriorly for posterior visualization of anterior tympanic structures.

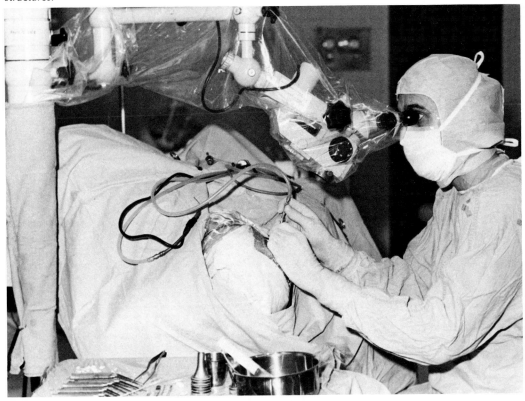

In our practice, local anesthesia is obtained by block injection of the ear canal using a lidocaine-epinephrine solution (Xylocaine, 1.5%, with epinephrine, 1:200,000). An initial injection of 0.2 cc is made at the inferior apex of the helicotragal junction with a 30-gauge 1.5-in needle (which is quite painless). Further circumferential injections are made at the external meatus with a 26-gauge 1.5-in needle so that a total of 2 cc is injected. Moistened applicators are used to "massage" the anesthetic fluid from the injection site medially to the region of the annulus. This accomplishes a partial elevation of the posterior skin flap and also encourages more complete anesthesia in the region of the annulus.

The operation is performed through an ear speculum, using the operating microscope for illumination and magnification. The incision is endomeatal, but in rare instances, such as in the presence of partial congenital canal atresia or in the presence of obstructive osteophytes, a modified endaural incision may be necessary. This is also carried out under local anesthesia.

Endomeatal Incision and Exposure of the Middle Ear

Angulated circumferential scalpels (large) are used for the incision. Bleeding is usually minimal. In some instances it may be persistent, calling for control by pressure or by electrocoagulation with a small cautery suction. Suction is obtained through blunt, curved, modified spinal puncture needles of various diameters (gauges 15, 18, and 22).

The incision in the posterior half of the canal skin is omega-shaped, starting at the inferior aspect of the annulus and ending superior to the short process of the malleus (see Ch. 12, Basic Otosurgical Procedures). The posterior flap, consisting of skin and periosteum, is dissected from the bone with the same large circumferential scalpel. The elevation is facilitated by gentle blunt dissection, using cotton balls. When canal suture lines are exposed, sharp dissection is used. The elevation is carried medially until the posterior margin of the annular sulcus is reached. The fibrous annulus is separated from the bony sulcus.

Enucleation of Fibrous Annulus, Opening of Middle Ear, and Exposure of Incudostapedial Joint

When the margin of the tympanic annular bony sulcus is reached, the small, round, circumferential scalpel is used to enucleate the fibrous annulus from the bony sulcus. This enucleation is best started at about the midpoint of the posterior margin, usually slightly superior to the iter chordae posterius. Following the enucleation, penetration of the tympanic air space is accomplished by penetration of the "veil" of the mucosal lining between the chorda and the annulus fibrosus. The enucleation of the fibrous annulus from the sulcus is continued superiorly and inferiorly until exposure of the entire posterior half of the middle ear is obtained. This exposure will be limited superiorly by the junction of the pars tensa and pars flaccida. When the exposure is completed, the incudostapedial joint, the chorda tympani, the stapedial tendon, the entire stapes, the long process of the incus, the oval and round window niches, and the horizontal portion of the seventh nerve are all in clear view (Fig. 19–52). The posterior aspect of the handle of the malleus will also be seen. The promontory and the round window niche will usually appear prominently in the field. If such clear visualization is not easily accomplished, it is necessary to obtain more adequate exposure by the removal of sufficient bony annular quadrant to make this possible (Fig. 19–53). This may be done in most cases by the use of a sharp curet. Such bone removal should be

FIG. 19–52. Elevation and enucleation of canal-tympanic flap.

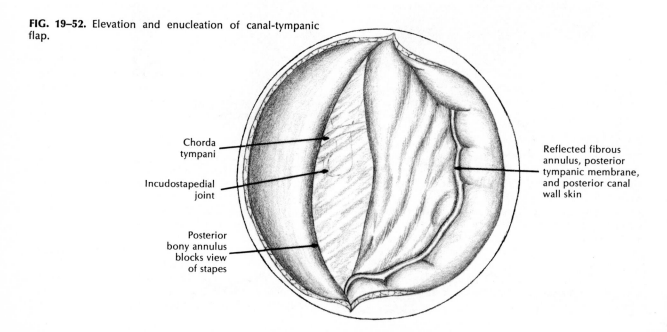

Chorda tympani

Incudostapedial joint

Posterior bony annulus blocks view of stapes

Reflected fibrous annulus, posterior tympanic membrane, and posterior canal wall skin

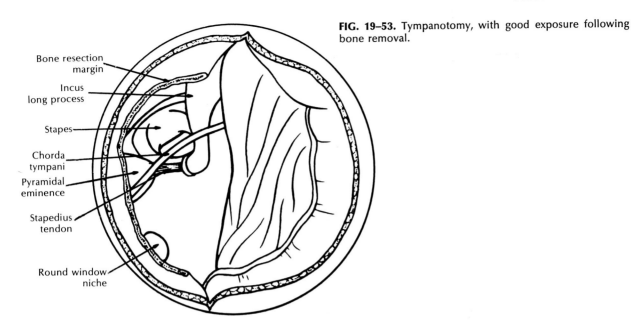

Bone resection margin

Incus long process

Stapes

Chorda tympani

Pyramidal eminence

Stapedius tendon

Round window niche

FIG. 19–53. Tympanotomy, with good exposure following bone removal.

done gently without trauma to the chorda tympani, which can usually be pushed aside with little difficulty. Sufficient posterior bone should be removed to give an adequate surgical approach. It is only occasionally necessary to cut the chorda so as not to jeopardize surgical access.

Exposure of Anterior Crus and Anterior Peribasal Region

It is necessary to obtain excellent exposure of the anterior as well as the posterior crus. Inasmuch as the otosclerotic lesion usually occupies the anterior peribasal region, this area must be adequately exposed to allow visualization and instrumentation.

Because of the curvature of the promontory and normal angulation of the stapes, the anterior crus can be seen only from its superior aspect in the usual posterior view. This angulation is frequently accentuated by the otosclerotic bony deformation of the anterior third of the footplate and the anterior crus. The anterior or frontal surgeon's position, previously described, obviates this difficulty. In this anterior approach, both posterior and anterior crura are adequately exposed.

Palpation of Incudomalleal Joint

With a probe, the incus is gently tested for mobility. Even in the presence of a rigidly ankylosed stapes, there is a degree of mobility of the incus that is easily determined by such palpation. A fixed incus usually is pathognomonic of a fixed incudomalleal joint. If the incudomalleal joint is fixed, as it may be in the fixed malleus syndrome, congenital anomalies, or in adhesive otitis media, this diagnosis is all-important. Such incudomalleal fixation may well account, by itself, for the entire conductive loss or it may coexist with the stapediovestibular fixation and cause failure if its presence is not realized.

Palpation of Incudostapedial Joint

The integrity of the incudostapedial joint is then assessed by palpation. Incudostapedial joint rigidity is pathologic and requires special attention.

Examination of Stapes

When the stapes is reached, three pledgets of compressed gelatin sponge (Gelfoam), dipped in a lidocaine solution are placed around the stapes (anterior, posterior, and inferior) for topical anesthesia of the tympanic plexus. They are removed before definitive stapedial manipulation begins.

The next very important step is to test the degree of footplate ankylosis via the capitulum and by palpating each crus. Occasionally, one encounters some apparent mobility. This may be real and should be followed by palpation of the pericrural footplate area. If there is indeed true mobility and if a round window reflex is noted, the diagnosis of stapedial otosclerosis is incorrect, and one is obviously dealing with some other problem such as a fixed malleus. Mobility may be false, either due to crural fracture or atrophy or to mobility of the mucoperiosteum only and not of the footplate *per se*.

Inspection of the footplate region requires an unimpeded view, particularly anteriorly. (An anterior approach by the surgeon has previously been stressed.) The majority of lesions predominate anterior to the anterior crus in the focus of predilection. Concomitantly, the mucoperiosteum in this region will be somewhat thicker and may obscure the extent and nature of the anterior lesion.

In the present stage of our experience, it seems prudent to use a rational selectivity of techniques based upon morphologic and functional differences. Thus, having inspected the lesion and evaluated all the data, usually one of three stapes procedures may be selected, keeping always in mind the possibility of a rare fourth subsequent procedure—*viz,* the semicircular canal fenestration. The three possible stapes procedures are 1) mobilization (pericrural stapediolysis, occasionally advisable); 2) partial stapedectomy (stapedioplasty or interposition); and 3) total stapedectomy (prosthetic stapedectomy).

MOBILIZATION (PERICRURAL STAPEDIOLYSIS)

There are limited indications for mobilization as follows: 1) the child or young adult with highly vascular mucoperiosteum ("juvenile" otosclerosis) with anterior ankylosis but definite mobility of the posterior footplate, 2) adults with excessive mucoperiosteal bleeding of vascular otospongiosis, and 3) congenital anomalies of the stapes, stapedial tendon, oval window niche, or facial nerve. There is a higher risk of labyrinthine complications when a stapedectomy is performed in such cases. Thus, in occasional situations pericrural stapediolysis is indicated.

Pericrural fracture (Fig. 19–54) is accomplished, utilizing either a chisel or a gouge. A gentle tap with a mallet is all that should be required for such a fracture. Usually, not more than one or two mallet taps are required to create the fracture line, with immediate rapid mobilization of the fixed stapes, a slight displacement into the vestibule, and an escape of perilymph. There should be no disruption of the stapedial

FIG. 19–54. Pericrural gouge cut in mobilization (stapediolysis).

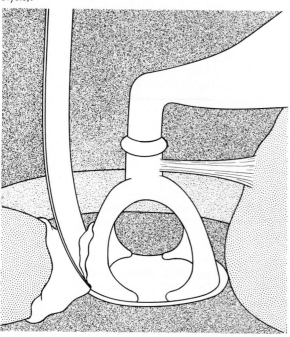

tendon or the incudostapedial joint. Probe palpation of the medial aspect of the manubrium should demonstrate a completely mobile ossicular chain with a good round window reflex.

Partial or complete hearing restoration can follow mobilization operations. If refixation occurs, secondary stapedectomy may be considered.

Many mobilizations were done between 1954 and 1960, and some of those patients still show hearing improvements lasting 15–20 years. However, the majority of mobilizations have subsequently refixed. Such patients are usually candidates for stapedectomy surgery.

There are thus two classes of patients who had operations for otosclerosis prior to the present era of stapedectomy: those who underwent fenestration and those who had mobilization. Many of these patients (fenestration and mobilization) are still seen in otologic clinics for postoperative follow-up care, and may be candidates for revision or modified stapedectomy.

THE "TEN COMMANDMENTS" FOR STAPEDECTOMY AND POSTERIOR ARCH STAPEDIOPLASTY

Ten basic commandments are advocated for consideration in any approach to stapedectomy, either in posterior arch stapedioplasty or in total stapedectomy with prosthesis techniques. In the following ten commandments, the term columella is used in an acoustical sense. It may be the retained posterior stapedial arch or a wire or plastic prosthesis.

1. *The first operation should be the only operation anticipated for that ear.*
     The procedure should restore the ossicular system to a near normal physiological state.
2. *Oval window technique should be designed to prevent osteogenic stimulation, periostitis, and granulomatosis.*
     Foot-plate removal should be atraumatic. The oval window should be sealed immediately with a mesodermal graft.
3. *Variations in pressure gradients of vestibular perilymph must be respected in oval window "sealing" techniques.*
     The major cause of early or late perilymph fistulas is an abnormally high perilymph pressure. This may be due to abnormal cochlear aqueduct "patency" or unusual cerebrospinal (CSF) pressure transmission through the area of the internal auditory meatus (see Ch. 37, Sudden Hearing Loss Syndrome).
     Thus, 1) a tissue graft is advisable, and 2) the patient should be placed immediately with the head elevated 30° to maintain low CSF pressure during the immediate oval window healing process and kept in that position 18–24 hours.
4. *The oval window seal should be mucosally in con-*

tinuity with the incudal mucoperiosteum (colu-mellar envelope).

An intact periosteum is assured by reconstitution of the incudostapedial joint and immediate contact of posterior crural mucoperiosteum with the perichondrial graft.

5. *The columella should be selected with the realization that it may be needed for many decades.*

The columella remains virtually the same one present at the patient's birth—namely, most of the stapedial arch. We must remember that in a 20-year-old patient, the columella may be needed for 70 or 80 more years.

6. *The survival of the long process of the incus should be considered in the choice of columella to avoid ischemic pressure.*

If possible, prostheses should be avoided to prevent inadvertent "crimping" forces.

7. *The stapedial tendon should be preserved (if possible) to minimize acoustic trauma.*

The tendon is not cut in 80% of cases.

8. *The columella should be an effective impedance-matching transducer in terms of mass.*

The mass of the posterior arch and perichondrial graft is virtually the same as that of a total arch and footplate, in the posterior arch stapedioplasty technique.

9. *Saccule and utricle should not be vulnerable to possible sequelae of delayed columellar pressures or barotrauma.*

In this technique, the oval window healing process is expedited by the rather thick canoe-shaped perichondrial graft that is seated in the oval window. The posterior crus contact with the concavity of the "canoe" is the same as that with a normal footplate.

10. *Tympanic mucosa and air space should not be compromised by techniques tending to produce fibrosis.*

The avoidance of foreign bodies and absorbable gelatin sponge (Gelfoam) probably minimizes tympanic fibrosis.

STAPEDECTOMY TECHNIQUES

The difference between mobilization (stapediolysis) and stapedectomy is removal of the fixed footplate (stapes base) in part or *in toto.* Two basic types of stapedectomy are in use: 1) posterior arch stapedioplasty (subtotal stapedectomy), in which footplate removal is followed by a tissue graft seal to the oval window and restoration of part of the stapedial arch; and 2) total stapedectomy, in which removal of the stapedial footplate is accompanied by the *removal of the entire stapedial arch* ("superstructure") with *substitution of a prosthesis* linking the incus to the oval window. The oval window is sealed with a tissue graft or covered with absorbable gelatin sponge.

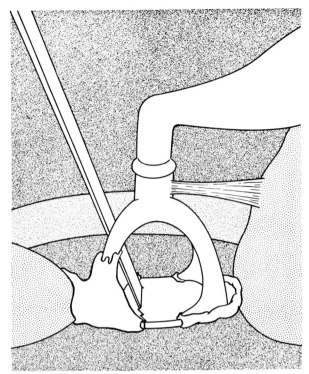

FIG. 19–55. Footplate fracture with chisel close to anterior fixation.

STAPEDECTOMY TECHNIQUES DETAILS

POSTERIOR ARCH STAPEDIOPLASTY (SUBTOTAL STAPEDECTOMY)

Stapedioplasty using the posterior arch (stapedial capitulum, neck, and posterior crus) is a conservative procedure eliminating the use of a prosthesis, but nevertheless it involves adequate removal of the fixed footplate. Stapedioplasty can be accompanied in 80% of cases with stapedial tendon preservation and allows for close to normal mass preservation. Stapedioplasty can be accomplished in 85% of all stapedectomy cases.

The first definitive maneuver is footplate fracture with a microchisel for the purpose of vestibular perilymph decompression (Fig. 19–55). This fracture allows for precise elevation of footplate fragments and diminishes the possibility of "floating footplate." (In the partially obliterative footplate, a fracture is not usually possible, and a partial drillout with cutting and diamond microburrs is necessary.)

The incudostapedial joint is sectioned with an angulated 0.5-mm knife (Fig. 19–56), and the junction between the posterior crus and footplate is scored (Fig. 19–57) to prepare a proper fracture line.

The arch is then fractured in a *superior direction* (toward the seventh nerve), blunt pressure being ap-

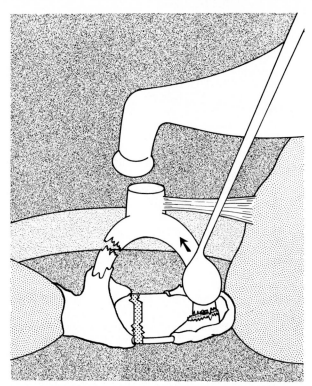

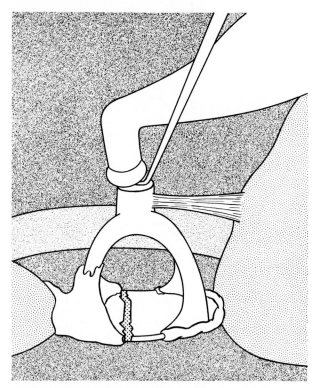

FIG. 19–56. Incudostapedial joint section.

FIG. 19–57. Scoring of posterior crus–footplate junction.

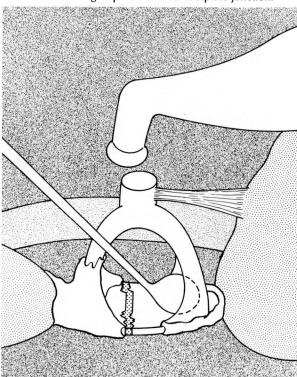

FIG. 19–58. Upward fracture of arch toward facial nerve.

plied to the caudal surface of the posterior crus (Fig. 19–58). This technique makes it possible to salvage the entire posterior crus in 95% of cases. Following the fracture, the arch is lifted out of the niche and rotated onto the promontory, with the tendon still intact.

The arch is stabilized on the promontory with two temporary absorbable gelatin sponge (Gelfoam) squares surrounding the anterior crus. The anterior crus is then amputated and removed (Fig. 19–59).

Attention is now directed toward the footplate. It is possible to remove most (75%) of the posterior footplate, with a 90° "hook" and a microalligator forceps (Fig. 19–60A). Anterior footplate fragment removal is optional (Fig. 19–60B), depending upon ease of elevation. If undue instrumentation is required, or if bleeding is excessive, the anterior footplate fragment need not be disturbed.

When an adequate oval window opening is achieved, it is sealed with an autogenous graft, preferably tragal perichondrium. Perichondrium is obtained from the tragus as illustrated in Figure 19–61. A canoe-shaped piece of perichondrium measuring 1.5–3.75 mm, on the average, is prepared from the dome portion of the tragus. The exact size of the graft depends upon appropriate measurement (Figs. 19–62, 19–63). The posterior arch of the stapes, still attached to the stapedial tendon is rotated gently back into the oval window niche, directing the posterior crus medially into the concavity of the perichondrial graft canoe. The incus

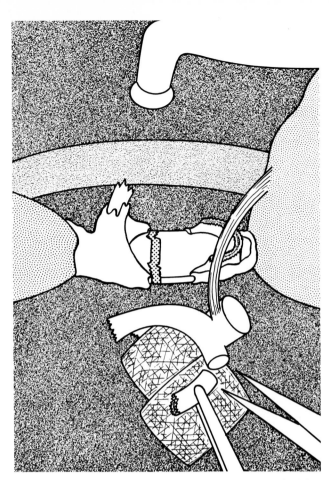

FIG. 19–59. Amputation of anterior crus.

FIG. 19–60. A. Removal of major posterior footplate. **B.** Removal of anterior footplate fragment (optional).

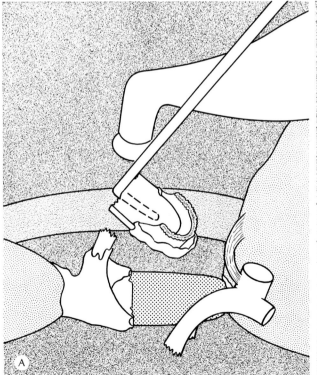

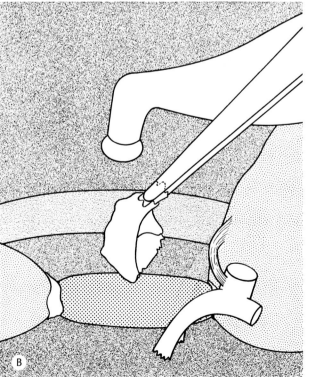

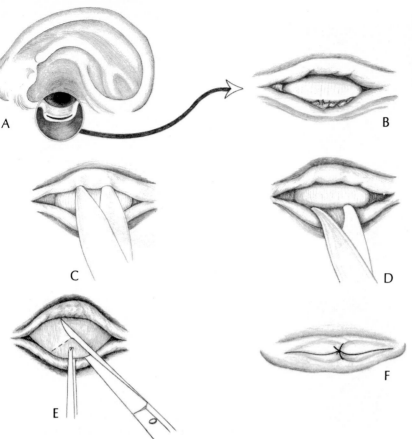

FIG. 19–61. A. Incision over tragal dome. **B.** Exposure of tragal perichondrium and cartilage. **C.** Elevation of subcutaneous posterior lip. **D.** Elevation of subcutaneous anterior lip. **E.** Resection of composite cartilage-perichondrium dome triangle. **F.** Closure of tragal incision.

FIG. 19–62. A. Excision of canoe-shaped segment of cartilage-perichondrium. **B.** Removal of cartilage. **C.** Final perichondrial canoe for oval window seal.

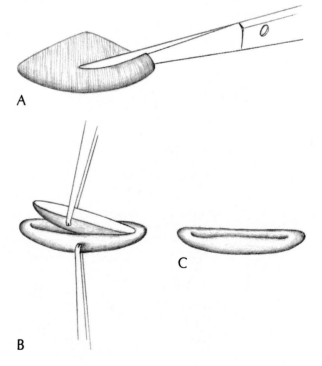

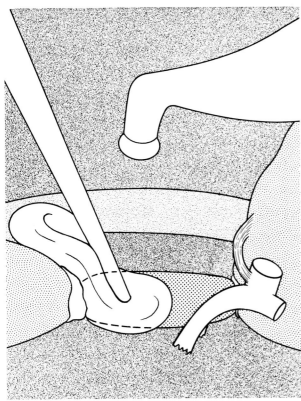

FIG. 19–63. Placement of oval window perichondrial graft with immediate seal.

FIG. 19–64. Posterior arch readaptation to incus. Repositioned posterior arch in intimate contact with concavity of perichondrial graft.

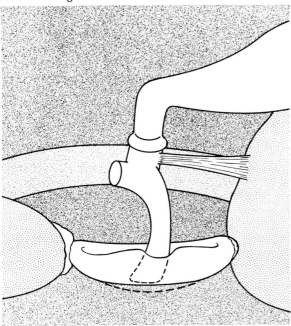

is gently lifted to expedite the approximation of the incudostapedial joint. Such readaptation occurs adequately in most cases (Fig. 19–64).

It is interesting to note the virtually immediate surface-tension effect allowing restoration of push-pull dynamics to this joint, which can be demonstrated by lifting the manubrium. This is probably due to the "tissue glue" effect, a synovial surface bioadhesive phenomenon. The head of pressure in the vestibular perilymph pool serves to act as a medial "clamp," keeping the reconstructed stapes arch snugly held between the oval window perichondrium and the incudal lenticular process.

In 20% of cases a short stapedius tendon may prevent complete joint readaptation, and in such cases, the tendon is cut.

TOTAL STAPEDECTOMY (PROSTHETIC)

Total removal of the stapes arch and all or most of the footplate is the standard approach of many otosurgeons. It is an optional technique in our practice (in less than 15% of cases) and is used when anatomic or pathologic conditions contraindicate partial stapedectomy.

Among the absolute indications for total stapedectomy are 1) obvious otosclerotic involvement of the posterior crus, 2) narrowing of the oval window niche by otosclerotic coronas in areas around the footplate in the otic capsule, or 3) in obliterative otosclerosis requiring a drillout. In instances of a congenitally narrow oval window niche, even an early otosclerotic lesion may deform the stapedial crura so that the crura come into immediate direct contact with the promontory. This is followed by torsional deformation and fibrous or bony fusion between crura and promontory. Such crural fusion may be the primary fixating lesion rather than the otosclerotic footplate invasion per se.

When stapedial arch removal is necessary, it follows incudostapedial joint section, stapedius tendon section, and footplate decompression. The arch is fractured in a cephalic or caudal direction and removed from the footplate. The posterior two-thirds to three-fourths of the footplate is then removed, as in posterior arch stapedioplasty. A perichondrial graft canoe is used to seal the newly opened oval window. In most total stapedectomy procedures, a tantalum ribbon prosthesis is used. In certain cases, a braided wire piston is used.

Tantalum Ribbon Prosthesis

In primary procedures in which the oval window niche is normal in size and it is not possible to utilize the posterior arch, a tantalum ribbon prosthesis is an excellent substitute, since it can be used as a precise substitute for the arch in contact with the perichondrial canoe. The ribbon is fashioned from Ethicon surgical foil tantalum, 0.0025 in. thick, and 0.8 mm wide × 4–5 mm long. It is easily crimped to the long process of the incus without excessive tension and its medial aspect

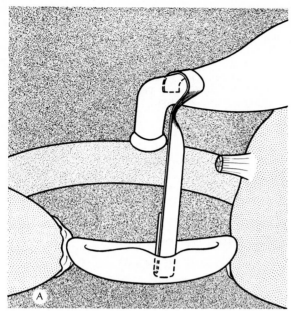

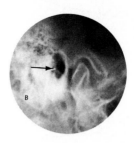

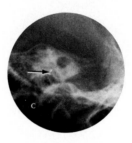

FIG. 19–65. A. Tantalum prosthesis in contact with perichondrial graft. **B.** Schuller films. **C.** Stenver films. These show tantalum prosthesis in position, poststapedectomy **(arrows).**

FIG. 19–66. Twisted-strand piston prosthesis, no medial loop, in contact with perichondrial grafts.

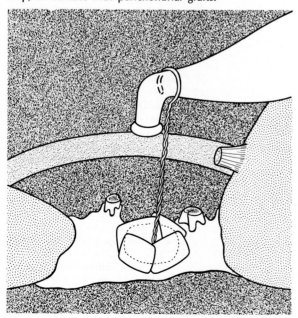

fits precisely into the ready-made cavity of the perichondrial canoe (Fig. 19–65).

Braided Wire Piston—Perichondrium Technique

A fine piston prosthesis of braided stainless steel wire without a medial loop is used when there is a very small niche, a drillout, or when revision is being done. It is crimped to the long process of the incus, its medial end in contact with perichondrium (Fig. 19–66), covering the newly opened oval window. Tragal perichondrium may be used as a single canoe or used in 1 × 1.5 mm segments applied in layers to seal the oval window.

SURGICAL PROBLEMS

OPERATIVE VERTIGO

In reflection of the chorda tympani following removal of fibrous annulus and the bony annulus, there may be momentary dizziness. It is of no significance.

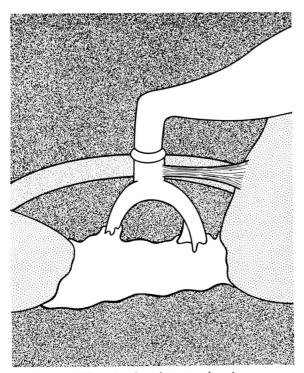

FIG. 19–67. Obliterative footplate otosclerosis.

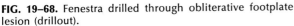

FIG. 19–68. Fenestra drilled through obliterative footplate lesion (drillout).

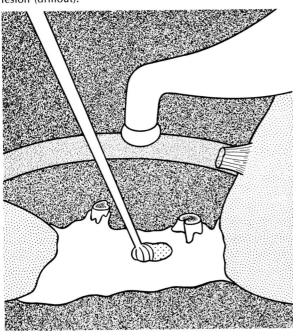

Upon footplate fracture, momentary dizziness is noticed by some patients. This is usually a sense of instantaneous imbalance, which disappears quickly. Individual vestibular hypersensitivity is variable. Care should be taken to avoid undue intravestibular manipulation. Vertigo can follow manipulation in close proximity to the utricle or saccule.

TYMPANIC MEMBRANE PERFORATION

The tympanic membrane is occasionally traumatized or perforated in the posterosuperior quadrant, particularly in a thin monomeric membrane. Postoperative healing of the tear or perforation occurs spontaneously in most cases and can be hastened by filling in the defect with a small perichondrium graft or square of absorbable gelatin sponge.

OVAL WINDOW—PROBLEM LESIONS

Obliterative Otosclerosis

Otosclerosis of the oval window occurs in a wide spectrum of severity, varying from the tiny anterior pericrural fixating lesion to an extensive obliterative involvement, in which the footplate and medial crural regions are replaced by an amorphous mass of otosclerotic bone filling the oval window niche (Fig. 19–67). Geographic as well as racial factors are reflected in this pleomorphism. Both Gristwood (18) and Willis (46) have described a higher incidence of obliterative otosclerosis in Australia than was hitherto reported from other areas.

The management of the obliterative lesion has been far from satisfactory. In general, the approach has been that of a drillout procedure. After removal of the arch, careful saucerization (Fig. 19–68) with cutting and diamond burrs allows for definition of the footplate region, followed by refenestration of the oval window. Occasionally, it is possible to create a fairly spacious fenestra. In some cases, it is possible only to create a small opening 2–2.5 mm in diameter (Fig. 19–69), into which a piston type of prosthesis may be inserted, surrounded by perichondrium. In rare cases, the lesion not only fills the niche but also occupies most of the vestibule so that no perilymph space can be identified.

When an adequate opening can be achieved and a prosthesis introduced, there is a fairly high predictability of a good hearing result immediately. However, regressions occur frequently, sometimes rather quickly. Cochlear losses are more frequent in drillouts. Revisions rarely are permanently effective and carry an even higher probability of cochlear loss following the operation.

Other Problems

Oval window surgical failures have been experienced not only in obliterative otosclerosis but also in such lesions as congenital fixation of the stapes, anomalies of the facial nerve, persistent stapedial artery, agenesis of the stapedial footplate, non-otosclerotic fixation of the footplate, tympano-sclerotic stapedial fixation, osteoarthritis at the stapediovestibular area, and a number of other diseases.

CEREBROSPINAL FLUID OTORRHEA

Minor variations in vestibular perilymphatic pressures are not unusual, and an increased perilymph flow usually subsides spontaneously.

Cerebrospinal fluid otorrhea or "gusher" may occur as soon as the footplate is fractured in very rare instances. In such gushers, the middle ear is almost immediately flooded with clear fluid (Fig. 19–70), which is not perilymph but cerebrospinal fluid, probably coming from an abnormally wide patent cochlear aqueduct. The cerebospinal fluid may be under such pressure that it will fill the external auditory canal and stream over the surgical drapes. If it occurs, absorbable gelatin sponge is placed in the middle ear, the endomeatal flap is replaced immediately, and a snug mastoid dressing is applied. The fluid may continue to seep out onto the mastoid dressing. Such fluid escape may continue for hours and, in some cases, for as long as 6–7 days. The patient is maintained at absolute bed rest with head elevated 35°. Prophylactic antibiotic therapy (ampicillin or tetracycline) is administered. There is little discomfort other than mild vertigo, which may be controlled with an antivertigo sedative. After a few days the flow of cerebrospinal fluid will stop and the dressings can be removed. The posterior tympanic skin flap is inspected and replaced if necessary. The hearing in most cases remains unchanged, with persistence of the conductive loss. Some patients will show an additional cochlear loss. No further surgery is advisable in such cases.

DEHISCENT SEVENTH NERVE AND SEVENTH NERVE PARALYSIS

The facial nerve (seventh nerve) will frequently be found dehiscent in its horizontal portion. Such a dehiscence may be minimal, moderate, or extreme. It may be possible to literally compress the entire facial nerve with a palpating probe in any

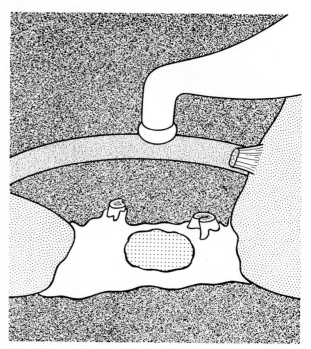

FIG. 19–69. Adequate, open, drillout footplate fenestra.

FIG. 19–70. Perilymph fistula with unusual flow and pressure which rapidly refills the oval window niche. This is due to cerebrospinal fluid (CSF), rather than perilymph *per se.*

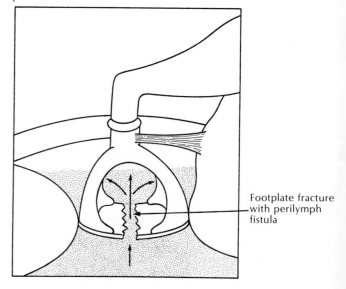

Footplate fracture with perilymph fistula

segment of the horizontal portion or along its entire extent.

Usually a dehiscent facial nerve does not create any major surgical problem.

It is not unusual to note a temporary postoperative paresis of the seventh nerve that is due to the effect of local anesthesia in the middle ear, but it usually lasts only a few hours. In postoperative seventh nerve paralysis, the middle ear should be explored if there are no signs of recovery within a few days. A bone chip will usually be found compressing the seventh nerve perineurium. Removal of the bone chip and removal of the prosthesis from contact with the seventh nerve usually is followed by recovery of function in the nerve.

SURGICAL AUDIOMETRY AND NOMOGRAPH USES IN STAPEDECTOMY

Columellar continuity in stapedectomy with prosthesis involves lateral and medial articulation considerations. Incudomalleal fixation or incudal atrophy (unrecognized bone necrosis) may occur with transmission failures. The incus-union prosthesis (crimping) may be inadequate. Thus, it may move medially on medial incus pressure (push effect) but remain stationary on lateral incus pull (pull effect).

The vestibular margin of the prosthesis may be caught in the superior or inferior margin of the oval window and prevent good *pull excursion* even though *push excursion* is normal. This may require repositioning and reorientation of the prosthesis on the incus or repositioning of the reconstructed incudostapedial joint in stapedioplasty techniques. In some prosthetic techniques the prosthesis may be too short and not reach the oval window membrane, either created by a tissue graft, or one which forms following gelatin sponge cover.

The experienced stapedectomy surgeon who performs such procedures regularly and frequently will have developed a number of visual and tactile guidelines to assure evidence of good mobility and good push-pull dynamics in the reconstructed ossicular system and in the remobilized scala vestibuli perilymph. However, the otologic surgeon who does stapedectomy surgery only occasionally will undoubtedly be greatly assisted by the utilization of surgical audiometry (see Ch. 12, Basic Otosurgical Procedures). This is also true of ossiculoplasty under local anesthesia.

CLOSURE AND PACKING

When the procedure is completed, the operative wound is closed. Prior to closure, all blood is gently suctioned from the tympanic cavity, particularly from the recess of the round window, as well as from the hypotympanic area, in which a blood clot may occasionally lie hidden. The tympanic membrane—posterior skin flap is gently replaced into position after removal of bone fragments, with care being taken that the fibrous annulus is approximated as closely as possible to the region of the tympanic annular sulcus from which it was enucleated. Skin edges are brought back as close as possible to the site of incision. Extraneous blood is suctioned from the canal and the cavity is packed. Nylon gauze strips saturated with an antibiotic ointment are used to keep skin margins in place.

A conventional mastoid dressing is applied. This is removed on the following morning before the patient is discharged from the hospital.

POSTOPERATIVE CARE

PROPHYLACTIC ANTIBIOTIC THERAPY

Although there are differences of opinion regarding prophylactic antibiotics in "clean" surgery, we use antibiotics orally for two reasons. First, middle ear surgery cannot always be considered clean surgery, since the middle ear mucosa is contiguous with the mucosa of the nasopharynx, a potentially infected area. Secondly, so-called "orthopedic" antiseptic preparation of ear canal skin frequently results in edema and hyperemia, which is counterproductive. Thus, one cannot be certain about the avoidance of bacterial infections introduced from the skin of the external auditory canal.

Our incidence of postoperative infections has been negligible since we have employed antibiotic prophylaxis almost routinely, using either ampicillin or one of the tetracyclines, depending upon the patient's history relative to antibiotic hypersensitivity. In occasional cases of history of allergic reactions to many antibiotics, such prophylactic treatment will be omitted.

Usually, prophylactic antibiotics will be started 1 day before the operation and then continued for 5 days after the operation. Ampicillin, 250 mg qidac, will be used, or tetracycline, 250 mg qidpc.

BED REST WITH HEAD ELEVATED

Our experiences with poststapedectomy fistulas (12), the rare "gusher" cases, and the phenomenon of labyrinth window ruptures in "sudden hearing loss" have prompted us to keep poststapedectomy patients in bed for 18–24 hours with the head elevated 30°. This prophylactic measure to lower intracranial pressure of cerebrospinal fluid will cause a decrease in cochlear aqueduct–scala tympani cerebrospinal fluid-perilymph pressure gradients. Such lowered gradients may facilitate definitive rapid healing and minimize the occurrence of persistent perilymph fistulas.

AMBULATION AND ACTIVITIES

Patients are usually allowed to ambulate and leave the hospital on the morning after surgery.

REMOVAL OF PACKING FROM THE EXTERNAL CANAL

The packing is usually removed on or about the fifth day. When removed, the flap is found to be well healed and is mobile. Hemotympanum and/or serous effusion are encountered only rarely and may be associated with temporary lack of hearing improvement. No further dressing is employed after packing has been removed.

POSTOPERATIVE HEARING

The hearing level in the operated ear, which may be subjectively improved immediately following surgery, may drop in the early postoperative period. It may remain unchanged or even lower than the preoperative level until the packing is removed. Upon removal of packing, there is usually immediate subjective hearing improvement. A Rinne test usually is positive with 250-Hz and 500-Hz forks. Formal audiometric testing is deferred for 2 weeks.

TRAVEL AND OTHER RESTRICTIONS

We advise patients not to travel by air for 3 weeks after the operation, but exceptions are made in individual cases. Water in the external auditory canal should be avoided for 4 weeks. Swimming is permitted at that time, but diving is discouraged for several months after the operation.

POSTOPERATIVE PROBLEMS

VERTIGO

Postoperative vertigo is most commonly due to temporary postoperative labyrinthine hydrops, which will respond to bed rest, oral antivertigo drugs, and a low-sodium diet.

For severe postoperative vertigo, promethazine, 50 mg, or dimenhydrinate, 50 mg, is given intramuscularly. If the vertigo is accompanied by nausea or vomiting (rare), intramuscular chlorpromazine, 10 mg, or prochlorperazine, 10 mg, is administered intramuscularly.

If the vertigo persists and is accompanied by further hearing loss, distortion of sound, or increased tinnitus, prompt surgical reexploration may be necessary. Such reexploration may reveal a persistent postoperative fistula, an excessively long prosthesis, a "slipped" prosthesis, or a postoperative tympanic and/or vestibular granuloma, or fibrosis.

TINNITUS

In the vast majority of patients, the "visceral" tinnitus of otosclerosis due to conductive block of ambient noise disappears with improvement in hearing. Thus, in the simple conductive lesion of otosclerosis, when the patient regains hearing, the tinnitus disappears. However, the cochlear tinnitus of the patient who has had otosclerosis with labyrinth involvement may not disappear, even if hearing improvement is excellent.

COCHLEAR HEARING LOSS

Instances of labyrinthine degeneration affecting the cochlea and occasionally the vestibular system occur in about 1–2% of patients. In the absence of fistula, prosthetic problems, or granuloma, it is difficult to explain such cochlear losses, which may happen immediately or later. Some are due to vascular phenomena, others may be due to utriculosaccular or to other intralabyrinthine disruptions.

FACIAL PARALYSIS

Facial paralysis in stapes surgery may occur in three categories.

1. Temporary paresis, which is not uncommon immediately after operation, may be due to anesthetic injection via the stylomastoid foramen or to the use of intratympanic topical anesthesia affecting the tympanic horizontal, or genu area. Such paresis usually clears spontaneously in a few hours.
2. Persistent immediate paralysis is rare and may be due to surgical trauma, to a dehiscent horizontal seventh nerve, or occasionally it is due to inadvertent bone chip penetration. Immediate facial paralysis which persists 5–7 days, with no evidence of improvement calls for surgical exploration. The prognosis for return of function is excellent, if the problem was caused by a bone chip. However, if major instrumental damage occurred, the prognosis depends upon the extent of trauma (see Ch. 30, Seventh Nerve Lesions and Injuries).

3. Delayed paralysis is also rare and may be due to an upper respiratory infection with secondary edema of a dehiscent seventh nerve, or to pressure on such a dehiscence by the surgical prosthesis. If spontaneous resolution does not occur within 5–7 days, surgical middle-ear exploration is indicated.

TUBOTYMPANITIS

Tubotympanitis with or without serous otitis may occur occasionally in the postoperative period. If this does not clear spontaneously on medical therapy, gentle tubal inflation by the Politzer technique or catheter is carried out. This is rarely necessary before the 14th postoperative day. Inflation is done gently with low pressure and visual observation of the tympanic membrane to avoid displacement of the recently healed posterior skin-tympanic membrane flap. Dramatic hearing improvement and closure of the air–bone gap frequently follows one such inflation.

OTITIS MEDIA

Immediate postoperative otitis media is encountered occasionally and is undoubtedly due to concomitant acute upper respiratory infection. Prophylactic antibiotic use (either ampicillin or tetracycline) has almost eliminated postoperative otitis media secondary to upper respiratory infections. An occasional case of post-operative *Pseudomonas* otitis media may be attributable to a latent low-grade *Pseudomonas* infection in the external auditory canal, especially in a long-term user of a hearing aid.

Otitis media is treated intensively by decongestants and antibiotics. Myringotomy is performed if intratympanic fluid does not respond to antibiotic therapy. A permanent perforation is rare and may require a myringoplasty. Occasionally, acute secondary labyrinthitis may follow a fulminating otitis media and may result in serious cochlear damage. Persistent, low-grade secretory otitis media following an acute otitis media is uncommon, but when it occurs, it may mimic perilymphatic fistula.

Delayed otitis media, years after stapes surgery, can be serious. For this reason, stapedectomy patients are advised to have a high respect for the possible dangers of otitis media. Although in general it is inadvisable to advocate routine antibiotic therapy for acute respiratory infections, this rule is abandoned in dealing with patients who have had previous ear surgery. The danger of postoperative otitis media involves not only possible disruption of the reconstructed ossicular chain and oval window membrane, but, more seriously, it carries with it the threat of labyrinthitis and/or meningitis. Labyrinthogenic meningitis (post stapedectomy) usually responds to antibiotic therapy and indicated temporal bone surgery.

EXTERNAL OTITIS

Occasionally, external otitis due to *Pseudomonas aeruginosa* or other organisms may occur. This is not uncommon in patients who have worn a hearing aid in the operated ear. Dermatitis of streptococcal or staphylococcal origin also occurs. Such external otitis is best treated by adequate cleansing with alcohol and local application of appropriate antibiotic preparations, weak acetic acid, or gentian violet. If necessary, systemic antibiotic therapy or chemotherapy may be required, as guided by culture and sensitivity tests.

CHORDA TYMPANI SYMPTOMS

Temporary unpleasant taste sensations may occur regardless of whether the chorda tympani nerve has been cut, but they usually disappear within a few months.

PERILYMPH FISTULA

Persistent vertigo most commonly takes the form of utricular vertigo. It is characterized by a feeling of falling rather than by a subjective feeling of rotation. The first cause is perilymph fistula (13). The second cause is the use of a prosthesis that is too long. Such vertigo will usually be immediate and will persist until surgically corrected. A third cause may be a slipped prosthesis that either is slowly drawn into the vestibule by fibrous tissue or literally penetrates the mucoendosteal membrane and contacts the utriculosaccular region producing delayed vertigo.

One must also consider the possibility of a temporary labyrinthine hydrops in the unoperated, as well as in the postoperative, otosclerotic patient. When the vertigo is not too severe and when there are no other ominous signs of labyrinthine penetration, medical therapy for hydrops including sodium chloride restriction, rest, and diuretics is advisable. When a patient does not respond promptly to such medical therapy, persistent vertigo calls for surgical exploration.

A fluctuating conductive hearing loss following stapes surgery should be considered to be a sign of perilymph fistula. A recurrent or persistent conductive loss may be attributed to a mechanical problem in the middle ear with special reference to the ossicular system or to the stapes substitute. Other explanations include 1) recurrent oval window otosclerosis, 2) prosthetic dislocations, 3) incus necrosis, 4) incudomalleal fixation, and 5) tympanic fibrosis or other middle ear lesions. However, the fact that a "leaking vestibule" can produce a simple mechanical loss of coupling at the air-fluid interface frequently eludes the attention of the surgeon.

It is crucially important, not only from the point of view of prevention of cochlear losses but also from the point of view of complications such as meningitis, that a fluctuating, persistent, or progressive conductive loss following stapedectomy be considered a manifestation of perilymphatic fistula, unless disproved by exploration.

Many otologists have noted that simple removal of the fixed stapes may improve hearing significantly even if the ossicular chain of the malleus and incus remains discontinuous with the oval window perilymph pool. This has been observed in surgical audiometry. Hearing levels remain higher in such instances when the drum membrane is still reflected open; they drop when the drum membrane is replaced and the middle ear is closed.

When a prosthesis is connected from the incus to the oval window and when a blood clot, a tissue graft, or a piece of gelatin sponge covers the window, a significant hearing gain occurs, although a hermetic seal does not yet exist and a temporary fistula of variable size is present. Such a hearing gain increases when the drum membrane is replaced and the middle ear is closed. Studies by preoperative audiometry utilizing the nomograph technique showed such immediate hearing gains consistently in several types of stapes operations.

The "backsplash" of a leaking vestibular perilymph space may be small mechanically when compared to the effect of the newly recreated transducer mechanism following stapedectomy. We know, therefore, that a significant gain in hearing with almost complete air–bone gap closure can occur in the presence of a small fistula. Physiologically, the ideal poststapedectomy result is the completely hermetically sealed "oval window-to-incus" unit with an adequate central compression lid surrounded by a sufficiently elastic "novo-annular" ligament. However, it is highly probable that there are hundreds—possibly thousands—of patients with incompletely healed oval windows following stapedectomy. Some of these patients, despite the presence of a small fistula, may indeed, have excellent hearing levels. When the seal is incomplete, the ratio of transducer effect to the perilymph spillage effect is less than ideal, and varying degrees of conductive loss may occur; thus, in these cases, primary conductive losses may be found. Such a primary lack of hearing improvement due to a fistula may be partial or complete, depending upon degree of transducer backsplash.

Primary Fistulas

The cause of a primary perilymphatic fistula is the operation itself (Fig. 19–71). If the particular technique is not designed to favor the creation of a mucosal seal between the oval window and the incus, the fistula created by every stapedectomy on the operating table may remain a fistula; thus, the first cause is iatrogenic (physician-induced). A patient with such a fistula may remain asymptomatic and may even show significant improvement in hearing. Symptoms occur only if the fistula is large, if the prosthesis drops or is forced into the vestibule, or if it is followed by extravagant tissue response resulting in fibrosis within either the vestibule or the middle ear, or both. Intravestibular reactions produce severe endolymphatic labyrinthine complications in most cases.

Most stapedectomy techniques rely purely upon chance and statistical probability insofar as provision of a hermetic seal is concerned. Actually, there is no such thing as a primary gelatin sponge seal, nor does connective tissue seal the medial aspect of a Teflon piston. Mucous membrane or endosteum will not form an immediate seal with stainless steel, with tantalum, with Teflon, or with polyethylene. A seal can occur only with viable cellular tissue; thus, the only seals that can occur following stapedectomy are 1) oval window tissue to intact stapedial crus, or 2) oval window tissue to incus (periprosthetic envelope).

Fortunately for most patients, there is enough surgical trauma to the oval window mucoendosteum and to the incus mucoperiosteum that an inflammatory repair "envelope" does indeed form between oval window and incus. In those procedures in which it is possible to preserve an intact stapedial crus, with or without a tissue graft, envelope formation is likely to occur rapidly, and little if any chance inflammation for stimulation of a seal formation is required. In procedures involving plastic or metal prostheses, it is absolutely essential for inflammatory reaction stimulation to create a mucosal periprosthetic oval window-to-incus envelope. Such mucosal envelopes may be thick or may consist of only one or two

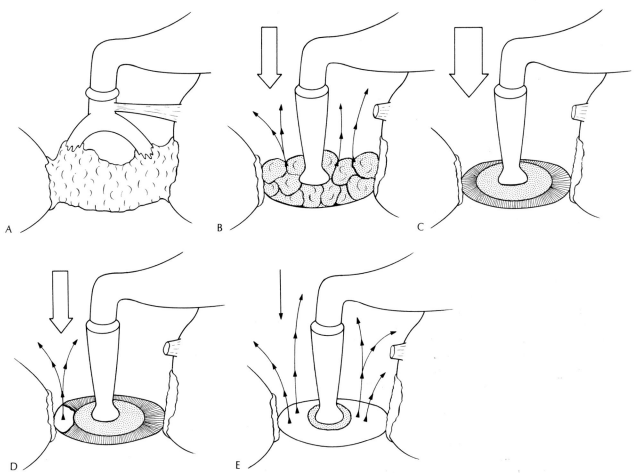

FIG. 19–71. Sequence of events from preoperative otosclerotic state (fixed stapes) **(A)** to first postoperative day **(B)**, in which a fistula is always present, to final ideal result with completely hermetically sealed oval window-to-incus strut **(C).** Partial and major perilymph leaks, causing backsplash and partial conductive loss **(D)** and major backsplash with major conductive loss **(E),** indicate relationship between size of fistula and extent of conductive hearing loss. (Goodhill V: Surgery for otosclerosis: stapedectomy, stapedioplasty, and fenestration. In English GM (ed): Otolaryngology, Volume II. Hagerstown, Harper and Row, 1976)

cell layers. We have noted their presence in revisions without fistulas as intact mucosal structures surrounding prostheses.

Fistulas definitely are most common with plastic prostheses, less common with wire, and least common with interposition (partial stapedectomy) techniques.

Primary persistent postoperative fistulas are not rare. We tend to forget that patients do not remain in a fixed position in which the oval window is dependent. As the patient leaves the operating table, there may be changes of 90–180° in the orientation of the oval window; furthermore, there is a head of pressure in the vestibular perilymph space. This is not a stagnant pool. The perilymphatic pressure in the vestibule varies from person to person and is affected by changes in blood pressure, intrathoracic pressure, posture, and by relative patency relationships between cochlear aqueduct and cerebrospinal subarachnoid space. We cannot assume that a perfect seal will always occur immediately around the prosthesis from oval window to incus. Indeed, the evidence is rapidly accumulating that such seals frequently are imperfect, especially when foreign bodies penetrate into the vestibule; thus, an operative fistula may remain open with no hearing gain or only a partial hearing gain.

Secondary or Acquired Fistulas

Secondary or acquired fistulas may be due to barotrauma, infection, or both. Barotrauma may break a fragile mucosal seal and create a secondary fistula at any time after operation. We must keep in mind the loss of the protective function of the stapes tendon and the subsequent possibility of the "bayonet stab" effect of an unrestrained wire or piston with sudden intratympanic pressure changes, particularly when the spontaneous muco-endosteal oval window membrane is very thin. Postoperative otitis media may create sufficient intratympanic pressure to break through a thin oval window seal with a resultant fistula. That this is not more common is due to the relatively rare instance of concomitant aditus and eustachian orifice closure.

Recognition

A high index of suspicion must be the rule with all stapedectomy patients. Because of anatomic variations, such as size or location of fistula, physiologic variations such as pressure variables in the vestibular perilymph, and pathologic variations in responses of bone, endosteal, and mucosal surfaces to surgical trauma, there is much variability in the otoaudiologic symptoms of perilymphatic fistulas.

The size of the fistula, the intrinsic vestibular pressure, and the topography of the middle ear may be such that occasionally one can actually see fluid in the middle ear. A pseudoserous otitis with bubbles and with moving meniscus line may be present. *In most instances, however, no such intratympanic perilymph evidence exists otoscopically.*

The only complaint may be that of fluctuating hearing loss of minor or major degree. This may be accompanied audiometrically by no bone conduction losses, no speech discrimination losses, and no other signs of a cochlear lesion. The only finding may thus be purely audiometric evidence of a conductive loss.

It is possible for a small leak to be present for years with no loss of hearing. This has been determined by the presence, in some patients, of intermittent vertigo with no hearing loss for 2 or 3 years, followed finally by a conductive hearing loss and operative diagnosis.

Cochlear Losses

An early sign of fistula may be nothing more than a slight high-frequency BC–AC dip with good speech discrimination scores.

A later sign is either a midfrequency, high-frequency, or combined BC–AC dip, with a drop in speech discrimination scores. At these levels, it is difficult to make a differential diagnosis between fistula and serous labyrinthitis or hydrops.

As fibrosis or infection supervenes, a flat curve may present with further deterioration in speech discrimination.

Labyrinthine (vestibular) fibrosis usually produces a rapidly deteriorating audiogram with further drops in pure tone and speech discrimination.

The terminal labyrinthine audiologic picture is that of anacusis.

The chief cochlear symptom is progressive deterioration of speech discrimination scores.

Tinnitus may be sudden in onset, mild to severe, and fluctuating. The speech discrimination score also may fluctuate. This is almost pathognomonic.

Nonauditory Labyrinth

Equilibrium disturbances usually are present but need not be. They may be of semicircular canal type (rotatory) or may be of utricular origin (falling). They may be violent, with nausea and vomiting, or mild with slight giddiness on positional change only. If nystagmus is present, it may be spontaneous with direction either to the left or to the right, as recorded electronystagmographically.

However, if the equilibrium disturbance is entirely utricular, it may be difficult to elicit directional eye movements.

Many combinations of audiologic and vestibular findings are possible, and keen diagnostic alertness is necessary in order to detect an early fistula. It is possible to save a distressed cochlea by prompt surgical intervention; thus, early recognition is extremely important.

Treatment of Fistula

Great care must be taken not to confuse a transitory hydrops (especially in a patient with coexistent labyrinthine otosclerosis) with a fistula. Conversely, excessively prolonged treatment of a presumptive hydrops may be responsible for surgical delay resulting in a permanently damaged labyrinth. Thus a mild, persistent poststapedectomy dysequilibrium with speech discrimination drop calls for exploratory tympanotomy.

A *sudden major loss* of hearing, either pure tone or in speech discrimination score, with or without equilibrium symptoms, is a surgical emergency.

In deciding whether to explore an ear, one must not be guided by excessive consideration of the technique originally used in the stapes operation. Although it is a fact that infinitely more fistulas are seen following use of plastic prostheses, we

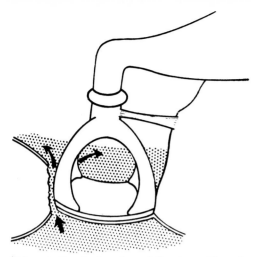

FIG. 19–72. Peribasal mobilization. The chronic perilymphatic fistula may follow a simple peribasal mobilization. **Cross-hatched area,** perilymph; **arrows,** its direction of flow. This has been observed in several cases, in one case almost 10 years after operation. (Goodhill V: Surgery for otosclerosis: stapedectomy, stapedioplasty, and fenestration. In English GM (ed): Otolaryngology, Volume II. Hagerstown, Harper and Row, 1976)

FIG. 19–73. Displaced polyethylene prosthesis that has perforated a tissue graft and is now in contact with the utricle, producing a positional type of equilibrium disturbance along with a conductive hearing loss. **Cross-hatched area,** perilymph pooling at site of penetration of the prosthesis. **Arrows,** direction of flow. There is scar tissue between the top of the prosthesis and the lenticular process of the incus, also extending down along the lumen of the tube into the vestibule in current contact with the utricle. This is a common type of perilymphatic fistula and can be seen not only with polyethylene prostheses, but also with various types of Teflon pistons and other plastic prostheses. (Goodhill V: Surgery for otosclerosis: stapedectomy, stapedioplasty, and fenestration. In English GM (ed): Otolaryngology, Volume II. Hagerstown, Harper and Row, 1976)

FIG. 19–74. Chronic perilymphatic fistula following penetration of a stainless steel wire prosthesis through a vein graft with a relatively small fistulous opening. **Cross-hatched area** and **arrows,** perilymph escaping from vestibule into oval window niche. (Goodhill V: Surgery for otosclerosis: stapedectomy, stapedioplasty, and fenestration. In English GM (ed): Otolaryngology, Volume II. Hagerstown, Harper and Row, 1976)

FIG. 19–75. A rather large perilymphatic fistula following the use of a prosthesis of wire and absorbable gelatin sponge. In this instance, probably because of greater than normal perilymphatic pressure, the usual production of a mucoendosteal membrane did not occur, thus leaving an open oval window, in which the vestibule was in direct continuity with the tympanic air space. **Cross-hatched area,** open perilymph pool, with wire prosthesis actually sitting in the pool, with no evidence whatsoever of tissue closure. (Goodhill V: Surgery for otosclerosis: stapedectomy, stapedioplasty, and fenestration. In English GM (ed): Otolaryngology, Volume II. Hagerstown, Harper and Row, 1976)

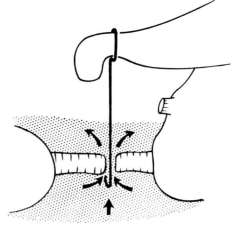

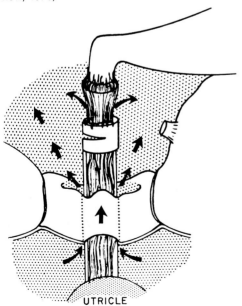

UTRICLE

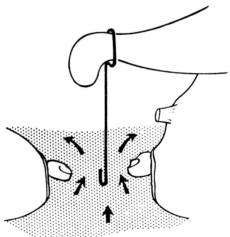

have recorded cases of fistulas following simple mobilization and all varieties of stapedectomy. Thus, we have seen fistulas following peribasal mobilization (Fig. 19–72), displaced plastic prosthesis (Fig. 19–73), wire-vein prosthesis (Fig. 19–74), prosthesis of wire and gelatin sponge (Fig. 19–75), and perforated or poorly sealed grafts (Figs. 19–76, 19–77). *Surgical repair should not be unduly delayed.*

1. Remove prosthesis carefully but completely.
2. Locate fistula and its mucosal tract (Fig. 19–78).
3. Remove mucosal tract, avoiding saccule and utricle.
4. Close with tissue—fat, cartilage, or perichondrium (11, 23, 24), or fascia—not with gelatin sponge, which may absorb allowing refistulization.
5. Leave oval window disconnected from incus temporarily or connect oval window to incus with cartilage autograft, which will expedite a mucosal seal from oval window to incus (Fig. 19–79).
6. Control with *antibiotic* and *steroid* therapy.

INCUDAL DISCONTINUITY AND NECROSIS PROBLEMS

The incus is connected to the oval window following stapedectomy either through posterior arch stapedioplasty or by the use of a columellar prosthesis made of either plastic, metal, or a combination.

In the early days of polyethylene prosthetic techniques, discontinuity was a very common problem, usually associated with incus necrosis, associated also with tympanic fibrosis, and frequently with perilymph fistula.

Discontinuity is rare in stapedioplasty, with or without necrosis, but rather common following use of prostheses made of plastic or metal. Discontinuity may be due to poor attachment but may also be due to recurrent otosclerosis, which can produce torsion forces upon the prosthesis.

POSTOPERATIVE OTOMASTOIDITIS

Occasionally an acute postoperative otitis media will not show evidence of complete resolution even after adequate antibiotic therapy and myringotomy. Mastoid x-rays will usually show evidence of a serous otomastoiditis. Myringostomy, aspiration, and middle ear ventilatory tubes are indicated and a simple mastoidectomy with prolonged drainage

and aeration through an endaural drain may be necessary.

A postoperative otomastoiditis can be purulent, with a quiescent development detectable on serial Schuller x-ray views of the mastoid process. An atticomastoidectomy and long-range antibiotic or chemotherapy may be required.

TYMPANIC FIBROSIS

Tympanic fibrosis is not an uncommon poststapedectomy problem. It may result from unusual reactions to absorbable gelatin sponge, to foreign body material from rubber-glove powder, or to posterior annular bony wall bone chips, but it also may be related to sensitivities to plastic and wire prostheses. An endomeatal tympanolysis is frequently followed by partial recovery of hearing.

Localized tympanic fibrosis which produces fixation of a wire prosthesis to the promontory may be dealt with by sharp dissection of the fixating fibers and replacement of the prosthesis on the intact oval window membrane. Such fixation superiorly causes wire prosthesis fixation to the horizontal seventh nerve bony canal. Sharp dissection in such cases must be extremely delicate in view of the possibility of dehiscence.

Pantympanic total fibrosis fills the entire middle ear. Meticulous section of scars is usually followed quickly by recurrences. Utilization of cortisone or other steroids in the middle ear has not been helpful.

The incidence of tympanic fibrosis is lower in cases in which tissue grafts are used instead of absorbable gelatin sponge. The posterior arch stapedioplasty technique in which neither gelatin sponge nor artificial materials are used has been characterized by a lowered incidence of poststapedectomy tympanic fibrosis.

GRANULOMA—TYMPANIC AND/OR VESTIBULAR

Poststapedectomy granuloma is uncommon but may be a very serious problem. Its recognition is primarily facilitated by a high index of suspicion. Granulomas may be limited to either the middle ear or the vestibule but can involve both. In most instances it is not possible to make the diagnosis otoscopically. A myringitis may indicate a middle ear granuloma. Granuloma should be suspected if there is either no significant postoperative hearing gain or if there is a severe or total hearing loss following surgery, accompanied by tinnitus and/or vertigo.

The term "serous labyrinthitis" is used fre-

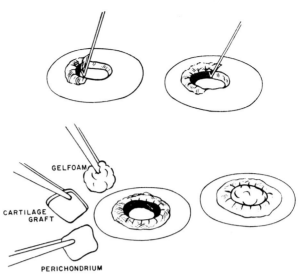

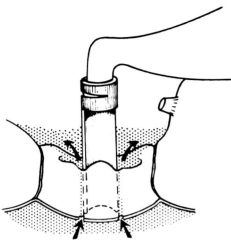

FIG. 19–76. Polyethylene prosthesis that has perforated its tissue graft, causing fistulas and allowing escape of perilymph through site of penetration. (Goodhill V: Surgery for otosclerosis: stapedectomy, stapedioplasty, and fenestration. In English GM (ed): Otolaryngology, Volume II. Hagerstown, Harper and Row, 1976)

FIG. 19–77. Fistula peripheral to poorly sealed graft, illustrating danger of inadequate seal. (Goodhill V: Surgery for otosclerosis: stapedectomy, stapedioplasty, and fenestration. In English GM (ed): Otolaryngology, Volume II. Hagerstown, Harper and Row, 1976)

FIG. 19–78. Surgical repair, with removal of the mucosal tract out of the fistula. This must be done with great care, but it is necessary if closure of the fistula is to be secured. If the mucosal tract is not removed, a fistula will continue to exist, regardless of the type of material used in an attempt to close it. Either cartilage graft or perichondrium may be used to seal the denuded fistulous tract from which the mucosa has been carefully removed. (Goodhill V: Surgery for otosclerosis: stapedectomy, stapedioplasty, and fenestration. In English GM (ed): Otolaryngology, Volume II. Hagerstown, Harper and Row, 1976)

FIG. 19–79. Autogenous cartilage graft in place over a sealed fistulous tract. The seal may have been obtained by the use of perichondrium. In some instances, cartilage itself may act very effectively as a seal and also as an effective transducer from incus to oval window. Cartilage autografts of this type are obtained from the tragus. (Goodhill V: Surgery for otosclerosis: stapedectomy, stapedioplasty, and fenestration. In English GM (ed): Otolaryngology, Volume II. Hagerstown, Harper and Row, 1976)

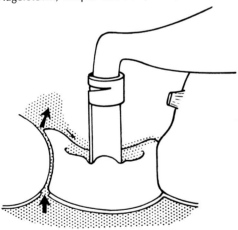

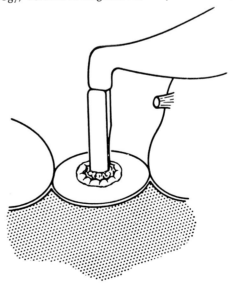

quently to describe such postoperative cochlear hearing losses with or without vertigo. However, there is need for clinical validation of such a lesion.

Urgent surgical exploration is indicated. Prompt removal of a granuloma may allow for subsidence of the process and significant return of hearing. The granuloma should be suspected of being intravestibular in location if absorbable gelatin sponge has been used as an oval window cover. An intravestibular granuloma is frequently related to persistent fistula. Reasons for granuloma formation are not known. They may represent abnormal immunologic responses of tympanolabyrinthine tissues to surgical manipulation, to gelatin sponge, or to graft tissue.

POSTOPERATIVE LABYRINTHITIS

The term "serous labyrinthitis" as used in stapedectomy reports is a clinical term not documented pathologically. It is a clinical impression rather than a definitive diagnosis in many instances. It is quite likely that the term "postoperative serous labyrinthitis" frequently is used mistakenly in cases of undiagnosed fistulas or granulomas or both. Reexploration of an ear with a diagnosis of serous labyrinthitis will almost always reveal such a discrete pathologic lesion to explain either lack of hearing gain, major cochlear hearing loss, and/or postoperative vertigo.

A true labyrinthitis of microbiologic etiology may follow poststapedectomy otitis media. When otitis media comes on immediately after operation, it may frequently be considered iatrogenic in origin, in terms of preexisting otitis media, inadvertent contamination of instruments, or in preexisting untreated or unrecognized external otitis. Labyrinthitis is usually manifested by a marked loss of cochlear function, nystagmus, and vertigo.

In rare instances labyrinthitis may be a late poststapedectomy complication as a result of fulminating otitis media following a respiratory infection. The labyrinth penetration route is commonly through a delicate oval window membrane after the use of gelatin sponge. It is possible, however, for labyrinthitis and labyrinthogenic meningitis to occur via the round window membrane and not be related to the stapes surgery.

MENINGITIS

Postoperative delayed meningitis is rare. It is always secondary to acute otitis media with or without barotrauma and is usually related to an occult or suddenly acquired perilymphatic fistula. The onset is relatively rapid in most cases, occurring within 36–48 hours after the onset of the earache. Immediate hospitalization, myringotomy, and adequate antibiotic therapy is the primary treatment of choice. If there is no immediate improvement, tympanotomy and search for a fistula is necessary. If there is x-ray evidence of mastoiditis, mastoidectomy with removal of posterior and middle fossa dural plates is necessary.

Palva, Palva, and Karja (36) recently reported the case of a patient with bilaterally operated otosclerosis, in whom fatal meningitis occurred, originating from one ear. Temporal bone studies showed that infection spread from an ear that had been operated upon in 1966, using a polyethylene strut technique. Retraction of the drum had probably allowed the strut to be drawn slightly into the vestibule. The pathway to the meninges was through the cochlear aqueduct.

Although meningitis is exceedingly rare post stapedectomy, it must be carefully considered as a possible problem. For this reason, patients who have had ear surgery should be warned to cultivate a very high respect for any upper respiratory infection of bacterial origin. The patient's general physician is well advised to treat the upper respiratory infection with broad-spectrum prophylactic antibiotics along with antihistamines and decongestants as soon as the infection is recognized. Such prophylactic antibiotic therapy is certainly not indicated as a routine in ordinary patients with colds, but it is indicated in patients who have had either stapedectomy, mastoidectomy, or tympanoplastic surgery at some time in the past.

RECURRENT OTOSCLEROSIS

Oval Window Problems

Footplate fragment impactions from previous mobilization surgery may become adherent to oval window margins and produce fixation.

New otosclerotic bone may invade footplate fragments, most commonly anteriorly but occasionally posteriorly, and create regrowth and footplate fixation.

Obliterative changes may occur in an unremoved footplate that was previously mobilized and left as a mobile-hinged footplate.

New otic capsule disease, most commonly originating from an anterior corona in the oval window niche itself may spread to close an entire oval-window niche area, even if total footplate removal was possible at the original operation. Such coronal otic capsular otosclerosis may actually be defined as a form of labyrinthine otosclerosis in that it may also involve other areas of the otic capsule in relation to saccule, utricle, and cecum vestibulare of the cochlea. Coronas may come from the anterior footplate region, from the facial canal region superiorly, and from the promontory region. All three areas may participate in the obliterative otosclerotic process requiring possible further surgery.

Revision surgery in otosclerosis recurrence requires a great deal of consideration and extremely meticulous and conservative surgical approaches. Impacted footplate or footplate fragments that are partially invaginated into the vestibule and held in place by fibrous tissue should be very carefully examined before an attempt at removal is made. In some instances it is wiser not to remove such a recurrent footplate fixation area. A simple fracture at the junction of the posterior two-thirds and anterior one-third may sufficiently mobilize the footplate or pseudofootplate so that a prosthesis (stainless steel or tantalum piston) may then be placed in contact with the mobile area. Danger to intravestibular viscera by excessive manipulation may thus be avoided.

Occasionally, a secondary drillout may be considered if there is still excellent cochlear function in the opposite ear and if the ear under consideration is very definitely the poorer ear by both speech reception threshold and speech discrimination score considerations. In general, secondary drillouts are usually advisable only in carefully selected cases.

In patients with rapidly progressive "juvenile vascular otosclerosis" with beginning obliterative changes, very conservative footplate removal is advocated. If there is rapid regression of hearing gain, it is necessary to explore the ear to make sure there is no fistula. If no fistula is encountered, additional removal of footplate bone should be undertaken with great care. Cochlear damage may follow footplate manipulation in some cases.

Round Window Niche Obliteration

In some cases of demonstrative postoperative air and bone conduction hearing regressions, exploration reveals no further oval window lesion, but a round window niche obliterative change. This is usually accompanied by what might be described as the "fat promontory," in which the promontory actually bulges and is greater than normal in both anteroposterior and superoinferior dimensions, a classic gross sign of cochlear otic capsule otosclerosis. Drillouts of round-window niche otoscle-

rosis are rarely successful. If useful cochlear function for hearing aid use can be demonstrated, it is advisable to avoid any round window surgical procedure.

BILATERAL STAPEDECTOMY

Bilateral stapedectomy is not a simultaneous surgical procedure but sequential operations.

In the early years of surgery for otosclerosis (fenestration), many otologic surgeons hesitated to perform bilateral operations. This hesitation was due to 1) preference of avoiding the creation of two fenestration cavities, and 2) lack of appreciation of advantages of binaural hearing. In the past there was a cavalier attitude toward the advantages of binaural hearing and stereophony. At the present time, most otologic surgeons believe that bilateral stapedectomy is desirable in affording the possibility of restoring stereophony and other obvious advantages of binaural hearing. In the present stapedectomy era, bilateral surgical procedures are usually recommended, usually following a 6-month to 1-year interval.

EVALUATION OF STAPES SURGERY RESULTS

The degree of "closure of the air–bone gap" is the only method available for measuring the efficacy of physiologic reconstruction in the surgery for conductive hearing loss (see Ch. 13, External Ear Diseases). This is true of stapes surgery, fenestration, tympanoplasty, ossiculoplasty, and other reconstructive procedures. **Closure of the air–bone gap** means "upward closure," obviously. (If bone conduction drops, along with air conduction, to a simultaneous lower level, the air–bone gap may certainly be closed in a "downward" direction, as a result of cochlear loss.) Any objective measure of surgical efficacy, in contrast to subjective improvement in communication, or in psychosocial adequacy of hearing, must involve a percentage of air–bone gap closure.

THE PERCENT IMPROVEMENT CONCEPT

If the difference between preoperative AC and postoperative AC (the gain) is divided by the preoperative air–bone gap (the maximum gain that could normally be expected), the result would be a percentage indicating the degree to which the air–bone gap has been closed and, therefore, the degree of surgical efficacy. This percentage can then be termed **percent improvement.**

This method of measuring surgical efficacy can be

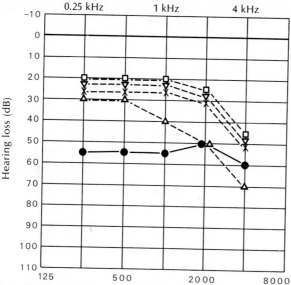

FIG. 19–80. Postoperative changes over time in air conduction thresholds. ●—●, preoperative; △---△, 1 week postoperative; □—□, 3 months postoperative; ▽—▽, 6 months postoperative; x---x, 1 year postoperative test. (Goodhill V: Surgery for otosclerosis: stapedectomy, stapedioplasty, and fenestration. In English GM (ed): Otolaryngology, Volume II. Hagerstown, Harper and Row, 1976)

FIG. 19–81. Preoperative and three months postoperative thresholds for the operated ear of all subjects. ●—●, AC, unmasked, RE, preoperative test; [—[, BC, masked, RE, preoperative test; ●--●, AC, unmasked, RE, postoperative; [- - -[, BC, masked, RE, postoperative. (Goodhill V: Surgery for otosclerosis: stapedectomy, stapedioplasty, and fenestration. In English GM (ed): Otolaryngology, Volume II. Hagerstown, Harper and Row, 1976)

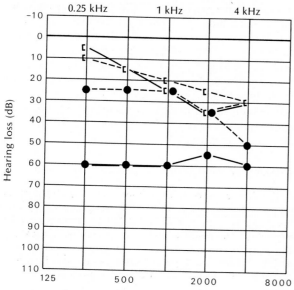

applied to individual cases as well as to averages of multiple case series.

Thus, it is possible to discuss in ratio form the relative gain or loss in the physiologic potential of each patient. Similarly, it is possible to combine such percentage data for group studies, since the information will always pertain to a relationship between theoretic possibility and therapeutic accomplishment, rather than to an artificial dB level unrelated to inherent dB potential. Thus the 30-dB postoperative level was used as an arbitrary lower limit of normal in many otosclerosis studies in the past. Results should be measured on physiological grounds. Any arbitrary postoperative level, such as a 20-dB or 30-dB level, tells nothing about the comparative efficacy of reconstructive otologic surgical procedures.

The following study on stapes surgery results was conducted with the collaboration and audiologic supervision of Laura M. Wilbur, Ph.D. (14). The study, which was conducted at University of California Los Angeles, is presented to illustrate approaches and specific findings, and involved both retrospective and prospective patient groups.

AUDIOLOGIC FINDINGS IN THE NONOPERATED EAR

Since otosclerosis is usually a progressive disease, it is difficult to consider the nonoperated, or contralateral ear as a true control ear. The rate of progression of otosclerosis is not constant, nor does it maintain the same pattern of change in both ears. In a preliminary study, carried out as a guide with normal hearing subjects, the average standard deviation of the test/retest difference scores was found to be approximately 5 dB. Therefore, we had reason to consider any change less than 5 dB to represent normal variability.

There was no change in hearing in the contralateral ear after the operation, regardless of etiology.

The negligible changes in hearing in the contralateral ear indicated that it could be used as a control for the operated ear.

AUDIOLOGIC CHANGES IN THE OPERATED EAR OVER A PERIOD OF TIME

Although results were obtained at several postoperative periods in the study, the postoperative results are based on 3-month data. This time period was selected because, in a substudy of a group of 50 consecutive patients tested after operation at intervals up to at least 1 year, there was an average drop in hearing of only about 2 dB between the 3-month and later postoperative results (Fig. 19–80). Thus, the 3-month period was found to be quite stable.

For purposes of comparison the preoperative and 3-month postoperative AC and BC thresholds for the operated ear in all subjects were combined in one audiogram. The average preoperative AC threshold for this group was an essentially flat 60-dB hearing level. The improvement in the operated ears averaged ap-

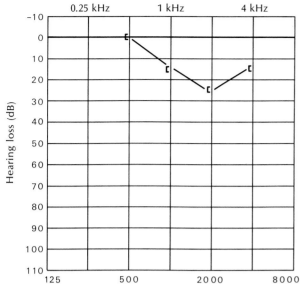

FIG. 19–82. Preoperative bone conduction thresholds (corrected for age differential). [—[, BC, masked, RE. (Goodhill V: Surgery for otosclerosis: stapedectomy, stapedioplasty, and fenestration. In English GM (ed): Otolaryngology, Volume II. Hagerstown, Harper and Row, 1976)

FIG. 19–83. Three months postoperative change in bone conduction thresholds for all subjects. •- - -•, operated ear; △- - -△, nonoperated ear. (Goodhill V: Surgery for otosclerosis: stapedectomy, stapedioplasty, and fenestration. In English GM (ed): Otolaryngology, Volume II. Hagerstown, Harper and Row, 1976)

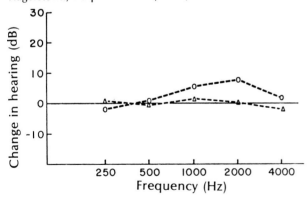

TABLE 19-1. Speech Reception Thresholds and Speech Discrimination Scores for Subjects Who Had Stapes Surgery

	Preoperative findings (dB)	3-Months postoperative results (dB)
Speech reception threshold	51.1	26.0
Speech discrimination at +8 SL*	72.2	72.3
Speech discrimination at +30 SL	95.3	95.5

*SL, sound level.

(Goodhill V: Surgery for otosclerosis: stapedectomy, stapedioplasty, and fenestration. In English GM (ed): Otolaryngology, Volume II. Hagerstown, Harper and Row, 1976, p 107)

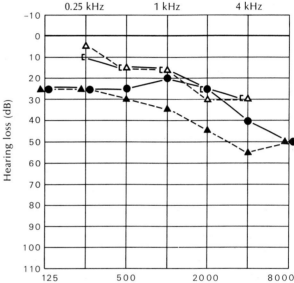

FIG. 19–84. Three months postoperative AC-BC for all subjects. •—•, interposition stapedioplasty, AC; [—[, interposition stapedioplasty, BC; ▲- - -▲, wire prosthesis, AC; △- - -△, wire prosthesis, BC. (Goodhill V: Surgery for otosclerosis: stapedectomy, stapedioplasty, and fenestration. In English GM (ed): Otolaryngology, Volume II. Hagerstown, Harper and Row, 1976)

proximately 30 dB from 250 through 1000 Hz, with lesser gains at 2000 and 4000 Hz. It is interesting to note that there is a very substantial gain in hearing even at 4000 Hz (Fig. 19–81).

The 1-week postoperative results reflect a temporary loss at 4 kHz, which could be due to one of several factors—temporary threshold shift due to acoustic trauma, a mass effect tilt created by postoperative edema, and the possible effect of temporary perilymph fistula. The ultimate improvement is discernible in the 3-month postoperative test, especially at 1000, 2000, and 4000 Hz.

Bone Conduction Results

Preoperative bone-conduction thresholds in otosclerotic patients are not true reflections of "cochlear reserve." Carhart (4) pointed out that patients with preoperative otosclerosis showed BC thresholds that were characterized by a notch in the middle frequencies: The BC thresholds gradually increased from 500–2000 Hz and then came upward at 4000 Hz (Fig. 19–82). This notch, corrected for age, is 2 dB at 500 Hz, 15 dB at 1000 Hz, 25 dB at 2000 Hz, and 15 dB at 4000 Hz.

Figure 19–83 illustrates the postoperative change in

BC thresholds for all subjects. There is virtually no change in hearing for the nonoperated ear of these subjects; however, there is a distinct gain in BC thresholds for the patients who had surgery, especially at 2000 Hz. This improvement in BC threshold reflects the surgical elimination of the Carhart notch.

The preoperative and 3-month postoperative SRT and SDS for the group (Table 19–1) show quite clearly that there was no change in speech discrimination that could be attributed to the surgery.

Bekesy Audiometry Results

Examination of the Bekesy tracing types before and after operation showed very few changes from type I to type II, a change that would probably be expected if cochlear damage had occurred as a result of stapes surgery.

Stapedioplasty Versus Wire Techniques

The 3-month postoperative audiometric results for the two groups of patients (Fig. 19–84) reveal that the BC curves still remain essentially equivalent, an indication that there was no demonstrable postoperative sensorineural hearing loss related to either type of surgical technique. The AC curve for the stapedioplasty interposition group tends to be quite close to the postoperative BC curve, especially in the three middle frequencies, indicating virtually complete air–bone gap closure by this technique. There is, however, an AC difference at every frequency (except at 250 Hz) between the interposition and metal prosthetic (wire) groups. The difference, which approaches 18 dB at 2000 Hz, is significant between the air–bone gap closure potential of the two techniques.

These findings tend to confirm audiologically the fact that the stapedoplasty technique with tissue—*i.e.*, perichondrium—is a physiologically desirable technique.

Audiologic Result Variations Dependent Upon Age

Patients in the prospective study group were divided into double decade age groups: group 1, 20- to 40-year-old subjects with a mean of 32.9 years; group 2, 40- to 60-year-old subjects with a mean of 49.5 years; and group 3, 60- to 80-year-old subjects with a mean of 65.7 years.

Superimposition of the three double-decade age groups on the same graph (Fig. 19–85) shows that although there is considerable interweaving of AC thresholds from 250 through 1000 Hz, the AC thresholds begin to differentiate sharply at 2000 Hz and especially at 4000 Hz. The relative changes in thresholds are probably due to the addition of a presbycusis sensorineural component, which would be expected on the basis of age.

The preoperative air–bone gap, which would be expected to influence the postoperative gain in hearing, is essentially the same for the three groups of subjects: group 1, 27.5 dB; group 2, 28 dB; and group 3, 24.8 dB.

The pure-tone averages for the three age groups *1 year after surgery* by the AC tests were 29.9 dB for group 1, 29.6 dB for group 2, and 29.5 dB for group 3. This is a rather remarkable superimposition of almost identical gains.

During a 5-year period in which the investigation was conducted, 95 patients over the age of 70 years had stapes operations. Their preoperative pure-tone average was 74.5 dB; their average gain was 28.1 dB, resulting in an average postoperative level of 46.4 dB.

Elderly patients with profound cochlear stapedial hearing loss constituted another interesting group. A group of 44 patients over the age of 70 years with an average hearing level of 89.9 dB was compared with a younger group of profoundly deaf patients under the ago of 70. In this younger group, there were 124 patients with an average loss of 89.6 dB. Surprisingly, gain in hearing for the patients over 70 averaged 34.6 dB, whereas the younger group averaged only 24.7 dB. Certainly the results of this study suggest that there is no oto-audiologic reason to deny the elderly patient the benefit of surgery. In fact, this may be an extremely important rehabilitative consideration. Elderly people generally do not do well with high-gain hearing aids. A rehabilitative prognosis is much more favorable if a useful hearing level can be obtained with a moderate-gain hearing aid with less distortion and greater likelihood of utilization.

Audiologic Results Dependent Upon Sex

It was not surprising that women outnumbered men approximately 2:1 in our sample, because of the gen-

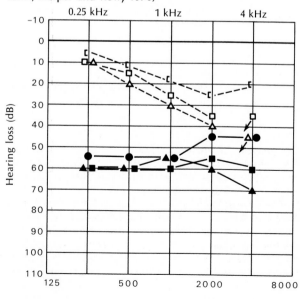

FIG. 19–85. Preoperative threshold measurements. ●—●, AC, [—[, BC, 20- to 40-year-old group; ■—■, AC, □- - -□, BC, 40- to 60-year-old group; ▲—▲, AC, △- - -△, BC, 60- to 80-year-old group. **Arrows,** no response at maximum output. (Goodhill V: Surgery for otosclerosis: stapedectomy, stapedioplasty, and fenestration. In English GM (ed): Otolaryngology, Volume II. Hagerstown, Harper and Row, 1976)

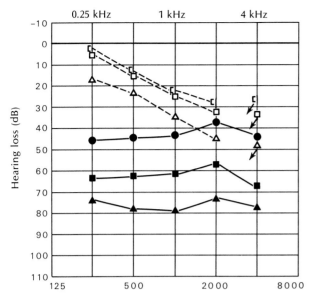

FIG. 19–86. Preoperative thresholds for all subjects, grouped according to initial hearing loss. ●—●, AC, unmasked, RE; [- - -[, BC, mild-to-moderate hearing loss (0–5 dB); ■—■, AC, unmasked, RE; □- - -□, BC, masked, RE, moderate-to-severe hearing loss (50–70 dB loss); ▲—▲, AC, △- - -△, BC, severe-to-profound loss (70–110 dB loss); **arrows,** no response at maximum output. (Goodhill V: Surgery for otosclerosis: stapedectomy, stapedioplasty, and fenestration. In English GM (ed): Otolaryngology, Volume II. Hagerstown, Harper and Row, 1976)

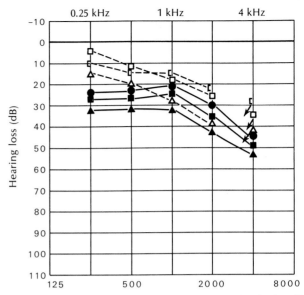

FIG. 19–87. Three months postoperative thresholds for all subject groups according to initial hearing loss. ●—●, AC, [- - -[, BC, mild-to-moderate (0–5 dB loss); ■—■, AC, □- - -□, BC, moderate-to-severe (50–70 dB loss); ▲—▲, AC, △- - -△, BC, severe-to-profound (70–110 dB loss); **arrows,** no response at maximum output. (Goodhill V: Surgery for otosclerosis: stapedectomy, stapedioplasty, and fenestration. In English GM (ed): Otolaryngology, Volume II. Hagerstown, Harper and Row, 1976)

eral preponderance of otosclerosis in females. In a prospective study of 75 women and 39 men, both groups had virtually the same preoperative AC threshold—*i.e.*, 56.2 dB for men, 58.2 dB for women. The BC thresholds were also similar—*i.e.*, 26.8 dB for men and 30.8 dB for women. There was a postoperative gain in hearing of 27.9 dB for the men and 28.7 dB for the women. There was no difference in surgical results on the basis of sex.

Audiologic Results Dependent Upon Degree of Initial Hearing Loss

Subjects were divided into three groups: 1) those with mild-to-moderate losses of 50 dB or less; 2) those with moderate losses of 50–70 dB; and 3) those with severe losses of 70 dB or more.

In the preoperative AC and BC thresholds for the three groups of subjects (Fig. 19–86) revealed that the BC thresholds were similar in the low frequencies for the three groups, although they did begin to differentiate at 2000 and 4000 Hz. The AC thresholds, however, differed consistently for the three groups. The preoperative AB gap for the three groups of subjects was as follows: Group 1 (mild-to-moderate loss) showed relatively small air–bone gaps, varying from 37–10 dB, which reflected a very definite Carhart notch for this population. Group 2 (moderate-to-severe loss)

showed air–bone gaps varying from 57–24 dB. Group 3 (severe to profound loss) had preoperative air–bone gaps of 63–32 dB.

In the 3-month postoperative thresholds (Fig. 19–87) for these three groups, the BC differences present before operation were still present, but the AC differences had been virtually eliminated.

The potential gain in hearing was virtually equivalent for all three groups of subjects. However, those who had the least amount of initial hearing loss (group 1) also had the smallest air–bone gap and, thus, had the smallest gain in hearing. It is not so much the initial hearing loss level that determines gain in hearing as it is *the potential as evidenced by the air–bone gap.* It was greatest for group 3 with the greatest hearing loss, therefore, this group showed the greatest average gain in hearing.

The magnitude of a profound hearing loss *per se* should not negate a recommendation for surgery. The average postoperative hearing level in the profoundly deaf group was 62 dB. Although this loss is obviously great enough to require the use of a hearing aid, it is possible to consider a better hearing-aid rehabilitation program. If there is a measurable air–bone gap of sufficient magnitude, the degree of the severity of the hearing loss should not preclude surgical intervention, all other factors being considered.

SUMMARY

This statistical review of stapedectomy surgery clearly points to the possibility of a high percentage of successful stapedectomy results, both in patients with moderate degrees of fixation and in patients with far advanced otosclerosis.

A number of problems have been solved as technical improvements have been applied to stapedectomy surgery. Thus, the heightened appreciation and early recognition of perilymph fistula has resulted in changes in technique to prevent fistula, and recognition and prompt management of early fistulas. Competent audiologic evaluations, improved microsurgical technology, and careful differential diagnosis have contributed to the presently stable status of stapedectomy as an effective therapeutic procedure in otosclerosis.

THE LEMPERT FENESTRATION OPERATION

No discussion of otosclerosis surgery can be complete without serious consideration of the late Dr. Julius Lempert's semicircular canal fenestration for otosclerosis (28, 29). Such consideration is essential not only for its historic importance but also for the role it may play in future otosurgery. Otologists must be familiar with the procedure since many patients undergoing fenestration require postoperative care and observation.

It is interesting to reflect upon Lempert's theoretical basis for fenestration surgery:

Clinical otosclerosis can be cured by ignoring the otosclerotic tumor in the region of the oval window which immobilized the stapedial footplate; a new oval window can be created in the surgical dome of the vestibule, which is not a site of predilection for otosclerosis and in which otosclerotic foci have been observed histologically only in the fulminating type of otosclerosis. Such a newly created window in the bony capsule of the vestibular labyrinth replaces the functionally impeded oval window and extablishes a new air conduction mechanism which permits the perilymph and the endolymph to be freely mobilized again by air borne sound. Clinical otosclerosis is thus converted into symptom-free otosclerosis.

Lempert approached fenestration via an endaural approach. The following surgical steps were used, as modified by Goodhill:

1. Single endaural incision is made.
2. Limited mastoidectomy exenteration is performed sufficient to expose the dome of the horizontal semicircular canal.
3. Removal of the posterosuperior bony canal wall is carried out with preservation of canal wall skin.

4. The short process of the incus, the incudomalleal joint, the head and neck of the malleus, the anterior malleal ligament, the long process of the incus, the incudostapedial joint, the tendon of the stapedius muscle, and the chorda tympani nerve are exposed to view.
5. The incus is separated from the head of the malleus and removed.
6. The head and neck of the malleus is severed from the malleus handle and removed.
7. A tympanomeatal flap is created, as a pedicle flap, composed of skin and periosteum lining the external auditory canal and tympanic membrane.
8. The flap is manipulated so that it will adapt itself to every elevation and depression within the postoperative mastoid wound, with its thinnest portion covering the fenestra to be created.
9. The bony capsule of the dome of the horizontal semicircular canal is gradually worn down to the endosteal bony layer until it is thinned to a bluish gray transparency, and a bluish gray cupola of endosteal bone is created. The bone dust thus formed is constantly removed by irrigating with saline solution and applying suction.
10. The bony endosteal cupola is removed.
11. The endolymphatic labyrinth, without having been disturbed from its normal position, is exposed to view (Fig. 19–88). The fenestra should be made as wide as possible—about 2 mm wide and about 6 mm long.
12. The tympanomeatal flap is positioned so that its thinnest portion will cover the fenestra gap.

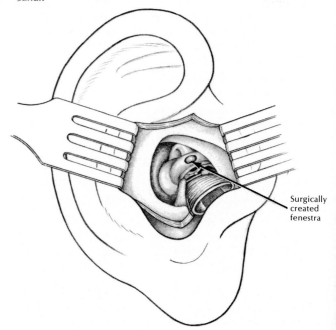

FIG. 19–88. Lempert fenestration of horizontal semicircular canal.

Surgically created fenestra

13. The flap is packed and the wound closed.
14. All packing is removed on tenth postoperative day.

RESULTS OF FENESTRATION SURGERY

The reader is referred to Lempert's classic papers (28, 29) on results of fenestration surgery.

POSTOPERATIVE CARE OF FENESTRATION CAVITIES

Many patients still appear for care who have had fenestration operations during the years 1938–1958. Some of these patients have dry, healed fenestration cavities. Others require periodic cleansing of the fenestration cavity, which resembles the radical mastoidectomy "cavity," or "stoma."

Since the fenestration operation was performed through an endaural incision, the external canal is larger and deeper than an ordinary ear canal. It includes an area of the previous mastoid pneumatized cellular area now contiguous with the original ear canal.

Periodic removal of cerumen and epithelial debris is carefully performed under magnification by gentle use of suction and blunt instruments. Such cavities should not be irrigated for cerumen removal. Special care should be taken in the region of the fenestra in the horizontal semicircular canal.

Vertigo may occur in a patient who has undergone fenestration. It is usually due to pressure of cerumen and debris in the region of the fenestra, producing a classic "fistula response" with nystagmus.

Otitis media may occur after fenestration, as it may in any patient. One must remember that the tympanic membrane is a "hemidrum" since both malleal head and incus have been removed. Prompt treatment is urgent in such a case to prevent labyrinthitis and labyrinthine meningitis.

POSTFENESTRATION STAPEDECTOMY

Patients who have had excellent immediate postfenestration results, with secondary hearing loss, or who never had any hearing gain following fenestration surgery may seek consultation regarding the possibility for further ipsilateral ear surgery. If audiologic studies indicate evidence of good cochlear function and a reasonable air–bone gap, it may be possible to consider a specialized type of stapedectomy procedure in the fenestrated ear.

Since the fenestrated ear is rather unusual, it is necessary to describe it. It is characterized by what appears to be a rather classic radical mastoidectomy cavity with a mastoid bowl (open mastoidostomy or stoma). The tympanic membrane however, is intact, but modified in appearance. It actually consists of the lower two-thirds of pars tensa. The malleal head and the incus have been removed during the fenestration operation, and the upper third of the pars tensa and the pars flaccida have been reflected, along with posterosuperior canal wall skin, to cover the previously made semicircular canal fenestra, which is usually obliterated at the time of the later examination. If the fenestra is wide open and a test for fistula is positive, the consideration of stapedectomy would be questionable.

There is a need to accomplish two surgical objectives: 1) stapedectomy, and 2) columellization between the modified hemi-tympanic membrane and the newly reopened oval window, since there is no incus.

It is possible to restore hearing to a significant number of patients who have had previously unsuccessful fenestration or one in which postoperative regression has occurred.

The operation is performed under local anesthesia, utilizing an endaural block. A modified omega incision is made, taking great care to avoid damage to the superficial position of the horizontal semicircular canal and facial nerve. The middle ear is opened and the normal remaining landmarks are identified. The distance between the oval window and the malleal manubrium is carefully measured and an appropriate prefabricated homograft of an extended "golf-tee" type is obtained from the ear tissue bank.

Following removal of the stapes, the oval window is closed with a fairly thick canoe-shaped tragal perichondrial graft. The rod end of the golf-tee homograft is then placed within the concavity of the perichondrial graft medially. The lateral aspect of the homograft, slightly modified to a crutch shape, is then placed laterally in contact with the malleal manubrium area, from which the mucosal and periosteal layers have been previously gently elevated to provide a raw surface. Following completion of the columellization, the flap is replaced and packed with absorbable gelatin sponge and gauze. The postoperative course is similar to that following ordinary stapedectomy.

Such a columellization may provide sufficient restoration of hearing to close the air–bone gap to within 10–15 dB. In some instances, this restoration of hearing may be extremely valuable, especially if the patient has bilateral otosclerosis.

SUMMARY

Otosclerosis, a common cause of conductive hearing loss, occurs in possibly 10% of the population of the world. It is a complex disease of the temporal bone, characterized histologically both by spongiosis and sclerosis, especially in the region of the oval window.

Otospongiosis-otosclerosis is a complex disease, which will continue to challenge the scientific imagination and ingenuity of physicians in the foreseeable future.

Stapedectomy surgery, developed to a high degree of success since 1945, has been of great rehabilitative value to the majority of patients.

REFERENCES

1. Barany E: A contribution to physiology of bone conduction. Acta Otolaryngol [Suppl] (Stockh) 26: 1938

2. Bast TH, Anson BJ: The Temporal Bone and the Ear. Springfield, IL, CC Thomas, 1949

3. Bekesy G: Zur Theorie des Hörens bei der Schalaufnahme durch Knochenleitung. Ann Physik 13:111–136, 1932

4. Carhart R: Clinical application of bone conduction audiometry. Arch Otolaryngol 51:798–807, 1950

5. Dirks D, Malmquist C: Comparison of frontal and mastoid bone conduction thresholds in various conductive lesions. J Speech Hear Res 12:725–746, 1969

6. Floderus B: Bidrag till stigbygelankylosens operativa Radikalbehandling. Nord Med Ark 32:1, 1899

7. Friedmann I: Pathology of the Ear. Oxford, Blackwell Scientific, 1974, p 247

8. Gapany-Gapanavicius B: Otosclerosis: Genetics and Surgical Rehabilitation. New York, John Wiley & Sons, 1975, pp 177–178

9. Goodhill V: The use of cortisone in otosclerosis. Trans Am Acad Ophthalmol Otolaryngol 56:635–646, 1952

10. Goodhill V: Pseudo-otosclerosis. Laryngoscope 70:722–757, 1960

11. Goodhill V: Tragal perichondrium as oval window graft. Laryngoscope 71:975–983, 1961

12. Goodhill V: The conductive loss phenomenon in post-stapedectomy perilymphatic fistulae. Laryngoscope 77:1179–1190, 1967

13. Goodhill V: Variable oto-audiologic manifestations of perilymphatic fistulae. Rev Panameric Otorrinolaringologia y Broncoesofagologia 1:100–109, 1967

14. Goodhill V: Surgery for otosclerosis: stapedectomy, stapedioplasty, and fenestration. Otolaryngology, Vol II, loose leaf series. Hagerstown, Harper & Row, 1973

15. Goodhill V, Dirks D, Malmquist M: Bone conduction thresholds: relationship of frontal and mastoid measurements in conductive hypacusis. Arch Otolaryngol 91:250–256, 1970

16. Goodhill V, Moncur JP: The low-frequency air bone gap. Laryngoscope 73:850–867, 1963

17. Gray A: Otosclerosis treated by local application of thyroxine. J Laryngol 50:729, 1935

18. Gristwood RE: Obliterative otosclerosis. J Otolaryngol-Soc Aust 2:40–48, 1966

19. Guggenheim LK, Gunther L, Goodhill V et al.: Reversal of halisteresis in the mammalian ear. Arch Otolaryngol 34:501–522, 1941

20. Gussen R: The labyrinthine capsule: normal structure and pathogenesis of otosclerosis. Acta Otolaryngol [Suppl] (Stockh) 235:1–38, 1968

21. Gussen R: Plugging of vascular canals in the otic capsule. Ann Otol Rhinol Laryngol 78:1305–1316, 1969

22. Gussen R: The stapedeovestibular joint: normal structure and pathogenesis of otosclerosis. Acta Otolaryngol 248:1–38, 1969

23. Harris I, Goodhill V: Functional viability of tragal cartilage autografts in tympanic surgery. Laryngoscope 77:1191–1203, 1967

24. Harris I, Weiss L: Granulomatous complications of oval window fat grafts. Laryngoscope 72:870–885, 1962

25. Holmgren G: Some experiences in surgery of otosclerosis. Acta Otolaryngol (Stockh) 5:460, 1923

26. Jenkins GJ: Otosclerosis. Certain Clinical Features and Experimental Operative Procedures. Trans 17th Int Congr Med (Lond) 16:609, 1913

27. Kessel J: Uber das Mobilisieren des Steigbügels durch Ausschneiden des Trommelfelles, Hammers und Ambosses bei Undurchgängigkeit der tube. Arch Ohrenheilk 13:69, 1878

28. Lempert J: Endaural, antauricular surgical approach to temporal bone; Principles involved in this new approach. Arch Otolaryngol 27:555, 1938

29. Lempert J: Improvement of hearing in cases of otosclerosis: new one stage surgical technique. Arch Otolaryngol 28:42–97, 1938

30. Mayer O: Untersuchungen über die otosklerose. Vienna, Holder-Pichler-Tempsky, A-G, 1917

31. Mayer O: Uber die Entstehung der Spontanfrakturen der LabyrinthKapsel. Hals-Nasen-Und Ohrenheilkunde 26:262, 1930

32. Mayer O: Die Ursache der Knochen—neubildung bei der Otosklerose. Acta Otolaryngol 15:35, 1931

33. The Medical Letter 18 (465): 100, Nov 5, 1976

34. Mendoza D, Ruis M: Histology of the enchondral layer of the human otic capsule. Acta Otolaryngol (Stockh) 62:93, 1966

35. Miot C: De la mobilisation de l'étrier. Rev Laryngol 10:49, 1890

36. Palva T, Palva A, Karja J: Fatal meningitis in a case of otosclerosis operated bilaterally. Arch Otolaryngol 96:130–137, 1972

37. Passow KA: Operative Anlegung einer offnung in die mediale paukenhohlenwand bei Stapesankylose. Verh Dtsch Otol Ges 6:141, 1897

38. Rosen S: Palpation of the stapes for fixation. Arch Otolaryngol 56:610, 1952

39. Schuknecht H: Pathology of the Ear. Cambridge, Harvard University Press, 1974, p 353

40. Sercer A, Krmpotic J: Thirty years of otosclerosis studies. Arch Otolaryngol 84:598, 1966

41. Shambaugh GE, Causse J, Petrovic A et al.: New concepts in management of otospongiosis. Arch Otolaryngol 100:419–426, 1974

42. Shambaugh GE, Scott A.: Sodium fluoride for arrest of otosclerosis. Arch Otolaryngol 80:263–270, 1964

43. Siebenmann F: Sur le traitement chirurgical de la sclerose otique. Congr Int Med Sect d'otol 13:11, 1900

44. Soifer N, Weaver K, Endahl GL, Holdsworth E: Otosclerosis: A review. Acta Otolaryngol (Stockh) [Suppl] 269, 1970

45. Sourdille M: Résultats primitifs et secondaires de quatorze cas de surdité par otospongiose opérés. Rev Laryngol 51:595, 1930

46. Willis R: The Tef—Wire piston in otosclerosis. J Otolaryngol Soc Aust 2:2, 1967

47. Wittmaack K: Betrachtungen Zum Otosklerose-problem. Acta Otolaryngol (Stockh) 18:215, 1933

48. Wolff D, Bellucci RJ: Otosclerosis. Arch Otolaryngol 79:571, 1964

SUGGESTED READING

Bretlau P: Otosclerosis electron microscopic studies of biopsies from the labyrinthine capsule. Arch Otolaryngol 93:551–561, 1971

Burtner D, Goodman ML: Etiological factors in post-stapedectomy granulomas. Arch Otolaryngol 100:171–174, 1974

Causse J, Bel J, Michaux P et al.: Systematisation des parametres d'otospongiose. Ann Otolaryngol Chir Cervicofac 91:21–40, 1974

Clairmont AA, Nicholson WL, Turner JS: Pseudo-monas Aeruginosa meningitis following stapedectomy. Laryngoscope 85:1076–1083, 1975

Goodhill V: Stapes Surgery for Otosclerosis. New York, Paul B Hoeber, 1961

Goodhill V: Stapedectomy revisions and "command-ments"—Posterior arch stapedioplasty. Trans Pac Coast Otoophthalmol Soc 55:35–59, 1974

Goodhill V: Posterior arch stapedioplasty. Arch Otolaryngol 100:460–464, 1974

Goodhill V: Surgical management of hearing loss. In Tower DB (ed): The Nervous System, Vol 3, Human Communication and Its Disorders. New York, Raven Press, 1975

Gristwood RE, Venables WN: Otosclerotic obliteration of oval window niche: an analysis of the results of surgery. J Laryngol 89:1185–1217, 1975

Gussen R: Hereditary deafness and otosclerosis. J Laryngol 84:1027–1031, 1970

Gussen R: Otosclerosis and vestibular degeneration. Arch Otolaryngol 97:484–487, 1973

Gussen R: Labyrinthine otosclerosis and sensorineural deafness. Arch Otolaryngol 101:438–440, 1975

House HP: Panel discussion: incidence and manage-ment of complications of stapes surgery. Arch Otolaryngol 97:35, 1973

House H, Linthicum FH: Sodium fluoride and the oto-sclerotic lesion. Arch Otolaryngol 100: 427–430, 1974

House HP, Linthicum FH, House JW: Stapes surgery: foot plate fragmentation in otosclerosis surgery. Laryngoscope 80:1256, 1970

Hughson W, Westlake H: Manual for program outline for rehabilitation of aural casualties both military and civilian. Trans Am Acad Ophthalmol Otolaryn-gol [Suppl] 48, 1949

Jerger J: Bekesy audiometry in analysis of auditory disorders. J Speech Hear Res 3:275–287, 1960

Lim DL, Saunders WH: Active otosclerotic foci in the stapes. Acta Otolaryngol (Stockh) 80:255–268, 1975

Linthicum FH, Schwartzman JA: An Atlas of Micro-pathology of the Temporal Bone. Philadelphia, WB Saunders 1974

McCandless GA, Goering DM: Changes in loudness after stapedectomy. Arch Otolaryngol 100:344–350, 1974

McConnell F, Carhart R: Influence of fenestration surgery on bone conduction measurements. Laryngo-scope 62:1267–1292, 1952

Tonndorf J: Bone conduction studies in experimental animals. Acta Otolaryngol (Stockh) [Suppl] 68:213, 1966

Vase P, Prytz S, Pedersen PS: Congenital stapes fix-ation, symphalangism and syndactylia. Acta Oto-laryngol (Stockh) 80:394–398, 1975

20

LATERAL OSSICULAR FIXATION

Lateral ossicular fixation is a cause of hearing loss and is due to fixation of the malleus-drum cone unit, not usually associated with other middle-ear lesions or with window occlusions. It may be very specific, as in the fixed malleus syndrome, the fixed incus syndrome, or the fixed incudomalleal syndrome. The basic lesion is idiopathic fixation of the malleus head (caput mallei), with or without accompanying incus fixation, producing variable audiologic sequelae. It is more common than hitherto realized. Most cases have been accidentally diagnosed during a surgical procedure originally planned for a stapedectomy. After finding no evidence of oval window otosclerosis, the surgeon will palpate the malleus and incus and then discover the correct diagnosis of lateral fixation.

Many unexplained poor stapedectomy results are due to nonrecognition of lateral ossicular fixation at the time of surgical exploration because the surgeon did not palpate for malleus and incus mobility prior to the removal of the stapedial arch and footplate, and did not carefully look for evidence of oval window otosclerosis. Recent developments in impedance audiometry, tympanometry, and the conductive loss test battery now make it possible to diagnose most lateral ossicular fixation cases before operation.

This preoperative diagnostic capability will undoubtedly improve with refinements in audiologic studies, polytomography, and quantitative pneumatic otoscopy. Total tympanic-membrane–malleal fixation can exist without an air–bone gap. The clinical audiologic findings are variable, and indicate need for further investigations of tympanic-membrane–ossicular physiology.

PATHOPHYSIOLOGY

More than a century ago, in a monumental study of otologic observations in autopsy dissections, Toynbee (8) described fixation of the ossicles as a cause of hearing loss, definitely differentiating fixation of the lateral ossicle (malleus and incus) from fixation of the stapes. A number of other observers corroborated Toynbee's findings throughout the century, but the concept was ignored. It is only in the past two decades that modern otologic microsurgery has been applied to the management of lateral ossicular fixation.

Malleal fixation to the tegmen tympani, which represents the epitympanic bony roof (floor of anterior cranial fossa) has been observed in temporal bone sections (Fig. 20–1). Of historic interest is the recent discovery of a malleus fixed to the tegmen in a 1600-year-old skull discovered in Israel (1). A very common finding is that of joint incudomalleal fixation (Fig. 20–2).

A rigidly fixed malleal head produces a change in the impedance and in the acoustic energy transfer capacity of the tympanic membrane. It is also responsible for similar interference with acoustic energy transfer through the incus. The secondary incus effect is due primarily to the nature of the incudomalleal joint (a modified cog-type saddle joint), which normally permits incus motion closely geared to that of the malleus. In cases of true incudomalleal osteoarthritis with joint capsule obliteration, this physiologic continuity with the malleus rigidity is virtually identical.

Fixation of the stapes, either by otosclerotic or pseudo-otosclerotic lesions, is one of the most common causes of *medial conductive hearing loss*. Otosclerotic stapedial fixation is due usually to a footplate fixation lesion or occasionally to crural fixation and should be described as *medial stapedial fixation*. A less common cause of stapedial conductive hearing loss is *lateral stapedial fixation* secondary to incus immobilization. Such incudal rigidity almost always accompanies malleal fixation. Malleal fixation can thus produce not only tympanic membrane fixation but also secondary stapes immobilization, in contrast to the usual medial fixation at the vestibular window. The stapes, therefore, becomes fixed—not medially (as in otosclerosis or in tympanosclerosis by footplate annular ligamental fusion or by crural promontory fusion) but laterally, by a restrictive displacement transmitted to the stapedial capitulum from the lateral ossicular chain.

Under certain circumstances, one could con-

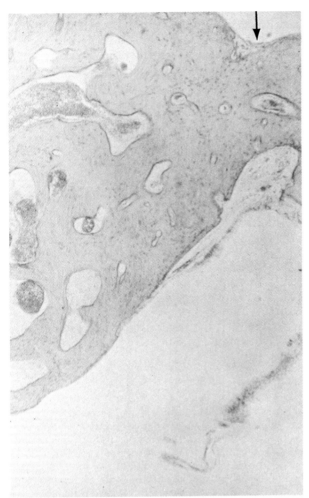

FIG. 20–1. Malleal fixation to tegmen tympani from a temporal bone section. **Arrow** indicates solid fixation between malleal head and epitympanic roof (floor of anterior cranial fossa). (Courtesy of Dr. R. Gussen)

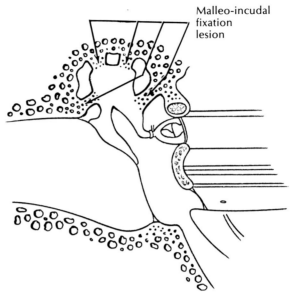

FIG. 20–2. Malleo-incudal fixation.

sider the fixed malleus syndrome to be within the category of pseudootosclerosis, a term applied to a number of conditions that mimic otosclerosis. However, less than complete malleal fixation, accompanied by a relatively mobile incudomalleal or incudostapedial joint will not produce stapes fixation. A different physiologic and a different audiologic sequel occurs.

CLINICAL DIAGNOSIS

The diagnosis in the past has usually been made when the condition was encountered accidentally during tympanotomy for a planned stapedectomy. It may or may not accompany true otosclerosis. It can be congenital or acquired. It may coexist with true or apparent sensorineural (cochlear) hearing loss. It usually appears as an idiopathic lesion, although the fixation can be a sequel of tympanosclerosis or keratoma (cholesteatoma), or as a component of ossicular panosteoarthritis, in which all three ossicles are fixed. Lateral ossicular fixation accompanying true oval window otosclerosis with identifiable histologic malleal or incudal otosclerosis is rare.

"Quantitative" pneumatic otoscopy (3) prior to operation can reveal a differential restriction in mobility of malleal short process. Compression-rarefaction of tympanic membrane with a calibrated pneumatic otoscope will demonstrate mobility differences between the circumumbo region of the tympanic membrane and the posterior-inferior pars tensa. Although, in normal tympanic membranes manubrium mobility is less than that of the pars tensa, this difference may be greatly increased with relative or complete immobilization of the umbo region.

AUDIOLOGIC FINDINGS

The classic air–bone gap may be the only audiologic feature of a completely fixed malleus when it produces lateral stapedial fixation. However, in subtotal fixation there is diminished malleal head mobility, and the incus, incudostapedial joint, and stapedial arch are still reasonably mobile. In such subtotal fixation the audiologic findings differ from the classic air–bone gap. Variable audiologic pictures occur in cases of partial tympanic membrane fixation. The bone conduction curve is usually depressed and slopes downward in the higher frequencies, producing a "mixed" hearing loss. The depressed high-frequency bone-conduction patterns may be incorrectly attributed to a cochlear lesion.

The conductive loss battery and acoustic impedance evaluation (see Ch. 6, Audiologic Assessment, Functional Hearing Loss, and Objective Audiometry) provide additional information to aid in the diagnosis of lateral ossicular fixation. Seven patients with ossicular fixation, other than stapedial, have been seen for pre- and postsurgical evaluations. Pure-tone audiometric findings typically consisted of minimal air–bone gaps in the low frequencies, generally no greater than 20 dB, and a sensorineural component in the high frequencies. The initial evaluation revealed that each patient had excellent speech discrimination ability. Conductive loss battery findings consistently confirmed good agreement between mastoid bone conduction and frontal bone conduction results (Fig. 20–3). Acoustic impedance results were as follows: All seven patients exhibited negative acoustic reflexes; five of these patients had restricted tympanometry with high acoustic impedance (low compliance); one patient had normal tympanometry and normal impedance; and one patient had hypermobile tympanometry and low impedance.

In general, clinical findings revealed that patients who have lateral ossicular fixation display small, low-frequency air–bone gaps with an apparent sensorineural component in the high frequencies. Acoustic impedance results consistently reveal negative acoustic reflexes, and generally demonstrate restricted tympanometry and high total impedance (low compliance). After operation, tympanometry falls within the normal range (Fig. 20–4).

SURGICAL DIAGNOSIS

Differential palpation of the stapes, as compared with the incus, is important. It is easy to miss a mobile stapes if attention is limited to palpation via the incudostapedial joint or via the neck or crura. A mobile stapes may be completely fixed laterally by fixed incus rigidity. Only palpation via the central footplate or via the pericrural footplate regions will demonstrate stapedial mobility. Such palpation usually will elicit a brisk round window reflex. A dramatic difference is thus noted between footplate palpation and incudostapedial joint or capitulum palpation. In doubtful cases, careful incudostapedial joint section will be followed by immediate dramatic evidence of stapedial mobility and incudal fixation.

SURGICAL MANAGEMENT

Surgical management of lateral fixation depends to some extent upon the etiologic and anatomic factors. Principles of management are similar in most cases.

Mobilization of the fixed malleal head by arthrolysis, applying pressure through the manubrium or the incus, is usually of only transitory value. Surgical restoration of mobility is best achieved by deliberate malleal neck transsection as a first step. The fixating lesion may be ligamentous, it may represent an exostotic connection with the lateral attic wall or with the tegmen tympani, or it may be due to some other ossifying process, such as replacement of the tensor tympani tendon by bony union of malleus and the processus cochleariformis.

Step 1. Lateral Atticotomy

When the diagnosis of incudomalleal fixation is made, a lateral atticotomy is necessary. Removal of lateral epitympanic wall (scutum) is necessary to obtain adequate exposure of the incudomalleal joint. This atticotomy is accomplished either with a curet or with a cutting burr. It should be sufficient for surgical access to the incudomalleal joint throughout its extent (Fig. 20–5).

Step 2. Incudostapedial Joint Section

The next step consists of incudostapedial joint section with an angulated 0.5-mm circumferential knife. This liberates the mobile stapes from transmitted incudal pressure to protect the cochlear perilymph from undue "pumping" forces. It also liberates the incus sufficiently to allow for more precise palpation of the incudomalleal joint (Fig. 20–6).

Step 3. Incudomalleal Joint Section

The incudomalleal joint can usually be sectioned with a 1-mm angulated knife (Fig. 20–7). In some cases, however, the incudomalleal joint may be fused because of arthropathy. In such cases, a sharp cutting burr is used to cut the joint. In instances of total incudomalleal joint obliteration, it may be necessary to abandon attempts at incudomalleal joint section because of potential danger to epitympanic tegment.

Step 4. Incus Rotation and Removal

Following incudomalleal joint section, the incus usually becomes freely mobile. It is elevated in a superior

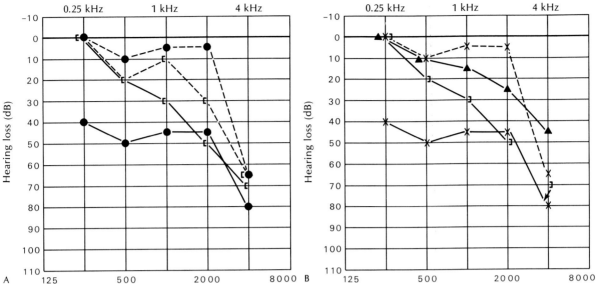

FIG. 20–3. A. Malleal fixation in a 71-year-old patient. Preoperative bone conduction level (mastoid placement) indicates probability of significant high-frequency hearing loss and only fair prognosis for hearing improvement surgically. However, postoperative air conduction level reveals almost normal hearing (see Fig. 20–4). ●—●, AC, unmasked, RE, before operation; [—[, BC, masked, RE, before operation; ●- - -●, AC, unmasked, RE, after operation; [- - -[, BC, masked, RE, after operation. B. Audiogram of left ear of same patient. Bone conduction by both mastoid and frontal placements. Note major differences at 500 Hz, 1000 Hz, and 2000 Hz. Postoperative AC level is in closer agreement with frontal BC measurements. x—x, AC, unmasked, LE, before operation;]—], BC, masked, LE, before operation; ▲—▲, BC, frontal, before operation; x- - -x, AC, unmasked, LE, after operation; **arrow,** no response at maximum output.

FIG. 20–4. Ossicular fixation tympanometry curve.

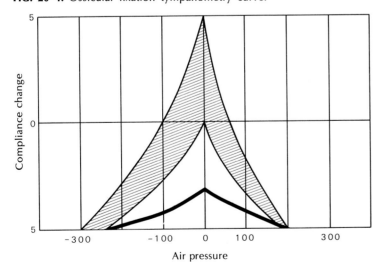

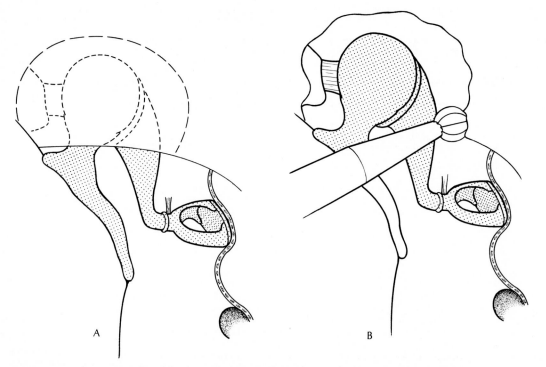

FIG. 20–5. Lateral atticotomy. **A.** Diagrammatic view of epitympanic area visualized before bone removal. **B.** Removal with cutting burr of a portion of the inferior aspect of the epitympanic wall to permit adequate exposure of the incudomalleal joint. (In this figure and in those following, the incus short process has been omitted, for purposes of simplification.)

FIG. 20–6. Incudostapedial joint section liberates the stapes from transmitted incudal pressure and thus protects the cochlear fluids.

FIG. 20–7. Incudomalleal joint section mobilizes the incus and prepares it for removal.

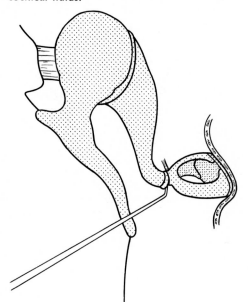

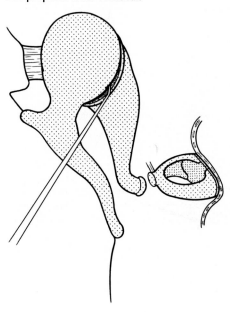

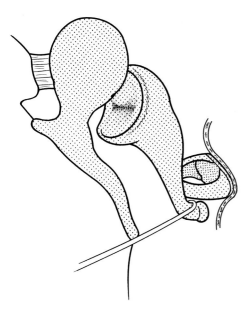

FIG. 20–8. Rotation of incus away from the stapes.

FIG. 20–9. Delivery of incus from middle ear cavity.

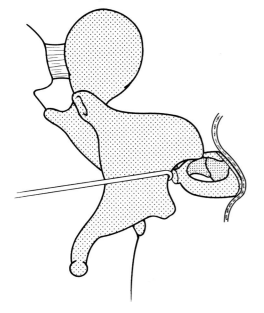

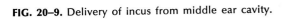

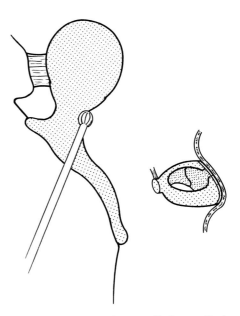

FIG. 20–10. Cutting burr applied to malleal neck.

FIG. 20–11. Malleal neck transection completed, allowing complete separation of the manubrium from the malleal head.

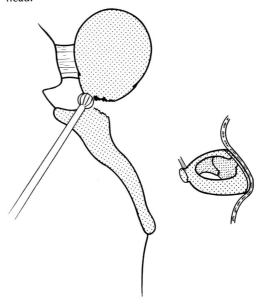

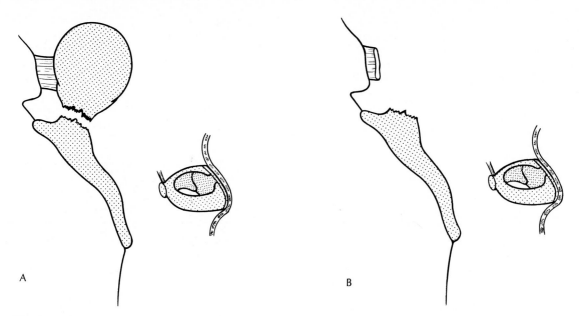

FIG. 20–12. Mobile manubrium. **A.** Malleal head *in situ*. **B.** Malleal head removed.

direction away from the stapes, using a 90° hook or similar instrument (Fig. 20–8). After preliminary elevation, a rotation maneuver lowers the articulating surface of the incus away from the malleal articulation, and the incus body is then rotated out of its fossa incudis (Fig. 20–9) and removed. It may be placed in a covered, moist container for subsequent remodeling into a hemiincus autograft.

FIG. 20–13. Mobile malleal manubrium trough with homograft ossicular connection to mobile stapes.

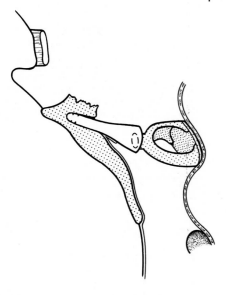

Step 5. Malleal Neck Transsection

Transsection of the malleal neck is the crucial step in the surgical procedure. It is necessary to separate the malleal manubrium completely from the malleal head to liberate the manubrium and its attached tympanic-membrane pars tensa. The primary lesion of the fixed malleus syndrome is tympanic membrane immobilization. Malleal neck transsection is the liberating maneuver, using a 1.5-mm cutting burr (Fig. 20–10). Pledgets of absorbable gelatin sponge (Gelfoam) saturated with Ringer's solution are placed in the epitympanum and medial to the tympanic membrane manubrium to protect mucosa and to trap bone dust. It is necessary to cut through the malleal neck and to sever all periosteal and submucosal tissue connections completely so that the manubrium is completely separated from the malleal head (Fig. 20–11).

Step 6. Management of the Malleal Head

The malleal head should be removed, but may be left *in situ* in the epitympanum (Fig. 20–12). If the osteophytic malleal head connection with epitympanic tegmen is extremely firm, removal may be hazardous to the tegmen and its overlying dura.

Step 7. Preparation of Hemiincus or Cartilage Autograft

In some instances, ossicular reconstruction following tympanic membrane liberation is accomplished by the use of a hemiincus autograft created from the previously removed incus. The incus is grasped with a "diamond" forceps, and a saw is used to resect the short process and a portion of the body of the incus, thus leaving only the articular surface, the long process, and the lenticular process as a hemiincus auto-graft. The processed hemiincus measures approximately 6.5 mm in length. If a shorter hemiincus is necessary, the superior half of the articular surface is resected, thus reducing the hemiincus length to 5 mm.

When it is impossible to remove the incus because of extensive incudomalleal osteoarthritis, as in some cases, the incudal long process is resected close to the body and removed. A tragal cartilage autograft (5) or a prefabricated "golf-tee" allograft (homograft) (6) is used to connect the malleal manubrium to the stapes capitulum or to the oval window (Fig. 20–13).

Step 8. Elevation of Manubrial Periosteum

The periosteum of the manubrium on its medial aspect is elevated from the cut end of the malleal transsection and a trough is created in the superior manubrium. The hemiincus "locks" into this trough (see Ch. 17, Otomastoditis Surgery—Mastoidectomy and Tympanoplasty).

Step 9a. Ossiculoplastic Reconstruction

The hemiincus autograft or allograft is articulated between the trough and the capitulum if the stapes is mobile.

In instances in which the arch does not adapt well to such a reconstruction, the crura are carefully removed and the bone graft is placed directly on the mobile footplate, after footplate periosteal elevation.

In coexisting true otosclerosis or stapediovestibular arthritis, the arch and footplate are removed, the oval window is sealed by a perichondrial graft, and the hemiincus or allograft is placed on the oval window graft (see Ch. 17).

Following accurate placement of the graft, the middle ear is closed in the usual manner and the external auditory canal is packed as in normal post-stapedectomy procedures.

Step 9b. Prefabricated Allografts

Recent developments in the use of prefabricated ossicular allografts, make it advantageous in some cases to use a modified golf-tee allograft to extend from the region of the transsected malleal-neck soft tissues to the stapedial capitulum. In most instances, since the stapes is mobile and the stapedial tendon is intact, the utilization of a golf-tee allograft is a more feasible procedure than an autograft.

LATERAL OSSICULAR FIXATION—A CAUSE OF CONDUCTIVE PRESBYCUSIS?

Presbycusis (see Ch. 41) is defined as a progressive, bilaterally symmetrical perceptive hearing loss occurring with age. The word is derived from the Greek *presby*, meaning "old," and Greek *akousis*, meaning "hearing." Thus, the derivation of the word itself simply indicates that it describes the hearing loss of old age, as a result of the aging process in hearing. Dorland's definition (2) contains the word "perceptive," implying only a sensorineural lesion. Thus, the classic concept of presbycusis has been a hearing loss in older people that is due to cochlear or other sensorineural etiologic factors.

Schuknecht (7) described several types of presbycusis, one of which he termed "mechanical presbycusis," and hypothesized that it "may be due to stiffening of the basilar membrane or some other mechanical disorder, the functional manifestation of which is a descending audiometric curve."

In an earlier paper on malleal fixation, Goodhill stated: "It may well be that one type of presbycusis previously considered sensorineural is, indeed, conductive and is due to a lesion or lesions of the epitympanic ligaments attached to the incudomalleal mass" (4).

We cannot exclude other possibilities, such as shortening and decreased elasticity of the tensor tympani and stapedius muscles. Such considerations may begin to explain the condition in patients with lateral ossicular fixation with a diagnosis of presbycusis who show descending audiometric patterns with slight or absent air–bone gaps and with disproportionately high speech-discrimination scores. It is necessary now to study not only the cochlea but also the ossicular coupler and other middle ear structures for additional explanations of presbycusis. In addition, CNS degeneration must be considered (see Ch. 41, Presbycusis).

SUMMARY

Lateral ossicular fixation (malleus, incus, or malleoincudal) causes a conductive hearing loss resembling that seen in otosclerosis. It occasionally accompanies true otosclerosis. However, it more frequently is mistaken for otosclerosis. It is also accompanied by true, as well as apparent, cochlear hearing losses. It poses difficult preoperative and operative diagnostic problems. When recognized, it can be corrected surgically by malleal neck transsection and ossiculoplasty.

REFERENCES

1. Arenberg B, Nathan H, Ziv M: Malleus fixed (ossified) to the Tegmen tympani in an ancient skeleton in Israel. Ann Otol Rhinol Laryngol 86:75–79, 1977

2. Dorlands Illustrated Medical Dictionary, 24th ed. Philadelphia, WB Saunders, 1965

3. Eviatar A, Goodhill V: Myringo-manometry: observations in normal and pathologic ears. Laryngoscope 80:1847–1858, 1970

4. Goodhill V: External conductive hypacusis and the fixed malleus syndrome. Acta Otolaryngol (Stockh) [Suppl] 217:1–43, 1966

5. Goodhill V: Tragal perichondrium and cartilage in tympanoplasty. Arch Otolaryngol 85:480–491, 1967

6. Goodhill V, Westerberg AM, Davis C: Prefabricated homografts in ossiculoplasty. Trans Am Acad Ophthalmol Otolaryngol 78:ORL 411–422, 1974

7. Schuknecht HF: Further observations on the pathology of presbycusis. Arch Otolaryngol 80:369–382, 1964

8. Toynbee J: Diseases of the Ear. Philadelphia, Blanchard & Lea, 1860

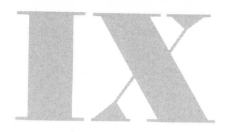

DYSTROPHIES AND TUMORS

21

TEMPORAL BONE GRANULOMAS AND DYSTROPHIES

A number of specific granulomas and osteodystrophies that involve the skull produce temporal bone lesions with characteristic syndrome profiles.

Histiocytic granuloma (histiocytosis X) and Wegener's granuloma are two relatively common temporal bone granulomas with special diagnostic and therapeutic features.

Paget's disease of bone, Van der Hoeve's syndrome (brittle bone syndrome) and monostotic fibrous dysplasia are three relatively common osteodystrophies that involve the temporal bone and that, in common with the granulomas, require differential diagnostic, as well as therapeutic, considerations in otologic practice.

HISTIOCYTIC GRANULOMA OF THE TEMPORAL BONE

In 1950 (5) I recommended that the triphasic clinicopathologic syndrome previously termed Letterer-Siwe disease, Hand-Schüller-Christian disease, and eosinophilic granuloma be considered as a single pathologic entity: histiocytic granuloma. Several years later Lichtenstein (9) suggested the term *histiocytosis X*, which is widely used today.

The disease is basically characterized by the abnormal production of large numbers of histiocytes with normal mitotic figures (Fig. 21–1).

The group of three diseases occurs most commonly in children. The most serious and frequently fatal category of Letterer-Siwe disease is the reticulum-cell stage for what might be termed *acute histiocytic granuloma*. Hand-Schüller-Christian disease is the xanthomatous lipid-storing phase, or *subacute histiocytic granuloma*. The

solitary chronic lesion of eosinophilic granuloma characterizes *chronic histiocytic granuloma*.

These distinctions are not sharply delimited. They have a rather random anatomic distribution of lesions in the skull and extremities, but all three forms can involve the temporal bone.

There are no regular sequential or chronologic patterns. The response of the histiocytic system is bizarre and unpredictable. Thus, acute cases can occur with and/or without bone or lymph node lesions. Subacute cases occur with and without proptosis or skin lesions. Chronic cases occur with and without skeletal or skull involvement. In various patients, visceral lesions have been seen in every stage of the disease and have been absent in every stage of the disease.

The pathological findings in the varying lesions are related to pressure phenomena produced by the granulomatous process. It is interesting to note the relative resistance of the capsule of the bony labyrinth to invasion by the granuloma. All other bones in the body, including the tympanic ossicles, the annulus tympanicus, and the entire mastoid and petrous pyramid can be destroyed by this disease, but the labyrinthine bony capsule appears to be resistant.

PATHOPHYSIOLOGY OF HISTIOCYTIC GRANULOMA

Letterer-Siwe Disease—Acute Phase

The classic reticulum cell phase, or the acute non-lipoid-storing phase, occurs in the infant who develops a rapidly progressing lesion characterized by multiple skeletal lesions, proptosis, and visceral involvement, with early and quickly spreading cutaneous manifestations accompanied frequently by diabetes insipidus, profound anemia, and high mortality (Fig. 21–2). The pathologic picture on biopsy of the various tissues involved usually reveals a widespread reticulum cell growth with occasional xanthoma cells in which there is no evidence of lipid storage. This stage will very frequently fuse almost imperceptibly with the subacute xanthomatous phase.

Hand-Schüller-Christian Disease—Subacute Stage

This subacute xanthomatous stage is characterized by slower growth and less noticeable skin lesions. There is little visceral involvement, and the diabetes insipidus is controllable in the vast majority of cases by the use of pituitary extracts and sella turcica radiation. The skull lesions—all of which are identical in all three phases of the disease—respond rather rapidly to x-ray therapy.

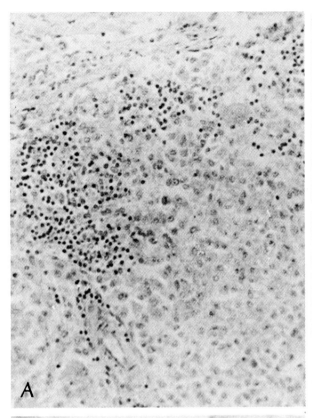

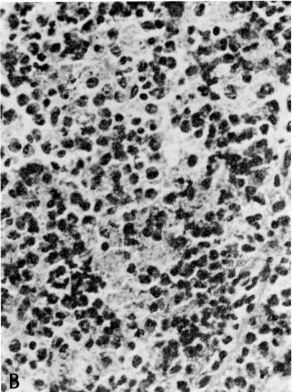

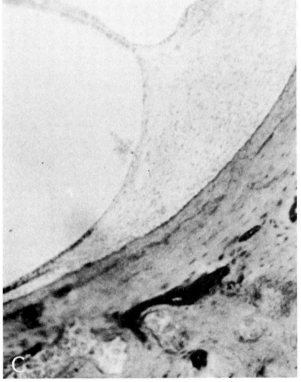

FIG. 21–1. A. Section from skull base with many pale foam or xanthoma cells characteristic of subacute histiocytic granuloma (Hand-Schüller-Christian disease). **B.** Temporal bone mastoid tissue section showing many eosinophiles, histiocytes, plasma and xanthoma type cells. Case of chronic histiocytic granuloma. **C.** Reticulum cell involvement of temporal bone pneumatic cell area. The bony capsule of the labyrinth apparently prevented labyrinth invasion.

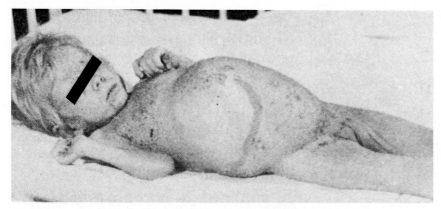

FIG. 21–2. Premortem photograph, showing characteristic purpuric seborrheic skin rash over forehead, scalp, palms, chest, and abdomen. Note also the enlarged abdomen, enlarged liver, and enlarged spleen as indicated by markings on abdomen.

FIG. 21–3. A. Very large skull erosions in eosinophilic granuloma. **B.** Smaller multiple skull erosions in subacute histiocytic granuloma.

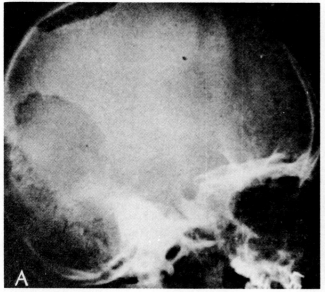
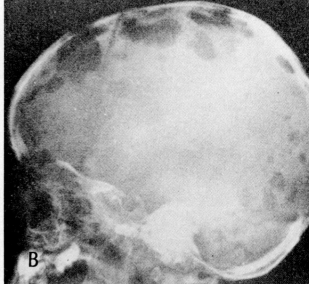

The response to x-ray therapy in the acute Letterer-Siwe reticulum-cell type is usually poor.

Eosinophilic Granuloma—Chronic Stage

This final chronic stage is characterized most usually by monolocular lesions, but they may be skeletal as well as calvarial. The lesions will respond to either surgery or x-ray; many patients have had uneventful recoveries with surgical removal of the lesions. Diabetes insipidus is usually not demonstrable, and skin lesions occur only occasionally. Although there may be recurrences in other parts of the skeletal system, temporal bone lesions respond well to surgical and/or deep x-ray therapy.

From the radiographic diagnostic standpoint (Fig. 21–3), there is practically no difference between the three phases, illustrating again the unity of the clinicopathologic picture. Thus Caffey (2) states:

In the skeleton, the radiolucent granulomatous proliferations replace radiopaque bone and appear roentgenographically as areas of diminished density in the flat bones of the skull, pelvis, and shoulder girdle, and also in the tubular bones of the thorax and extremities. Involvement of the bones distal to the elbows and knees is practically unknown. These bony defects may be single or multiple; they are usually sharply demarcated and rounded or scalloped, and are of variable size.

In cholesterol reticulosis (Schüller-Christian's disease and Letterer-Siwe's disease) the roentgenographic findings are identical.

Under "eosinophilic granuloma," Caffey states: "Roentgenographically, the skeletal changes are identical with those of cholesterol reticulosis" (2).

DIFFERENTIAL DIAGNOSIS

The first differential diagnosis must be made from the standpoint of the skull lesions. The skull lesions are frequently confused with those of multiple myeloma and metastases from carcinoma. Lues and tuberculosis will occasionally produce this type of skull lesion. The outstanding feature in the behavior of this group of skull lesions is the usually quick response to deep x-ray therapy. Large tumor masses will disappear quickly and almost melt away within days following administration of deep x-ray therapy to the calvarium, to the orbit, or to the long bones.

The second differential diagnosis is that of the temporal bone lesion, frequently mistaken clinically for keratoma (cholesteatoma). The fetid discharge, frequent attic perforation, evidence of bone destruction, conductive hearing loss and radiographic evidence of trabecular destruction resemble findings in keratoma (cholesteatoma). What confuses the picture still further is that a smear taken for cholesterol crystals will almost always demonstrate them in histiocytic granuloma, particularly of the xanthomatous type, as well as in keratoma (cholesteatoma). The differential diagnosis is best made by radiography of the skull, by a close search for diabetes insipidus in urine concentration studies, and by careful study for evidence of early proptosis. "Granulation" tissue biopsy is extremely valuable and will frequently make the diagnosis. The response of the temporal bone to x-ray therapy is as dramatic as the response to x-ray of the other cranial bones. The otorrhea will frequently cease and the tympanic perforation will frequently heal entirely, following adequate deep x-ray therapy.

TREATMENT

Inasmuch as the basic cause of the production of the histiocytic proliferation characteristic of the three phases of histiocytic granuloma is unknown, no specific therapy exists.

The acute reticulum-cell type of Letterer-Siwe disease usually does not show a good response to x-ray therapy. The response may be temporary or partial, but it rarely is of sufficient value to completely control the disease, and the patient usually succumbs to widespread granulomatous lesions that eventually interfere with pulmonary, hepatic, or cerebral function.

The subacute xanthomatous stage of Hand-Schüller-Christian disease shows an excellent response to x-ray therapy in many cases but not in all.

The chronic low-grade eosinophilic granuloma phase very quickly responds to roentgen therapy but is equally responsive to surgical extirpation. The judgment as to which to employ depends a great deal upon the site, mechanical factors, and size of lesion. An extremely large lesion might better be treated surgically, with radiation reserved for the treatment of any residual swellings or recurrences.

WEGENER'S GRANULOMATOSIS

The special type of granuloma described by Wegener (14) is characterized by respiratory tract granulomatosis, necrotizing vasculitis, and glomerulitis. The "rhinogenic" granuloma is also accompanied frequently by temporal bone involvement.

Otalgia, otorrhea, and mixed conductive and sensorineural hearing losses occur, accompanied by systemic pulmonary and renal lesions. Temporal bone surgical exploration show diffuse granulomatous disease. Friedmann and Bauer (4) reported characteristic Wegener type multinucleated giant cells with compact hyperchromic nuclei. Grossly the lesion resembles cholesterol granuloma, as seen in type A chronic otomastoiditis, but clinically this lesion is much more serious, with a poor prognosis.

PAGET'S DISEASE—OSTEITIS DEFORMANS OF TEMPORAL BONE

Paget's disease of bone is a systemic heritable disease involving principally skull and axial skeleton. It is manifested by dystrophic bone strongly resembling the otospongiosis stage of otosclerosis, when it occurs in the temporal bone. The two diseases have in common the presence of large vascular marrow spaces. The skull and temporal bones are involved in two-thirds of cases. The head becomes progressively enlarged, and the tibiae become bowed. In the skull, the pathologic process may encroach upon vital structures such as blood vessels, cranial nerves, and even portions of the central nervous system. It does invade the temporal bone and can mimic otosclerosis. It may cause softening of the crura with ossicular discontinuity, or it may involve the internal auditory canal with pressure upon the auditory nerve. The vestibular portion of the labyrinth may be involved. If discontinuity occurs between the stapes crura and the footplate, or if the footplate becomes fixed, surgical intervention is possible, but the prognosis is guarded inasmuch as a growth of dystrophic bone may reclose the oval window.

Nager (12) described Paget's disease (osteitis deformans) as a chronic heritable bone disease of undetermined etiology. Recurrent bone resorption phases are followed by repair periods. The result is increased bone mass with skeletal deformity. It is an inherited abiatrophy of collagen bone matrix (10) which is inherited as an incomplete dominant gene carried on an X chromosome (1), or as a simple autosomal Mendelian dominant gene (10).

In its solitary monostatic form it may be undiagnosed. As a disseminated polyostotic lesion it becomes recognizable as clinical Paget's disease.

The disease affects 3% of the population over 40, more frequently males. Skull radiographs show classic thickening of diploe and outer table, with areas of decreased and increased density (Fig. 21–4).

The early temporal bone changes (6) produced by Paget's disease start with an increase in cellular perivascular bone. This occurred as an exaggeration of the normal remodeling repolymerization of the bone about the vascular canals, spreading from adjacent periosteal surfaces into the labyrinthine capsule and eventually reaching the endosteum of the membranous labyrinth. As these areas become confluent they spread into and replace interstitial bone (Fig. 21–5).

Recent reports of medical treatment of Paget's disease of bone are encouraging. Khairi and colleagues (8) report significant improvement in levels of serum alkaline phosphatase and urinary hydroxyproline in addition to clinical improvement and bone-scan improvement following treatment with sodium etidronate. However, Menzies and co-workers (11) report treatment with calcitonin in four patients, who showed improvement in those biochemical parameters that reflect skeletal disease but did not show hearing improvement.

Finerman and associates (3) reported their results with diphosphate (EDHP, disodium etidronate) treatment. Their study shows striking biochemical, bone scan, and systemic clinical improvement, with evidence of remission following cessation of therapy.

Thus, with developments in diphosphonate therapy, some optimism regarding the fate of Paget's disease of the temporal bone seems warranted.

VAN DER HOEVE'S SYNDROME— OSTEOGENESIS IMPERFECTA

Fragilitas ossium, or "brittle bones" is a rare disease, usually hereditary in nature, characterized by marked bone fragility (Fig. 21–6). A peculiarity of the sclerae, which robs them of pigment, is described as "blue sclerae." In this disease, multiple fractures occur and it is not unusual for a patient to have as many as 40–50 fractures during a 10- to 15-year period, resulting in many deformations. Similar lesions may occur in the ossicular chain, in the tegmen mastoidei, tegmen tympani, and in the otic capsule. Lesions that simulate otosclerosis have occurred in this area, but true otosclerosis can also occur in conjunction with the disease. Stapedial fixation may occur with or without concurrent otosclerosis. Stapes surgery may be performed, but as with Paget's disease, the prognosis must be guarded (see Ch. 19, Otosclerosis).

FIBROUS DYSPLASIA OF THE TEMPORAL BONE

Fibrous dysplasia of the temporal bone usually represents the monstatic form of the disease (13). Fibrous tissue forms within the temporal bone trabeculae with variable degrees of cellularity. Bone expansion and bone erosion occur irregularly. Mastoid and middle ear involvement are common, with secondary keratoma development in some cases. It can occur in association with *en plaque* meningioma with temporal bone involvement. Surgical removal is not always successful, with frequent recurrence reported.

SARCOIDOSIS

Among the many granulomas that can affect the temporal bone is sarcoidosis. This chronic disease of lymph nodes, lung, liver, spleen, and skin can affect the eyes and the ears, nose and throat.

Noncaseating tubercules are found, unlike those of tuberculosis. Kane (7) reported a recent case with tinnitus, hearing loss, and facial paralysis.

FIG. 21–4. A. Lateral view of skull, 78-year-old male. Enlargement and change in configuration are the result of thickening of the diploe and outer table. The close association of areas of radiolucency (osteoporosis) and increased density (osteosclerosis) produces a "cotton wool" pattern, most prominent in the frontal and parietal region. Alteration of the hypophyseal fossa and bulging of the base of the skull into the cranial cavity are apparent. (Nager GT: Ann Otol Rhinol Laryngol [Suppl 22] 84: July–August 1975). **B.** Postero-anterior view of skull, 63-year-old male. Involvement and enlargement of the calvaria are symmetrical. The outer table and diploe exhibit the most characteristic changes. Progressive softening of the base resulted in platy- and convexobasia with elevation of the petrous apices and a downward slanting of the petrous crests. Note partial obliteration of the frontal sinuses. (Nager GT: Ann Otol Rhinol Laryngol [Suppl 22] 84: July–August 1975)

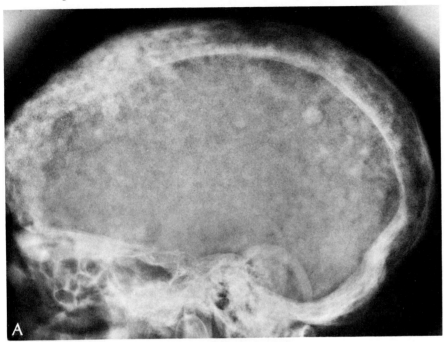

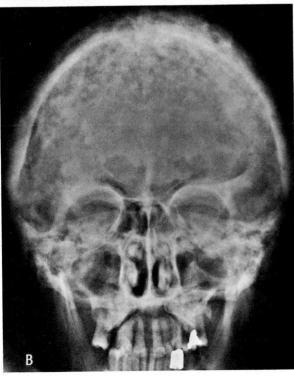

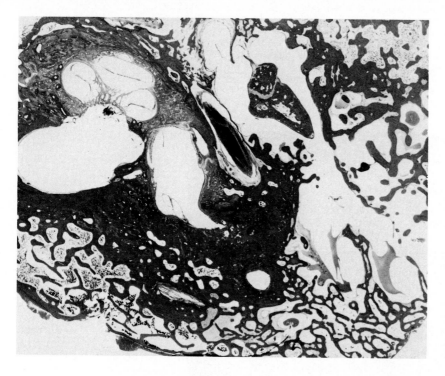

FIG. 21–5. Paget's disease of right temporal bone. Note increase in bone trabeculae with marrow and cellular fibrovascular tissue in mastoid and posterolateral regions, as well as along medial aspect of temporal bone. Wave of confluent repolymerizing perivascular bone in internal auditory canal, one reaching endosteum of cochlea. Perivascular foci in cochlear capsule. (Gussen R: Arch Otolarygol 91:341–345, 1970. Copyright 1970, American Medical Association)

FIG. 21–6. A. Normal neonatal stapes (× 49). **B.** Very thin stapes of neonate who suffered from osteogenesis imperfecta (× 52). (Bergstrom L: Laryngoscope [Suppl 6] 87: Sept, 1977)

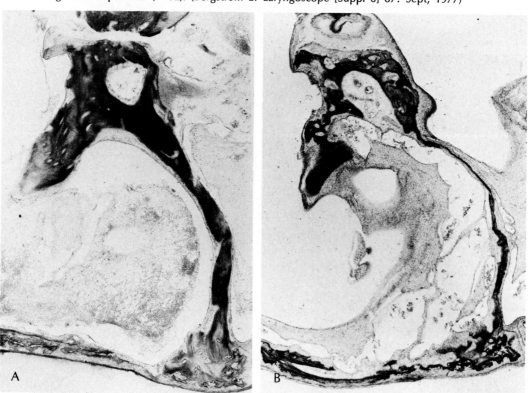

REFERENCES

1. Ashley-Montague MF: Paget's disease (osteitis deformans) and heredity. Am J Hum Genet 1:94–95, 1947
2. Caffey J: Pediatric X-Ray Diagnosis. Chicago, Year Book Medical, 1945, pp 71–73
3. Finerman GA, Gonick HC, Smith RK et al.: Diphosphonate treatment of Paget's disease. Clin Orthop 120:115–124, 1976
4. Friedmann I, Bauer F: Wegener's granulomatosis causing deafness. J Laryngol 87:449–464, 1973
5. Goodhill V: Histiocytic granuloma of skull. Laryngoscope 60:1–54, 1950
6. Gussen R: Early Paget's disease of the labyrinthine capsule. Arch Otolaryngol 91:341–345, 1970
7. Kane K: Deafness in sarcoidosis. J Laryngol 90:531–537, 1976
8. Khairi MR, Johnston CC, Attman RD et al.: Treatment of Paget disease of bone (osteitis deformans). JAMA 230:562–567, 1974
9. Lichtenstein L: Histiocytosis X. Arch Pathol Lab Med 56:84–102, 1953
10. McKusick VA: Heritable Disorders of Connective Tissues. St Louis, CV Mosby, 1972, pp 718–723
11. Menzies MA, Greenberg PB, Joplin GF: Otological studies in patients with deafness due to Paget's disease before and after treatment with synthetic human calcitonin. Acta Otolaryngol (Stockh) 79:378–383, 1975
12. Nager GT: Paget's disease of the Temporal bone. Ann Otol Rhinol Laryngol [Suppl] 22:1–32, 1975
13. Sharp M: Monostostic fibrous dysplasia of the temporal bone. J Laryngol 84:697–708, 1970
14. Wegener F (1936) from Friedmann I, Bauer F: Wegener's granulomatosis causing deafness. J Laryngol 87:449–464, 1973

SUGGESTED READING

Badrinas F, Bruguera M, Reitg de Llobet L et al.: Histiocitosis X. Rev Clin Esp 32:209–218, 1971

DeSa JV: Eosinophilic granuloma of the temporal bone. Arch Otolaryngol 70:593–596, 1959

Lindsay JR, Suga F: Paget's disease and sensorineural deafness. Temporal bone histopathology of Paget's disease. Laryngoscope 86:1029–1042, 1976

Lopez-Rios G, Benitez JT, Vivar G: Histiocytosis: histopathological study of the temporal bone. Ann Otol Rhinol Laryngol 77:1171–1180, 1968

Rao PB: A case record of eosinophilic granuloma and its pathology. J Laryngol 79:62–65, 1965

Smoler J, Rivera-Camacho R, Vivar G et al.: Otolaryngologic manifestations of histiocytosis X. Laryngoscope 81:1903–1911, 1971

Toohill RJ, Kidder TM, Eby LG: Eosinophilic granuloma of the temporal bone. Laryngoscope 83:877–889, 1973

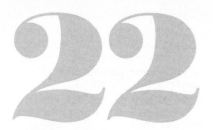

TEMPORAL BONE TUMORS

Benign, intermediate, and malignant tumors occur within the temporal bone, or may invade it from neighboring structures. These include tumors of the auricle, external canal, and middle ear, as well as those of the mastoid process and petrous pyramid. Intracranial tumors contiguous to the temporal bone can involve the temporal bone secondarily. Salivary gland, nasopharyngeal, and neck tumors may similarly spread to the temporal bone. Metastases may also involve the temporal bone from abdominal, thoracic, or other regions.

Ear tumors can be masked by other findings. It is thus possible for carcinoma of the middle ear to masquerade as otomastoiditis. A glomus jugulare tumor may be mistaken for secretory otitis media. It is also possible for an aberrant jugular bulb or internal carotid artery to be mistaken for a glomus jugulare tumor.

Benign tumors may include any skin or cartilage tumor involving the auricle and the cartilaginous external ear canal. Common tumors in the external auditory canal are osteomas and osteophytes. In the middle ear, the glomus jugulare (glomus tympanicum), usually histologically benign, may be malignant. Meningiomas (usually benign) arise either in the middle or posterior fossa dural regions of the temporal bone. They may be *en plaque*, solid, or pleomorphic in character.

"Intermediate" tumors can behave in benign or malignant fashion and can occur in the external auditory meatus or external auditory canal as ceruminous adenomas and in the middle ear or mastoid as glomus tumors and carcinoids.

Malignant tumors may occur in the auricle, external canal, tympanic membrane, middle ear, and anywhere in the temporal bone. Squamous-cell carcinomas may start in the external auditory canal or middle ear and extend to other parts of the temporal bone. Rhabdomyosarcoma is rare and is seen most commonly in infants and young children. Metastatic carcinomas and malignant lymphomas may involve any portion of the temporal bone.

The so-called "acoustic neurinoma" is a benign neurilemmoma, or schwannoma of the vestibular nerve, starting usually within the internal auditory canal where it is designated as an intracanalicular tumor. Infrequently the origin is from the vestibule, as a precanalicular lesion, or it may start in the cerebellopontine angle as an extracanalicular tumor. It may arise also from cochlear nerve or from facial nerve. Symptoms similar to those seen in acoustic neurinoma may occur from various benign and occasionally malignant lesions in the cerebellopontine angle. Vascular anomalies and meningiomas in the cerebellopontine angle can produce symptoms comparable to those of acoustic neurinoma (see Ch. 23, Lesions of the Eighth Nerve, Petrous Apex, and Cerebellopontine Angle).

BENIGN TUMORS

OSSEOUS EXTERNAL AUDITORY CANAL TUMORS

Benign bony growths of the external auditory canal occur frequently. The most common external auditory canal osseous lesions are osteophytes. (See Color Fig. 2.) Less commonly, osteomas (osteochondromas or exostoses) are found.

Osteophytes, the more common bony growths found in the medial external auditory canal, are usually multiple, bilateral, and variable in size. They are not true tumors, but irregular nodular masses or ledges of periosteal bone (Fig. 22–1) arising through periosteal irritation or stimulation. In contrast to lateral osteomas, they are medial and are frequently found closer to bony annular tympanic membrane margins. They may be posterior, anterior, superior, or inferior to the bony annulus. Osteophytes have been attributed etiologically to cold-water swimming; however, they occur in nonswimmers also. When they enlarge, they may entrap epithelial debris and cerumen, producing external otitis. When totally obstructive, a conductive hearing loss results. Occasionally a canal keratoma (cholesteatoma) may develop medial to obstructive osteophytes.

Osteoma (exostosis osteochondroma) of the ex-

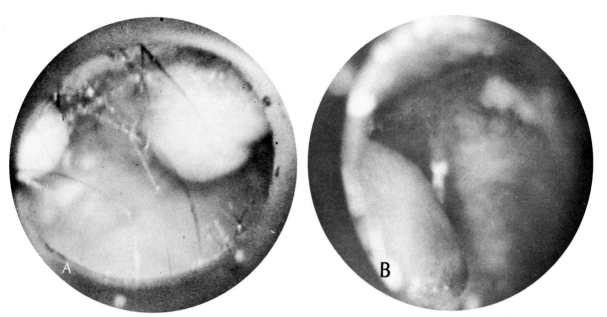

FIG. 22–1. A. Nonobstructive canal osteophytes. **B.** Large canal osteophytes in contact (obstructive).

FIG. 22–2. Lateral meatal osteoma—completely obstructive.   **FIG. 22–3.** Lateral meatal osteoma—partially obstructive.

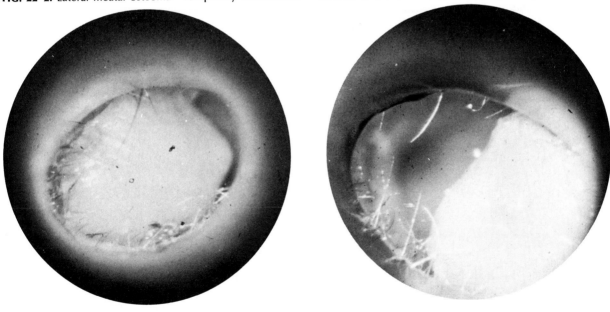

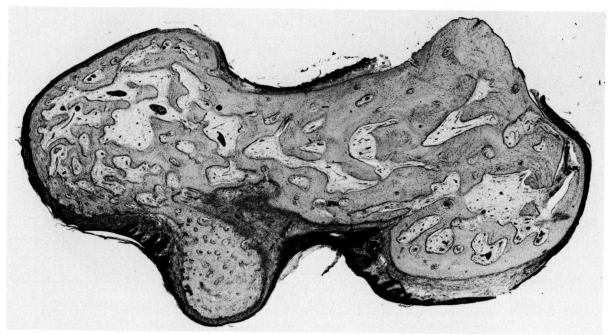

FIG. 22–4. Osteoma. Note wide trabeculae of mature bone with loose fibro-vascular inter-trabecular tissue. Prominent osteoblasts are present along bone surfaces in some areas. (Gussen R: Pathology of eighth nerve tumors. In Tower DB (ed): The Nervous System. Human Communication and Its Disorders, Volume 3. New York, Raven Press, 1975)

FIG. 22–5. Superior and inferior osteophytes almost obstructing tympanic membrane.

FIG. 22–6. Posterosuperior bone removal to enlarge canal.

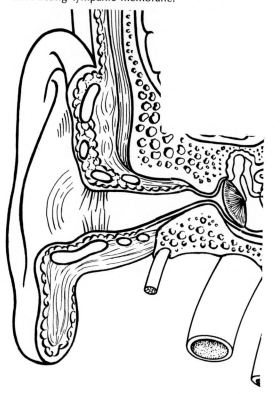

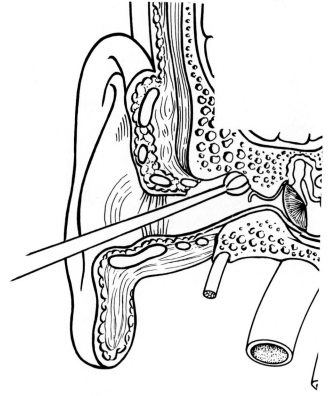

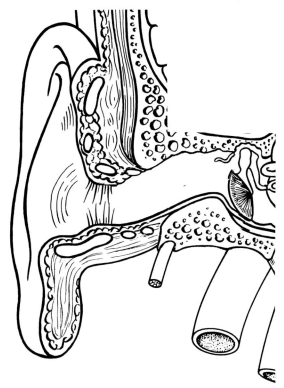

FIG. 22–7. Removal of posterosuperior osteophyte and enlarged canal.

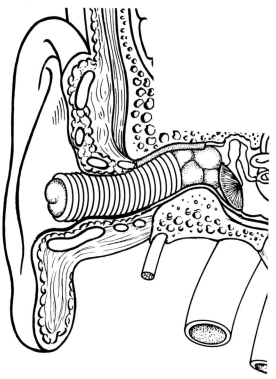

FIG. 22–8. Perichondrial graft lines raw bony surface. Dacron arterial tube used for packing.

ternal auditory meatus usually starts at the chondro-osseous junction in the external auditory canal floor or meatus and may enlarge to occlude the external auditory meatus laterally (Figs. 22–2, 22–3). (See Color Fig. 1.) Histologically, it is composed of irregular wide trabeculae of mature bone. The intertrabecular tissue is sparse and may be fibrous and vascular and may contain hematopoietic elements (Fig. 22–4).

SURGICAL MANAGEMENT OF MEDIAL CANAL OSTEOPHYTES

Multiple obstructive osteophytes (Fig. 22–5) sometimes described as "kissing osteophytes," frequently produce intermittent or permanent total occlusion of the external canal because of epidermal or ceruminous collections between them. External otitis is a common sequel. Canal keratoma occurs occasionally.

Surgical removal is carried out under local, general, or combined anesthesia. An endomeatal or endaural incision is used. Attention is usually directed only to the posterosuperior osteophytes, since it is possible to obtain space more feasibly by removal of posterosuperior canal wall bone alone

(which is anterior mastoid cortex bone). Removal of anterior canal wall bone may involve the temporomandibular joint space.

Posterosuperior canal wall skin is reflected medially, and bone removal proceeds microsurgically with cutting and diamond burrs (Fig. 22–6) to enlarge the canal adequately. An anterior osteophyte is removed only if it is attached by a slender bony trabeculum.

When an adequate canal enlargement has been attained with posterosuperior osteophyte removal, there should be good visualization of at least the posterior three-fourths of the tympanic membrane (Fig. 22–7). A perichondrial graft from the tragus is used to line the bony defect, and the canal is packed with absorbable gelatin film and gelatin sponge medially. A Dacron arterial tube filled with antibiotic-soaked gauze is used as packing (Fig. 22–8), which can be removed in 10–14 days.

SURGICAL MANAGEMENT OF LATERAL MEATAL OSTEOMA

The surgical approach is similar to that for osteophytes, except that the incision is in the medial aspect of the meatus, at the medial cartilaginous

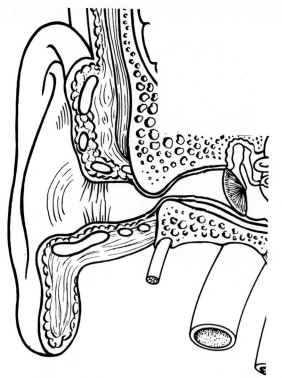

FIG. 22–9. Superior and inferior osteomas almost occluding external auditory meatus.

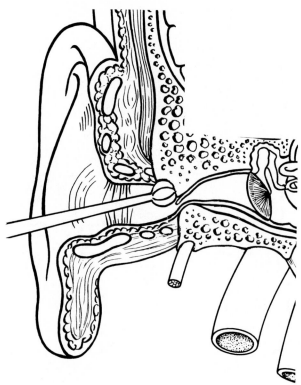

FIG. 22–10. Posterosuperior osteoma is removed.

FIG. 22–11. Meatal enlargement with skin preservation.

FIG. 22–12. Meatus enlarged following osteoma removal. Dacron arterial tube used for packing.

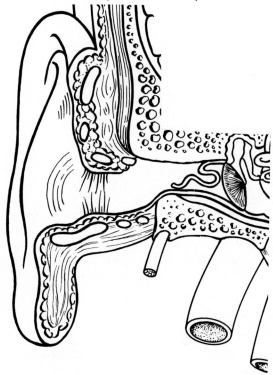

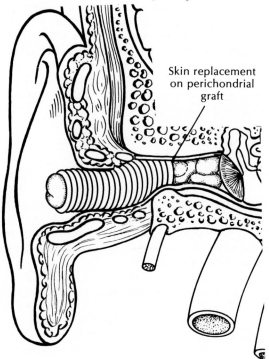

Skin replacement on perichondrial graft

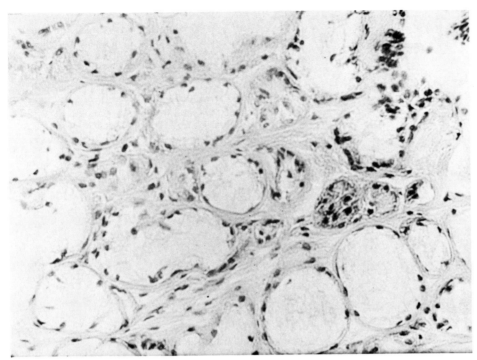

FIG. 22–13. Choristoma of middle ear and mastoid.

FIG. 22–14. Meningioma invading temporal bone.

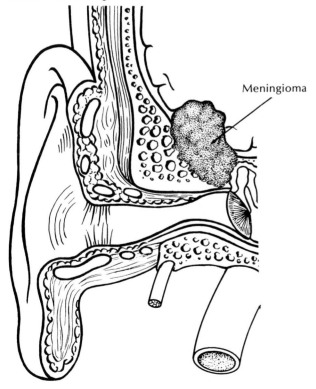

Meningioma

border; the incision is either posterior or anterior, depending upon the origin of the osteoma. If there are two "kissing osteomas" (Fig. 22–9), it is advisable to remove the posterosuperior one. Canal enlargement is obtained, as in osteophyte surgery, by removal of posterior canal bone (anterior mastoid cortex) (Fig. 22–10) rather than risking the more vulnerable area of the temporomandibular joint space region. Raw bony surfaces (Fig. 22–11) are covered by perichondrium if there is inadequate remaining skin (Fig. 22–12). Packing is similar to that used in osteophyte surgery.

CHORISTOMA—ABBERANT SALIVARY GLAND IN MIDDLE EAR

Choristoma is an uncommon benign middle-ear tumor that represents an ectopic presence of salivary gland tissue (submaxillary or parotid) in middle ear. The saliva secreted within the middle ear gives the appearance of secretory otitis media. The tympanic membrane slowly bulges into the external auditory canal, and there is an accompanying conductive hearing loss. Surgical exposure reveals a glandular middle ear mass with biopsy findings of salivary gland tissue (Fig. 22–13).

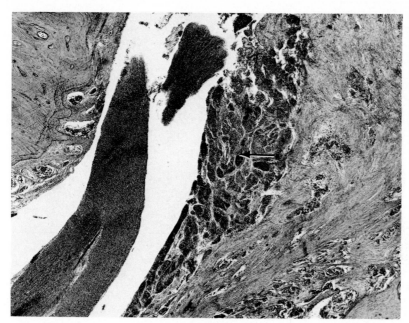

FIG. 22–15. *En plaque* meningioma **(arrow)** extending within the internal auditory canal, in meningeal lining, and within adjacent marrow spaces. Note erosion of bony wall. (H&E × 20) (Gussen R: Pathology of eighth nerve tumors and petrosal meningiomas. In Tower DB (ed): The Nervous System. Human Communication and Its Disorders, Volume 3, pp 245–252. New York, The Raven Press, 1975)

Surgical removal through an endaural wide field mastoid approach is advisable. In advanced cases, a modified or complete radical mastoidectomy may be necessary to assure total removal with preservation of the facial nerve and labyrinth.

MENINGIOMA

Intracranial meningiomas can invade the temporal bone. Nager (10) has described the different types of invasion of the temporal bone by meningiomas. They are accompanied by variable temporal bone symptoms and findings. Occasionally, meningiomas represent phases of von Recklinghausen's disease and may be accompanied by neurinomas. Nager (10) considers the term meningioma as anatomical rather than pathological, and attributes it to Cushing who first introduced it to describe a group of hamartomas that were not considered truly neoplastic tumors of the meninges. The present conception regarding the genesis of meningiomas is that they arise in the dura from arachnoid villi. Thus, meningiomas really represent neoplasia of arachnoid lining cells. They can occur in the middle ear as well as in the internal auditory meatus and cerebellopontine angle regions (Fig. 22–14).

Because of nonspecific sites of origin, a variety of otologic symptoms and signs may occur. A meningioma can be a hidden cause of other lesions, such as fibrous dysplasia of bone with secondary secretory otitis media producing inter-

mittent collections of middle ear fluid. Other symptoms may involve various cranial nerves, depending upon tumor size and location. Most hearing losses with meningiomas are conductive because of middle-ear involvement, although sensorineural hearing loss does occur.

Gussen (5) describes circumscribed as well as diffuse tumors that may grow *en plaque* with cranial nerve and vessel involvements at the base of the skull, including the internal auditory meatus and internal auditory canal (Fig. 22–15). Hyperostosis can follow marrow space involvement. Although a meningioma can spread actively, it is rarely considered malignant and metastases are rare.

EPIDERMOID—PRIMARY KERATOMA (CHOLESTEATOMA)

Keratoma (cholesteatoma) is a major acquired (secondary) lesion within the category of chronic otomastoiditis and constitutes a common problem in type B chronic otomastoiditis lesions (see Chs. 16, 17, and 18).

Primary keratoma is frequently designated as an epidermoid. Nager (11) considers it to be a blastomatous malformation arising from aberrant epithelial remnants. Predilective sites are the intracranial cavity, skull diploë, and, rarely, the spinal canal, with the base of the skull (temporal bone) the chief site (Fig. 22–16). They are found in the cerebellopontine angle and in the chiasmal

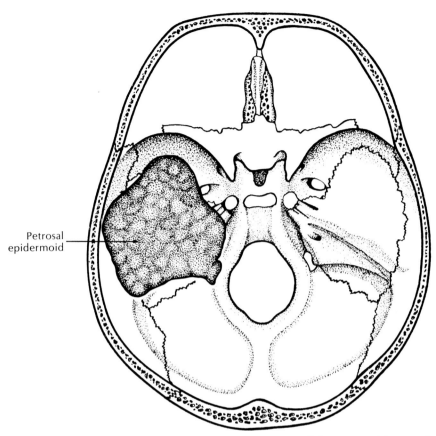

FIG. 22–16. Large intracranial epidermoid occupying most of the temporal bone petrosa.

regions. Frontal and parietal bones are less common sites than the temporal bone.

A middle ear keratoma may not be primary but can represent the medial aspect of a large congenital intracranial epidermoid, rather than the more common result of otitis media or mastoiditis.

Signs and symptoms can mimic those of chronic otomastoiditis, cerebellopontine angle lesions, and those of any intracranial or skull tumors.

Plain and polytome radiographs may delineate the lesions; however, it is not uncommon for an epidermoid to be discovered during a tympanomastoid surgical exploration for what appears to be more common type B otomastoiditis (secondary or acquired) keratoma lesion.

Temporal bone epidermoids can give rise to a host of symptoms, primarily involving hearing loss, tinnitus and vertigo. Removal frequently requires joint otosurgical–neurosurgical procedures and staged operations.

INTERMEDIATE TUMORS

A useful classification of intermediate neoplasms has been proposed by Friedmann (3). Within this classification are tumors arising in the apocrine ceruminous glands of the external auditory canal (ceruminoma) and middle ear chemodectomas (glomus tumors or paragangliomas). Both of these share benign and malignant characteristics, determinable only on long-range observation. It appears that the carcinoid would also belong in this intermediate category.

GLOMUS TUMORS (CHEMODECTOMA, NONCHROMAFFIN PARAGANGLIOMA)

Guild (6) reported a structure located in the jugular bulb adventitia, which he described as the "glomus jugulare." Rosenwasser (16) first described a tumor of the middle ear, related to the

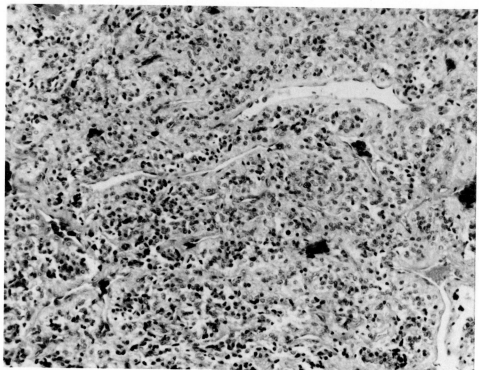

FIG. 22–17. Glomus jugulare tumor. Note nests and cords of uniform cells associated with vascular stroma and, at times, bulging into vascular channels. (Gussen R: Pathology of eighth nerve tumors and petrosal meningiomas. In Tower DB (ed): The Nervous System. Human Communication and Its Disorders, Volume 3, pp 245–252. New York, The Raven Press, 1975)

glomus jugulare and histologically comparable to carotid body tumors. The terms chemodectoma, paraganglioma, and nonchromaffin ganglioma have also been used to describe glomus tumors.

These tumors were originally considered to be always benign. However, glomus tumors may show evidence of malignant cytologic character with extensions and metastatic behavior. The usual site of a glomus jugulare tumor is in the dome of the jugular bulb, along the course of Jacobson's nerve (tympanic branch of the ninth nerve), and Arnold's nerve (auricular branch of the tenth nerve). Glomus tumor confined to the middle ear is commonly termed **glomus tympanicum,** in contrast to glomus jugulare.

A glomus may occur and begin to grow wherever there is glomus tissue. Therefore, the tumors may also occur in the bone between the jugular bulb and the hypotympanum, in the hypotympanum, on the cochlear promontory, in the medial layer of the tympanic membrane, or in the bony external auditory canal, and they may spread to all parts of the temporal bone.

Although metastases are rare, they have been recorded in the base of the skull, the upper cervical jugular lymphatics, in the nose, in thoracic vertebrae, and in liver, spleen, and lungs.

The microscopic picture of glomus jugulare tumor or glomus tympanicum is similar to that of the glomus itself. There is a rich network of vascular spaces lined by large epithelioid cells arranged in cordlike structures. The cells are usually uniform in size, with vacuolated cytoplasm and small, regular nuclei. Mitotic figures are rarely seen (Fig. 22–17).

The blood supply to a glomus tumor usually comes from the ascending pharyngeal branch of the external carotid artery and occasionally from the vertebral-basilar system. Only rarely does it come from the cavernous branches of the internal carotid artery.

The most common glomus, the glomus tympanicum, starts in the floor of the tympanic cavity and slowly grows into the middle ear, displacing the pars tensa of the tympanic membrane laterally.

A glomus tumor in the ear may be very slow in asserting its presence. The most common first symptom is that of ear pulsation. Occasionally the first symptom may be a conductive hearing loss. Pain is rare. The diagnosis is frequently missed

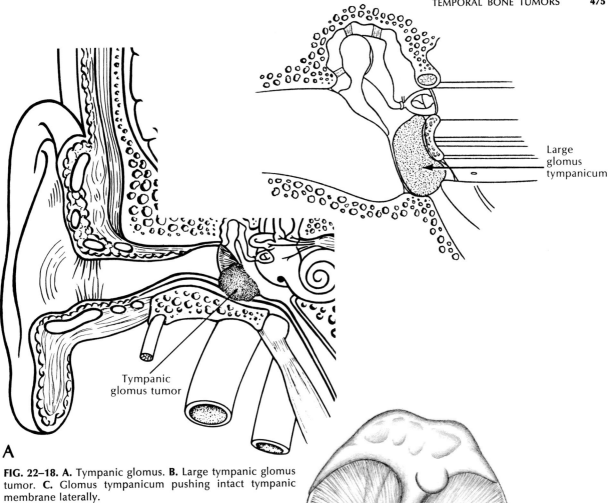

Large
glomus
tympanicum

Tympanic
glomus tumor

A

FIG. 22–18. A. Tympanic glomus. **B.** Large tympanic glomus tumor. **C.** Glomus tympanicum pushing intact tympanic membrane laterally.

Tympanic membrane
intact but bulging
from tympanic
glomus tumor

C

since the slightly prominent tympanic membrane may resemble the slight bulging of otitis media (Fig. 22–18). The tumor is occasionally mistaken for a middle-ear polyp, if it has broken through the tympanic membrane. In more advanced cases, there may be partial or complete occlusion of the entire external auditory canal by a slightly pulsating bluish tumor mass (Fig. 22–19). Occasionally the first sign will be spontaneous ear bleeding or otorrhea due to bone necrosis. With growth of the tumor, symptoms may include vertigo, profound sensorineural hearing loss, seventh nerve (facial) paralysis, and involvement of other cranial nerves, especially the ninth, tenth, and eleventh. Such findings are more common in glomus jugulare, with glomus tumor masses in the chain of anatomic glomus jugulare-glomic tissue distribution.

The most serious pseudoglomus is the presence of internal carotid artery as a congenital anomaly in the middle ear. Similarly, a highly placed jug-

ular bulb may produce otoscopic findings comparable to the bluish bulge that is seen usually in the lower portion of the tympanic membrane in the glomus tympanicum.

In a recent study of 75 patients with head and neck glomus tumors, Spector, Ciralsky, and Ogura (19) reported a 37% incidence of cranial nerve paralysis and a 14.6% incidence of intracranial

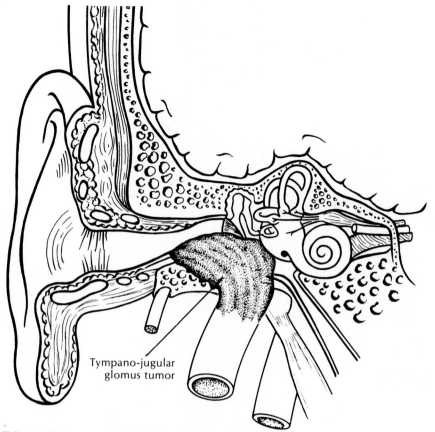

FIG. 22–19. Tympano-jugular glomus tumor.

Tympano-jugular
glomus tumor

extension. Jugular foramen syndrome signs, hypoglossal nerve involvement, posterior fossa invasion, Horner's syndrome, and middle cranial fossa tumor invasion were relatively common. According to their analysis, neither otologic findings nor seventh nerve paralysis alone correlated with tumor resectability, CNS extension, and prognosis (Fig. 22–20).

Prior to planning management, it is extremely important to define the size and ramifications of the tumor, by skull x-rays, conventional mastoid x-rays (Schuller and Stenver views) and polytomography. But in many cases it is also helpful to obtain subtraction angiography studies with selective internal, external carotid, and vertebral artery injections. Retrograde jugular venography is very useful in delineating all possible extensions of the glomic tissue. Computerized tomography scans will undoubtedly be of diagnostic value.

The preferred treatment of glomus tympanicum or jugulare is surgical excision. However, it is necessary to consider surgery with postoperative radiation, or radiation therapy alone in some cases.

The surgical treatment for the small tumor—the glomus tympanicum—is best accomplished by an endaural approach to the middle ear. In a small tumor, it is not necessary to open the mastoid cells. The tumor can be exposed with careful elevation of a posterior canal flap, care being taken to separate the tympanic membrane only to the point of tumor involvement. Bleeding may be minimized and tumor tissue removed with the use of a small cryoprobe. A microunipolar coagulator serves a similar purpose. It is possible in many cases to excise the tumor completely without disturbing the ossicles or the labyrinthine windows and without significant trauma to the tympanic membrane. In larger tumors a mastoid cavity approach is advisable, and it may be necessary to perform a radical mastoidectomy to get adequate exposure. In very extensive lesions, surgical removal will require large-vessel ligations, neck dissection, and possibly a middle fossa approach.

Postoperative irradiation may be considered 3–4 weeks after surgery, if only subtotal removal was pos-

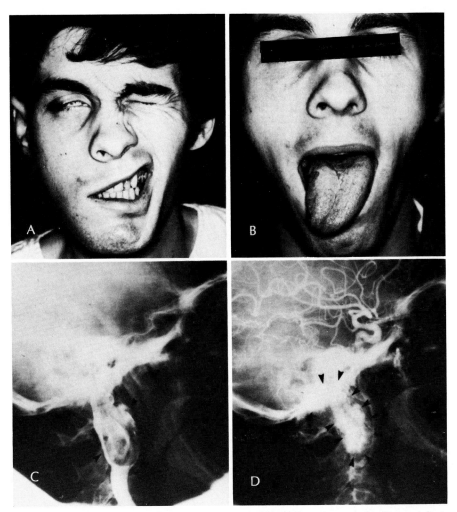

FIG. 22–20. Patient with seventh **(A)** through twelfth **(B)** nerve paralysis. Retrograde jugular venogram **(C)** demonstrates large glomus jugulare filling vein lumen **(arrow)**. Carotid arteriogram **(D)** outlines large jugulare tumor **(arrows)**. All paralyses were peripheral, without CNS invasion. The tumor was successfully resected. (Spector GJ, Ciralsky RH, Ogura JH: Ann Otol Rhinol Laryngol 84:73–79, 1975)

sible. Silverstone (18) recommended supervoltage radiation, either from the 2-mev generator, cobalt 60, the linear accelerator, or the betatron, with dosage in the 4000–5000 rad range over a period of 4–6 weeks. Therapy should be started, when indicated, only after complete surgical wound healing has occurred. Silverstone recommends the wedge–pair radiation technique comprised of two angled beams (with compensating filters) that converge on the tumor area with the least effect on adjacent brain stem. Postoperative radiation carries a significant possibility of delayed radionecrosis of the temporal bone, producing sloughing of external auditory canal bone and skin and occasional secondary infection. Long-term postoperative follow-up is advisable. Late recurrences are not unusual, and metastases occur occasionally.

In the authoritative experience of Dr. Harry Rosenwasser (17), "surgery, when feasible is the method of choice in treatment of this lesion. . . . Irradiation is a potent modality of treatment and has been most valuable, especially when recurrences occur after surgery."

Recently, a new approach to the management of extensive glomus tumors has been advanced by R. W. Rand and J. Bentson at University of California Los Angeles (14). In very far advanced large glomus tumors involving several cranial nerves in addition to the temporal bone, the approach of ferromagnetic silicone vascular occlusion in a superconducting magnetic field appears to be very promising.

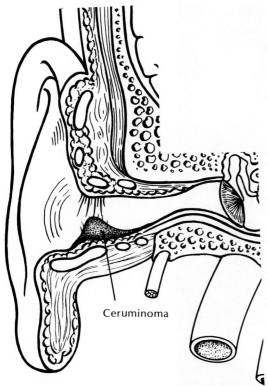

FIG. 22–21. Ceruminoma of lateral (cartilaginous) external ear canal.

The basic technique consists of mixing microspheres of iron, which are less than 5μ in size, with Silastic 382, which is then diluted with silicone diluent 360. Once the proper mixture is made so that it can be injected through small catheters that have been placed into the tumor bed, then a catalyst of stannous octoate is added to bring about vulcanization. This vulcanization occurs within the tumor bed, in the capillary vessels, without producing noxious substances. The material is held in place by a magnet system, which can be placed adjacent to the tumor tissue. Both electric magnets and superconducting magnets have been used. Once the material has vulcanized, the catheter in the feeding vessels is removed. This technique of literally "starving" a tumor is a great advance and may well make it unnecessary to use heroic surgical procedures as well as x-ray therapy in some cases.

CERUMINOMA, HIDRADENOMA, CERUMINOUS ADENOMA

A number of varieties of ceruminous gland tumors have been identified. Harrison and co-workers (8) defined a benign form of "ceruminous adenoma"

as a well-differentiated localized neoplasm, occasionally cystic, which may show papillary proliferation of glands resembling the histologic characteristics of normal ceruminous glands.

The term **hidradenoma** has also been used to describe tumors arising from the modified apocrine ceruminous glands in the external auditory meatus and external auditory canal (12).

The term **ceruminoma** has been used in both specific and general manners, to describe specifically a benign ceruminous adenoma, or hidradenoma, or more generally a group of external auditory meatus and cartilaginous external auditory canal tumors that may be benign or that may present as adenoid cystic carcinoma (Fig. 22–21).

Ceruminoma, in the specific benign sense, is defined as a tumor that arises from the modified cerumen-secreting apocrine sweat glands in the cartilaginous portion of the external auditory canal. It is basically a two-layer structure resembling the normal ceruminous gland, with an inner columnar layer and an outer myoepithelial layer with varying amounts of interglandular stroma (Fig. 22–22). If stoma predominates, the histologic features resemble those of a mixed tumor of the skin, and it is usually classified as benign, on histologic grounds. Local recurrences are common following excision. In some instances, however, there are histologic signs of adenoid cystic carcinoma, either in the primary or recurrent tumor. Thus, long-range observations are wise even in histologically and clinically benign ceruminomas.

Adenomatous tumors of the middle ear and mastoid were reported by Derlacki and Barney (2). Histologically, two cell type patterns were noted: 1) cuboidal cells arranged in rudimentary glandlike patterns and 2) angular cells forming irregular nests. Clinical findings were characterized by middle-ear origin, intact but bulging tympanic membrane, lack of pain, lack of bony erosion, and occurrence in young people. Surgical excision was carried out in these cases.

Ceruminous adenocarcinoma is an invasive form of ceruminoma, frequently cytologically indistinguishable. The two-layered eosinophilic gland pattern appears as in other adenocarcinomas.

Adenoid cystic carcinoma resembles salivary-gland carcinoma with frequent clinical evidence of osseous and/or neural invasion. Metastases can occur in lung and kidney. Hageman and Becker (7) reported a case of delayed intracranial invasion by a ceruminous gland adenocarcinoma following excision and postoperative radiation.

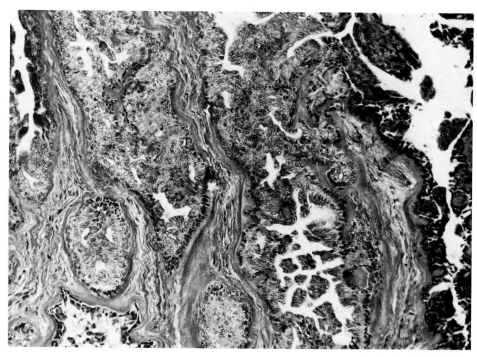

FIG. 22–22. Ceruminoma of external auditory canal. Note irregular inner columnar cell layer and outer myoepithelial layer of glands. Small amounts of interglandular stroma are present. (Gussen R: Pathology of eighth nerve tumors and petrosal meningiomas. In Tower DB (ed): The Nervous System. Human Communication and Its Disorders, Volume 3, pp 245–252. New York, The Raven Press, 1975)

FIG. 22–23. Trichoepithelioma of external auditory meatus before excision.

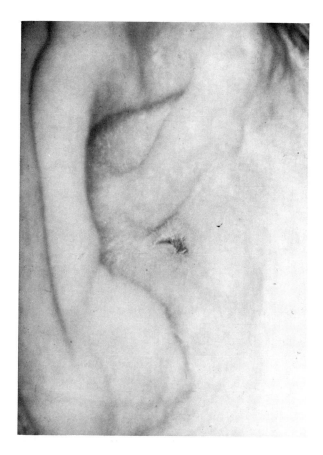

MALIGNANT TUMORS

CANCER OF THE EAR

AURICLE CANCER

In a study of 273 cases of ear malignancies by Conley and Schuller (1), primary auricular malignancies were present in 187 patients, accounting for 69% of the entire group. Auricle cancer is the most common ear malignancy, with helix and postauricular regions as primary sites. There was a male preponderance of 82.9% in the group. Predominant cell types in the entire group were basal cell cancer (41%), malignant melanoma (34.4%), and squamous cell carcinoma (22.9%).

Basal cell carcinoma, which occurs so frequently in the head and neck, is also found in the

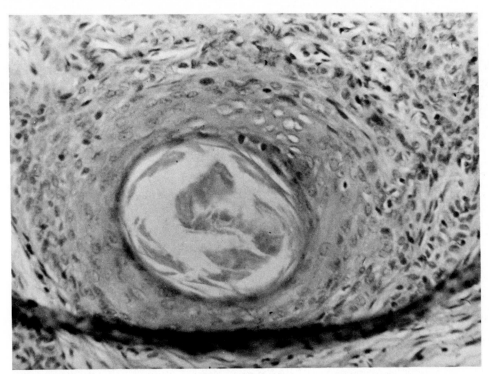

FIG. 22–24. Histologic section of trichoepithelioma, a variant of basal cell carcinoma (section of lesion seen in Fig. 22–23).

FIG. 22–25. Malignant melanoma of auricle.

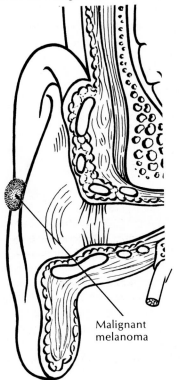

Malignant melanoma

FIG. 22–26. Squamous cell carcinoma of auricle.

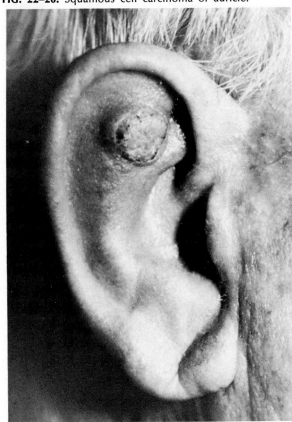

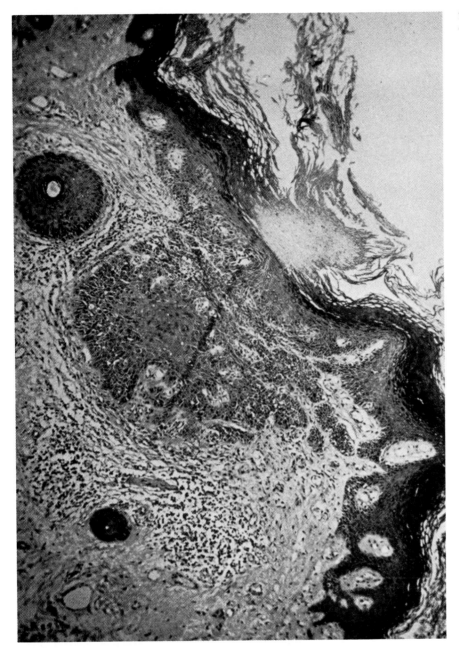

FIG. 22–27. Squamous cell carcinoma of the pinna. (× 54) (Friedmann I: Pathology of the Ear. Oxford, Blackwell Scientific Publications, 1974)

auricle. When it occurs in the external auditory meatus, it can take the form of a trichoepithelioma (Figs. 22–23, 22–24). Local excision is usually adequate although radiation and/or chemotherapy may be necessary. Basal-cell carcinoma can result in extensive spread, with skull penetration in some cases.

Melanoma is a common auricular malignancy (Fig. 22–25). Wide excision, chemotherapy, ir-

radiation, and electrodesiccation may be necessary with long-range follow-up for possible recurrences and/or metastases.

Squamous cell carcinoma in the auricle takes the form of a classic skin cancer (Fig. 22–26) but is complicated by cartilaginous invasion. It may be proliferative, polypoid, or "warty" in appearance (Figs. 22–27, 22–28).

Cancer limited to the auricle requires radical

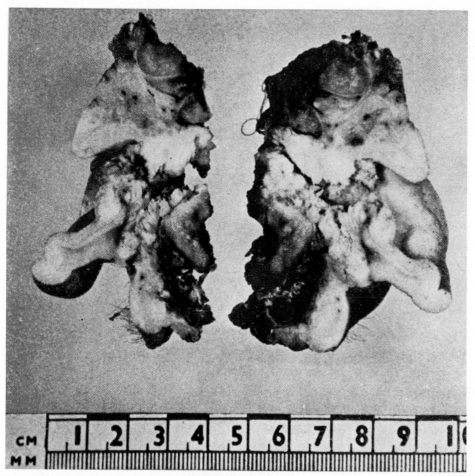

FIG. 22–28. Surgical specimen of entire external ear removed for squamous cell carcinoma of external auditory meatus invading the middle ear. (× 2) (Friedmann I: Pathology of the Ear. Oxford, Blackwell Scientific Publications, 1974)

excision (frequently total auriculectomy), followed in many cases by radiation therapy and/or cryosurgery.

EAR CANAL AND MIDDLE-EAR CANCER

Cancer in the external auditory canal and middle ear is difficult to detect, frequently appearing as either a "simple" external otitis or otitis media. The diagnostic and management problems of ceruminous tumors have been discussed earlier in this chapter.

Squamous cell cancer of the osseous external ear canal usually produces severe otalgia. A "stubborn external otitis" involving the bony canal (Fig. 22–29) should be considered cancer unless ruled out by repeated biopsies, polytomography,

and/or clinical improvement following topical therapy.

Squamous cell carcinoma of the middle ear and mastoid is a serious lesion, which can spread rapidly, destroying the tympanic membrane and middle-ear contents, and invade any portion of the temporal bone, ranging from the mastoid process to the petrous apex. The invasive tumor may encompass the eustachian tube, labyrinth, facial nerve, temporomandibular joint, the jugular bulb, mandible, parotid gland, and meninges (Figs. 22–30, 22–31). Early diagnosis is based upon a high index of suspicion of any middle-ear discharge that is not explained by customary findings of otomastoiditis. Persistent polypoid growths, even if histologically benign, which do not respond to surgical removal of underlying bone disease,

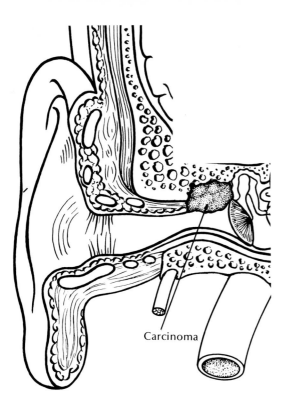

FIG. 22–29. Cancer of bony canal "masquerading" as external otitis.

Carcinoma

FIG. 22–30. Mastoid bone infiltrated by well-differentiated squamous cell carcinoma. Patient had had chronic otitis media of 40 year's duration. (× 112) (Friedmann I: Pathology of the Ear. Oxford, Blackwell Scientific Publications, 1974)

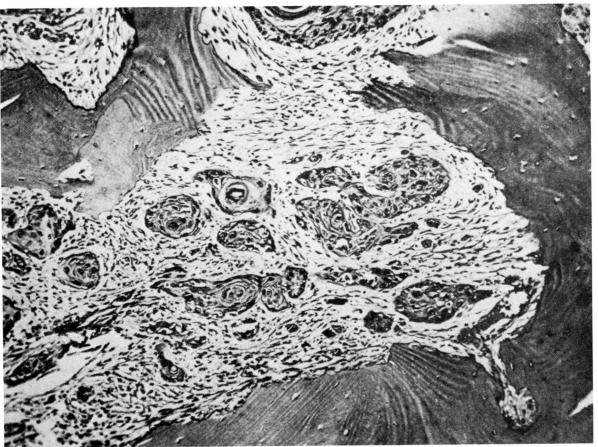

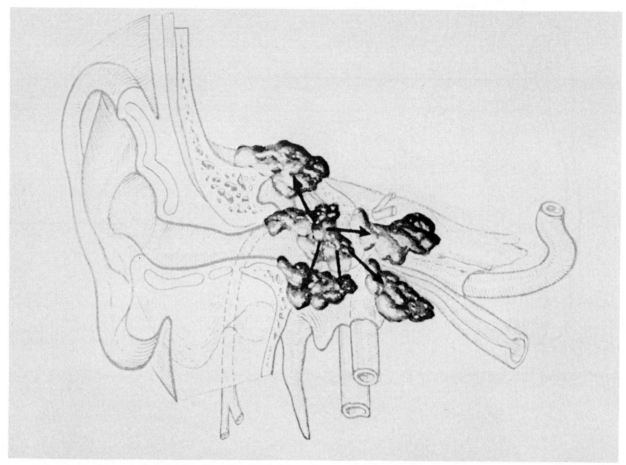

FIG. 22–31. Pernicious extensions of cancer of the middle ear may involve dura, petrous apex, base of the middle fossa, and may extend along the eustachian tube. (Conley J: Concepts in Head and Neck Surgery. New York, Grune & Stratton, 1976, p 76. By permission)

and which continue to recur, with or without bleeding, should be suspected of being carcinomatous. Polyps removed from the external auditory canal or middle ear should be repeatedly biopsied. Recurrent middle-ear "granulation tissue" (Fig. 22–32) should also be biopsied since it is in such "polypoid" tissue or "granulation" tissue that an external canal or middle ear carcinoma may be hidden.

Carcinoma of the middle ear and mastoid may occur at any age, although it is more common in the older age groups. It may be a late development in a chronic otomastoiditis, or it may begin as what appears to be nothing more than chronic otomastoiditis. As in any other cancer, the etiology is obscure. It is not possible to state categorically that chronic otomastoiditis may predispose to carcinoma, but neither can that possibility be excluded.

Squamous-cell carcinoma may start within the posterior wall of the bony external ear canal and then spread into the middle ear through the bony and fibrous annulus. However, the tumor can start from within the middle-ear tympanic mucosa and spread to the mastoid. Radical mastoidectomy, followed by radiation, is followed occasionally by "cures." However, there are both local and remote recurrences, frequently with extension from the temporal bone into the cranial nerves, middle fossa, or posterior fossa. Thus, surgical excision requires a more radical approach than that of classic radical mastoidectomy.

Conley and Schuller (1) divide cancer of the auricle, external auditory canal, and middle ear into two main groups, from the point of view of surgical management—the first involving the auricle, external auditory meatus, and cartilaginous external auditory canal, and the second

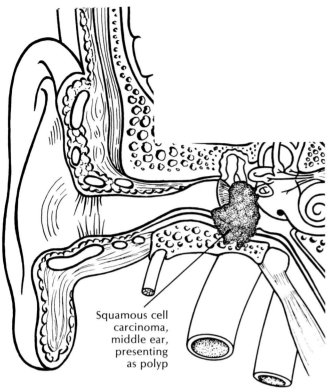

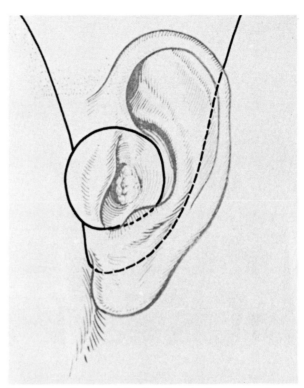

FIG. 22–34. Cancer originating deep in the ear canal, tympanic membrane intact. (Conley J: Concepts in Head and Neck Surgery. New York, Grune & Stratton, 1976. By permission)

FIG. 22–32. Cancer of middle ear "masquerading" as chronic otitis media with polyposis.

FIG. 22–33. Small cancer of membranous ear canal resected and cavity dressed with skin graft **(A).** Cancer of inner ear canal resected with bony meatus and tympanum **(B).** Cavity dressed with skin graft. (Conley J, Schuller D: Laryngoscope 86:1147–1268, 1970)

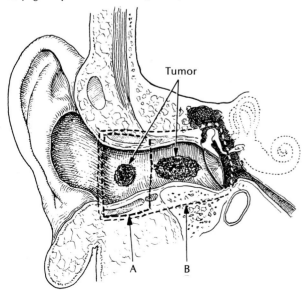

(much more serious) involving the osseous external auditory canal, middle ear, and mastoid. Most of these lesions are squamous cell cancers.

The management of cancer of the ear involves limited or extensive surgical resection, depending upon extent.

A limited surgical resection can be considered, in cancer, limited to the external auditory meatus and cartilaginous external auditory canal (Fig. 22–33).

In bony external auditory canal lesions with intact tympanic membrane, Conley and Schuller advise mastoidectomy, with removal of the external auditory canal (membranous and bony), tympanic annulus, and tympanic membrane *en bloc*, with preservation of the seventh nerve (Figs. 22–34 to 22–36).

In middle ear and mastoid cancer a temporal bone resection is necessary. An ear flap is elevated (Fig. 22–37), and this step is followed by removal of the temporal bone squama, an upper neck dissection, a temporal bone neck dissection, a temporal bone resection medial to the arcuate eminence, with a hypoglossal nerve crossover with

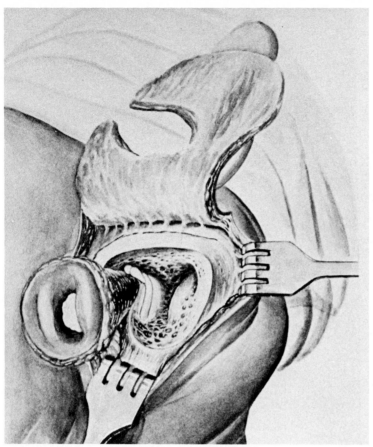

FIG. 22–35. Mastoidectomy and exposure of the facial nerve. (Conley J: Concepts in Head and Neck Surgery. New York, Grune & Stratton, 1976. By Permission)

FIG. 22–36. Membranous and bony canal, annulus tympanicus and tympanic membrane removed *en bloc* with preservation of the facial nerve (Conley J: Concepts in Head and Neck Surgery. New York, Grune & Stratton, 1976. By permission)

FIG. 22–37. Elevation of ear flap and exposure of anatomy about temporal bone. (Conley J: Concepts in Head and Neck Surgery. New York, Grune & Stratton, 1976. By permission)

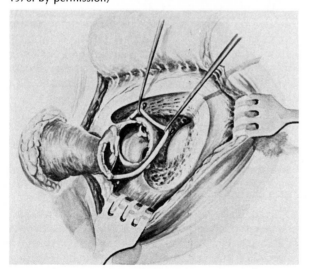

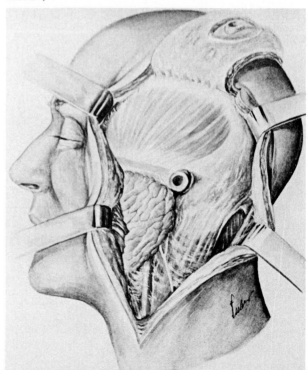

striation, as well as large anaplastic cells and truly differentiated neoplastic rhabdomyoblasts on light microscopy. Electron microscopic studies may be helpful in differentiating the various stages of malignant rhabdomyoblasts synthesizing cytoplasmic fibrils during various periods of the tumor growth (9).

The treatment of rhabdomyosarcoma up to the present time has been tragically unsuccessful. There have been few confirmed cases of cure from radical surgery, radiation, or chemotherapy.

However, a 1976 report from the 50-center Intergroup Rhabdomyosarcoma Study seems to indicate a more favorable prognosis, through a program of complete surgical excision followed by treatment with vincristine, dactinomycin, cyclophosphamide, and radiation (15).

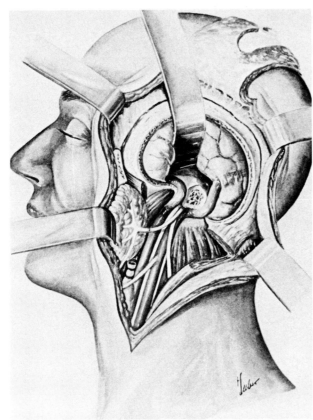

FIG. 22–38. Temporal bone resected just medial to arcuate eminence. Hypoglossal nerve crossover has been made with facial nerve. (Conley J: Concepts in Head and Neck Surgery. New York, Grune & Stratton, 1976. By permission)

the seventh (facial) nerve (Fig. 22–38). In some cases it may also be necessary to resect the head and neck of the mandible and the parotid gland.

EMBRYONAL RHABDOMYOSARCOMA

This uncommon neoplasm occurs primarily in very young children. The very first sign can be a painless swelling behind the auricle, followed by massive outward, forward, and downward squamal displacement by involvement of the squamous and mastoid portions of the temporal bone, with extension to the parietal and occipital bones (Fig. 22–39).

The tumor, in some patients, may start out as an apparent otitis media, and the first sign may be a polypoid mass presenting through the tympanic membrane. It is not unusual for such a polypoid mass to be biopsied with the primary report of "granulation" tissue. An adequate surgical biopsy will show strap-shaped cells with cross-

FIG. 22–39. Rhabdomyosarcoma of temporal bone squama.

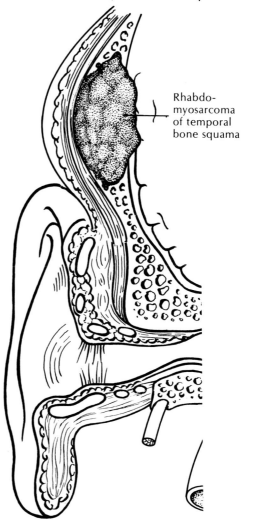

Rhabdo-myosarcoma of temporal bone squama

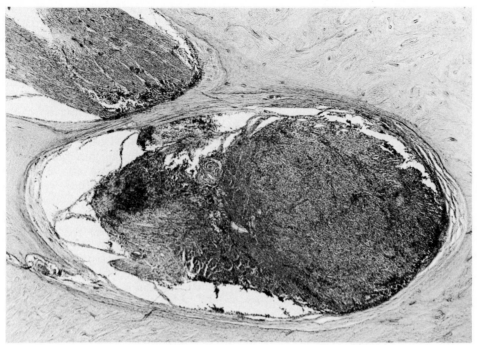

FIG. 22–40. Malignant melanoma tumor mass in medial portion of internal auditory canal, invading facial and superior vestibular nerves. Facial nerve and superior vestibular branch, **upper left.** (H&E, original magnification ×26) (Gussen R, Adkins W: Arch Otolaryngol 99: 132–135, 1974. Copyright 1974, American Medical Association)

METASTATIC TUMORS OF THE TEMPORAL BONE

Metastatic malignant tumors of the temporal bone may follow cancer of the breast, kidney, lung, stomach, neck, and prostate. The most likely route of spread is that of hematogenous dissemination to the bone marrow. Direct invasion from nearby tumors is seen in malignancies of the nasopharynx and parotid gland. There are rare meningeal metastases with tumor cells that occupy the internal auditory canal invading the seventh and eighth nerves. This type has been seen in malignant melanoma.

Among the signs and symptoms of metastatic temporal bone tumors are otorrhea, hearing loss, otalgia, facial paralysis, periauricular swelling, and occasional sudden profound inner ear hearing loss along with vestibular symptoms. Many primary tumors, including malignant melanoma, may metastasize to the temporal bone. In a recent report, Gussen and Adkins (4) described temporal bone changes in a 25-year-old patient with a history of removal of a primary malignant melanoma of the skin 2 years before death. Both temporal bones contained metastatic melanoma within the internal auditory canals. There was an unusual finding of unilateral saccule degeneration and displacement with encapsulation of the otolithic membrane. Fibrous nodules containing clumps and otoconia were present, obliterating the cochlear portion of the ductus reuniens, with marked distention of the cochlear cecum vestibulare. The tumor in the medial portion of the internal auditory canal invaded facial and superior vestibular nerves (Fig. 22–40).

MALIGNANT LYMPHOMA

A number of lymphomas can occur in the temporal bone. Paparella and El Fiky (13) have recently reported temporal bone findings of eight patients with malignant lymphoma invasion, including lymphosarcoma, reticular cell sarcoma, and Hodgkin's disease. The metastases may occur anywhere in the temporal bone, including the middle ear, ossicles, eustachian tube, internal auditory meatus, labyrinth, and facial nerve (Fig. 22–41).

FIG. 22–41. Disseminated lymphosarcoma, extensively invading the middle ear. Note the lymphoblastic infiltration **(arrows)** surrounding the lateral mallear process. **TM,** tympanic membrane (lateral mallear process); **CT,** chorda tympani; **ME,** middle ear. (H&E × 40) (Paparella M, El Fiky FM: Ann Otol Rhinol Laryngol 81:352–363, 1972)

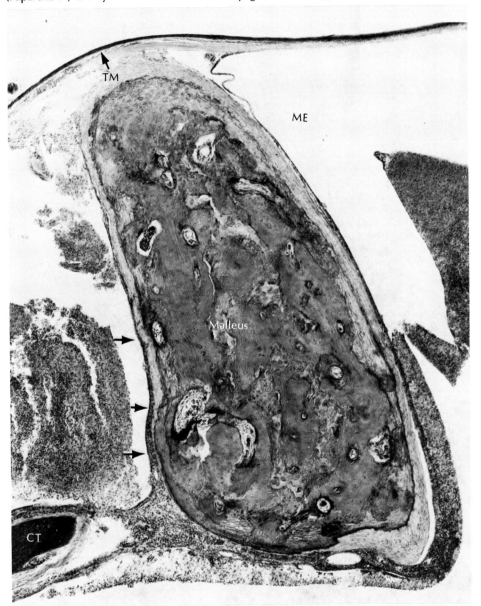

REFERENCES

1. Conley J, Schuller D: Malignancies of the ear. Laryngoscope 86:1147–1268, 1976
2. Derlacki EL, Barney PL: Adenomatous tumors of the middle ear and mastoid. Laryngoscope 86:1123–1135, 1976
3. Friedmann I: Pathology of the Ear. Oxford, Blackwell Scientific, 1974
4. Gussen R, Adkins W: Saccule degeneration and ductus reuniens obstruction. Arch Otolaryngol 99:132–135, 1974
5. Gussen R: Pathology of eighth nerve tumors and petrosal meningiomas. In Tower DB (ed): The Nervous System, Vol 3, Human Communication and Its Disorders. New York, Raven Press, 1975, pp 245–252
6. Guild SR: A hitherto unrecognized structure, the Glomus Jugularis, in Man. Anat Rec [Suppl] 79 (2):28, 1941
7. Hageman MEJ, Becker AE: Intracranial invasion of a ceruminous gland tumor. Arch Otolaryngol 100:395–397, 1974
8. Harrison K, Cronin J, Greenwood N: Ceruminous adenocarcinoma arising in the middle ear. J Laryngol 88:363–368, 1974
9. Hosada S, Suzuki H, Kawabe Y et al.: Embryonal rhabdomyosarcoma of the middle ear. Cancer 27:943–947, 1971
10. Nager GT: Association of bilateral VIIIth nerve tumors with meningiomas in Von Recklinghausen's disease. Laryngoscope 74:1220–1261, 1964
11. Nager GT: Epidermoids involving the temporal bone: clinical, radiological and pathological aspects. Laryngoscope 85 (2):1–22, 1975
12. Pahor AL, O'Hara MD: Hidradenomata of the external auditory meatus. J Laryngol 89:707–720, 1975
13. Paparella M, El Fiky FM: Ear involvement in malignant lymphoma. Ann Otol Rhinol Laryngol 81:352–363, 1972
14. Rand R: Personal communication
15. Rhabdomyosarcoma: survival nears 80%. Medical World News, June 14, 1976, p 31
16. Rosenwasser H: Carotid body tumor of the middle ear and mastoid. Arch Otolaryngol 41:64–67, 1945
17. Rosenwasser H: Long-term results of therapy of Glomus Jugulare tumors. Arch Otolaryngol 97:49–54, 1973
18. Silverstone SM: Radiation therapy of Glomus Jugulare tumors. Arch Otolaryngol 97:43–48, 1973
19. Spector GJ, Ciralsky RH, Ogura JH: Glomus tumors in the head and neck. III. Analysis of clinical manifestations. Ann Otol Rhinol Laryngol 84:73–79, 1975

SUGGESTED READING

Conley JJ, Schuller DE: Reconstruction following temporal bone resection. Arch Otolaryngol 103:34–37, 1977

Fernandez–Blasini N: Glomus Jugulare tumors of the middle ear and mastoid: diagnosis and surgical treatment. Laryngoscope 86:1669–1678, 1976

Gotay V: Unusual otologic manifestation of chronic lymphocytic leukemia. Laryngoscope 86:1856–1863, 1976

Neely JG, Britton BH, Greenberg SD: Microscopic characteristics of the acoustic tumor in relationship to its nerve of origin. Laryngoscope 86:984–991, 1976

Shanon E, Samuel Y, Adler A et al.: Malignant melanoma of the head and neck in children. Arch Otolaryngol 102:244–247, 1976

Steel A: Secretory otitis media due to a hair—bearing dermoid of the mastoid cavity. J Laryngol 90:979–989, 1976

Valvassori GE, Buckingham RA: Middle ear masses mimicking glomus tumors: radiographic and otoscopic recognition. Ann Otol Rhinol Laryngol 83:606–612, 1974

Lesions of the eighth nerve, petrous pyramid apex, and cerebellopontine angle are characterized by similar symptoms and clinical findings. These include unilateral tinnitus, sensorineural (retrocochlear) hearing loss, mild vertigo with canal paresis, and associated cranial nerve lesions in some patients. Although a number of tumors and vascular lesions can produce these clinical findings, the classic lesion is the so-called "acoustic neuroma."

Acoustic neurinoma is a benign tumor that is frequently also called "acoustic neuroma." These terms are inaccurate, since the tumor's origin is rarely of the acoustic eighth nerve division, nor is it a neuroma. The tumor is a vestibular eighth nerve schwannoma. Approximately 8% of all intracranial tumors are schwannomas. A vestibular schwannoma usually arises in the internal auditory canal within the petrous portion of the temporal bone (Fig. 23–1). In this position it is usually designated as an intracanalicular tumor. Occasionally it arises as an extracanalicular tumor either in the internal auditory meatus (Fig. 23–2) or in the region of the cerebellopontine angle (Fig. 23–3). Its origin is usually from one of the branches of the vestibular division of the eighth nerve. It may arise, uncommonly, from the cochlear division of the eighth nerve; however, the cochlear division of the nerve usually becomes involved as the tumor grows. For the purpose of brevity, the term **eighth nerve tumor** will be used.

Eighth nerve tumors are usually unilateral, although in the Recklinghausen form of multiple neurinomatosis (a mendelian disorder) the lesions may be bilateral, particularly in young people. The tumor may start at any age, and its growth rate is usually slow. However, in young patients, the growth may be rapid. It is possible for an eighth nerve tumor to remain relatively sessile, as an intracanalicular, extracanalicular, or cerebellopontine angle lesion that is relatively asymptomatic for years.

Although the tumor usually starts in the vestibular branch of the eighth nerve, the slow compression of vestibular nerve fibers does not commonly produce vertigo. It is not until there is tumor compression or vascular compression of the cochlear nerve that the most common first symptom—tinnitus—occurs. Thus, unilateral tinnitus rather than vertigo is probably the most common first symptom of early vestibular schwannoma. As the tumor grows within the internal auditory canal and cochlear nerve encroachment occurs, specific auditory findings in addition to tinnitus may be elicited. These auditory findings are usually retro-

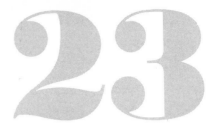

23

LESIONS OF THE EIGHTH NERVE, PETROUS APEX, AND CEREBELLOPONTINE ANGLE

cochlear in audiologic characteristics. However, the tumor may grow into the cochlea and produce cochlear audiologic findings.

With further growth, an intracanalicular tumor usually becomes extracanalicular, invading the internal auditory meatus, and eventually becomes a cerebellopontine angle lesion with symptoms and findings similar to primary tumors of the cerebellopontine angle or vascular lesions. Such symptoms are due to other cranial nerve involvement. Fifth nerve symptoms are manifested by absence of an ipsilateral corneal reflex and by facial hypesthesia and trigeminal pain. When the seventh (facial) nerve becomes involved, seventh nerve motor and sensory branch symptoms appear. A growing schwannoma can also affect the anterior-inferior cerebellar artery.

The auditory symptoms of eighth nerve tumor include tinnitus and increasing high-frequency hearing loss. Sudden occlusion of a branch of the internal auditory artery by tumor pressure may produce severe or total sudden cochlear hearing loss.

Vestibular symptoms may vary from a sudden attack of vertigo to subacute dysequilibrium. Later developments may include spontaneous nystagmus and ataxia.

Facial (seventh) nerve symptoms in eighth nerve tumors are manifested by varying degrees of facial nerve motor weakness. Prior to motor fiber involvement, however, there may be afferent seventh nerve symptoms, as manifested by loss of taste in the anterior two-thirds of the tongue.

Pressure from eighth nerve tumors may eventually also produce symptoms from the fifth, sixth,

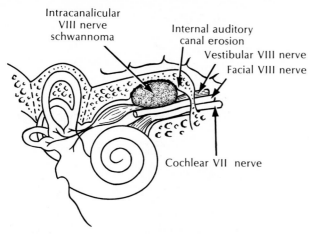

FIG. 23-1. Primary intracanalicular eighth nerve schwannoma with internal auditory canal bone erosion.

FIG. 23-2. Primary extracanalicular eighth nerve schwannoma beginning to erode internal auditory meatus bony wall as it grows laterally to become secondarily intracanalicular.

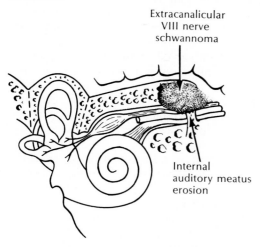

ninth, tenth, eleventh, and twelfth cranial nerves. These multiple cranial nerve findings may be accompanied by internal hydrocephalus, papilledema, and signs of supratentorial and cerebellar pressure. The treatment of eighth nerve tumors is surgical.

PATHOLOGY

SCHWANNOMA

Schwannomas are tumors of peripheral nerves and cranial and spinal nerve roots. Gussen summarized the two schools of thought regarding the cell of origin of these tumors, the Schwann cell theory and the fibroblast theory (11).

The Schwann cell theory stresses that the zone of transition from central myelin to the peripheral type of myelin (the Obersteiner-Redlich area) is the vulnerable area. This zone of transition lies within the internal auditory canal.

Microscopically, two patterns occur, Antoni type A and Antoni type B. In Antoni type A, interlacing spindle cells with long oval nuclei are parallel (Fig. 23-4). Characteristic palisading is due to parallel clusters of cells. The Antoni B type is characterized by cells widely separated by a watery, poorly staining matrix.

Schwannomas do not contain nerve fibers; the tumor grows into the nerve rather than displacing it (Figs. 23-5, 23-6).

Schwannomas rarely, if ever, become malignant. One pediatric case was described by Schuknecht (22) as a rare instance of malignant schwannoma transformation.

An eighth nerve tumor can grow into the cerebellopontine recess with displacement and compression of adjacent cranial nerves, vessels, and brain stem as described by Dublin (6) (Fig. 23-7).

MENINGIOMA

Meningioma of the temporal bone or cerebellopontine angle occurs in several forms (see Ch. 22, Temporal Bone Tumors). In comparison with

FIG. 23-3. Primary cerebellopontine angle tumor (such as meningioma or schwannoma) beginning to erode internal auditory meatus bony wall.

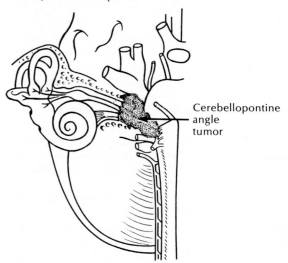

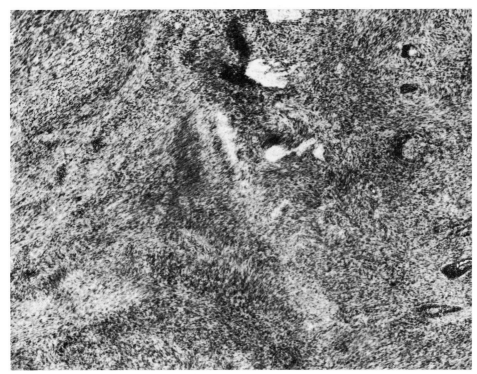

FIG. 23–4. Acoustic schwannoma, Antoni type A. (H&E × 45) (Gussen R: Pathology of eighth nerve tumors and petrosal meningiomas. In Tower DB (ed): The Nervous System. Human Communication and Its Disorders, Vol. 3. New York, Raven Press, 1975)

FIG. 23–5. Internal auditory meatus completely occupied by eighth nerve tumor (vestibular schwannoma, **arrow**). (Gussen R: Pathology of eighth nerve tumors and petrosal meningiomas. In Tower DB (ed): The Nervous System. Human Communication and Its Disorders, Vol. 3. New York, Raven Press, 1975)

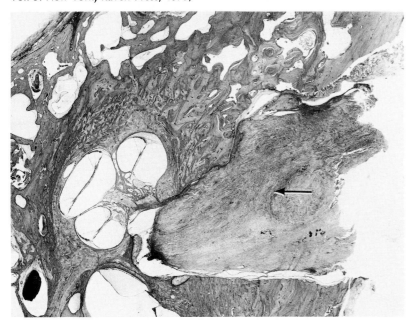

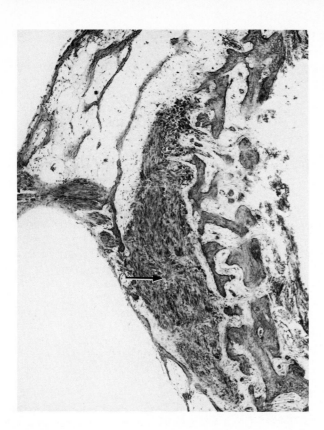

FIG. 23–6. Vestibular schwannoma within modiolus **(arrow)** (eighth nerve tumor—so called acoustic neuroma). (Gussen R: Pathology of eighth nerve tumors and petrosal meningiomas. In Tower DB (ed): The Nervous System. Human Communication and Its Disorders, Vol. 3. New York, Raven Press, 1975)

FIG. 23–7. A. Acoustic neurofibroma growing as left cerebellopontine recess tumor with displacement and compression of adjacent structures. **B.** Normal right inner auditory meatus. **C.** Left inner auditory meatus, showing destruction of the osseous wall. (Dublin WB: FUNDAMENTALS OF SENSORINEURAL AUDITORY PATHOLOGY, 1976. Courtesy of Charles C Thomas, Publisher, Springfield, Illinois)

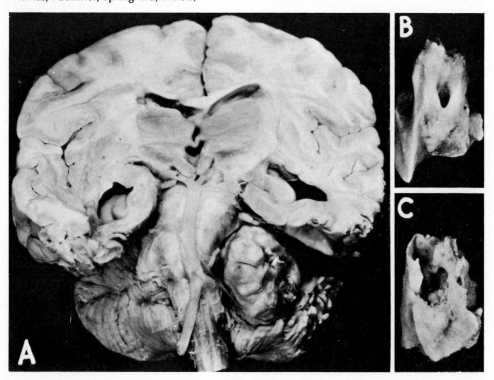

eighth nerve schwannomas in these areas, they are rare. As with eighth nerve schwannomas, they can occur as part of Recklinghausen's disease.

PRIMARY PETROUS APEX LESIONS

Gacek (8) described the occurrence of congenital epidermoids, chondromyxosarcomas, and neurofibroma as primary lesions of the petrosal apex. The origin of these tumors may be developmental with reference to the foramen lacerum. Congenital epidermoids resemble keratoma (cholesteatoma) grossly and histologically (see Ch. 16, Chronic Otomastoiditis—Diagnosis and Management).

LESIONS OF THE CEREBELLOPONTINE ANGLE

In a study of 44 lesions of the cerebellopontine angle, Rosomoff reported 23 eighth nerve tumors of the 38 mass lesions encountered (21). Other lesions with diagnostic findings simulating eighth nerve tumors included meningioma, pontine glioma, multiple (neurinoma-glioma, etc.), trigeminal neurinoma, malignant tumors, epidermoid tumors, hydrocephalus, aneurysm, and arachnoidal cyst.

Basilar artery ectasia can simulate eighth nerve tumor. Gibson and Wallace report two such cases (9). In both, hemifacial spasm was a concomitant clinical finding.

CLINICAL ASPECTS OF LESIONS IN THE INTERNAL ACOUSTIC MEATUS, PETROUS APEX, AND CEREBELLOPONTINE ANGLE

Unilateral tinnitus and sensorineural hearing loss can be due to a number of lesions. In a discussion of "nerve deafness and brain tumors" in 1960, I stated:

The patient with the label of pseudo-Meniere's disease, or the Meniere syndrome, should be kept under long-term surveillance and the possibility that his symtoms are caused by retrocochlear neoplasm should not be dismissed until ruled out by appropriate studies. Every case of unilateral nerve deafness deserves a caloric study and a roentgen examination of the porus acusticus region (10).

A patient who presents with the primary symptoms of unilateral tinnitus and unilateral sensorineural hearing loss without other symptoms would be considered a candidate for an eighth nerve tumor study. Such a diagnostic study will involve not only a complete otologic, audiologic,

and vestibular examination but will also include a neurologic examination and Stenver and transorbital radiograms of the internal auditory canal and meatus, in addition to Schuller radiographs of the mastoid. Polytomography is frequently necessary and may require posterior fossa Pantopaque contrast studies, air studies, and angiography. Computerized axial tomography (CAT) isotope brain scans are becoming increasingly useful (see Ch. 4, Otoradiology).

The first nonauditory finding of clinical significance is that of unilateral vestibular paresis. The triad of unilateral sensorineural hearing loss, unilateral tinnitus, and unilateral vestibular paresis is sufficiently significant to warrant the diagnosis of eighth nerve tumor until disproved. Such findings require a continuous high index of suspicion in terms of longitudinal follow-up studies of such patients, even though primary studies may be inconclusive and not diagnostic.

AUDIOLOGIC FINDINGS

There are significant variations in audiologic test findings. In general, the classic picture includes unilateral high frequency pure tone loss with no air–bone gap, low speech discrimination score, absence of loudness recruitment, as determined by the alternate loudness balance test, a low score (less than 30%) on the short-increment sensitivity index (SISI) test, and variable Bekesy type tracings (types II, III, IV). As diagnostic refinements improve, a number of variations in audiologic findings are reported. The original stress on predominant types II and IV Bekesy tracings has been modified. More and more type II tracings are being found, apparently as the result of earlier diagnoses. Thus, a type II or even a type I Bekesy tracing does not, by itself, rule out a retrocochlear lesion.

In the type III Bekesy responses, continuous and interrupted tracings may be superimposed for low frequencies (100–500 Hz), followed by a marked drop for continuous tracings as higher frequencies are tested. It is necessary to do both continuous and interrupted frequency studies at octave or semi-octave bands. In type IV Bekesy tracing, there is a characteristic separation of continuous from interrupted tracings at all frequencies. In contrast to type II Bekesy responses, the continuous tracing is not as narrow but may have the same height of excursion.

Temporary threshold drift may be a significant audiologic finding. Fixed frequency Bekesy tracings are uniquely suited to measure this phenomenon. A steady (continuous) tone presented over a period of time (2–3 min) may result in rapid deterioration of threshold sensitivity in the patient with an eighth nerve tumor or any other retrocochlear lesion. One may note threshold drift downward to the maximum audiometer output.

Recent studies of "backward Bekesy" tracings advocated by Jerger and Jerger (15) have added further audiologic differential diagnostic information of value in studies of eighth nerve tumor and other retrocochlear lesions.

Tone decay is a frequent finding in eighth nerve tumor, as is stapedius reflex decay. The acoustic reflex test is a sensitive clinical sign. Reflex decay or total absence of it is a very important finding in eighth nerve lesions. There also appears to be an increasingly useful diagnostic input from electric response audiometry (ERA), especially from brain stem audiometry.

Audiologic studies require the use of a total auditory test battery, components of which should be repeated at intervals. Changing auditory site-of-lesion results are normative in most eighth nerve tumors. Thus, repeated tests are advisable, if other clinical findings remain unclear. In a recent study, Johnson (16) pointed out that inconsistent audiologic patterns occurred in more than half of cases.

Pure-tone losses in high frequencies and speech discrimination score deficits along with other audiologic variants are illustrated in the two following cases.

In one patient, a 53-year-old woman (Fig. 23–8), initial pure-tone and speech audiometric studies were characterized by moderate loss of hearing in the left ear and tinnitus, which had been noted 4 months prior to the initial examination. There were no other complaints. Bekesy tracings were type II for the left ear, and SISI scores were low for both ears at 4000 Hz and positive in the left ear at 2000 Hz. Complete recruitment was present at 1000 Hz and 2000 Hz. Caloric studies were normal. The SISI score 3.5 years later was negative at 500 Hz. There was no recruitment at 500 Hz. The patient complained of transient imbalance, dizzy episodes, and headache. There was an elevation of protein in the CSF. Internal auditory meatus polytomography suggested tumor. Total removal of a large acoustic neurinoma with preservation of seventh nerve function was accomplished through a suboccipital approach.

The second patient was a 27-year-old man who began to notice decreased hearing in the right ear and tinnitus. He had periodic nausea and vomiting, some numbness in the left hand, and some lack of coordination in gait. He underwent audiologic testing (Fig. 23–9) a week after the onset of symptoms. Fixed-

frequency Bekesy tests revealed a 30-dB gap between tracings for continuous and interrupted stimuli at 250 Hz. Tracings at other frequencies showed no separation of more than 10–15 dB between continuous and interrupted. Also significant was the marked drop (60 dB) in sensitivity for the fixed continuous tone at 1500 Hz. Sweep frequency Bekesy tracings revealed extremely rapid adaptation to continuous tonal stimuli, extending to frequencies at least as low as 100 Hz. The gap between continuous and interrupted was as great as 60 dB or more at the low and mid frequencies and then gradually closed at 1500 Hz. Both interrupted and continuous tracings then dropped sharply, but the continuous tracings continued to show a separation of 15–20 dB for frequencies 2000 Hz and above. This tracing was atypical and could not be clearly classified as type IV. A large eighth nerve schwannoma was completely removed from the cerebellopontine angle via a suboccipital approach, with preservation of the seventh nerve.

VESTIBULAR STUDIES BY ELECTRONYSTAGMOGRAPHY

Vestibular studies usually reveal hypoactive responses on the affected side (vestibular paresis), as manifested by contralateral labyrinthine preponderance. Such hypoactivity may first appear on the warm caloric test and later become apparent also on the cold caloric test. Vestibular findings may vary from slight labyrinthine contralateral preponderance (reduced vestibular response [RVR]) on the affected side, to total vestibular paralysis on the affected side. Spontaneous or positional nystagmus in several positions is a variable finding.

In a recent study of confirmed eighth nerve tumors by Tos and co-workers (26), optokinetic nystagmus abnormalities were found to be significantly diagnostic in relationship to the size of the tumor and its relation to the brain stem. Abnormal optokinetic nystagmus is due to pressure by the tumor upon the pontine optokinetic center.

Impaired ocular pursuit movements when the eyes were moving toward the side of the lesion, as detected by eye tracking and optokinetic studies, were reported as significant diagnostic signs in eighth nerve tumors. Benitez and Bouchard (3) reported unilateral diminution of optokinetic response toward the side of the tumor (moving target toward the unaffected side). The presence of saccades (jerking movements) during optokinetic response provided additional diagnostic information. Caloric abnormalities usually indicate the site of the lesion but relatively little information as to the size of the tumor.

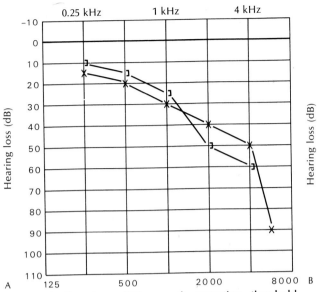

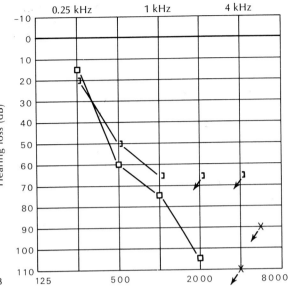

FIG. 23–8. Pure-tone **(PT)**, speech reception threshold **(SRT)**, and speech discrimination score **(SDS)** changes in eighth nerve tumor audiologic findings in a 53-year-old woman. **A.** Initial pure-tone and speech audiometric studies indicated moderate loss of hearing in left ear. Bekesy tracings were type II for left ear. **x—x,** AC, unmasked, LE; **]—],** BC, masked, LE. **B.** The SDS dropped from 70% to 8% 3.5 years later; SRT was 75 dB. Bekesy tracings remained primarily type II, but there is an emerging separation of the continuous from the interrupted tones at frequencies below 1000 Hz. **□—□,** AC, masked, LE; **]—],** BC, masked, LE; **arrows,** no response at maximum output.

FIG. 23–9. Audiologic findings in a 27-year-old patient with a 1-week history of hearing loss. **●—●,** AC, unmasked, RE; **△—△,** AC, masked, RE; **[—[,** BC, masked, RE; **arrows,** no response at maximum output. **SRT,** 16 dB; **SDS,** 38% at 46 dB.

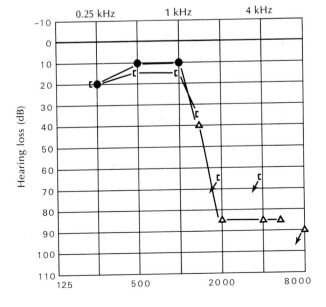

RADIOLOGIC STUDIES

Radiologic examination of the skull may or may not be informative. However, radiologic examination of the internal auditory canal and meatus by transorbital and Stenver's views may definitely show 1) differences in size with a larger internal auditory canal and/or meatus on the affected side, 2) erosion of superior or inferior walls of the internal auditory canal, and 3) haziness or disappearance of the transverse crista. However, normal transorbital or Stenver's views do not rule out the possibility of a tumor originating in the cerebellopontine angle. Polytomography is more informative, and posterior fossa myelography and air studies are usually diagnostic. Computerized axial tomography (CAT) scans are proving useful. Rarely is angiography indicated. However, in cases with conflicting findings, angiography and subtraction studies may be necessary.

Asymmetry of the internal acoustic meatuses may represent normal variants. Lin and colleagues (17) recently reported five such cases proved normal by iophendylate-injection tomographic studies. They pointed out that tomographic findings reportedly can be correct in 78% of cases by simple polytomography. Their studies indicated the great significance of the use of contrast in radiologic studies in the differential diagnosis of eighth nerve tumor.

Hanafee, Gussen, and Rand (12) pointed out that the use of the basal projection in polytomography is of great importance and may well be the method of choice for early visualization of eighth nerve tumors.

Etter (7) reported the value of conventional radiography in the diagnosis of eighth nerve tumors. His observations have been confirmed in our own clinical experience, in which eighth nerve tumors have been clearly demonstrable on conventional Stenver projections, frequently confirmed by transorbital projections.

Brain scanning has recently come into diagnostic use in eighth nerve tumor problems. Baum and associates (1) reported identifying 18 of 22 tumors with the use of Tc-sodium pertechnetate brain scans. They reported improved visualization of the posterior cranial fossa with technetium 99m and delayed scans. With the latter, they found that the optimum time for scanning eighth nerve tumors was 2.5 hours following radionuclide administration. The study points out that eighth nerve tumors 2 cm or greater in diameter can be detected in a high percentage in both primary and recurrent lesions.

For a detailed description of otoradiologic findings in eighth nerve tumors, see Chapter 4, Otoradiology.

NEUROLOGIC STUDIES

A complete neurologic examination is indicated in the patient with significant otologic, audiologic, vestibular, and radiographic findings pointing to the possibility of a lesion in the internal auditory canal or meatus or in the cerebellopontine angle. Differential diagnostic neurologic screening is necessary to rule out other CNS lesions that can produce similar findings.

BIOCHEMICAL STUDIES OF CEREBROSPINAL FLUID

Spinal fluid studies show elevated protein in a majority of cases of eighth nerve tumors. The normal protein level in spinal fluid is 50 mg or less per 100 ml. Protein levels can reach 75 to over 100 mg/100 ml in eighth nerve tumors. Protein elevations are proportional to tumor size. Frequently, such spinal fluid studies are done when Pantopaque contrast studies are made.

Silverstein and Griffin (23) reported the use of diagnostic labyrinthotomy as a diagnostic technique, particularly in the differential diagnosis between eighth nerve tumors and advanced Meniere's disease. This involves the use of microchemical determinations of vestibular perilymph obtained through a tympanotomy procedure. In this study, a perilymph protein concentration of over 1,000 mg/100 cc is considered good evidence for eighth nerve tumors. A potassium concentration of 100 mEq/liter or greater is considered good evidence for endolymphatic hydrops.

Palva and co-workers (19) reported eighth nerve diagnostic findings by disk electrophoresis studies based upon immunoelectrophoresis and immunodiffusion techniques.

MANAGEMENT

MANAGEMENT OF EIGHTH NERVE SCHWANNOMA

The treatment for eighth nerve vestibular schwannomas (acoustic neuroma) which is a benign but space-occupying lesion, is surgical removal, if there is no contraindication. Although nonsurgical management, with the substitutive use of steroid therapy, has been advocated, such treatment is not in common use at the present time, except in extremely large tumors and/or in patients who are not safe candidates for surgery.

A number of surgical techniques are in current use, including 1) the translabyrinthine approach, 2) the suboccipital approach, and 3) the middle fossa approach.

The **translabyrinthin approach** (13) is based upon a mastoidectomy followed by complete exenteration of the three semicircular canals with their endolymphatic contents, including the vestibule. It is this labyrinthectomy which offers a useful surgical approach to the internal auditory meatus, especially in cases with major hearing loss. The labyrinthectomy destroys any remaining hearing and vestibular function in that ear, obviously. The relatively small surgical opening is adequate for the removal of a large percentage of eighth nerve tumors. However, problems encountered in larger tumors may require either concomitant or secondary approaches through one of the other routes.

The **suboccipital approach** (20) combined with a microsurgical petrous bone dissection yields a high percentage of successful one-stage total tumor removals. It has the advantage of wider exposure and visualization not only of the internal auditory canal, the internal auditory meatus and its contents, but also of the cerebellopontine angle, the cerebellar vessels, and contiguous cranial nerves. It is possible to maintain the integrity of the facial nerve in the majority of cases (whether by translabyrinthine or suboccipital approach) unless the tumor itself has infiltrated the facial nerve. The suboccipital approach does carry with it the possibility not only of saving facial nerve function in extensive tumors but also of saving useful residual hearing since the labyrinth need not be destroyed in the surgical access.

The **middle fossa** approach carries with it the possibility of wide exposure, comparable to that in the suboccipital approach. It also obviates the necessity of a labyrinthectomy and thus a more conservative, function-saving advantage is readily apparent. Recent reports of results with both the suboccipital and the middle fossa approaches offer hopes of saving hearing in the affected ear. This becomes extremely critical in the young person with multiple neurofibromatoses (Recklinghausen's disease) who already has evidence of bilateral lesions or who may indeed develop a lesion of the contralateral ear within a matter of a few years.

Surgical removal of eighth nerve tumors, while obviously the desirable goal, cannot be considered an absolute necessity in every case. Some patients with small, intracanalicular, slowly growing tumors may have no symptoms except for slow auditory loss over a period of decades. Acoustic neurinoma is not cancer. Only one malignant acoustic neurinoma has been reported (22). We really do not know how many patients go through decades of adult life with small eighth nerve tumors that are relatively asymptomatic except for hearing loss.

Continuous investigation of a suspected tumor is necessary over a period of years. There are no simple guidelines. Variations in growth, in size, and in extent are great. Sudden increases in size are not unusual.

Internal acoustic meatus asymmetry on radiographic studies does not always indicate eighth nerve tumor. In addition to eighth nerve tumors and vascular anomalies, a number of other lesions may occur, including meningioma, intrapetrosal keratoma, and other intracranial benign and malignant lesions.

With the rare exception of a microscopic eighth nerve tumor that may occur primarily as an intralabyrinthine lesion, the eighth nerve tumor is a lesion that occurs within the borderlines of the disciplines of otology and neurosurgery. The management of an eighth nerve tumor requires a team approach, in which the otosurgeon and neurosurgeon have the benefit of neuroradiologic, neuroaudiologic, and vestibular electronystagmographic expertise.

Smith, Miller, and Cox (24) point out that the ideal goals of eighth nerve tumor surgery are total tumor removal, preservation of facial and cochlear function, and low morbidity and mortality. The suboccipital microsurgical approach is recommended as fulfilling the criteria of good acoustic tumor surgery. They point out the advantages of the unilateral suboccipital approach with microsurgical unroofing of the internal auditory meatus, which permits rapid, total removal of small and medium-sized tumors of the eighth nerve. In some instances maintenance of preoperative hearing levels is possible with such small and medium-sized tumors. Surgical decompression and staging are recommended by these investigators in the removal of large tumors when decompensations by increased intracranial pressure are present.

Rand (20) recommends suboccipital transmeatal microneurosurgical resection of eighth nerve tumors. He initially reported on 31 cases and more recently on a series of 79 cases with DiTullio and Malkasian in 1978 (5a). In small-sized tumors (2 cm or less) and medium-sized tumors (2–4 cm), there were no deaths and total tumor removal was accomplished in 100% and 93% of the cases respectively. Residual tumor tissue firmly attached to the brain stem was destroyed by cryosurgery in the remaining 7% of medium-sized tumors. Total removal was performed in 91% of large to massive tumors (greater than 4 cm), again destroying any residual tumor capsule by cryosurgical temperatures of at least −80° C. The overall mortality was 3.7%.

In the small tumors, the facial nerve was preserved perfectly in all instances. In the medium tumors, it was preserved in 93% of cases, and in the tumors greater than 4 cm, in 84%.

Montgomery (18) advocates a one-stage translabyrinthine procedure for small eighth nerve tumors.

Montgomery (18a) in 1978 reported the case of a 17-year-old patient who had two years previously undergone suboccipital posterior fossa surgery for removal of a 4.5 cm left acoustic neurinoma. This was followed by total left hearing loss and a left facial paralysis which was corrected by hypoglossal facial anastomosis. The onset of right hearing loss two years later (20 dB SRT and 96% SDS) was followed by diagnosis of a right acoustic neurinoma. This difficult dilemma was solved by a right suboccipital craniotomy and removal of a 1.5 cm tumor. Two months postoperatively there was normal right facial nerve function and the hearing in the right ear remained at a 30 dB SRT level with 100% SDS. This case report exemplifies the management challenges of eighth nerve tumors.

Rosomoff (21) describes a subtemporal transtentorial approach to the cerebellopontine angle, which he feels is the most versatile of all the approaches because of delineation of cranial nerves and the ventrolateral brain stem with its blood supply from the middle fossa to the foramen magnum.

Dawes and Curry (5) recommend the suboccipital route because of its wider exposure, the possibility of varying technique according to the size of the tumor, the accessibility of the antero-inferior cerebellar artery, and the possibility of avoiding entrance into the tympanomastoid air system.

Very small intravestibular eighth nerve tumors may be encountered and removed through an endomeatal stapedectomy type approach. Storrs (25) reported an eighth nerve tumor which was present only in the labyrinthine vestibule.

There are enormous differences in the growth aspects of eighth nerve schwannomas. This fact must constantly be weighed in the difficult decision-making task of management. In the past few years, advances in neuro-audiology, neuro-radiology, and vestibulometry have led to an enormous increase in early diagnoses of such tumors. Concurrently, there have been advances in microsurgical techniques for removal of such tumors. These have been described earlier in this chapter. As a result, a great sense of urgency has been introduced into the question of timing of surgery.

Some investigators have advocated very prompt surgical removal as soon as a positive diagnosis has been made. Unfortunately, in spite of improved techniques, there is still a significant morbidity and mortality in the removal of these **benign tumors.** Many urgent directives in the literature have created a fear that a small tumor, with only eighth nerve involvement and no evidence of brain stem pressure, may indeed be an ominous lesion which may grow rapidly and, although benign, can create cerebellopontine angle and brain stem problems unless removed immediately. Indeed, there is evidence that such rapid growth has occurred in some cases, especially in young adults.

However, there is also evidence that such tumors may remain unchanged in size for years and even decades. We have such patients under care in our clinic with positively identified eighth nerve tumors who have refused surgery. Continuous diagnostic observations of a significant number of such patients have failed to reveal tumor growth over long periods of time. Some patients whose only symptom is unilateral hearing loss may and do decline surgical intervention.

A dilemma thus exists in the management of such cases, and it appears that longer range considerations are necessary regarding timing of surgery. This is particularly characteristic of eighth nerve tumors in middle or later decades. Constant diagnostic vigilance is necessary, and careful evaluation must be constantly reviewed. We have no final answers on the eighth nerve tumor surgery problem.

A new nonsurgical method of destroying eighth nerve tumors involves the use of gamma rays. The stereotaxic cobalt "gamma knife" has 179 sources of cobalt which can be columnated to a point in space approximately 1–1.5 cm in circular diameter. At this point the irradiation turns out to be approximately 300 rads/min.

In a recent personal communication, Dr. Robert Rand, Professor of Neurosurgery at UCLA, reported to me that Professor Lars Leksell of the University of Stockholm "has treated a variety of diseases including cerebral aneurysms (subcortical), arteriovenous malformations, pinealomas, and acoustic neuromas." In 1971, Leksell published a series of seven cases of acoustic neuroma, and five of them showed improved hearing. All the tumors were 2 cm or less in size. Since that time he has treated an additional 23 cases and in my correspondence with Professor Leksell I understand that over 80% of the patients have shown improvement in function, both of cochlear and vestibular nerves; and the tumors were substantially reduced in size by the focal radiation. In one instance there was a transient facial palsy which recovered. It is now the policy of the Department of Neurosurgery at the Karolinska Institute to treat acoustic tumors that are 2 cm or less in size by the stereotaxic gamma knife radiation technique provided the patient has useful hearing. The total radiation given at one time is approximately 3000 rads. This is equivalent to the 6000 rads which would be given by other techniques over a period of weeks. The procedure is done basically on an outpatient basis with the patient coming to the unit, having the stereotaxic instrument fitted onto his head by means of applying a plaster or plastic band around the head and then setting the stereotaxic instrument into the band. The coordinates of the acoustic neoplasm are then calculated by taking x-rays and the stereotaxic instrument is adjusted so that when the patient is placed on the table which slides into the unit holding the cobalt sources, the target to be radiated is aligned to the point where the 179 sources are columnated. It is an especially unique design, and after the radiation the patient simply is removed from the unit, the stereotaxic device is dismantled, and he is sent home.

MANAGEMENT OF MENINGIOMA

Because of the variations in size and the pleomorphism of temporal-bone meningiomas, surgical management requires wide-field approaches such as obtained with the suboccipital and middle fossa procedures.

MANAGEMENT OF LESIONS IN THE PRIMARY APEX AND CEREBELLOPONTINE ANGLE

Although some lesions of the petrous pyramid apex and cerebellopontine angle can be removed via middle fossa or suboccipital approaches, others require more extensive anatomic exposure. House and Hitselberger (14) describe a transcochlear approach to the skull base by a forward extension of the translabyrinthine approach into the cerebellopontine angle.

Bochenek and Kukwa (4) suggest a submeningeal approach through the middle cranial fossa after cutting the tentorium cerebelli.

Nonsurgical management may be advisable for some cases, as pointed out by Bender (2), who advises steroid therapy in special situations.

SUMMARY

1. Eighth nerve vestibular schwannoma may be an entirely asymptomatic lesion for years.
2. Unilateral tinnitus is the first symptom in many patients.
3. Unilateral hearing loss (usually high frequency), a concomitant symptom, is usually characterized by slow onset, which may be delayed following the onset of tinnitus. However, sudden hearing loss may be the first symptom.
4. Vestibular symptoms (vertigo and/or ataxia) are present in only one-third of cases even though the primary lesion starts from the vestibular branch of the eighth nerve. Vestibular abnormalities are usually present even in the absence of vestibular symptoms. The most common vestibular finding is unilateral depressed caloric response, which may or may not be accompanied by spontaneous or positional nystagmus.
5. Conventional Stenver radiographs will show internal auditory meatus abnormalities in 75% of cases.
6. Polytomography with the frequent supplementary information from computerized axial tomography (CAT) scans or pantopaque posterior fossa myelography will yield a positive diagnosis in more than 90% of cases.
7. Multiple and longitudinal studies may be necessary in diagnosis. The primary ingredient is a high index of suspicion.
8. The treatment of choice is surgical removal, via translabyrinthine, suboccipital, or middle fossa approaches.
9. In older patients, slowly growing intracanalicular tumors need not be considered urgent indications for surgery, but regular, frequent examinations are advisable.

REFERENCES

1. Baum S, Rothballer A, Shiffman F et al.: Brain scanning in the diagnosis of acoustic neuromas. J Neurosurg 36:141–147, 1972
2. Bender MB: Cerebellopontine angle tumors or acoustic neuromas: long range management. Arch Otolaryngol 97:160–165, 1973
3. Benitez JT, Bouchard KR: Electronystagmography: significant alterations in tumors of the cerebellopontine recess. Ann Otol Rhinol Laryngol 83:399–402, 1974
4. Bochenek Z, Kukwa A: An extended approach through the middle cranial fossa and the internal auditory meatus and the cerebellopontine angle. Acta Otolaryngol (Stockh) 80:410–414, 1975
5. Dawes JDK, Curry AR: Surgical aspects of acoustic neurinoma. Acta Otohinolaryngol Belg 25:784–792, 1971
5a. DiTullio MV Jr, Malkasian D, Rand RW: A critical comparison of neurosurgical and otolaryngological approaches to acoustic neuromas. J Neurosurg 48:1–12, 1978
6. Dublin WB: Fundamentals of Sensorineural Auditory Pathology. Springfield, IL, CC Thomas, 1976
7. Etter LB: Plain film demonstration of acoustic nerve tumors. Arch Otolaryngol 98:414–416, 1973
8. Gacek RR: Diagnosis and management of primary tumors of the petrous apex. Ann Otol Rhinol Laryngol [Suppl] 84 (18), Jan.–Feb., 1975
9. Gibson WPR, Wallace D: Basilar artery ectasia (an unusual cause of a cerebellopontine lesion and hemifacial spasm). J Laryngol 89:721–731, 1975
10. Goodhill V: Nerve deafness and brain tumors. Trans Am Acad Ophthalmol Otolaryngol 65:241–245, 1961
11. Gussen R: Pathology of eighth nerve tumors and petrosal meningiomas. In Tower DB (ed): The Nervous System, Vol 3, Human Communication and Its Disorders. New York, Raven Press, 1975
12. Hanafee WN, Gussen R, Rand R: Laminography of the mastoid in the basal projection. Am J Roentgenol 110:111–118, 1970
13. House WF: Evolution of transtemporal bone removal of acoustic tumors. Arch Otolaryngol 80:731–741, 1964
14. House WF, Hitselberger WE: The transcochlear approach to the skull base. Arch Otolaryngol 102:334–342, 1976

15. Jerger J, Jerger S: Audiologic comparison of cochlear and eighth nerve disorders. Ann Otol Rhinol Laryngol 83:275–285, 1974

16. Johnson EW: Auditory test results in 500 cases of acoustic neuroma. Arch Otolaryngol 103:152–158, 1977

17. Lin SR, Lee F, Stein G et al.: Asymmetrical internal auditory canals. Arch Otolaryngol 98:164–169, 1973

18. Montgomery WW: Surgery for acoustic neurinoma. Ann Otol Rhinol Laryngol 82:428–440, 1973

18a. Montgomery WW: Bilateral acoustic neurinomas: a case report. Ann Otol Rhinol Laryngol 87:135–137, 1978

19. Palva T, Silverstein H, Forsen R et al.: Disc electrophoresis in acoustic neurinoma. Ann Otol Rhinol Laryngol 81:106–113, 1972

20. Rand RW: Suboccipital transmeatal microneurosurgical resection of acoustic tumors. Ann Surg 174:663–671, 1971

21. Rosomoff HL: The subtemporal transtentorial approach to the cerebellopontine angle. Laryngoscope 81:1448–1454, 1971

22. Schuknecht HF: Pathology of the Ear. Cambridge, MA, Harvard University Press, 1974

23. Silverstein H, Griffin W: Diagnostic labyrinthotomy in otologic disorders. Arch Otolaryngol 91:414–423, 1970

24. Smith MFW, Miller RN, Cox DJ: Suboccipital microsurgical removal of acoustic neurinomas of all sizes. Ann Otol Rhinol Laryngol 82:407–414, 1973

25. Storrs LA: Acoustic neurinomas presenting as middle ear tumors. Laryngoscope 84:1175–1180, 1974

26. Tos M, Rosborg J, Adser J: Optokinetic nystagmus in acoustic neurinomas. Acta Otolaryngol (Stockh) 76:239–243, 1973

SUGGESTED READING

Clemis JD, Mastricola PG: Special audiometric test battery in 121 proved acoustic tumors. Arch Otolaryngol 102:654–656, 1976

Fisch UP, Nedzelski J, Wellauer J: Diagnostic value of meatocisternography. Arch Otolaryngol 101:339–343, 1975

Jahrsdoerfer RA, Sweet DE, Fitz-Hugh S: Malignant fibrous xanthoma with metastasis and cerebellopontine angle. Arch Otolaryngol 102:117–120, 1976

Lin SR: Radiologic evaluation of acoustic neurinoma. ORL 11–16, 1975

Neely JG, Britton BH, Greenberg SD: Microscopic characteristics of the acoustic tumor in relationship of its nerve or origin. Laryngoscope 87:984–991, 1976

Olsen WO, Noffsinger D, Kurdziel S: Acoustic reflex and reflex decay. Arch Otolaryngol 101:622–625, 1975

Ozsahinoglee C, Harrison MS: The symptoms of neurofibroma of the 8th nerve. Br J Audiol 8:61–65, 1974

Sheehy JL, Inzer BE: Acoustic reflex test in neurootologic diagnosis. Arch Otolaryngol 102:647–653, 1976

Thomsen J, Zilstorff K: Intermedius nerve involvement and testing in acoustic neuromas. Acta Otolaryngol (Stockh) 80:276–282, 1975

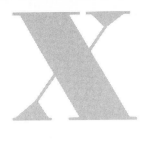

X

TRAUMA

24

TRAUMATIC DISEASES OF THE EAR AND TEMPORAL BONE

JOEL B. SHULMAN

Injuries to the ear and temporal bone are ubiquitous, and proper early management is crucial. Signs may be obvious or very subtle, and may be either isolated or associated with multiple injuries involving both open and closed head trauma inflicted by sharp or blunt objects.

EXTERNAL EAR TRAUMA

AURICLE

Lacerations of the cartilaginous framework are repaired by absorbable sutures placed in the perichondrium or through cartilage. Soft tissues are then closed meticulously with fine (6–0) monofilament nylon with debridement of only obviously nonviable tissue. Because of the exceptionally good blood supply, tenuous flaps will usually survive and even completely amputated portions may often be successfully replaced as free autografts.

Hematomas must be promptly evacuated (by aspiration or incision and drainage) to prevent a severe deformity (cauliflower ear). A bolster dressing affixed with through-and-through sutures is the most satisfactory dressing (Fig. 24–1), but alternatively, moistened cotton may be molded to the auricle as a "cast" and a standard mastoid pressure dressing applied.

EXTERNAL AUDITORY CANAL

Abrasions, small lacerations, and hematomas generally require no treatment other than topical antiseptic or antibiotic. If flaps of canal skin are elevated, an attempt should be made to replace them with absorbable gelatin foam (Gelfoam), or packing of petroleum-impregnated fabric of viscose filament (Adaptic) may be inserted into the canal for several days to hold the flaps in place. If blunt trauma to the head has produced bleeding from the ear or laceration of the external auditory canal, middle ear damage or temporal bone fracture must be strongly suspected (see section on Ossicular Chain Injuries–Middle Ear Trauma later in this chapter).

The most commonly implicated traumatic tool is the cotton applicator, wielded by patients with the mistaken notion that regular cleaning of the external auditory canal with a cotton-tipped applicator is an important part of personal hygiene. The cerumen often becomes impacted more deeply in the canal. Since the delicate skin of the canal is easily damaged, infection is thus promoted. Reports of tympanic membrane perforations are numerous, sometimes with ossicular or facial nerve injury.

Consequently, the cotton applicator has no use in the ear. The outer ear may be cleansed with a washcloth wrapped over the finger, and in those few individuals with troublesome cerumen accumulation, periodic careful cleansing under direct vision with a cerumen loop and/or the external auditory canal irrigator should be carried out by a physician or trained and supervised assistant. However, if the patient has a history of past otorrhea or tympanic membrane perforation, irrigation must be avoided when the entire membrane cannot be visualized; debris may be washed into the middle ear through an unseen perforation or the delicate neomembrane of a healed perforation may be ruptured by the irrigating stream.

TRAUMATIC TYMPANIC MEMBRANE PERFORATIONS

ETIOLOGY

Perforation of the tympanic membrane is the most common serious ear injury and may result from a wide variety of causes: 1) direct injury by such "weapons" as cotton applicators, pencils, paper clips, flying objects (slag), irrigation of the external auditory canal, etc.; 2) concussive injury from an explosion or from a blow to the ear, which

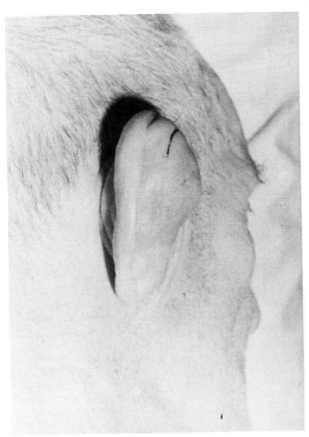

FIG. 24–1. Hematoma of auricle.

suddenly compresses the air within the external auditory canal; 3) various types of barotrauma; 4) tears from temporal bone fractures; and 5) lightning injury and other miscellaneous causes. Any of these may produce varying types and sizes of perforations, ranging from tiny tears of the pars tensa to massive injuries involving not only the tympanic membrane and the ossicular chain, but even the labyrinthine windows and facial nerve.

DIAGNOSIS

Accurate and early diagnosis is important in the proper management of traumatic tympanic membrane perforations. General principles of evaluation and management of the patient with head trauma are followed. The mechanism of injury is usually readily apparent from the history, unless multiple injuries add confusion. Careful examination of the external auditory canal and tympanic membrane with good lighting and magnification (see Ch. 3, Ear Examination) will identify the type and extent of the perforation. Blood and debris may be removed from the canal with sterile suction but never by irrigation. Particular attention is paid to facial nerve and audiovestibular function.

The hearing status as determined by adequate audiologic studies will give information about possible concomitant injury to the ossicular chain or cochlea. Mastoid radiographs are essential to evaluate the extent of injury as well as the possibility of preexisting ear disease. Laminography will enhance radiographic information regarding the site of injury in some cases.

MANAGEMENT

Management of the Small Tympanic Membrane Perforation

The small perforation occupying no more than one quadrant of the tympanic membrane area, with less than 30 dB conductive hearing loss, no radiographic abnormalities, and no other sequelae, can be dealt with in many instances by simple "patching" of the perforation as an outpatient procedure.

It is advisable to delay such patching for several days following the injury to make sure that there is no foreign body in the middle ear. A sterile piece of cotton is kept in the external auditory canal. No water is allowed in the ear, and repeat examinations are carried out every few days.

Because of the high risk of introducing contaminated material from the external auditory canal into the middle ear through the perforation, prophylactic broad-spectrum systemic antibiotics are recommended.

Very small perforations (less than 2 mm), the edges of which are not curled inward, will often close spontaneously without any special treatment. If the perforation remains dry but shows no signs of closing after several days, and if the margins can be easily seen, patching may be carried out. A 3- to 4-mm disk of clean cigarette paper is moistened with 10% $AgNO_3$ and picked up simply by touching it with a fine, cotton-tipped, metal applicator, which has also been dampened with $AgNO_3$. Handled in this way the paper patch may be easily introduced through a speculum and manipulated into exact position so that it covers the perforation completely with a margin of at least 1.5 mm. The mildly irritating effect of the $AgNO_3$ stimulates proliferation of the squamous layer of the tympanic membrane, and the piece of paper acts as a "scaffolding," under which the epithelium will tend to grow. A disk of absorbable gelatin film (Gelfilm) may also be used as a patch. This type of simple management will be effective in approximately 50% of cases without further procedures (Fig. 24–2). If the postoperative audiogram reveals nearly complete closure of the air-bone gap,

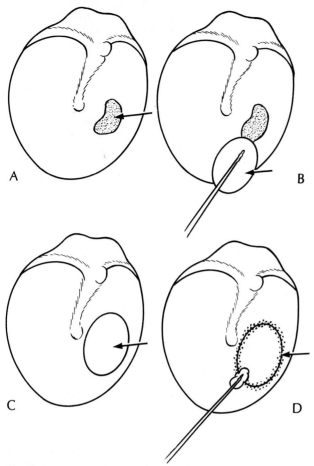

myringoplasty or another form of tympanoplasty. Thorough preoperative evaluation cannot be over-emphasized. If there is evidence of mastoid disease on radiography, or if there is significant conductive hearing loss, then myringoplasty (type I tympanoplasty) may be inadequate. Evaluation of such lesions, surgical planning, and techniques are described in Chapter 12, Basic Otosurgical Procedures.

If there is no evidence of mastoid or middle ear disease, a type I tympanoplasty is successful in the majority of cases. Using an endomeatal approach (under local or general anesthesia) a posterosuperior tympanomeatal flap is elevated, and an exploratory tympanotomy is performed so that the ossicular chain and the medial aspect of the tympanic membrane can be carefully inspected. Frequently the torn membrane actually invaginates into the middle ear and attaches to the medial surface of the tympanic membrane (Fig. 24–4). If this is not recognized, tympanoplastic reconstruction may actually cause more harm than good by enclosing viable squamous epithelium within the middle ear, thus creating the potential for development of a keratoma (cholesteatoma). If such an invaginated piece of tympanic membrane is found, the treatment of choice is to carefully release fibrous adhesions between the infolded flap and the medial surface of the tympanic membrane and gently but completely unfold the torn edges toward the central portion of the perforation. Occasionally it will be possible to

FIG. 24–2. Technique of paper patching of small, thin, traumatic perforation. **A. Arrow,** small central perforation. **B. Arrow,** thin paper patch advanced to cover perforation. **C. Arrow,** patch in position. **D. Arrow,** patch margins moistened with 10% AgNO₃.

FIG. 24–3. Audiogram in a case of a small, uncomplicated traumatic perforation, showing a mild conductive hearing loss before patching and complete closure of the air–bone gap with the patch in place. ●—●, AC, unmasked, RE, prepatching; [—[, BC, masked, RE, prepatching; ●- - -●, AC, unmasked, RE, postpatching.

then one can be fairly certain of the absence of significant concomitant ossicular injury (Fig. 24–3). Careful observation is important to detect secondary infection of the external auditory canal or middle ear. Repeat patching may be necessary if the patch migrates off the tympanic membrane before healing is complete. If application of a patch is followed by purulent middle ear drainage, the patch is immediately removed with suction and not replaced until the infection is controlled. Appropriate systemic antibiotic therapy is preferred.

Persistent perforations are treated by myringoplasty as described in the following section.

Management of Large Tympanic Membrane Perforations by Myringoplasty—Tympanoplasty

When the perforation is large or when simple patching has failed, surgery is necessary—namely,

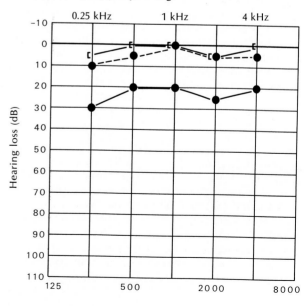

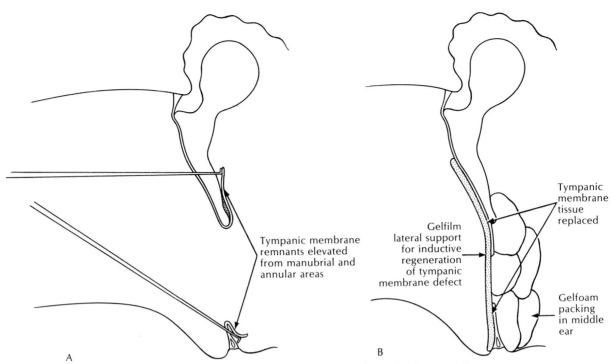

FIG. 24–4. Repair of traumatic TM perforation. The inwardly curled edges of this traumatic TM perforation are carefully released and unfolded **(A)** and then supported medially with pledgets of gelatin foam and splinted laterally with gelatin film **(B)**.

completely close the perforation using the patient's own reflected tympanic membrane splinted by a laterally placed piece of absorbable gelatin foam (Gelfoam) or film (Gelfilm). Even if a small gap remains, as is usually the case, it may be bridged by a gelatin film disk (Fig. 24–5).

If the perforation is large and there is no available tympanic membrane tissue for reflection from the medial surface, then a definitive graft is necessary. Tragal perichondrium is our choice of tissue for this purpose. After denudation of the squamous epithelium surrounding the perforation, perichondrial graft is placed externally to cover the deepithelialized area. The special shape of the tragal perichondrium graft allows it to be tailored to fit the concavity of the tympanic membrane and thus it has an advantage over other tissues (see section on type III tympanoplasty, in Ch. 12, Basic Otosurgical Procedures). The type of reconstruction described is shown in Figure 24–6. Sometimes the surgeon may prefer to place the graft medial to the tympanic membrane remnant, supported by a bed of absorbable gelatin sponge (Gelfoam).

Slag Injuries of the Tympanic Membrane

Certain occupations, such as welding, involve the hazard of injury from flying beads of hot metal, which will produce perforations accompanied by burns of the tympanic membrane and the middle ear mucosa. Since small bits of metal may be hidden within the middle ear, neither patching nor simple type I tympanoplasty suffices. A careful middle ear exploration, and in some instances, mastoid exploration should precede grafting. Graft "takes" are not so satisfactory in slag injuries as they are in uncomplicated perforations. A fairly common sequel of slag injuries is chronic otomastoiditis and may be either type A or type B in character (see Ch. 16, Chronic Otomastoiditis—Diagnosis and Management).

COMPLICATIONS

Infection

Penetration of the tympanic membrane with a contaminated instrument or by a blast inevitably introduces pathogenic bacteria into the middle ear with or without gross foreign matter. However, as long as prophylactic ear drops or canal irrigations are avoided in the presence of a dry traumatic perforation, the incidence of infection is surprisingly low. When otorrhea develops, spontaneous *Staphlococcus aureus* or *Pseudomonas aeruginosa*

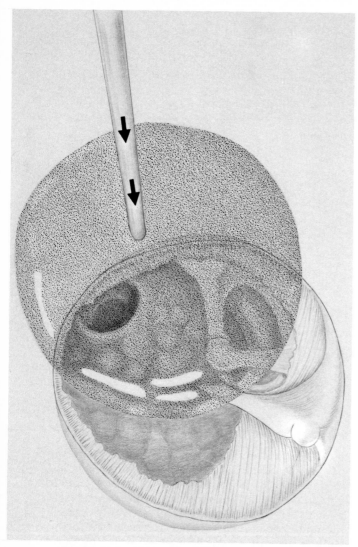

FIG. 24–5. A gelatin film disk (cut to size with an ear speculum) is being inserted to cover a tympanic membrane perforation.

with a dry perforation, minimal hearing loss, and well-pneumatized mastoid. Unsuspected epitympanic keratoma has been encountered in several cases and is most likely due to the proliferation of squamous epithelium from an undetected inwardly rolled-up piece of tympanic membrane. For this reason, exploratory tympanotomy must be accom-

FIG. 24–6. Repair of traumatic perforation by myringoplasty. **A.** Area of tympanic membrane to be covered by the lateral graft is deepithelialized **(arrow). B.** The edge of the perforation is trimmed **(arrow)** to remove any remaining fragments of squamous epithelium which would inhibit healing or possibly develop into keratoma. **C.** Tragal perichondrial graft in place on lateral surface of tympanic membrane **(arrow).** Alternatively, graft may be placed medial to the TM remnant and supported on a bed of gelatin foam, thus eliminating the need for deepithelialization.

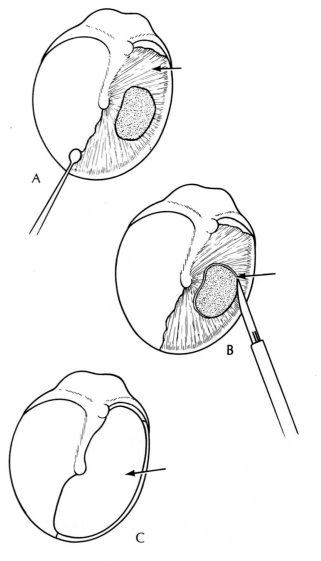

are the most common organisms cultured. Systemic antibiotic treatment alone is preferable unless organisms are resistant to oral preparations. In such cases, carefully selected topical antibiotics as drops or powder may be used with caution. Otorrhea that is not controlled by these measures may require hospitalization for parenteral antibiotic therapy and/or otomastoid surgery.

Keratoma (Cholesteatoma)

One must be alert to the possibility of silent keratoma occurring as a sequel to an apparently uncomplicated traumatic perforation, particularly in children. This complication may be present even panied by adequate removal of posterosuperior canal wall bone to allow visualization of the epitympanum. In blast injuries, fragments of viable squamous epithelium may be blown into the middle ear and proliferate as isolated implants. If the tympanic membrane then heals or is grafted early, keratoma may develop behind the intact membrane.

OSSICULAR CHAIN INJURIES—MIDDLE EAR TRAUMA

All the various mechanisms described in connection with traumatic tympanic membrane perforations may be associated with injuries to the ossicular chain, occasionally even without actual rupture of the membrane. Violent, closed-head injuries, especially if the temporal bone is fractured, also commonly cause ossicular chain disruption. In such instances bleeding from the ear and a period of unconsciousness frequently occur. Significant ossicular chain damage usually produces a major conductive hearing loss (30–60 dB), which does not improve when the associated tympanic membrane perforation is patched. When the tympanic membrane is intact, impedance audiometry is helpful in detecting ossicular discontinuity (Fig. 24–7).

The most common traumatic ossicular chain lesion is incudostapedial joint dislocation with or without a fracture of the long process of the incus. However, virtually any imaginable ossicular fracture or displacement may be found.

Surgical exploration and ossicular repair is not urgent and, in fact, is best delayed at least several days until soft-tissue reaction has subsided and any infection ruled out. The various tympanoplastic techniques are discussed in Chapter 12, Basic Otosurgical Procedures.

TEMPORAL BONE FRACTURES

ANATOMY

Fractures involving the temporal bone are the most common fractures of the base of the skull. Because of the special architecture of the temporal bone, fractures tend to follow one of two general pathways through the bone, producing relatively predictable clinical effects (Fig. 24–8). Approximately 80% of these fractures run parallel to the petrous ridge coursing through the middle ear and tympanic ring, sparing the labyrinth. These are termed **longitudinal fractures** and usually result from a blow to the side of the head.

About 15% of temporal bone fractures are produced by blows to the occiput. The fracture line begins in the posterior fossa, at or near the foramen magnum, crosses the petrous ridge through the internal auditory canal and/or the otic capsule, and it is thus called a **transverse fracture.** A small minority of fractures combine features of both longitudinal and transverse types.

DIAGNOSIS

The clinical features of temporal bone fractures are presented in Table 24–1. On the basis of history and physical examination alone, the type of fracture and likely otologic consequences can usually be determined.

In the case of a longitudinal fracture there is usually a bloody discharge in the external auditory canal with or without cerebrospinal fluid issuing from a posterosuperior tympanic membrane perforation. Often a fracture line can be seen in the tympanic ring, extending into the external auditory canal posterosuperiorly. When the facial nerve is involved, paralysis is often delayed in onset or is incomplete and, rarely, goes on to neurotmesis; lacrimation is usually intact. Hearing loss is predominantly conductive, resulting from tympanic membrane perforation, hemotympanum, or ossicular damage. Vestibular symptoms are seldom severe, although positional vertigo may persist for many months.

A transverse fracture, on the other hand, exhibits a hemotympanum with an intact tympanic membrane. Facial paralysis, when present, usually appears immediately, with diminished tearing in the ipsilateral eye as a result of disruption of the facial nerve in the internal auditory canal; recovery is often incomplete. Generally, hearing loss is sensorineural and profound because the otic capsule is fractured, but the loss may occasionally be mixed. As expected, vertigo with spontaneous nystagmus is commonly severe until compensation for the destroyed labyrinth is achieved. Transverse fractures may also be bilateral.

The radiologic diagnosis of temporal bone fractures is often difficult. Transverse fractures generally can be seen on plain films of the skull and mastoid. Tomography is usually necessary to clearly delineate longitudinal fractures; if anteroposterior, lateral, and basilar projections are taken, a very adequate preoperative visualization of the otic capsule, fallopian canal, and ossicular chain

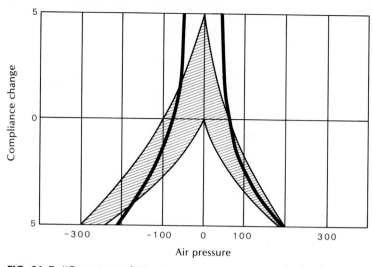

FIG. 24–7. "Open-topped" tympanogram suggesting ossicular discontinuity.

FIG. 24–8. Temporal bone fractures. **A.** Lateral view demonstrating course of longitudinal fracture **(L)**. **B.** View of skull base, showing longitudinal **(L)** and transverse **(T)** fracture lines.

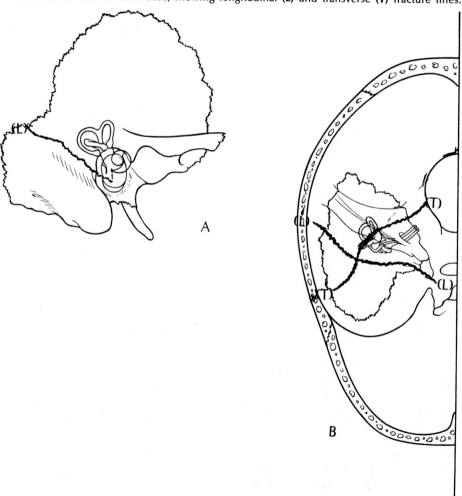

TABLE 24-1. Occurrence of Clinical Features With Temporal Bone Fractures

Clinical condition	Occurrence and extent of condition on basis of fracture type	
	Longitudinal	Transverse
Hearing loss	Conductive	Sensorineural or mixed
Bleeding from EAC*	Usual	Seldom
Hemotympanum	Usual	Usual
TM† perforation	Usual	Rare
CSF‡ otorrhea	Frequent	Seldom
Facial nerve injury	25% (usually transient)	50% (often permanent)
Vertigo (nystagmus)	None or positional	Severe, long-lasting, until compensation

*External auditory canal
†Tympanic membrane
‡Cerebrospinal fluid

can be achieved. Nevertheless, radiography has severe limitations in this area and can never be depended upon completely to rule out a fracture if one is strongly suspected on clinical grounds.

Audiometry is, of course, an essential diagnostic procedure. Vestibular testing is of some value in assessing the extent of labyrinthine or vestibular nerve damage.

MANAGEMENT

The acute management of the patient with head trauma ideally involves a multidisciplinary team approach with collaboration between emergency-room physician, general surgeon, neurosurgeon, otolaryngologist, ophthalmologist, and others. Establishment of airway, maintenance of vital signs, evaluation and treatment of intracranial injuries, and management of major injuries to other parts of the body will always take precedence over strictly otologic problems.

If blood or cerebrospinal fluid is draining from the ear, a temporal bone fracture should be presumed. A sterile bandage is applied and further evaluation deferred until the general condition is stabilized. Facial nerve function should be evaluated as early as possible since the time of onset of a traumatic facial paralysis will dictate subsequent treatment (see Ch. 30, Seventh Nerve Lesions and Injuries). As soon as practical, it is best to examine the affected ear under the microscope, using a sterile speculum and instruments for cleansing (see Ch. 3, Ear Examination). Part of the initial examination should include gross assessment of hearing (whispered voice, rubbing the fingers together, and tuning-fork tests) and a check for nystagmus. Audiometric, vestibular, and special radiographic studies are obtained as soon as the patient's condition allows.

The specific management of traumatic perforation of the tympanic membrane, ossicular damage, facial paralysis, and post-traumatic vertigo are discussed elsewhere. The special problem of cerebrospinal fluid otorrhea requires close cooperation between the otologist and neurosurgeon. Even when mixed with blood, cerebrospinal fluid otorrhea can be detected by allowing a drop of the discharge to fall on a piece of filter paper (a paper towel or bed linen will also suffice). The cerebrospinal fluid will migrate faster than the blood, leaving a characteristic double ring. Strict sterile procedures should be followed when the ear is examined, and a dry sterile mastoid dressing or head dressing should be in place continuously for protection. At the risk of offending the aesthetic sensibilities of some hospital personnel, we have even affixed a colostomy bag around the auricle to maintain sterility while at the same time enabling measurement of the amount of discharge.

Most cases of cerebrospinal fluid otorrhea due to fractures of the temporal bone will respond to conservative management, consisting of bed rest with head elevation (when possible), drainage of cerebrospinal fluid by twice daily lumbar punctures or indwelling subarachnoid catheter, and dehydrating agents such as acetazolamide (Diamox). Prophylactic antimeningitis doses of antibiotics are given until the otorrhea ceases.

Approximately 2 weeks should be allowed before resorting to surgical intervention. Sometimes an intracranial approach is necessary, guided by the location of the fracture or by the presence of herniated brain tissue as seen on tomography. However, before craniotomy is carried out, an exploratory tympanotomy should be performed to rule out a traumatic perilymphatic fistula from the oval window (avulsed stapes), from the round window, or from a promontory fracture. Such a fistula may be undetected unless the middle ear is explored. It is possible for such a fistula to be an etiologic factor in postfracture otitic (labyrinthogenic) meningitis.

Fractures of the tegmen tympani (roof of the middle ear) or tegmen mastoideum (roof of the aditus ad antrum mastoideum) may result in small but steady cerebrospinal fluid leaks with secondary cerebrospinal fluid rhinorrhea (via the eustachian tube), or otorrhea or both. In these cases exploratory tympanotomy will reveal clear fluid slowly entering the middle ear from the epitympanum or aditus region. Then, through a mastoidectomy approach, the source of the cerebrospinal fluid leak can usually be found and sealed with a tissue graft, thus avoiding a craniotomy. A high index of suspicion must be maintained in every patient who has sustained a temporal bone fracture, for the possibility of a postoperative quiescent and unrecognized cerebrospinal fluid or perilymph leak, both of which require exploration and closure by appropriate connective-tissue grafting (Fig. 24–9).

Following this systematic approach, most cases of traumatic cerebrospinal fluid otorrhea can be successfully managed conservatively or by low-risk otologic surgical procedures. Craniotomy, with its greater attendant mortality, is then reserved for refractory or complicated cases (e.g., those with herniated brain tissue).

Ossicular and tympanic membrane injuries lend themselves to surgical correction only if there is evidence of adequate cochlear function. Nothing will be gained by elaborate ossiculoplastic procedures if the patient has no measurable cochlear function as determined by adequate special audiologic procedures. In general, absence of bone-conduction responses on the affected side, with careful masking, points to absent cochlear function and militates against consideration of ear surgery for correction of hearing loss.

COMPLICATIONS

Despite the prophylactic use of antibiotics in all patients with hemotympanum or cerebrospinal fluid leaks, meningitis or intracranial abscesses may still occur. Otorrhea containing cerebrospinal fluid may escape detection by draining through the eustachian tube if the tympanic membrane is intact or healed. Late meningitis may occur in transverse fractures because of the inability of the otic capsule to undergo substantial osseous regeneration. This risk is much less in longitudinal fractures, which have a greater tendency to heal,

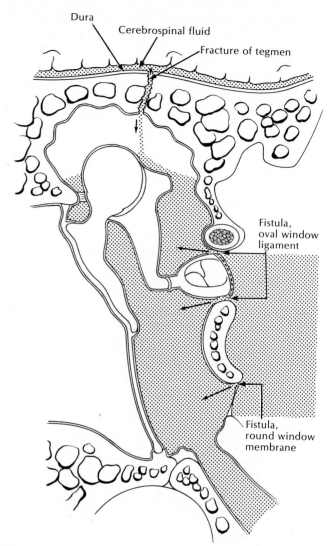

FIG. 24–9. Diagrammatic representation of the most common potential pathways for posttraumatic CSF otorrhea: through a tegmental fracture, OW or RW rupture.

although dura or mucosa may interpose itself in the fracture line to prevent bony union. Thus, in any case of meningitis, the possibility of previous head injury must be considered and the appropriate history elicited.

BAROTRAUMA

A special category of otologic trauma is caused by relatively gradual changes in ambient pressure, as opposed to the sudden change occurring in blast injuries. Because of the frequency of airplane travel and the increased popularity of deep-sea diving, barotrauma has become an important clinical problem.

EXTERNAL EAR

Obstruction of the external auditory canal by cerumen or tight-fitting ear plugs during a dive may produce canal hemorrhage or blood-filled blebs, sometimes with a bloody discharge. These injuries may be painful, with distressing symptoms, but are rarely serious and require no treatment.

MIDDLE EAR—BAROTITIS MEDIA

When extratympanic pressure decreases in aircraft ascent or after diving, the expanding air in the middle ear passively escapes through the eustachian tube to equalize the pressure. This is experienced as faint clicking sensations in the ears as altitude increases or depth decreases. Thus since the buildup of relative positive pressure in the middle ear is self-limiting, few problems occur during ascent. However, during descent, the eustachian tube must actively open by muscular contraction or forced inflation (modified Valsalva maneuver or politzerization) to prevent a sustained pressure gradient across the tympanic membrane. When the pressure differential exceeds 90 mm Hg, a muscular action can no longer open the eustachian tube, and it is said to become "locked." If inflation is not achieved, the tympanic membrane retracts. The subsequent vascular engorgement, edema, and ecchymosis of the middle ear with transudate of fluid, which is sometimes bloody, result in barotitis media. The tympanic membrane may even rupture. This process is encouraged by preexisting eustachian tube dysfunction from mucosal congestion (URI's, allergy, etc.), otitis media, mechanical obstruction (mucosal polyps, surgical scarring), or simply congenital variations in eustachian tube size and patency. Symptoms of "fullness" in the ear and decreased hearing accompany pain, which is more transient. The tympanic membrane appears retracted and hyperemic or hemorrhagic, with a serous middle ear effusion or hemotympanum.

Treatment of barotitis is based on the use of systemic and intranasal decongestants, antibiotics if infection is present in the ears or nasopharynx, and gentle politzeration as long as the nasopharynx is free of infection. Myringotomy, with or without intubation, is performed when medical management fails.

Prevention of this condition is, or course, more desirable. Patients should be discouraged from flying or diving with URI or during severe nasal allergy episodes. Airplane passengers should remain awake during descent and actively engage in maneuvers to exercise the eustachian tube (chewing, swallowing, yawning). Gentle Valsalva maneuver (forcible expiration against closed mouth and nose) or the safer but more difficult Frenzel maneuver (contracting muscles of floor of mouth and pharynx with the glottis, mouth and nose closed) may be added if necessary. Systemic decongestants or topical intranasal vasoconstrictors used 0.5–1 hour before descent are helpful. When barotrauma is recurrent, special attention should be paid to correction of obstructive nasal and pharyngeal lesions (polyps, septal deviations, etc.), allergies, and chronic sinus infections. The occasional patient who must continue to fly despite recurrent aerotitis resistant to the foregoing measures may require the chronic insertion of a transtympanic ventilation tube.

A special type of barotitis media may occur 2 or more hours after breathing high concentrations of oxygen. As the oxygen in the middle ear is absorbed, a relative negative pressure develops, resulting in the typical syndrome of barotitis unless the ears are adequately ventilated. This is most commonly seen in the flier who has gone to sleep shortly after returning from a flight and awakens with ear pain.

INNER EAR

Problems During Compression (Diving or Aircraft Descent)

When extratympanic pressure increases during descent, the tympanic membrane moves inward, the stapes is depressed into the oval window, and the displacement or perilymph bulges the round window membrane outward. As has been mentioned, passive opening of the eustachian tube readily equalizes positive intratympanic pressure. However, if this pressure change occurs rapidly or with great force, damage may be inflicted upon the membranous structures within the otic capsule, producing sensorineural hearing loss and/or vertigo. The round-window or oval-window membranes themselves may be ruptured, resulting in a perilymph fistula (see Ch. 37, Sudden Hearing Loss Syndrome). A modified Valsalva maneuver, performed to "clear the ears" very rapidly, pulls the stapes outward, reversing the perilymph flow. This is more likely to produce inner ear damage than a more gradual change in ambient pressure. In fact, forceful Valsalva maneuver alone may produce perilymph fistula. Symptoms may include a sense of fullness in the ear, decreased hearing (immediate or delayed as much as several days, complete or merely high frequency loss, particularly with loss of speech discrimination), and vertigo of varying degrees.

Treatment of inner ear compression barotrauma is essentially that for perilymph fistula and is well outlined in Chapter 37. Prompt repair (either spontaneous or surgical) may bring about a dramatic return of hearing although recovery is usually incomplete.

Problems at Stable Pressures

Nitrogen narcosis and oxygen poisoning occur as a result of increased partial pressures of nitrogen and oxygen, respectively, in the blood and other body tissues and therefore occur only in super-atmospheric pressure situations (diving). The danger of developing these conditions is directly related to the depth and time of exposure.

Nitrogen narcosis produces an effect similar to that of alcohol intoxication, with euphoria, giddiness, impaired judgment, and confusion, as well as dysequilibrium. To prevent this syndrome, nitrogen is replaced by the less toxic gas helium during deep dives (4).

The precise cause of oxygen toxicity is unknown, but it may result in nausea, vertigo, muscle twitching, auditory and visual disturbances, and sudden convulsions. The minimum depth at which oxygen poisoning may occur is about 40 feet (4). Some toxic symptoms may develop from breathing 100% oxygen at a total pressure as low as 380 mmHg in subatmospheric pressure situations for prolonged periods (e.g., space flight) but data are incomplete (7).

The equilibrium disturbances noted with nitrogen narcosis and oxygen toxicity appear to be related to their CNS effects rather than to any vestibular end-organ dysfunction, but these conditions must be kept in mind by the physician and the diver when dizziness occurs while on the bottom or during descent.

Sudden changes in inspired inert gases at deep depths also may result in vertigo secondary either to end-organ damage or to CNS disturbance (2).

Problems During Decompression (Diving or Aircraft Ascent)

As the diver or flier ascends, gases in the middle ear (and other body cavities) expands, increasing the relative middle ear pressure. If equalization of pressure via the eustachian tube occurs asymmetrically in the two ears, so-called alternobaric

vertigo and nystagmus may result. The precise mechanism for this phenomenon is not clear (5).

Cerebral air embolism is a major CNS catastrophe, in which vestibular symptoms play a minor role. This is caused by the diver failing to exhale adequately during ascent; expanding gasses rupture alveoli, allowing air bubbles to escape into the arterial circulation. Immediate recompression may prevent permanent CNS damage or death.

Inner ear injuries with hearing loss, tinnitus, and/or vertigo may be the major or only manifestation of decompression sickness or the "bends," a condition related to the release of nitrogen bubbles into the bloodstream and other body tissues as its solubility is exceeded during decreasing pressure (2). The greater the depth and the longer the diver remains at that depth, the more nitrogen becomes dissolved and the more slowly the diver must ascend, to allow the bubbles to dissipate and be expired in the lungs; special tables are used to gauge the safe rate of ascent. Other symptoms include itching, paresthesias, joint pain, CNS disturbances (visual problems, paralysis, seizures), and dyspnea (4). Should symptoms occur, prompt recompression is critical if permanent damage is to be avoided. It must be remembered, however, that decompression sickness does not occur in shallow dives (less than 30 feet) no matter how long the submersion or how rapid the ascent, and other causes must be sought for symptoms developing under these conditions. Furthermore, inner ear injury that may have been suffered during descent should bring to mind the possibility of labyrinthine window rupture and recompression is contraindicated (2).

Decompression sickness may occur during aircraft ascent but it is usually less severe than the diving counterpart and rarely produces long-lasting symptoms. Several factors influence the development of subatmospheric "bends." The rate of ascent is less critical than the rate in diving, but the altitude attained and duration of exposure are quite important. For example, decompression symptoms are rare below 20,000 feet, and over 90% of young healthy people can tolerate 1 hour at 35,000 feet without symptoms. After 1 hour at 40,000 feet 20% become symptomatic, and 45% cannot tolerate 35,000 feet for 4 hours (3). Tolerance diminishes with age and with obesity. Exercise increases susceptibility to decompression sickness as does reexposure within 24 hours. This syndrome is effectively prevented by cabin pressurization to less than 25,000 feet. Denitrogenization by breathing 100% oxygen before flight is also helpful. If the syndrome does occur, recompression by simple descent is curative in the great majority of instances. In severe cases compression to pressures greater than one atmosphere may be necessary.

MISCELLANEOUS TRAUMATIC CONDITIONS

BLAST

Blast trauma is defined as injury sustained from a sudden explosion and is dependent on the rate of pressure wave buildup, the intensity of the pressure, and the duration of the pressure wave. Tympanic membrane perforations and middle-ear damage commonly occur, but some degree of sensorineural hearing loss with tinnitus is almost universal. The high frequencies are most severely affected, with a surprisingly strong tendency toward rapid spontaneous improvement over the first few hours. The major recovery is complete within a few days, but some improvement may continue to take place over a period of 6 months. Beyond that time, any residual loss should be considered permanent. Attempts have been made to reduce the amount of permanent hearing loss following blast injury by using steroids, vasodilation, or low molecular weight dextrans, but compelling evidence for their effect is lacking. Vertigo is unusual following exposure to blast and, if present, should raise the suspicion of perilymph fistula.

CLOSED HEAD INJURY WITHOUT TEMPORAL BONE FRACTURES—CONCUSSION

Significant hearing loss and/or vestibular damage may result from head trauma, even without a demonstrable fracture of the temporal bone. The degree of functional impairment is quite variable, depending upon the location and force of the blow. A sensorineural hearing loss maximal around 4 kHz is observed in nearly 50% of patients with skull fractures not involving the temporal bone. In cerebral concussion without skull fractures, the incidence of hearing loss is smaller. Occasionally the loss is purely conductive or mixed. Special audiometric studies may indicate cochlear, retrocochlear, or central pathology. Some improvement may take place in many patients up to 6 months after injury. Fluctuating hearing loss and/or vertigo should always raise the suspicion of perilymph

fistula. The precise mechanisms responsible for the auditory and vestibular depression are unknown. Theoretic proposals include inner ear hemorrhage, with or without pressure waves transmitted through the inner ear fluids to damage the sensory cells.

Vertigo caused by a stretching of the vestibular nerve fibers in the internal auditory meatus is a very common complaint following head injury, and postural nystagmus with or without canal paresis is observed in many cases. Positional vertigo and nystagmus generally disappear within 1 year, and even canal paresis resolves in about half the cases.

Studies correlating histopathology with audiometric and vestibular function data are sparse. Degenerative changes occur in the organ of Corti and cochlear neurons, most marked in the midbasal coil, the area which is responsible for 4–8 kHz. Chronic hyperplastic inflammation and osteogenesis are found in perilymphatic spaces, presumably secondary to intralabyrinthine hemorrhage (8, 6).

LIGHTNING INJURY

The devastating force of lightning may cause temporal bone injury by mechanisms that are as yet unknown. Surviving victims often sustain burns of the external auditory canal, tympanic membrane rupture, ossicular damage, sensorineural hearing loss, vestibular disturbances, and facial nerve injury. In the only lightning-damaged temporal bone to be studied pathologically, Bergstrom (1) found hemorrhage and inflammatory exudate in the middle ear and mastoid, tympanic membrane perforation, rupture of Reissner's membrane, degenerative changes in the stria vascularis, and facial nerve edema within the internal auditory meatus. Such injuries are treated initially by aural hygiene and management of complications such as cerebrospinal fluid otorrhea or infection. Tympanic membrane perforations may be patched with paper or absorbable gelatin film (Gelfilm) after elevation of infolded edges. However, because of the compromised vascularity secondary to the burning of local tissues, definitive tympanoplasty should be deferred for at least 6 months to allow for revascularization. Otherwise, a high percentage of graft failures would be expected. Similar reasoning dictates that cautery of perforation margins be avoided as well. Facial nerve palsy is managed as are other traumatic facial nerve injuries.

REFERENCES

1. Bergstrom L, Neblett L, Sando I et al.: The lightning-damaged ear. Arch Otolaryngol 100:117–121, 1974

2. Farmer JC, Thomas WG, Youngblood DG et al.: Inner ear decompression sickness. Laryngoscope 86:1315–1327, 1976

3. Gillies JA (ed): A Textbook of Aviation Medicine. New York, Pergamon Press, 1965

4. Henry FR: Hyperbaric problems as they relate to divers. Trans Am Acad Ophthalmol Otolaryngol 75: 1322–1332, 1971

5. Ingelstedt S, Ivarsson A, Tjernström O: Vertigo due to relative over-pressure in the middle ear. Acta Otolaryngol (Stockh) 78:1–14, 1974

6. Lindsay JR, Zajtchuk J: Concussion of the inner ear. Trans Am Acad Ophthalmol Otolaryngol 58: 19–103, 1970

7. Randel HW (ed): Aerospace Medicine, 2nd ed. Baltimore, Williams & Wilkins, 1971

8. Schuknecht HF: Pathology of the Ear. Cambridge, MA, Harvard University Press, 1974

SUGGESTED READING

Ballantyne J: Traumatic conductive deafness. In Ballantyne J, Groves J (eds): Scott-Brown's Diseases of the Ear Nose and Throat, 3rd ed. London, Butterworths, 1971

Bauer F: Dislocation of the incus due to head injury. J Laryngol 72:676–682, 1958

Blagoveschenekaya NS, Leushkina LN: Otoneurological symptoms in patients with partial transverse and longitudinal fractures of the pyramids of the temporal bone at the residual period of the craniocerebral trauma. Vestn Otorhinolaringol 34:60–67, 1972

Chalat NI: Middle ear effects of head trauma. Laryngoscope 81:1286–1303, 1971

Dietzel K: Traumaschäden am Hörorgan ohne Fraktur des knöchernen Schädels. Zentralbl Chir 96:1039–1044, 1971

Dudley JP: Cotton applicator: friend or foe? Conn Med 37:187, 1973

Escher F: Funktionelle Ohr Chirurgie traumatischer Mittelhor läsionen. Fortsch Hals Nasen Ohrenheilk 11:1–50, 1964

Farmer JC: Diving injuries to the inner ear. Ann Otol Rhinol Laryngol [Suppl] 86 (36), 1977

Glaninger J: Zur operativen wiederherstellung einer durch Schädeltrauma unterbrochenen Gehörknöchelchenkette. Z Laryngol Rhinol Otol 43:184–190, 1964

Guerrier Y: Le mécanisme des lésions ossiculaires dans les traumatismes fermés du crâne. Acta Oto-Rhino-Laryng Belg. 25:607–614, 1971

Kerr AG: Blast Injury of the Ear. ORL Aug. 11–17, 1975

Marquet J: Considérations sur le diagnostic des surdités de transmission par traumatisme de l'oreille. Acta Otorhinolaryngol Belg 25:641–652, 1971

Martin R, Yonkers AJ, Yarington CT: Perichondritis of the ear. Laryngoscope 86:664–673, 1976

Meunier J-L: Les accidents audiculaires barotraumatiques chez les plongeurs sous-marins. Rev Laryngol Otol Rhinol (Bord) 93:586–594, 1972

Murphy KWR: Head injury and fractures of the ankylosed stapes. J Laryngol 86:169–171, 1972

Pearson BW, Barber HO: Head injury: some otoneurologic sequelae. Arch Otolaryngol 97:81–84, 1973

Podoshin L, Fradis M: Hearing loss after head injury. Arch Otolaryngol 101:15–18, 1975

Tos M: Fractura ossis Temporalis. Ugeskr Laeger 133:1449–1456, 1971

Tos M: Prognosis of hearing loss in temporal bone fractures. J Laryngol 85:1147–1159, 1971

Tos M: Course of and sequelae to 248 petrosal fractures. Acta Otolaryngol (Stockh) 75:353–354, 1973

Ziv M, Philipsohn NC, Leventon G et al.: Blast injury of the ear: treatment and evaluation. Milit Medicine 138:811–813, 1973

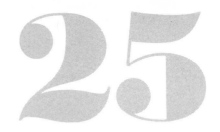

ACOUSTIC TRAUMA AND NOISE-INDUCED HEARING LOSS

The auditory sensitivity of the normal human cochlea is remarkable. However, this extraordinary auditory capability is vulnerable to the effects of acute acoustic trauma and to chronic environmental noise.

In the Middle Ages, people working with metal crafts (cannoneers and blacksmiths) frequently noted hearing loss and tinnitus. A century ago, "boilermaker's deafness" was well known, and its high-tone hearing loss characteristics were recognizable with tuning-fork tests. During the past half-century, increased mechanization and its accompanying noise have caused an inevitable increase in damage to the human ear.

Noise may be simply defined as unwanted sound.

The auditory organ is unable to withstand either acute acoustic trauma or continued or repeated exposures to high-intensity sound without eventual organic damage to the inner ear and the sequelae of hearing loss, tinnitus, occasional vertigo, and occasional nonauditory systemic effects.

The hearing loss produced by acute noise exposure is referred to as **acute acoustic trauma.** The hearing loss produced by chronic noise exposure is referred to as **noise-induced hearing loss.**

Acute acoustic trauma may be unilateral or bilateral. In chronic noise-induced hearing loss, the loss is almost always symmetrical unless modified by some other unrelated otologic problem.

PATHOLOGY

TEMPORAL BONE PATHOLOGY

Haberman (6), in 1890, described the findings in the temporal bones of a metalsmith with hearing loss of high-pitch tones, who was struck and killed by a train because he was unable to hear it. The microscopic study showed absence of hair cells, nerve fibers, and ganglion cells in the cochleas, especially in the basal turns. These classic observations have recently been refined only in details.

Light Microscopy Findings

The primary lesion is in the 8- to 10-mm region of the cochlea within which the 4-kHz pitch area is located. Loss of external hair cells and radial nerve fiber damage are noted (Fig. 25–1).

Electron Microscopy Findings

Lim and Melnick (12) reported a series of guinea-pig noise-exposure experiments utilizing scanning and transmission electron-microscopic studies. They described basal and apical turn lesions due to noise exposure as follows: 1) an increase in the formation of blebs on the surface of sensory cilia; 2) vesiculation proceeding through vacuolization of the smooth endoplasmic reticulum system; 3) heavy accumulation of lysosomal granules in the subcuticular region; 4) deformation of cuticular plates; and 5) eventual cell rupture and lysis (Fig. 25-2). Lim and Melnick pointed out that the space occupied by the destroyed sensory cells was immediately sealed off by processes from neighboring Deiters cells.

Phase Microscopy Findings

The degeneration patterns in human ears exposed to noise were shown by Johnsson and Hawkins in microdissection studies (10). The most common lesion associated with the classic 4-kHz audiometric dip was diffuse degeneration in the 9- to 13-mm area of the basal turn of the cochlea (Fig. 25-3).

Vasoconstriction Factors

Hawkins (7) clarified the role of vasoconstriction in noise-induced hearing loss in terms of hair-cell damage, dissolution of supporting structures of organ of Corti, replacement by a flat, undifferentiated epithelium, and subsequent transganglionic degeneration of afferent cochlear nerve fibers (Fig. 25–4). With only 8 hours of noise exposure at 118–120 dB, a permanent impairment with hair-cell loss was noted. Prolonged hypoxia causes degeneration of capillaries and hair cells.

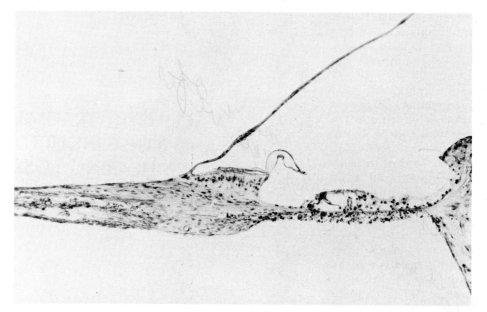

FIG. 25–1. Acoustic trauma. Note loss of outer hair cells in organ of Corti from basal turn. (Gussen R: Ann Otol Rhinol Laryngol 81:235–240, 1972)

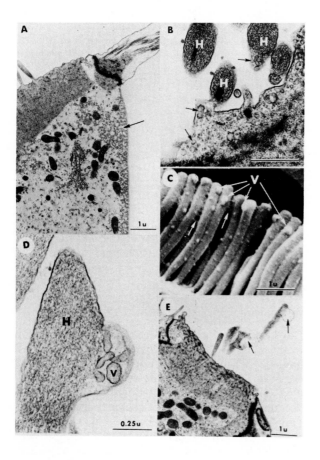

FIG. 25–2. A. Scanning electron micrograph showing vesicles **(V)** in sensory hairs of inner cells at apex of cochlea. **Arrow,** string-like structures connecting sensory hairs (300–600 Hz, 4-hour exposure). **B.** Transmission electron micrograph showing vesicles in sensory hairs of inner hair cell in basal turn (300–600 Hz, 6-hour exposure). **C.** Ruptured sensory hairs of inner cell **(arrows)** in basal turn (300–600 Hz, 24-hour exposure, 17 days' recuperation). **D.** Transmission electron micrograph of upper part of outer hair cell **(H)** showing early state of vesiculation at basal turn **(arrow)** (300–600 Hz, 4-hour exposure). **E.** Trapped vesicles **(arrows)** in cuticular plate and also inside sensory hairs at apical turn (300–600 Hz, 4-hour exposure). (Lim DJ, Melnick W: Arch Otolaryngol 94:294–305, 1971. Copyright 1971, American Medical Association)

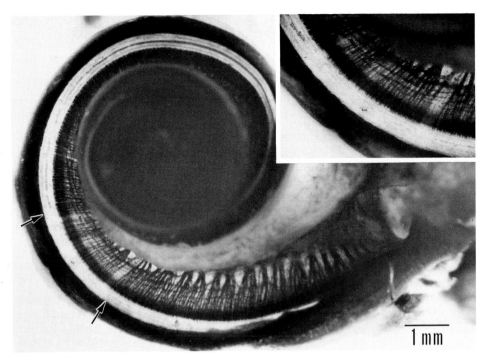

FIG. 25–3. Left cochlea. Note lesion in second quadrant between **arrows (insert)** with three small sectors of nerve degeneration corresponding to three areas of complete absence of organ of Corti (OsO$_1$). (Johnsson L-G, Hawkins JE: Trans Am Otol Soc 64:52–66, 1976)

FIG. 25–4. Capillary vasoconstrictions in outer spiral vessel, with trapped red cells **(arrow)** directly beneath the hair cells. Noise exposure, 188–120 dB for 8 hours. (Hawkins JE: Ann Otol Rhinol Laryngol 80:903–913, 1971)

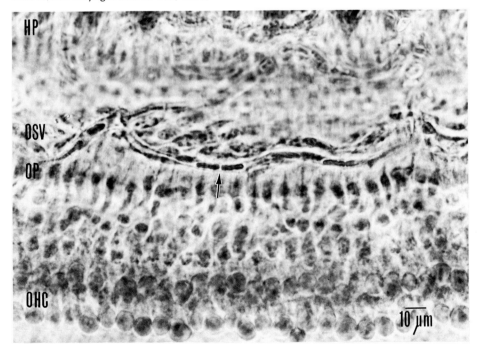

AUDITORY PATHOPHYSIOLOGY

Acute Acoustic Trauma

One of two things may happen as a result of high-level intensity acute-noise exposure. If it is of great magnitude, as exemplified by blast or percussive noise, a tympanic membrane rupture will occur. In such instances, the very rupture may act as a "safety valve" to prevent what would otherwise have been greater damage to the cochlea. In acute acoustic trauma without tympanic membrane rupture, cochlear losses may be total, severe, or moderate.

In acute acoustic trauma resulting from short intense exposures, the basic changes are due to mechanical damage caused by excessive vibration of the organ of Corti by high-amplitude noise levels, and consist of outer hair-cell damage in the basal turn, close to the oval window. In longer exposures, there will be total destruction of the organ of Corti, with rupture of Reissner's membrane.

Chronic Noise-Induced Hearing Loss

In chronic noise-induced hearing loss, the mechanism of a progressive series of traumatic excitations results in an asymmetrical amplitude of displacement of the basilar membrane, which conforms to the basic traveling-wave hypothesis of Von Békésy (18). The 4-kHz region in the basal turn of the cochlea is the most vulnerable area. According to Lehnhardt (11), the phenomenon is due to the fact that those regions of the basilar membrane whose characteristic vibration frequencies are higher than the frequency of the stimulating tone are shaken more vigorously than regions having a lower characteristic frequency —namely, those at the cochlear apex. Therefore, all components of a mixed-frequency noise source below the 4-kHz region will contribute and add their effects to that area. The same may not be true for higher-frequency noise sources.

In the early phase of chronic noise-induced hearing loss, the patient may not be aware of hearing loss subjectively, with the exception of speech discrimination problems in the presence of background noise. The first audiometric finding is usually a 4-kHz "notch." With progression of the hearing loss, this early notch begins to spread into lower frequencies (3 kHz, 2 kHz, and 1 kHz), and into higher frequencies (5 kHz and 6 kHz). As the degree of hearing loss increases in speech reception threshold decibel levels, the hearing capability for ordinary speech, even in quiet areas, decreases. The loss is noticed particularly in consonant identification and in increasing communication difficulties in noisy environments.

CLINICAL ASPECTS

ACUTE ACOUSTIC TRAUMA

The history of the patient with acute acoustic trauma is chronologically definitive. The onset of the sudden hearing loss and tinnitus is related to a single incident or to a short-time episode, which may be exposure to sudden intense noise with or without blast, explosion, or direct cranial or ear trauma. Vertigo may be mentioned as a transient symptom at a time of the acute acoustic trauma.

In acute acoustic trauma, the patient is usually examined in a matter of hours or a few days after onset. There may be otoscopic evidence of vascular congestion in the tympanic membrane. In acute acoustic trauma associated with blast injury there may be tympanic membrane perforation and possible ossicular damage, as well as cochleovestibular damage. A labyrinth window (oval or round window) fistula can result from acute acoustic trauma, and will be characterized by perilymph leak surrounded by fibrous webs.

The audiologic sequelae of sudden acoustic trauma may range from a 4-kHz notch to major losses in all frequencies above 500 Hz. This pure tone loss will be accompanied by concomitant losses in speech reception threshold and speech discrimination score. In some instances there will be total loss (anacusis). Spontaneous nystagmus may be present, and caloric electronystagmography responses may be greatly diminished.

In the differential diagnosis of acute acoustic trauma, the history of sudden hearing loss following exposure to intense noise or blast is of primary importance. In differential diagnosis all of the etiologic factors included in the sudden hearing loss syndrome must be considered (see Ch. 37, Sudden Hearing Loss Syndrome). If the acute acoustic trauma incident is accompanied by obvious damage to the tympanic membrane, appropriate management of the injury is indicated (see Ch. 17, Otomastoiditis Surgery—Mastoidectomy and Tympanoplasty).

In total anacusis, immediate surgical exploration is indicated to locate a possible round window or oval window perilymph fistula (see Ch. 37). If such a fistula is present, early surgical intervention with fistula repair may result in some hearing gain. Even if there is a long delay (4–8 weeks) between onset and time of examination in total anacusis dating from acute acoustic trauma, middle ear exploration is indicated. While hearing improvement is unlikely in late fistula repair, it is important to explore and repair a fistula, even at a late date, from the point of view of preventing possible subsequent intracranial infection.

CHRONIC NOISE-INDUCED HEARING LOSS

The history of a patient with chronic noise-induced hearing loss may be vague. The presenting complaint may be tinnitus with a secondary complaint of hearing loss. This is especially true in a patient with classic bilateral 4-kHz notch losses with relatively good hearing in the other frequencies. Vertigo is a rare complaint, and nonauditory symptoms are uncommon. Otoscopic findings are usually normal unless there is another unrelated otologic disease.

Auditory sequelae of noise-induced hearing loss are 1) specific 4-kHz notch hearing loss; 2) speech reception threshold changes; 3) recruitment of loudness; and 4) diplacusis.

Tota and Bocci (17) reported a correlation between eye color and auditory fatigue. Blue-eyed subjects showed greater noise fatigability than brown-eyed subjects. Hood, Poole, and Freedman (8) have confirmed these findings. Their studies suggest that for stimulus intensities below 110 dB such iris melanin relationships apply to auditory adaptation and that fatigue effects become apparent at noise levels above 110 dB.

There is a variation in individual susceptibility to noise-induced hearing loss. Temporary auditory fatigue produced by brief noise exposures produces a **temporary threshold shift,** the term now used to describe such auditory effects that produce no permanent damage. Long duration of exposure to noise produces a permanent hearing loss, described as **permanent threshold shift.**

Many studies have been made in attempts to relate temporary threshold shift measurements with eventual permanent threshold shift sequelae. There are differences of opinion with reference to such relationships numerically. The development of permanent threshold shift changes, however, is almost always due to repetitive temporary threshold shift episodes.

The earliest audiometric finding may be a slight notch at 4 kHz (Fig. 25–5A). With further noise-induced hearing damage, the audiologic findings change with widening and deepening of the 4-kHz notch (Fig. 25–5B). However, there are variations in this susceptibility area in patients whose major noise-induced hearing loss notches occur at

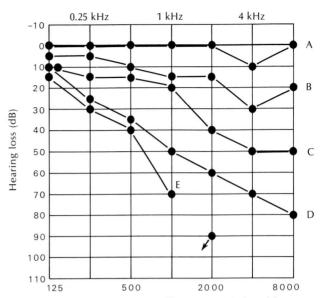

FIG. 25–5. Five audiometric profiles in noise-induced hearing loss. **A.** Slight notch at 4 kHz (**SDS,** 96%). **B.** Widening and deepening of 4-kHz notch (**SDS,** 80%). **C.** Major hearing loss at 5 or 6 Hz (**SRS,** 70%). **D.** Deepening loss over period of years with shift to left (**SDS,** 60%). **E.** Complete loss of high-frequency perception (**SDS,** 30%).

5 kHz, or 6 kHz, and occasionally at 3 kHz, or 2 kHz (Fig. 25–5C).

With longer exposures to noise, usually over a period of years, the 4-kHz notch not only deepens, but there is a shift to the left of the audiometric profile with losses at 3 kHz, 2 kHz, and 1 kHz (Fig. 25–5D). The shift to the left in the lower frequencies is also accompanied by a lesser shift to the right, with losses at the 5-kHz, 6-kHz, and 8-kHz regions. As the losses increase and the notch shifts into the shape of a "valley," eventually all high-frequency perception may be completely lost (Fig. 25–5E).

The diagnosis of noise-induced hearing loss is based primarily upon the history of exposure to noise with a 4-kHz notch and its variants. Such bilateral audiologic findings, unaccompanied by other significant otoscopic or x-ray findings, usually are diagnostic. However, differential diagnostic considerations are extremely important in patients with noise-induced hearing loss. Too frequently the false assumption is made that a history of noise exposure and a high frequency audiometric notch constitutes clear evidence of noise-induced hearing loss. It is possible for other conditions to coexist and be missed, unless a high index of suspicion regarding differential diagnosis accompanies the diagnosis of noise-induced hearing loss.

A number of causes other than noise can produce comparable notches. Head injuries with or without fractures or concussion may produce comparable hearing losses. A number of both congenital and postnatal genetic and acquired cochlear lesions (rubella, rubeola, influenza, mumps, etc.) can produce high-frequency notches in a person who also may have a history of noise exposure. Consideration should be given also to exposure to industrial chemicals, and to effects of ototoxic drugs (see Ch. 39, Ototoxicity). The quantification of the contributions of other possible etiologic factors is extremely difficult.

The presbycusis problem poses serious differential diagnostic responsibilities in relative assessment of hearing loss due to noise and hearing loss due to age (see Ch. 40, Systemic Adult Sensorineural Hearing Losses, and Ch. 41, Presbycusis).

Both urban and agricultural community environmental noise (sociocusis) can produce hearing losses, and must be reckoned with in all differential diagnostic considerations.

A patient may appear for examination and report a clear-cut noise-exposure history. However, a careful assessment of the audiologic findings may show asymmetry. Radiographic studies may show an ipsilateral enlarged or eroded internal auditory canal on Stenver's or polytome views. Thus, as an example, a patient may have a coexistent eighth nerve schwannoma that plays a role in ipsilateral tinnitus accentuation. Similarly, a patient with noise-induced hearing loss and tinnitus may also have recently received an ototoxic drug, which has added to the hearing loss and tinnitus. Thus, a history of noise-induced hearing loss does not eliminate the need for a complete oto-audiologic study. A patient with a clear-cut history, typical audiometric findings, and negative otoscopic findings all indicating noise-induced hearing loss still deserves a complete otologic examination. This should include temporal bone x-rays (mastoid and internal auditory canal views). In cases of audiometric asymmetry, electronystagmographic vestibular studies and polytome radiographs are also indicated, even if there are no complaints of vertigo.

There is no treatment for noise-induced hearing loss. While a temporary threshold shift is spontaneously reversible, a permanent threshold shift is irreversible. There is no effective medication for either the hearing loss or tinnitus. The primary management lies in prevention or reduction of further noise exposure and measures designed to assist in habilitation. The individual with far advanced hearing loss may require amplification through using a hearing aid and training in speech (lip) reading.

The tinnitus problem in noise-induced hearing loss requires careful clinical judgment and management (see Ch. 42, Tinnitus). There is no specific treatment for tinnitus.

The patient with a diagnosis of noise-induced hearing loss should be counseled regarding further noise exposure, not only from the basic cause (industrial or military), but with reference to other causes of such loss unrelated to the patient's occupation. Thus, the patient should avoid exposure to loud music, to motorcycle noise, firearm use, and to the noise of hobby workshop machinery.

Additional cochlear insult possibilities should be explained to the patient, and the patient should recognize a personal responsibility for assuming prevention of additional cochlear damage. The high-risk aspect of the cochlear lesion should be thoroughly explained, since most patients are completely ignorant of the irreversible effects of noise upon hearing.

Hearing "protectors" have been in use for a number of decades, in industry and in the military. There are no devices that offer complete protection from the ubiquitous noise sources in our society.

The two major types of protectors are muffs and plugs. Ear plugs are most commonly in use in industry, military exposure, and sports. Variable degrees of acoustic attenuation are provided by plugs, and greater attenuation by muffs. The combination of plugs and muffs affords the best possible protection from unavoidable high noise levels.

INDUSTRIAL NOISE

Occupational hearing loss can be defined as a hearing impairment of one or both ears, partial or complete, arising in or during the course of one's employment. Both acoustic trauma and noise-induced hearing loss may be due to industrial noise.

In 1969 the US Department of Labor established noise criteria guidelines in industry under the Walsh-Healy Act. The Occupational Safety and Health Act (OSHA) became effective in April 1971 and applies to all safety and health aspects of workers producing supplies, services, and materials in interstate commerce. Both the OSHA and the Walsh-Healey Act define hazardous noise exposure and make recommendations for noise reduction measures, personal ear protection, and the establishment of hearing testing programs.

MEGAAMPLIFICATION OF MUSIC

A change in our music culture during the last decade has produced a new problem in terms of noise-induced hearing loss—namely, that related to "hard rock" music, "pop" groups, and "discotheque" music. These problems have been encountered and studied in all parts of the world.

In a recent study from Norway, Flottorp (2) pointed out that the typical feature of modern pop music is its very narrowed dynamic range. The level of the average rock group is one that exceeds the normal maximum level of a symphony orchestra. Loud speakers which may be as close as 1 m to the listeners result in a sound pressure level at the listener's ear of 120–130 dB.

Both temporary threshold shifts and permanent threshold shifts have been measured not only in rock musicians but in members of the audience.

Reddell and Lebo (13) pointed out in a recent study of the ototraumatic effects of hard rock music that in some instances it is possible to prevent serious cochlear damage by the use of attenuation of amplification to safe levels and by the use of appropriate ear-protection devices.

Jathko and Hellman (9) studied the problem of acoustic trauma in orchestra musicians and found significant hearing losses, primarily in those professional musicians playing in loud-music orchestras utilizing powerful amplifiers and speakers. Such high-frequency losses also may occur in musicians in vulnerable orchestral positions, in which they are subjected to acoustic trauma from brass instruments (trumpets and trombones) and percussion instruments.

ENVIRONMENTAL AND COMMUNITY NOISE

A study by Rosen and co-workers (14) among the Mabaans, a primitive African tribe living in an environment of low psychic stress and extremely low sound pressure levels, has indicated singular freedom from presbycusis, even among the very aged (also significant is the low incidence of coronary arteriosclerotic heart disease in this tribe). Rosen and colleagues hypothesize that the presbycusis seen in civilized countries may well be the cumulative result of a lifetime of exposure to sound pressure levels that, in the ordinary sense, we would not consider traumatic.

Noise pollution has become a common concern of all members of society, and noise abatement methods have received a great deal of attention from public health authorities, acoustic physicists, and audiologists. The noise problem is complex and is related to the increase in labor-saving machinery and in transportation. The control of noise at the source—e.g., design of buildings and in community planning—is the primary approach to noise abatement in community life.

In a recent study of sound power and mechanical power, Shaw (16) compared the relative effects of some transportation vehicles, recreational machines, and power tools.

In dealing with the problem of monitoring community noise, Branch, Gilman, and Weber (1) described the significance and requirements of monitoring outdoor noise pollution of urban environments and identified the potentialities of using regular telephone networks for noise monitoring with electronic and data-processing components.

Such studies illustrate the enormity of the problem of environmental noise and its effect upon society.

CONSTITUTIONAL NONAUDITORY EFFECTS OF NOISE

Schiff (15) pointed out that noise can alter EEG patterns during sleep. The rapid-eye-movement stage of sleep patterns can be interrupted by noise levels as low as 50 dB.

Physiological nonauditory effects of noise include peripheral vaso-constriction and increased depth and diminished rate of respiration. There may also be endocrine and glandular stress responses to environmental noise. Increase in urinary catecholamines have been reported as a response to loud and long noise exposure with resultant blood pressure elevation and decreased peripheral circulation. Geber (3, 4) reported that noise stress produced developmental anomalies following exposure of the gravid woman, apparently related to maternal hormone changes producing reduced fetal blood flow and biochemical disturbances that result in teratogenic changes.

In a summary of multiple aspects of noise exposure, Glorig (5) pointed out that undesirable nonauditory effects can occur in sound fields with sound pressures of 120–150 dB or higher, which cannot be prevented by ear protection. In addition, intense noise with a spectrum primarily in the area below 1 kHz can be felt (tactile) as well as heard. The respiratory system is affected in the 40- to 60-Hz range because of resonant characteristics of the chest. In spite of these findings, Glorig (5) states: "As far as we can determine from industrial records, we can find no increase in cardiovascular problems or ulcers, or both, and no increase in fatigue or irritability or tendencies to nervousness."

It appears, therefore, that nonauditory effects are not always clearly defined. The effects of stress, fatigue, and vertigo are difficult to quantify. In noise sources unrelated to industry, an enormous range of environmental noises can affect all individuals in our contemporary noise filled society.

SUMMARY

The human ear and its neural pathways are susceptible to damage by noise, resulting either in acute acoustic trauma or noise-induced hearing loss.

Noise-induced hearing loss is an increasingly frequent problem for the individual as well as for society.

The essential management is prevention.

Sociocusis, a new term identifying the societal sequelae of noise "pollution," indicates the pervasiveness of the problem.

REFERENCES

1. Branch M, Gilman S, Weber C: Monitoring community noise. AIP Journal 10:266–273, 1974
2. Flottorp G: Music—a noise hazard? Acta Otolaryngol (Stockh) 75:345–347, 1973
3. Geber WF: Developmental effects of chronic maternal audiovisual stress on the rat fetus. J Embryol Exp Morphol 16:1–16, 1966
4. Geber WF: Vascular and Tetratogenic Effects of Chronic Intermittent Noise Stress. Presented at the AAAS Symposium on Non-Auditory Effects of Noise, Boston, Dec. 28–30, 1969
5. Glorig A: Noise exposure—Facts and myths. Trans Am Acad Ophthalmol Otolaryngol 75:1254–1262, 1971
6. Haberman J: Ueber die Schwerhörigkeit der Kesselschmiede. Arch Ohrenheilk 30:1–25, 1890
7. Hawkins JE: The role of vasoconstriction in noise induced hearing loss. Ann Otol Rhinol Laryngol 80:903–913, 1971
8. Hood JD, Poole JP, Freedman L: The influence of eye color upon temporary threshold shift. Audiology 15:449–464, 1976
9. Jathko K, Hellman H: Zur Frage des Larm—und Klangtraumas des Orchestermusikers. HNO 20:21–29, 1972
10. Johnsson L-G, Hawkins JE: Degeneration patterns in human ears exposed to noise. Trans Am Otolaryngol Soc 64:52–66, 1976
11. Lehnhardt E: The C^5-dip: its interpretation in the light of generally known physiological concepts. Int Audiol 6:86, 1967
12. Lim DJ, Melnick W: Acoustic damage of the cochlear. Arch Otolaryngol 94:294–305, 1961
13. Reddell R, Lebo C: Ototraumatic effects of hard rock music. Calif Med 116:1–4, 1972
14. Rosen S, Bergman M, Plester D et al.: Presbycusis study of a relatively noise-free population in the Sudan. Ann Otol Rhinol Laryngol 71:727–743, 1962
15. Schiff M: Non-auditory effects of noise. Trans Am Acad Ophthalmol Otolaryngol 77:ORL 348–ORL 398, 1973
16. Shaw E: Noise pollution—What can be done? Physics Today; Jan. 46–58, 1975
17. Tota G, Bocci G: The importance of the color of the iris on the evaluation of resistance to auditory fatigue. Rev Otoneurooftalmol (Bologna) 42:183–192, 1967
18. Von Békésy G: Experiments in Hearing. New York, McGraw-Hill, 1960

SUGGESTED READING

Altman MM, Shenhav R, Schaudinischky LH: Semi-objective method for auditory mass screening of neonates. Acta Otolaryngol (Stockh) 79:46–50, 1975

Ollendorff F, Schaudinischky LH, Rosenhouse G: Noise level threshold for wakening and wake-up dependence on noise level. Acustica 32:100–103, 1975

Shaudinischky LH: About the effect of high-frequency-audio-sound on the hearing and wellbeing of people. Inter-Noise 75 Sendai, Aug, 27–29, 1975, pp 191–198

Schaudinischky LH: Sound, Man and Building. Essex, England, Applied Science Publishers, 1976

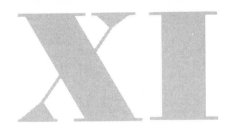

XI

DIZZINESS AND VERTIGO

26

PERIPHERAL VERTIGO, LABYRINTHITIS, AND MENIERE'S DISEASE

VICTOR GOODHILL
IRWIN HARRIS

Peripheral vertigo is due either to intralabyrinthine or extralabyrinthine causes. Lesions that are either intralabyrinthine or extralabyrinthine may involve 1) both cochlear and vestibular sense organs, (cochleovestibular) or 2) vestibular sense organs alone (vestibular disorders) (Fig. 26–1).

The general term labyrinthitis is frequently used to describe labyrinthine vertigo or peripheral vertigo. Labyrinthitis, however, is not always a correct term since many of the lesions are not inflammatory. True labyrinthitis does occur and will be discussed under the heading of Otomastoiditis and Labyrinthine Complications. True labyrinthitis may also occur following surgical procedures and/or trauma involving the labyrinth.

Meniere's disease, a common intralabyrinthine cause of episodic peripheral vertigo and fluctuant cochlear hearing loss is discussed separately.

COCHLEOVESTIBULAR DISORDERS

Cochleovestibular disorders, which usually produce auditory symptoms and findings (hearing loss and tinnitus), in addition to vestibular symptoms and findings (vertigo and nystagmus), may occur in the labyrinth (intralabyrinthine) or may occur medial to the labyrinth (extralabyrinthine, retrolabyrinthine).

The prototype intralabyrinthine auditory-vestibular disorder is Meniere's disease. A number of other lesions can mimic Meniere's disease.

Because the facial nerve accompanies the eighth nerve through the petrosa of the temporal bone, the internal auditory canal, and the cerebellopontine angle, seventh nerve symptoms and findings may accompany either intralabyrinthine or extralabyrinthine lesions.

The most significant extralabyrinthine lesions causing cochleovestibular disorders are eighth nerve tumors and lesions of the cerebellopontine angle.

Vestibular disorders producing only vertigo and nystagmus consist also of intralabyrinthine lesions (uncommon) and extralabyrinthine lesions such as viral vestibular neuronitis.

INTRALABYRINTHINE LESIONS

MENIERE'S DISEASE

Meniere's disease is a very common cause of peripheral labyrinthine vertigo. It is an intralabyrinthine disease of the endolymphatic vestibular viscera, accompanied by endolymphatic hydrops of the scala media and very frequently of the saccule, utricle, and semicircular canal systems. It is characterized by episodic attacks of vertigo, fluctuating cochlear hearing loss, and fluctuating tinnitus. (Details are given in a special section on the disease later in this chapter.)

OTOSCLEROSIS AND COMPLICATIONS OF OTOSCLEROSIS SURGERY

Otosclerosis and/or the complications of otosclerosis surgery may produce cochleovestibular syndromes comparable to those of Meniere's disease.

In the early stage of otosclerosis, the most common two symptoms are tinnitus and slowly developing hearing loss. In some patients, vertigo is present. Occasional vestibular abnormalities will be demonstrated on electronystagmographic examination. As the disease matures in time and in severity, vertigo usually disappears.

The primary surgery for otosclerosis is stapedectomy, which may be accompanied by peroperative and postoperative vertigo. In most instances, however, such vertigo is transitory. Persistent vertigo following otosclerosis surgery or delayed sudden vertigo occurring at any time following otosclerosis surgery is almost always a sign of labyrinth fistula or a granuloma. This calls for

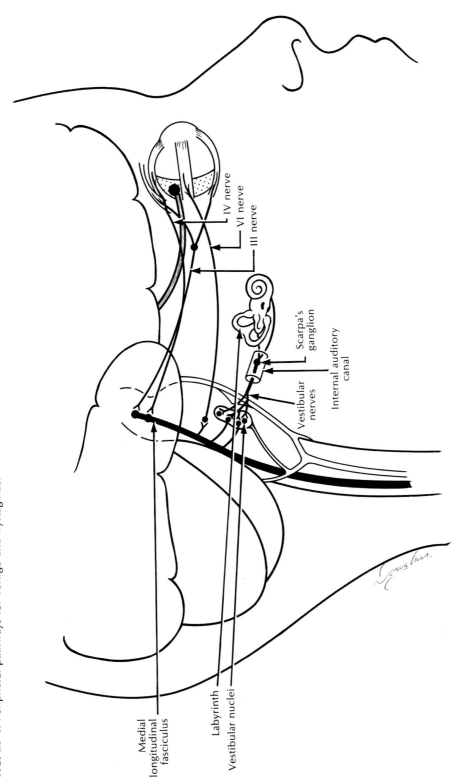

FIG. 26–1. Peripheral pathways for vertigo and nystagmus.

IV nerve

VI nerve

III nerve

Scarpa's
ganglion

Internal auditory
canal

Vestibular
nerves

Medial
longitudinal
fasciculus

Labyrinth

Vestibular nuclei

consideration of immediate exploratory surgery since cochlear function may well depend upon prompt surgical intervention.

Vertigo (usually mild) following stapes surgery (with removal of stapedial footplate and disturbance of the vestibular fluid system) is a routine expectation in stapes surgery. In the absence of complications, such vertigo subsides within 48 hours.

A persistent oval window fistula can result in persistent positional vertigo caused by utricular and/or saccular irritation.

Infrequently a middle ear granuloma forms and can extend into the vestibule. The diagnosis of an oval window fistula or a granuloma is made by prompt surgical reexploration of the operated ear (see Ch. 19, Otosclerosis).

OTOMASTOIDITIS AND LABYRINTHINE COMPLICATIONS

Tubotympanitis

The acute tubotympanitis accompanying an upper respiratory infection usually causes only fullness and conductive hearing loss, but can cause vertigo. Such vertigo is probably due either to vestibular response asymmetry or to asymmetry in degree of left/right tubotympanitis. Negative middle ear air pressure can change labyrinth window pressures and provoke vestibular response. Such vertigo subsides promptly upon treatment of the eustachian tube blockade.

Acute Otomastoiditis

Acute otomastoiditis is not a common cause of vertigo, but it does occur. More commonly, mild vertigo will accompany secretory otitis media rather than acute otomastoiditis.

Chronic Otitis Media (Perforata)

Otitis perforata (quiescent or draining) can cause vertigo as a result of the caloric effect of cool air upon the exposed oval and round window regions. Such vertigo usually stops when the ear canal is occluded with cotton or when the patient is away from wind or air conditioning. If it persists, labyrinthitis must be considered.

Otomastoiditis and Labyrinthitis

Labyrinthine vertigo can follow either acute or chronic otomastoiditis. Invasion of the labyrinth can occur directly through the oval or round windows, through erosion of the bony otic cap-

sule, or via retrograde thrombophlebitic routes. Diffuse or circumscribed types of labyrinthitis occur, and a continuum between "serous" (nonpurulent) and purulent varieties produces varying pathologic lesions and symptoms.

Invasion of the labyrinth by an inflammatory reaction is usually manifested by vertigo, nystagmus, hearing impairment, nausea, and vomiting. The vertigo is rotatory-horizontal, accompanied by manifest or occult nystagmus.

A clinical differentiation between serous and suppurative labyrinthitis is the return of normal auditory and vestibular function in the serous form of labyrinthitis, a reversible inflammation with recovery of function. In suppurative labyrinthitis there is a permanent loss of function. (Since the pathology of serous labyrinthitis has not been well documented by temporal bone pathology studies, the term nonsuppurative will be used).

NONSUPPURATIVE LABYRINTHITIS. In acute otomastoiditis the inflammatory process in mastoid air cells and bone can extend to labyrinthine structures, producing an inflammatory labyrinthitis. This will frequently subside following antibiotic therapy and/or appropriate mastoid surgery. If the process localizes within the bony labyrinth, a circumscribed labyrinthitis develops. A circumscribed labyrinthitis due to bony capsule osteitis can produce irritative labyrinthitis, with similar symptoms. If the disease continues, an erosion of the bony capsule of the labyrinth occurs, producing labyrinthine fistula, an uncommon sequela of acute nonsuppurative labyrinthitis.

SUPPURATIVE LABYRINTHITIS. Suppurative labyrinthitis may follow acute or chronic otomastoiditis and usually is due to antibiotic-resistant otomastoiditis. Purulent exudate in vestibular and cochlear labyrinths results in a partial or total nonresponsive cochlea. Vestibular testing similarly reveals a nonresponsive vestibular labyrinth.

Intensive antibiotic therapy and mastoid surgery are described in Chapter 18, Complications of Otomastoiditis. Intralabyrinthine surgery is indicated in the presence of concomitant meningitis or epidural abscess.

LABYRINTHINE FISTULA. Labyrinthine fistula due to erosion of the bony capsule presents the characteristic findings of a positive fistula sign. This is an evoked nystagmus induced by pressure change as transmitted through the external auditory canal to the middle ear. It can be produced (most efficiently) with positive or negative pneumatic otoscopy. The direction and form of the nystagmus depends upon the lesion. The size and position of the fistula in relation to labyrinth structures, and the presence of granulations, keratoma, polyps, etc., will influence electronystagmographic findings. A positive fistula sign in the presence of otomastoid disease is an indication for surgical intervention (see Ch. 18, Complications of Otomastoiditis).

TUMORS

Tympanic glomus tumors usually produce pulsating tinnitus, hearing loss, and occasional pain. Vertigo may be a primary symptom in some patients, but it is not a common problem in glomus tumors. However, an acute hemorrhage in a glomus tumor can be accompanied by sudden episodic vertigo.

External and middle ear carcinoma can produce vertigo in addition to otorrhea, pain, and hearing loss if there is invasion of the labyrinthine windows or fistulization.

Intralabyrinthine tumors are less common than extralabyrinthine (internal auditory meatus) tumors. A slowly growing neurolemmoma (schwannoma) or meningioma within the vestibule will cause hearing loss, but only occasionally will vertigo occur.

The common "acoustic (eighth nerve) neurinoma" (vestibular schwannoma) produces vestibular findings but rarely produces severe vertigo. However, it may produce symptoms clinically similar to those of labyrinthitis or Meniere's disease.

EAR TRAUMA

Barotrauma

Barotrauma, due either to airplane travel or to water sports, produces labyrinthine symptoms under a number of conditions. Nitrogen embolization in scuba diving will produce auditory and vestibular labyrinthine symptoms, usually temporary, occasionally permanent. Labyrinthine window ruptures may accompany nitrogen embolization or may occur separately. In aircraft flight, under conditions of either rapid descent or "clear air turbulence" or in the presence of tubotympanitis, barotrauma may affect the middle ear with or without rupture of the tympanic membrane. It may produce inner ear membrane ruptures with acute vertigo. The vertigo is frequently accompanied by hearing loss and constitutional symptoms of nausea and vomiting. Both hearing loss and vertigo can be transitory or permanent (see Ch. 24, Traumatic Diseases of the Ear and Temporal Bone and Ch. 37, Sudden Hearing Loss Syndrome).

Spontaneous Labyrinthine Window and Labyrinthine Membrane Ruptures

Physical stress-induced labyrinthine window and/or intralabyrinthine membrane ruptures have been described recently (13, 14). Hearing loss and vertigo may occur simultaneously or separately. The vertigo may be as severe as that seen in acute episodic Meniere's disease, accompanied by nausea and vomiting and brisk manifest nystagmus. Spontaneous healing of membranes may occur with bedrest. In some instances prompt surgical intervention and repair of an obvious oval or round window fistula will be effective in control of the vertigo. Hearing improvements are variable (see Ch. 37, Sudden Hearing Loss Syndrome).

Temporal Bone Fractures

In transverse fractures of the temporal bone, due to automobile accident or other causes of head injury, the labyrinth will be involved more frequently than in longitudinal fractures. Severe vertigo with severe or total hearing loss is not uncommon with such injuries. In milder injuries, labyrinthine "concussion" may occur, with transitory auditory-vestibular symptoms (see Ch. 24, Traumatic Diseases of the Ear and Temporal Bone).

Traumatic Rupture of the Tympanic Membrane

Traumatic tympanic membrane ruptures produced by self-inflicted manipulation of cotton-tipped wooden applicators, hairpins, and other foreign bodies, or trauma produce hearing loss and vertigo in many cases. The vertigo severity is related to the extent of middle ear and inner ear damage in addition to the tympanic membrane defect itself (see Ch. 24, Traumatic Diseases of the Ear and Temporal Bone).

Acute Acoustic Trauma and Chronic Noise-Induced Hearing Loss

Acute severe acoustic trauma such as produced by gunfire close to the external auditory canal can cause major hearing loss, frequently accompanied by severe vertigo.

Chronic noise-induced hearing loss may occur either as a result of industrial or community environmental noise, but in some patients, varying degrees of vertigo are also present (see Ch. 25, Acoustic Trauma and Noise-Induced Hearing Loss).

OSTEODYSTROPHIES AND GRANULOMAS

A number of granulomas and bony dystrophies can invade any portion of the temporal bone. Paget's disease, histiocytosis X, osteogenesis imperfecta, and other granulomatous and osteolytic lesions involving the middle ear, labyrinthine windows, or the labyrinth itself can produce the triad of hearing loss, tinnitus, and vertigo. Acute vertigo is not common, but electronystagmographic responses to caloric tests may be abnormal.

VIROPATHIES

Postmumps labyrinthitis is the prototype of all other labyrinthine viropathies. Hearing loss, tinnitus, and vertigo in varying degrees accompany minor and major viral invasions of the labyrinth.

A nonspecific "viral labyrinthitis" is frequently described clinically and is often confused with viral vestibular neuronitis or with benign paroxysmal positional vertigo. It is possible, however, that true viral "serous" labyrinthitis may accompany certain upper respiratory infections. There is scant histopathologic confirmation for such a diagnosis. Clinically, however, episodic vertigo may occur in the course of a viral upper respiratory infection or shortly thereafter. Most commonly, the symptoms are confined to vertigo; hearing loss and tinnitus are relatively uncommon. It is quite likely that most of these "viral labyrinthitis" cases are probably not true labyrinthine lesions but represent inflammatory lesions related either to tubotympanitis and asymmetric middle ear intratympanic pressures or to viral vestibular neuronitis.

SYPHILIS

Neither congenital nor acquired syphilis is rare. Syphilis, the "great imitator," can produce vertigo with hearing loss and tinnitus similar to that seen in Meniere's disease. However, acute attacks are not common. A subacute dysequilibrium is more commonly the accompaniment of luetic temporal bone lesions. Bilateral peripheral vestibular end organ paralysis is frequently found on electro-nystagmographic studies in temporal bone syphilis, in spite of the facts that the vertigo may be completely absent and the patient may never have had a history of vertiginous episodes.

DRUG OTOTOXICITY

A number of antibiotics, diuretics, and antioncologic chemicals have ototoxic properties, frequently with accompanying renal sequelae. Aminoglycosides can act on vestibular and cochlear sensory cells. Toxicity is related to high concentration and long half-life in perilymph as compared with blood.

The antibiotic drugs that may cause ototoxicity when given parenterally include streptomycin, dihydrostreptomycin, gentamicin, neomycin, paromomycin—all of which belong to the aminoglycoside group. Vancomycin, which is chemically similar to the aminoglycosides, viomycin, and capreomycin are being investigated as to ototoxicity. Vertigo may occur alone or may be accompanied by tinnitus and hearing loss with many of these drugs.

HEREDITARY OR ACQUIRED CONGENITAL COCHLEOVESTIBULAR SYNDROMES

A number of congenital hereditary or acquired cochleovestibular lesions can produce varying degrees of hearing loss, tinnitus, and vertigo.

The vertigo is probably related etiologically to a Tullio-like effect produced by high-level hearing-aid amplification in some instances. Such acute vertiginous episodes may be accompanied by spontaneous nystagmus.

Such episodes of vertigo can also occur sporadically, unrelated to hearing aid use, in both pediatric and adult cases. They are due either to progression of the endolabyrinthine lesion (e.g., hydrops, vascular occlusions or hemorrhages), or to associated otitis media. The vertigo may simulate that of Meniere's disease in such cases.

HERPES ZOSTER OTICUS

Herpes zoster oticus (the Ramsay Hunt syndrome) is an intrapetrosal lesion involving a viropathy of the geniculate ganglion, its neural distribution, and its spread into neighboring auditory and vestibular nerve fibers.

The usual symptoms of herpes zoster oticus are severe otalgia and seventh nerve paralysis. However, in addition to herpetic auricular and periauricular lesions, vertigo, hearing loss, and tinnitus can also be present (see Ch. 28, Seventh Nerve Diagnostic Techniques).

EXTRALABYRINTHINE LESIONS

INTRACANALICULAR TUMORS AND ANOMALIES

The most common intracanalicular eighth nerve tumor is acoustic neurinoma, which actually starts in the vestibular nerve within the internal auditory canal (vestibular schwannoma). Because of the slow-growing nature of the tumor, vertigo is not a common finding, although hearing loss and vertigo may both be present and may mimic Meniere's disease. Acute vertigo may be superimposed upon a mild dysequilibrium in a patient with an intracanicular tumor when there is a sudden change of blood supply in the tumor. Similarly, vascular anomalies without tumors in the internal auditory meatus will be responsible for episodic vertigo in some patients. Electronystagmographic findings usually demonstrate canal paresis on caloric tests.

CEREBELLOPONTINE ANGLE TUMORS AND VASCULAR ANOMALIES

Cerebellopontine angle tumors (meningioma, congenital keratomas, neurilemmoma) and vascular anomalies produce both hearing loss and vertigo, along with seventh, fifth, and other cranial nerve symptoms. Episodic severe vertigo is not a common symptom of cerebellopontine angle lesions. Vestibular asymmetry or canal paresis will be noted upon caloric electronystagmographic studies.

VESTIBULAR DISORDERS (VERTIGO AND NYSTAGMUS ONLY)

INTRALABYRINTHINE LESIONS

MOTION SICKNESS: CONGENITAL VESTIBULAR END ORGAN ASYMMETRY

Motion sickness is a term frequently used as a synonym for dizziness or vertigo. It should be reserved for those categories of dysequilibrium or vertigo that are definitely related to motion. The most common varieties of motion sickness are seasickness, airsickness, and carsickness. Carsickness is usually increased when the passenger is not the driver and is in the back seat. In patients who complain of any one or all three of these categories of motion sickness, spontaneous or positional nystagmus may occasionally be elicited. Vestibular asymmetry is frequently found on caloric studies, noted as labyrinthine preponderance. Hearing is usually normal. Asymmetric congenital vestibular responses are probably enhanced by constitutional or psychogenic factors (See Ch. 27, Central Nervous System Vertigo and Motion Sickness). It may be a maladaptation syndrome.

No definitive treatment other than the use of vertigo sedatives is of value. Dimenhydrinate and similar drugs, administered orally or intramuscularly, are useful in management. A combination of promethazine hydrochloride, 25 mg, and dextroamphetamine, 10 mg, is useful. Diazepam, 10 mg, may also give symptomatic relief, as well as prophylactic therapy.

BENIGN PAROXYSMAL POSITIONAL VERTIGO— OTOLITHIC VERTIGO

Benign paroxysmal positional vertigo is paroxysmal vertigo that occurs only on positional change. The self-limited vertigo is unaccompanied by hearing loss or tinnitus. It has variously been attributed to labyrinthine anomalies or to metabolic or psychogenic problems.

Barany drew attention to this type of positional vertigo in 1921 (4), in describing the symptoms of a 27-year-old woman, stating: "The attacks only appeared when she lay on her right side. When she did this there appeared a strong rotatory nystagmus to the right. The attack lasted about 30 seconds and was accompanied by violent vertigo and nausea. If immediately after the cessation of the symptoms the head was immediately turned to the right, no attack occurred, and in order to evoke a new attack in this way the patient had to lie for some time on her back or on her left side."

Thus, benign paroxysmal positional vertigo is characterized by the following syndrome:

1. The attack occurs when the patient assumes a supine position with the head turned so that the involved ear is undermost.
2. There is almost always a latent period, 5 or 6 sec, before the onset of symptoms.
3. The nystagmus is chiefly rotatory, the direction being toward the undermost ear.

Schuknecht (29, 30) attributed benign paroxysmal positional vertigo to cupulolithiasis. Gacek (12) demonstrated temporal bone evidence of otolith displacement in severe cases of the vertigo.

Degenerative otoliths from the utricular macula gravitate down and become embedded in the cupula of the posterior canal crista. Benign paroxysmal positional vertigo occurs at infrequent intervals in most patients, and in most instances the condition is self-limited. However, in some patients it is a handicapping vertigo lesion. In such cases Gacek (12) recommends surgical section of the posterior ampullary (singular) nerve by transsection via the round window niche.

In addition to the cupulolithiasis theory, it must be pointed out that benign paroxysmal positional vertigo accompanied by benign positional nystagmus, can be something other than "benign." It can be found in association with CNS lesions. Consequently, repetitive neurologic studies should be considered in such cases.

EXTRALABYRINTHINE (RETROLABYRINTHINE) LESIONS

VESTIBULAR VIRAL NEURONITIS

Dix and Hallpike (8) described the viral vestibular neuronitis syndrome in 1952. It is an acute lesion unaccompanied by hearing loss, frequently following a viral upper respiratory infection. It is characterized by severe episodic vertigo with spontaneous nystagmus, usually manifest. There may be moderate or severe canal paresis on caloric electronystagmographic studies. Auditory tests usually show normal hearing.

The disease is usually self-limited. The episodic attacks decrease in frequency, and in most instances the symptoms disappear in 6–9 months. In some patients there is a return to normal caloric vestibular function following subsidence. The clinical picture closely resembles that of benign paroxysmal positional vertigo.

Morgenstein and Seung (24) described the histopathologic changes in a case of vestibular neuronitis, which showed degeneration of Scarpa's ganglion and its central and peripheral neurons, as well as semicircular canal and utricle changes.

The management of this lesion is purely symptomatic, with administration of dimenhydrinate or similar antivertigo sedatives. Small doses (25 mg) once or twice daily offer some relief until spontaneous subsidence occurs.

A great problem of the presumptive diagnosis of vestibular neuronitis is its nonspecificity and the danger that the clinical findings represent early signals of undetected labyrinthine or CNS lesions. Long-term follow up is, therefore, advisable.

TOXIC VESTIBULAR NEURONITIS

Episodic vertigo, unaccompanied by auditory symptoms, with variable caloric electronystagmographic findings, without the positional features of benign paroxysmal positional vertigo and without a history of viral infection, has been termed toxic vestibular neuronitis in some texts. This designation is purely a clinical concept, unconfirmed by current neuro-otologic studies.

MENIERE'S DISEASE—ENDOLYMPHATIC HYDROPS

HISTORY OF MENIERE'S DISEASE

In 1861 Prosper Meniere (23) gave the classic description of the symptom complex of 1) vertigo, 2) hearing loss, and 3) tinnitus. This combination of three symptoms characterized by episodic attacks of fluctuating severity was attributed to the inner ear and has since become known as Meniere's disease. Hallpike and Cairns (18) clearly described endolymphatic hydrops as the basic histopathologic lesion associated with Meniere's disease. Although "endolymphatic hydrops" has become a clinical synonym for Meniere's disease, the cause-and-effect relationships between the hydrops and the clinical findings remain unclear.

PATHOPHYSIOLOGY OF MENIERE'S DISEASE

Temporal bone studies from patients with clinical diagnoses of Meniere's disease usually show hydrops of the cochlear scala media, less frequently of the utricle, and of one or more of the semicircular canal ampullas. The extent, severity, and duration of the hydrops, presumably determine such secondary complications as rupture of membranes, herniations of vestibular organs, and eventual degeneration of the organ of Corti and loss of spiral ganglion cells.

The occasional changes noted histologically, other than hydrops, involve the endolymphatic sac and its surrounding loose tissue, and, more recently, studies implicate significance to the length and development of the vestibular aqueduct itself.

Occasional case reports have described fibrosis of the normally loose or potentially loose tissue surrounding the intermediate portion of the endolymphatic sac (1, 2, 17, 18). This, however, has not been a consistent finding.

Maldevelopment, or anomalies, involving the vestibular aqueduct have been described in some

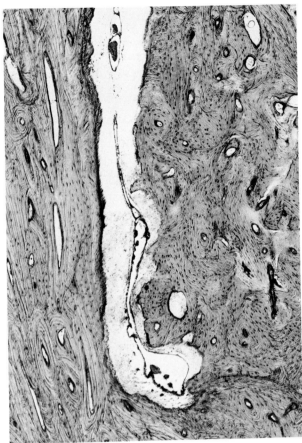

FIG. 26–2. Vestibular aqueduct—normal. (Gussen R: Laryngoscope 81:1695–1707, 1971)

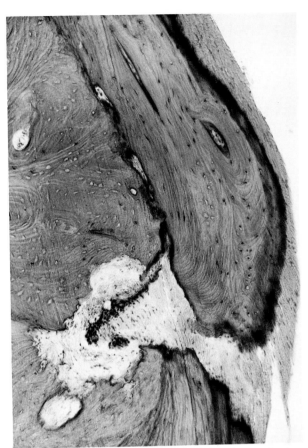

FIG. 26–3. Abnormal vestibular aqueduct. (Gussen R: Ann Otol Rhinol Laryngol 81:235–240, 1972)

patients with Meniere's disease, predominantly on tomographic study or at surgery (7). One temporal bone study has demonstrated partial atresia of the vestibular aqueduct (15, 16) (Figs. 26–2, 26–3). Occasional temporal bone studies have described a more direct course of the vestibular aqueduct from the vestibule to the posterior surface of the temporal bone, and other studies have demonstrated a shorter vestibular aqueduct in some patients with Meniere's disease (5, 28, 32). Whether or not these findings relate to decreased function of the endolymphatic sac and its surrounding loose fibrovascular tissue, as in cases with perisac fibrosis, and decreased amounts of functioning endolymphatic sac and perisac tissue, as in vestibular aqueduct anomalies is not clear.

ETIOLOGIC THEORIES

The cause of Meniere's disease is unclear. Many hypotheses are used operationally in treatment, but the exact etiopathologic factors involved in the disease are unknown.

Our concept is that there are at least two basic coexisting and interacting etiologic factors: 1) an anatomicophysiological basic factor; and 2) a constitutional secondary-factor group.

PRIMARY ANATOMICOPHYSIOLOGICAL FACTORS

Most present evidence points to some dysfunction of the endolymphatic duct and sac system in conjunction with endolymphatic hydrops (Fig. 26–4). In addition, evidence of involvement of the vein of the vestibular aqueduct is accumulating, with venous "lakes" surrounding the vein and the endolymphatic duct system. Thus, vascular factors probably play a role in endolymphatic dysfunction. There is radiologic and surgical evidence of fibrous and/or bony closure of the endolymphatic sac and duct (Fig. 26–5); actual obliteration of the vestib-

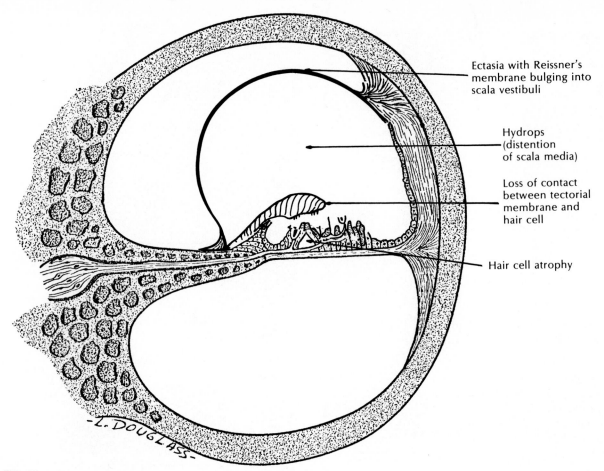

Ectasia with Reissner's
membrane bulging into
scala vestibuli

Hydrops
(distention
of scala media)

Loss of contact
between tectorial
membrane and
hair cell

Hair cell atrophy

FIG. 26–4. Diagrammatic representation of hydrops of scala media in Meniere's disease.

ular aqueduct has been noted on polytomography in some cases of Meniere's disease. However, these findings are not consistently present. The fact that Meniere's disease is more often unilateral than bilateral supports the theory of a basic anatomicophysiological primary cause.

In a review of anatomic, tomographic, and microanatomic studies (3), it was concluded that there is a decrease in the periaqueductal and opercular air-cell pneumatization in Meniere's disease, with a concomitant shorter and straighter vestibular aqueduct. This seems to correlate with decreased endolymphatic sac patency and a more inferiorly positioned sac.

CONSTITUTIONAL SECONDARY FACTORS

Therapeutic experiences indicate that a number of secondary constitutional factors play roles in the clinical course of Meniere's disease. These factors are vascular, infectious, metabolic, allergic, neurogenic, and psychologic.

Vascular hypotheses have been based upon observation of capillary sludging and have been reinforced by therapeutic responses to intravenous, intradermal, and other forms of histamine use.

Allergic hypotheses have been strongly advanced by allergy studies and allergy therapy, as described by Wilson (34).

Metabolic relationships have been variously attributed to thyroid, pituitary, ovarian, and other endocrine deficiencies.

Psychosomatic aspects of Meniere's disease have been stressed in a number of reports. Fowler and Zeckel reported significant psychosomatic aspects in many Meniere's disease patients (11). Hinchcliffe (20) concluded that there was a special psychosomatic type personality profile that could be identified on the Minnesota Multiphasic Personality Inventory.

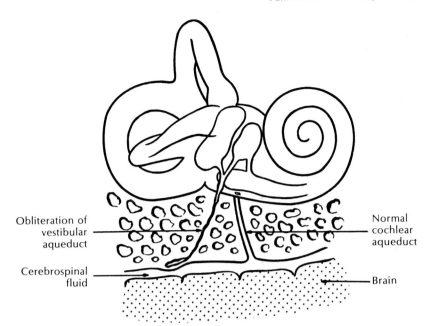

Obliteration of vestibular aqueduct

Cerebrospinal fluid

Normal cochlear aqueduct

Brain

FIG. 26–5. Obliterative changes in vestibular aqueduct in Meniere's disease.

A recent study by Brightwell and Abramson (6) using the Eysenck Personality Inventory and Cornell Medical Index does not implicate emotion as an etiologic agent but suggests that psychological vulnerability exists in some patients. The study indicates that emotional factors be seriously considered in patients with Meniere's disease.

In similar studies Stephens (33) concluded: "The most notable finding was an elevated obsessionality score in the patients with Meniere's disorder as compared with other groups."

CLINICAL ASPECTS OF MENIERE'S DISEASE

In addition to the episodic vertigo, cochlear hearing loss, and tinnitus, patients will frequently complain of intermittent feelings of pressure or stuffiness in the involved ear.

VERTIGO AND VESTIBULAR FINDINGS

The vertigo of true Meniere's disease occurs in severe sudden attacks and in intermittent milder episodes. The sudden attack is frequently accompanied by nausea and/or vomiting, perspiration, or even mild shock. It lasts minutes to hours and may require one or several days of complete bedrest with the use of antivertigo sedatives before there is a return of stable equilibrium. The patient is not unconscious, and there are no neurologic abnor-

malities. The vertigo attack may be followed by a prolonged chronic state of imbalance sometimes called "giddiness." This chronic, mild, giddy state may be punctuated by recurrent acute vertigo attacks. Great variations exist in the vertigo patterns, in severity, and in side effects.

During an acute sudden attack, manifest spontaneous and/or positional nystagmus is present. In some cases it may be noted with +20 lenses or recorded on the electronystagmogram. It is labyrinthine (end-organ) in type, definitely directional, usually horizontal or horizontal-rotary.

During the postattack period which may last a number of days, there is usually a subsidence of manifest nystagmus. However, on electronystagmographic studies in the dark, spontaneous and/or positional nystagmus may be recorded. During the postattack period, the patient may complain of positional vertigo, and occasionally ataxia. Constant vertigo is not characteristic of Meniere's disease.

When examined by electronystagmographic techniques at intervals between acute attacks, the patient will most commonly show evidence of positional nystagmus in several positions. Spontaneous nystagmus may or may not be present. There will usually be evidence of labyrinthine preponderance in the opposite ear usually indicative of a hypofunction (canal paresis) in the diseased labyrinth. Occasionally "hyperfunction" may be recognized by labyrinthine preponderance of the affected ear, rather than the usual recording of labyrinthine preponderance of the opposite ear (which presumably indicates hypofunction in the involved ear). This "hyperfunction" is at the present time a debatable electronystagmographic concept. Some investigators believe that hyperfunction does not exist as a real entity and that the opposite is true—mainly that the uninvolved ear may reveal depressed vestibular activity. However, we have seen many instances of labyrinthine preponderance with the involved ear as the preponderant ear. Such findings may be indicative of what might be considered vestibular recruitment. "Decruitment" (see Ch. 10, section on Special and Unusual Electronystagmographic Findings) has also been described as a finding in some varieties of Meniere's disease. Recruitment may be described as "exaggerated response" and decruitment as "diminished response" to standard stimuli.

In essence, the vestibular findings in Meniere's disease are usually abnormal and variable (see Ch. 10, Examination of the Dizzy Patient), depending upon time factors with reference to either the preceding acute attack or to a possible impending new acute attack.

HEARING LOSS, TINNITUS, AND AUDIOLOGIC FINDINGS

The hearing loss of Meniere's disease is characteristically a unilateral sensorineural loss with audiologic findings that are primarily cochlear. In most instances, the condition is unilateral, although bilateral hearing loss occurs in 10–20% of cases. The low frequencies may be involved first, a feature which may mimic early otosclerosis. The low frequency hearing loss usually shows an upward slope with a close to normal response in the higher frequencies. The major difference between early Meniere's disease and early otosclerosis is that there is no *true* air–bone gap in Meniere's disease. The hearing loss in Meniere's disease fluctuates, whereas the hearing loss in otosclerosis is usually steady and progressive. The hearing loss following the fluctuating period can stabilize for months or years. The audiometric pattern eventually changes from an upward sloping curve to a flat curve and eventually slopes downward for the higher frequencies (Fig. 26–6).

Although major fluctuations in hearing can occur in Meniere's disease, with hearing returning almost to normal in early cases, the eventual pattern is that of slowly progressive major cochlear hearing loss. Occasionally there may be permanent return to normal hearing (Fig. 26–7).

Site-of-lesion audiologic findings are distinctive of disease in the organ of Corti in the differential diagnostic auditory test battery. Loudness recruitment on alternative binaural loudness balance testing is present, speech discrimination scores are low, and short-increment sensitivity index scores are high. There may be diplacusis. There is no pathologic tone decay, and Bekesy findings are characteristically type II. The audiologic findings may change to mixed patterns late in the disease with the development of type IV Bekesy patterns, probably as a consequence of slow retrocochlear degenerative changes (Fig. 26–8).

Subjectively, the hearing loss is frequently accompanied by fullness and feelings of pressure in the affected ear. Tinnitus may be roaring, buzzing, whistling, or mixed in character.

RADIOGRAPHIC FINDINGS

No significant radiologic findings occur in the labyrinth *per se*, either in the cochlear or in the semicircular canal systems. However, varying degrees of abnormality may be seen in polytomographic examinations of the vestibular aqueduct. There may be total absence of the vestibular aqueduct in the affected ear. Indeed, such absence has been also noted in the surgical findings of patients with Meniere's disease who have been subjected to endolymphatic sac decompression procedures. Instances have been reported where neither endolymphatic sac or duct could be visualized surgically. There are recent studies relating pneumatization variations in temporal bone radiographs of patients with Meniere's disease. However, at the present time, the radiologic aspects of Meniere's disease are still in the data-gathering stage, with no clear-cut definitive radiologic findings that either rule in or rule out Meniere's disease.

CLINICAL COURSE

The course of the disease, untreated or even with "treatment," is progressively downward in the majority of cases, interspersed with plateaus of latency. Usually there will be progressive deterioration in hearing, with decreasing intensity and frequency of vertigo attacks. Because of spontaneous favorable and unfavorable fluctuations in hearing loss and in vertigo, great caution must be exercised in evaluating any medical or surgical treatment.

DIFFERENTIAL DIAGNOSIS OF MENIERE'S DISEASE

Differential diagnostic aspects of Meniere's disease are exceedingly important. Meniere's disease may mimic or may be mimicked by a number of otologic lesions, including otosclerosis, labyrinthine fistula, intracanalicular eighth nerve schwannoma, meningioma, cerebellopontine angle lesions, intermittent tubotympanitis, multiple sclerosis, syphilis, and barotrauma with sudden hearing loss.

The audiologic and vestibular findings that have been described in Meniere's disease are subject to many variations. Almost identical findings may occur in tumors involving the eighth nerve or in labyrinthine fistulas. For example, the audiologic findings of a unilateral Bekesy type II and a high short-increment sensitivity index score does not always rule out the diagnosis of an eighth nerve tumor. Radiographs of the temporal bone are necessary in every patient with a clinical diagnosis of Meniere's disease, not to find radiographic evidence of Meniere's disease specifically, but because of the need to rule out other lesions in differential diagnosis. Thus, a minimal radiologic study requires a Schuller mastoid radiograph to consider the possibility of otomastoiditis, and a Stenver radiograph to rule out an enlargement or erosion of the internal acoustic meatus. An otherwise asymptomatic meningioma or keratoma may show up on a Schuller radiograph view with tegmen and mastoid cell changes. An eighth nerve schwannoma may be revealed on a Stenver radiograph view. In questionable cases, polytomography and/or contrast studies and computerized axial tomography (CAT) scans may be advisable.

Otosclerosis in its early stages may be accompanied by vertigo, thus leading frequently to an erroneous diagnosis of Meniere's disease. However, there is only rare fluctuation of hearing in otosclerosis (otospongiosis phase) when the hearing loss is less than 25 dB, and the air–bone gap is minimal.

Unrecognized syphilis must always be considered. The fluorescent treponemal antibody-absorption test is now the most reliable diagnostic guide in syphilis detection. Thus, critical differential diagnostic techniques are essential to rule out other diseases that may be characterized by the syndrome of fluctuating cochlear hearing loss, tinnitus, and episodic vertigo.

THE HISTORY OF TREATMENT FOR MENIERE'S DISEASE

Because of many etiopathologic theories, the treatment of the patient with Meniere's disease has been largely empirical and has included both medical and surgical therapeutic approaches. Scores of drugs, operations, and other treatment modalities have been advanced for decades with controversial therapeutic debates detailed in hundreds of papers.

MEDICAL

Medical management has included psychotherapy, allergic hyposensitization, diuretics, low sodium diets, specific antivertigo drugs, antihistamines, vasodilators, vasoconstrictors, and steroids. Histamine has been used empirically and administered intravenously, subcutaneously, intracutaneously, and sublingually. The same patient may be receiving mutually antagonistic drugs with no real rationale for diverse empirical therapeutic approaches.

A number of "vertigo sedatives" have been in use with reasonably effective responses. These include dimenhydrinate, meclizine, cyclizine hydrochloride, and other similar antihistamine derivatives.

Recently droperidol, fentanyl (19, 21), and lithium carbonate have been suggested as effective nonspecific vertigo-suppression drugs.

SURGICAL

Two types of surgical approaches have been advanced for decades. The first group of surgical procedures is directed to conservation or improvement of labyrinth function (hearing, vertigo, and tinnitus). The second group is directed to destruction of labyrinth vestibular function in cases of intractable disabling vertigo.

Conservation Surgery in Meniere's Disease

Because of evidence of involvement of the endolymphatic duct and sac system, a number of surgical endolymphatic sac approaches have been tried. Surgical sac decompression of the endolymphatic sac, advocated more than half a century ago (27), was abandoned, only to be revived subsequently in a number of versions. Simple sac decompression, sac incisions, vascular and muscular grafts to the sac, sac "shunts," with shunt tubes introduced between the sac lumen and the cerebrospinal fluid system (subarachnoid space), and sac obliterations have all been tried and are still in use (10,

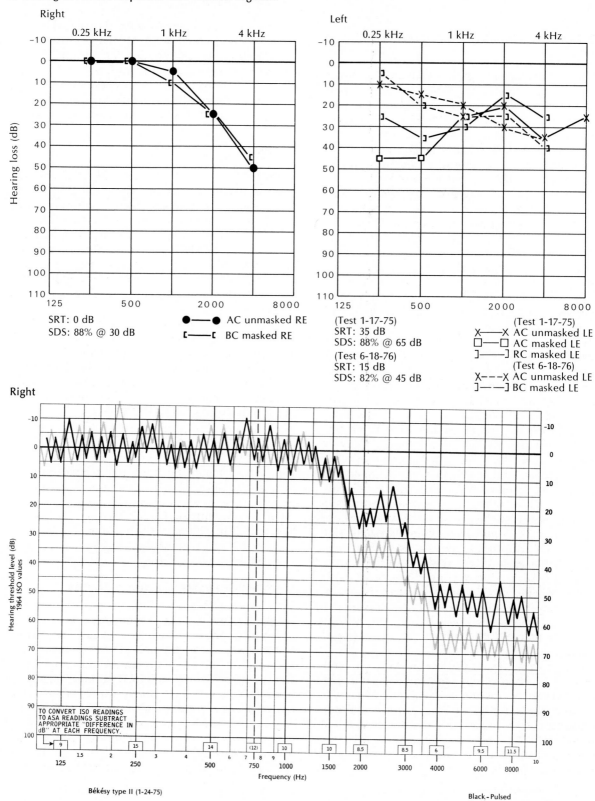

FIG. 26–6. Meniere's disease (reversible) in left ear. Note restricted tympanometry, mixed conductive-cochlear loss before treatment, positive reflex, type II Bekesy patterns in both ears (although left ear showed low-frequency and high-frequency separation). Note return of hearing in AC–BC responses after medical regimen.

Right

SRT: 0 dB
SDS: 88% @ 30 dB

●——● AC unmasked RE
[——[BC masked RE

(Test 1-17-75)
SRT: 35 dB
SDS: 88% @ 65 dB
(Test 6-18-76)
SRT: 15 dB
SDS: 82% @ 45 dB

(Test 1-17-75)
X——X AC unmasked LE
□——□ AC masked LE
]——] RC masked LE
(Test 6-18-76)
X---X AC unmasked LE
]——] BC masked LE

Right

TO CONVERT ISO READINGS TO ASA READINGS SUBTRACT APPROPRIATE "DIFFERENCE IN dB" AT EACH FREQUENCY.

Békésy type II (1-24-75)

Black – Pulsed
Gray ⊢ Continuous

FIG. 26–6 (continued)

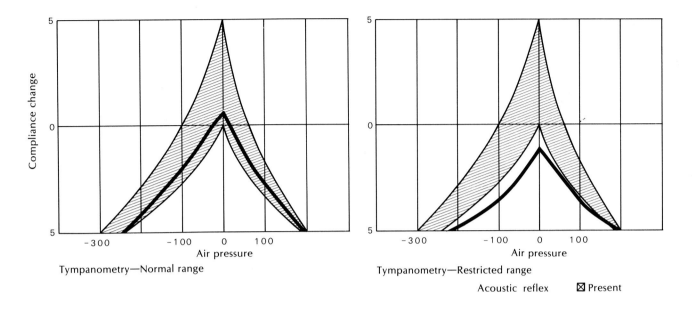

Tympanometry—Normal range

Tympanometry—Restricted range

Acoustic reflex ⊠ Present

Left

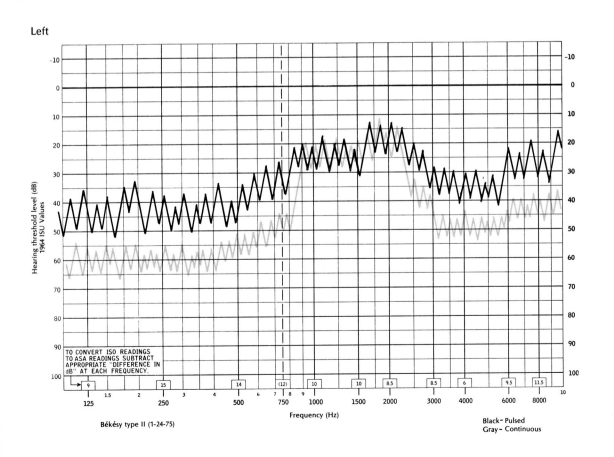

TO CONVERT ISO READINGS TO ASA READINGS SUBTRACT APPROPRIATE "DIFFERENCE IN dB" AT EACH FREQUENCY.

Frequency (Hz)

Békésy type II (1-24-75)

Black- Pulsed
Gray - Continuous

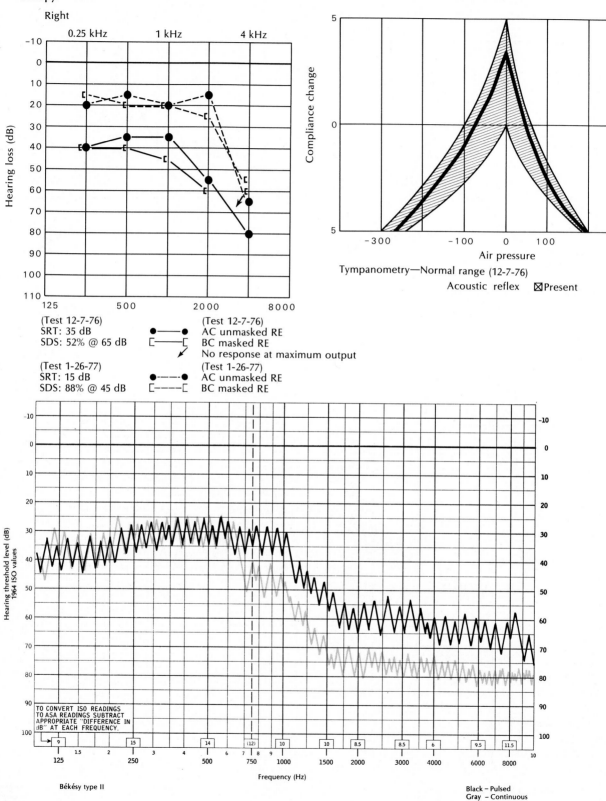

FIG. 26–7. Meniere's disease (reversible) in right ear. Note low-, middle-, and high-frequency AC–BC loss before treatment, normal tympanometry, and type II Bekesy with middle- and high-frequency separation. Note dramatic AC–BC hearing improvement following medical therapy.

Right

Compliance change

Air pressure

Tympanometry—Normal range (12-7-76)

Acoustic reflex ☒Present

(Test 12-7-76)
SRT: 35 dB
SDS: 52% @ 65 dB

(Test 12-7-76)
●——● AC unmasked RE
⊏——⊏ BC masked RE
↙ No response at maximum output

(Test 1-26-77)
SRT: 15 dB
SDS: 88% @ 45 dB

(Test 1-26-77)
●----● AC unmasked RE
⊏----⊏ BC masked RE

Hearing threshold level (dB) 1964 ISO values

TO CONVERT ISO READINGS TO ASA READINGS SUBTRACT APPROPRIATE "DIFFERENCE IN dB" AT EACH FREQUENCY.

| 9 | | 15 | | 14 | (12) | 10 | | 10 | 8.5 | | 8.5 | | 6 | | 9.5 | 11.5 | |

Frequency (Hz)

Békésy type II

Black – Pulsed
Gray – Continuous

25, 26). Widely disparate reports of results have appeared in the literature.

Other conservation surgical procedures in use are saccule decompression (tack operation) and ultrasonic irradiation of the semicircular canals, round window and/or cochlear promontory. Freezing of these areas has also been advocated. A number of intralabyrynthine otic–periotic shunt procedures have been tried. Sodium chloride crystals have been applied to the round window membrane in an effort to deal with the hydrops by direct osmolarity reversal.

Lability in serum osmolarity as a factor has prompted the use of glycerol dehydration orally, both for diagnosis and treatment. Results are still inconclusive (31).

Myringostomy with collar-button (grommet) tubes has been advised. Cervical ganglion block with production of a temporary Horner's syndrome has been in use for several decades.

Destructive Surgery in Meniere's Disease

In some patients with disabling vertigo and poor hearing, destructive surgical procedures have been found necessary. Two types of destructive surgery are in use: labyrinthectomy and intracranial vestibular nerve section.

LABYRINTHECTOMY. Labyrinthectomy procedures have been used with significantly good results in carefully selected patients with unilateral Meniere's disease who have no useful hearing in the involved ear and who are incapacitated by the vertigo.

Both transmastoid exenteration of the three semicircular canals and/or trans-oval-window and/or trans-round-window exenteration of the utricle and saccule have been used with good results. Such surgery is probably less advisable in elderly patients because of difficulties in adjustment to the postoperative ataxia.

VESTIBULAR NERVE SECTION. The first approach to vestibular nerve section was the neurosurgical suboccipital approach to the cerebellopontine angle for intracranial vestibular nerve neurectomy. This major surgical procedure, attended by significant morbidity and occasional mortality, has been effective in many patients.

Recent techniques include translabyrinthine or middle cranial fossa approaches to Scarpa's ganglion. "Scarpectomy" is a rather precise procedure that is performed without labyrinthectomy, thus offering the possibility of hearing conservation in cases with salvageable residual cochlear function (9).

MANAGEMENT OF THE PATIENT WITH MENIERE'S DISEASE IN OUR CLINIC

When one surveys the many hundreds of papers dealing with medical and surgical techniques, it is interesting to note that in almost all reports, the same type of result is reported: Approximately 70% of patients are reported as being "improved." The term "improvement" is usually directed to the symptom of dizziness. Rarely do the reported data indicate significant permanent improvement in hearing or subsidence of the hearing fluctuations that are so characteristic of the disease. Few reports have included significant changes in vestibular findings, other than canal paresis following vestibular neurectomy or labyrinthectomy. Most therapeutic reports emphasize purely subjective results, such as relief from "fullness," less distracting tinnitus, and primarily lessened dizziness. Hearing improvements reported are usually within the fluctuating changes so characteristic of Meniere's disease.

Jongkees (22) stated: "I feel sure that here, as in every treatment for these . . . patients, the doctor has success with the treatment he really believes in, whether it is combating water and sodium retention (Perlman, Goldinger, and Coles), antiallergic, giving prismatic glasses, psychiatric support, some kind of shunt operation, or another of the numerous possibilities."

As one reviews the enormous data compiled in such widely disparate approaches to the treatment of the patient with Meniere's disease, it becomes obvious that *management*, rather than "treatment" of Meniere's disease is the appropriate term, in view of present knowledge concerning etiology. Management must be based on two considerations, the primary anatomicophysiological factor, and a number of possible secondary factors.

The following management plan is used in our clinic and is based on fluctuating physiologic changes in a dynamic organ, the endolymphatic labyrinth, with osmotic, vascular, and endocrine interrelationships. Our management of Meniere's disease is primarily medical. We prefer, wherever possible, to collaborate with the patient's general physician, outlining certain basic principles in medical management. Basic constitutional problems, *i.e.*, thyroid disease, diabetes, hypertension, etc., are left to the care of the general physician.

We usually advise moderate restrictions on sodium intake. Caffeine (coffee and tea) is restricted. Smoking is discouraged, as is alcohol.

Allergy is a significant secondary factor in many patients. Common allergenic foods (milk products,

FIG. 26–8. Advanced Meniere's disease, right ear, recurrent. In 1971, the onset was accompanied by a 40-dB cochlear hearing loss, which responded to a medical regimen with return of hearing (in April 1976) to the same level as shown at top. A recurrence, accompanied by only transient mild vertigo was followed by marked decrease in hearing, accompanied by tinnitus. The recurrence followed fatigue and emotional stress. Note major change in hearing acuity and speech discrimination ability. Bekesy tracing shows a mixed pattern—type II and type IV. Acoustic reflex is absent when right ear is stimulus ear, probably as a result of the severe degree of hearing loss.

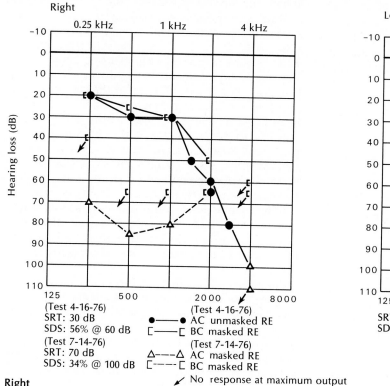

Right

(Test 4-16-76)
SRT: 30 dB
SDS: 56% @ 60 dB
(Test 7-14-76)
SRT: 70 dB
SDS: 34% @ 100 dB

● ——— ● AC unmasked RE
⊏ ——— ⊏ BC masked RE
(Test 7-14-76)
△ – – – △ AC masked RE
⊏ – – – ⊏ BC masked RE
↙ No response at maximum output

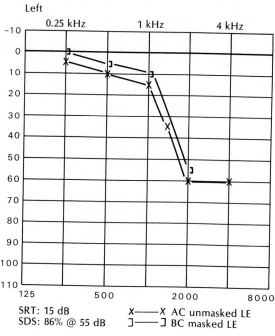

Left

SRT: 15 dB
SDS: 86% @ 55 dB

X ——— X AC unmasked LE
⊐ ——— ⊐ BC masked LE

Right

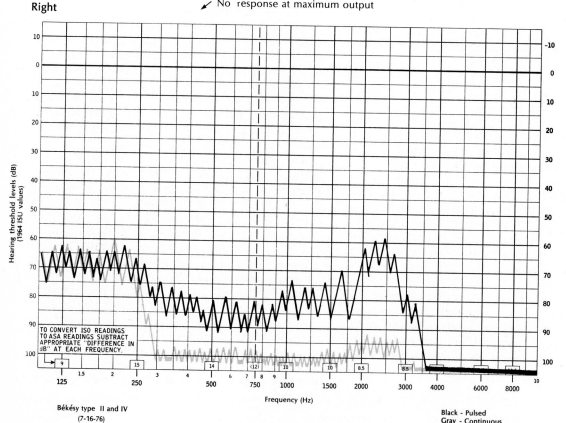

TO CONVERT ISO READINGS TO ASA READINGS SUBTRACT APPROPRIATE "DIFFERENCE IN dB" AT EACH FREQUENCY.

Békésy type II and IV
(7-16-76)

Black - Pulsed
Gray - Continuous

FIG. 26–8 (continued)

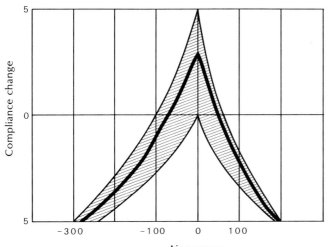

Tympanometry (7-14-76)—Normal range

Acoustic reflex
(monitor ear)   ⊠ Present

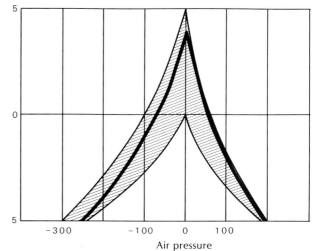

Tympanometry—Normal range

Acoustic reflex (monitor ear) ⊠ Absent

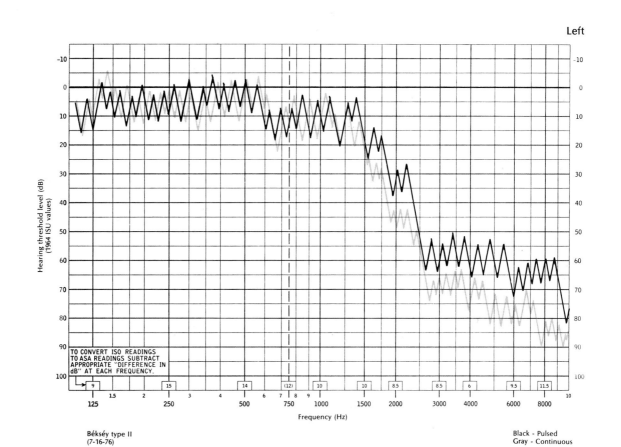

Béksèy type II
(7-16-76)

Black - Pulsed
Gray - Continuous

corn, chocolate, pork, nuts, shellfish, and eggs) are usually eliminated or decreased in the patient's diet. In addition to diminished sodium intake, non-ototoxic diuretics are advised for limited periods of time. On the basis of the principles cited, the following management schedule is suggested:

Management of Mild Attack
1. Bed rest in position of greatest comfort
2. Bland, low-sodium diet with only moderate intake of fluids, and distilled water
3. Dimenhydrinate, 50 mg every 3 hours, or diazepam, 5 mg. If nausea is present, substitute promethazine hydrochloride, 50-mg suppository
4. No smoking, no coffee, no tea, no "Cokes," no alcohol

Management of Severe Attack
1. Bed rest
2. Dimenhydrinate, 50 mg IM, repeated every 3–4 hours as necessary
3. Prochlorperazine, 25-mg suppository, if severe nausea is present, accompanied by vomiting; or diazepam, 10 mg every 4 hours; or droperidol, 25 mg IM every 4 hours
4. If attack has been prolonged and the patient is dehydrated, I-V fluids may be necessary

Long-range Management Between Attacks
1. Complete review of detailed history of patient's way of life, contacts, stresses, etc., in an effort to find precipitating causes and possible allergies
2. Careful review of audiologic, vestibular, and radiographic findings to rule out possibility of a cerebellopontine angle tumor, other intracranial disease, FTA-abs serology, etc
3. Eliminate smoking, coffee or tea, and stimulating drugs. Control habits and environmental factors which produce fatigue and stress
4. Low-sodium diet with use of distilled water rather than spring water or tapwater for all cooking and drinking purposes. Empirical hypoallergenic diet, eliminating milk, eggs, chocolate, shellfish, corn, pork, nuts, and their products
5. Periodic utilization of diuretics such as hydrochlorothiazide, 50 mg once or twice daily. Such therapy frequently will relieve the feeling of fullness in the ear, relieve the vertigo and the tinnitus, and will occasionally be accompanied by significant hearing improvement. Choice of diuretics will depend upon prudent evaluation of the general medical status of patient
6. Intermittent use of diazepam, phenergan, or dexedrine
7. Consultations with other physicians will be necessary if there are significant signs of special problems, such as allergy, emotional stress, and neurologic problems

Most patients with Meniere's disease will respond, insofar as vertigo is concerned, to medical therapy as outlined, provided it is accompanied by good physician-patient relationship and is given over a reasonable period of time. The functional component in Meniere's disease is a great one, although the lesion itself is a clear-cut organic entity —namely, endolymphatic hydrops. Surgical treatment is indicated in the nonresponsive patient who is disabled by the vertigo and whose hearing is seriously impaired.

INDICATIONS FOR SURGERY

None of the vast spectrum of surgical procedures in use for the treatment of Meniere's disease have fulfilled all the requirements for validity, since there are such profound emotional and systemic factors to be considered in treating Meniere's disease, and in addition, spontaneous remissions are quite frequent. The only indication for surgery in which there is complete agreement is found in a patient whose vertiginous episodes are completely disabling and whose hearing level, by discrimination tests as well as threshold tests, has dropped almost to the useless level in the affected ear. Such a patient is a candidate for vestibular neurectomy or labyrinthectomy. The simplest technique for labyrinthectomy that is quite effective is an endomeatal transstapedial approach to the vestibule with ablation of the utricle (Fig. 26–9) and saccule and replacement of the stapes. This is a relatively benign surgical procedure under local anesthesia, with relatively short hospitalization, and results in a high incidence of vertigo cures. Under special circumstances, more drastic semicircular canal destructive procedures are occasionally necessary.

BILATERAL MENIERE'S DISEASE

The management of Meniere's disease must always be tempered by the knowledge that the disease can occur bilaterally. The exact incidence is debated at the present time, with figures ranging from 10–40% for bilateral involvement. This emphasizes the seriousness of any treatment that carries with it the possibility of placing the contralateral labyrinth at risk as a result of the sequelae to the first labyrinth. Thus, surgical procedures that might possibly result in total hearing loss in a patient with apparently unilateral Meniere's disease may place the patient in an untenable position if the disease develops in the contralateral ear some years later.

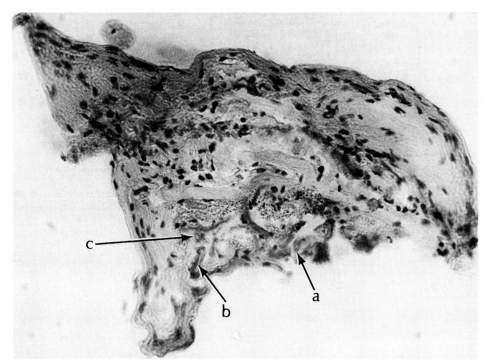

FIG. 26–9. Utricular biopsy following trans-footplate surgery. **(a)** Cluster of otoliths; **(b)** one large otolith in longitudinal section; **(c)** cluster of small otoliths. (Eviatar A, Goodhill V: Ann Otol Rhinol Laryngol 77:264–274, 1968)

REFERENCES

1. Altmann F, Fowler EP: Histological findings in Meniere's symptom complex. Ann Otol Rhinol Laryngol 52:52–80, 1943

2. Altmann F, Zechner G: The pathology and pathogenesis of endolymphatic hydrops: new investigations. Arch Ohren Nasen Kehlkopfheilkd 192:1, 1968

3. Arenberg IK, Rask-Andersen H, Wilbrand H et al.: The surgical anatomy of the endolymphatic sac. Arch Otolaryngol 103:1–11, 1977

4. Barany R: Diagnose von Krankheitser-Scheinungen im Pereische des Otolithenapparates. Acta Otolaryngol (Stockh) 2:434–437, 1921

5. Black FO, Sando I, Hildyard VH et al.: Bilateral multiple otosclerotic foci and endolymphatic hydrops. Ann Otol Rhinol Laryngol 78:1062–1073, 1969

6. Brightwell DR, Abramson M: Personality characteristics in patients with vertigo. Arch Otolaryngol 101:364–366, 1975

7. Clemis JD, Valvassori GE: Recent radiographic and clinical observations on the vestibular aqueduct. Otolaryngol Clin N Am 1968, pp 339–346

8. Dix R, Hallpike CS: The pathology, symptomatology and diagnosis of certain common disorders of the vestibular system. Ann Otol Rhinol Laryngol 61:987–1016, 1952

9. Fisch U: Neurectomy of the vestibular nerve. Surgical technique. Indications and results in 70 cases. Acta Otorhinollaryngol Belg 25:729–732, 1971

10. Fisch U: Surgical treatment of vertigo. J Laryngol 90:75–86, 1976

11. Fowler EP, Zeckel A: Psychosomatic aspects of Meniere's disease. JAMA 148:1265–1268, 1938

12. Gacek RR: Transection of the posterior ampullary nerve for the relief of benign parosysmal positional vertigo. Ann Otol Rhinol Laryngol 83:596–605, 1974

13. Goodhill V: Sudden deafness and round window rupture. Laryngoscope 81:1462–1474, 1971

14. Goodhill V, Harris I, Brockman SJ et al.: Sudden deafness and labyrinthine window ruptures. Ann Otol Rhinol Laryngol 82:2–12, 1973

15. Gussen R: Meniere's disease: new temporal bone findings in two cases. Laryngoscope 81:1695–1707, 1971

16. Gussen R: Abnormalities of the endolymphatic sac system. Ann Otol Rhinol Laryngol 81:235–240, 1972

17. Gussen R: Meniere syndrome. Compensatory collateral venous drainage with endolymphatic sac fibrosis. Arch Otolaryngol 99:414–418, 1974

18. Hallpike CS, Cairns H: Observations of the pathology of Meniere's syndrome. J Laryngol 53:625–654, 1938

19. Harris I, Eviatar A, Goodhill V: Droperidol and Fentanyl Citrate compound as a vestibular depressant. Arch Otolaryngol 89:482–487, 1969

20. Hinchcliffe R: Personality profile in Meniere's disease. J Laryngol 81:477–486, 1967

21. Johnson WH, Fenton RS, Evans A: Effects of Droperidol in management of vestibular disorders. Laryngoscope 86:946–954, 1976

22. Jongkees LBW: Some remarks on the patient suffering from Meniere's disease. Trans Am Acad Ophthalmol Otolaryngol 75:374–378, 1971

23. Meniere P: Mémoire sur des lésions de l'oreille interne donnant lieu à des symptomes de congestion cérébrale apoplectiforme. Gaz Med Paris 16:597–601, 1861

24. Morgenstein KM, Seung HI: Vestibular neuronitis. Laryngoscope 81:131–139, 1971

25. Morrison AW: The surgery of vertigo: saccus drainage for idiopathic endolymphatic hydrops. J Laryngol 90:87–93, 1976

26. Paparella MM, Hanson DG: Endolymphatic sac drainage for intractable vertigo (method and experiences). Laryngoscope 86:697–703, 1976

27. Portmann G: Vertigo: surgical treatment by opening the saccus endolymphaticus. Arch Otolaryngol 6:209–319, 1927

28. Sando I, Holinger LD, Balkany TJ et al.: Unilateral endolymphatic hydrops and associated abnormalities. Ann Otol Rhinol Laryngol 85:368–376, 1976

29. Schuknecht HF: Positional vertigo: clinical and experimental observations. Trans Am Acad Ophthalmol Otolaryngol 66:319–331, 1962

30. Schuknecht HF: Cupulolithiasis. Arch Otolaryngol 90:765–778, 1969

31. Synder JM: Extensive use of diagnostic test for Meniere's disease. Arch Otolaryngol 100:360–365, 1974

32. Stahle J, Wilbrand H: The vestibular aqueduct in patients with Meniere's disease. Acta Otolaryngol (Stockh) 78:36–48, 1974

33. Stephens SDG: Personality tests in Meniere's disease. J Laryngol 89:479–496, 1975

34. Wilson WH: Antigenic excitation in Meniere's disease. Laryngoscope 82:1726–1735, 1972

In central nervous system lesions involving the central vestibular system, true vertigo can occur (Fig. 27–1). The problems of vertigo and dysequilibrium as components of dizziness have been discussed (see Ch. 9, Equilibrium and Dizziness and Ch. 10, Examination of the Dizzy Patient). The term dizziness is frequently used to describe minor seizures, lightheadedness, cerebellar ataxia, mental confusion, and other nonvertiginous conditions.

Eighth nerve tumors are not always associated with vertigo as a major symptom. Acoustic neurinoma (vestibular schwannoma) or the less common internal auditory meatus or cerebellopontine angle meningiomas or epidermoid cysts rarely give rise to vertigo because of their slow-growing characteristics. However, cerebellopontine angle lesions involving arterial or venous malformations may produce severe prolonged and sometimes incapacitating attacks of vertigo, which may very easily be confused with Meniere's disease.

The most common causes of vertigo arising from the brain stem are vascular lesions, such as thrombosis of the posterior inferior cerebellar artery or basilar artery insufficiency. Localized brain-stem encephalitis produces vertigo, but primary tumors of the brain stem or cerebellum less frequently give rise to true vertigo. A type of systemic imbalance—dysequilibrium—is more commonly noticed with such tumors of the brain stem or cerebellum. Metastatic tumors of the brain stem or cerebellum, however, may be accompanied by true vertigo. Although multiple sclerosis does produce vertigo, its most common vestibular symptom is dysequilibrium or systemic imbalance.

The association of hearing loss and tinnitus with vertigo becomes less common as one deals with lesions in the upper portion of the CNS. In addition to dissociation between vestibular and audiologic symptoms in higher CNS lesions, there are frequent involvements of other cranial nerves. Thus, there may be alterations in facial sensation (fifth nerve), ocular paralyses (third, fourth, and sixth nerves), conjugate ocular deviation, difficulty in swallowing, and hoarseness (tenth nerve).

In cerebellar lesions, arm or leg ataxia, intention tremors, and unsteady gait may be noted.

Vertiginous lesions of the CNS can be divided into vascular and nonvascular etiologies. A number of "steal" syndromes, vertebral-basilar system lesions, and other vascular phenomena, especially transient ischemic attacks (TIA), characterize vascular etiology. Disseminated sclerosis, cerebellar tumors, and head injuries are included in the nonvascular group.

Motion sickness, a maladaptation syndrome in-

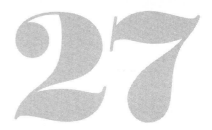

CENTRAL NERVOUS SYSTEM VERTIGO AND MOTION SICKNESS

volving the vestibular system, as well as the ocular, proprioceptive, and various CNS centers, is the all-inclusive category for seasickness, air sickness, car sickness, and related dizziness problems associated with motion.

As experience with electronystagmographic (ENG) measurements increases, a number of cardinal ENG findings are significant in CNS diseases. Spector (23) emphasized hyperexcitability on caloric stimulation tests, and persistent spontaneous nystagmus in spite of normal caloric tests. Abnormal pendulum tracking with eyes open is a very common finding in many CNS lesions. Of importance also in eyes-open testing are the frequent findings of calibration overshoot and failure of fixation suppression.

Kimm and MacLean (18) point out that disconjugate eye movements occur in certain CNS lesions. By studying independent eye movements during ENG tests, they found that disconjugate eye movements could be demonstrated even with extraaxial lesions that spared the medial longitudinal bundle.

Baloh, Honrubia, and Sills (1) in a recent UCLA study, found dramatic differences between peripheral and CNS lesions in eye tracking and optokinetic (OKN) studies. In acute peripheral labyrinthine lesions OKN deficits are temporary. But in patients with cerebellopontine angle tumors, there are progressive eye-pursuit and OKN deficits with tumor enlargements. Cerebellar lesions result in severe saccadic impairments of accuracy. Relationships of such ENG abnormalities in focal CNS lesions are presented in Figure 27–2.

Posturally evoked vomiting dissociated from

FIG. 27-1. Vascular and tumor lesions of the CNS, responsible for nystagmus and vertigo.

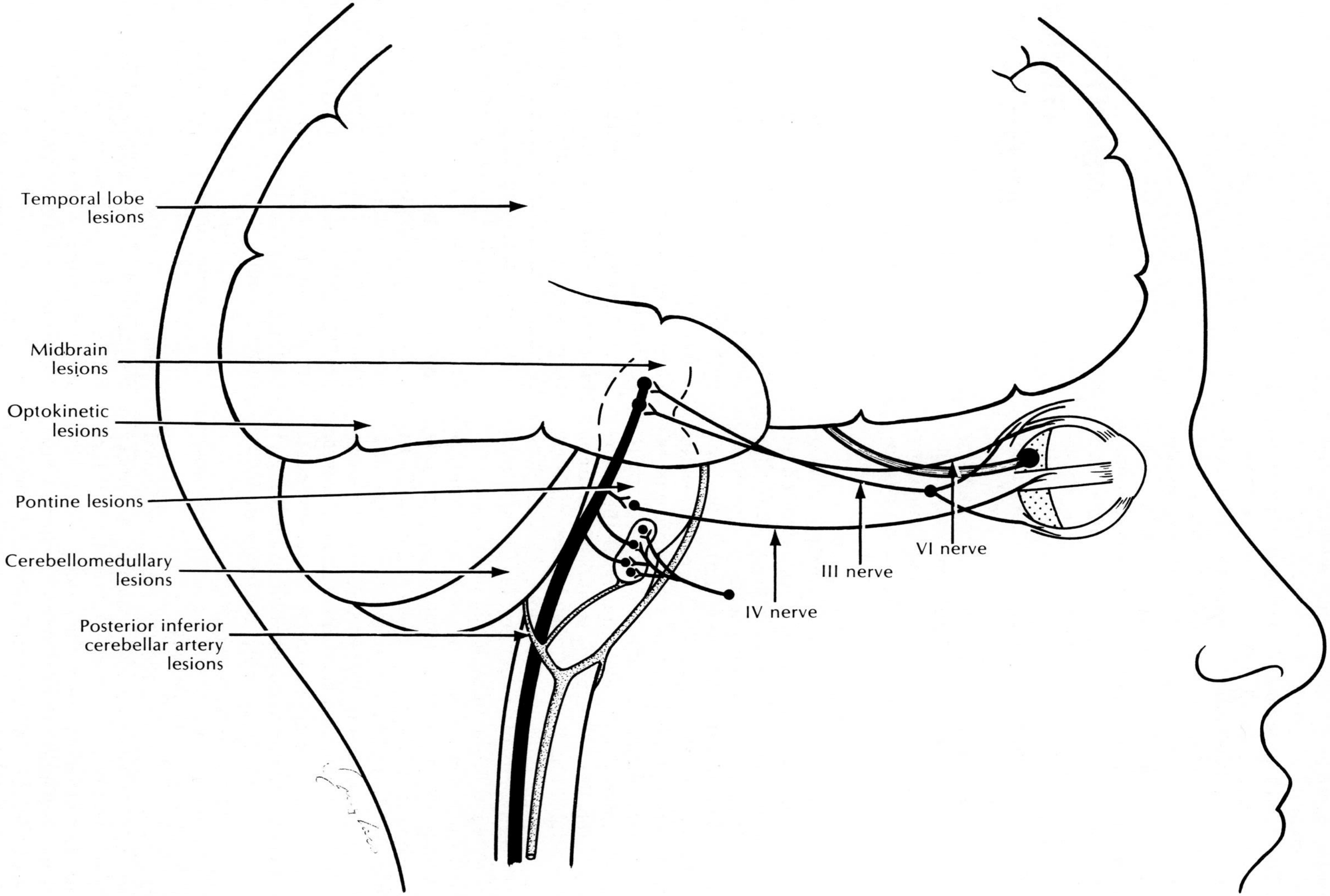

VI nerve

III nerve

IV nerve

Temporal lobe lesions

Midbrain lesions

Optokinetic lesions

Pontine lesions

Cerebellomedullary lesions

Posterior inferior cerebellar artery lesions

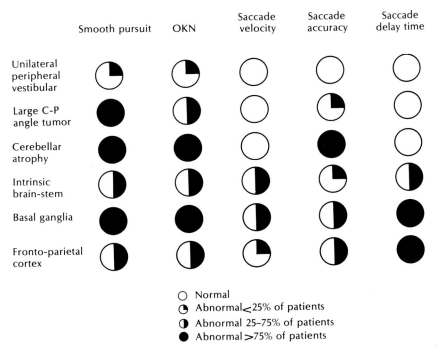

FIG. 27–2. Tracking and optokinetic abnormalities seen with focal nervous system lesions. The percentages were determined on a minimum of five patients in each category. (Baloh RW, Honrubia V, Sills A: Ann Otol Rhinol Laryngol 86:108–114, 1977)

vertigo was reported in posterior fossa (infratentorial) masses by Drachman, Diamond, and Hart (6). This is a differential observation between the so-called "benign positional nystagmus" of certain peripheral vestibular lesions and posterior fossa CNS lesions.

In a number of cerebellar lesions, Takemori (25) reported differential visual suppressions of caloric-induced vestibular nystagmus. Variations were noted in flocculus, nodulus, dentate, and other intracerebellar lesions.

VASCULAR CENTRAL VERTIGO LESIONS

A number of microcirculatory CNS problems may produce vertigo or dysequilibrium, or a combination of the two, depending upon location of lesion and severity of vascular occlusion. Extracranial arterial lesions primarily affect the vertebral-basilar system. The two major arteries involved in this system are the anterior inferior cerebellar artery, which is a branch of the basilar artery, and the posterior inferior cerebellar artery, which is a branch of the vertebral artery. Symptoms are due either to TIA or to actual occlusive syndromes. Intermittent vertebral basilar insufficiency involving the entire

system may produce a constellation of syndromes. One of the most common problems is the insufficiency secondary to vertebral artery compression by cervical spondylosis, with vertigo due to arterial compression upon turning of the neck.

In patients suffering occlusive syndromes, the vertigo attack is sudden and usually severe. The "drop" attack throws the patient to the ground, is accompanied by nausea, and lasts for hours.

Patients with this syndrome have cochlear hearing loss only if the anterior inferior cerebellar artery is involved. (This artery supplies the cochlea.) The vestibular findings are usually those of positional nystagmus without vestibular paresis. An evoked positional nystagmus is elicited by neck torsion or sudden change of posture. The normal cochlear findings and absence of contralateral labyrinthine preponderance (canal paresis) point to a vertebral basilar system lesion.

In vertebrobasilar disease, there are four characteristic symptoms. Barber (2) has suggested a very useful "4D" mnemonic approach. The 4D's include dizziness, diplopia (transient), dysphasia (speech slurring), and drop attacks.

In some cases, these are potentially prestroke lesions. There may be visual disturbances, *i.e.*, diplopia, blurred vision, or transient blindness. Vertigo is the most common symptom in intermittent vertebral insufficiency, occurring in about 45% of cases and usually provoked by postural changes. Occasionally, there will also be ataxia, seventh nerve paralysis (upper motor neuron) and hemiparesis.

Arteriography is indicated unless there is a specific contraindication. Arteriographic studies may point to the need for definitive surgical treatment, such as endarterectomy or arterial bypass, or for orthopedic surgical procedures, such as removal of cervical osteoarthritic spurs.

The most significant finding on neurootologic examination is the presence of evoked postural nystagmus with or without caloric abnormality and without cochlear hearing loss.

Treatment is basically medical, neurologic, and/or orthopedic. No definitive otologic therapy is indicated.

CERVICAL VERTIGO

Cervical vertigo is a clinical term describing vertiginous episodes, occasionally accompanied by fluctuating sensorineural hearing loss and tinnitus due to any one of several neck lesions, with mechanisms attributed variously to vertebral-basilar insufficiency, to disorders of the sympathetic vertebral plexus with secondary labyrinthine circulatory effect, or to lesions in sensory afferent neck nerves.

The cranial form of the cervical syndrome is characterized by myalgia and neuralgia in the neck and arm, and labyrinthine symptoms. A stiff neck, with tense muscles, guarded motion, and tenderness, frequently occurs in cervical vertigo. Fluctuant sensorineural hearing loss with tinnitus occurs in some patients.

Cervical vertigo usually responds rapidly to local therapy, *i.e.*, massage with heat, traction, and muscle relaxants. Local anesthetic block can produce dramatic cessation of symptoms. However, it is possible for massage and/or local anesthetic block to exacerbate symptoms.

Jongkees (17) stated: "In every case of vertigo, in combination with pain in the neck or in the back of the skull, particularly when the vertigo is related to the pain or is reproduced only by certain movements, the physician must remember the possibility of a cervical origin. X-rays are sometimes misleading. Persons over 60 all show osteoarthritic spurs or other changes in the X-ray picture of the nuchal vertebrae."

BENIGN POSITIONAL VERTIGO

Benign postional vertigo is closely allied symptomatically to cervical vertigo, with transient symptoms on position change. There is latency of onset and it is of short duration, moderately severe, and accompanied by systemic symptoms. Both the vertigo and nystagmus show adaptation and fatigability. The nystagmus is direction-fixed.

CENTRAL POSITIONAL VERTIGO

Central positional vertigo, in contrast to the benign type, shows no latency. Onset of nystagmus and vertigo is sudden, the nystagmus does not adapt but persists, and the nystagmus direction changes.

OTHER VASCULAR CENTRAL VERTIGO LESIONS

The subclavian steal syndrome is due to occlusion of the proximal subclavian artery, in which the more distal vertebral artery acts as a collateral to the arm. The blood is thus siphoned from the vertebral-basilar system into the distal subclavian bed. The low pressure in the arm and the low peripheral resistance of arterial arborization causes reversal of blood flow in the vertebral system, and results in symptoms of vertebral basilar insufficiency by exercise of the involved arm. In addition, fatigue or claudication of the involved forearm is noted on exercise. A systolic bruit may be heard in the supraclavicular fossa, and there is quite frequently a disparity of arm blood pressures of 30 mm Hg or more. Blood pressure differences and a bruit would call for the consideration of arteriography. There may be indication for subclavian endarterectomy or a supraclavicular carotid–subclavian graft.

Vertigo, with or without ataxia, accompanied by systolic cervical bruit points to the possibility of extracranial arterial insufficiency, a possible prestroke lesion.

The occipital steal syndrome, as a variant of the subclavian steal syndrome may produce unilateral vestibular abnormalities and a concomitant cochlear hearing loss similar to that of Meniere's disease. An abnormal communicating anastomosis between the vertebral and occipital arteries may produce a shunt away from the vertebral circulation.

Posterior inferior cerebellar occlusion will produce a lateral superior medullary infarct, known as the Wallenberg or lateral superior medullary syndrome. This is characterized by a rather abrupt onset. The patient may be thrown to the ground with nausea and vomiting that may last hours, days, or weeks, and is exaggerated by movement. The lateral medullary syndrome has associated neurologic symptoms including gait difficulty, Horner syndrome, facial analgesia, and palate weakness.

Internal auditory artery occlusion (vestibular and/or cochlear branch) is not a common lesion. The entire internal auditory artery, a branch of the anterior inferior cerebellar artery, may occlude, with sudden hearing loss as well as sudden vertigo. The symptoms and findings resemble peripheral labyrinthine lesions.

According to Fisher (7), the region of the confluence of the vertebral arteries to form the basilar artery is therefore a very major "vascular theatre of dizziness."

He reported that of 112 patients with basilar occlusion, 86 (77%) had "dizziness." He pointed out that in patients with dizziness as an unaccompanied first symptom, the dizzy attacks could occur hours, days, or even months before the next neurologic sign occurred. In most patients, a stroke occurred less than 6 weeks after the onset of the initial attack of dizziness. The next most common event was dysarthria, followed in short order by facial numbness, hemiparesis, headache, and diplopia.

The patient with an isolated complaint of sudden dizziness should be carefully questioned for these other symptoms since they may well be prodromas of an impending stroke that might be averted by appropriate anticoagulant therapy in time. The presence of coarse nystagmus between dizzy spells, excessive imbalance, and the Horner syndrome would also point to basilar ischemia. Nausea, vomiting, diarrhea, sweating, chills, and chilly feeling, pallor, faintness, a sense of limbs floating in the air, generalized weakness, staggering, ataxia, blurred or dim vision may all be signs linked to a potential transitory ischemic attack or a true stroke when they accompany dizziness that cannot be explained on any other grounds.

GUIDE TO DIFFERENTIAL DIAGNOSIS

In evaluating the entire group of syndromes involving the vertebral-basilar system, a simple guide in differential diagnosis is the question of associated symptoms. A patient with unilateral tinnitus and hearing loss accompanying an acute episode of vertigo should be considered to have a peripheral labyrinthine lesion if there are no signs of brain stem involvement. If such a patient, however, has concomitant ipsilateral Horner's syndrome, facial analgesia, palatal weakness, limb ataxia, contralateral analgesia of the body and limbs, a definite central lesion exists unless proved otherwise. Differential diagnosis calls for careful cochlear and vestibular studies by quantitative audiologic techniques and by quantitative vestibular studies utilizing electronystagmography, in addition to neurologic examination.

NONVASCULAR CENTRAL VERTIGO LESIONS

In multiple sclerosis, the very first symptom may be acute vertigo in about 15–25% of patients. Eventually acute vertigo occurs in 50–75% of patients with multiple sclerosis. Diagnosis is based on evidence of disseminated nervous system demyelinating lesions and/or ocular dysmetria. The young patient with acute vertigo and vertical nystagmus that persists after the vertigo ceases is a multiple sclerosis suspect.

Otherwise unexplained vertigo and vertical nystagmus can be attributed to acute demyelination or chronic gliosis in the lower pons or upper medulla, affecting the vestibular nucleus and/or its connections. Vertical nystagmus, in combination with pendular or jerking horizontal nystagmus, with a rapid component in the direction of gaze, is a common finding in multiple sclerosis. Persistent vertical nystagmus is relatively rare in peripheral labyrinthine disease, except in utricular lesions without semicircular canal involvement.

Ocular dysmetria is due to CNS lesions. Vertical nystagmus may also be due to drug therapy, which points up the need to postpone vestibular examinations until sedative, diphenylhydantoin (dilantin), or tranquilizer therapy has been discontinued.

Auditory abnormalities in multiple sclerosis are characterized by diversity. Noffsinger and colleagues (19) reported subtle audiologic findings, and only challenging speech and pure tone tests yielded abnormal responses. Most of the findings were elicited by responses to sustained stimuli, speech discrimination in competing environments, and binaural masking tests. Their electronystagmographic findings in multiple sclerosis patients included positional nystagmus, caloric hyperresponse, abnormal optokinetic tracking, and abnormal pendular tracking.

Command

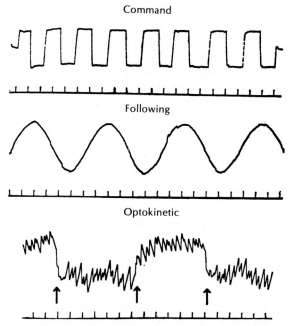

Following

Optokinetic

FIG. 27–3. Command, following, and optokinetic responses in a normal subject. **Arrows,** drum reversal. (Dix MR: Proc R Soc Med 64:857–860, 1971)

MEDIAL LONGITUDINAL FASCICULUS SYNDROME

The medial longitudinal fasciculus syndrome produces nystagmus and internuclear ophthalmoplegia. Studies by Stroud and co-workers (24), however, also report abducting nystagmus, in addition to supranuclear paresis of the ipsilateral medial rectus muscle.

CEREBELLAR LESIONS

Vertigo and nystagmus can occur in a number of cerebellar lesions. The dizziness is linked to gait, with a description of "dizzy on my feet." The classic observations of Holmes (12) in traumatic cerebellar hemispheric lesions were ipsilateral gaze paralysis followed by gaze-paretic nystagmus on gaze toward the side of injury. This gaze-paretic nystagmus subsides spontaneously as a result of oculomotor adaptation.

Recently, Hood, Kayan, and Leech (13) have described "rebound nystagmus" in cerebellar lesions. This nystagmus is evoked by changes in direction of gaze and is inhibited by eye closure. Each shift of gaze determines the direction of rebound nystagmus.

Cerebellar ectopia produces pressure pain in occiput and neck. There are cerebellar signs, in

addition to headache and abnormal vestibular findings, due to compression of vestibular nuclei and the vestibulospinal tract by the ectopic cerebellar tonsils. The vestibular abnormalities, according to Bertrand and Montreuil (3), do not conform to any precise pattern. There may be abnormal spontaneous or postural nystagmus and abnormal caloric responses.

BASAL GANGLIA AND ANTERIOR MIDBRAIN LESIONS

Lesions central to the brain stem and the cerebellum cause certain classic electronystagmographic findings. Dix (4) has described essential "command," "following," and optokinetic electronystagmographic responses in basal ganglion lesions. Normal saccades on command, normal following movements, and normal optokinetic responses with drum reversals (Fig. 27–3) contrast with those in a patient with basal ganglion disease (Fig. 27–4) in whom the saccadic responses are slow and irregular, the following movements are stepped up, and optokinetic tracings are deranged.

AGING CHANGES AND DIZZINESS (PRESBYVERTIGO AND PRESBYATAXIA)

Aging phenomena in the auditory system, usually termed **presbycusis** have analogies in the vestibular system, which I suggest should be termed **presbyvertigo** and **presbyataxia.**

FIG. 27–4. Command, following, and optokinetic responses in a patient with basal ganglion disease. (Dix MR: Proc R Soc Med 64:857–860, 1971)

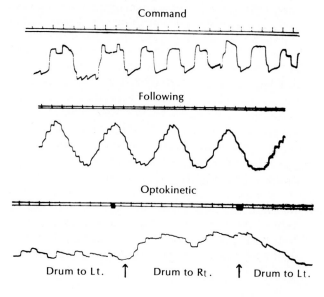

Command

Following

Optokinetic

Drum to Lt.   Drum to Rt.   Drum to Lt.

Schuknecht (22) has suggested a useful classification of four types of aging phenomenon in the vestibular system—three peripheral and one central.

CUPOLOLITHIASIS PRESBYVERTIGO

Cupular deposits in the posterior semicircular canal produce a gravity type of response which causes episodes of sudden, short attacks of falling.

AMPULLAR PRESBYVERTIGO

This vertigo is associated with angular head movements, without falling, which may last for several hours. (It may be difficult to dissociate this from cervical vascular vertigo.)

MACULAR PRESBYVERTIGO

Vertigo upon getting out of bed may be related to saccular macular atrophy described in 1965 by Schuknecht, Igarashi, and Gacek (21). In 1969 Johnsson and Hawkins (16) stated that, as in ampullar vertigo, it is not possible to eliminate cervical circulatory factors from this type of vertigo. An interesting senile saccula change has been reported by Johnsson (15a) (Fig. 27–5).

PRESBYATAXIA

This dysequilibrium syndrome is probably of CNS origin and is an ataxia that occurs primarily upon walking.

MOTION SICKNESS (SEASICKNESS)

HISTORICAL ASPECTS

Although seasickness has been known for centuries and was described in ancient Greek literature, its relationship to vertigo and dysequilibrium has been unclear until recently. The term **motion sickness** has come into current usage during the last few decades, which witnessed the growth of many new forms of rapid transport in addition to sea travel. Military and civilian aviation, submarine and space travel are examples of new modes of locomotion.

Seasickness may be defined as a repetitive syndrome of "dizziness," nausea, and vomiting, accompanied by pallor and cold sweating. These symptoms can occur upon real or simulated motion.

The term **nausea** is derived from the Greek word *naûs* (ship). Hippocrates reportedly stated that "sailing on the sea proves that motion disorders the body." Nonvestibular as well as vestibular theories have been advanced to explain motion sickness. The predominance of the nausea and vomiting symptoms gave rise to the so-called "gut shift" etiologic theory in motion sickness. Most contemporary observers agree that the vestibular system must be implicated basically in motion sickness phenomena.

The vestibular basic matrix of motion sickness dates to observations made following the recognition of Meniere's disease. Thus, Irwin, in 1881 (14), was able to deduce the fact that equilibrium is related to the cerebellum, the ocular system, and other related portions of the CNS, but he definitely attributed the primary pathologic lesion to the semicircular canals. The later recognition of the significance of the separate neuroanatomic and neurophysiologic functions attributable to the semicircular canals and to the otolith system has resulted in some of our present conceptions regarding the etiology of motion sickness.

VESTIBULAR SYSTEM INVOLVEMENT

William James, in 1882 (15), reported that 36% of deafmutes in a study conducted in institutions for the deaf were not made dizzy—*i.e.,* did not show vestibular responses to rotating stimuli—on a turning chair.

The vestibular overstimulation theory that resulted from studies following the second world war implicated only the vestibular system in the etiology of motion sickness. More recent studies point to a more complex concept. The vestibular system is involved, but there is also a "sensory conflict" phenomenon. Reason and Brand (20) in a major contribution to the subject, stress the etiologic importance of sensory rearrangement, in which motion information resulting from vestibular receptors, eyes, and nonvestibular proprioceptive mechanisms, conflicts with previously experienced inputs from these systems.

Thus, a number of competing etiologic parameters can explain basic mechanisms in motion sickness. These include an intermodality conflict between ocular and vestibular receptors, and an intramodality (intralabyrinthine) conflict between semicircular canals and otolith systems.

The development of extremely high speed aircraft and developments in astronautics have brought to the fore the consideration of symptoms

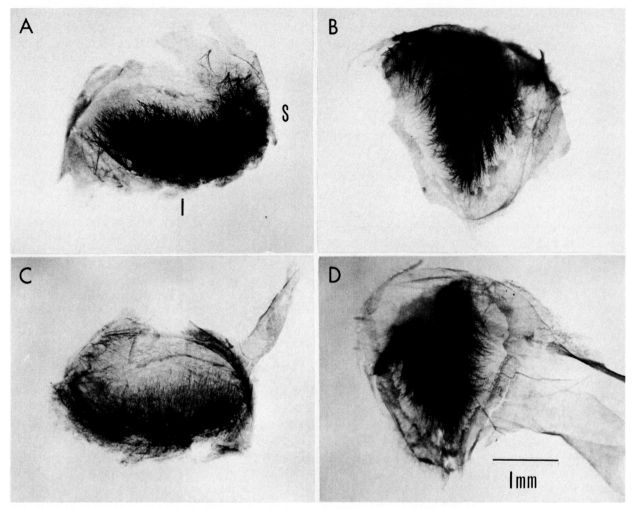

FIG. 27–5. A. Right saccule; **B.** utricle from a white 17-year-old male; **C.** left saccule; and **D.** utricle from a white 77-year-old male. The statoconial membrane and the neuroepithelium have been removed from the maculae so that the myelinated nerve fibers are displayed. In the older patient there is a severe nerve degeneration in the saccule, but only a mild degeneration in the utricle. There was an almost complete loss of saccular statoconia in the older patient. Note the innervation of the saccule. **I,** the saccular nerve from the pars inferior of the vestibular nerve; and **S,** Voit's nerve from the pars superior. In **C,** the saccular duct is seen at the upper right. Fixation, 5 hours and 14 hours, respectively, post mortem, OsO₄. (Johnsson LG: Laryngoscope 81:1682–1694, 1971)

that result from unexpected interactions of major differences between semicircular canal and otolithic inputs. Constant rotation about an off-vertical axis, as in the "barbecue-spit" rotation, when the body is spun around an earth-horizontal axis, create symptoms that arise as a result of continuously changing otolithic signaling inputs without expected confirmatory signals from the semicircular canal system.

Reason and Brand conclude that the underlying factor in all provocative motion sickness situations is that of sensory rearrangement, in which information to the vestibular receptors is artificially distorted by unusual stimuli. There is either an incompatibility between otoliths and semicircular canal-system inputs or between vestibular system and the ocular system inputs or both (20).

Motion sickness is, therefore, a complex peripheral and central vestibular problem with systemic visceral memory-pattern components. It is a definite vestibular syndrome rather than a form of dysequilibrium in which the vestibular system is uninvolved.

The interactions of cerebrum, cerebellum, extra-

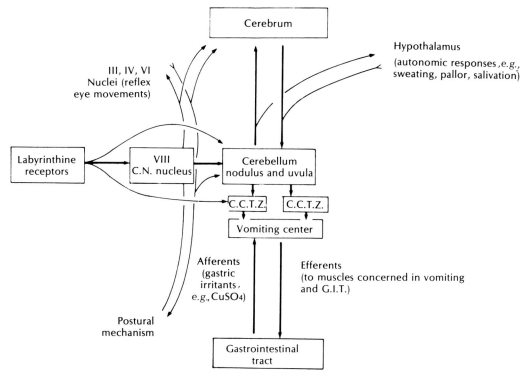

FIG. 27–6. Principal structures involved in motion sickness syndrome. (Reason JT, Brand JJ: Motion Sickness. London, Academic Press, 1975)

ocular muscles, labyrinthine receptors, chemo-receptive trigger zone factors, vomiting center, and the gastrointestinal tract are diagrammed in Figure 27–6.

CLINICAL ASPECTS OF MOTION SICKNESS

The dizziness of motion sickness is primarily characterized by extraordinary emphasis on nausea and vomiting, accompanied by pallor and cold sweating. The sweating occurs in the absence of an adequate thermal stimulus. Prodromas of increased salivation, sighing, and yawning are probably indications of drowsiness, which is commonly seen as a response to repetitive vestibular stimulation.

Headache, hyperventilation, anxiety, and other symptoms, are common to many of the symptoms of dysequilibrium, but it is the presence of vestibular phenomena that definitely separates motion sickness from dysequilibrium.

In addition to vertigo and nystagmus and/or counterrolling of the eyes, other post-vestibular-stimulation phenomena can occur. They include the oculogyral illusion (OGI) (10), the Coriolis

oculogyral illusion and the oculogravic illusion (8). The Coriolis OGI illusion is that of apparent motion of stationary objects elicited by tilting motions of the head about axes other than the axis of bodily rotation (11).

So-called "chronic motion sickness" is a persistent unsteadiness and associated symptoms long after the provocative motion-stimulating experience on land, sea, or in the air has ceased. This is probably related to biochemical factors concerned with fluid and electrolyte losses following the vomiting of the acute motion sickness episode.

VESTIBULAR PHENOMENA IN MOTION SICKNESS

The intensive studies of Graybiel and Clark (9) resulted in the conclusion that motion sickness must indeed be characterized as "vestibular sickness."

Although the semicircular canals appeared to be the primary loci of involvement in motion sickness, the dominant contribution of the otolithic system is now established. In most recent studies the primacy of otolithic stimulation in the production of motion sickness has been summarized by Reason and Brand (20) as due to four factors: 1) Linear accelerations in both ships and aircraft are well in excess of thresholds for otolithic stimulation in contrast to those for angular acceleration. 2) Nystagmus has rarely been observed during seasickness or airsickness. 3) It is possible to elicit motion-sickness symptoms experimentally by linear acceleration. 4) The adoption of the supine position by the patient or a simple tilting of the head backwards will either prevent or relieve symptoms of motion sickness in many instances.

There are conflicting opinions regarding the elicitation of nystagmus following linear (otolithic) stimulation. However, nonnystagmoid eye movements (counterrolling) have been recorded and are recognized as sequelae of otolithic stimulation by either horizontal or vertical linear acceleration.

The Coriolis effect is provoked by delivery of an unusual stimulus to the semicircular canal system. It results in the illusion of spinning about an axis which is orthogonal to both the head-tilt axis and the body-rotation axis. The weightless or zero gravity state can also produce symptoms of motion sickness.

VESTIBULAR FINDINGS IN MOTION SICKNESS

Motion sickness is rare in individuals with no measurable vestibular response. This has been noted in the vestibular nonresponse of both congenitally deaf patients and in patients with acquired vestibular paralysis. The ataxia that frequently occurs in acquired bilateral vestibular paralysis differs in symptoms and in findings on neurologic and vestibular examination from the findings in motion sickness.

Most studies in people prone to motion sickness have centered most recently upon abnormalities of linear acceleration rather than on abnormal findings on rotation or caloric stimulation.

In my own clinical experience, I have noted the frequent presence of caloric response asymmetry unaccompanied by hearing loss in a number of patients whose histories include a propensity to motion sickness throughout their lifetimes. In those with histories of being carsick (especially in the rear seat) ever since childhood or who become nauseated and vomit during or following sea or air travel, vestibular findings rarely show true canal paresis. Instead, there is a significant difference in caloric response (labyrinthine preponderance following warm and/or cold caloric stimulation). In our clinic we have not been able to gather sufficient

evidence regarding linear acceleration to draw any comparative conclusions from the otolith systems.

PREVENTION AND MANAGEMENT OF MOTION SICKNESS

In motion sickness–prone individuals a number of drugs have been considered to be of significant value in prevention and protection. Among these drugs are hyoscine, cyclizine, diphenhydramine, promethazine, and meclizine.

Many conflicting reports have resulted from studies of drug effectivity, including such objective measurements as cupulometry and the Dial test (26).

The Dial test, as conducted by Wood and co-workers (26), indicates the rather significant effectiveness of a combination of scopolamine and amphetamine as a superior protective approach to motion sickness when compared with antihistamines and other drugs.

In summarizing observations on effective anti-motion-sickness drugs, it appears that they must be drugs that block the vestibulomedullary emetic pathway at the level of the chemoreceptive trigger zone. This prevents or delays a recruitment phenomenon which would otherwise trigger medullary emetic mechanisms.

In the prevention of so-called "intractable airsickness," an adaption program was recommended by Dobie (5), which involves "turntable" component therapy.

The patient sits within an enclosed cabin aboard a rotating table. The chair is tilted through 90° in the fore and aft plane and can be tilted through 90° in the lateral plane. By combinations of such rotatory stimuli, it appears possible to obtain adaptation by some subjects who have had problems. The method has proved particularly useful in the management of recruits in flight training.

Reason and Brand (20) have suggested a working hypothesis for motion sickness mechanisms in demonstrating relationships of the cerebrum, cerebellum, vomiting center, and gastrointestinal tract to both peripheral and central labyrinthine receptors and to ocular and proprioceptive mechanisms. Motion sickness is thus defined as a self-inflicted maladaptation phenomenon. The presence of pallor, cold sweating, nausea, and vomiting, which occur at the onset of motion sickness episodes, is related at both onset and cessation to conditions of sensory rearrangement, when the pattern of inputs from the vestibular system, of other proprioceptors and of vision is at variance with the stored patterns derived from recent transactions with the spatial environment.

REFERENCES

1. Baloh RW, Honrubia V, Sills A: Eye-tracking and optokinetic nystagmus. Ann Otol Rhinol Laryngol 86:108–114, 1977

2. Barber HO: Diagnostic techniques in vertigo. J Vertigo 1:1–16, 1974

3. Bertrand R, Montreuil F: The role of nystagmography in the evaluation of cochleo vestibular function in cases of cranial trauma. Proc Can Otolaryngol Soc 20:47–77, 1966

4. Dix MR: Disorders of balance: a recent clinical neuro-otological study. Proc R Soc Med [Biol] 64:857–860, 1971

5. Dobie TG: Airsickness in Aircrew. AGARDograph No. 177, London, Technical Editing and Reproduction Ltd, 1974

6. Drachman DA, Diamond ER, Hart CW: Posturally-evoked vertigo association with posterior fossa lesions. Ann Otol Rhinol Laryngol 86:97–101, 1977

7. Fisher CM: Vertigo in cerebrovascular disease. Arch Otolaryngol 85:529–534, 1967

8. Grady FE, Montague EK: Quantitative evaluation of the vestibular coriolis reaction. Aerospace Med 32:387–550, 1961

9. Graybiel A, Clark B: Perception of the horizontal or vertical with head upright, on the side, and inverted under static conditions and during exposure to centripetal force. Aerospace Med 33:147, 1962

10. Graybiel A, Clark B: Validity of the oculogravic illusion as a specific indicator of otolith function. Aerospace Med 36:1173–1181, 1965

11. Graybiel A, Hupp I: The oculogyral illusion. A form of apparent motion which may be observed following stimulation of the semicircular canals. J Aviat Med 17:3–27, 1946

12. Holmes G: The symptoms of acute cerebellar injuries due to gunshot injuries. Brain 40:461–535, 1917

13. Hood JD, Kayan A, Leech J: Rebound nystagmus. Brain 96:507–526, 1973

14. Irwin JA: The pathology of seasickness. Lancet 2:907–909, 1881

15. James W: The sense of dizziness in deafmutes. Am J Otolaryngol 4:239–259, 1882

15a. Johnsson LG: Degenerative changes and anomalies of the vestibular system in man. Laryngoscope 81:1682–1694, 1971

16. Johnsson LG, Hawkins J Jr: Nerve Degeneration and Vascular Changes in Corti's Organ Based on Surface Preparations of the Human Cochlea. Proc IX Int Congr Oto-Rhino-Laryngol, Mexico, 1969. Amsterdam, Excerpta Medica Int Congs Ser No. 206

17. Jongkees LBW: Cervical vertigo. Laryngoscope 79: 1473–1484, 1969

18. Kimm J, MacLean JB: Disconjugate eye movements during electronystagmographic testing in patients with known central nervous system lesions. Ann Otol Rhinol Laryngol 84:368, 1975

19. Noffsinger D, Olsen W, Carhart R et al.: Auditory and vestibular aberrations in Multiple Sclerosis. Acta Otolaryngol [Suppl] (Stockh) #303:1, 1972

20. Reason JT, Brand JJ: Motion Sickness. London, Academic Press, 1975

21. Schuknecht HF: Pathology of the Ear. Cambridge, MA, Harvard University Press, 1974

22. Schuknecht HF, Igarashi M, Gacek R: The pathological types of cochleo-saccular degeneration. Acta Otolaryngol (Stockh) 59:154–170, 1965

23. Spector M: Electronystagmographic findings in central nervous system disease. Ann Otol Rhinol Laryngol 84:374, 1975

24. Stroud MH, Newman NM, Keltner JL et al.: Abducting nystagmus in the medial longitudinal fasciculus (MLF) syndrome: internuclear ophthalmoplegia (INO). Arch Ophthalmol 92:2–5, 1974

25. Takemori S: Visual suppression of vestibular nystagmus after cerebellar lesions. Ann Otol Rhinol Laryngol 84:318–326, 1975

26. Wood CD, Graybiel A, McDonough R et al.: Evaluation of some antimotion sickness drugs on the Slow Rotation Room. (No. 1) NSAM—922 Pensacola, Florida Naval School of Aviation Medicine, 1965

SUGGESTED READING

Altmann F: Otologic aspects of vertigo. Med Science, Feb, 43–49, 1966

Bergan JJ, Levy JS, Trippel OH et al.: Vascular implications of vertigo. Arch Otolaryngol 85:78–83, 1967

Eviatar L, Eviatar A: Vertigo in childhood. Clin Pediatr 13:940–941, 1974

Sharpe JA: Rebound nystagmus—A cerebellar sign JAMA 227(6): 648–649, 1974

Torok N: Vestibular decruitment in central nervous system disease. Ann Otol Rhinol Laryngol 85:131–136, 1976

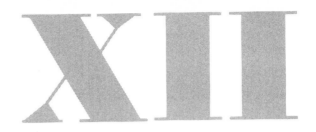

SEVENTH NERVE
LESIONS

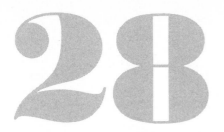

SEVENTH NERVE DIAGNOSTIC TECHNIQUES

Facial nerve (seventh nerve) paralysis may be caused by many types of lesions and may occur in a number of locations along the nerve's extensive course. Lesion locations may range from brain centers, the entire temporal bone, the parotid gland, and related neck and facial areas. The terms **facial nerve palsy** and **facial nerve paralysis** (which are not true synonyms) are used frequently interchangeably. The very common term **Bell's palsy** or **Bell palsy** identifies a special type of facial paralysis, which is treated separately in Chapter 29, Bell's Palsy.

Although the facial nerve is primarily a motor nerve, its sensory and secretory fibers accompany its motor divisions through most of its course. Differentiations of functions between specific motor groups and between sensory and secretory responses are used in tests for site-of-lesion diagnosis. Special quantitative and qualitative motor and sensory tests for determination of neural fibers' functional status provide valuable management information.

In addition to evaluations of facial nerve function involving motor, sensory, and secretory fibers, the contiguity of the facial nerve to both the vestibular and auditory branches of the eighth nerve make it necessary also to include vestibular and auditory function tests in the evaluation of most facial nerve lesions. Precise radiographic studies are also essential. Facial nerve paralysis may be due to an intracranial neurologic problem, to an intratemporal otologic problem, or to an extratemporal head and neck problem.

Upper and lower motor neuron lesions produce different symptoms and findings.

The very common lower motor neuron paralyses are most frequently due to lesions of the temporal bone. Because of the long and the intricate temporal bone course of the facial nerve, facial paralysis is primarily an ear disease and an otologic problem.

CLINICAL ANATOMY AND PHYSIOLOGY OF THE FACIAL NERVE

The facial nerve nucleus in the pons may be divided into upper and lower motor neuron divisions. Upper motor neuron lesions cause central facial nerve paralyses, and are usually due to intracerebral diseases, most commonly hemiplegia. Lower motor neuron lesions cause peripheral facial nerve paralyses, most commonly associated with temporal bone diseases.

UPPER MOTOR NEURON (CENTRAL) ANATOMY

Supranuclear fibers from frontal lobe areas (precentral gyrus) come from both (right and left) cerebral hemispheres to innervate the frontalis and orbicularis oculi muscles (Fig. 28–1). Because of this bilateral innervation, a unilateral cortical lesion will paralyze the lower face but not the forehead or eyelids. Three different cortical tracts are involved in upper motor neuron lesions.

1. *The crossed pyramidal (corticobulbar) tract* is the major frontal-lobe motor pathway to the facial nerve motor nucleus in the pons and is the primary tract for *contralateral* facial-muscle function.
2. *The uncrossed pyramidal tract* is the additional tract for *ipsilateral* facial muscle motion. However, this ipsilateral branch innervates only the three forehead muscles—the frontalis, orbicularis palpebralis, and corrugator supercilii muscles. Therefore, these three muscles have bilateral cortical representation.
3. *Extrapyramidal tracts* are related to *involuntary* functions. Two important tracts are a) the thalamic and associated pathways for muscles of expression related to emotional stimuli; and b) the reflex pathways associated with trigeminal, optic, and acoustic nuclei. These extrapyramidal pathways are responsible for blinking (optical and tactile palpebral reflexes) and the stapedius muscle reflex, which responds to acoustic stimuli.

LOWER MOTOR NEURON (PERIPHERAL) ANATOMY

The main trunk of the facial nerve is composed of motor fibers originating in the pontine nucleus and distributed to the periphery. Three special fiber

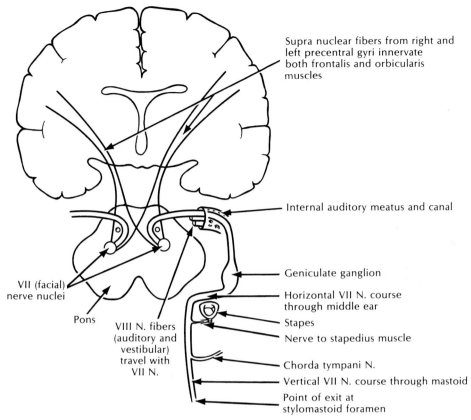

FIG. 28–1. Schematic drawing of seventh (facial) nerve pathway from origins in precentral gyri, to pontine nuclei, through internal auditory canal, middle ear, and mastoid, to exit at stylomastoid foramen.

tracts are associated with the main motor trunk and enter and leave the trunk at different levels. This variable anatomic relationship within the course of the facial nerve makes possible a rather precise topodiagnostic approach to the diagnosis of facial nerve lesions.

The three special tracts are "neighbors" originating from other nuclei. They include the following:

1. Motor fibers from the hypoglossal nucleus to the orbicularis oris muscle
2. Preganglionic secretomotor fibers—sphenopalatine (lacrimation) and submaxillary (salivation)
3. Sensory fibers for tactile sensation and for taste

Basically four portions of the facial nerve are differentiated by functionally separate nerve-fiber characteristics. There are two efferent portions (motor and secretomotor) and two afferent portions (tactile sense and taste). The afferent portions constitute the *nervus intermedius* or *nerve of Wrisberg.*

The main trunk of the facial nerve consists of motor fibers originating in the pontine motor nucleus. This major trunk leaves the pons at the cerebellopontine angle and enters into the internal auditory meatus of the temporal bone along with the nervus intermedius and the eighth cranial nerve (auditory and vestibular). At the lateral end of the internal auditory canal the facial nerve enters the fallopian canal within the petrous pyramid. It bends horizontally and passes through the geniculate ganglion (Fig. 28–2) located at the site of the first (anterior-superior) genu. It then courses posteriorly through the tympanic cavity (middle ear) (Fig. 28–3A) within the horizontal portion of the facial bony canal (Fig. 28–3B). It bends inferiorly at the second (posterior-inferior) genu and extends vertically through the mastoid portion of the temporal bone, leaving the temporal bone through the stylomastoid foramen. At this point the nerve trunk turns anteriorly to enter the

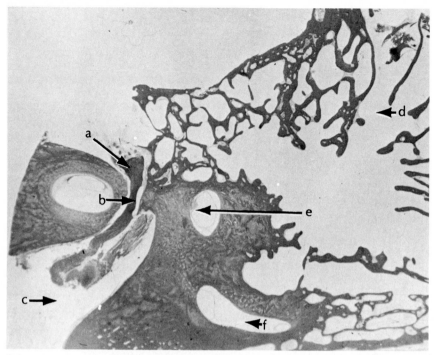

FIG. 28–2. Right ear section showing seventh nerve and geniculate ganglion (**a** and **b**), internal auditory canal (**c**), mastoid air cells in antrum region (**d**), superior semicircular canal with ampulla (**e**), and crus commune (**f**). (Gussen R: Ann Otol Rhinol Laryngol 81:235–240, 1972)

FIG. 28–3. Seventh nerve course. **A.** Intratympanic course. **B.** Intratemporal course.

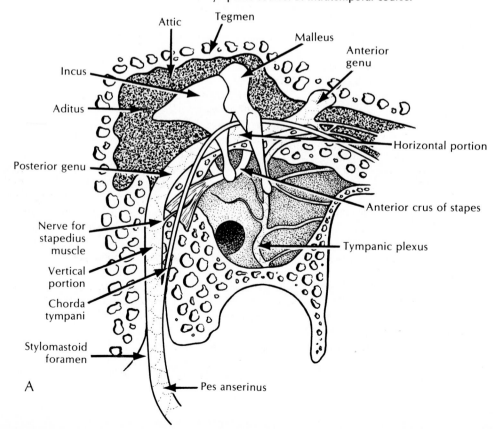

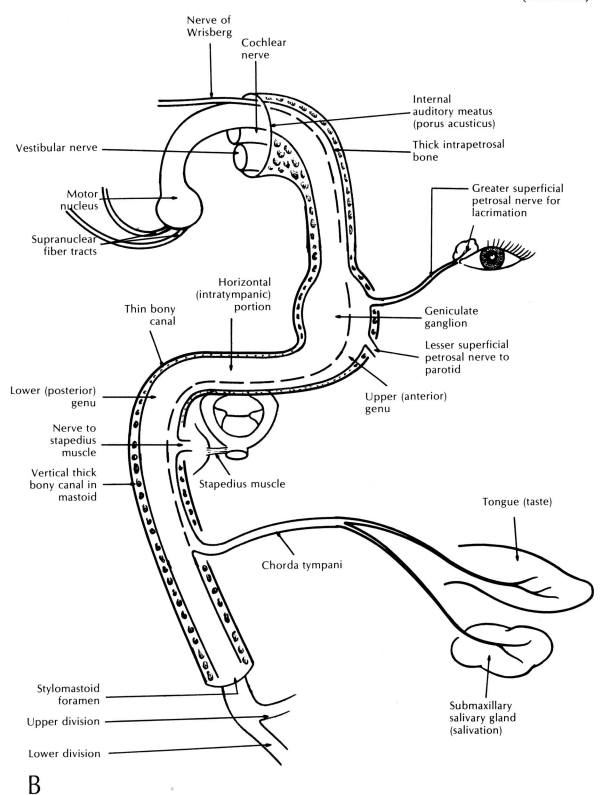

Nerve of Wrisberg

Cochlear nerve

Internal auditory meatus (porus acusticus)

Thick intrapetrosal bone

Vestibular nerve

Greater superficial petrosal nerve for lacrimation

Motor nucleus

Supranuclear fiber tracts

Horizontal (intratympanic) portion

Thin bony canal

Geniculate ganglion

Lesser superficial petrosal nerve to parotid

Upper (anterior) genu

Lower (posterior) genu

Nerve to stapedius muscle

Vertical thick bony canal in mastoid

Stapedius muscle

Tongue (taste)

Chorda tympani

Stylomastoid foramen

Upper division

Lower division

Submaxillary salivary gland (salivation)

B

FIG. 28–4. Peripheral distribution of seventh nerve branches.

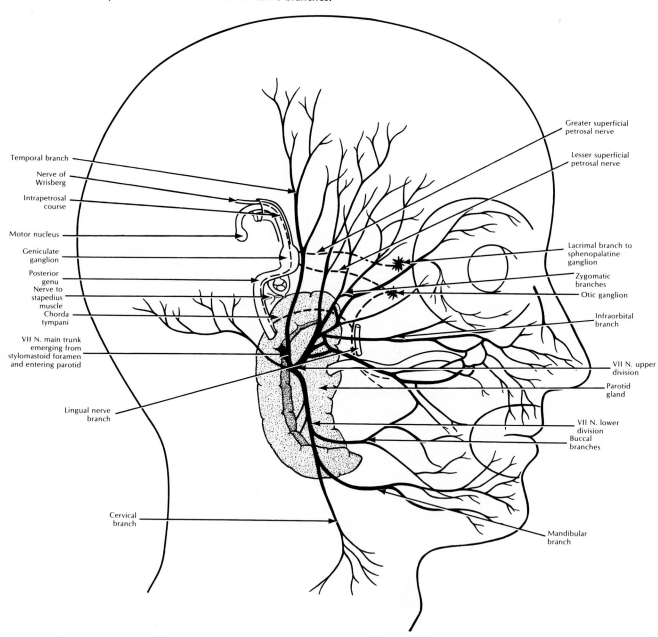

parotid gland. Within the parotid gland (Fig. 28–4) it bifurcates into upper and lower divisions, with a number of subdivisions, prior to final distribution to the entire facial area (pes anserinus). A number of major variations occur in this peripheral distribution of the branches of the facial nerve.

The greater superficial petrosal nerve, which innervates the lacrimal gland, usually leaves central to the geniculate ganglion. The first nerve branch to arise below the geniculate ganglion is that for the stapedius muscle, which comes off just below the inferior (posterior or second) genu within the vertical course of the seventh nerve through the mastoid bone. Shortly below, the chorda tympani nerve arises. Its fibers are described later in this chapter in the section on Infrastapedial Lesions.

FIG. 28–5. Eight topodiagnostic seventh nerve divisions.

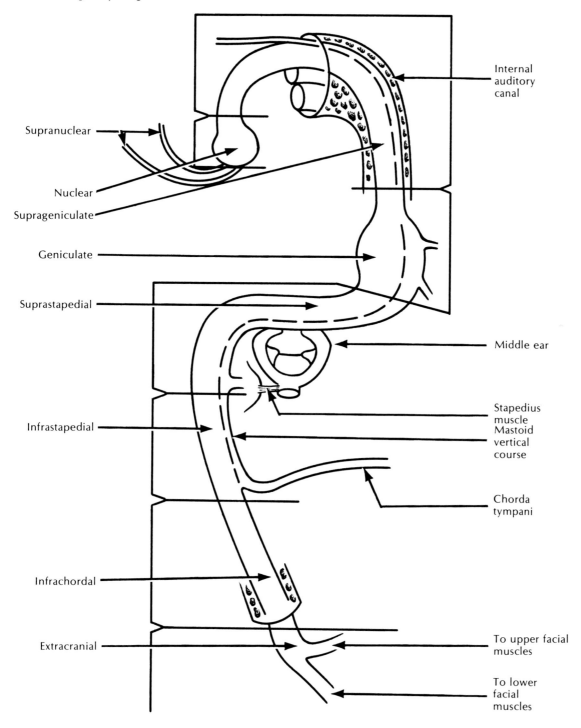

TABLE 28-1. Various Facial Nerve Findings at Eight Different Sites of Lesion

Site of lesion	Upper face movement	Bell's phenomena	Emotional movements	Blinking reflex	Stapedius reflex	Orbicularis oris movement	Tears	Taste	Deviation of chin on opening mouth
Upper motor neuron									
Supranuclear	Yes	No	Yes	Yes	Yes	Yes	Yes	Yes	Yes
Nuclear	No	Yes	No	No	No	Yes	Yes	Yes	Yes
Lower motor neuron									
Suprageniculate	No	Yes	No	No	No	No	No	Yes	Yes
Geniculate	No	Yes	No	No	No	No	No	No	Yes
Suprastapedial	No	Yes	No	No	No	No	Yes	No	Yes
Infrastapedial	No	Yes	No	No	Yes	No	Yes	No	Yes
Infrachordal	No	Yes	No	No	Yes	No	Yes	Yes	Yes
Infraforaminal	No	Yes	No	No	Yes	No	Yes	Yes	No

FACIAL NERVE PARALYSIS

Eight topodiagnostic divisions in seventh nerve anatomy may be considered, two for upper motor neuron paralysis lesions, and six for lower motor neuron lesions (Fig. 28–5 and Table 28–1). The two topodiagnostic upper motor neuron lesions deal with supranuclear and nuclear lesions.

CHARACTERISTICS OF UPPER NEURON PARALYSIS

Supranuclear Lesions

Crossed corticobulbar tract lesions are accompanied by the following clinical findings:

1. Unilateral paralysis of lower facial muscles is evident with voluntary stimuli.
2. Voluntary movements are normal in the three forehead muscles—orbicularis palpebralis, frontalis, and corrugator supercilii. The eyelids can be closed, the forehead can be wrinkled, and it is possible for the patient to frown.
3. Facial muscle response to emotional stimuli is normal.
4. Blinking and stapedial reflexes are preserved.
5. Orbicularis oris function is normal. The patient may produce labial sounds "B" and "P."
6. Lacrimation and taste sensations are normal (5).

Nuclear (Pontine) Lesions

A lesion due to the facial nerve nucleus itself (pons lesion) is usually flaccid rather than spastic and involves the entire face, including the forehead muscles. Although taste, lacrimation, and saliva are normal, the stapedius reflex is usually lost because there are separate nuclei involved in these functions. Frequently, pontine lesions that produce nuclear central paralysis are vascular or neoplastic and are associated with abducens paralysis due to sixth nerve involvement, with associated diplopia.

General Characteristics of Upper Motor Neuron Lesions

In upper motor neuron lesions, the most common cause is either a vascular lesion such as hemiplegia or a cerebral neoplasm. Lacrimation, taste, and salivation are normal in upper motor neuron lesions.

Hemiplegia is the most common associated neurologic lesion with upper motor neuron facial paralysis. This is ipsilateral when the lesion is above the pontine decussation. It is contralateral when the lesion is below the pontine decussation. A lesion limited to the decussation area may cause a bilateral upper motor neuron facial paralysis.

There are a number of difficult differential diagnostic aspects to upper motor neuron lesions. Only the emotionally induced lability of the facial muscles of expression is truly diagnostic. Many of the other signs that are regularly present in upper motor neuron lesions may also be occasionally seen in lower motor neuron lesions. Thus, lower facial paralysis alone may occur in peripheral lesions under the following conditions:

1. A lesion may be limited to the cervical branch of the facial nerve. When there is damage by trauma or tumor to the cervical branch of the facial nerve, such as follows radical neck dissections, the angle of the mouth may appear to be raised when the patient is asked to show his teeth. This is due to the isolated paralysis of the

triangularis oris muscle, which is an upper extension of the platysma muscles innervated by the cervical branch of the facial nerve.

2. Recovery from peripheral paralysis is incomplete. Branches innervating the lower face around the angle of the mouth are usually the last fibers to recover in diseases such as Bell's palsy and may remain permanently paralyzed.

CHARACTERISTICS OF LOWER MOTOR NEURON PARALYSIS

Six lower topodiagnostic divisions may be considered for clinical purposes.

Suprageniculate Lesions (Intracranial—Cerebellopontine Angle)

Lesions below the motor nucleus, either within the cerebellopontine angle or intrapetrosal but central to the geniculate ganglion produce similar topodiagnostic findings.

Lesions of the cerebellopontine angle produce varying sequelae. There may be diminished lacrimation and salivation. Taste may or may not be affected because of variations in distributions of chorda tympani fibers. Muscles controlled by the facial nerve are involved throughout the face including frontalis. Lesions of the cerebellopontine angle will involve neighboring cranial nerves, such as the eighth and/or fifth nerves.

Geniculate Ganglion Lesions

The greater superficial petrosal nerve leaves the main trunk at the geniculate ganglion. Postganglionic fibers to the sphenopalatine ganglion supply parasympathetic nerves to the lacrimal gland. The significance of this innervation is related to the Schirmer test for tearing. Lacrimation is absent.

Suprastapedial Lesions

The suprastapedial area is that part of the nerve above the origin of the motor branch to the stapedius muscle, and involves the intratympanic horizontal facial nerve in its bony canal, which extends from the anterior (superior) genu to the region below the posterior (inferior) genu within the vertical segment of the facial nerve in the temporal bone—a rather long course.

The stapedius nerve innervates the stapedius muscle, and is responsible for the stapedius reflex, which is activated by strong acoustic stimuli, ipsilaterally or contralaterally. A suprastapedial lesion produces a paralysis of the stapedius reflex, manifested by hyperacusis (increased sensation of loudness), and/or phonophobia (painful sensation of sound). It may be measured and recorded by tympanometry and stapedius reflex registration (see Chs. 6, 7, and 8).

Infrastapedial Lesions

The infrastapedial area is that part of the nerve within the vertical portion below the branch for the stapedius muscle and above the origin of the chorda tympani. Stapedius reflex is present, and salivation and taste are normal, indicating normal chorda tympani function. The chorda tympani nerve contains three different types of fibers: 1) fibers responsible for taste in the anterior two-thirds of the tongue; 2) fibers for tactile sensation in the intraoral part of the geniculate zone of the mouth and in the temporomandibular joint area; and 3) preganglionic secretomotor fibers that innervate the salivary glands at the floor of the mouth and are responsible for salivation from the submaxillary duct.

Chorda tympani function can be measured by taste sensation—gustometry—and by salivary flow studies.

Infrachordal Lesions

The infrachordal area is the most peripheral part of the nerve. In an infrachordal lesion, taste, salivation, and tactile sensations are preserved. An infrachordal lesion may be divided into infradigastric and supradigastric segments. This lowest branch of the nerve, the digastric nerve (close to the stylomastoid foramen) innervates the posterior belly of the digastric muscle and the stylohyoid muscle, both of which are involved in the act of opening the mouth. Paralysis of the digastric branch produces deviation of the chin to the opposite side on the attempt of maximal mouth opening.

Infraforaminal Lesions

In an infraforaminal lesion (in the neck) there is no such deviation. This is, of course, an extratemporal lesion.

DIAGNOSTIC APPROACHES TO FACIAL NERVE PARALYSIS

The first diagnostic task in a patient with facial paralysis is determination of the site and nature of the lesion. In addition, it involves a careful history, general physical and neurologic examination, and should also include an assessment of all cranial nerve functions, especially eighth nerve (auditory and vestibular).

Temporal-bone radiographs (Schuller's for the mastoid and Stenver's for the internal auditory meatus) are necessary in every patient with facial paralysis. In many cases additional helpful information is obtained by polytomography.

AUDIOLOGIC STUDIES

A basic standard audiogram is necessary, consisting of pure tone air conduction and bone conduction studies, speech reception threshold, and speech discrimination scores. A special auditory test for stapedial reflex function is an essential part of the site-of-lesion testing technique in facial paralysis (see Chs. 6, 7, and 8).

VESTIBULAR STUDIES

A screening vestibular examination is necessary and should include observations for spontaneous and positional nystagmus, adiadochokinesia, and observation for gait abnormalities. In special problems, a complete electronystagmographic vestibular and neurootologic investigation may be advisable.

Facial Nerve Studies

Two types of facial nerve studies are necessary: site-of-lesion tests, and motor neuron physiology (nerve conduction) studies.

FACIAL NERVE SITE-OF-LESION TEST TECHNIQUES

Lacrimation Test

The Schirmer tearing test (for geniculate ganglion lesions) is a simple test and is very informative. A small piece of litmus paper is placed in the lower fornix of the eye. The nasal lacrimal reflex is elicited either by stimulation of the nasal mucosa with an applicator or by inhalation of ammonia or some other aromatic. A difference between the degree of tearing in the two eyes would indicate a diminished lacrimation reflex and would point to a lesion proximal to or in the geniculate ganglion.

Stapedial Reflex Test

The stapedial reflex test is performed along with tympanometry. The stapedius reflex is monitored on one ear while the contralateral ear is stimulated (see Ch. 6).

Taste Sensation Test

This test of the chorda tympani nerves is useful both in site-of-lesion diagnosis and in nerve-conduction physiology studies.

Taste may be tested by simple methods utilizing sugar, salt, and other standard taste-excitation stimuli. More precise methods of testing taste involve the use of electrogustometry.

Impairment of taste in the anterior two-thirds of the tongue may carry an unfavorable prognosis for patients with Bell's palsy. Afferent fibers from the anterior two-thirds of the tongue are transmitted through the chorda tympani nerve. Gustometry equipment is usually based on an apparatus consisting of a 120-v dry battery connected to a circuit which delivers up to 300 μamp. The cathode is held in the patient's hand and the stimulating electrode, the anode, is applied to the lateral aspect of the tongue, first to the normal side with gradually increasing stimulus strength until the patient becomes aware of a metallic taste. The same procedure is repeated on the affected side and changes in threshold are noted. Normal responses agree within 30 μamp.

A normal electrogustometry response on the affected side usually carries with it a good prognosis for a full recovery in Bell's palsy or other facial nerve lesions. High thresholds on the affected side are usually associated with more severe lesions and a poorer prognosis. Prognostic aspects of Bell's palsy can be determined with electrogustometry in some cases before nerve conduction is affected. There may be an alteration in taste within the first few days of the paralysis.

In most cases of Bell's palsy there is some degree of taste involvement at onset. Recovery of taste in the first 8 days is invariably followed by satisfactory recovery (2). Impairment of taste lasting more than 2 weeks is usually associated with motor denervation. Quantitative electrogustometry is important if there is a critical difference of more than 100 μamp.

Salivation Tests (Secretomotor Fibers)

Precise salivation quantitative studies may be made by cannulation of the salivary gland ducts to compare salivary flow from the affected and the normal sides. As in gustometry, salivary flow studies are useful in both site-of-lesion diagnosis and in nerve conduction physiology studies (4).

TSCHIASSNY EIGHT LEVEL SITE OF LESION TEST SCHEMA

Tschiassny (6) described a useful eight-level site-of-lesion test schema.

In upper-motor-neuron lesions, two topodiagnostic divisions exist, supranuclear and nuclear, as described.

In lower motor neuron lesions, there are six topodiagnostic divisions.

MOTOR-NEURON FUNCTION TESTS

Several quantitative tests are used to measure motor-neuron facial-nerve physiology. Each test furnishes special information regarding neuromuscular function. Combinations of tests are used to determine functional status during the course of Bell's palsy and in traumatic and neoplastic lesions.

Nontraumatic facial-nerve lesions within the temporal bone are related to its bony canal course. In Bell's palsy, the nerve is compressed by bony canal entrapment. The first sequel of this edematous compression is a physiological block (neuropraxia). This temporary and potentially completely reversible conductivity loss is of short duration—usually a few days or a week. Reversal of neuropraxia results in total recovery of nerve function. Neuropraxia varies in severity of nerve involvement, depending somewhat upon lesion location. Continuation of edema is followed by axon degeneration (axonotmesis) and death of the axon. If the entire nerve trunk dies, the result is neuronotmesis. Nerve degeneration is partial at first, and then progresses to complete Wallerian neural degeneration.

Posttrauma axonotmesis can result in delayed regeneration of the facial nerve, with a disorderly regenerative process resulting in *synkinesis* (associative movements). Delayed regeneration also causes *mass movements* and *hemifacial spasm* which can accompany synkinesis.

Major clinical electrodiagnostic tests of the facial nerve include 1) the nerve excitability test; 2) the conduction latency test; 3) the intensity duration curve; 4) electromyography; and 5) electrogustometry.

Nerve-Excitability Tests

The nerve-excitability test is designed to differentiate neuropraxia (simple physiological block) from axonotmesis (degeneration) and is based upon comparative stimulation thresholds of the two sides of the face. The instrument used is a battery-operated square-wave generator (3). With physiological block (neuropraxia) there is no significant difference in stimulation thresholds. As axonotmesis begins, a decreased response is noted on the affected side.

A complete lack of response to stimulation on the affected side at high intensity indicates probable complete nerve degeneration (neuronotmesis).

The stimulating current from the square-wave generator is applied with a ball-end probe to the skin in the region of the stylomastoid foramen at the mastoid tip and along the proximal course of the facial nerve. A reference electrode is applied to the nape of the neck with electroconductive cream to improve surface conductivity. Current intensity is increased until the facial muscles begin to twitch. At this point, the relative current intensity is read from the dial as measured in milliamperes.

The square wave of negative polarity is 600 μsec in duration, with a repetition period of 166 msec. In square-wave studies a 3-mamp threshold seems to be the norm, although there are variations. In most cases the change between the affected side and the normal side becomes dramatic as nerve degeneration sets in. There are no important precise numerical values. The critical aspect is one of comparison (Fig. 28–6A).

The same device can be used with a triangular-wave form to produce muscle stimulation. Such tests are usually not valid until adequate time has elapsed for loss of motor end plate excitability. Prior to this time a normal muscle will not respond to the direct triangular-wave stimulation (Fig. 28–6B).

Electromyography

Electromyography is an older electrodiagnostic test used in facial-nerve function studies. Equipment for electromyography includes a pickup electrode, a stimulating electrode to determine motor nerve conduction time, and a cathode ground electrode. The electromyographic coaxial needle is the pickup electrode. It is inserted into each muscle under study, and it is placed approximately 2.5–2.75 cm away from the stimulating skin electrode. The cathode ground electrode is placed over the stylomastoid region. Stimulus intensity is varied until the muscle under study responds, producing a cathode-ray scope spike response. Muscles are explored at rest and during attempts at voluntary motion.

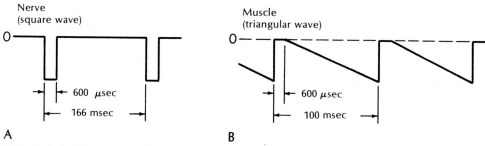

FIG. 28–6. A. Nerve excitability test—square wave. **B.** Muscle stimulation test—triangular wave. (Adapted from Hilger J: Trans Am Acad Ophthalmol Otolaryngol 68:74–76, 1964)

FIG. 28–7. A. Electromyography tracings for denervation and reinnervation studies. (Adapted from Alford B: Arch Otolaryngol 85:259–264, 1967. Copyright 1967, American Medical Association). **B.** Intensity duration curves for denervation diagnosis. (Adapted from Yanagihara N, Kishimoto M: Arch Otolaryngol 95:378, 1972. Copyright 1972, American Medical Association)

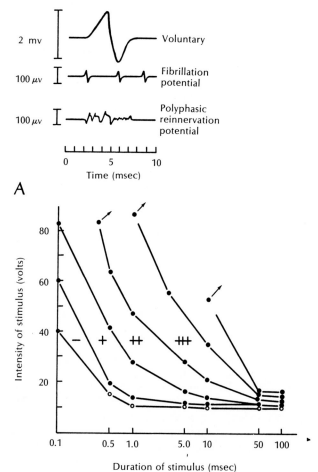

In neuropraxia (conduction block) the conduction time is usually less than 4 msec. The conduction time may remain normal during the first week of complete axonotmesis (nerve degeneration). Following this period there is absence of response. It is thus possible to establish the presence of a functional neuromuscular unit with electromyographic studies when nerve-excitability tests show evidence of apparent complete degeneration. Electromyography is a more precise test in monitoring the prognosis for neural recovery and in distinguishing voluntary-muscle-action potentials from fibrillations and from polyphasic reinnervation potentials.

In traumatic facial-nerve lesions, electromyography is a precise and valuable electrodiagnostic test (1). Voluntary-action-potential recordings (evoked electromyographic responses) would indicate anatomic continuity, even though there are no responses to external stimulation. True denervation potentials with electromyography are short in duration, smooth, and triphasic. Polyphasic potentials usually indicate some degree of reinnervation. True nerve degeneration will be displayed on electromyographic studies by fibrillation responses, which rarely occur prior to 2 weeks after onset of paralysis (Fig. 28–7A).

Since electromyography involves the use of needle electrode implantations into individual muscle groups, it is not used as frequently at the present time as the nerve-excitability test. However, it is a valuable and informative test and has an important place in diagnosing long-duration facial-nerve paralysis.

Intensity-Duration Studies

Intensity-duration studies are made at the motor points of the orbicularis oculi and oris muscles. A curve plotting the intensity of stimulus against duration of stimulus gives information regarding the extent of denervation. Three types of straight duration curves may usually be found in a series of facial-nerve paralysis cases. A normal curve is a smooth continuous curve. In partial denervation a discontinuous curve is noted. In denervation a steep sloping curve is observed. The intensity-duration curve studies are useful only after 7 or more days have elapsed (Fig. 28–7B).

Nerve-Conduction Latency Studies

Facial nerve stimulation with square waves as in the nerve-excitability technique is accompanied by recording of a midline muscle response. The time required for impulse travel is recorded as conduction latency. If conduction latency remains normal when nerve-excitability test responses decline, a favorable prognosis can be made.

REFERENCES

1. Alford B: Electrodiagnostic studies in facial paralysis. Arch Otolaryngol 85:259–264, 1967
2. Groves J, Gibson W: Significance of taste and electrogustometry in assessing the progress of Bell's (idiopathic) facial palsy. J Laryngol 88:855–861, 1974
3. Hilger J: Facial nerve stimulator. Trans Am Acad Ophthalmol Otolaryngol 68:74–76, 1964
4. May M, Harvey JE: Salivary flow. A prognostic test for facial paralysis. Laryngoscope 81:179–192, 1971
5. Tschiassny K: The method of locating the lesion in facial nerve paralysis. Am Acad Ophthalmol Otolaryngol, Instruction Course #492, Instruction Section, 1952
6. Tschiassny K: Eight syndromes of facial paralysis and their significance in locating the lesion. Ann Otol Rhinol Laryngol 62:677–691, 1953

29

BELL'S PALSY

VICTOR GOODHILL
SEYMOUR J. BROCKMAN

The term **Bell's palsy** applies to primary idiopathic facial paralysis that appears spontaneously—the most common facial paralysis in clinical practice. It is a peripheral (lower motor neuron) facial nerve paralysis, and in most instances the site of lesion is infrageniculate.

ETIOLOGY AND PATHOLOGY

Since Bell's palsy is characterized by neural conduction interference, it probably can be produced by several causes. Etiologic theories include viremia, allergy, vascular lesions, chilling, and systemic diseases. The herpes simplex virus has been implicated as a possible "reactivation" lesion of Bell's palsy. In a recent study of 41 patients with Bell's palsy (1), it was reported that serums from all 41 patients contained antibodies to herpes simplex virus.

Diabetes, pregnancy, and heredity are significant etiologic factors. Korczyn (7) reported an incidence of diabetes in 45% of children ages 10–19, increasing with age. In a series of 130 patients with diabetes, 66% had Bell's palsy with no other evidence of diabetic neuropathy. Bell's palsy tends to occur quite frequently in pregnant women. It may be inherited, as noted in several recent reports of family aggregates. Recent studies by Willbrand and co-workers (15) would suggest an autosomal dominant inheritance.

Abnormal spinal fluid findings were reported in 13 of 35 cases studied by Stien and Tonning (14). They concluded that Bell's palsy may be part of a generalized CNS lesion, even though no other abnormalities can be detected.

Bell's palsy is usually considered a mononeuropathy. In a recent report of vestibular findings, Rauchbach, May, and Stroud (13) reported 5 of 14 patients with classic Bell's palsy who had vestibular symptoms, 3 of whom had definite vestibular abnormalities on electronystagmographic studies. They concluded that Bell's palsy may be a polyneuropathy.

The multiple factors in etiology and in management make it difficult at the present state of knowledge of the disorder to evaluate epidemiology, recovery, and the therapeutic effectiveness of the various treatment modalities. Climatic, metabolic, genetic, and other factors play roles in incidence of the disorder. It appears that there is a higher incidence of Bell's palsy in colder climates and a lower incidence in tropical climates, although these observations have been disputed. Moreover, the vast majority of patients are seen by primary physicians rather than by otologists or neurologists, a factor complicating the evaluation of incidence in various populations and in different geographic regions. The fact that spontaneous recovery occurs in most patients compounds the problems of statistical analysis, especially in relation to the effectiveness of various medical and/or specific surgical therapies.

According to a recent study by Gussen (5), the pathogenesis of Bell's palsy is a retrograde epineurial compression edema resulting in facial nerve ischemia. The compression force results in either reversible or irreversible ischemic degeneration of myelin sheaths and axons, with varying degrees of cellular reaction to myelin breakdown. The resorption of the edema may leave either reversible or irreversible nerve damages, or it may stimulate collagen formation within the epineurium, resulting in persistent fibrous compression and entrapment neuropathy of the facial nerve (Figs. 29–1, 29–2).

CLINICAL ASPECTS

HISTORY

The history is usually a rather sudden awareness of unilateral facial weakness, frequently upon

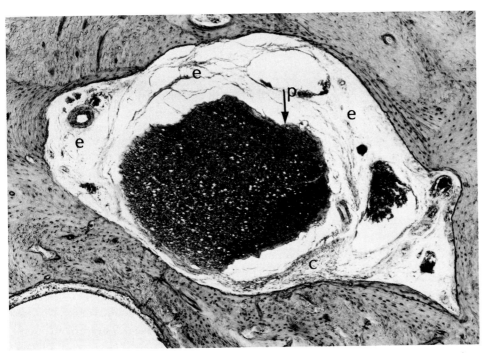

FIG. 29–1. Left normal side. Upper vertical descending facial nerve canal. Note loose areolar epineurial tissue **(e)** containing arteries and veins, and perineurial sheath **(p)** immediately surrounding the nerve. Individual collagen bundles **(c)** in cross-section can be seen in the epineurium below the nerve. (H&E, × 59) (Gussen R: Ann Otol Rhinol Otolaryngol. In press)

FIG. 29–2. Right side. Note dense fibrous tissue replacement of epineurium **(e)**. Arteries appear normal, but only rare slitlike venous channels **(v)** are present. Note dense fibrous tissue surrounding stapedius nerve **(s)**. Spaces are shrinkage artifact. Nerve appears normal but stains paler than on left side. (H&E, × 59) (Gussen R: Ann Otol Rhinol Otolaryngol. In press)

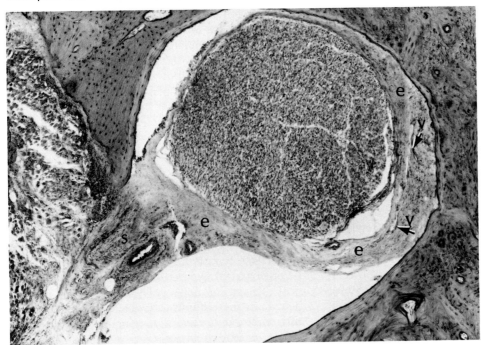

awakening in the morning. It is unassociated with other symptoms or findings. The patient is aware of a feeling of numbness and stiffness on the affected side of the face and frequently experiences discomfort in and around the ear. The discomfort may increase to severe pain in some patients, and when it does so, it is usually an indication of poor prognosis. As the condition progresses, the patient is unable to wrinkle the forehead, raise the eyebrows, or close the eye completely. There is difficulty in retracting the angle of the mouth and an inability to pucker the lips or to whistle.

EXAMINATION

The face, upon examination, is usually asymmetrical. There may be difficulty in drinking, and the patient may drool saliva. There may or may not be a loss of unilateral taste sensation, diminished lacrimation, and/or salivation on the affected side.

Bell's palsy is usually a unilateral (peripheral) lower motor neuron lesion of the facial nerve, affecting the frontalis and eye muscles and resulting in forehead paralysis and inability to close the eye on the affected side. By contrast, in upper motor neuron (central) lesions, the frontalis and eye muscles are spared, but upper and lower limb muscles on the affected side may be involved.

Diagnostic steps involve otologic and neurologic studies. In addition to a complete general medical examination, a systematic otologic examination, including otoscopic, ENT, audiologic, and radiographic studies are carried out. A facial nerve topodiagnostic survey (six topodiagnostic facial nerve divisions), facial nerve site-of-lesion tests, and appropriate motor-neuron physiology tests are performed as described in Chapter 28, Seventh Nerve Diagnostic Techniques.

It is extremely important in all cases of unilateral lower motor neuron facial nerve paralysis to rule out one of the most common causes of such paralysis—namely, otitis media. Otitis media and otomastoiditis may exist with little evidence of pain or other symptoms. Thus not only are careful otoscopic and mastoid x-ray examinations essential, but basic audiometric and vestibular examinations are frequently crucial in differential diagnosis. Other possible causes that must be considered are previous skull trauma, granulomatous and neoplastic diseases of the skull, temporal bone tumors, and lesions of the parotid gland, external auditory canal, and stylomastoid foramen.

MANAGEMENT OF BELL'S PALSY

MEDICAL MANAGEMENT

Once the diagnosis of Bell's palsy is made, basic medical therapy is primary. Ideally, the patient should remain at rest indoors. The patient should avoid chilling and exposure to drafts and winds. There is usually no need for hospitalization.

Protection of the involved eye from inadvertent corneal damage is necessary. The wearing of a protective eye-shield is advisable, especially at night. Five drops of 0.5% methylcellulose should be instilled every 4 hours. Conjunctivitis or keratitis may develop. The eye should be protected to avoid undue corneal drying and ulceration. Ophthalmologic consultation is advisable in cases of long duration, and tarsorrhaphy may be necessary.

Medical examination to rule out such metabolic conditions as diabetes is necessary.

The patient should have the nerve-excitability test at once and repeated every 24–48 hr to monitor the status of the nerve. The patient with physiological block (neurapraxia) and a clinically confirmed diagnosis of mild incomplete Bell's palsy without otalgia needs no specific medication during the first 3–4 days.

In most instances the patient with incomplete neurapraxia has an excellent chance for spontaneous recovery without treatment. If there is no spontaneous improvement after 3 days, in incomplete neurapraxia without otalgia, corticosteroid therapy is indicated.

Such therapy is indicated immediately in the patient with complete paralysis–neurapraxia as soon as the diagnosis is made unless there is medical contraindication to corticosteroid therapy.

A course of oral prednisone is started in a dosage of 60 mg daily for 5 days, 40 mg for 2 days, 20 mg for 2 days, and 10 mg for 1 day. A low-sodium intake and antacids are advised. Stools should be tested for blood at the beginning and at the end of the treatment.

The utilization of steroids in the medical therapy of Bell's palsy is widespread but not routine. In a double-blind study, May and associates (9) used steroids in one group and vitamin complex capsules in the others. No significant differences in results were reported.

Controversial aspects of other medical and surgical therapy for Bell's palsy are not new. Nevertheless, in most clinics steroid therapy is in use. Only time and carefully designed studies will produce definitive answers.

Physical therapy has been employed in Bell's palsy for years. Its therapeutic value, however, is still unclear. Some patients receive comfort from simple gentle massage of the muscles around the eye and mouth. Some physiatrists and neurologists recommend mild galvanic stimulation therapy, but the actual efficacy of such therapy is unknown.

SURGICAL DECOMPRESSION INDICATIONS

Beginning axonotmesis (nerve degeneration) is shown by diminished responses to the nerve-excitability test or to conduction latency tests and is an indication for consideration of early surgical decompression of the facial nerve, especially if otalgia is present. In such cases, electromyographic studies are advisable for more precise neurophysiological information. Electrogustometry and salivation studies can also contribute to the decision-making process concerning facial nerve decompression.

Paparella (12) lists the following indications for surgical decompression:

1. Electrical evidence of complete degeneration (axonotmesis)—facial muscles which cannot be stimulated with 20 mamp in the nerve-excitability test
2. Evidence of neurapraxia changing to axonotmesis (when additional 3.5 mamp are required to stimulate facial function)
3. Facial paralysis (neurapraxia) that persists without evidence of recovery in 6–8 weeks

Relative indications for decompression should be considered in the following special situations:

1. Severe otalgia (usually retroauricular) that persists from onset of paralysis
2. Recurrent Bell's palsy, especially if the first attack was followed by residual weakness
3. Immediate complete paralysis (gradual paralysis carries a much better prognosis for spontaneous recovery)

Although surgical decompression of the facial nerve in Bell's palsy has been accepted widely for a number of decades, some recent differences of opinion have been expressed. In 1972 Manning and Adour (8) stated that "experience with 504 patients of all age groups seen within four years has led the authors to abandon facial nerve decompression in the treatment of 'Bell's palsy'."

In 1969, Jongkees (6) expressed the more classic opinion for decompression surgery in Bell's palsy as follows:

We can be sure of only one thing: A paralysis which is complete after a fortnight will never recover completely; whether or not we operate at this moment. Some rests will always be found: asymmetries at rest or during movements, synkinesis, or contractures. This is especially true if electromyography shows the presence of fibrillations; but this test also requires a fortnight to appear.

In our opinion, there are very definite places for both steroid therapy and decompression surgery of the facial nerve in the management of Bell's palsy. The patient who shows definitive evidence of axonotmesis (denervation) in spite of a course of steroid therapy should be considered a candidate for decompression if there has been no evidence of improvement in 12–14 days.

We are well aware of the fact that excellent spontaneous improvements have occurred in many patients after long waiting periods. The bulk of the evidence, however, is in agreement with the opinion of Jongkees and others and indicates that when such improvement does occur, it is accompanied by asymmetries at rest, synkineses, or muscle contractures. These findings point to the advisability of decompression surgery when there are definite signs of denervation (axonotmesis) or when neurapraxia persists for 2 weeks following onset.

TECHNIQUES FOR SURGICAL DECOMPRESSION OF THE FACIAL NERVE

The traditional technique for facial-nerve decompression is a transmastoid exposure of the seventh nerve vertical segment's bony canal, followed by removal of bone from the region of the posterior genu to the stylomastoid foramen. This is usually followed by splitting of the perineural sheath, which reveals evidence of a "bulging" nerve. However, such bulging is not always present. In many instances, surgical decompression is a formal anatomical procedure without surgical microscopic evidence of abnormality in the nerve sheath or in the nerve itself. Surgical decompression is not always successful although, in general, decompression surgery has been followed by favorable responses in many patients, depending upon the duration of denervation prior to the surgery and depending also to some degree upon the experience and skill with which the decompression was performed. The traditional decompression operation has been limited to the vertical temporal bone segment.

A number of observations have been made in our clinic pointing to a variety of preexisting anatomical lesions discovered in the seventh nerve in surgical decompression.

We have observed that neural edema may not be present in the vertical segment but may be confined to the horizontal intratympanic course of the nerve. Thus, limited vertical segment decompression alone may be an anatomically inadequate surgical procedure.

Congenital dehiscences of the horizontal portion of the facial canal are present in 50% of temporal bones. In a number of our cases, the nerve edema was found to be located in, and restricted to the intratympanic horizontal part of the facial nerve immediately posterior to the posterior limit of a horizontal dehiscence. Such an edematous area may extend only into the posterior genu. Decompression limited (by traditional teaching) to the vertical segment in such a case is not only inadequate but inappropriate since it may cause unnecessary trauma to a basically normal portion of the facial nerve.

Precise site-of-lesion tests will frequently point to suprastapedial lesions, which may or may not be located in the vertical suprastapedial segment of the nerve. The lesion may well be within the posterior genu, within the horizontal portion, and in some instances anterior to the anterior boundary of a dehiscence, or close to the geniculate ganglion. Edematous lesions certainly occur where there are no dehiscences. Unnecessarily extensive decompressions based upon empirical rather than on microsurgically visualized decisions may be counterproductive. Splitting of a normal sheath in a nonedematous nerve may be an iatrogenic reason for incomplete recovery, synkinesis, and other undesirable postoperative sequelae.

The conventional posterior (vertical segment) decompression technique was undoubtedly based upon the traditional postauricular mastoid surgical approach, in which the facial nerve canal could be visualized only below the region of the horizontal semicircular canal. In order to visualize the posterior genu completely and to gain access to the horizontal portion of the canal, a wider exposure is necessary than that of a conventional posterior mastoid approach. This will involve greater epitympanic dissection and the need for removal of the incus. In the very small, contracted mastoid, such visualization via the standard postauricular technique is impossible without a facial recess dissection.

Through the circumnavigation surgical technique, and anterior position of the surgeon (see Ch. 17, Otomastoiditis Surgery—Mastoidectomy and Tympanoplasty, and Ch. 19, Otosclerosis) as used in stapes surgery, it is possible to visualize the horizontal portion of the facial nerve completely, to detect dehiscences, and to decompress the peridehiscent area through an intratympanic and antromastoid approach (via endomeatal or endaural incisions). In some instances it is necessary to section the incudostapedial joint and incudomalleal joint and temporarily remove the incus so that the region between the horizontal facial nerve portion and the posterior genu will be adequately exposed. It is possible to complete the entire dissection via the anterior approach without opening into mastoid cells, with total exposure of the facial nerve from the geniculate ganglion to the stylomastoid foramen.

Nerve sheath incision need not be total and may well be confined only to the area of obvious edema. In many instances the nerve exposure is limited to the horizontal portion and to the posterior genu. In some instances it is necessary to do a traditional vertical segment decompression. All of these anatomic options are easily available through an anteroposterior approach with circumnavigation of the patient's head (Fig. 29–3).

It is our practice to decompress only that portion of the nerve in which there is obvious edema and vascular injection of the perineural capillaries. In our experience, it appears to make little or no difference whether the sheath is split. Frequently, immediate return of function to the facial nerve is noted following anesthesia, particularly if the lesion has been confined to the region of the posterior third of the horizontal segment and the posterior genu.

If the incus has been removed it may be replaced in good contiguity with both malleus and stapes (2). In certain instances it is advisable to sculpt the incus into a hemiincus of the "golf-tee" type and place it between the stapedial capitulum and a malleal manubrium trough as an ossiculoplastic reconstruction (3). In the vast majority of cases, excellent hearing is maintained. As an alternative to replacement of the incus and difficult exposures, a prefabricated homograft ossiculoplastic procedure may be used (4).

The decompression procedure should include meticulous and delicate microsurgical removal of bone, followed by identification of the nerve sheath with adequate decompression, both proximally and distally, to secure visualization of normal nonedematous nerve.

The exposed decompressed nerve may be left alone, covered by blood clot, by absorbable gelatin sponge or film (Gelfoam or Gelfilm) or by a thin silicone (Silastic) sheet.

ADVERSE RESULTS FROM FACIAL NERVE DECOMPRESSION

In a recent study of 21 patients (11) who had surgical decompression of the facial nerve for Bell's palsy, seven patients showed evidence of cochlear or vestibular postoperative lesions. Three of the seven patients had tinnitus and hearing loss, one had tinnitus and intermittent vertigo, two had hearing loss, and one patient had transitory vertigo. This study seems to indicate that surgical decompression of the facial nerve is not an innocuous procedure and should not be carried out without serious awareness of possibility of such postoperative complications.

In our own experience with the anterior surgical

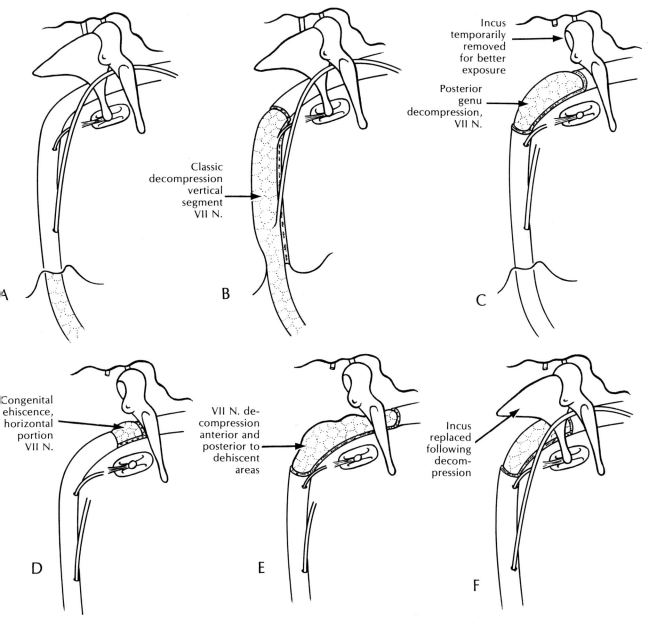

FIG. 29–3. A. Middle ear and mastoid segment of seventh (facial) nerve. **B.** Classic vertical segment decompression. **C.** Limited posterior (inferior) genu decompression following temporary removal of incus. **D.** Frequent (30–50%) dehiscences of horizontal portion. **E.** Peridehiscence decompression. **F.** Incus replacement.

approach, the number of adverse labyrinthine lesions is virtually nil. Such complications can occur in facial-nerve paralysis associated with surgery for either gram-negative type A lesions or type B otomastoiditis lesions. In uncomplicated Bell's palsy with the excellent surgical visualization provided by head circumnavigation and availability of the anterior position of the surgeon,

untoward labyrinthine trauma occurs exceedingly rarely.

A DUAL-TRACK MANAGEMENT PHILOSOPHY

McNeill (10) reported a group of 19 patients who underwent surgical decompression for idiopathic Bell's palsy and who were compared to a similar group of 11 patients to whom no treatment was given. According to this study, surgical decompression did not appear to improve the outcome of the disease and actually the results were slightly worse in the patients who underwent surgery as compared to the control group. There appeared to be a definite relationship between the age and the outcome of the disease, with better results in younger patients.

In the current debate between the advocates of steroid therapy alone and advocates of early decompression surgery, it is obvious that there is a place for both medical therapy and surgical therapy in the management of Bell's palsy. There are no "final answers" in the treatment of Bell's palsy, any more than there are in the treatment of any other complex disease. Both corticosteroid therapy and facial nerve decompression in the management of Bell's palsy should be considered in the management approach to the patient with Bell's palsy.

PEDIATRIC BELL'S PALSY

Bell's palsy occurs in children, but in the majority of pediatric cases of facial nerve paralysis, the cause is not true Bell's palsy. Unrecognized otitis media, birth injury, histiocytosis, skull fracture, and other lesions may be responsible for the facial paralysis. In true pediatric Bell's palsy the therapy of choice is prednisone therapy. In children above the age of 10, 40 mg daily in divided doses may be given for 4 days tapering off to 5 mg daily for a total of 8 days (8). In the absence of a favorable response to such corticosteroid therapy, surgical decompression should be considered, as in adults.

REFERENCES

1. Adour K, Bell D, Hilsinger R: Herpes simplex virus in idiopathic facial paralysis (Bell's palsy). JAMA 233:527–530, 1975
2. Brockman S: The anterior surgical approach in facial paralysis: the neglected horizontal position. Laryngoscope 84:1918–1924, 1974
3. Goodhill V: Hemi-incus and Tragal Cartilage Autographs in Ossiculoplasty. Proc IX Int Cong Oto-Rhino-Laryngol, Mexico. Amsterdam, Excerpta Medica Int Congr Ser No. 206, 1969
4. Goodhill V, Westerbergh A, Davis C: Prefabricated homografts in ossiculoplasty. Trans Am Acad Ophthalmol Otolaryngol ORL 411–422, 1974
5. Gussen R: The pathogenesis of Bell's palsy. Ann Otol Rhinol Laryngol 86:549–558, 1977
6. Jongkees LBW: The timing of surgery in intratemporal facial paralysis. Laryngoscope 79:1557–1561, 1969
7. Korczyn A: Bell's palsy and diabetes mellitus. Lancet 1/7690:108–110, 1971
8. Manning JJ, Adour K: Facial paralysis in children —diagnosis and treatment. Pediatrics 49:102, 1972
9. May M: Study casts doubt of efficacy of corticosteroids against Bell's palsy. JAMA 232:1203–1204, 1975
10. McNeill R: Facial nerve decompression. J Laryngol 88:445–455, 1974
11. Olson N, Goin D, Nichols R et al.: Adverse effects of facial nerve decompression for Bell's palsy. Trans Am Acad Ophthalmol Otolaryngol 77:ORL 67–71, 1973
12. Paparella M: Forum: Bell's palsy: drugs or decompression? Mod Med, Aug, 37–38, 1974
13. Rauchbach E, May M, Stroud M: Vestibular involvement in Bell's palsy. Laryngoscope 85:1396–1398, 1975
14. Stien R, Tonning FM: Acute peripheral facial palsy. Arch Otolaryngol 98:187–190, 1973
15. Willbrand J, Blumhagen J, May M: Inherited Bell's palsy. Ann Otol Rhinol Laryngol 83:343–346, 1974

Although Bell's palsy (primary idiopathic facial nerve paralysis, Ch. 29) is a major cause of facial (seventh) nerve paralysis, a number of other conditions are implicated etiologically. Indeed, the diagnosis of Bell's palsy is frequently made incorrectly because of a lack of awareness of many secondary lesions of the facial nerve that can mimic Bell's palsy.

Otitis media and otomastoiditis frequently cause facial nerve paralysis, and the surgery for otomastoiditis may also cause occasional iatrogenic facial nerve paralysis. Surgery for other ear conditions, too, may lead to injuries to the facial nerve.

Trauma from birth injuries and/or from skull and external ear injuries causes facial nerve paralysis also.

Viral infections, tumors, and vascular lesions are among other causes of secondary facial nerve paralyses. Aberrant anatomical courses of the seventh nerve can be responsible for surgical or other damage (5).

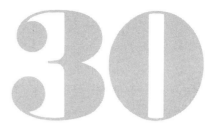

SEVENTH NERVE LESIONS AND INJURIES

FACIAL NERVE PARALYSIS IN OTITIS MEDIA, OTOMASTOIDITIS

Peripheral paralysis of the facial nerve may occur as a secondary lesion during the course of pediatric acute otitis media. The nerve paralysis may be present even before otalgia, fever, or otorrhea are manifested. Adequate treatment by immediate myringotomy and appropriate antimicrobial therapy will usually be followed by subsidence of the acute otitis media and return of facial nerve function.

Such secondary facial nerve lesions can also occur in adults, in association with either viral or bacterial acute otitis media or in chronic otomastoiditis. It must be differentiated, both in children and in adults, from the acute facial nerve paralysis specifically due to herpes zoster, or to its special variant, Ramsay Hunt's syndrome.

In facial nerve paralysis occurring in association with acute otitis media, special attention should be given to the possibility of concomitant unrecognized mastoiditis. Prompt and repeated mastoid radiographs, audiometric studies, and vestibular examinations are indicated. An unrecognized or untreated subacute or chronic otomastoiditis infection, especially in children, may be responsible for persistence of facial nerve paralysis. Facial nerve paralysis accompanying acute otitis media calls for prompt atticomastoidectomy. This may be performed either through a postauricular or an endaural incision. It is usually not

necessary to decompress the facial nerve in every case. If there is clearcut evidence of suppurative disease, bone necrosis, and/or polypoid or hyperplastic mucositis, then mastoid exenteration, removal of the basic lesion, and exposure of the entire bony vertical segment as well as posterior genu is required. Unnecessary decompression of the facial nerve in such cases may do more harm than good.

However, following an adequate indicated myringostomy and/or mastoidectomy and appropriate antibiotic therapy, if the facial nerve function tests show no evidence of recovery within 7–14 days following surgery, decompression should be considered. In such cases, the same criteria are used as those considered for decompression in Bell's palsy. The nerve-excitability test, electromyography, and site-of-lesion and other tests such as electrogustometry are useful in prognosis. If there is no evidence of improvement of neurapraxia and/or if there is evidence of definitive axonotmesis (denervation), a secondary procedure will be necessary for facial nerve decompression. In most cases of acute otitis media with facial nerve paralysis, immediate decompression of the nerve is unnecessary. Accordingly, it should not be considered a routine procedure during mastoidectomy in such cases.

In chronic otomastoiditis, facial nerve paralysis may occur in type B disease (keratoma-cholesteatoma) and/or tympanosclerosis, or in type A polypoid granulomatous temporal bone lesions. Most commonly, facial nerve paralysis in chronic otomastoiditis is a sign of extension of bone necrosis to some portion of the tympanic or mastoid course of the nerve. Bone necrosis in the posterior genu region, accompanied by fistulization of the horizontal semicircular canal is not uncommon, especially in cholesteatoma.

There is only one treatment for facial paralysis that appears during the course of chronic otomastoiditis—*i.e.*, adequate and prompt surgery. Such "adequate surgery" usually will involve removal of the incus, either temporarily or permanently, to be able to visualize adequately the horizontal segment of the facial nerve, the posterior genu, and the vertical segment. The circumnavigation technique and combined anteroposterior approach is very helpful in surgical access. Cell groups in the sinus tympani region, in the anterofacial, and in the retrofacial cell areas may all be implicated in the facial nerve paralysis. In some cases, a classic radical mastoidectomy may be essential, although an intact-canal-wall procedure suffices in most cases. In many instances it is necessary to decompress the facial nerve completely in its course from geniculate ganglion to stylomastoid foramen. It is advisable to preserve the perineurium (facial nerve sheath) in the presence of active suppurative otomastoiditis. In extensive keratoma or other type B otomastoid lesions or in nonresponsive, spreading, gram-negative type A otomastoiditis lesions with evidence of geniculate ganglion involvement, a radical primary decompression may require a subsequent middle fossa approach to deal with facial nerve lesions in the intrapetrous apex. However, routine decompression from stylomastoid foramen to internal auditory meatus is not a necessary procedure except in extremely rare cases.

IATROGENIC FACIAL NERVE TRAUMA

FACIAL PARALYSIS FOLLOWING TYMPANOMASTOID SURGERY

Prevention

Facial paralysis not infrequently is a complication of tympanomastoid surgery and may occur in surgery for either type A disease (chronic granulomatosis with extensive polyposis) or type B disease (keratoma-cholesteatoma, or tympanosclerosis). In incarcerated keratoma (cholesteatoma), tympanosclerosis, or granulomatous polyposis, the aditus ad antrum area connecting the mastoid antrum and major cell groups with the middle ear may be so occluded and compressed that adequate visualization of landmarks becomes difficult.

Extensive edema of the periosteum, accompanied by hyperostotic areas due to bone repair, may make it extremely difficult to recognize the normal landmarks of the short process of the incus, the horizontal semicircular canal, the genu of the facial nerve, and the tegmen tympani. Extremely meticulous microsurgical dissection under adequate magnification is essential. Sharp curets should not be used. Polishing or "diamond" burrs should be used with adequate irrigation to avoid undue heating of bone. The anteroposterior surgical approach is of tremendous help in such cases in that the tympanic landmarks may be viewed simultaneously with mastoid landmarks, thus facilitating identification of posterior tympanic contents (stapes, stapedial tendon, chorda tympani nerve) and providing adequate visual guides to identify crucial tympanomastoid structures. The relatively avascular chronic keratoma (cholesteatoma) mastoiditis is rarely a dissection problem with reference to the facial nerve. Operations during the course of a fulminating subacute otomastoiditis carry a high risk of facial nerve injury or postoperative facial nerve inflammatory neurapraxia. Not every facial paralysis following mastoid surgery is due to definitive facial nerve trauma. The paralysis is usually neurapraxic and temporary and subsides within a few days. On the other hand, the paralysis may be due not only to cutting of the nerve but to actual avulsion of several millimeters of nerve.

Repair of Postsurgical Paralysis of the Facial Nerve

It is imperative that facial nerve paralysis observed immediately following mastoid surgery be explored at once. If it is noted on the operating table, the operation should be resumed, following resterilization as necessary. Complete surgical preparation for a secondary procedure should be started immediately, provided there is no contraindication to continued anesthesia.

In reexploration, the surgeon must consider a possible lesion anywhere from the geniculate ganglion to the stylomastoid foramen. In extensive mastoid cellular disease, exposure of the nerve may be difficult. It is helpful to stimulate the facial nerve above and below the surgically exposed area, with a surgical electrode used with a square wave generator. Such diagnostic information is helpful in decision-making regarding simple decompression versus resection of an injured segment, rerouting, or nerve graft.

A careful search must be made for all of the tympanomastoid landmarks and the facial nerve's bony canal should be immediately decompressed. No significant harm will be done to the facial nerve if it has not been cut. If a bone chip that sharply penetrates through the nerve sheath is not immediately removed, neurapraxia will be quickly followed by axonotmesis (denervation). If there has been definitive trauma to the facial nerve with loss of a nerve segment, immediate repair is advisable. Such repair may be carried out by an end-to-end anastomosis or by rerouting the vertical segment from the facial bony canal. In some instances it is more expeditious to repair loss of facial nerve by the use of a nerve autograft taken from the posterior auricular nerve, a branch of the cervical plexus (Fig. 30–1).

FACIAL PARALYSIS FOLLOWING TRAUMA AND TEMPORAL BONE FRACTURE

The basic principles of facial nerve repair are based on precise microsurgery. "Accurate and meticulous apposition of cleanly transected distal and proximate epineurium" is one of the important aspects described by McCabe (7).

In longitudinal fractures of the temporal bone, facial paralysis is relatively uncommon and spontaneous recovery occurs in the majority of cases.

In transverse fractures of the temporal bone, facial paralysis occurs in 50% of cases, and is usually due to penetrating bone chips within the nerve trunk. Usually such fractures are accom-

panied by other aspects of skull fracture, which may require prior urgent management. In addition, there may be accompanying fractures of the labyrinth, cerebrospinal fluid leaks, and oval-window or round-window fractures with perilymph fistulas, all of which will require management. It is frequently possible to combine the facial nerve repair with repair of these other postfracture lesions.

Early diagnosis is extremely important in temporal bone fractures. Thus, electrodiagnostic tests of facial nerve function are necessary immediately after the injury. If there is delayed onset of the paralysis, the prognosis is usually good for spontaneous recovery. If electrical tests demonstrate beginning axonotmesis (denervation), facial nerve exploration should be scheduled as soon as possible, taking into consideration the general condition of the patient and other needs for more urgent surgical procedures. In most instances the facial nerve will have been traumatized in the horizontal and posterior genu regions rather than within the petrous pyramid. Usually a conven-

FIG. 30–1. Traumatic seventh nerve lesion produced during tympanomastoid surgery and management. **A.** Cutting burr used in removal of granuloma or specific lesion (type A or type B) inadvertently damages vertical seventh nerve canal and nerve. **B.** Excision of traumatized nerve segment. **C.** Proximal and distal segments freed and resutured. **D.** Nerve graft used to repair defect.

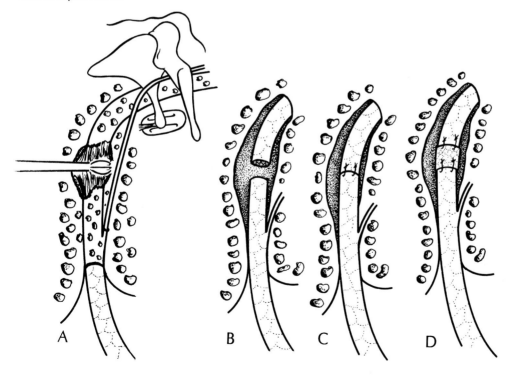

tional surgical approach to the tympanomastoid area via a postauricular or endaural incision will yield adequate exposure to deal with the facial nerve lesion. In some instances all that is necessary is removal of bone chips and appropriate decompression of the nerve sheath. In other cases a definitive repair of injured segments may be necessary.

Facial nerve reparative surgery should be undertaken when the patient's general condition is stable enough to allow for an orderly surgical procedure that may be time-consuming. Additional tympanomastoid problems should be dealt with surgically at the same time. Thus it is necessary that the labyrinth be carefully explored for a fracture, the tegmen be explored for a cerebrospinal fluid leak, and the oval-window and round-window niches be explored for the possibility of concomitant perilymphatic fistulas. All of these injuries should be promptly repaired at one surgical sitting.

Occasionally the fracture may be related to a middle fossa lesion. If there is evidence of impaired integrity of the greater superficial petrosal nerve with a loss of lacrimal gland function, it may be necessary to consider a middle fossa approach as well as a mastoidectomy. If there is no other indication for a middle fossa approach than the lacrimal gland observation, preliminary classic tympanomastoid exploration should be planned and middle fossa exposure deferred or undertaken as a second phase of the original temporal bone exploration. In most instances middle fossa exploration is not essential when the findings are confined to the facial nerve, middle ear, and labyrinth.

FACIAL PARALYSIS DUE TO BIRTH INJURY

Occasionally, peripheral facial paralysis will be noted immediately following delivery. This may be traumatic because of an unusually superficial stylomastoid foramen in the incompletely developed temporal bone. Forceps pressure may result in trauma to the distal portion of the facial nerve. In many instances there will be spontaneous return of function following subsidence of the edema. If there is no spontaneous return of function, as evidenced by electrodiagnostic tests, surgical decompression should be considered, utilizing the criteria previously described.

Occasionally, facial paralysis at birth may be central rather than peripheral in type and may be accompanied by other neurologic findings. This calls for serial neurootologic examinations for definitive diagnosis.

RAMSAY HUNT'S SYNDROME—HERPES ZOSTER OTICUS

The Ramsay Hunt syndrome is a herpetic viral infection primarily involving the geniculate ganglion, with sensory, and/or motor involvement. It may be associated with auditory, vestibular, and CNS symptoms and findings. Herpetic lesions may occur in the auricle or in the external auditory canal and may either precede or follow the onset of the facial nerve paralysis. Severe otalgia, malaise, fever, and weakness may accompany the other symptoms. The paralysis is usually complete and lacrimation is usually absent. The Schirmer test shows little or no tearing on the involved side.

The course of the disease is comparable to that of any severe herpes zoster infection. There is no specific medical therapy at the present time, although steroid therapy may be useful at the onset. Satisfactory spontaneous return of facial nerve function occurs in most cases. The question of conventional surgical decompression in this syndrome has not been resolved. Neither is there agreement on the necessity for middle fossa and transpetrosal decompression. At the present writing, no definitive medical or surgical management has been agreed upon. Supportive measures and physiatric muscle stimulation are helpful symptomatically.

FACIAL NERVE NEURILEMOMA AND MENINGIOMA

Neurilemomas and meningiomas may occur in the facial nerve, although they are rare. They are benign tumors and have usually been encountered during decompression operation for what had appeared to be ordinary Bell's palsy. They may appear with pain only and no paralysis; they may simulate acoustic tumor; they may appear as parotid masses with or without paralysis; they may simulate Bell's palsy; and they may be accompanied only by neurapraxia for periods of several years (Fig. 30–2). Neely and Alford described multiform variations in the extent of such tumors (9).

FACIAL HYPERKINESIA: HEMIFACIAL SPASM AND BLEPHAROSPASM

Abnormal facial movements may occur in two types. Hemifacial spasm is characterized by an

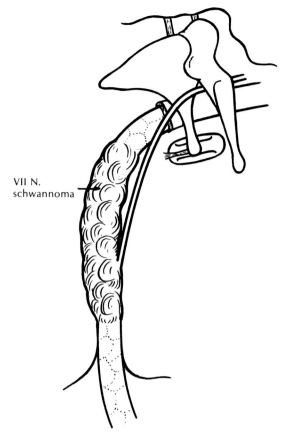

VII N.
schwannoma

FIG. 30–2. Seventh nerve schwannoma.

irregularity of unilateral twitches and spasms, involving especially the perioral, perinasal, and periorbital muscles. Occasionally the frontalis muscle may participate. Blepharospasm is almost always a bilateral phenomenon, with involvement of both orbiularis oculi muscles. In the initial stages of blepharospasm there is no other muscle group involvement, but in later stages other muscle groups may be involved.

Etiologic factors in facial hyperkinesia are not clearly understood. In general the treatment is not very favorable. A number of procedures have been utilized and include peripheral facial nerve branch block, excision of peripheral facial nerve branches, and partial nerve trunk excision. Posterior fossa craniotomy has been recommended by Janetta (6) for identification and ligation of possible anomalous vessels in the cerebellopontine angle. Although there are temporary improvements with many of these treatments, recurrence rates are unfortunately high.

MELKERSSON SYNDROME

This syndrome consists of recurrent facial nerve peripheral paralysis accompanied by swelling of the ipsilateral face and upper lip. It has been considered due to a vasomotor lesion involving the facial nerve, accompanied by neurotropic edema. In some cases there is associated tongue fissuring.

The syndrome, which may be bilateral, is not common. Surgical decompression has been performed in some cases with variable success (2).

SPONTANEOUS REINNERVATION AFTER FACIAL NERVE EXCISION

The phenomenon of "spontaneous" reinnervation of the facial nerve has been described periodically (3). The interpretation of apparent return of facial nerve function following radical excision of the nerve for such conditions as carcinoma is problematic. Reinnervation as studied by electromyography indicates homolateral rather than contralateral dominance in reinnervation.

The basic issue relates to fifth nerve motor fiber roles in such reinnervation, which may be from the masseteric nerve. Buccal branches of the fifth and seventh nerves may run together above the buccinator muscle.

Much additional investigation is required for clarification of facial nerve motor fibers and trigeminal motor branch relationships.

BILATERAL FACIAL NERVE PARALYSIS— FACIAL DIPLEGIA

Bilateral facial paralysis is relatively rare and usually occurs in neurologic lesions such as multiple sclerosis, viral polyneuritis, and midline brain tumors.

THE MANAGEMENT OF CHRONIC IRREVERSIBLE FACIAL PARALYSIS

Chronic irreversible facial paralysis may be due to a number of causes. It can be due to delayed treatment of Bell's palsy or lack of response to medical treatment or to surgical decompression. It may be due to trauma or to tumors. Regardless of etiology, it is a serious, deforming condition.

Facial nerve repair may be successful in some cases, and is effective even in a major loss of facial nerve trunk fibers. Encouraging results are being reported from even large seventh nerve grafts. The posterior auricular nerve provides excellent nerve graft tissue. Microsurgical apposition to the cut ends of the injured facial nerve is followed by some degree of function return in almost every case. In some instances the function is of the mass movement type, which can sometimes be improved by exercise techniques. If there is severe facial muscle involvement, it is not possible to hope for major functional repair with nerve grafts.

In rare cases spontaneous partial return of facial movement has been reported, and the movement is apparently due to unusual aberrant neural pathways involving the fifth nerve motor division.

Nerve crossover operations have been used for many years and have demonstrated a fairly significant degree of efficacy. This has been particularly true in cases of major head injury and in removal of large acoustic neurinomas in which the facial nerve was deeply involved within the tumor and had to be removed. The spinal accessory nerves—hypoglossal nerves—are used in crossover repairs. Excellent results can be expected in most patients. Movement may be noticed within 3–6 months after operation but may not appear for 12 months. This, of course, is mass movement; it is occasionally hypertonic and may be accompanied by a tic. However, the degree of response is worth while in most patients.

In very late cases with severe facial muscle atrophy, some rehabilitation successes follow facial support (face-lifting) operations, sling procedures, muscle rotations, and rhytidectomy.

Recent reports on cross-face innervation transplantation surgery are encouraging. It is possible to sacrifice several branches of the peripheral facial nerve without functional loss. Millesi (8), Scaramella (10) Anderl (1) and Fisch (4) have reported favorable findings in such cross-face facial nerve transplantations. The largest buccal and orbitozygomatic facial nerve branches of the normal side are anastomosed to mandibular and orbitozygomatic branches of the paralyzed side via double sural nerve grafts threaded across the face.

This procedure does offer new hope for certain types of irreversible facial paralysis.

REFERENCES

1. Anderl H: Cross-face nerve transplantation in facial palsy. Proc R Soc Med [Biol] 69:781–783, 1976
2. Canale T, Cox R: Decompression of the facial nerve in Melkersson syndrome. Arch Otolaryngol 100:373–374, 1974
3. Cerny L, Steidl L: Reinnervation after resection of the facial nerve. Acta Otolaryngol (Stockh) 77:102–107, 1974
4. Fisch U: Cross-face grafting in facial paralysis. Arch Otolaryngol 102:453–457, 1976
5. Greisin O: Aberrant course of the facial nerve. Arch Otolaryngol 101:327–328, 1975
6. Janetta P: The cause of hemifacial spasm: definitive microsurgical treatment at the brainstem in 31 patients. Trans Am Acad Ophthalmol Otolaryngol 80:319–322, 1975
7. McCabe B: Injuries to the facial nerve. Laryngoscope 82:1891–1896, 1972
8. Millesi H: Wien Med Wochenschr 9/10, 182, 1968
9. Neely J, Alford B: Facial nerve neuromas. Arch Otolaryngol 100:298–301, 1974
10. Scaramella LF: Arch Ital Otol Rinol Larngol 82:209–218, 1971

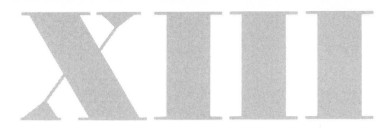

PEDIATRIC
OTOLOGIC
SYNDROMES

31

CONGENITAL HEARING LOSSES

EMBRYOLOGIC ASPECTS

The embryologic principles underlying the development of the human ear (as described in Ch. 1) provide a conceptual matrix for many ear anomalies. Congenital malformations of the auricle and external ear are related to developmental defects of the first and second branchial arches and to lesions of the branchial groove, which joins with the endoderm of the first pharyngeal pouch to form the external auditory canal.

Common auricular anomalies include aplasias, such as anotia and microtia, and auricular malpositions due to first and second branchial arch malformations.

External auditory meatus and external auditory canal aplasias, partial or complete, are due to first branchial groove malformations. Combined external auditory canal and middle ear aplasias are due to concomitant defects of branchial arch, branchial groove, and the first pharyngeal pouch, the latter being responsible for eustachian tube, middle ear, and mastoid cell differentiation.

The ectodermal otocyst develops independently from external and middle ear primordia; it is the auditory placode that eventually differentiates into the complex inner-ear cochleovestibular system. Because of the separate development of the inner ear from that of the external auditory canal and middle ear, combined external, middle, and inner ear lesions are not very common, but they are not rare. Combined lesions do occur. A number of special syndromes have been identified and are described in this section.

SEMANTIC PROBLEMS

The terms "hearing loss" and "deafness" are not true synonyms (see Ch. 5, "Hearing Loss" and "Deafness"). Nor are the terms "congenital" and "hereditary" (genetic) synonymous. **Congenital** is a chronologic, time-linked term meaning *present at birth, natal,* or immediately *postnatal.* **Hereditary** is a term meaning *inherited* or *genetic,* in relation to cause. Congenital (at birth) hearing losses may be hereditary or acquired.

Congenital hereditary hearing losses may be due to intrauterine lesions (prenatal), birth lesions (natal), or to immediately postnatal lesions. Congenital acquired hearing losses may be due to prenatal lesions (as in maternal rubella), to natal lesions (as in the Rh factor—hyperbilirubinemia group), or to immediate postnatal lesions (as in infantile meningitis).

Both hereditary and acquired hearing losses may be due to a number of morphologic abnormalities in the auditory system.

The term "congenital nerve deafness" is very commonly used by otologists, pediatricians, audiologists, teachers of hearing-impaired and deaf children and others. Although it has been useful, it is a confusing term. The following three factors must be considered: 1) Many patients are not born (congenitally) with a hearing loss. The hearing loss may have started in early childhood or later but was not recognized at birth. Thus, "congenital" may be chronologically incorrect in such cases. 2) The hearing loss may not be entirely due to nerve deafness. There are many patients who have combined (mixed) conductive and sensorineural hearing losses. In some cases it is possible surgically or medically to correct the conductive hearing loss component of the lesion. 3) The hearing loss may be completely correctable either medically or surgically alone, through the use of a hearing aid alone, or through the combination of medical treatment, surgery, and amplification. The patient with a corrected hearing loss may function as well as a person with normal hearing. The term "deafness," when used indiscriminately, is inappropriate sociologically and educationally and can be very damaging both to patients and their families.

MEDICAL AND ANCILLARY SPECIALIST ROLES

The child with a communicative disorder is first a patient and only secondarily a client or student needing therapy, habilitation, and education. The responsible professionals in such cases are physicians—*i.e.,* pediatricians and/or family physicians, otologists (otolaryngologists)—and audiologists. The first requirement is diagnosis, as made by the *otologist,* interacting with other physicians, and by the *audiologist*. The two, in effect, constitute an *ad hoc* diagnostic team. The final result is an otologic-audiologic diagnosis. Subsequently, a dual medical and audiologic team will be responsible for the infant or child with a communicative defect. The pediatrician as well as the otologist is intimately involved in the overall management of the child with a communicative disorder; in addition the neurologist, the child psychologist, the child psychiatrist, the radiologist, and other specialists, may have important roles. Finally, the habilitation and educational team that will be responsible for guidance, habilitation, and educational planning, will constantly interact with the otologic-audiologic team (8).

The next several chapters deal with developmental malformations (both hereditary and acquired) that may create external, middle ear, and/or inner ear lesions. In addition, pathology and clinical findings in the many lesions causing serious hearing losses are described. Habilitation and education of hearing-impaired and deaf children are covered in the closing chapters of this section.

Sensorineural hearing losses in children are pleomorphic. In spite of sharp embryologic demarcations between external, middle, and inner ear developments, mixed lesions do occur and must be considered in diagnosis and management.

CLASSIFICATIONS OF CONGENITAL HEARING LOSS SYNDROMES

Some congenital lesions (hereditary or acquired) are primarily of external or middle ear origin and usually associated primarily with conductive hearing losses. In congenital sensorineural hearing losses the major problem is cochlear (inner ear). In some syndromes, concomitant external and/or middle-ear conductive components accompany cochlear and/or neural lesions.

Conductive Lesions

In dealing with congenital malformations producing primarily conductive hearing losses, it is useful to use the following classification.

1. Auricle malformations
2. Combined malformations of the auricle, and external auditory canal
3. Combined malformations of auricle and/ or external auditory canal and middle ear
   A. Atresia with mobile lateral ossicular system
   B. Atresia with fixed lateral ossicular system
   C. Atresia with congenital stapes fixation
4. Malformations limited to ossicles

5. Combined external-ear and/or middle-ear and associated malformation syndromes

In the conductive lesion malformation group, concomitant cochlear and/or neural lesions may coexist.

Sensorineural Lesions

A large group of patients with congenital hearing losses have no external or middle ear lesions. The presenting lesion is sensorineural hearing loss with or without associated malformations.

Several classifications are useful in considering the patterns of congenital sensorineural hearing loss, *i.e.*, site-of-lesion (cochlear, eighth nerve, and CNS) and special or combined syndrome classifications.

Cochlear lesions may be hereditary or acquired. Either may be present at birth or manifested after birth.

Neural lesions limited to the auditory nerve (eighth nerve) or cochlear nuclei alone, are rare, on either hereditary or acquired bases.

Infantile meningitis, in which the auditory (and usually vestibular) nerves in the cerebellopontine angle and in the internal auditory meatus are involved, may spare the membranous labyrinth and cause purely neural hearing loss, but usually the inflammatory process is diffuse, with combined cochlearneural lesions.

Rhesus incompatibility and similar diseases of the hyperbilirubinemia type probably involve only the cochlear nuclei in some cases, but the auditory nerve and cochlea may also be involved by pigment deposition and subsequent hypoxic changes.

Congenital CNS lesions in the auditory system without cochlear or neural components have not been verified. A presumptive congenital CNS auditory lesion is that seen in autism. However, no definitive correlated otopathologic, neuropathologic, and/or audiologic studies are available in autism. Autism may not even be a truly auditory problem.

Acquired CNS auditory lesions are seen primarily in certain brain tumors and in cerebrovascular lesions.

Congenital hereditary cochlear lesions consist of prenatal aplasias or dysgeneses. Heredodegenerative lesions may be manifested at birth, after birth, or delayed into childhood or adult periods.

Congenital acquired cochlear lesions producing sensorineural hearing loss may also be divided into prenatal, natal, or postnatal. They exhibit greater etiologic diversity than hereditary lesions, as follows:

1. Prenatal
   A. Toxic causes (ototoxicity)
   B. Infections
      1) Maternal rubella
      2) Congenital syphilis
2. Natal
   A. Trauma
   B. Hypoxia and anoxia
   C. Rh factor (primarily cochlear nucleus)
   D. Prematurity
3. Postnatal (infantile and childhood)
   A. Mumps
   B. Rubella, rubeola, and related viremias
   C. Bacterial diseases

SYNDROME CLASSIFICATIONS OF HEREDITARY SENSORINEURAL LESIONS

A number of syndrome classifications of sensorineural hearing loss hereditary lesions are in use. Many are designated by eponyms. The late Dr. Bruce Konigsmark introduced an orderly syndromal classification of types of hereditary hearing loss lesions (9). Five criteria were used for the classification: 1) mode of hereditary transmission; 2) anatomic characteristics of the lesion; 3) age of onset; 4) audiologic characteristics; and 5) associated nonotologic lesions.

Mode of Hereditary Transmission in Deafness Due to Mendelian Inheritance

The mode of hereditary transmission can be 1) autosomal dominant, 2) autosomal recessive, and 3) sex-linked.

Anatomic Characteristics

The anatomic characteristics may be pleomorphic, *i.e.*, external ear, middle ear, and/or cochlear lesions. Thus, it is possible for a patient to have a congenital auricular lesion on one side, combined with complex middle ear and inner ear deformities. On the other side, there may be a normal auricle and external canal with a middle ear abnormality and a normal cochlea.

Four basic morphologic temporal bone patterns may be recognized. Histopathologic lesions in both hereditary and acquired congenital hearing loss cases are complex. The pathologic patterns are not necessarily characteristic of either origin. The following simplified classification starts with the most severe and proceeds to milder lesions.

AGENESIS OF BONY LABYRINTH. This lesion, the most severe, is characterized by total or partial absence of the bony labyrinth, involving either cochlear or vestibular portions, or both. Fragmentary membranous structures may be present. The auditory and vestibular nerves may or may not be present. There is no hearing response. The disorder is commonly known as the Michel lesion.

VARIABLE MALFORMATIONS OF BONY AND/OR MEMBRANOUS LABYRINTH. A variety of malformations of the bony labyrinth occur. The cochlea may be partially developed and the basal turn is usually present. The middle or apical cochlear turns, however, may be defective. There may be developmental anomalies in saccule, utricle, and semicircular canals. Auditory and vestibular ganglia and nerves are usually present, at least in part. In these lesions, commonly known as Mondini lesions, there may be measurable hearing for pure tones in the low or middle frequencies, but there is rarely significant measurable or useful hearing for speech.

MEMBRANOUS LABYRINTHINE MALFORMATION. Normal to close-to-normal bony labyrinth formation is accompanied by variable cochleovestibular membranous integrity. There is partial degeneration of both cochlea and saccule. Audiograms in patients with this malformation, commonly known as the Scheibe lesion, show varying degrees of pure tone hearing response in the low and middle frequency ranges, and speech-hearing responses may be within significantly useful ranges.

MODERATE MEMBRANOUS LABYRINTH MALFORMATION/DEGENERATION. This lesion is characterized by delayed onset type of hearing loss. The bony labyrinth is usually completely normal. The gradual onset of cochlear hearing loss is due to mild-to-moderate degrees of cochlear membranous degenerative changes and has been commonly called the Alexander lesion.

The classic audiologic finding is that of the so-called "dishpan" audiogram, with predominant pure-tone hearing losses in the middle frequencies. Such losses may be slowly progressive or may stop at undetermined levels during adult life (Figs. 31–1, 31–2).

Age of Onset

The age of onset of hereditary hearing loss may vary from *congenital* (prenatal, perinatal, and early postnatal lesions, as noted in dominant congenital severe cochlear lesions) to *delayed onset* in the young adult (as noted in Alport's disease—

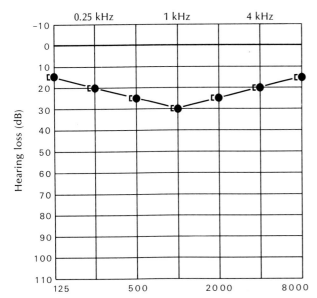

FIG. 31–1. "Dishpan" audiogram with major loss at 1 kHz seen in a young adult with Scheibe type hearing loss. ●—●, AC, unmasked, RE; [—[, BC, masked, RE.

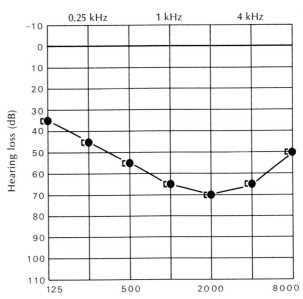

FIG. 31–2. Modified "dishpan" audiogram in a 55-year-old man with Scheibe type hearing loss. Note major loss at 2 kHz. ●—●, AC, unmasked, RE; [—[, BC, masked, RE.

congenital renal lesions), to *the older adult* with hereditary otosclerosis. Age of onset distinguishes a number of the classic syndrome types.

Audiologic Characteristics

There is a misconception that hereditary (genetic) hearing losses involve primarily the higher frequencies. While this is true in many cases, it is certainly not an absolute pattern. Dominant low-frequency hearing loss varieties occur and dominant mid-frequency ("dishpan" varieties) occur along with the more frequently encountered high-frequency losses. There may be symmetrical losses bilaterally, or asymmetrical losses. There may be mixed lesions characterized by both conductive and cochlear components. The presence of a rather obvious external ear deformity does not preclude the possibility of a concomitant cochlear lesion. Thus, surgical management of external ear deformities must be carefully evaluated in terms of the strong possibility that the external canal or the tympanic-ossicular defect may also be accompanied by malformation of the cochlea and/or a lesion of the spiral ganglion and other components of the auditory system.

"Mixed" conductive-cochlear hearing losses have been described. In a study of "congenital pseudo-mixed deafness," Anderson and Barr (1) pointed out the complex diagnostic problems in cases where there is a low-frequency bone conduction

response in deaf children, as further analyzed by Dayal, Wortzman, and Hands (3). In most instances such audiologic findings represent neither the hearing responses nor so-called "vestibular hearing." Our own studies turned up such cases, in which surgical exploration revealed either concomitant ossicular fixation or anomalous oval and round window findings (6). Such findings included normal stapes mobility with absent round window reflexes, or pulse-synchronous pulsation of round window membranes. No instances of surgically correctable hearing loss were encountered.

Associated Nonotologic Congenital Hereditary Abnormalities

In many cases of hereditary hearing loss there are accompanying abnormalities in other parts of the body. Such accompanying lesions may include the integument, the eyes, the nervous system, the skeletal system, the endocrine system, and the urinary system.

NEONATAL SCREENING AND HIGH-RISK REGISTRIES FOR CONGENITAL DEAFNESS

Early diagnosis of deafness is obviously desirable in the management of an infant with either hereditary or acquired congenital hearing loss. The success in acquiring communicative skill is largely related to early diagnosis and prompt habilitation programs (see Chs. 34, 35, and 36)

Neonatal screening programs have been instituted in a number of communities with testing of neonates shortly after delivery. In a 1967 editorial Goodhill (7) pointed out disagreements as to the practicability and reliability of such testing. In commenting on the advisable studies of Downs and Steritt (4), exception was taken to the statement that: "the number of false positives does not represent any real problem for the physician, who can determine often by simple tests ... whether a true loss exists."

Even to the experienced pediatric otologist and audiologist, these "failed" babies present a real problem. The process of auditory maturation and the variability from child to child are still largely uncharted and unknown. It is a common experience for the otologist to have referred to him infants who at 2–4 months are suspected of having hearing losses, but who several months later, with additional maturation, are found to be responding quite normally.

Recognition of a significant hearing loss in an infant is extremely important from the point of view of early educational management. Their simple testing technique does afford a practical method for demonstrating normal hearing in the newborn and possibly for detecting those infants who have a hearing impairment.

Workers in the field of pediatric audiology are well aware of the outstanding capability of Mrs. Downs and her group in the assessment of hearing in infants. Such capability, however, is not widespread. Therefore, we urge a conservative approach to mass screening programs for neonates (7).

In a 1976 report by Feinmesser and Tell (5) of a longitudinal study of 17,731 newborns tested by an acoustic signal generator hearing test (Apriton), 25 children were identified as deaf, 14 with severe or profound hearing loss, and 11 with moderate or moderately severe hearing loss.

They concluded in their summary: "The screening hearing test did not prove to be sensitive enough for detection of deafness in newborns, and, therefore, is not considered valid for screening purposes. The 'at risk for deafness,' register, which in our program covered 20% of the entire newborn population, proved to be too expensive and impractical; a restricted register, including approximately 7% of the newborns, is suggested."

As experience in high-risk registries increases, it becomes obvious that *selective neonatal screening is very important.* Thus, it appears most desirable that neonatal screening be instituted in such categories. Bergstrom, Hemenway, and Downs (2) recommended a "two tier" screening procedure be adopted: "The first 'tier' involves selection of the 'at risk' population, a group in which the likelihood of the handicapping disorder is apt to be significantly greater than in the general population. For this first stage of the procedure to be feasible a minimal sensitivity level of 80 per cent must be achieved. This means that the prevalence of the disorder being sought must be at least 16 times greater in the high risk group than in the general population. Therefore, in setting up a high risk register it is first imperative that we establish that such increased prevalence for congenital deafness does occur in the high risk group."

The "second tier" in the screening process is the actual neonatal audiometric test. When findings point to need for formal evaluation of an infant who has "failed" a screening test and in whom a hearing loss is diagnosed, a study should include a complete pediatric examination, with family genetic and audiologic surveys. Special studies may include antibody titers, viral cultures, and a number of other diagnostic studies, as recommended by Stewart (10).

REFERENCES

1. Anderson H, Barr B: Congenital pseudo-mixed deafness. Laryngoscope 77:1825–1839, 1967
2. Bergstrom L, Hemenway WG, Downs M: A high risk registry to find congenital deafness. Otolaryngol Clin North Am 4 (2):369–399, 1971
3. Dayal VS, Wortzman G, Hands C: Low frequency bone conduction response in deaf children. Ann Otol Rhinol Laryngol 81:429–432, 1972
4. Downs MP, Sterritt GM: A guide to newborn and infant hearing screening programs. Arch Otolaryngol 85:37–44, 1967
5. Feinmesser M, Tell L: Neonatal screening for detection of deafness. Arch Otolaryngol 102:297–299, 1976
6. Goodhill V: External conductive hypacusis and the fixed Malleus syndrome. Acta Otolaryngol [Suppl] (Stockh) 217:1–33, 1966
7. Goodhill V: Editorial. Arch Otolaryngol 85:23, 1967
8. Goodhill V: The Otologic-Medical Team Relationship With the Audiologist in the Field of Communication Defects. Proc IX Int Congr, Oto-Rhino-Laryngology, Mexico, 1969. Amsterdam, Excerpta Medica Int Congr Ser No. 206
9. Konigsmark BW: Syndromal approaches to the nosology of hereditary deafness. In Birth Defects: Original Article Series, Vol 7, #4. Baltimore, Williams & Wilkins, 1971, pp 2–17
10. Stewart JM: The pediatric management of the congenitally deaf child. Otolaryngol Clin North Am 4(2):337–369, 1971

A large variety of congenital ear syndromes are determined by mendelian inheritance. According to Fraser (11), autosomal recessive deafness is a heterogeneous entity determinable at different gene loci by homozygosity for distinct pathologic alleles. The mutations that result are probably responsible for specific enzyme deficiencies. A number of syndrome groups have been identified.

CONDUCTIVE SYSTEM MALFORMATIONS

Auricular malformations may occur without associated external canal or middle ear abnormalities. A large variety of combined lesions, however, are seen in pediatric populations. In addition, special syndromes involving systemic malformations are encountered.

AURICLE MALFORMATIONS

Congenital malformations limited to the auricle are defects in branchial arch differentiation. They are usually not associated with anomalies of the tympanic membrane, middle ear, and ossicles. Thus, normal bone-conduction thresholds and normal speech discrimination scores (indicating normal cochlear function) will be found in most patients with congenital defects limited to the auricle.

A large variety of "abnormal" auricles occur with no associated external ear canal or middle ear lesions. Such malformations primarily constitute cosmetic problems, with the exception of conchal collapse and Reger effect (see Ch. 13, External Ear Diseases). They include ears that are larger or smaller than normal, ears that lack cartilaginous adequacy (lop ears), and ears with gross differences in shape (Figs. 32–1, 32–2, 32–3). They are brought to the attention of the patient either by family or friends or by personal self-assessment.

Malformations that are limited to the auricle and do not involve the external ear canal or middle ear basically require aesthetic and cosmetic considerations. The management is surgical and includes a number of auriculoplasty approaches (many of which are successful), as well as prosthetic techniques. Details regarding cosmetic auricular problems are well covered in texts on reconstructive and plastic head and neck surgery.

COMBINED MALFORMATIONS OF THE AURICLE, EXTERNAL CANAL AND MIDDLE EAR

Much more serious are the problems of anotia, microtia, and auricle malposition, which are fre-

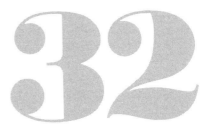

HEREDITARY CONGENITAL EAR SYNDROMES

VICTOR GOODHILL
RUTH GUSSEN

quently combined with malformations of the external auditory meatus, canal, and middle ear and are usually accompanied by conductive hearing losses. Even greater challenges are those combined lesions in which eighth nerve (cochlear) and seventh nerve malformations accompany external ear problems.

Major auricular deformities are aplasia, which may range from partly formed auricles to small shapeless cartilaginous or soft-tissue appendages on the side of the head (Fig. 32–4). They very frequently are low-set in position, below the normal auricular level. They vary tremendously and may be unilateral or bilateral. In most instances they are accompanied by audiologic evidence of good cochlear function, as measured by normal or close to normal bone-conduction studies. They may be associated with radiographic evidence of well-developed and well-pneumatized temporal bones or with contracted nonpneumatized temporal bones. Usually, there is no true external canal, the canal region being represented by a noninvaginated area. A so-called atresia plate of solid bone (32) replaces the tympanic membrane. There may be a vestigial tympanic membrane, represented only by the medial fibrous layer, and a mucous membrane layer. Incudomalleal fusion may be

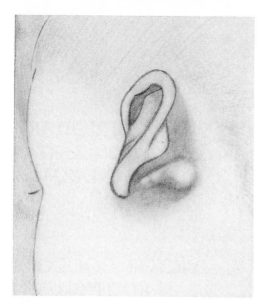

FIG. 32–1. Lop ear with supernumerary posterior tag.

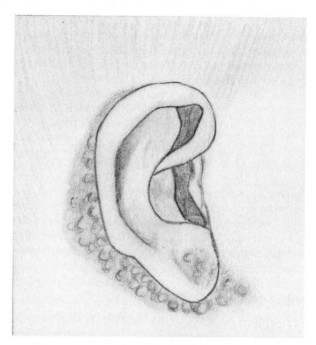

FIG. 32–2. Anterior auricular accessary tags.

FIG. 32–3. Malformed concha and tragus.

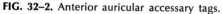

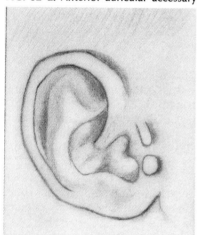

FIG. 32–4. Cartilaginous auricular appendage.

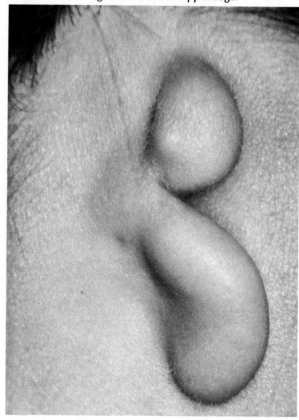

present. The incus and malleus may be represented by one anomalous ossicle. The stapes is also malformed in most instances, frequently monopodal, and not infrequently the footplate is fixed. This major anomaly has both cosmetic as well as auditory implications.

Frequently, major auricular anomalies are associated with other embryologic problems and are described under the Special Syndromes section later in this chapter.

Some basic concepts regarding management of auricular aplasia must be considered prior to any surgical planning. Two surgical problems require solution: 1) cosmetic surgical auricular reconstruction, which requires a multistaged surgical approach; and 2) tympanoplastic surgical correction of anomalies of the external canal, tympanic membrane, and middle ear.

With reference to the first problem, many difficulties still exist in the surgical creation of a cosmetically acceptable auricle. Under ideal circumstances, several surgical stages are necessary with utilization of cartilage and skin grafts.

With reference to the second problem, which is discussed in some detail later in this chapter, staged surgery is also necessary in most cases, and the ongoing development of the growing temporal bone must be considered in the surgical planning. In general, postoperative auditory results are not always satisfactory. Moderate improvements are frequently obtained. "Normal" hearing is usually the exception, because of the complex anomalous structures encountered.

It is not always advisable to consider surgery in unilateral aplasia. If the hearing in the contralateral ear is normal, the desirability of obtaining hearing improvement in the abnormal ear is primarily a consideration regarding the advantage of binaural hearing and stereophony. Since normal hearing does not always result from surgery, an asymmetrical hearing level may be obtained even under ideal circumstances. The potential benefit from reconstructive surgery must be carefully weighed, especially since multiple staged surgical procedures may be necessary.

The major cosmetic rehabilitation problem is in the male child, and even that problem has changed in recent years with the change to long hair styling. It was a major cosmetic problem in the days of short haircuts when a malformed auricle was conspicuous.

Most patients with bilateral auricular aplasia are good candidates for satisfactory hearing through the use of bone-conduction hearing aids. When it is possible to conceal the auricular lesion by long hair, there is no urgent necessity for reconstructive surgery in any patient at the present time.

In bilateral aplasia, early surgical intervention may be necessary if bone conduction utilization is unsatisfactory for some reason (7). In general, the closer the age of the patient approaches that of the adult skull development, the better is the outlook for surgical reconstruction. The reconstruction of the external canal, tympanic membrane, and middle ear requires surgical space "borrowed" from the mastoid cellular area. Pneumatization of the temporal bone usually increases with skull growth. The course of the seventh nerve through the temporal bone is also an important consideration in surgical planning. Such factors are crucial in surgical reconstruction, not to mention the problems of surgical aftercare in very young children.

The consideration of tympanoplasty should include polytomographic radiography to assess middle ear and cochlear relationships, as well as the course of the seventh nerve. It is obviously assumed that careful audiologic assessment has preceded any surgical planning. The problems of postoperative contraction and stenosis of the reconstructed external canal are not rare, requiring multiple staged procedures especially in children.

If cosmetic correction of a major auricular anomaly is urgently desired by parents, the question of surgical correction versus the use of a plastic prosthesis must be considered. Auricular reconstructions require a number of surgical stages, multiple anesthetics, and multiple incisions in the region of the temporal bone as well as in other parts of the body. The benefits to be gained must be seriously weighed against the cosmetic advantage of a well-made prosthetic auricle. The present availability of cosmetically excellent auricular prostheses and the contemporary longer hair styling require consideration before cosmetic auricular surgical procedures are undertaken.

In bilateral microtia, with malformations of the external canal, tympanic membrane, and middle ear requiring both cosmetic auricular reconstruction and tympanoplasty, the tympanoplastic procedure should be performed prior to auricular plastic surgery. The creation of an adequately healed external auditory meatus, external canal, and tympanic membrane, and a mobile ossicular system in a well-healed tympanic cavity should be the first consideration. If a plastic auricular surgical reconstruction has preceded tympanoplasty, it is frequently very difficult to obtain surgical access to the tympanum without some possible injury to the previous plastic surgical auricular reconstruction. Therefore, joint otologic-plastic surgical consultation is advisable prior to consideration of surgery in these cases.

Congenital malformations of the external auditory canal with or without auricular malformations may range from small canals or canals with pinpoint openings to complete lateral and/or medial aplasia of cartilaginous and/or bony external canal.

In the rare lateral cartilaginous aplasia with an adequate bony canal and normal tympanic membrane and middle ear, a simple lateral canal plasty repair follows the same principles as those in the repair of acquired atresia of the external canal.

In partial asplasia of the cartilaginous and bony external canal, combined with a normal mucosal and fibrous layer of the tympanic membrane, it is not unusual to find keratoma (cholesteatoma) filling that aplastic portion of the canal lateral to the tympanic membrane. The congenital canal keratoma is probably produced by desquamating epithelial rests from the tympanic membrane. The medial portion of the keratoma is usually in continuity with the abnormal squamous epithelial layer of the tympanic membrane.

This type of congenital aplasia of the ear canal lends itself to surgical correction via an endaural surgical approach. Excision of the entire aplastic soft-tissue region with removal of anomalous cartilage, subcutaneous tissue, posterolateral bone, and squamous epithelium from the exterior canal is necessary until the tympanic membrane landmarks are reached. If there is a congenital keratoma, it is usually encountered lateral to the medial (fibrous) layer of the tympanic mem-

brane. Anterior mastoid cortex bone is removed with diamond burrs, with care to avoid opening into mastoid cells. Such bone removal (confined to the posterior external canal–anterior mastoid cortex) allows for creation of a spacious canal. The anterior external canal bone (contiguous to the temporomandibular joint space) should not be disturbed.

The middle ear is explored, necessary tympanic and/or ossicular lesions are repaired and the newly created external canal is lined with a split-thickness skin graft. The graft is covered with a thin Silastic sheet, and an arterial dacron tube is placed into the reconstructed and widened external auditory canal, its medial aspect close to the tympanic membrane and its lateral aspect sutured to the endaural incision margins. The endaural incision is closed and the dacron tube is packed with lubricated gauze to give it some degree of stiffness. After adequate epithelialization occurs (3–6 weeks) the Dacron tube is removed.

In many instances the congenital aplasia which involves the bony external canal is frequently as-

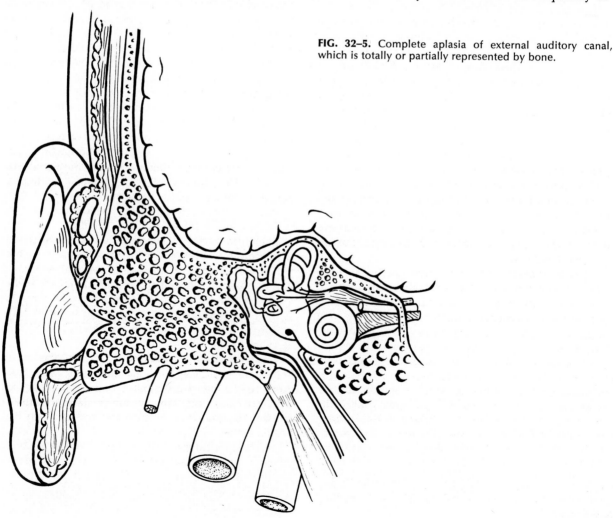

FIG. 32–5. Complete aplasia of external auditory canal, which is totally or partially represented by bone.

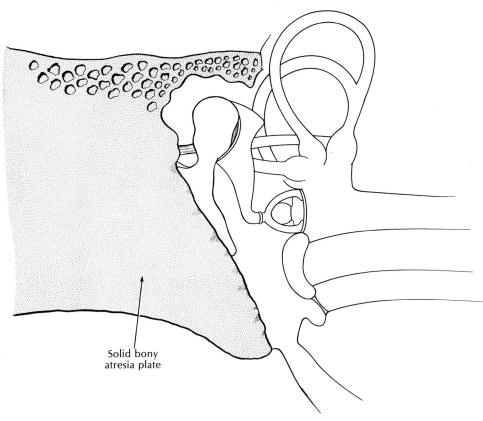

Solid bony
atresia plate

FIG. 32–6. Thick atresia plate with fusion to malleus.

sociated with absence of the tympanic membrane
and an abnormal middle ear.

The absent tympanic membrane is represented
by a primitive tympanic bony plate, the so-called
"atresia plate" (Figs. 32–5, 32–6). Malleus, incus,
and/or stapes may be absent or deformed in a
multiplicity of variations.

Careful preoperative polytome radiographic
studies of the temporal bone will show the extent
of pneumatization and middle ear, ossicle, labyrinth, and seventh nerve details.

Following an endaural or postauricular incision with
removal of skin, subcutaneous tissue, and cartilage, a
transmastoid approach follows mastoid cell groups in
an orderly fashion to identify antrum, aditus ad
antrum, and middle and posterior fossa tegmen plates.
The atresia plate is removed with diamond burrs, the
new, surgically created external auditory canal is lined
with a split-thickness skin graft, the middle ear is explored, and necessary ossiculoplastic reconstruction
completed. Skin is not placed directly over the tympanic air space and its contents. A mesodermal connective tissue graft (*i.e.*, perichondrium, fascia temporalis, or vein) is used to create a new tympanic
membrane.

Individual surgical procedures are employed to
deal with the following different anomalous intratympanic lesions.

Aplasia with Normal Mobile Ossicular Chain

When tympanic exploration reveals a normal ossicular
chain without fixation, fusion, or discontinuity, no
definitive intratympanic procedure is necessary. A
canal plasty is performed. The mesodermal graft (Fig.
32–7) is then placed in direct contact with the exposed malleal manubrium, thus creating a neotympanic membrane in place of the tympanic atresia
plate.

Aplasia with Fixed Malleus and Mobile Incus and Stapes

In a number of cases, the tympanic "atresia plate" is
fused with an abnormal malleus, associated with a
combined fusion of tympanic atresia plate, scutum,
and malleoincudal fusion. However, the stapes may be
mobile. Following lysis of the fused incudomalleal
joint, which is usually fused to the tympanic atresia
plate, the malleal head is removed in continuity with
the tympanic atresia plate, following transsection of
the malleal neck. The mobile malleal manubrium is
usually left *in situ*. It may be possible to mobilize or to
rotate the long process of the incus so that it is in good

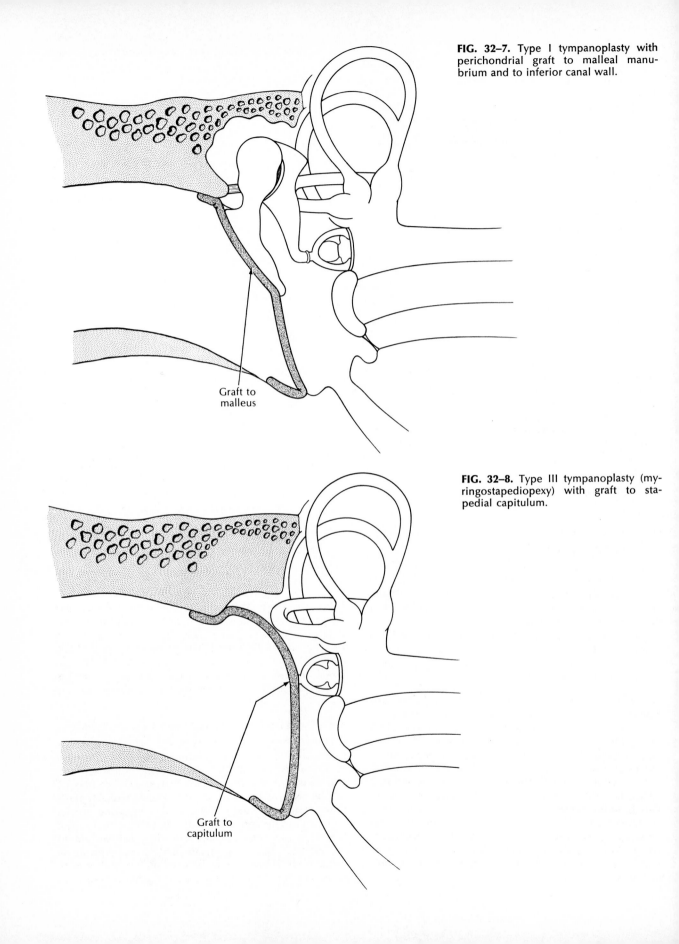

FIG. 32–7. Type I tympanoplasty with perichondrial graft to malleal manubrium and to inferior canal wall.

Graft to
malleus

FIG. 32–8. Type III tympanoplasty (myringostapediopexy) with graft to stapedial capitulum.

Graft to
capitulum

anatomic contiguity with the malleal short process and manubrium. If this is not feasible, an autograft or homograft sculptured columella is "locked" to the malleal short process or to the manubrium to connect with the stapedial capitulum (see Ch. 17, Otomastoiditis Surgery—Mastoidectomy and Tympanoplasty).

Aplasia with Fixed Malleus, Incus, and/or Stapes

In these rather common anomalies, the malleus and incus constitute one deformed double ossicle that is attached either completely or partially to the tympanic atresia plate. In many instances the stapes is mobile, although it may have atypical architecture—*e.g.*, monopod. If the stapes is mobile with a good round window reflex, the procedure of choice is the removal of the fused incudomalleal mass followed by myringostapediopexy (Fig. 32–8) or by a columellization-myringostapediopexy. A "double saddle" prefabricated homograft is placed between the stapedial capitulum and the perichondrial graft, which is used with its natural convexity in medial position so that it contacts the lateral saddle of the homograft snugly. The lateral concavity of the perichondrial graft has a partial cone shape which resembles the tympanic membrane cone and is more ideally suited to this type of reconstruction than a formless fascia temporalis or vein graft. Split-skin grafts are used to line the newly created external auditory canal and meatus and may consist of separate grafts or the ingenious "skin bag" described by Livingstone (25).

If the deformed malleoincudal mass is associated with abnormal stapedial crura, but if the stapedial footplate is mobile, a similar approach is advisable. The abnormal stapedial arch is removed along with the incudomalleal mass. A modified double-saddle prefabricated homograft (4–4.5 mm) is placed on the mobile stapedial footplate. The convexity of a perichondrial graft is placed medially to contact the homograft for a columellar myringostapediopexy reconstruction.

The malformation of the stapes very frequently takes the form of a monopod columella-like stapes, without an arch and without an obturator foramen (Fig. 32–9). If it is mobile, it may be used with or without an extension provided by a homograft.

If panossicular fixation is accompanied by a fixed footplate, the possibility of an abnormal cochlear aqueduct and increased pressure by perilymph and cerebrospinal fluid must be considered in all such anomalies. Stapedectomy is not an innocuous procedure even under ideal circumstances in otosclerosis. In congenital anomalies it may be hazardous. An exploratory mini-puncture of the footplate is made prior to footplate removal. Preoperative assessment of the cochlear aqueduct relationships by polytomography is valuable, but it does not replace careful exploratory puncture by a probe prior to footplate removal.

If the oval-window niche architecture is anomalous, there is usually evident or potential abnormal position of the horizontal portion of the seventh nerve. In some instances it is a split nerve, encircling the oval window

niche. It is inadvisable to attempt any type of "drill-out" procedure because of danger to the facial nerve branches either by the drillout itself or by subsequent adhesive fibrosis. The alternatives in such cases are either 1) no attempt at surgical reconstruction, or 2) a horizontal semicircular canal fenestration (Fig. 32–10), which may be performed in one or two stages (see Ch. 19, Otosclerosis).

If preoperative polytomography shows no vestibular or cochlear aqueduct abnormalities and if the oval window is anatomically in normal position, the stapedial footplate may be removed if the lesion is not obliterative. A perichondrial graft "canoe" is placed into the oval window niche, snugly sealing the niche. A 4.5-mm rod-saddle homograft prosthesis is placed into the perichondrial canoe medially. Its lateral extremity is placed in contact with a perichondrial concave reconstruction of the extended columellar type III tympanoplasty.

In summary, basic tympanoplastic principles (see Ch. 17) can be used in surgical reconstruction of most congenital lesions of the external auditory canal and middle ear. In some instances anatomic problems may dictate the advisability of staging such surgery. In cases of major anomalies of the round window niche and/or oval window niche, tympanoplasty should rarely be considered. Inadequate round window function would also contraindicate fenestration of the semicircular canal.

Surgical correction of combined external canal and middle ear anomalies will depend upon 1) the status of the auricle, 2) osseous and soft tissue conditions of the external auditory meatus and external canal region, pneumatization of the temporal bone, and polytome radiographic evaluation of the middle ear and labyrinth.

FIG. 32–9. Monopod stapes.

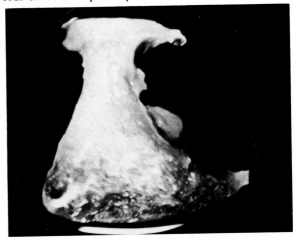

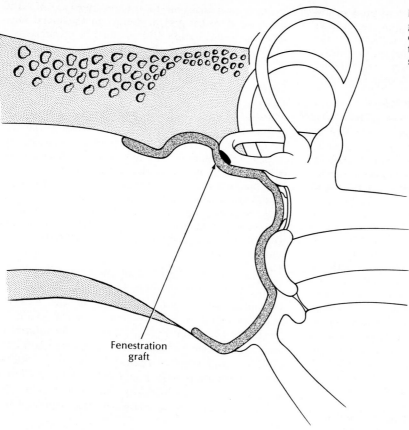

FIG. 32–10. Type V tympanoplasty with graft applied to promontory (round window and eustachian tube in aerial continuity) and to fenestra in horizontal semicircular canal.

Fenestration graft

MALFORMATIONS OF THE MIDDLE EAR

A number of congenital intratympanic anomalies may occur in cases with otherwise normal external ear and normal tympanic membrane. In some cases there may be a normal canal on one side and an abnormal, small, oblique canal or total canal aplasia on the other side. Surprisingly, in some cases there may be no real correlation between the external canal anomalies and those of the middle ear.

Intratympanic anomalies with normal canal and normal tympanic membrane are not rare. The lesions usually mimic otosclerosis and are discussed under the differential diagnosis of otosclerosis (see Ch. 19, Otosclerosis).

SPECIAL SYNDROMES OF THE EXTERNAL EAR, MIDDLE EAR, AND/OR INNER EAR

Preauricular Pits and Fistulas, and Related Anomalies

Preauricular fistulas may occur with and without auricular anomalies. They are usually due to defective dedifferentiation of the auricular hillocks, which originate from first and second branchial arch mesenchyme. Fistulas may be unilateral or bilateral. Most commonly they are located immediately in front of the helix. They may be insignificant superficial pits or dimples, but they may also be major fistulas (10) communicating with the middle ear, temporomandibular joint, and with deep asymptomatic branchial arch neck fistulas (see Ch. 13, External Ear Diseases). Minor superficial preauricular fistulas that are uninfected require no treatment. Infected preauricular fistulas require thorough excision.

Surgical approaches should be preceded by preoperative contrast radiographic studies. Both plain and polytome radiographs will be of value in pointing to multiform tracts of fistulas. Familial genetic malformations of auricles accompanied by congenital fistulas, with or without hearing losses, are not uncommon. Such auricular anomalies with fistulas are not infrequently accompanied by partial or complete facial nerve paralysis present at birth. Staged surgical management may be necessary. In general, if the fistula is unilateral, not infected, unaccompanied by seventh nerve paralysis, and if the contralateral ear is normal, it is probably wise to defer surgery until adulthood unless there is a complicating infection that requires earlier intervention.

Another variety of hereditary congenital hearing loss with external ear malformations is that of thickened auricles, accompanied by various abnormalities of the incudostapedial joint. This dominant malformation may also include absence of the obturator foramen in the stapes. The hearing loss is usually entirely conductive in character.

A dominant ear malformation accompanied by a conductive hearing loss is characteristic of the Wildervanck syndrome. There are deformed auricles, marginal pits, and frequent preauricular appendages in this group. The hearing loss is almost always conductive and in many cases surgically correctable.

A variety of hereditary syndromes of conductive hearing loss with associated external ear malformations occur in certain communities where there is a good deal of marriage between close relatives. Such syndromes have been reported from Mennonite communities in Pennsylvania and from regions of central Europe. The hearing loss is most commonly conductive and due to various ossicular malformations.

Treacher-Collins Syndrome (Mandibulofacial Dysostosis of Franceschetti)

This autosomal dominant hereditary condition is characterized by external ear and other multiple anomalies. The facial appearance is characteristically described as birdlike or fishlike, with antimongoloid palpebral fissures (Fig. 32–11). In addition to micrognathia and undeveloped mandibles and maxillas; bilateral microtia, aplasia of the external auditory canal, malformed ossicles with conductive hearing loss and occasional sensorineural hearing loss are encountered.

The microtia varies in degree and appearance. The auricles are usually low, frequently asymmetrically set, and the external canals, in addition to being underdeveloped, frequently are curved in inferiorly slanting courses. Pretragal pits and accessory appendages are common. There may be complete or partial bony aplasia.

Not infrequently there are seventh nerve anomalies. The malformed epitympanum and mesotympanum may be filled with collagenous fibrous tissue, and the tympanic membrane will frequently be absent.

Surgical reconstruction may be considered in some cases, and in general should precede surgical auricular reconstruction. An alternative to auricular reconstruction may be a prosthetic auricle.

Surgical reconstruction, if considered, should be postponed beyond childhood if possible, unless there is infection in the abnormal external auditory canal or some other indication for earlier intervention. Congenital or acquired keratoma may exist lateral to a bony atresia plate. If there is evidence of suppuration or if there are infected fistulas, surgical intervention is necessary at any age.

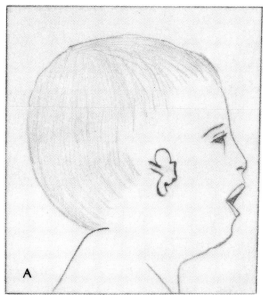

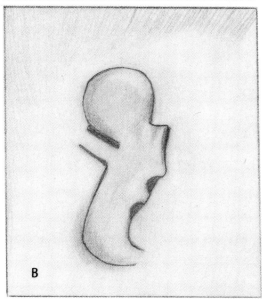

FIG. 32–11. A. Treacher-Collins syndrome facies with micrognathia and microtia. **B.** Auricular microtia malformation detail.

FIG. 32–12. A, B, C, D. Ocular proptosis, parrot nose, strabismus, hypoplasia of maxilla, and syndactyly are present in acrocephalosyndactyly. (Bergstrom L, Neblett LM, Hemenway WG: Arch Otolaryngol 96:117–123, 1972. Copyright 1972, American Medical Association)

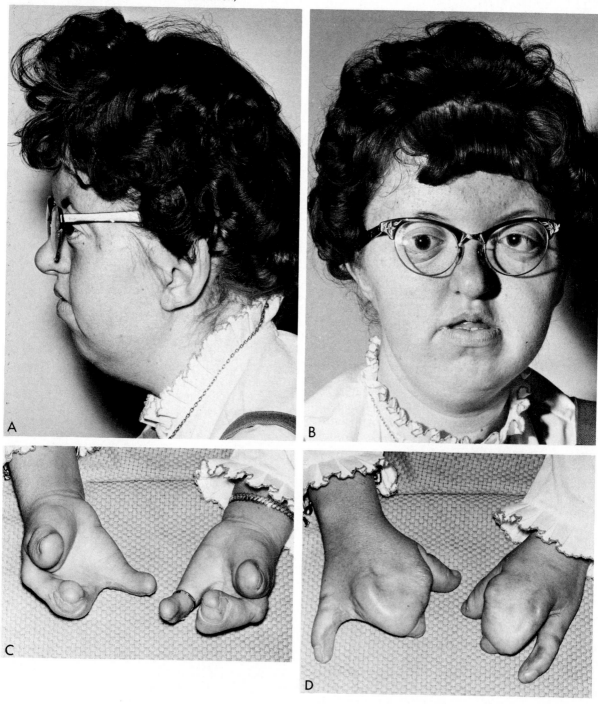

Acrocephalosyndactyly (Apert's Disease)

This middle ear malformation is accompanied by craniofacial dysostosis (brachycephaly and hypocephaly), occipital flattening, prominent forehead, hypoplastic maxillas, and flattened face. The nose is parrot-shaped and there is a high palate. The eyes slope outward and downward and are frequently proptosed. There may or may not be abnormal auricles (Fig. 32–12).

The primary otologic lesion is stapedial fixation, although other ossicular abnormalities may also be present. A conductive hearing loss is the presenting otologic symptom. The possibility of an abnormally patent cochlear aqueduct must be considered. Removal of the stapedial footplate may be accompanied by a perilymph "gusher." Surgical management of such cases must be undertaken with great care and with recognition of possibility of poor results (2, 24).

Crouzon's Disease (Craniofacial Dysostosis)

Crouzon's disease resembles Apert's disease (acrocephalosyndactyly), the primary finding being a displacement of the petrous pyramid as part of cranial-basal dysplasia involving the base of the skull. There is abnormal pneumatization of the petrous pyramid (35).

It is characterized by parrot-beaked nose accompanied by exophthalmos, squint, a short upper lip, a small maxilla, and mandibular prognathism. It is also accompanied by cranial synostosis, hypertelorism, aplasia of the external auditory canal, and abnormalities of the tympanic membrane and the ossicular system. The cochlea is usually uninvolved but may be minimally involved in some patients. There may be pseudocochlear hearing loss due to anomalies of the oval and round windows. In some instances hearing correction may be obtained through ossiculoplastic-tympanoplastic procedures.

Turner's Syndrome

Turner's syndrome is characterized by a short "webbed" neck, shortness of stature, and sexual underdevelopment. It is apparently limited to females. The abnormal ear findings are primarily those of low-set and anteriorly placed auricles. No major middle ear malformations are present; however, frequent otitis media and mastoiditis is a major characteristic of this syndrome. In Szpunar and Rybak's studies (34) of more than 30 patients, most of the cases were characterized by maldevelopments of the pneumatic air-cell systems. Hypocellularity of the mastoid is probably the primary otologic lesion, with secondary otitis media as a superimposed problem.

The frequency of otomastoiditis in these girls is probably related to morphologic skull changes, major metabolic deficiencies, and poor immunologic responses to infections.

Klippel-Feil Syndrome

The Klippel-Feil deformity includes congenitally short neck, head deviation, low-set auricles, and "butterfly" vertebrae with fusions. Hearing loss is usually conductive although cochlear defects have also been described (19).

The Klippel-Feil syndrome is closely related to Turner's and to Wildervanck's syndromes, including abducens (sixth nerve) paralysis, eyeball retraction, and hearing loss; the term **cervicooculoacoustical syndrome** has also been used in these cases. Polytomography may show underdeveloped labyrinths in addition to nonpneumatized mastoids. The term **cleidocranial dysostosis** has also been used for the group of anomalies involving shoulder, neck, skull, and ears (18) (Fig. 32–13).

Madelung's Deformity with Hearing Loss

Madelung's deformity, related to the dyschondrosteosis of Leri-Weill, is characterized by short stature, short forearms, and short lower extremities. There are multiple abnormalities of carpal bones, tibia, and fibula. The condition is familial, with autosomal dominance, and is more common in females with a ratio of 4:1. A number of related orthopedic abnormalities are found in this syndrome.

The hearing loss is primarily conductive, although it may be partially cochlear. The lesions are usually ossicular and may involve any or all three ossicles. Hearing improvement frequently follows ossiculoplasty and tympanoplastic repair (27).

Otopalatal-Digital Syndrome and Related Syndromes

The otopalatal-digital syndrome, frequently accompanied by dwarfism includes middle ear anomalies with mild to moderate conductive hearing loss. It is characterized by a broad nasal bridge, hypertelorism, and frontal bossing. The hands and feet are widely spaced, and the first digits are usually shortened.

Recessive absence of tibias with relatively severe mixed cochlear and conductive hearing losses is another variety of hereditary hearing loss with skeletal disease. There may be congenital absence of one or both tibias and malformations of the fibula.

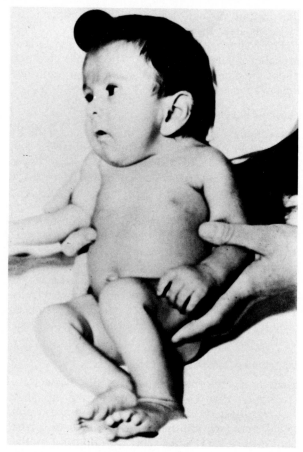

FIG. 32–13. Infant with Klippel-Feil syndrome. Note short neck giving impression that head is set directly on shoulders. (Black FO, Bergstrom L, Downs M, Hemenway WG: Congenital Deafness. Boulder, Colorado Associated University Press, 1971)

The recessive split-hand-and-foot syndrome is exceedingly rare and is characterized by moderate to severe mixed hearing loss and absence of phalanges, accompanied by syndactyly.

Dominant proximal symphalangia and hearing loss is a prenatal lesion of dominant transmission characterized by symphalangia, especially in the lateral digits, and mild to moderate conductive hearing loss. The conductive hearing loss may be related to the meatus, the eardrum, the lateral ossicles, or to the stapediovestibular region. In some cases the hearing loss may be correctable surgically.

Albers-Schönberg Disease—Osteopetrosis (Marble Bone Disease)

Albers-Schönberg disease is a recessively transmitted disease characterized by brittle or sclerotic skull bones due to failure of resorption of calcified cartilage and primitive bone. Cranial nerve palsies, especially seventh nerve paralysis, are not infrequent and may be present in childhood. Cochlear lesions are secondary to changes in labyrinthine windows, accompanying ossicular malformations, but the auditory lesions are primarily conductive.

Pyle's Disease

Pyle's disease (cranial-metaphyseal dysplasia) is characterized by dominant conductive loss although occasional cochlear components may be present. The femurs are splayed. Occasionally there are changes in the skull comparable to those in osteopetrosis. The disorder is also characterized by occasional episodes of cranial nerve paralysis.

Craniotubular bone dysplasias usually are accompanied by visual losses as well as by hearing losses. Polytomography (21) shows characteristic constriction of optic foramens and internal auditory canals. The middle-ear cavities are also malformed, with accompanying ossicular anomalies. The otic capsule is usually thickened.

Van der Hoeve's Disease (Osteogenesis Imperfecta)

Van der Hoeve's disease, a dominant hereditary lesion, may start in childhood but is commonly noticed in the second and third decades. It is also known as "fragile bone disease" (fragilitas ossium). The characteristic finding is that of blue sclerae and conductive hearing loss. The patients frequently give a history of multiple fractures of long bones. Tympanic findings are variable. Some patients have atypical stapedial fixation due to pseudootosclerosis. Surgical correction of the hearing loss is possible but is not usually obtained by classic stapedectomy. Very frequently, additional ossiculoplastic procedures are necessary because the ossicular lesion may be quite varied (see Ch. 17, Otomastoiditis Surgery—Mastoidectomy and Tympanoplasty, and Ch. 19, Otosclerosis).

Paget's Disease (Osteitis Deformans) and Related Diseases

Paget's disease, a deforming skeletal disease involving the skull, occurs through dominant transmission.

The onset is usually in adult life, and the progression is usually slow. The characteristic skull involvement is accompanied by narrowing of the cranial nerve foramina and changes in the otic capsule, as well as in the ossicular chain. The internal auditory meatus apertures may be narrowed, and the auditory, vestibular, and seventh nerves may be compressed by encroachment of the deforming bony lesion. Frequently the hearing loss is

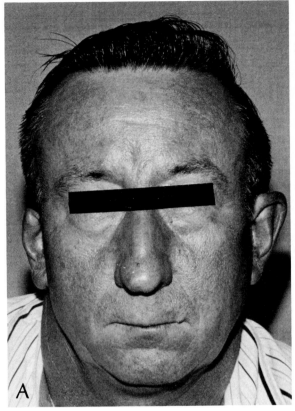

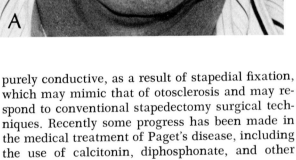

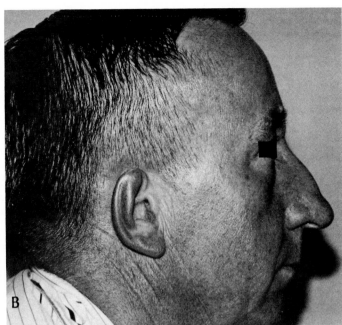

FIG. 32–14. Low-set auricles and ossicular anomalies. **A.** Frontal view. **B.** Lateral view.

purely conductive, as a result of stapedial fixation, which may mimic that of otosclerosis and may respond to conventional stapedectomy surgical techniques. Recently some progress has been made in the medical treatment of Paget's disease, including the use of calcitonin, diphosphonate, and other drugs.

Englemann's Disease (Progressive Diaphyseal Dysplasia)

Englemann's disease is a delayed adult lesion of skeletal nature that produces hearing loss. The limb bones are characterized by thickening of the diaphyseal cortices. Occasionally there will also be accompanying skull thickening, with cranial nerve palsies and cochlear, or conductive, or mixed hearing losses.

Van Buchem's Disease (Hyperostosis Corticalis Generalisata)

This disorder is characterized by thickening of the entire skull, including the mandible. The clavicles and ribs are also involved. The onset is most commonly noticed during puberty. The lesion is recessive in transmission. The hearing loss that accompanies this lesion may be conductive, but more commonly it is a cochlear loss due to encroachment by deformation of bone in the internal auditory meatus and in the bony cochlea.

Pierre Robin Syndrome (Cleft Palate, Micrognathia, and Glossoptosis)

The Pierre Robin syndrome is characterized by auricular deformities consisting of cupped or low-set ears, palatal malformations, and eustachian tube obstruction accompanied by glossoptosis and micrognathia. Both a middle and inner ear anomaly (15) has been reported in this syndrome. Conductive hearing loss will usually be found as a result of the palate and eustachian tube obstruction.

Gargoylism (Hurler's Syndrome)

Gargoylism is a genetic mucopolysaccharidosis, the lesions of which become manifest at approximately 12 months of age. The primary middle-ear anomalies are in the lateral ossicular chain. Apparent persistent mesenchyme, which appears as "gargoyle cells," may obliterate the labyrinthine windows. The auricles may also be low-set. Urinary findings of mucopolysaccharides (chondroitin sulfate B and heparitin sulfate) may be diagnostic (31).

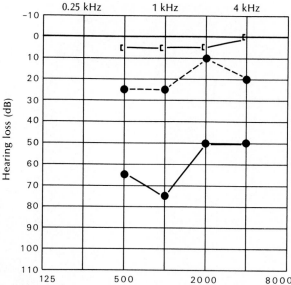

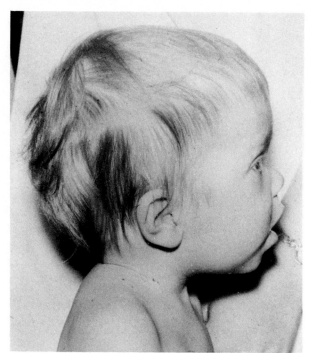

FIG. 32–15. Preoperative and postoperative audiograms of same patient whose ear is shown in Figure 32–14. He had undergone ossiculoplastic repair of congenital ossicular lesion, with accompanying low-set auricles. ●——●, AC, unmasked, RE, before operation; [——[, BC, masked, RE, before operation; ●- - -●, AC, unmasked, RE, after operation; **SRT**, 60 dB before operation, 17.5 dB after operation; **SDS** 94%.

FIG. 32–16. Microcephaly, hypertelorism, epicanthic folds, carp-shaped mouth, flat nasal bridge, hypoplasia of midface, and somewhat low-set but otherwise normal appearing pinnae with external meatuses. (Bergstrom L, Stewart J, Kenyon B: Laryngoscope 84:1905–1917, 1974)

FIG. 32–17. Same patient as in Figure 32–16. Frontal view. (Bergstrom L, Stewart J, Kenyon B: Laryngoscope 84:1905–1917, 1974)

Low Set Auricles and Ossicular Anomalies

A possible recessive syndrome of conductive hearing loss and malformed low-set ears has been reported (26). This is similar to cases with thickened but normally positioned auricles, described as a dominant syndrome (9).

This auricular-ossicular anomaly syndrome is exemplified by the case of a 41-year-old male with a family history of deafness (mother and maternal uncle). He had a small, low-set right auricle, with a conductive hearing loss due to an absent incudal long process and absent stapes arch. The posterior one-fourth of the footplate was mobile. Prosthetic ossiculoplasty was followed by hearing gain from a 60-dB level to 25-dB level (Figs. 32–14, 32–15).

External Auditory Atresia and the Deleted Chromosome

A new syndrome of external auditory atresia and partial deletion of chromosome 18 was reported by Bergstrom, Stewart, and Kenyon (3). The major features are external auditory atresia with an atresia plate, associated with a number of other defects, including epicanthic folds, strabismus, microcephaly, hypertelorism, short stature and congenital heart disease. Chromosome analysis

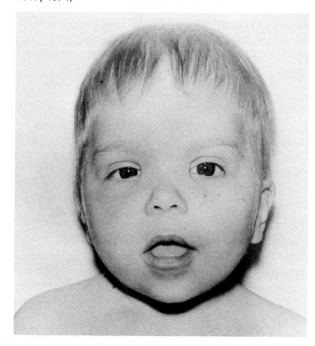

showed deletion of the long arm or a ring formation of chromosome 18 (Figs. 32–16 to 32–20).

First Branchial Cleft Syndromes with Conductive Hearing Loss

Cavo, Pratt, and Alonso (8) have reported the combination of first branchial cleft syndromes (submandibular cervical fistula) and ossicular anomalies. The hearing losses are primarily conductive. The anomaly is probably related to maldevelopment of the first and second arches and the first groove (see Ch. 1, Clinical Anatomy and Physiology of the Peripheral Ear).

DiGeorge Syndrome—Third and Fourth Pharyngeal Pouch and Ear Malformations

Congenital absence of thymus and parathyroid glands in the DiGeorge syndrome can be accompanied by middle and inner ear malformations.

Adkins and Gussen (1) reported temporal bone findings of a bilateral cochlear anomaly and otitis media. The hypoparathyroid state is associated with cellular immune deficiencies. Black, Spanier, and Kohut (5) reported auricular and other craniofacial malformations in their studies.

SENSORINEURAL SYSTEM MALFORMATIONS

Eight groups of syndromes can be classified within the known varieties of hereditary lesions that cause sensorineural hearing loss (22). These groups include, in addition to a syndrome with 1) no associated abnormalities, those that are associated with 2) external ear malformations, 3) integument diseases, 4) ophthalmic lesions, 5) CNS lesions, 6) skeletal malformations, 7) renal disease, and 8) miscellaneous defects.

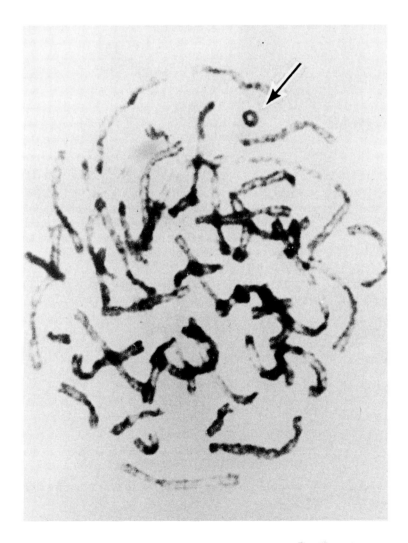

FIG. 32–18. Ring type of 18 chromosome deletion **(arrow),** as shown in karyotype (see Fig. 32–20), same patient as in Figure 32–16. (Bergstrom L, Stewart J, Kenyon B: Laryngoscope 84:1905–1917, 1974)

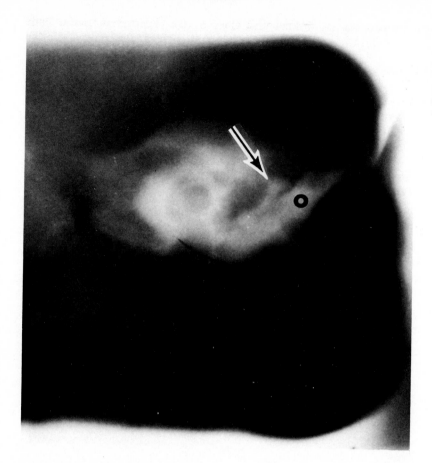

FIG. 32–19. Petrous pyramid polytomography, left ear, frontal view, same patient as in Figure 32–16. Note heavy ossification **(O)** in area of tympanic membrane just lateral to an ossicle, probably the malleus **(arrow).** (Bergstrom L, Stewart J, Kenyon B: Laryngoscope 84:1905–1917, 1974)

HEREDITARY SENORINEURAL HEARING LOSS WITH NO ASSOCIATED ABNORMALITIES

Dominant Bilateral Severe Loss

This type of loss is relatively frequent. The lesion is cochlear, and pathologically it is either of the Mondini or of the Scheibe form.

Dominant Unilateral Severe Loss

This type of loss is uncommon and resembles the bilateral form.

Recessive Severe Loss

The loss is cochlear and not as common as the dominant variety of bilateral loss.

Sex-Linked Severe Loss

Present in a relatively small number of cases, the lesions are usually bilateral.

Dominant Mild to Moderate Autosomal Low-Frequency Loss

In contrast with the severe lesions, a form of mild to moderate sensorineural hearing loss occurs relatively commonly, characterized only by low-frequency loss, with normal hearing in higher frequency regions (Fig. 32–21). It is bilateral, probably cochlear, and is frequently diagnosed in older children or even in young adults. In most instances it appears to be congenital and either of prenatal or natal origin (36).

However, it is quite likely that the lesion can appear in later childhood as well as in adult life.

Dominant Mid-Frequency Loss

This lesion can be congenital but can also appear in later childhood or in adults (Fig. 32–22) (23). Because of good low- and high-frequency responses, the hearing problem may not be recognized early in life (6).

HEREDITARY SENSORINEURAL HEARING LOSSES ASSOCIATED WITH EXTERNAL EAR MALFORMATIONS

These lesions have been described earlier in this chapter.

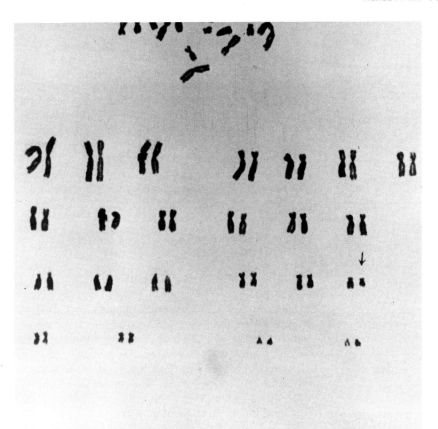

FIG. 32–20. Karyotype of deletion of long arm of chromosome 18, same patient as in Figure 32–16. **Arrow** indicates deletion. (Bergstrom L, Stewart J, Kenyon B: Laryngoscope 84:1905–1917, 1974)

FIG. 32–21. Audiogram in low-frequency dominant auto-somal sensorineural hearing loss (ears were identical). ●—●, AC, unmasked, RE: [—[, BC, masked, RE; **SRT,** 20 dB; **SDS,** 90%.

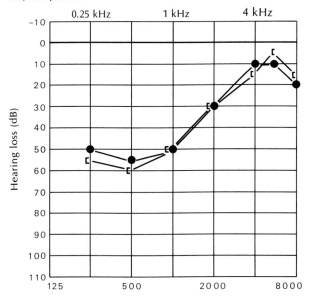

HEREDITARY LESIONS CAUSING SENSORINEURAL HEARING LOSS ASSOCIATED WITH INTEGUMENTARY SYSTEM DISEASE

Waardenburg's disease, which may account for 2–3% of all cases of congenital deafness in the United States, is the primary example of this pre-natal group and is characterized by rather typical facial findings. These are widely spaced medial canthi, flat nasal shape, and confluent eyebrows. In most instances there will also be different colored irides (heterochromia), as well as the very typical "white forelock" (Fig. 32–23). Not all per-sons with these characteristics will have hearing losses. Neither the heterochromia nor the white forelock is always present. The lesion should not be confused with mongolism or with hypertelorism. The genetic transmission is dominant, with pre-natal onset, occasionally recessive, or sex-linked. A mixed hearing loss of moderate to severe degree is usually bilateral and may vary from a mild to a profound cochlear hearing loss, with multiple audiometric configurations.

Waardenburg's syndrome may occur in a num-

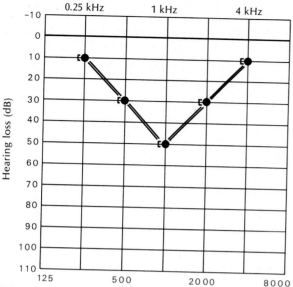

FIG. 32–22. "V"-shaped mid-frequency autosomal-dominant sensorineural hearing loss (ears were identical). ●—●, AC, unmasked, RE; [—[, BC, masked, RE.

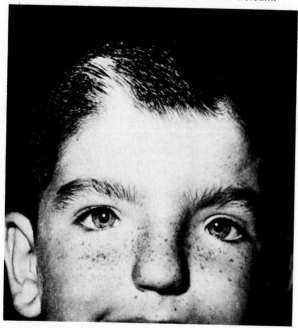

FIG. 32–23. Waardenburg's syndrome. Note white forelock, widely spaced medial canthi, flattened nasal dorsum.

ber of generations, and as many as six generations in one family have been reported (29).

Other genetic cochlear lesions with integumentary diseases comparable to Waardenburg's syndrome have been reported. Among these are dominant albinism, the leopard syndrome, hereditary piebaldness, sex-linked pigmentary abnormalities, recessive congenital atopic dermatitis, dominant keratopachydermia, digital constrictions, recessive pili torti, dominant knuckle pads, leukonychia, dominant or recessive onychodystrophy and coniform teeth, all accompanied by congenital cochlear hearing loss.

HEREDITARY SENSORINEURAL HEARING LOSS ASSOCIATED WITH OPHTHALMIC LESIONS

Usher's Syndrome—Hearing Loss with Retinitis Pigmentosa

Usher's syndrome is a prenatal genetic autosomal recessive combined lesion of cochlear hearing loss and retinitis pigmentosa. The hearing loss varies from moderate to severe and is due to a cochlear lesion of the Mondini type. There are no associated vestibular abnormalities. The visual loss is rarely present at birth but begins at any age and may progress to any degree of severity.

Hallgren's Syndrome and Related Otoophthalmic Anomalies

Hallgren's syndrome is characterized by autosomal recessive cochlear hearing loss and progressive atypical retinitis pigmentosa, with constricted visual fields and night blindness. It is accompanied by other neurologic lesions such as polyneuropathy, cerebellar ataxia, and ocular nystagmus, and by muscle wasting. The cochlear hearing loss is usually severe, and is accompanied by abnormal vestibular changes. The pathologic findings in the cochlea are Mondini/Scheibe in type.

The term **Hallgren's syndrome** is used to describe cochlear hearing loss with ophthalmic lesions accompanied by CNS involvement, whereas the term **Refsum's syndrome** applies more accurately to cases with peripheral nervous system lesions.

Other prenatal genetic lesions of cochlear hearing loss combined with ophthalmic disease include a number of relatively infrequent combinations of hereditary lesions, in which both hearing and vision are involved, such as recessive myopia and retinitis pigmentosa with spastic diplegia.

Among the postnatal combined ophthalmic and cochlear lesions is that of infantile polyneuropathy and optic atrophy that begins in early childhood, accompanied by a second-decade onset of cochlear hearing loss.

Other lesions and combinations of lesions that are all associated with cochlear hearing loss are those of dominant saddle nose, myopia, and cataract; dominant myopia; peripheral neuropathy, skeletal lesions, and recessive retinal degeneration, diabetes and obesity (Alstrom's disease); retinal detachment, telangiectasia, and mental retardation; opticocochleodentate degeneration, which is characterized by early onset of progressive spastic quadriparesis, optic atrophy, and dementia; and finally the adult lesion of dominant corneal dystrophy. In the latter lesion a ribbon-like corneal degeneration occurs in late adult life, accompanied by abnormal calcium metabolism and a cochlear hearing loss of moderate degree.

HEREDITARY SENSORINEURAL HEARING LOSS ASSOCIATED WITH CNS DISEASES

Prenatal, Natal, or Postnatal Lesions

A few combined lesions of cochlear hearing loss with CNS disease begin in the infant period. They include 1) recessive cochlear hearing loss, truncal ataxia, hypogonadism, with decreased estrogen and 17-ketosteroids, and 2) Hurler's disease, characterized by mucopolysaccharoidosis type 1, in which the hearing loss starts in infancy, the progression is moderate, and the cochlear loss may vary from mild to moderate. There may be associated progressive mental deterioration, bony deformities, and corneal opacities.

Sanfilippo disease is characterized by moderate mental deterioration, bony deformities, and mild recessive cochlear hearing loss.

Hunter's disease is characterized by mental retardation, dwarfing, and hepatosplengomegaly, along with cochlear hearing loss.

Other lesions include prenatal dominant photomyoclonus, cochlear hearing loss, diabetes, and nephropathy; and the Richards-Rundle syndrome of recessive cochlear hearing loss, mental deficiency, ataxia, and hypogonadism.

Postnatal Delayed Lesions

Dominant acoustic neurinoma (vestibular eighth nerve schwannoma) associated with generalized neurofibromatosis (von Recklinghausen's disease) is the most common delayed postnatal lesion involving sensorineural hearing loss with CNS disease. The hearing loss is neural (eighth nerve), not cochlear. Cochlear involvement may occur secondarily. The tumor is a benign schwannoma that starts most commonly in the vestibular branch

of the eighth nerve and involves the cochlear branch secondarily by pressure. Thus, while this is a syndrome of genetic dominance that starts in early life, most frequently in the second or early third decade, the progression is variable and the hearing loss is moderate to severe. Bilateral lesions are common. Vestibular paralysis is the first finding, although usually the first symptom is tinnitus. The lesion is very often associated with the skin lesions of neurofibromatosis.

HEREDITARY LESIONS CAUSING SENSORINEURAL HEARING LOSS AND ASSOCIATED WITH SKELETAL DISEASES

There are a number of classic otoskeletal lesions, in which skeletal deformities are of many varieties and the hearing losses primarily involve external ear and middle ear. Usually the hearing loss is conductive, but it is occasionally combined with cochlear loss. In addition to cochlear components, eighth nerve lesions can also occur as a result of ossification of the internal auditory meatal region, producing in the meatus and internal auditory canal.

These syndromes (Crouzon, Treacher-Collins, Paget's, van der Hoeve's, Pyle's, and others) are discussed earlier in this chapter.

HEREDITARY LESIONS CAUSING SENSORINEURAL HEARING LOSS WITH ACCOMPANYING RENAL DISEASE

Prenatal Lesions

There are only a few prenatal combined renal and cochlear lesions, which are characterized by recessive transmission, and a combination of middle ear and renal and genital anomalies. There may be unilateral or bilateral renal agenesis and vaginal atresia. The hearing loss is primarily conductive, but it may be mixed.

Postnatal Lesions

An uncommon syndrome is that of postnatal dominantly transmitted combined sensorineural hearing loss and renal disease, the characteristics of which are nephritis, ichythyosis with prolinuria, and hearing loss. The hearing loss is usually cochlear and the renal lesions are variable, occasionally accompanied by renal cysts.

Delayed Lesions in the Adult—Alport's Disease

Alport's disease is the one major lesion in which there is a dominant hereditary cochlear hearing loss with accompanying renal disease. Nephritis or nephrosis may begin in the first decade. Occa-

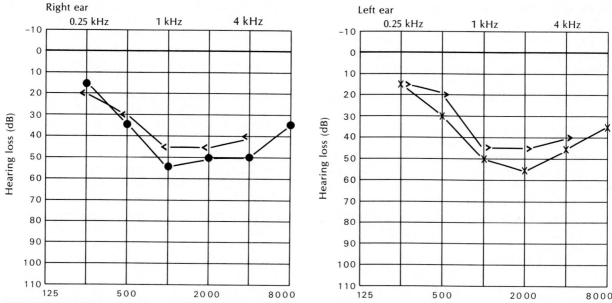

FIG. 32–24. Audiogram of Alport's disease, 18-year-old patient. **At left,** ●—●, AC, unmasked, RE; <—<, BC, unmasked, RE; **At right, x—x,** AC, unmasked, LE; >—>, BC, unmasked, LE. (Gussen R: Ann Otol Rhinol Laryngol 82:871–875, 1973)

sionally there are lens abnormalities. The hearing loss is primarily cochlear in nature and usually bilaterally symmetrical. It is transmitted as a dominant and is more common in males (37).

The pathologic findings in Alport's disease are pleomorphic. Since many of the patients who come to autopsy have been treated with extracorporeal hemodialysis or have been recipients of renal homografts, it is difficult to relate temporal bone findings precisely to the kidney lesion. Of special interest is a recent case in a male, reported by Gussen (14). Hematuria started at age 5, and at age 18, audiologic studies showed a bilateral cochlear hearing loss with a dominant midfrequency characteristic (Fig. 32–24). At age 23 he had bilateral congenital lenticonus (congenital lens defects) and was hospitalized for severe uremia. He received a renal transplant and was maintained on immunosuppressive therapy for 4 years, finally dying of primary malignant lymphoma of the brain and cryptococcal meningitis, probably related to the immunosuppressive therapy. The temporal bone findings showed spiral ligament projections partitioning the beginning of the scala vestibuli bilaterally. There were also spongy spiral ligament changes, strial atrophy, and decreased spiral ganglion cells in the basal and middle cochlear turns (Figs. 32–25, 32–26).

In addition to Alport's disease there are a number of other combined renal-auditory lesions which include that of dominant urticaria, amyloidosis, nephritis, and cochlear hearing loss. There is also a rare category of recessive renal acidosis with progressive cochlear hearing loss, starting occasionally in childhood but usually in adult life. Hyperuricemia with ataxia and deafness has been reported by Rosenberg *et al.* (28).

HEREDITARY SENSORINEURAL HEARING LOSS ASSOCIATED WITH OTHER ABNORMALITIES

Pendred's Disease—Thyroid Abnormality

Pendred's disease is relatively common, prenatal in origin, and is characterized by recessive transmission, cochlear hearing loss (bilaterally symmetrical), accompanied by depressed thyroid function and goiter. There also may be concomitant depressed vestibular function. The hearing loss varies from relatively mild loss to severe cochlear loss. The pathologic findings are usually limited to the cochlea.

There are reports of patients with cochlear hearing loss associated with depressed thyroid function coming on in later life, in which the hearing losses are relatively minor and fluctuant. There are questionable reports of improvements in hearing with thyroid replacement therapy. Illum *et al.* (17) reported 15 patients with sensorineural hearing loss, goiter, abnormal results in perchlorate tests, and cochlear defects on radiographic studies. The basal cochlear turn is normal, but the apical turns form a common cavity. This defect is related to a fault in modiolus development in the

FIG. 32–25. A. Right ear (vertical section) with spiral ligament partition **(arrow)** overlying collapsed Reissner's membrane. Note spongy appearance of spiral ligament and decreased numbers of spiral ganglion cells in descending basal cochlear turn, as well as strial atrophy above spiral prominence. **SV,** scala vestibuli; **R,** round window membrane; **ME,** middle ear; **ST,** scala tympani. (H&E, × 16) **B.** High-power view of spiral ligament partition. **SV,** scala vestibuli; **ST,** scala tympani. (H&E, × 50) (Gussen R: Ann Otol Rhinol Laryngol 82:871–875, 1973)

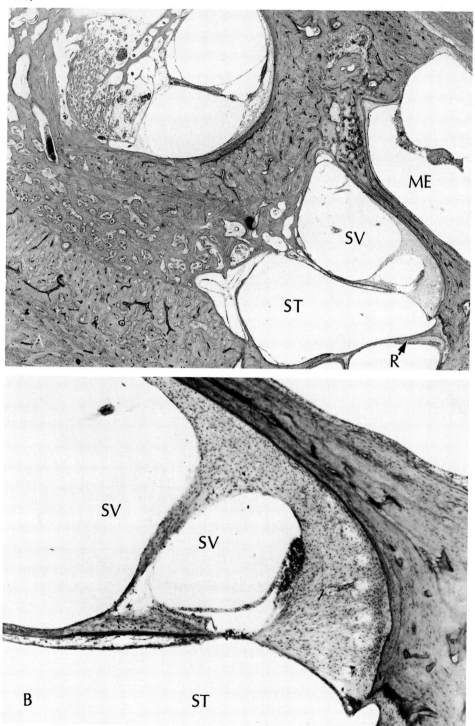

FIG. 32–26. A. Left ear (vertical section) with spiral ligament partition **(arrow),** overlying and attached to Reissner's membrane a short distance from limbus. **FP,** footplate; **R,** round window membrane; **V,** vestibule; **SV,** scala vestibuli; **ST,** scala tympani. (H&E, × 20) **B.** High-power view of spiral ligament partition; **SV,** scala vestibuli; **ST,** scala tympani. (H&E, × 50) (Gussen R: Ann Otol Rhinol Laryngol 82:871–875, 1973)

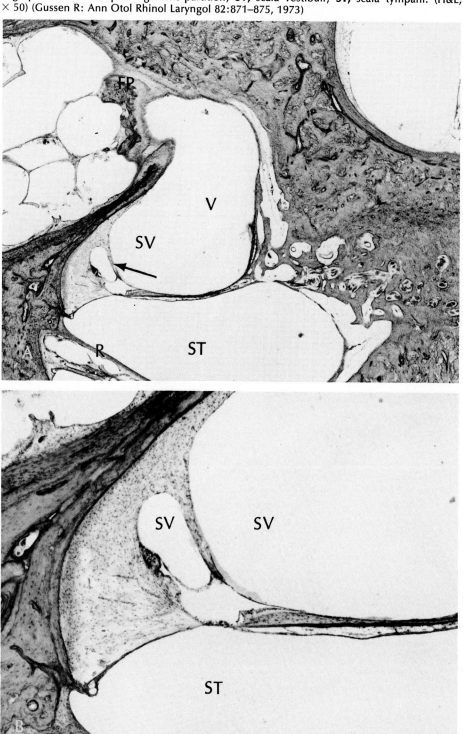

seventh fetal week. In one patient available for histologic study there was a bilateral cochlear Mondini malformation. The cochlear lesions are considered the results of a deficiency in the peroxidase enzyme system.

Jervell–Lange-Nielson Syndrome

This syndrome (20) comprises congenital profound cochlear hearing loss accompanied by a cardiac syndrome characterized by prolongation of the QT interval. There may be recurrent Stokes-Adams attacks, and occasionally the disorder results in sudden death. Pathologically there is marked atrophy of the organ of Corti, fibrosis and atrophy of the stria vascularis, and adhesion of Reissner's membrane to the tectorial membrane. Autosomal recessive transmission, the congenital severe sensorineural hearing loss, and the prolonged QT intervals are characteristic.

Trisomy Syndromes—Down's Syndrome (Mongolism)

The term **trisomy** indicates the presence of an extra chromosome in the cell nucleus. Instead of the normal 22 pairs of autosomes and 2 sex chromosomes making a total of 46, a trisomy patient has an additional chromosome, making the number 47. The classic trisomy syndrome is that of mongolism, otherwise known as Down's syndrome, which is a trisomy 21 or 22.

Another trisomy version is that of trisomy 18, which is characterized by multiple anomalies— mental retardation, hypertonicity, low birth weight, low-set auricles, and other skeletal deformities, including a prominent occiput and a small mouth. These patients frequently die at birth and rarely can be evaluated audiologically.

Both middle and inner ear abnormalities may occur in trisomy 13–15 (D1). In a recent case reported by Black and co-workers (4), the classic findings were small, low-set auricles accompanied by other congenital defects, including cleft lip and palate, undescended testes, and cardiac lesions. The temporal bone findings showed multiple anomalies of middle ear structures derived from the second branchial arch, accompanied by otic capsule abnormalities. A shortened but otherwise well-formed organ of Corti was present in a distorted and incompletely developed bony cochlea. Cochlear hair cells were fairly well preserved. The stapes was malformed, the incudostapedial joint was abnormal in its position, and there was an abnormal middle ear course of a partially dehiscent facial nerve.

The stapedial artery may be persistent in the 13–15 trisomy syndrome (trisomy D1 or Patou's syndrome) as reported by Sando and associates (30). A persistent stapedial artery may be encountered as a completely isolated finding, without other temporal bone lesions, and has been reported also in Paget's disease, otosclerosis, and in thalidomide deformities.

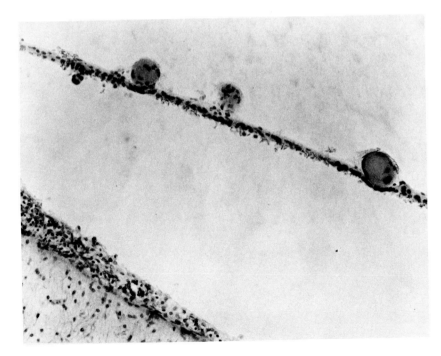

FIG. 32–27. Hyaline (PAS-positive) globules abutting on scala vestibular surface of Reissner's membrane. (H&E, × 180) (Gussen R: J Laryngol 82:41–45, 1968)

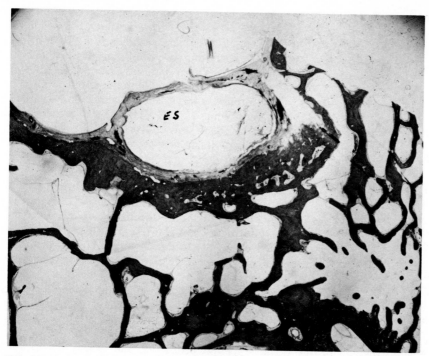

FIG. 32–28. Markedly distended endolymphatic sac **(ES).** (H&E, × 5) (Gussen R: J Laryngol 82:41–55, 1968)

FIG. 32–29. Erosion of bone along lateral surface of enlarged endolymphatic sac **(ES).** Medial portion of sac was torn off with dura. Note enlarged endolymphatic duct **(ED).** (H&E, × 9) (Gussen R: J Laryngol 82:41–45, 1968)

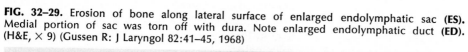

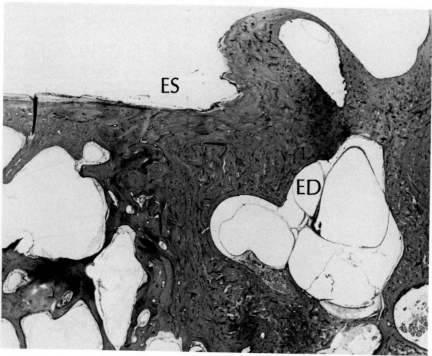

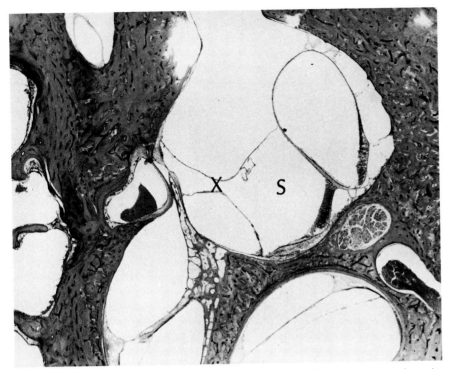

FIG. 32–30. Distended saccule **(S)** and ductus reuniens **(X).** Note fresh hemorrhage in utricle and saccule. (H&E, × 15) (Gussen R; J Laryngol 82:41–45, 1968)

Congenital Cochlear Malformation (Mondini Defect)

Gussen (12) described the Mondini malformation as due to a dominant hereditary trait with an involvement of the cochlear bony structure as well as of the length of the membranous cochlea. The most common defect is considered to be the absence of the interscalar septum in the upper part of the cochlea, with the formation of a common scala (scala communis). In most of the reported cases there has also been the description of a marked distention of the endolymphatic duct and sac. A 31-year-old patient with bilateral Mondini congenital hereditary deafness was reported. The microscopic features included periodic acid-schiff–positive globules (Fig. 32–27), which may be considered the result of a break-up of basement membrane layer secondary to the attempt to transport large amounts of intracochlear fluids across membranous walls. Other distinctive features are shown in Figures 32–28 to 32–31.

In a review of Mondini cochlear malformations, Illum (16) recently reported tomographic demonstration of the Mondini defect. The axial pyramidal projection demonstrates the defect. Only the basal turn of the cochlea can be identified; the remaining part of the cochlea forms a common cavity.

Illum considers that the Mondini defect is an arrest malformation in the development of the cochlear modiolus (Fig. 32–32) in the seventh fetal week. This defect can be spontaneous or hereditary, either autosomal recessive or autosomal dominant. It may be due to Pendred's syndrome, as a result of a defect in the peroxidase enzyme system. It may also be related to chemical damage in thalidomide poisoning or to infections, as in rubella. Thus, the Mondini defect may occur as a result of a number of lesions.

Delayed Progressive Hereditary Cochlear Hearing Loss

Delayed onset, post infancy, of cochlear hearing loss was reported in 13 children by Brockman (6). Two of the children were brothers. Both had normal hearing at birth and in early childhood (Figs. 32–33, 32–34).

Gussen described the temporal bone findings in the grandmother of these two children (13). She had had normal hearing until the age of 65 when she developed rather rapid onset of bilateral hear-

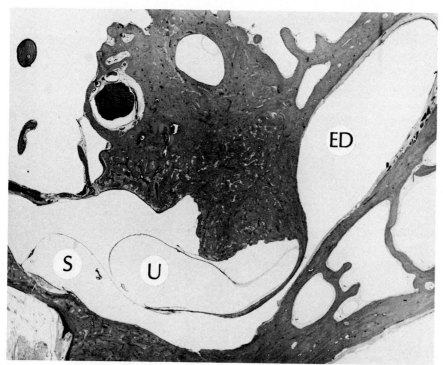

FIG. 32–31. Moderately distended saccule **(S)** opening into markedly distended endolymphatic duct **(ED).** (H&E, × 9) (Gussen R: J Laryngol 82:41–45, 1968)

FIG. 32–32. A preparation from the Ibsen-Mackeprang collection. The cochlea has been opened so carefully that the general impression has been retained. The Mondini defect with hypoplasia of the modiolus can clearly be seen. (Illum P: Arch Otolaryngol 96:305–311, 1972. Copyright 1972, American Medical Association)

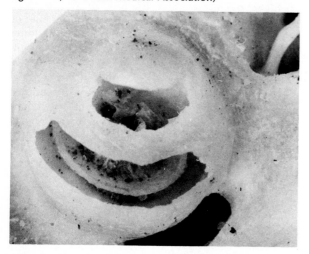

ing loss (Figs. 32–35, 32–36). When the temporal bones were studied, this 80-year-old woman showed findings characteristic of cochleovestibular degeneration of the Siebenmann-Bing type. Among the unusual features were hydrops, periodic acid-schiff–positive globules, and obstruction of the cerebral aperture of the cochlear aqueduct, with fibrotic dura accompanied by aqueduct wall erosion and fistula formation into the internal auditory canal (Figs. 32–37, 32–38, 32–39).

Sensorineural Hearing Loss and Familial Hand Abnormality

Stewart and Bergstrom (33) reported five generations of a family with arthrogrypotic types of hand abnormalities; 7 of 12 affected members had associated sensorineural hearing loss. The Stewart-Bergstrom syndrome is another example of the many unusual combinations of hereditary congenital sensorineural hearing loss and associated malformations.

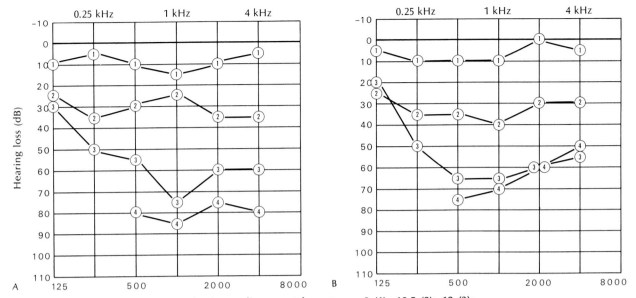

FIG. 32–33. Serial pure-tone air-conduction audiograms taken at ages 8 (1); 10.5 (2); 12 (3); and 17 (4) years. **A.** Right ear. **B.** Left ear. (Brockman SJ: Arch Otolaryngol 70: 340–356, 1959. Copyright 1959, American Medical Association)

FIG. 32–34. Serial pure-tone air-conduction audiograms taken at ages 4 (1), 5 (2), 6 (3), and 10 (4) years. **A.** Right ear. **B.** Left ear. (Brockman SJ: Arch Otolaryngol 70:340–356, 1959. Copyright 1959, American Medical Association)

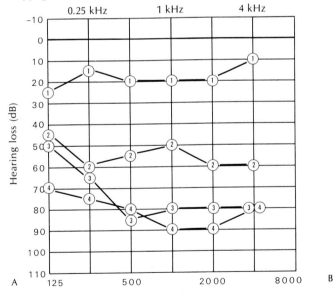

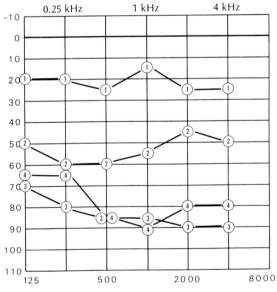

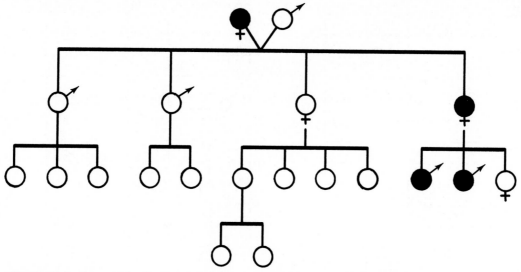

FIG. 32–35. Pedigree of family. **Open circles** mean normal hearing; **solid circles** indicate decreased hearing. (Gussen R: Arch Otolaryngol 90:429–436, 1969. Copyright 1969, American Medical Association)

FIG. 32–36. Audiogram of grandmother 4 years prior to death. (Gussen R: Arch Otolaryngol 90:429–436, 1969. Copyright 1969, American Medical Association)

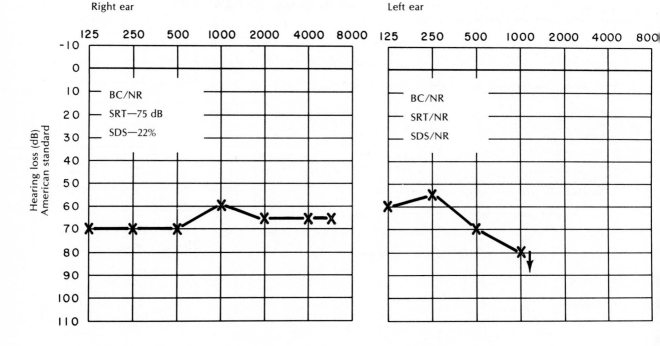

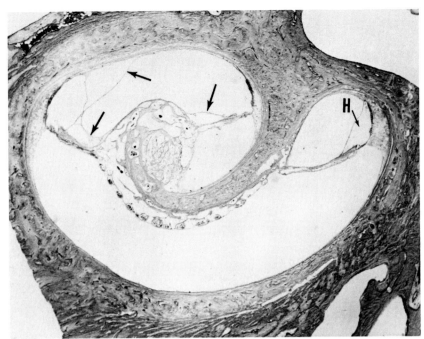

FIG. 32–37. Right cochlea. Note marked hydrops of cochlear duct of superior horizontal portion of basal turn. **Arrows,** Reissner membrane distention in this area. Proximal part of cochlear duct in the hook region **(H)** appears normal. Note marked decrease of spiral ganglion cells in modiolus. (H&E, × 5) (Gussen R: Arch Otolaryngol 90:429–436, 1969. Copyright 1969, American Medical Association)

FIG. 32–38. Right cochlear aqueduct **(CA)** with erosion of wall **(arrows)** and proliferation of arachnoid elements into adjacent bone and marrow, forming fistulous tract **(F)** into internal auditory canal. (H&E, × 9) (Gussen R: Arch Otolaryngol 90:429–436, 1969. Copyright 1969, American Medical Association)

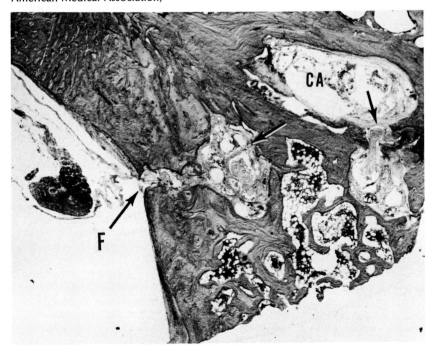

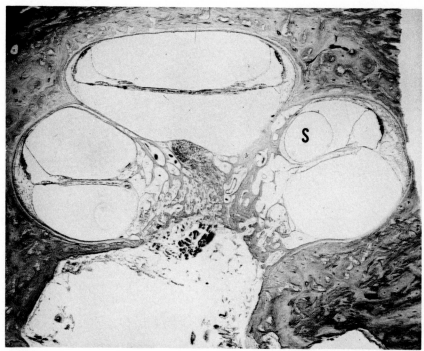

FIG. 32–39. Left cochlea. Note herniated saccule (**S**) in ascending limb of basal turn. Cochlear duct is moderately compressed beyond this level. There is marked loss of ganglion cells and nerve fibers in proximal basal turn, increasing somewhat progressively distalward. (H&E, × 16) (Gussen R: Arch Otolaryngol 90:429–436, 1969. Copyright 1969, American Medical Association)

REFERENCES

1. Adkins WY, Gussen R: Temporal bone findings in the third and fourth pharyngeal pouch (DiGeorge) syndrome. Arch Otolaryngol 100:206–208, 1974

2. Bergstrom L, Neblett LM, Hemenway WG: Otologic manifestations of acrocephalosyndactyly. Arch Otolaryngol 96:117–123, 1972

3. Bergstrom L, Stewart J, Kenyon B: External auditory atresia and the deleted chromosome. Laryngoscope 84:1905–1917, 1974

4. Black FO, Sando I, Wagner J et al.: Middle and inner ear abnormalities. Arch Otolaryngol 93:615–619, 1971

5. Black FO, Spanier SS, Kohut RI: Aural abnormalities in partial DiGeorge syndrome. Arch Otolaryngol 101:129–134, 1975

6. Brockman SJ: An exploratory investigation of delayed progressive neural hypacusis in children. Arch Otolaryngol 70:340–356, 1959

7. Carver WF: An unusual application of a cross hearing aid. Laryngoscope 86:1712–1713, 1976

8. Cavo JW, Pratt LL, Alonso WA: First branchial cleft syndromes and associated congenital hearing loss. Laryngoscope 86:739–745, 1976

9. Escher F, Hirt H: Dominant hereditary conductive deafness through lack of incus stapes junction. Acta Otolaryngol (Stockh) 65:25–32, 1968

10. Fitch N, Lindsay JR, Srolovitz H: The temporal bone in the preauricular pit, cervical fistula, hearing loss syndrome. Ann Otol Rhinol Laryngol 85:268–275, 1976

11. Fraser GR: The Causes of Profound Deafness in Childhood. London, Bailliere Tindall, 1976

12. Gussen R: Mondini type of genetically determined deafness. J Laryngol 82:41–55, 1968

13. Gussen R: Delayed hereditary deafness with cochlear aqueduct obstruction. Arch Otolaryngol 90:429–436, 1969

14. Gussen R: Scala vestibuli partition with deafness and renal disease. Ann Otol Rhinol Laryngol 82:871–875, 1973

15. Igarashi M, Felippone M, Alford B: Temporal bone findings in Pierre Robin syndrome. Laryngoscope 86:1679–1687, 1976

16. Illum P: The Mondini type of cochlear malformation. Arch Otolaryngol 96:305–311, 1972

17. Illum P, Kiaer HW, Hvidberg-Hansen J et al.: Fifteen cases of Pendred's syndrome. Arch Otolaryngol 96:297–304, 1972

18. Jaffe IS: Congenital shoulder-neck-auditory anomalies. Laryngoscope 78:2119–2139, 1968

19. Jarvis JF, Sellars SL: Klippel-Feil deformity associated with congenital conductive deafness. J Laryngol 88:285–289, 1974

20. Jervell A, Lange-Nielsen F: Congenital deaf-

mutism, functional heart disease with prolongation of Q-T interval and sudden death. Am Heart J 54: 59–68, 1957

21. Kim BH: Roentgenography of the ear and eye in Pyle disease. Arch Otolaryngol 99:458–461, 1974

22. Konigsmark BW: Syndromal approaches to the nosology of hereditary deafness. In Birth Defects: Original Article Series, Vol 7, #4. Baltimore, Williams & Wilkins, 1971, pp 2–17

23. Konigsmark BW, Salman S, Haskins H et al.: Dominant mid frequency hearing loss. Ann Otol Rhinol Laryngol 79:42–53, 1970

24. Lindsay JR, Black FO, Donnelly WH: Acrocephalosyndactyly (Apert's syndrome): temporal bone findings. Ann Otol Rhinol Laryngol 84:174–178, 1975

25. Livingstone G: The establishment of sound conduction in congenital deformities of the external ear. J Laryngol 73:231–241, 1959

26. Mengel MC, Konigsmark BW, Berlin CI et al: Conductive hearing loss and malformed low set ears, as a possible recessive syndrome. J Med Genet 6:14–21, 1969

27. Nassif R, Harboyan G: Madelung's deformity with conductive hearing loss. Arch Otolaryngol 91:175–178, 1970

28. Rosenberg AL, Bergstrom L, Troost T et al.: Hyperuricemia and neurologic deficits. N Engl J Med 282:992–997, 1970

29. Rugel SJ, Keates EU: Waardenburg's syndrome in six generations of one family. Am J Dis Child 109: 579–583, 1965

30. Sando I, Leiberman A, Bergstrom L et al.: Temporal bone histopathological findings in Trisomy 13 syndrome. Ann Otol Rhinol Laryngol [Suppl] 84 (#21), 1975

31. Sando I, Wood R: Congenital middle ear anomalies. Otolaryngol Clin North Am 4:291–318, 1971

32. Schuknecht HF: Reconstructive procedures for congenital aural atresia. Arch Otolaryngol 101: 170–172, 1975

33. Stewart JM, Bergstrom L: Familial hand abnormality and sensorineural deafness: a new syndrome. J Pediatr 78:102–110, 1971

34. Szpunar J, Rybak M: Middle ear disease in Turner's syndrome. Arch Otolaryngol 87:52–58, 1968

35. Terrahe K: Das Gehörorgan bei den kraniofazialin Misbildungssyndromen nach Crouzon und Apert. Z Laryngol Rhinol Otol 50:794–802, 1971

36. Vanderbilt University hereditary deafness study group. Dominantly inherited low frequency hearing loss. Arch Otolaryngol 88:242–250, 1968

37. Winter LW, Cram BM, Banovitz JD: Hearing loss in hereditary renal disease. Arch Otolaryngol 88: 238–241, 1968

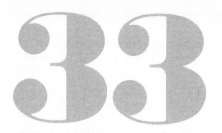

ACQUIRED CONGENITAL EAR SYNDROMES

PRENATAL ACQUIRED OTOTOXIC LESIONS

A number of mild and severe prenatal drug ototoxicity lesions produce changes in the temporal bone resulting in both conductive and cochlear hearing losses.

THALIDOMIDE OTOTOXICITY

Thalidomide ototoxicity is a serious iatrogenic lesion. It causes inner ear aplasia, accompanied by either total (Fig. 33–1) or partial agenesis of the auricle, external canal, and middle ear. Facial nerve lesions and severe cardiac and integumentary defects also occur.

Jorgensen, Kristenden, and Buch (18) reported a classic case of total labyrinthine aplasia caused by thalidomide ingestion during the first month of gestation. This was due to an ingestion of only one or possibly two tablets, corresponding to 100–200 mg thalidomide about 20 days after conception. The infant was asphyxiated at birth but responded to artificial respiration. There were major auricular defects, small external canals, but apparently normal tympanic membranes. There were no responses to neonatal tests with acoustic stimuli, and vestibular studies failed to elicit any reactions.

The infant was examined by polytomography, which showed abnormalities on both sides. There was a severe deformity of both external ears, along with facial paralysis and severe cardiac atrial septal defect.

Temporal bone studies following death at the age of 4 months showed abnormal middle ears and labyrinthine windows on both sides. Instead of the inner ear, there was a small spherical cavity within the temporal bone containing primordia of membranous labyrinth, probably the utricle. There were no nerve fibers, cochlea, saccule, or utricle. Only one inner ear struc-

ture could be identified—the ampulla of the superior semicircular canal.

This is probably the most severe form of thalidomide temporal bone damage. Other forms of thalidomide temporal bone lesions have been reported. In some cases, surgical reconstruction of external and middle ears has been possible, with hearing improvement following ossiculoplastic and tympanolabyrinthine window surgical procedures. In general, the prognosis for hearing improvement through reconstructive surgery in thalidomide hearing loss is poor, because of the high incidence of cochlear aplasia.

OTOTOXIC LESIONS CAUSED BY ANTIBIOTIC DRUGS ADMINISTERED TO THE PREGNANT WOMAN

There is evidence that administration of ototoxic antibiotics to a pregnant woman during any period of gestation, especially in the first and second trimesters, can produce cochlear lesions in the fetus. Streptomycin, dihydrostreptomycin, kanamycin, and other ototoxic antibiotics have been implicated in fetal ototoxic cochlear aplasia (see Ch. 39, Ototoxicity).

PRENATAL ACQUIRED VIREMIC LESIONS

Maternal rubella, a major cause of congenital hearing loss, is an acquired viremic lesion due to rubella in the first trimeter and is the prototype of this group of lesions.

SENSORINEURAL HEARING LOSS DUE TO MATERNAL RUBELLA

In 1941 Gregg (15) reported teratogenic effects of the rubella virus on the fetus. He showed that maternal prenatal rubella was responsible for a number of lesions, including profound sensorineural hearing loss.

Goodhill, in a study of rubella epidemiology in 1950 (13), reported that rubella accounted for at least 20% of the population of a school for the deaf.

Thus, rubella, which at one time was considered to be the mildest of all childhood diseases, became recognized as a very serious disease, if not the most serious of all the viral diseases for the pregnant woman who contracts it, because of its effects upon her unborn child.

Rubella, apparently one of the mildest of the communicable exanthemas, was shown to be an exceptionally virulent destructive agent to fetal

FIG. 33–1. A and **B.** Total bilateral agenesis, accompanied by mixed conductive cochlear hearing loss. Note micrognathia. Mother took one thalidomide tablet in first trimester of pregnancy.

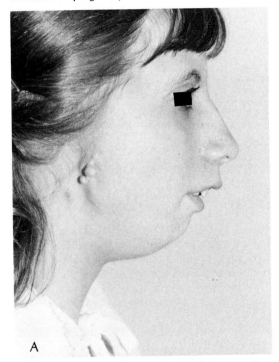

A

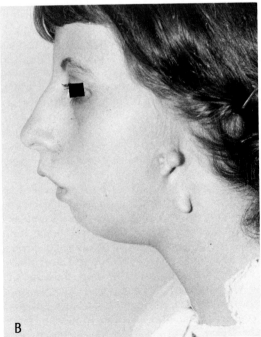

B

organs when it infected the mother, especially during the *first trimester of pregnancy*. Generally, the earlier in pregnancy the infection occurred, the more severe and numerous were the defects. Bordley and co-workers (2) reported that rubella in the second and third trimester may also be teratogenic; in the series were included two cases of rubella-deformed babies born of mothers who contracted rubella before conception.

In 1964–65, the rubella epidemic in the United States was exceptionally virulent and produced many newborn children with congenital defects. Estimates range from 30,000–50,000 deformed infants born to women in the United States who had rubella during pregnancy. Clinical auditory sequelae found in the Baylor University rubella study group in 1967 were summarized as follows: 29% were "deaf," and 17% were presumed to have hearing losses. Additional congenital defects reported were ocular (65%) cardiac (65%), thrombocytopenia (30%), bone changes (34%), hepatomegaly and/or splenomegly (81%). Studies by Bordley and Hardy (3) of 22 postrubella infants reported communicative defects in 35% and motor or developmental retardation in 32%. Another study (2) surveyed 165 children whose prenatal exposure to rubella was confirmed by laboratory studies, reported a high incidence of hearing loss. In children showing live virus at birth the investigators found a failure rate for the hearing test of 56.6%, and in the children with positive serology, a failure rate of 41.5%. The virus-positive group with hearing loss had a higher percentage of associated defects than those with hearing loss and positive serology. The most commonly associated defects were pulmonary stenosis and cataracts.

Typical temporal bone pathology in a child with positive virus culture and serologic evidence of maternal rubella was reported by Hemenway, Sando, and McChesney (16). Primary abnormalities were changes in the saccule, stria vascularis, tectorial membrane, and organ of Corti hair cells. The findings basically resemble those of the Scheibe cochleosaccular degeneration and have also been described in the temporal bones of patients following postnatal measles. Some pathologists have also described changes in the stapes, indicating the possibility of a combined conductive and cochlear hearing loss. Such stapedial findings have been uncommon.

The typical audiometric picture in rubella deafness may be described as symmetrical and flat, but sometimes unilateral (Fig. 33–2). Vernon

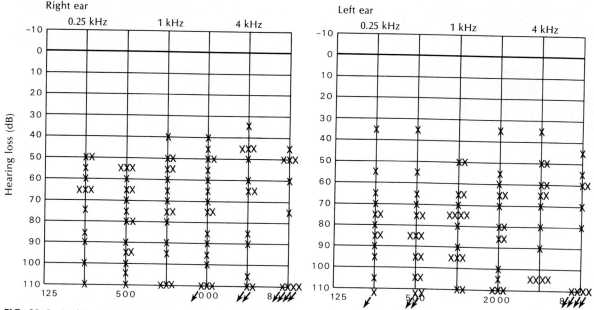

FIG. 33–2. Audiometric scattergram of 16 cases of rubella sensorineural hearing loss. Note wide spread in degrees of hearing loss. **X**, air conduction; **arrows,** no response at maximum output.

(31), reporting on 8.8% of the population of a school for the deaf, found the mean hearing loss to be 82.3 dB (American Standards Association) (500–2000 Hz) and the configuration to be flat. Vernon's psychodiagnostic data corroborates medical research indicating CNS dysfunction as one of the sequelae. A greater prevalence of learning disability (including aphasia) and severe emotional disturbance (poor impulse control, excitability, rigidity, emotional instability, distractibility, and emotional shallowness) was reported for the post rubella children.

In etiologic histories, maternal rubella is often lacking when, in fact, it was the etiologic factor. The infection may have been quite inapparent, the mother having had no clinical symptoms. The virus is recoverable from the young child for some time after birth, and it is believed that it is active in various organs, including the brain, where it causes a low-grade encephalitis. The rubella virus can be recovered from blood and various secretions and grown in tissue culture, and antibodies can be demonstrated. Following the age of 2 years, although viral cultures and antibodies may still be obtained, it becomes increasingly likely that the child contracted rubella on his own, so that the evidence becomes less conclusive for an in-utero infection.

As data accumulate, it is now possible to document far more diffuse sequelae to the rubella syn-

drome than were primarily recognized. Brookhauser and Bordley (4) list the following lesions under "the expanded rubella syndrome": deafness; eye defects, congenital heart defects, microcephaly, mental and/or motor retardation, hepatosplenomegaly in newborn period, thrombocytopenia, radiolucencies in long bones, interstitial pneumonitis, encephalitis, and low birth weight.

As studies are evaluated from various centers, it becomes clear that the hearing loss is primarily cochlear. The conductive components may be considered rare. The severity of the hearing loss varies greatly from patient to patient and to a lesser degree may vary from one ear to the other of the same patient.

At the present time the pathogenesis of congenital rubella deafness is not entirely clear. The distinct asymmetry in hearing acuity and temporal bone pathology seen in the ears of the same individual create problems in clarification of pathogenesis. There are changes in the stria vascularis, such as cystic dilation, and this may indicate the possibility that the stria is a portal of entry into the scala media. It is difficult to explain collapse of the cochlear duct and saccule. Anderson, Barr, and Wedenberg (1) propose the existence of a genetic predisposition for maternal rubella deafness, an intriguing hypothesis.

As public health measures and rubella immunization become more widespread, the incidence of rubella deafness will decrease, and it is to be hoped that it will become a rarity. In general, most rubella children who do not have severe CNS lesions do quite well with amplification, if there is a reasonable remnant of amplifiable hearing in one or both ears. Most rubella children do not show evidence of significant delayed deterioration but a rather static level of hearing loss.

From an educational standpoint, rubella deaf children, if they are not multiply handicapped, have no more difficulty in profiting from aural rehabilitation and education techniques than other deaf children. In the use of hearing aids they do not appear to have any more difficulty because of abnormal tolerance problems than other children with amplification. There are no more emotionally disturbed pupils among the rubella deaf population than the population of "normal deaf" in the schools for the deaf.

As in any type of congenital hearing loss, early diagnosis and early educational management are the key to success in rehabilitation, in development of language patterns, and in ultimate communicative educational skills developed by the rubella deaf child.

Advances in immunology are extremely encouraging. Immunologists consider children to be the primary target for immunization because they carry the bulk of virus pools in the community. Reducing this virus pool will indirectly protect women.

Immunization of women in the childbearing years is urged because it does offer immediate protection and it is a direct approach. One must be absolutely sure, however, that no pregnancy ensues for 2 months after vaccination. More effective vaccines with better antibody responses are being studied.

SENSORINEURAL HEARING LOSS DUE TO CYTOMEGALOVIRUS

Cytomegalovirus (CMV) is now considered to be a very common congenital viral infection (1.5% of all live births). Cytomegaloviral inclusion-body infection can cause liver disease and such neurologic sequelae as microcephaly, mental retardation, and—recently reported—loss of hearing.

Myers and Stool (26) reported changes in the temporal bones from an infant who died from CMV disease. They reported changes in the stria vascularis with cochlear duct and saccule hydrops. Davis (7) reported CMV inclusions in the cochlear duct and semicircular canals of a 1-week-old infant who had died from meningitis in whom

cytomegaloviral inclusions were found in kidneys and salivary glands. No hearing data were available in either of these two temporal-bone studies, obviously.

In a recent audiologic study of children (6) with history of subclinical congenital CMV infection, 9 of 18 infected subjects showed hearing losses ranging from slight high-frequency losses to severe unilateral loss.

CONGENITAL SYPHILIS

Congenital syphilis is a significant cause of cochlear hearing loss in the fetus. It has numerous manifestations, varying from relatively minor to severe losses. Specific details are discussed in Chapter 38, Syphilis of the Temporal Bone.

LESIONS ACQUIRED AT BIRTH

In lesions occurring at birth, the specific etiologic factor may be effective immediately before delivery, during delivery, or immediately following delivery. Acquired natal lesions include such causes as trauma, congenital hypoxia and anoxia, prematurity, and Rh factor bilirubinemia lesions.

TRAUMA

A number of traumatic lesions, either involving the mother prenatally, or during delivery, may cause congenital acquired hearing losses. Difficult prolonged deliveries may be accompanied by physical trauma to the infant skull. Actual skull lesions or presumptive lesions due either to a congenitally narrowed pelvic outlet or to unusual forceps procedures have been considered as possible, but unproven, causes of congenital acquired hearing losses.

HYPOXIA AND ANOXIA

Fetal hypoxia at delivery probably plays a significant role in the etiology of some otherwise unexplained cochlear hearing losses. These are instances in which there is no evidence of physical trauma to the skull but hypoxic change is indicated by fetal pulse abnormalities and by obvious "blue baby" observations at the time of delivery. Experimental work on fetal hypoxia in animals has shown that it is possible to produce definitive physiological cochlear lesions, which may or may not be accompanied by cerebral lesions.

PREMATURITY

Prematurity may be accompanied not only by constitutional lesions involving the CNS, but by cochlear lesions. The specific aspects of exact cochlear and CNS prematurity parameters have not been completely identified. Prematurity, however, is a probable cause of some instances of congenital acquired cochlear hearing loss.

The primary lesion in prematurity and natal hypoxia is atrophy of the organ of Corti, with degeneration of both sensory and supporting cells. The stria vascularis is almost completely atrophic. There are very frequent massive labyrinthine hemorrhages in newborn infants who are premature.

RH FACTOR ABNORMALITIES—HYPERBILIRUBINEMIA, NEONATAL HEMOLYTIC DISEASE

A number of hyperbilirubinemic lesions will produce the Rh factor type of congenital sensorineural hearing loss. The lesion may primarily involve the cochlear nuclei, rather than the cochlea *per se.*

A special type of sensorineural hearing loss occurs in neonatal hemolytic disease (NHD), due to hyperbilirubinemia, which can cause CNS diseases of the kernicterus type. Classic kernicterus produces athetosis, sensorineural hearing loss, and defective ocular supravergence. Rh factor incompatibility is the primary etiologic factor in NHD, although ABO incompatibility may also produce hyperbilirubinemia.

Orth in 1875 (27) described "brain jaundice," later termed kernicterus by Schmorl in 1903 (28) to designate cranial nuclear jaundice. Erythroblastosis fetalis (congenital hemolytic disease) was later linked to congenital fetal hydrops and icterus gravis neonatorum (32).

Following the designation of the Rh factor by Landsteiner and Wiener (20), the immunologic aspect of erythroblastosis fetalis became clarified.

Serologic incompatibility between fetus and mother (Rh or ABO) is responsible for a variety of hemolytic diseases of the newborn, in which red blood cells are destroyed and the resulting bilirubin circulates freely within the fetal circulation. The sequelae of hyperbilirubinemia are primarily noted in the CNS, the auditory system, and in other sensory organs. The prime example for serologic incompatibility is erythroblastotic kernicterus.

In 1949 Dublin (9) described in detail the neuropathologic sequelae of kernicterus, with delineation of golden yellow pigment in a number of CNS locations, including inferior olivary, dentate, and vestibular nuclei.

In 1950 Goodhill (14) reported a clinical study of 11 cases of bilateral sensorineural hearing loss with histories of NHD or erythroblastosis fetalis. In 8 of the 11 cases there was associated athetoid cerebral palsy. On the basis of relatively moderate sensorineural hearing losses with clear-cut bilateral symmetry (Fig. 33–3), the clinical assumption was made that the site of lesion was not primarily the cochlea, but more likely the cochlear nuclei. Thus, the term "nuclear deafness" was proposed as a designation for erythroblastotic (NHD) sensorineural hearing loss acquired at birth.

The results of a collaborative study of otologic and neuropathologic findings were reported in 1951 by Dublin (10).

It is quite likely that CNS hypoxia and anoxia, with or without icterus, may also produce cochlear nuclear hearing losses.

Studies of a large sample of children (17, 19) with hyperbilirubinemia showed that only sensorineural hearing loss and athetosis showed a significant association with neonatal high ($\geqq 20$ mg/100 ml) bilirubin exposure.

The mortality due to Rh disease has decreased greatly, largely because of the use of amniocentesis, and associated developments that are monumental in dealing preventively with a problem that would usually result in irreversible damage. In addition to exchange transfusions, the uses of phototherapy, phenobarbital and/or serum albumin and other modalities appear to offer therapeutic promise for the future.

Since CNS damage by bilirubin is irreversible, management must be directed toward *prevention.* The key is a team approach, with close communication and cooperation between the pregnant woman, the physicians handling the obstetric and pediatric aspects of her case, and the laboratory. Sensitization to the $Rh_o(D)$ factor can now be prevented by the proper use of anti-Rh immunoglobulin in those Rh-negative mothers who have not been previously immunized. For those who have been immunized and are pregnant with an Rh-positive fetus, the mortality and morbidity may be decreased with prenatal prediction of NHD, proper timing of delivery, and availability at the time of delivery of trained personnel and adequate facilities for the immediate care of the infant. The focus of neonatal therapy is directed toward controlling the serum bilirubin concentration below 20 mg/100 ml by means of exchange transfusion.

These advances of prevention and management give hope to the possibility that Rh nuclear deafness produced by this serious immunologic problem may eventually be entirely eliminated as a cause of hearing loss in children.

However, sophisticated obstetric and pediatric management of this problem is not available everywhere, and it is quite likely that Rh factor hearing loss may continue to be a problem requiring diagnosis and management for many years to come.

The audiologic aspects of kernicteric nuclear sensorineural hearing loss are provocative in relationships with other brain stem hearing loss lesions.

A number of investigators have found the usual pure-tone audiogram, in cases of children with kernicteric defects, to be bilaterally symmetrical with a mild to moderate loss in the low frequencies, increasing to a severe loss in the high frequencies.

Carhart (5) compiled group data obtained in major studies and reported the characteristic configuration with International Standards Organization 1964 thresholds as follows: about 30 dB for 125 and 250 Hz, about 40 dB for 500 Hz, about 60 dB for 1 kHz, about 70 dB for 2 kHz, about 75 dB for 8 kHz. These studies were limited to patients of sufficient maturity to respond consistently. Speech discrimination was variable, and good in many instances. Amplification was also of varying benefit. The triad of recruitment, type II Bekesy tracings, and positive SISI scores in the high frequencies was commonly seen.

Matkin and Carhart (25) attributed these findings to cochlear lesions but postulated a "dual dysfunction" involving both the cochlear and the central auditory system. However, there is postmortem evidence to show that kernicteric foci in the cochlear nuclei are common, and cochlear damage has not been proved. Carhart (5) theorized that auditory findings similar to those found in cochlear disorders may be produced by central lesions when "normal trains of information from the inner ear suffer disruption in transmission through damaged cochlear nuclei and/or associated basal centers en route to perceptual processing in higher center." He postulated that normal inner ear and eighth (cranial) nerve function may be present.

The shape of the audiogram (better hearing for low tones) may be attributed to a differential disruption in acuity located within the cochlear nuclei. Carhart utilized Wever's volley-place theory and considered that the place-sensitive mechanism operant for high tones may receive greater damage than the volley-analyzing mechanism (synchronous neural-discharging predominating in low-frequency sensitivity) but at a level within the cochlear nuclei where, he theorized, the first definitely separate coding may take place.

The evidence of recruitment could have occurred, according to Carhart, if a normal cochlea were present and a gating process were operating within the cochlear nuclei, which resulted in tonal stimulation at normal intensities. This could also account for positive SISI scores in that, through action of the gating function, the stimulus level is high enough to evoke a normal response (normal ears usually detect a 1-dB intensity increment at levels about 75 dB), despite the kernicteric subject's limited ability to perceive stimuli of less intensity.

Type II Bekesy tracings may be attributed to normal peripheral adaptation coupled with a centrally imposed drop in neural activity. Thus, a central auditory disorder (shown by postmortem evidence) may mimic a cochlear lesion and be misdiagnosed as a peripheral sensory impairment. Carhart's hypothesis is as warranted as other contrary ones and will await further clinical and histologic research.

In a recent study of symmetrical hearing loss and brain stem lesions, Dix and Hood (8) described symmetrical hearing losses exhibiting loudness recruitment in patients with known or suspected brain-stem lesions. They considered that this suggested that the derangement is not in the cochlea but in the cochlear nuclei. The auditory losses in patients with confirmed brainstem lesions resemble very closely the auditory symmetrical pattern seen in kernicteric sensorineural hearing loss.

There has been a paucity of temporal bone material in cases of Rh incompatibility. A recent study of a temporal bone in a case of Rh disease was reported by Lindsay (22) in a young person with a bilateral sloping sensorineural hearing loss. His report included the following information:

Examination of temporal bones showed normal cochleas with the hair cells well preserved except for slight postmortem changes. A population of ganglion cells was normal in number throughout.

The absence of a recognizable end organ or peripheral neuron lesion favors a nuclear lesion as a cause for deafness. The brain had unfortunately not been preserved in this case, hence confirmation is lacking.

In a recent neuropathologic study of a case of erythroblastosis, Dublin described degeneration in the ventral cochlear nucleus (especially in the superior division). There is a tonotopic pattern resembling that seen in animal (cat) studies that is suggested as relating a cochlear nucleogram with a pure-tone audiogram, in known cases of Rh nuclear "deafness" (11).

SUMMARY

Rh nuclear "deafness" is an example of the type of communicative lesion which transcends

FIG. 33–3. A, B, C, D. Varieties of Rh cochlear nuclear hearing loss audiograms. ●—●, AC, unmasked, RE; [—[, BC, masked, RE; x—x, AC, unmasked, LE;]—], BC, masked, LE; **arrow,** no response at maximum output.

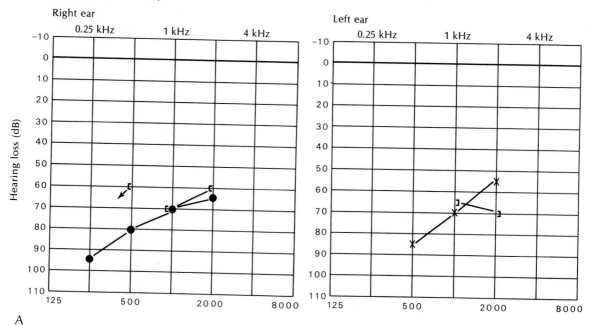

A

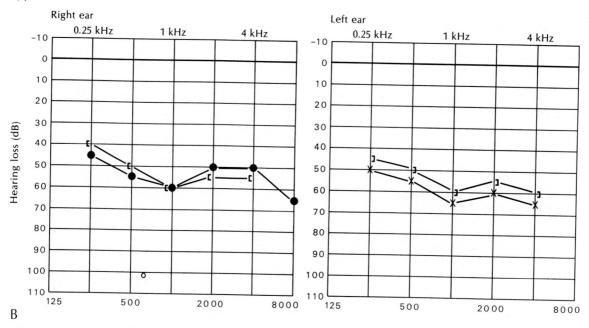

B

FIG. 33–3 (*continued*)

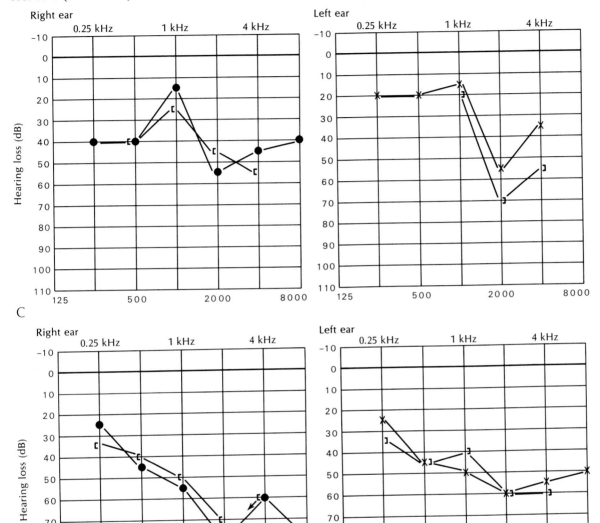

C

D

limited considerations of the peripheral auditory mechanism but involves complex analyses of central pathways, requiring immunologic, pediatric, obstetric, psychological and educational expertise. We have come a long way from pre-Rh "congenital hemolytic anemia" to cochlear nuclear "deafness," to amniocentesis, to exchange transfusion, to noninvasive phototherapy of hyperbilirubinemia, and, most important, to prophylaxis with the use of Rhogam vaccine. Nowhere is the role of the physician in deafness more dramatically portrayed than the role in this complex disease.

POSTNATAL (INFANTILE AND CHILDHOOD) ACQUIRED LESIONS CAUSING SENSORINEURAL HEARING LOSS

A number of postnatal infections in infancy and childhood are causes of acquired sensorineural hearing losses. Only those that occur during the very first few postnatal days can appropriately be termed congenital. Most of the lesions are not congenital.

BACTERIAL INFECTIONS

Bacterial diseases of childhood invade the CNS with resultant sensorineural hypacusis and anacusis. Meningitis and encephalitis are two chief examples, with meningitis the major offender. Epidemic or meningococcic meningitis is a cause, as is the meningitis complicating streptococcal, pneumococcal, or staphylococcal respiratory infections. Bacterial influenzal meningitis, often of otitic origin, is one of the more common varieties in young children. Tuberculous meningitis may also produce the same type of invasion with the same sequelae.

Most meningitic sensorineural losses are bilateral, and most of them are profound, primarily in the anacusic category. In some instances, there is also evidence of vestibular disturbance.

There is no satisfactory treatment for the sequelae of meningitic deafness, but meningitis, *per se*, can now be treated far more satisfactorily than it was one or two decades ago. Consequently, more survivals are reported than ever before. Many of these survivors will be left with neurologic sequelae, one of which will be sensorineural hypacusis. When the meningitis therapy is started very early in the course of the disease, and when the organism is particularly responsive to the antibiotic agent, avoidance of sensory defects may be expected. It is not too much to hope that early

intensive treatment of meningitis may eventually result in the virtual elimination of postmeningitic sensorineural hypacusis as a major cause of deafness. Labyrinthogenic meningitis and meningogenic meningitis lesions both occur, producing severe hearing losses in most cases.

VIRAL INFECTIONS

Most viral exanthemas may produce serious neurologic sequelae. These may be limited to one or another of the sense organs, or may involve the CNS. Thus, sensorineural hypacusis and anacusis may follow measles, mumps, chickenpox, whooping cough, herpes, rubella, and members of the virus influenza group. All of these diseases may attack the organ of hearing. Such invasion may be unilateral or bilateral, partial or complete. In general, cochlear involvement by viruses is relatively infrequent except in mumps, rubella, and rubeola, although the sudden hearing loss syndrome that occurs especially in adults can be viral in origin in a high percentage of cases, probably as the result of one of the influenzal viral strains.

The most common prenatal cochlear lesion due to viral infection is that seen in rubella (see section on Sensorineural Hearing Loss Due to Maternal Rubella, earlier in this chapter). Of the postnatal viral infections, rubeola (measles) has been a major cause of conductive hearing loss in the last, particularly because of secondary bacterial temporal-bone infections. Postnatal mumps is a relatively common cause of severe unilateral cochlear hearing loss.

Measles (rubeola), however, also continues to be a serious cause of profound cochlear hearing loss. The incidence of "deafmutism" attributed to measles has been reported as ranging from 3% -10% (21).

Measles (Rubeola)

The histopathology of temporal bone measles in a 7½-month-old child has been clearly defined by Lindsay and Hemenway (24). The primary changes were in the endolymphatic system, with limited secondary degeneration of peripheral cochlear neurons. The stria vascularis showed extreme degeneration, and the organ of Corti was entirely degenerated in the basal coil, with progressively less evidence of damage in the upper coils. All air cells were absent. Saccule and utricle damage was accompanied by degeneration of the crista ampullaris in two canals. In view of these findings, it appeared that the primary route of invasion was hematogenous. Therefore, the term

endolymphatic labyrinthitis was proposed to differentiate this lesion from the type of lesion seen in meningogenic bacterial labyrinthitis, which is primarily an involvement of the perilabyrinthine spaces. The characteristic detachment of the tectorial membrane was seen in many of these cases. It is rolled up and covered by cells and lies in the angle between Reissner's membrane and the limbus (Figs. 33–4, 33–5).

Mumps

Although mumps deafness was mentioned by Hinze (16a) in 1802, and described grossly by Toynbee in 1860 in temporal bone examination (30), the first definitive description of the viral lesion was that reported by Lindsay, Davey, and Ward, in 1960 (23). Everberg (12) states that "the frequency of deafness as a complication to mumps may be estimated to be about 0.05 per thousand."

In the typical case of unilateral post-mumps cochlear deafness, there is no unusual history. In almost every instance the hearing loss is accidentally discovered either by the patient or the family. Unilateral hearing loss does not manifest itself with dramatic symptoms, particularly in the absence of vestibular involvement. Vestibular involvement in mumps deafness is rare. Caloric tests usually reveal normal responses. Tinnitus is extremely rare. Consequently the diagnosis is frequently missed.

Frequently, the diagnosis of mumps cochlear hearing loss is first made on routine school audiometric tests. Occasionally a wrong diagnosis of conductive hearing loss is made because of inadequate masking for air and bone conduction, and for speech reception threshold and speech discrimination measurements. Patients are occasionally seen in consultation who have been advised to have middle ear surgery on the basis of a wrong diagnosis of an air–bone gap in the affected ear. Such a spurious air–bone gap can always be attributed to inadequate masking for bone-conduction studies. Similar inadequacies in masking result in inaccurately high speech discrimination scores. Usually the pure-tone air-conduction hearing loss in mumps, as illustrated in Figure 33–6, is severe in the high and middle frequencies. Occasionally, low-frequency air-conduction responses may exist with questionable bone-conduction responses at 250 Hz and 500 Hz, giving rise to a misconception regarding a conductive component. Although there may well be true air-conduction responses in the 60–70 dB range in the lower frequencies, speech discrimination scores usually vary from 0 to 12–15%. In effect, the mumps ear is usually a nonfunctioning ear and cannot be used for hearing-aid amplification.

There is usually no history of vertigo and there is rarely evidence of vestibular function impairment in mumps. The time of onset is difficult to determine because there is uncommon symptomatic evidence immediately following the disease, and hearing measurements are frequently delayed for years following the acute mumps illness.

Although mumps most frequently occurs in early childhood, older children and adults may also have the disease.

Mumps is probably the most frequent cause of unilateral severe cochlear hearing loss in children. The diagnosis of mumps hearing loss may be based upon the history of mumps, the presence of a profound unilateral cochlear hearing loss, no evidence of middle ear disease on otologic examination, and no radiographic abnormalities. In the absence of a family history of mumps, it is possible to get a positive complement fixation test and skin test for hypersensitivity in some cases, although such findings are only confirmatory and may not prove or disprove definitive etiologic relationship. Caloric studies in mumps cases usually reveal normal responses, but there may be hypoactive responses in some cases and, rarely, even entirely absent vestibular responses.

The definitive histopathic details described by Lindsay, Davey, and Ward (23) were cochlear duct collapse, and degeneration of stria vascularis and organ of Corti in basal and middle coils, collapse of Reissner's membrane, and degeneration of the tectorial membrane.

The pathogenesis is considered to be of viremic origin, with primary involvement of stria vascularis. Lindsay points out that the lesions of the tectorial membrane observed in the mumps labyrinth, as well as in the endolymphatic labyrinthitis due to rubella and rubeola, are characteristic but not necessarily diagnostic, since similar lesions are found in other pathologic states. It is not likely that mumps deafness is associated with meningoencephalitis.

It is difficult to evaluate the epidemiology of mumps deafness. Mumps epidemic parotitis may involve one or both parotid glands and occasionally the submaxillary salivary glands, testes, or ovaries. It is a highly communicable contagious disease of childhood and occasionally of adults. Occasionally mumps will produce otalgia during the acute course of the disease. Examination of the ears at this time will usually reveal no otoscopic abnormalities. The absence or presence of hearing loss during an acute episode may not be related to the

FIG. 33–4. Sections through cochlear duct of right ear. **A.** Upper basal coil. Note total degeneration of stria vascularis and organ of Corti. Tectorial membrane lies in inner sulcus, covered by cells **(arrow).** ($\times$ 129) **B.** Middle coil. Note remnants of stria vascularis, tectorial membrane detached from limbus, covered by cellular layer, attached to organ of Corti **(arrow).** Hair cells absent. (H&E, original magnification $\times$ 144) (Lindsay JR, Hemenway WG: Ann Otol Rhinol Laryngol 63:754–771, 1954)

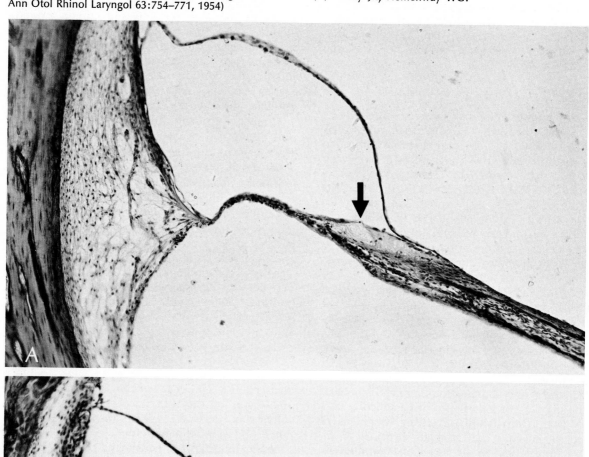

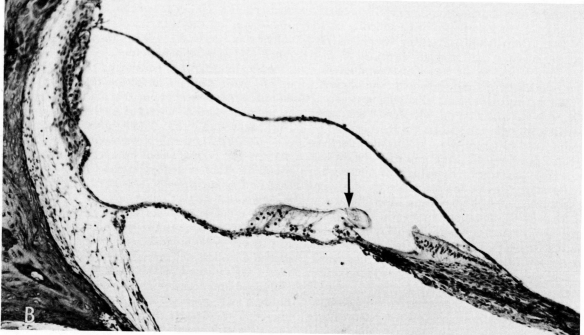

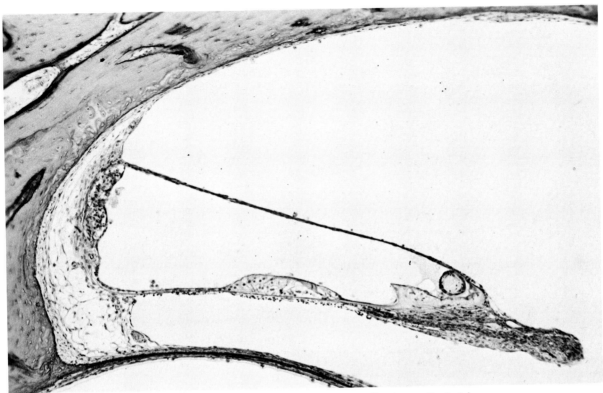

FIG. 33–5. Section through part of the apical coil, left cochlea. Hair cells absent. Tectorial membrane detached, rolled up, covered by cells, lying in angle between Reissner membrane and limbus. (H&E, original magnification × 130) (Lindsay JR, Hemenway WG: Ann Otol Rhinol Laryngol 63:754–771, 1954)

FIG. 33–6. Unilateral mumps sensorineural hearing loss. ●—●, AC, unmasked, RE; [—[, BC, masked, RE; **arrows,** no response at maximum output; **SRT,** 70 dB; **SDS,** 12%.

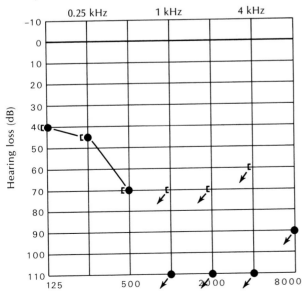

discovery of significant and frequently total sensorineural hearing loss later. The otalgia at the time of the acute disease may be due solely to referred pain from the parotid gland and have nothing to do with the ear *per se.*

Even if a severe hearing loss were diagnostically discovered during the acute mumps viremia, there is no known treatment that can be used to deal with such a viral cochleopathy.

Occasionally mumps deafness can be diagnosed only presumptively by a history of mumps in which the parotid glands are not involved (involvement of testes or ovaries). Patients have been seen with unilateral profound cochlear hearing loss of unknown etiology. Careful history however, reveals that one or two siblings in the family had mumps, even though the patient with the hearing loss did not have clinical parotitis or extraparotid mumps lesions.

There is no definitive treatment for mumps deafness and there is very little that can be done insofar as rehabilitation is concerned. Fortunately, a unilateral hearing loss, while inconvenient, is

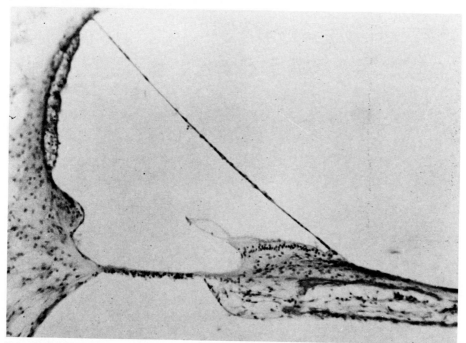

FIG. 33–7. High-power view, ascending basal turn. Note hyaline droplets at edges of tectorial membrane. (H&E, original magnification × 96) (Smith GA, Gussen R: Arch Otolaryngol 102:108–111, 1976. Copyright 1976, American Medical Association)

not handicapping. For special purposes a hearing aid with contralateral routing of signal (CROS) may be of value. Indications for the use of a CROS hearing aid rarely exist in the average schoolchild. In adults, however, who have postnatal unilateral mumps deafness, a CROS hearing aid may be indicated if there are special vocational or occupational needs.

Adult onset of mumps is not common. When it occurs in adults, it is more severe systemically than it is in children, and it is more frequently associated with meningitis. Smith and Gussen (29) reported temporal bone studies in an adult with a bilateral post-mumps cochlear hearing loss of moderate degree. There was absence of the organ of Corti in the ascending basal turn (Fig. 33–7).

SUDDEN COCHLEAR HEARING LOSS DUE
TO VIREMIA

Sudden hearing loss in children or adults (see Ch. 37, Sudden Hearing Loss Syndrome) occasionally is seen in intimate association with an upper respiratory tract infection. Various types of cochlear hearing loss have been recorded in such cases varying from minor high-frequency losses

to total cochlear hearing loss, most commonly unilateral.

In the temporal bone studies that have been made in patients with the history of sudden hearing loss following an apparent upper respiratory infection, the pathologic findings resembled those in endolymphatic labyrinthitis produced by maternal rubella, mumps, and measles. In general the perilymphatic system in these temporal bones appears to be normal. There is usually evidence of degeneration of the stria vascularis, especially in the basal coil, with changes in the tectorial membrane frequently comparable to those seen in measles and mumps.

Postnatal viral infections can affect the inner ear and the auditory nerve. The portal of entry may be through viremia or through the meningeal cerebrospinal fluid system. Viremic involvement is usually through the labyrinth via the stria vascularis, with subsequent involvement of the endolymphatic system. If there is invasion of the ear through the meningeal-subarachnoid system via the internal auditory meatus or the cochlear aqueduct or occasionally through the vestibular nerves, the modiolus is directly exposed to an inflammatory process that may then spread through the perilymphatic system. There has been little evidence regarding the potential role of the cochlear aqueduct. Theoretically, the cochlear aqueduct may also be a portal of entry of meningogenic viral infections, particularly if there is some degree of diminution of the barrier membrane between the cochlear aqueduct and the scala tympani.

REFERENCES

1. Anderson H, Barr B, Wedenberg E: Genetic disposition—a prerequisite for maternal rubella deafness. Arch Otolaryngol 91:141–147, 1970

2. Bordley JE, Brookhouser PE, Hardy J et al.: Prenatal rubella. Acta Otolaryngol (Stockh) 66:1–9, 1968

3. Bordley JE, Hardy JMD: Laboratory and clinical observations on prenatal rubella. Ann Otol Rhinol Laryngol 78:917–928, 1969

4. Brookhouser PE, Bordley JE: Congenital rubella deafness. Arch Otolaryngol 98:252–257, 1973

5. Carhart R: Audiological tests: questions and speculations. In McConnell F, Ward PH (eds): Deafness in Childhood. Nashville, Vanderbilt University Press, 1967, p 229

6. Dahle AJ, McCollister FP, Hammer BA et al.: Subclinical congenital cytomegalovirus infection and hearing impairment. J Speech Hear Dis 39:320–329, 1974

7. Davis G: Cytomegalovirus in the inner ear. Ann Otol Rhinol Laryngol 78:1179–1189, 1969

8. Dix MR, Hood JD: Symmetrical hearing loss in brain stem lesions. Acta Otolaryngol (Stockh) 75:165–177, 1973

9. Dublin WB: Pathogenesis of kernicterus. J Neuropathol Exp Neurol 8:119, 1949

10. Dublin WB: Neurological lesions of erythroblastosis fetalis in relation to nuclear deafness. Am J Clin Pathol 21:935, 1951

11. Dublin WB: Cytoarchitecture of the cochlear nuclei. Arch Otolaryngol 100:355–359, 1974

12. Everberg G: Deafness following mumps. Acta Otolaryngol (Stockh) 48:397–403, 1957

13. Goodhill V: The nerve deaf child. Significance of Rh, maternal rubella, and other etiologic factors. Ann Otol Rhinol Laryngol 59:1123–1147, 1950

14. Goodhill V: Nuclear deafness and the nerve deaf child: the importance of the Rh factor. Trans Am Acad Ophthalmol Otolaryngol 54:671–687, 1950

15. Gregg NM: Congenital cataract following German measles in the mother. Trans Ophthalmol Soc Aust 3:35, 1941

16. Hemenway WG, Sando I, McChesney D: Temporal bone pathology following maternal rubella. Arch Klin Exp Ohr Nas Kehlk Heilk 193:287–300, 1969

16a. Hinze A: Kleinere Schriften Medicinischen Chirurg und Hebärztl. Inh Erster Band, Liegnitz und Leipzig, Siegert, 1802

17. Hyman C, Keaster J, Hanson V et al.: C.N.S. abnormalities after neonatal hemolytic disease or hyperbilirubinemia. Am J Dis Child 117:395–405, 1969

18. Jorgensen MB, Kristensen HK, Buch NH: Thalidomide induced aplasia of the inner ear. J Laryngol 78:1095–1101, 1964

19. Keaster J, Hyman C, Harris I: Hearing problems subsequent to neonatal hemolytic disease or hyperbilirubinemia. Am J Dis Child 117:406–410, 1969

20. Landsteiner K, Wiener AS: An agglutinable factor in human blood recognized by immune sera for rhesus blood. Proc Soc Exp Biol 43:223, 1940

21. Lindsay JR: Histopathology of deafness due to postnatal viral diseases. Arch Otolaryngol 98:258–264, 1973

22. Lindsay JR: Profound childhood deafness. Inner ear pathology. Ann Otol Rhinol Laryngol [Suppl] 5, 1973

23. Lindsay JR, Davey PR, Ward PH: Inner ear pathology in deafness due to mumps. Ann Otol Rhinol Laryngol 69:918–935, 1960

24. Lindsay JR, Hemenway WG: Inner ear pathology due to measles. Ann Otol Rhinol Laryngol 63:754–771, 1954

25. Matkin ND, Carhart R: Hearing acuity and Rh incompatibility. Arch Otolaryngol 87:383–388, 1968

26. Myers EN, Stool S: Cytomegalic inclusion disease of the inner ear. Laryngoscope 78:1904–1915, 1968

27. Orth (1875): Cited by Zimmerman HM, Yannet H (Ref #32)

28. Schmorl (1903): Cited by Zimmerman HM, Yannet H (Ref #32)

29. Smith GA, Gussen R: Inner ear pathologic features following mumps infection. Arch Otolaryngol 102:108–111, 1976

30. Toynbee J: The Diseases of the Ear. Philadelphia: Blanchard and Lea, 1860

31. Vernon M: Characteristics associated with postrubella deaf children: psychological, educational, and physical. Volta Rev 69:176–185, 1967

32. Zimmerman HM, Yannet H: Kernikterus: jauntice of the nuclear masses of the brain. Am J Dis Child 45:740–759, 1933

34

THE "HARD OF HEARING" CHILD

D. M. STEIN

There has been considerable variability in describing children and adults with peripheral hearing loss. A multitude of terms (deaf, deafened, partially hearing, hard of hearing, hearing-handicapped, hearing-impaired, hypacusis, dysacusis, etc.), as well as definitions, have developed which have often led to more confusion than clarity about this population. With the advent of evaluative techniques that afford earlier diagnosis, modern technical advances medically and surgically, transistorized amplification, and individualized educational instruction, many of our present definitions and points of view about hearing loss have become obsolete.

Hearing impairment is a continuum. One can describe the extent of impairment in terms of several levels (Table 34–1) (13). These levels, however, do *not* necessarily define or describe the communicative abilities or educational functioning of an individual with peripheral hearing impairment. In fact, prejudging an individual's potential educational or social competence on the basis of audiometric data has led to overgeneralizations of abilities and limitations as well as inappropriate labeling, vocational, and educational placement. There are children and adults who function more poorly than one would guess upon examination of an audiogram (26), perhaps as a direct result of inappropriately low expectations of their teachers (28). Individuals with similar losses may process speech very differently from one another, as a result of a variety of factors. The differences in processing ability do not necessarily

relate directly to the audiometric configuration (2).

In this discussion, therefore, we will use the categories in Table 34–1 (13) to describe the **degree or extent of the physical impairment.** The term **hard of hearing** will be used *only* to describe *how* the child communicates and learns. A hard-of-hearing child is one who, with amplification and appropriate rehabilitative techniques (auditory training, speech reading, academic tutoring), can learn to assimilate verbal information auditorily—a child whose primary language- and speech-learning avenue is the auditory pathway (21, 26).

CHARACTERISTICS OF THE HARD-OF-HEARING CHILD

Although educational programs for hard-of-hearing children were provided in other countries as early as 1867 (32), programs in the United States have been sparse until recently. Many hard-of-hearing children have floundered in their neighborhood schools with minimal or no special help in speech and language or academics; others have been placed in classes in schools for the deaf when regular class placement has been prohibited because of their unsatisfactory achievement. Although there has been great progress in education for the *severely* hearing impaired, there has been a lag in providing meaningful and effective programs for hard-of-hearing children in the public schools (19). As a result, the hard-of-hearing child can be from 6 months to more than 2 years retarded in school achievement (3, 18, 33).

There are many factors that influence the success or failure of the hard-of-hearing child in educational or social situations. Included are the type, extent, and onset of the loss; the progression of the loss, if any; the onset of use of amplification; the onset of habilitation, especially auditory training; the expectations of family and teachers, as well as those of the hearing-impaired child; academic, perceptual, and cognitive potential; and opportunity for learning. These factors can account for varying degrees of communicative and adjustment problems: limited language, poor understanding of speech, and defective speech articulation, as well as academic, social, and vocational problems (1).

EXPRESSIVE SPEECH ABILITIES OF HARD-OF-HEARING CHILDREN

The expressive speech patterns of the hearing-impaired are often defective. The extent to which

TABLE 34-1. Degrees of Hearing Loss

Hearing level	Range (dB)
Normal limits	−10–25
Mild loss	26–40
Moderate loss	41–55
Moderately severe loss	56–70
Severe loss	71–90
Profound loss	91+

(Goodman AC: *ASHA* 7:262–263, 1965)

the speech is defective can be affected by the extent of loss, the auditory discrimination, and the perceptual abilities of the hearing-impaired child, fine motor abilities of the child, and particularly the extent to which the child has had training in monitoring his own vocal patterns. Speech articulation may be characterized by omissions of sounds ("too-brush" for "toothbrush"), distortions of sounds, or substitutions of sounds ("doddie" for "doggie"). Voice quality can be hyponasal or hypernasal, as well as harsh or strident. It can be monotonous or "flat" in affect, as well as too loud or too soft in intensity. Often, speech is arrhythmic. Intonation patterns are distorted, making the talker harder to understand. This is especially evident in children with more severe losses who have had poor speech training, inconsistent or poor use of amplification, or both. As children are often judged (by adults as well as their peers) on their abilities to express themselves and be understood, it becomes most important that early training include speech remediation, with particular emphasis on the rhythmic and tonal expressions of speech. An interesting, "alive," pleasant voice with much expression adds to the communication situation and fosters further social contact with teachers, peers, family, and future coworkers.

Although many hard-of-hearing children often develop some spontaneous language, others do not. A child with considerable residual hearing (*i.e.*, mild to moderate loss) may develop normal vocal patterns, some vocabulary, and sentence structure. However, by the time the child enters first grade, there may be a significant deficiency in language abilities, which will contribute to educational handicaps. The child with less residual hearing (*i.e.*, severe or profound loss) does not develop speech and language without amplification and professional help. It is extremely important that when parents first question a hearing loss, note a developmental delay (physical or linguistic), or report that the child is not talking when he should be, the child be evaluated audiologically and linguistically. Children do not outgrow their de-

velopmental delays; the effects come back to haunt them at a time in their school years when remediation cannot compensate for the educational and intellectual scars.

LINGUISTIC AND COGNITIVE ABILITIES OF HARD-OF-HEARING CHILDREN

In recent years, since the advent of special education programs, integrated programs, and supplementary services in the regular neighborhood classroom, there have been efforts to develop better tools that can be used to predict the hearing-impaired child's readiness to enter and succeed in a variety of educational programs. Hearing-impaired children, while appearing to function well on cursory examination, often have deficiencies in, and subtle problems with linguistic skills that do not allow them to compete effectively and successfully with their normally hearing peers. A child's capacity to learn language has been thought to be the major criterion of his success or failure in general learning and development (15). Intelligence appears to be a significant factor in processing and using connected language, while maturation and stress have an influence on daily language learning (15).

Vocabulary development and speech and language functioning of hearing-impaired children in regular classrooms, even those with mild to moderate losses, may be significantly retarded (12, 23, 30, 33).

Auditory discrimination abilities may be retarded as much as a year and, although they can improve, may never reach the levels attained by children without impairment (12).

Cognitive abilities can also be significantly impaired. Moderately to severely hearing-impaired (pure tone average* range, 35–70 dB) children's knowledge of basic concepts and their interpretation of complex sentences (sentences with similar vocabulary and structure though having different meaning) on a standardized test were compared with those of their normally hearing peers. Not only were the scores of the hearing-impaired children significantly lower, but the types and patterns of their errors differed significantly (4). Other data indicate that hearing-impaired children fall further behind in their knowledge of basic con-

* The pure tone average of thresholds in the better hearing ear, measured at 500, 1000, and 2000 Hz. All decibel references are American National Standards Institute (ANSI), 1969; all data reported in American Standards Association figures, 1951, have been converted to ANSI, 1969.

cepts as they progress from kindergarten to second grade, when compared with their normally hearing peers (3).

ACADEMIC ABILITIES OF HARD-OF-HEARING CHILDREN

Often, as a result of poor linguistic abilities, the academic achievement of hearing-impaired children is also significantly affected and hinders their successful competition with normally hearing peers. Although some data demonstrate scholastic achievement at an appropriate age level (5), other data are not as optimistic. Hard-of-hearing children may progress more slowly in the typical school situation than will normally hearing children (29). From second grade on, those children in regular classes may be from 1 to over 2 years behind in achievement compared with their peers (18). Educational lags may be obvious in reading and arithmetic skills and, to a limited degree, spelling skills (24, 30). Students in special education facilities are often found to be consistently below grade placement for their chronological age.

BEHAVIORAL AND PSYCHOLOGIC CHARACTERISTICS

Behavioral characteristics of hearing-impaired children without amplification vary in relationship to the amount of residual hearing in the better ear. Many children with very minimal but high-frequency losses (above 2000 Hz) go undiscovered, as their behavior is similar to that of the normally hearing child. Children with "ski-slope" losses (i.e., normal-range hearing in the lower frequencies and severely sloping losses in the mid and higher frequency range) have often been misdiagnosed as "aphasic" or "mentally retarded"; they may attend normally to voice and environmental sounds but may have difficulty understanding speech and following conversation. Often, their own speech articulation is poor. They may appear hyperactive, as they are monitoring their environments visually, while normally hearing youngsters can monitor their environments auditorily. The greater the loss, the greater the visual monitoring and use of visual cues without amplification. Children with hearing losses often watch faces carefully and can respond well to facial and situational cues. A bright child may "fool" the family as he participates well in group activities and seems to follow directions. Parents may complain that he is inattentive and restless, when, in fact, he observes what goes on around him and responds to those cues accordingly. He may be inattentive because he is not hearing enough of the message clearly or loudly enough, if at all. Many children attend and respond well in a one-to-one situation or when only a few feet from the talker, yet fail at distances, in group situations, and when there is background noise (high noise levels or several other people talking at once). This is common in children with chronic secretory otitis media or congenital mild-to-moderate conductive losses (e.g., Treacher-Collins syndrome). It is often true of children with unilateral losses (see Special Problems section in the latter part of this chapter).

The behavior of hearing-impaired children who use amplification can vary tremendously from child to child, even with those who have similar losses. Again, this is affected by the many factors mentioned earlier in this chapter. Particularly significant are the child's use of his residual hearing, his own self-image, and his communication skills. An educational program that emphasizes children's use of visual cues (speech reading, or finger spelling and sign language) will produce children who monitor their worlds visually. Educational programs that emphasize listening skills, regardless of the extent of the unaided loss, will produce children who are able not only to monitor their worlds auditorily but often to make better use of combined visual and auditory cues, as well.

Hearing-impaired children who may not have had the advantages of early intervention and training in good communication skills often behave peculiarly in a test situation; these behaviors, which are also common in social and educational settings, can often mislead the evaluator:

The child's flat affect, nonresponsive remarks, and apparent withdrawal may be based on the reality factors of the child not clearly understanding the examiner and/or a history of not being able to grasp spoken language. Often the child copes with this by either keeping quiet or by trying to dominate the conversation in order to avoid having to understand that which is unclear. Many of these children have learned to handle their hearing loss by becoming masters of the neutral response, smiling, saying yes, and periodically nodding their heads in the affirmative. The techniques are often remarkably effective in unintentionally misleading psychologists and others into thinking there has been understanding and full communication when actually the child has unknowingly used . . . reflective responses to conceal his inability to understand (31).

The social adjustment of many hearing-impaired children may be deficient. The hearing-handicapped as a group are not as well accepted by their normally hearing classmates, although there may be a wide range of acceptance of hearing-handicapped children as individuals (9). Poorer general classroom performance and social adjustment were noted by teachers for the hearing-impaired children in their regular classes, compared with the normally hearing peers, while pupils in special classroom programs (hard-of-hearing and oral-training units) generally are rated in the acceptable range of social adjustment by both special and regular classroom teachers. Parents of hearing-impaired children in regular classes judged their children to be less popular with other children, to strain more frequently in listening to conversation, to be less interested in conversation, to tire easily or appear more restless, to understand other children less frequently while playing, and to play the radio or TV too loudly. They noted their hard-of-hearing children tending to need more parental approval, interrupting others while talking, and using their hearing losses as the basis for their problems. Normally hearing children described their hearing-impaired peers as being quiet, not speaking plainly, and having problems that sometimes make school difficult (30).

SPECIAL PROBLEMS

THE CHILD WITH CHRONIC OTITIS MEDIA

For a long time many otologists, audiologists, and educators have assumed that a minimal (up to 30 dB) conductive or intermittent loss would pose minimal or no communication or academic problems for the child, provided preferential seating in the classroom were available. There is a considerable body of recent data that contradicts this notion and forces us to reevaluate our attitudes toward children who have histories of chronic conductive hearing loss, during the early language-learning years, that is due to otitis media as well as to congenital anomalies.

The effects of otitis media can linger on. Thresholds may be poorer for variable periods of time after the acute infection, even in children who are not subject to recurrent otitis media (22). Hearing losses up to 20 dB can be observed in children who had their last episode of otitis 5–10 years previously (10). Linguistic and verbal skills may be significantly deficient (16, 17). Educational achievement may be poorer by as much as 1–2 years as a result of chronic bilateral otitis media in infancy (17). It is highly probable that children with chronic upper respiratory allergies causing long-term poor eustachian tube function and concomitant conductive losses are equally handi-

capped. Although the medical problem may be resolved by school age, effects of the disease that interfere with normal receptive processes during the critical language-learning years can take their toll in many forms. The child, by school age, may, in fact, behave and function as if he were hearing-impaired:

The child who . . . has had hearing difficulties early in life, during those crucial stages in which one learns to listen to the speech of others, to pay attention, to respond with speech and to develop relationships with others, may never learn to do these things in a normal or adequate manner. He fails to make fine discriminations among sounds or to localize them. Lacking basic attitudes with regard to interpersonal communication, he fails to acquire the vocabulary and the general information acquired by the normal child who listens, pays attention, and attempts speech. As maturation proceeds, he does not have the necessary foundation out of which develops the use of implicit speech or thought. This in turn leads to inadequate development of higher order processes of abstraction and conceptualization. In school he may have difficulty learning to read (8).

It is estimated that middle ear disease occurs in 20–30% of children between birth and 6 years of age (6). With this enormous number of potentially handicapped children, communicatively, educationally, and socially, criteria for audiologic and medical care must be reevaluated. The audiometric data (hearing levels of 15 dB or more, fluctuating levels from 0 to over 15 dB for more than half the time for 1 year) and the medical history (indication of secretory otitis media in a child under 2 years for more than half the time for a period of 6 months) may signify a high-risk child (6). Continual audiologic and educational monitoring, with the possible use of mild-gain amplification until the medical problem is resolved (7), becomes a critical factor for those children if they are to progress with success both educationally and socially.

THE CHILD WITH A UNILATERAL HEARING LOSS

Another group of children who historically have been overlooked are those with moderate to severe unilateral hearing losses. Traditionally, educational recommendations have included preferential classroom seating, and sometimes, more recently, the use of amplification. The most successful fittings have been using contralateral routing of signal (CROS) hearing aids (see Ch. 43, Hearing Aids). Physicians and audiologists have counseled children and adults on the difficulties they may encounter in localizing sound sources and hearing in noisy and group situations. Recent data have suggested that these children, too, can have behavioral, psychological and academic problems (11, 24, 30). The presence of extraneous noise is the single most contributing factor in difficult listening situations, even when speech is directed toward the "good" ear (11).

THE HEARING-IMPAIRED CHILD WITH OTHER PROBLEMS

There is an abundance of literature describing learning problems in children, appropriate test instruments for evaluation, and various educational programs that have been found to be of benefit to these children. Diagnosis and evaluation become complex when the peripherally hearing-handicapped child is suspected of having learning, behavioral, or emotional problems. Standardized tests exist that can evaluate motor and visual perceptual problems in hearing-handicapped children. Psychologists and educators familiar with the hearing-handicapped may be able to evaluate behavioral and emotional problems of these children. Central auditory processing problems, however, are hard to diagnose when a peripheral problem exists. There are several tests now that can assess these abilities in children with peripherally normal hearing. However, the test results become invalid when used with the hearing-handicapped child. Often the presence of nonverbal perceptual problems (*i.e.,* visual or motor) suggests the possibility of central auditory perceptual problems, but not always. Etiology, however, can be a clue to the possible existence of subtle central problems. Hard-of-hearing children in whom the source of the problem is exogenous (*e.g.,* rubella, Rh incompatibility, prematurity, anoxia) have been shown to perform more poorly on short-term auditory memory tests when compared with children whose hearing losses are due to endogenous causes. Those with marked high-frequency hearing-loss configurations performed as well as those with flat hearing loss configurations, ruling out the slope of the loss as a contributing factor (20).

Peripheral visual problems can occur with hearing loss, as well as mental retardation, brain damage, and a variety of other sequelae. In fact, educationally, the child's major handicap may not be his peripheral hearing loss but another factor that inhibits learning. The physician, audiologist, and other professionals working with the child need to be aware of other factors that may contribute to academic, linguistic, behavioral, and social retardation, so that these problems may be investigated as early in the diagnostic and remedial process as possible, to plan an appropriate program for the child.

EVALUATION AND OPTIONS FOR EDUCATION

Audiologic evaluation has been discussed elsewhere in this book. The unaided audiogram does not necessarily give us information regarding all the residual hearing the child may have, the potential for speech understanding the child has when amplification is provided, or how the child will use his hearing in relation to his other abilities and his environmental milieu (25). It certainly gives us no information about the child's medical history. Aided audiometric and speech discrimination scores only give us information about the child's performance on these specific tests. How the child will *function* in a communicative—specifically a learning—situation, such as a classroom, depends on a variety of other factors previously discussed. The team approach concept becomes important here: the physician, the audiologist, the speech and language specialist, the educator, and the psychologist, working together *with* the child and the family to facilitate maximum growth by the child. Family expectations and attitudes can be crucial to the placement of the child in a specific educational setting; helping the parents accept and deal with the hearing-impaired child is of major importance.

Making broad assumptions on educational needs of a child on the basis of audiometric data is invalid. Psychological, educational, and linguistic evaluations can be better sources of data on which to base a child's placement—regular class placement with resource assistance (a resource teacher is a teacher of the hearing-impaired who is available to the child for tutoring in specific areas of weakness), or special or regular class placement with designated instructional services (*i.e.,* remedial speech therapy, audiology). A child's placement in terms of his linguistic functioning should not be restrictive (Table 34–2). Additional handicapping conditions may warrant different class placement.

CASE STUDIES

The following case studies illustrate the variety of audiometric configurations and functioning levels of several children seen in a pediatric set-

TABLE 34-2. Suggested Instructional Placement for Hearing-Impaired Children

Type of facility	Age range (yr)			
	0–3	3–5	5–19	19–21
Full-time special developmental language, speech, auditory training, and school subject assistance (language function: 3σ)				
Special class	x		x	x
Designated instructional services	x		x	x
Part-time special developmental language, speech, auditory training, and school subject assistance (language function: 2σ)				
Special class	x		x	x
Designated instructional services	x		x	x
Regular			x	x
Other		x		
Part-time special developmental language, speech, auditory training, and school subject assistance (language function: 1σ)				
Designated instructional services	x		x	x
Resource specialist			x	x
Regular class			x	x
Other		x		
Remedial speech, language, or physical education; hearing conversation; lipreading (language function: x̄ or better)				
Designated instructional services	x		x	x
Regular class			x	x
Other		x		

The type of instruction suggested and the facilities used apply to all levels of hearing disability, as proposed by the Conference of Executives of American Schools for the Deaf (CEASD), 1974: Level I, 35–54 dB; level II, 55–69 dB; level III, 70–89 dB; level IV, 90 dB and beyond; better ear, pure tone average.

(Adapted from Ellery Adams, consultant to hearing impaired program, office of the Los Angeles County Superintendent of Schools)

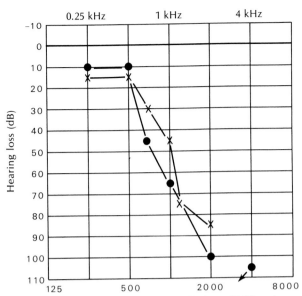

FIG. 34–1. Audiogram of 6.5-year-old boy (D.S.), whose severely sloping loss went undiscovered until first grade. ●—●, AC, unmasked, RE; x—x, AC, unmasked, LE; **SRT,** 20 dB, RE, 25 dB LE; **SDS,** 72% at 60 dB, RE; 76% at 55 dB, LE; **PTA,** 58 dB RE; 48 dB, LE; **arrow,** no response at maximum output.

ting. These children are particularly interesting in that factors other than the extent of loss contributed so significantly to how each child functions that educational placement based solely on audiometric data would have been inappropriate.

MISPLACEMENT FOR MISDIAGNOSED APHASIA. D.S. was referred for an audiologic evaluation after he failed a routine school screening test (Fig. 34–1). He was in a class for aphasic children at the time of referral. There was a history of neonatal hyperbilirubinemia (without transfusions) and respiratory distress with subsequent anoxia. The child's speech was characterized by multiple misarticulations and distortions. Although there was a significant vocabulary deficit, other language functioning was sufficiently adequate for him to return to the regular classroom with resource help, after the fitting of appropriate amplification.

DELAYED LANGUAGE SKILLS AND BEHAVIOR PROBLEMS. D.C. is an 8-year-old youngster with a moderate-to-severe flat loss in the better hearing ear (Fig. 34–2). The etiology is probably maternal rubella. D.C. comes from a bilingual home, in which the father is extremely unaccepting of the child's inability to "behave and do what I tell him." There's little, if any, language stimulation at home. Although the loss was diagnosed at age 2 years and school placement began at age 3, the child has worn amplification inconsistently in the home situation. He has demonstrated behavior problems at school that manifest themselves in tantrums and hostile behavior toward classmates. D.C. has been in a Total Communication program since age 4; receptive and expressive skills are severely delayed although his intelligence is normal and he appears not to have any perceptual problems. He functions as a "deaf" child, despite the considerable amount of residual hearing, probably as a result of his lack of opportunity. He is unable to recognize common spondaic words using audition only. Placement based on audiometric data (*e.g.,* oral program with hard-of-hearing children) would have been a disservice to this child.

COMMUNICATION DIFFICULTIES. D.R. is a youngster whose progressive, mixed loss went undiscovered until age 10 (Fig. 34–3A). Mentally gifted, with a reading

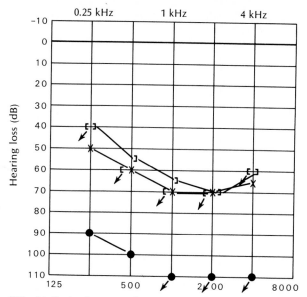

FIG. 34–2. Audiogram of 8-year-old moderately hearing-impaired child (D.C.). **PTA,** CNE, RE; 66 dB, LE; **SAT** (speech awareness threshold), 95 dB, RE, 55 dB, LE (unable to perform SRT); ●—●, AC, unmasked, RE; [—[, BC, unmasked, RE; x—x, AC, unmasked, LE;]—], BC, masked, LE; **arrows,** no response at maximum output.

level 4 years above grade level, D.R. has been able to function successfully without amplification although he has had a significant hearing loss bilaterally. Surgical exploration of the left ear revealed a non-correctable lesion. D.R. now wears binaural aids; his only communication difficulties occur in situations in which there is considerable background noise and poor lighting (*e.g.*, restaurants) (Fig. 34–3B).

ADJUSTMENT THROUGH TRAINING. In another child (Fig. 34–4), pure-tone average audiometric results reveal a profound bilateral sensorineural hearing loss despite the unusual configuration of the loss with considerable residual hearing in the very low and the very high frequencies. This child has had "all the opportunities": early diagnosis, early use of amplification with considerable auditory training, early integration on a part-time basis in kindergarten. She is now integrated into a regular fourth grade with resource help. Her speech is good, despite some articulation problems and a slightly hypernasal voice; vocabulary, concept development, and other linguistic skills are at grade level. The etiology is unknown; the loss, discovered at age 1 year, has not progressed. Despite the severity of the loss, this child is functionally "hard of hearing."

MENTAL RETARDATION AS A COMPLICATION. C.E. is a 12-year-old youngster in a Trainable Mentally Retarded classroom. She was one of a triplet pregnancy in which

FIG. 34–3. A. Test results of mentally gifted child (D.R.) in April 1971, at 10.5 years of age. ●—●, AC, unmasked, RE; [—[, BC, masked, RE; x—x, AC, unmasked, LE;]—], BC, masked, LE. **B.** Test results in same child at age 15, in August 1975. ●—●, AC, unmasked, RE; [—[, BC, masked, RE; x—x, AC, unmasked, LE;]—], BC, masked, LE; **SRT,** 68 dB, RE, 58 dB, LE; **SDS,** 80% at 98 dB, RE; 60% at 88 dB, LE; **PTA,** 75 dB, RE; 63 dB, LE. With binaural aids in sound field, **SRT,** 20 dB, **SDS,** 86% at 50 dB.

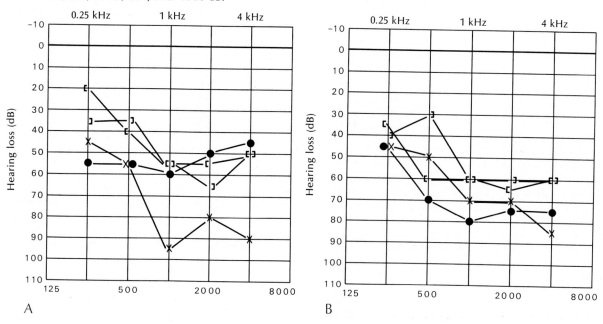

A

B

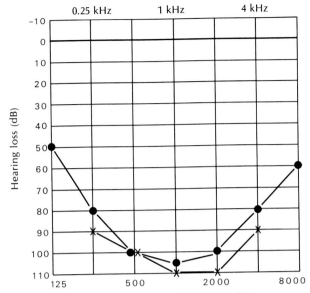

FIG. 34–4. Audiogram of 9-year-old child (A.B.) in a regular classroom, with early use of amplification. ●—●, AC, unmasked, RE; **x—x**, AC, unmasked, LE; **SRT,** 85 dB, RE; 100 dB, LE; **PTA,** 101 dB, RE; 106 dB, LE; **SAT,** 60 dB, RE; 95 dB, LE. Aided sound field: **SRT,** 45 dB, **SDS** (auditory only) 48% at 60 dB (PBK [phonetically balanced—kindergarten], 50's) lipreading plus audition, **SDS,** 78% at 60 dB (PBK, 50's).

one fetus died *in utero* and one paranatally. This child suffered severe anoxia at birth, which resulted in a multiplicity of handicaps, including spastic hemiplegia and retardation (IQ 50 on a nonverbal scale). Although audiometric screening at age 10 revealed hearing within normal limits throughout the speech frequency range (500 Hz through 4000 Hz) bilaterally, C.E.'s teacher continued to describe the child as "not hearing." In addition, there is a history of chronic middle ear problems. Closer examination of the child's linguistic functioning revealed essentially no verbal language, receptively or expressively; responses to her name were inconsistent even at close range. Visually alert, C.E. picked up situational clues when participating in class activities; she could read some of her classmates' names although she could not discriminate among them auditorily. An intensive auditory training program was initiated as well as the use of printed symbols and sign language. Within 6 months C.E. was using four- and five-word signed sentences. It was the first time she had had a language system for self-expression. Although hearing is peripherally normal, this mentally retarded child has auditory agnosia and functions as if severely hearing-impaired.

MULTIPLICITY OF PROBLEMS. G.S. is a 7½-year-old in a class for multiply handicapped children (Fig. 34–5). His severe congenital mixed loss, which will be surgically explored in a few years, was not discovered

until age 5. The etiology is unclear; however, the child has several physical anomalies. His receptive language functioning is approximately 4 years delayed; speech is unintelligible and usually consists of one-word utterances. He has had intensive auditory training over the last 2 years within the context of a Total Communication program. Intelligence is thought to be essentially within the normal range. The child's behavior (short attention span, hyperactivity, difficulty working in a group situation or independently) precludes his placement in a class for hearing-impaired children at this time.

SUMMARY

Historically, the term **hard of hearing** has been used to reflect hearing acuity represented by a decibel level. It is, in actuality, a reference to the auditory functioning ability of a hearing-impaired individual. Peripheral hearing impairment may manifest itself in a variety of audiometric configurations: mild, moderate, severe or profound; flat, U-shaped, sloping, or dropping precipitously; conductive, sensorineural, or mixed. A hearing-impaired individual will function as hard of hearing or deaf as a result of a variety of factors, the primary one being the extent to which the residual

FIG. 34–5. Audiogram of 7.5-year-old child (G.S.), with mixed congenital hearing loss and multiple handicaps. ●—●, AC, unmasked, RE; **x—x**, AC, unmasked, LE; [—[, BC, masked, RE; **PTA,** 78 dB, RE, 81 dB, LE; **SAT,** 65 dB, RE; 65 dB, LE. Aided soundfield results: **SRT** (selected pictured spondees), 30 dB; **SDS** (Peabody kit pictures), 25 single words, 96% at 55 dB.

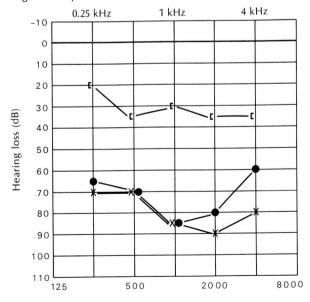

hearing is used for monitoring the environment, monitoring one's own speech, and listening to others in various communication situations. Many other factors influence the learning potential of the hearing-impaired individual. Although there are considerable data demonstrating deficient linguistic, speech, cognitive, academic, behavioral, and social adjustment abilities in the hearing-impaired population, this situation need not exist. There is substantial evidence to suggest that these problems have their roots in the child's preschool years (23). Early diagnosis and intervention and early amplification with training for the maximum use of one's residual hearing, regardless of the severity of loss, have been shown to be critical factors in children's successful learning of language (14, 25). Ongoing and consistent audiologic and educational monitoring becomes mandatory, once the medical and audiologic diagnoses are made. *There is no substitute for normal hearing.* However, those children who have had these opportunities demonstrate development of oral language, academic, social, and cognitive skills comparable to their normally hearing peers (5, 27). These skills allow them to be competitive educationally and vocationally. The need for education of normally hearing children regarding their peers' hearing losses can also be critical to hearing-impaired children's social adjustment. Hearing-impaired children who have not had these benefits may become academically, communicatively, and socially retarded.

REFERENCES

1. Berg FS: Breakthrough for the Hard of Hearing Child (pamphlet). Logan, Utah, JP Smith, 1971
2. Danaher E, Pickett JM: Some masking effects produced by low frequency vowel forments in persons with sensorineural hearing loss. Speech Hear Res 18:242–260, 1975
3. Davis J: Performance of young hearing-impaired children on a test of basic concepts. J Speech Hear Res 17:342–351, 1974
4. Davis J: Perceptual strategies in normal-hearing impaired children. Paper presented at annual meeting of the American Speech and Hearing Association, Las Vegas, NV, November, 1974
5. DiCarlo L: Speech, language and cognitive abilities of the hard-of-hearing. In Proceedings of the Institute on Aural Rehabilitation. University of Denver, 1968
6. Downs MP: Hearing loss: definition, epidemiology, and prevention. Public Health Rev, 1974 (in press)
7. Downs MP: Education sequelae of serous otitis media. Paper presented at Ninth Colorado Medical Audiology Workshop, Vail, CO, March, 1975
8. Eisen NH: Some effects of early sensory deprivation on later behavior: the quondam hard-of-hearing child. J Abnorm Psychol 65:338–342, 1962
9. Elser RP: The social position of hearing handicapped children in the regular grades. Except Child 25:305–309, 1959
10. Fry J, Dillane JB, Jones, RP, Kalton G, Andrew E: The outcome of acute otitis media. Br J Prev Soc Med 23:205–209, 1969
11. Giolas T, Wark DJ: Communication problems associated with unilateral hearing loss. J Speech Hear Dis 32:336–343, 1967
12. Goetzinger CP: Effects of small perceptive losses on language and on speech discrimination. Volta Rev 64:408–414, 1962
13. Goodman AC: Reference zero levels for pure-tone audiometers. ASHA 7:262–263, 1965
14. Hanners B: The role of audiologic management in the development of language by severely hearing impaired children. Paper presented at the annual meeting of the Academy of Rehabilitative Audiology, Detroit, MI, October, 1973
15. Hardy WG, Pauls M, Haskins H: An analysis of language development in children with impaired hearing. Acta Otolaryngol [Suppl] (Stockh) 141, 1958
16. Holm VA, Kunze LV: Effects of chronic otitis media on language and speech development. Pediatrics 43:833, 1969
17. Kaplan GJ, Fleshman JK, Bender TR, Baum C, Clark PS: Long-term effects of otitis media—A ten year cohort study of Alaskan eskimo children. Pediatrics 52:577, 1973
18. Kodman FJ: Educational status of hard of hearing children in the classroom. J Speech Hear Dis 28:297–299, 1963
19. Lawrence CJ, Kapfen MB: The potential of current trends in public education for the hard of hearing child. In Berg F, Fletcher S (eds): The Hard of Hearing Child. New York, Grune & Stratton, 1970
20. Lewis RG: Short-term auditory memory ability in hard of hearing children. Paper presented at the annual meeting of the American Speech and Hearing Association, Las Vegas, NV, November, 1974
21. Northcott W (ed): Hearing Impaired Child in a Regular Classroom: Preschool, Elementary and Secondary Years. Washington DC, Alexander Graham Bell Association for the Deaf, 1973
22. Olmstead RW, Alvarez MC, Moroney JD, Eversden M: The pattern of hearing following acute otitis media. J Pediatr 65:252–255, 1964
23. Owrid HL: Hearing impairment and verbal attainments in primary school children. Educ Re 12, 1970
24. Peckham CS, Sheridan M, Butler NR: School attainment of seven year old children with hearing difficulties. Dev Med Child Neurol 14:592–602, 1972
25. Pollack D: Educational Audiology for the Limited Hearing Infant. Springfield, Il, CC Thomas, 1970
26. Prokes JE: The audiometrically hard of hearing, deaf child. In Report of the Proceedings of the 46th

Meeting of the Convention of American Instructors of the Deaf, Indianapolis, IN, June, 1973. Washington DC, US Government Printing Office, 511–517, 1974

27. Reynolds LG: The school adjustment of children with minimal hearing loss. J Speech Hear Dis 20: 380–384, 1955

28. Ross M, Calvert D: The semantics of deafness. In Northcott E (ed): The Hearing Impaired Child in the Regular Classroom: Preschool, Elementary and Secondary Years. Washington DC, Alexander Graham Bell Association for the Deaf, 1973

29. Sprunt JW, Finger FW: Auditory deficiency and academic achievement. J Speech Hear Dis 14:26–32, 1949

30. Steer MD, Hanley TD, Spuchler HE, Barnes NS, Burk KW, Williams WG: The Behavioral and Academic Implications of Hearing Losses Among Elementary School Children. Purdue University, Project #PU 240, February, 1961

31. Vernon M: The psychological examination. In Berg FS, Fletcher S (ed): The Hard of Hearing Child, New York, Grune & Stratton, 1970

32. Watson TJ: The Education of Hearing-Handicapped Children, London, University of London Press, 1967

33. Young C, McConnell F: Retardation of vocabulary Development in hard of hearing children. Except Child 48:368–370, 1957

35

THE DEAF CHILD

RICHARD G. LEWIS

WHO IS THE "DEAF" CHILD?

The term *deaf* has been used educationally to describe varying characteristics in hearing-impaired children. In 1938, the Conference of Executives of American Schools of the Deaf (2) applied the term deaf to those "in whom the sense of hearing is nonfunctional for the ordinary purposes of life." In 1969 the Secretary of Health, Education, and Welfare's Advisory Committee on Education of the Deaf termed deaf those children "whose principal source for learning language and communication skills is mainly visual and whose loss of hearing, with or without amplification, is so great that it is of little or no practical value in learning to understand verbal communication auditorially, and whose loss of hearing was acquired pre-lingually" (3).

Both of these definitions take as a base the necessity of almost total visual functioning, with a very small part being played by audition. Following such definitions to a logical conclusion, it is not difficult to see why many professionals in the medical and educational field do not emphasize the early fitting and use of hearing aids for deaf children. This is a typical case of how a definition can determine to a large degree the attitudes toward the defined population.

Of a more realistic nature are those definitions based upon knowledge of amplification and its potential for benefiting deaf children. It was emphasized by Whetnall and Fry (15) that it is not possible to determine how much hearing a child has until after at least a year of auditory training, utilizing appropriate amplification. These investigators also believe that while a hearing-impaired child's degree of cochlear dysfunction will remain static, his ability to use his cochlear reserve will change with training, making possible a higher level of auditory functioning.

One is reluctant to dichotomize the hearing-impaired into the educational subdivisions "deaf" and "hard of hearing," since such categorization often results in lock-step education for those labeled deaf. Since these children are believed to have little or no usable hearing, development of the auditory function is often neglected in favor of more visual means, and amplification is applied only sporadically at best. Many children categorized with the initial impression of "total deafness" are later found to have usable hearing as a result of greater responsiveness obtained in subsequent testing.

DEVELOPMENT OF THE AUDITORY FUNCTION

Auditory development in any child must follow the same hierarchic order, whether the category is severe hearing loss or normal hearing. Deaf children do not follow a different system in learning to hear but only proceed at a different rate, with appropriate professional intervention and assistance.

The auditory continuum, in terms of stages of development of auditory function, and implementation of techniques to facilitate this development is briefly reviewed as follows (12, 13). Additional details will be applied in relation to levels of hearing-aid usage.

AUDITORY AWARENESS

This is the basic imperative underlying all other auditory abilities. In its earliest stage, it incorporates no learned behavior, only reflexive responses to stimuli of varying qualities and intensities. In the deaf child, unlike the normally hearing child, awareness must be taught. The deaf child typically does not receive amplification as a neonate, and therefore the opportunity for sound awareness is deferred until, at best, several months of age. After fitting for amplification, building of awareness activities is essential. Merely fitting a child with a hearing aid will not insure this development.

AUDITORY ATTENTION

Beyond simple awareness of sound when it is present, the deaf child must be guided to a differentiation of when sound is and is not present. Further, the fact that hearing aids amplify background noise as well as the desired signal requires that hearing-impaired children receive assistance in auditory figure–ground differentiation. Both behaviors necessitate the use of attentional abilities, *i.e.*, the ability to carry out selective listening as well as listening in the presence of a quiet condition (absence of competing sound).

AUDITORY LOCALIZATION

Localization behavior commences by 4 months of age and by 6 months is well developed on a lateral plane (10). Development of this ability is essential in establishing the social reward inherent in listening—mainly that it results in interpersonal contact. For the deaf child, localization is possible only through the use of binaural amplification and specific therapeutic training techniques.

AUDITORY DISCRIMINATION

In the hearing child, discrimination abilities become apparent only after performance has been established in the foregoing areas. Such is also the case for the deaf child. Too many so-called auditory training programs carried out in classes for the deaf begin at the level of discrimination, usually using noisemakers, with no attention having been paid to the development of the aforementioned requisite developmental abilities. Auditory discrimination in the deaf child is possible with stimuli other than noisemakers, even though linguistic understanding may not be present. It is essentially the same task to develop differentiation between "whee" and "uh-oh" as it is to establish discrimination between a bell and a drum. The point is that hearing children derive ultimate social reinforcement from speech stimuli, indicating that auditory development in the deaf child should follow the same lines of development.

Since sensorineural hearing loss imposes the dual impairment of decreased loudness and possible distortion, auditory discrimination is, for the deaf child, a major problem source. Even the most suitable amplification will deliver, at best, a distorted version of what a normally hearing person perceives. If the signal can never be perceived normally by the deaf child, how then may auditory discrimination take place in such an individual? This question can be answered (5) by pointing out that there is no standard set of acoustic cues for everyone to use in decoding a given phonologic system. In essence, the deaf child must form his own set of cues through training. The efficiency and extent of this cue system will determine the relative discrimination sophistication a deaf child can exhibit.

AUDITORY MEMORY

If auditory behavior is to be developed beyond the predicting of auditory responses as single units, storage ability must be developed in relation to both the span and sequence of auditory stimuli.

AUDITORY CONCEPTUALIZATION

This umbrella term is used to identify increasingly more complex levels of listening (8), including 1) following directions, 2) understanding a sequence of events through listening, 3) recalling details, 4) getting the main idea, 5) making inferences and drawing conclusions, and 6) critical listening.

LEVELS OF AWARENESS WITH AMPLIFICATION

The extent to which a deaf child develops his auditory function is determined by the level of usage he attains in regard to his hearing aids. Just as children with comparable audiograms can develop quite different auditory abilities, so can children with identical hearing losses attain differing levels of hearing-aid usage. These levels include

1. **Signal Warning.** This level involves the ability to use amplification only for the monitoring of sudden and unusual occurrences such as a dish falling, brakes squealing, and other relatively loud events. This level of usage can be attained by vibrotactile stimulation by any deaf child for whom amplification is not medically contraindicated.
2. **Speech Awareness.** Usage at this level enables the individual to be aware of the presence or absence of speech and can lead to gross localization skills.
3. **Temporal Perception.** Increasing sophistication in hearing-aid usage enables an individual to perceive such temporal features of speech as rate of utterance, number and accent of syllabication, and accents within a given utterance. Such perceptions deal mainly with in-

tensity differences within speech. This type of perception may be more significant in language learning than even the perception of frequency formats (10).

4. **Inflectional Perception.** This level of usage necessitates an ability to recognize pitch differences in speech. Competency in inflectional perception enables a person to differentiate spoken questions from statements.

5. **Phonemic Perception.** The ability to differentiate between even a few phonemes auditorially is of great help in the perception and development of language. It affords the individual an opportunity to function at the highest level of language performance with a hearing aid, which is cognitive processing. One having developed hearing-aid usage to this extent would utilize speech reading input only minimally for communication.

VARIABLES AFFECTING HABILITATION

The extent to which a deaf child will develop an auditory function and progress in hearing-aid usage is directly dependent upon the presence of certain essential variables: 1) early diagnosis, 2) expert therapy, 3) modifications allowing for any attendant learning disabilities, 4) an accepting supportive home environment, 5) well-fitted and scrupulously maintained binaural hearing aids (wherever possible).

The first three ingredients are self-evident and need no elaboration here (see Ch. 34, The "Hard of Hearing" Child, and Ch. 36, Parent Counseling). The fourth will be dealt with later. The fifth variable is important in that each term in the statement is crucial.

Well fitted means that the instrument should be chosen as the result of both clinical and therapeutic selection procedures. Both frequency response and behavioral manifestations are given weight in the decision as to which hearing aid should be fitted. **Scrupulously maintained** indicates that the hearing aid, regardless of its expense, is only as good as its functioning on a given day. Daily listening checks and trouble-shooting must be carried out at home and in school. **Binaural** means that each ear must have its own amplification instrument whenever possible.

VISION AS AN INPUT SYSTEM

Prior to the advent of present sophistication in binaural amplification, teaching a deaf child to speak relied mainly, if not solely, upon speech-reading. By this system, the person decodes the spoken message by observing mouth and lip configurations, together with facial expressions. The questionable efficacy of this mode of language input is demonstrated by the fact that less than 30% of English speech sounds are visible on the lips. Judgment regarding the unseen 70% must come from the receiver's "filling in" by guessing derived from his language base. With a prelingually deaf child (usually defined as a child deaf before age 18 months), the language base is non-existing, making such guesses improbable. It follows that speechreading as the main source of language input, even with minimal auditory supplement, will be insufficient for language development.

In any population of normally hearing children, there will be those who cannot learn to read by conventional means, and with whom a special technique must be employed, such as the Fernald method (4), the Peabody Rebus program (11), .etc. Likewise, there exists a small number of deaf children who, regardless of the presence of the five critical variables named earlier, will not develop auditory function to a point where it can act as the main avenue of communication input. For these children, visual input via speech reading will not suffice for language development. In such cases, a more concrete, more wholly visible symbol is required.

Historically the two means of representing ideas in a concrete visual manner in educating the deaf have been finger spelling and manual sign language. Finger spelling is an alphabetically intact rendition of English spelled with the hand. Currently at least five separate manual sign-language systems are in use in the United States. Finger spelling and sign language often are combined with speech, speech reading, and audition, into a program of **total communication.** It is probable that certain deaf children need the concrete visual input afforded by total communication, but just as not all children benefit from a Peabody Rebus approach in reading, a relatively small number of deaf children need or benefit from total communication.

Unfortunately, education of hearing-impaired children has suffered from educational polemics, as has many areas of education of handicapped youngsters. Little attention has been devoted to analysis of total communication components, to standardization of input techniques, and to examination of long-term results. So frequently, total communication, a seemingly viable concept for some deaf children, is merely adopted as a conveniently fashionable term by a poorly executed oral program, in which the teachers have learned to sign and finger spell. A poor total communication program is no better, and in many ways is worse than a poor oral program.

EDUCATIONAL PLACEMENT

Educational placement for the deaf can be discussed in two ways: the ideal and the real. Ideally, following early identification, the deaf child should be fitted with a hearing aid, and a program of home tutoring should be started. A trained professional can initiate a program of therapy through regular visits that involve all members of the family in an environment familiar to the child. This therapeutic program would be primarily auditory in nature and would prepare the child to enroll in a nursery school program with hearing children at the proper age. Individual therapy would also be continued when the child is enrolled in a regular class in his neighborhood public school, where he could continue through his academic years.

In reality, however, such ideal educational programs are, for the most part, more expensive than school districts can afford. Although deafness is considered a low-incidence handicap, 1 in 2000 births (10), the number, cost and quality of personnel to provide such individualized service are beyond the present budgetary limits of most school districts.

For this reason, many districts with sufficient population have established centers within public schools where deaf children are educated together in a self-contained class. These children are integrated within regular classes as their academic progress warrants. In 1966 approximately 49% of the school-age deaf population received their education in such classes (1).

Where large metropolitan school districts have a great number of deaf children, entire schools are devoted to their education.

In every state, public residential schools exist to serve a number of types of deaf children. In many areas there are no appropriate school programs for the deaf; thus a child must reside at such a state school. In other cases, the residential school offers programs to serve the multi-handicapped deaf child for whom no local program exists.

The problem of suitable placement should be considered in the light of several questions: 1) Can the deaf child integrate meaningfully within the local school program? 2) Is the home situation sufficiently supportive so as to provide adequate carryover of therapy from the school? 3) Are personnel available within the public school to serve the child audiologically, as well as to devise suitable curricular modifications to compensate for specific learning problems?

If the answer to any of these questions is "no," then residential placement should be considered. The task of educating the deaf child is too large to be assumed by the public schools alone. The active support and aid of the home is vital. This parental support is the critical ingredient for public school placement, and if it is not present, placement in a residential facility is a more reasonable alternative (see Ch. 36, Parent Counseling).

Integrated public school programs should serve those deaf children who can indeed integrate and who have the necessary linguistic, and cognitive competence to make such integration more meaningful. Integration should include the progressively greater involvement of the child in academic classes and not merely his or her inclusion in recess and physical education with normal-hearing children.

THE ROLE OF THE PARENT

As mentioned previously, a vital ingredient for the successful habilitation of the deaf child is the presence of an accepting and supportive home environment. Unfortunately, it is the very nature of deafness which makes such acceptance and support most difficult to achieve. In many ways the reactions of parents to having a deaf child are comparable to the emotions felt by the relative of a dead or dying person (9).

Kübler-Ross (7) identifies stages of the "mourning process" which typically surround the death of a loved one. This mourning is a process of separating oneself from the lost object or person. This same process appears to be in evidence with the parent of the deaf child, in this case being separation from the normal child who was not born (9). It is necessary to emphasize that this process is normal, natural, and necessary. It is sad that our culture discourages the verbalization and display of such emotions.

A parent who hears the diagnosis of deafness in a child for the first time may break down in tears. The inclination of the professional at this point is to emphasize positive aspects, such as what a hearing aid will do, the availability of educational programs, etc. These suggestions tend to communicate the negation or denial of the feelings being experienced by the parent. It is any human being's right to feel whatever feelings present themselves. Professionals should create an atmosphere in which these feelings can be expressed freely.

The stages of "mourning" in this continuum are as follows:

1. **Shock.** The initial reaction of a parent after hearing a diagnosis of deafness in a child is for all "systems to shut down." The parent, at this point, is unable to incorporate any further information. It is not unusual for a physician or audiologist to communicate a deafness diagnosis to a parent and then to launch into a lengthy explanation of the operation of hearing aids, the proper things to do with the child at home, and the procedure for enrollment in an appropriate educational situation. The parents will report later that all they heard was "that their child was deaf."

2. **Denial.** This stage is familiar to professionals; it involves "shopping around" and/or a negation of the diagnostician's expertise. This stage typically is difficult for the professional to deal with, since the inclination is to become defensive and to try to convince the parent of one's expertise and of the accuracy of the diagnosis. Such efforts will be to no avail, and may actually further the denial process.

3. **Anger.** At this stage, the parent asks, "Why me?" The anger can be directed against any of a number of likely targets: the professional, the parent *per se*, and/or even the child. "Felt anger," as opposed to "acted-upon anger," is harmless and should not be denied. Indeed it is a reasonable reaction to the burdens imposed by deafness. In most cases, however, it is abhorrent to both professionals and parents to consider the possibility of anger directed toward a child.

4. **Guilt.** This stage follows closely upon anger and is an internalization of the concept of self as the ultimate cause of calamities. It is fruitless to attempt to reason with parents passing through this stage because guilt is, in essence, an unreasoning feeling, as are all emotions.

5. **Depression.** Depressed parents are the most difficult to deal with. They can do nothing to help the child. They are the parents for whom having a deaf child is an overwhelming, seemingly unsurmountable obstacle. One can outline for such parents a course of action in the simplest possible terms and have it completely disregarded. It is difficult to deal with because there is no clear-cut issue at least on the surface. The depressed parents will agree with all that the professional says regarding necessary action, but can and will do nothing. All the right answers are there, but still nothing is done. Nor can the professional do anything to move the parents until the depression has run its course. The only action the professional can take is to speak to the affect demonstrated by the parents rather than to the content in question.

6. **Bargaining.** The bargaining stage is considered to be very quiet, very personal, and a last desperate attempt to get back the normal child who was lost. Bargaining is expressed in the individual who says to himself, "If only my son's deafness is cured, I'll give all I have to charity" (9).

Once mourning has run its course, the parents are ready to begin the process of coping with the idea of having a deaf child. It would be a mistake to attempt to hurry mourning or to manipulate the parents into the next stage. As stated, the process is normal, natural, and necessary, and will happen in its natural progression if the professional only allows it.

Since there is no definitive time frame in which mourning is completed, the professional would be mistaken to sit by until it is completed before enlisting the help and support of the parents in facilitating the deaf child's education. The crucial issue is in drawing the line between the parent as teacher and the parent as parent.

In the deaf child's early years, as with normally hearing children, parents are the most important, if not the only, teachers. The parents of a deaf child must spend time specifically teaching common household concepts that the normally hearing infant and toddler learn incidentally. The amount of learning done by a normally hearing child before entering school constitutes an impossibly large number of concepts to expect a deaf child to learn in the preschool period. Clearly, most of this preschool learning must be the responsibility of the parents with the guidance and support of an educator of the deaf.

Given this solid conceptual foundation, the deaf child of elementary-school and later high-school age should require proportionately less teaching and more parenting, *i.e.*, emotional support. An unfortunate number of parents of deaf children feel it necessary to remain primarily teacher throughout their child's educational life, thereby creating another school at home. This type of undue pressure can result in any child's rejection of school, of parents, and ultimately of himself.

Clearly the parents have an important and indispensable role in the education of their deaf child. Their primary role, however, must be as parents—which is by far the more difficult.

HABILITATION TODAY AND TOMORROW

The past several years have witnessed a revolution in educating deaf children. Across the United States, programs which were once designated "oral" are now designated as so-called "total communication." This trend once again denotes a certain amount of educational polemics, in that use of total communication is applied without differential attention to a child's asset abilities. It is hoped, however, that some of these programs are practicing total communication in its truest sense, rather than merely adding a manual component to a weak oral program. If so, and if total communication as a teaching method lives up to the claims of its advocates, the next few years will hopefully reveal an improvement over the dismal record of the past, as illustrated by several research studies in which the highest reading comprehension scores in a population of deaf 19-year-olds was at the fourth-grade level (14).

It would be beneficial if more were known regarding how and what children process in the presence of total communication. Research tends to support the efficacy of successive rather than simultaneous processing of information presented via different sensory modalities (6). More knowledge is needed about how much auditory versus visual information is received by children in these classes. A better understanding of affective factors in relation to parents is clearly indicated, as is more attention to the deaf child as a human being with emotions of his own. The whole area of mental health in the deaf population has only recently begun to receive sorely needed attention. More competent professionals are desperately needed.

Training programs for teachers of the deaf must incorporate a higher level of preparation in parent counseling techniques. Greater awareness must also come about within the medical profession in regard to appropriate educational referrals for deaf children.

REFERENCES

1. Brill R: Administrative and Professional Development in the Education of the Deaf. Washington DC, Gallaudet College Press, 1971
2. Conference of Executives of American Schools. Report of the conference committee on nomenclature. Am Ann Deaf 83:1–3, 1938
3. Education of the Deaf. A Report to the Secretary of Health, Education, and Welfare by his Advisory Committee on the Education of the Deaf. Washington DC, Reproduced by the Department of Health, Education, and Welfare, February, 1965
4. Fernald G: Remedial Techniques in Basic School Subjects. New York, McGraw-Hill, 1943
5. Fry D: The development of the phonological system in the normal and the deaf child. In Smith F, Miller G (eds): The Genesis of Language: A Psycholinguistic Approach. Cambridge, MA, MIT Press, 1966
6. Gaeth J: Learning with visual and audiovisual presentations. In McConnell F, Ward PH (eds): Deafness in Childhood. Nashville, Vanderbilt University Press, 1967
7. Kübler-Ross E: On Death and Dying. New York, MacMillan 1969
8. Lerner J: Children with Learning Disabilities. Boston, Houghton Mifflin, 1971
9. Moses K: Issues of parent counseling: an introduction to mourning theory. A mini-seminar presented at the Convention of the American Speech and Hearing Association, Las Vegas, Nevada, 1974
10. Northern J, Downs M: Hearing in Children. Baltimore, Williams & Wilkins, 1974
11. Pollack D: Educational Audiology for the Limited Hearing Infant. Springfield, IL, CC Thomas, 1970
12. Pollack D: The development of an auditory function. Otolaryngol Clin North Am 4:319–335, 1971
13. Reis P: Academic Achievement Test Results of a National Testing Program for Hearing Impaired Students. Washington DC, Office of Demographic Studies, Gallaudet College, 1973
14. Whetnall E, Fry D: The Deaf Child. Springfield, IL, CC Thomas, 1971
15. Woodcock R, Clark C: Peabody Rebus Reading Program. Circle Pines, MN, American Guidance Service, 1969

36

PARENT COUNSELING

H. PATRICIA HEFFERNAN
MARSHA R. SIMONS

RATIONALE FOR EARLY DETECTION

The need for early detection becomes obvious in light of the considerations discussed previously, and in view of the desirability of prompt medical intervention where applicable. About 5% of the school-age population have a degree of hearing loss that requires special consideration. Unfortunately, there is a tendency to judge the severity of a hearing handicap by standards applicable to adults. Recent studies on hearing loss and language delay have revealed that many children with a hearing loss of 15–25dB demonstrated statistically significant delay in all language skills (1). This strengthens the need for early detection and complete assessment of any auditory handicap so that immediate audiologic and educational habilitative and rehabilitative measures can be instituted, regardless of concurrent medical care.

FACTORS AFFECTING SEVERITY OF HANDICAP

Problems in early detection such as parental attitudes, behavioral inconsistencies, and the presence of complicating multiple handicaps have been discussed in the previous two chapters. However, once a diagnosis has been made, habilitative management and educational placement may depend upon a variety of factors that affect the severity of the handicap. These factors follow.

The **degree** of hearing loss (which can range from mild to profound; see Table 34–1) has a significant effect on educational achievement, language, and speech capabilities, vocational potential, and social adjustment (Table 36–1).

The **type** of loss (whether conductive, cochlear, retrocochlear, or mixed) is significant. The effects of hearing loss are more pronounced as the locus of the lesion progresses from peripheral to more central mechanisms. Children with sensorineural lesions have poorer speech discrimination scores than those with middle-ear lesions alone. Although CNS auditory disorders also create discrimination problems, the findings differ from those of cochlear or cochlear nuclear lesions. As a matter of fact, in lesions central to cochlear nuclei there will be no reduction in hearing acuity.

The **configuration** of the hearing loss can influence the degree of communication handicap realized by the patient. Vowel sounds have most of their energy in the low frequencies (below 1000 Hz). They possess the greatest amount of intensity (*i.e.*, 60% of acoustic energy) and are most easily perceived, while consonants have the least amount of energy (5% of acoustic energy) and are less easily perceived. However, consonants contribute more significantly to speech perception than vowels, having a 60% intelligibility factor versus a 5% intelligibility factor (3). The consonants that occur most frequently in the English language and that contribute significantly to linguistic interpretation occur in the high-frequency spectrum (*e.g.*, s, f, v, sh, ch, etc.). Therefore, the patient with a high-frequency sensorineural hearing loss will have poorer discrimination ability with a more critical communication handicap than the patient with decreased auditory acuity in the low frequencies alone.

Causal factors must be considered: For example, does the hearing loss result from exogenous factors (nongenetic) or endogenous factors (genetic)?

Age at onset and/or discovery is a critical determinant of the significance of an auditory disability. Hearing loss may be differentiated as occurring on a congenital basis (present at birth) or on an adventitious basis (occurring after birth). Of more critical importance, however, is whether the hearing loss occurred before or after the advent of language and speech development (prelingual or postlingual).

It has been theorized that the basic elements of one's native language are mastered by 3.5–4 years of age (5). The child whose hearing loss is postlingual already has a reference for auditory stimuli

TABLE 36-1. Relationship of Degree of Loss to Linguistic and Educational Expectations

Degree of loss	Listening characteristics	Speech and language development (voice quality)	Educational needs and amplification considerations
40 dB Mild loss	Difficulty in hearing faint speech, speech at a distance, or speech in noise.	Generally within normal limits, but some children may have language and speech development delayed as much as 2–3 years.	Attend class for normal hearing; preferential seating in class; should be able to watch teacher's lips; may need speech and/or language tutoring. Amplification considered individually for each child.
41–55 dB Moderate loss	Without amplification can hear direct conversation at 3 feet; often have difficulty in understanding, especially in noise, even with hearing aids.	Language skills affected; have difficulty with infrequently used words and subtleties of meaning; articulation usually affected, but speech is intelligible; voice quality and inflection most often normal.	Can attend regular class, preferential seating; need teacher with patience; should be able to watch teacher's lips. Special attention to reading and writing skills, and vocabulary development; early language and speech instruction needed; require continual monitoring by speech and language therapist. Amplification definitely indicated. May wear postauricular hearing aids.
56–70 dB Moderately severe loss	Without amplification hear loud speech at 3 feet; with amplification, have difficulty understanding in many situations, particularly classroom.	Frequently confused by language; grammar is deficient and vocabulary limited; speech and language development significantly delayed, and early speech is usually unintelligible. Voice quality and intonation usually defective.	Some, with extensive assistance, can benefit from regular class placement; many require special education. In regular class, need preferential seating. Need extensive early assistance in basic language, reading, and writing skills. In later grades may only require tutorial assistance in special academic areas. Amplification needed early; auditory training may continue for many years.
71–90dB Severe loss	Aware of loud voices and some moderately loud sounds at 1 foot from the ear, without amplification.	Do not develop language and speech spontaneously; voice and intonation will be noticeably defective.	May be considered "educationally deaf"; need extensive early assistance in basic language, reading, and writing skills; enrollment in special preschool programs is essential; most require special education. Some few will have regular classroom placement in elementary grades; in later grades many integrate in regular classes. Amplification needed early; auditory training will continue for many years.
≥91 dB Profound loss	May respond to some very loud sounds without amplification, but in general do not rely on hearing as the primary channel for communication.	Language and speech develop only through consistent and prolonged training; voice quality and intonation noticeably defective.	Considered "educationally deaf"; need extensive early assistance in basic language, reading, and writing skills. Enrollment in special preschool programs essential. Because hearing may not be primary channel for communication, may be dependent on sign language. Most will need special classes or residential schools. Select few may integrate in regular classes. Amplification needed early; auditory training will continue for many years.

and an extensive auditory memory, which makes sound differentiation of many stimuli automatic. In addition, the child has learned the basic syntax of the language and can deduce more information from limited cues than one who lacks this familiarity. The hearing loss distorts the familiar auditory pattern of sound. As a result, the child will experience various degrees of difficulty identifying the message by the acoustic symbol alone. Children whose "deafness" is postlingual tend to require less extensive rehabilitative measures than those who have no prior language structure.

Individual characteristics influencing future capabilities are chronologic age, emotional maturity, current linguistic ability level, intellectual capacity, motor capacity, former educational instruction, and presence of additional handicapping disorders.

Parental attitudes can adversely affect future performance, initially by avoiding discovery, and later by failure to follow through on necessary medical, habilitative, and rehabilitative measures (see Ch. 34, The "Hard of Hearing" Child, and Ch. 35, The Deaf Child). Once diagnosis is made, it is imperative that thorough counseling be included as part of the evaluation process, since effective child care is contingent upon parental understanding of the problem and knowledge of the parent's role in remedial procedures.

Diagnostic "tunnel vision" can result when a diagnostician specializing in a single aspect of health care tends to view the child in a specific disorder category (*e.g.*, orthopedic disorder, auditory disorder), rather than *first* as a child, who *secondly* happens to have a handicap requiring special attention. In addition, in the zeal to diagnose all possible existing disorders and seek out etiology, the diagnostician may neglect to identify the primary handicap (that which creates the greatest need for remedial care) and thus may neglect to focus on the most effective rehabilitation program. A time-consuming quest for total diagnosis may delay the initiation of habilitation for inexcusably prolonged periods.

The audiogram itself is helpful in demonstrating degree and type of loss and the configuration, so the child can be educationally classified. Labeling the degree of hearing impairment is descriptive but provides a limited picture of the patient. A combination of factors determines the severity of the handicap. Therefore, rather than label a child as "mildly," "moderately," or "profoundly" handicapped, on the basis of decibels alone, it is more important to describe how a child actually functions and then decide upon the habilitative

and rehabilitative measures most appropriate for his needs.

MANAGEMENT AND COUNSELING

The need for complete diagnostic assessment includes medical, audiologic, linguistic, and psychological evaluation prior to educational placement. Audiologic habilitative measures must now concern amplification needs and then educational management guidance.

AMPLIFICATION

The hearing levels determining the necessity for amplification are presented in Table 36–2, which is based upon current thinking as to who can derive the most benefit from a hearing aid.

Special problems concern those children who have borderline sensorineural hearing losses (not more than 30 dB); "ski-slope" losses (essentially normal hearing through 500 Hz, or even 1 K Hz, with an abrupt drop thereafter); unilateral asymmetrical hearing losses (a mild or moderate loss in the better ear with a significantly greater loss in the opposite ear); and chronic middle ear problems.

Many of these children can be fitted successfully with hearing aids. New forms of earmolds, new types of circuitry (particularly CROS type), and limited power instruments are providing assistance to children who previously had to compensate for their hearing handicaps by their own ingenious methods.

Binaural Versus Monaural Amplification

Binaural versus monaural amplification has been often discussed. In our opinion most children perform better with binaural (two aids) than with monaural (one aid) amplification. In our clinical

TABLE 36-2. Usefulness of Amplification at Various Hearing Levels

Hearing level (dB)	Indications for amplification
0–25	Only in special circumstances
25–40	Useful for educational and professional situations
40–55	Generally used with success
55–85	Greatest benefit derived
85–110	Benefit limited without provisions for ongoing habilitative service

experience binaural aids improve localization, make understanding in noisy environments easier for most children, require less hearing aid gain necessary for each ear. Greater social ease is often noted in situations previously avoided by the child.

Binaural hearing aids are two separate amplifying systems. There are two separate microphones, two separate receivers, and two separate volume controls. The attempt to approximate binaural amplification through Y cords is not justified. Most often the purpose is to stimulate both ears with sound. However, most Y-cord setups reduce the intensity of the sound reaching both ears, thus possibly preventing either ear from receiving adequate sound stimulation.

Our practice is initially to fit all children with a monaural hearing aid, preferably the better hearing ear. If there does not appear to be a significant difference between ears, we will have the parent alternate the instrument from one ear to the other on a weekly basis. During this adjustment period (intended to last not more than 3 months), we monitor the hearing thresholds by regularly scheduled hearing tests to assure that there is no temporary reduction in hearing sensitivity. A temporary threshold shift (TTS) may occur following introduction of amplification; thus caution should be exercised in the selection procedure (Figs. 36–1 to 36–3). The fitting of a hearing aid for the second ear is done on an individual basis, only after acceptance of the first aid is completed, and only after the stability of hearing threshold levels has been determined.

The question of a body aid versus a postauricular aid is a major problem, especially in terms of amplification requirements of young children. The important consideration is to provide sufficient amplification for beginning language needs. The superiority of one or the other cannot be assumed without testing the children with both types of aids and observing performance differences. Physical problems must also be considered—the size of the auricle and/or cartilaginous structure of the auricle versus size and weight of the postauricular hearing aid and the motor skills of the child.

While frequency response curves of postauricular instruments appear to be essentially similar to those of body-worn aids, a more realistic consideration is that a hearing aid's optimum benefit depends upon its being *worn consistently* and remaining in *good working condition.* Therefore, even if the body aid might offer somewhat better quality amplification (as reported by some experienced teen-aged hearing aid users), the older child will rarely wear it. Most children over the age of 5 years much prefer postauricular hearing aids, wear them routinely, and perform exceptionally well with them even when a profound hearing loss exists.

There are power and gain limitations. Previously, it was common practice to attempt to fit children with a hearing aid offering gain essentially equal to the amount of loss. We now know that most children wear their hearing aids (particularly body-worn instruments) at approximately half of the available gain. This is true even for profoundly deaf children.

In addition, the noise environment to which we all are being exposed is of special concern for the child using amplification. In general, we limit all hearing aids fitted to our pediatric patients to no more than (an often less than) 128 dB sound pressure level (SPL). Some profoundly deaf youngsters require and insist on more power, and in those instances we may recommend a hearing aid with 132 dB SPL. This is our maximum limit.

BONE CONDUCTION VERSUS AIR CONDUCTION AMPLIFICATION

Bone-conduction hearing aids have benefited from space-age technology. It is now possible to provide adequate bone conduction amplification with a postauricular unit that is equal in capacity to many of the previously available body-worn units.

The majority of children with bilateral atresia, agenesis, and other external malformations should be fitted with bone-conduction amplification units as soon after birth as possible. In addition, some children with unilateral external malformations may also require amplification because of middle-ear abnormalities of the opposite ear. Since audiologic testing can reveal whether truly adequate bone conduction levels are present, we can easily determine if bone conduction hearing aids will be satisfactory for the child's needs.

In addition, we have found that multiply handicapped children with serious language delay and/or behavioral problems will often benefit from bone conduction amplification when persistent middle ear problems are present. These children may be found to have normal hearing on some occasions, and mild or even moderate conductive losses at other times. Obviously, with the already present burden of other handicaps, the presence of fluctuating hearing is a serious detriment to development of necessary communication skills. The use of bone conduction hearing aids can provide

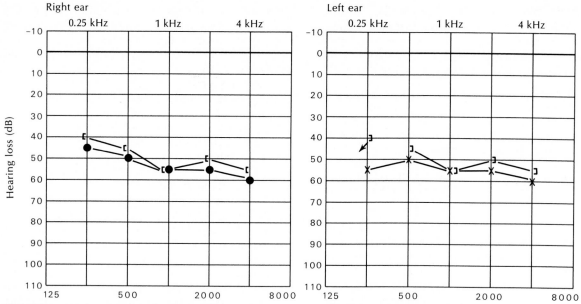

FIG. 36–1. Initial audiogram of patient 5.5 years old, before introduction of amplification to right ear. **At left,** ●—●, AC, unmasked, RE; [—[, BC, masked, RE; **At right, x—x,** AC, unmasked, LE;]—], BC, masked, LE; **SRT,** 50 dB RE and LE; **arrow,** no response at maximum output.

FIG. 36–2. Audiogram of same patient as in Figure 36–1, after hearing aid was used for 7 months. Note significant change in both AC and BC thresholds, right ear, while no change occurred in left ear. **At left,** ●—●, AC, unmasked, RE; [—[, BC, masked, RE; **At right, x—x,** AC, unmasked, LE;]—], BC, masked, LE; **arrow,** no response at maximum output; **SRT,** 70 dB, RE; 55 dB, LE.

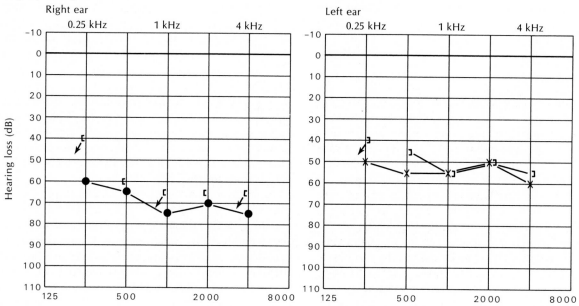

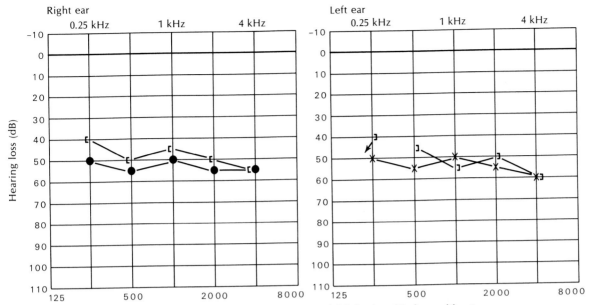

FIG. 36–3. Audiogram for same patient as in Figures 36–1 and 36–2 after 21 days without wearing hearing aid in right ear. Both AC and BC thresholds returned to preamplification levels, while thresholds for left ear continued unchanged. **At left,** ●—●, AC, unmasked, RE; [—[, BC, masked, RE; **At right, x—x,** AC, unmasked, LE;]—], BC, masked, LE; **arrow,** no response at maximum output; **SRT,** LE, 55 dB.

such children with consistent levels of auditory input from their daily environment.

AUDITORY TRAINING

Auditory training should represent a consistent, organized plan of exposure to auditory input for the development of auditory skills, with awareness and recognition of the signals and eventually of the symbolic elements of communication (see Ch. 34, The "Hard of Hearing" Child, and Ch. 35, The Deaf Child).

FINANCIAL AID

The types of financial aid that are available vary greatly from one community to another. Parents need to be aware of the expense of the procedures and prostheses needed for their children. A general awareness will lead to the understanding and recognition of whether they will need assistance in handling these costs. As an example, in the State of California the Crippled Children's Services assists where financial need exists. Medicaid provides the states with funds to assist children of families in financial need. Many local community service groups will assist in individual cases where needed, and local school districts often know of local agencies that can be helpful.

EDUCATIONAL ALTERNATIVES

Different geographic locations provide a variety of instructional alternatives for children with hearing impairments, ranging from regular classroom placement with part-time special instruction to full-time residential schools. Parents should be encouraged to explore all available programs in their area, and observe those schools being considered. The choice of systems or school district is not as important as that of parental agreement with and commitment to the system of their choice. Most parents do not have the experience and skills necessary to make these decisions independently. The best decisions for long-term management are made with a team approach. The team should include parents, physician, audiologist, educator, psychologist, and counselor. Some factors to consider are:

1. The type of program. Types of classroom arrangement and program alternatives vary significantly, depending on the geographic location (see Chs. 34 and 35).
2. The applicability of the program for the child's particular needs. The student enrollment within a specific district may consist primarily of one group of hearing-impaired children (*i.e.*, moderately hard of hearing, or profoundly deaf,

etc.). Obviously, if a child has a hearing loss of mild to moderate degree, we would not regard a classroom of profoundly deaf youngsters as an adequate language and speech model for him.

Conversely, a classroom consisting primarily of children with mild to moderate hearing loss may not be appropriate for a profoundly deaf child. Although the children may serve as good language models, they will be developing language and academic skills in a format primarily auditory in emphasis, which may not be sufficient for the profoundly deaf child's development.

In addition, when more than one handicap is believed to exist, it is imperative that educational assessment determine the approach that will be most effective for the child. For instance, the school diagnostic team must determine whether a child diagnosed as developmentally disabled with severe hearing loss and no verbal skills must be placed in a program emphasizing language development through aural rehabilitation and auditory training as the primary educational objective, with secondary emphasis on the effects of the developmental disability, or vice versa.

3. Method of instruction. **Oral/Aural** signifies a program utilizing amplification and hearing capability as the primary mode of educational development. This approach relies heavily on speech-reading as the primary approach for development of language skills and language input.

Manual communication is a program in which words and/or concepts are communicated via a system of organized signs (Ameslan) and in which each letter of the alphabet is represented by a finger symbol. Thus communication occurs through "finger spelling." Manual communication has a vocabulary of 500–1000 words, in contrast to the 5000 words known and used by the average kindergartener. One may quickly recognize the poverty of this method. In addition, this language technique requires interpreters for the general public. Finger spelling affords the use of a larger vocabulary at the expense of speed (imagine verbally spelling every word in a conversation). Semantics are also sacrificed with this technique. Very few programs of this type are found today in the United States.

American Sign Language (Ameslan or ASL) is used for general content, not specific intent. It consists of a basic conceptual vocabulary (signed and spelled) in its own language structure with heavy use of facial and body expressions. One major drawback is that its crude syntax is not conducive to development of acceptable English. It is difficult to express pronouns, verb tense is indicated only by context, and signs follow each other according to convenience and not necessarily in accepted English word order.

Total communication is a philosophy requiring the incorporation of appropriate aural, manual, and oral modes of communication to insure effective communication with and among hearing-impaired persons (2). Several varieties of sign language may be used. Some examples are:

1. Signed English (Siglish) is Ameslan vocabulary signed and some English vocabulary spelled in basic English syntax with no tense indicators. Emphasis is upon signing the meaning of what is said. It involves synonym signing and is used in college classrooms and by most interpreters with adults.
2. Manual English uses Ameslan vocabulary, new specific concept vocabulary, and English-bound morphemes all signed in English syntax. Meaning is conveyed primarily by the signs themselves.
3. Visual English (Seeing Essential English—SEE 1) represents word forms or word parts. It reflects English syntax by emphasizing normal word order. Verb tense and irregular verb forms are clearly indicated.
4. Visual English (Seeing Exact English—SEE 2) uses signs that represent words rather than roots. It is intended to be used by young children. Seventy-nine percent of SEE 2 is based on traditional Ameslan signs.

The audiologist and/or physician may make unwise decisions about an individual child's ability to function in an educational setting on the basis of a single examination, perhaps as infrequently as once a year. This is a major error, since this annual (or even semi-annual) visit, in which the child interacts individually with the audiologist and/or physician is hardly adequate as an indicator of the youngster's ability to deal with his peers and to participate in the learning process within a classroom.

Whatever personal preferences we may have developed over the years, whatever biases we may admit to regarding the education of the hearing-impaired, we cannot impose these attitudes on a family. The parents ultimately become the decision-makers—they become the managers of the early years of their child's education. They have to live daily with their decisions, and their attitudes and degree of cooperation will, to a large extent, determine the success or failure of their child in a particular program. Imposing one's personal professional preference fails to allow for individual differences and capabilities, both of parents and children. In addition, the infrequent services provided by the physician and audiologist are hardly adequate to lend support for parents in their never-ending struggle to cope with the variety and complexity of problems they must continually face.

PARENT COUNSELING

Parent Organizations

Once parents have accepted the diagnosis, they can become active forces of change (or support) for education of the hearing-impaired. They often express the need for communication with other parents of children with hearing impairment. Some schools have counseling services and organized parent groups for this purpose.

The Alexander Graham Bell Association International Parents Organization,* and the National Association for the Deaf† are active and intensely committed groups that welcome interest and involvement from parents. Unfortunately some parents may avoid true acceptance and adjustment to their child's hearing handicap by becoming actively involved in the issue of education, legal rights, etc. (see Ch. 35, The Deaf Child). Nevertheless, parents have been a major force in the improvement and the maintenance of education systems and should not be deterred from attempting these valuable efforts.

Correspondence Courses

Courses and suggestions for home carry-over and participation are available. The John Tracy Clinic‡ Correspondence Course, available by mail and through the clinic's regular services to parents, gives specific training suggestions for parents to use in the home with their child (see Ch. 44, The John Tracy Clinic Approach to Deaf Children and Their Families). In addition, most therapists working with the family of a hearing-handicapped child plan lessons and therapy approaches involving the parents both in structured and fairly unstructured situations in the home and daily living experiences.

* Alexander Graham Bell Association, 3417 Volta Place, N.W., Washington, DC 20007.
† National Association for the Deaf, 814 Thayer Ave., Silver Spring, MD 20910.
‡ John Tracy Clinic, 806 West Adams St., Los Angeles, CA 90007.

Establishment of Goals

Establishment of realistic educational and vocational goals is necessary. The parents' response to a diagnosis of hearing impairment in their child may result in a deep grief for the "loss" of their child (see Ch. 35, The Deaf Child). Often the parents abandon all hope for any of their "dreams" for the child's future. *Realism* is the key word in the approach to a discussion of the child's future.

As it is impossible to foretell the educational achievement of any child, the responsible audiologist will not attempt to tell the parents what to expect of their child's future and will avoid the "soothsayer's" role. On the basis of experience, the audiologist will explain what commonalities are found among the adult hearing-impaired. Although the parents cannot be assured that their child will "talk and sound just like everyone else," it is possible to encourage them by explaining that many children with impaired hearing develop good articulation skills and are easily understood by other people. Such encouragement should be qualified with a gentle reminder that others may remain unintelligible to the average listener.

OTOLOGIC-AUDIOLOGIC FOLLOW-UP CARE

Parents must be impressed with the need for regularly scheduled otologic-audiologic reevaluation. For instance, the deleterious effect of serous otitis media superimposed on a severe sensorineural hearing loss can be quickly ameliorated when a child is seen by his physician on a regular basis. However, all too often we find children returning for otologic examination only on a 2- to 3-year rotating basis. Some of these children have had decreases in hearing acuity during this period, and they may be wearing inadequate amplification devices. In addition, the amplification originally recommended may appear to be creating a temporary threshold shift. Regular monitoring of hearing acuity following hearing aid selection is essential to prevent potential permanent problems.

A recommended program for follow-up care is as follows:

1. During the first year after diagnosis, the child should be seen at least every 3 months. Hearing tests should be a regular part of these visits.
2. During the second year, if hearing sensitivity remains stable, the child should be seen every 6 months. If hearing changes are observed, the checkups should continue on a 3-month basis.
3. Once stability of hearing threshold is estab-

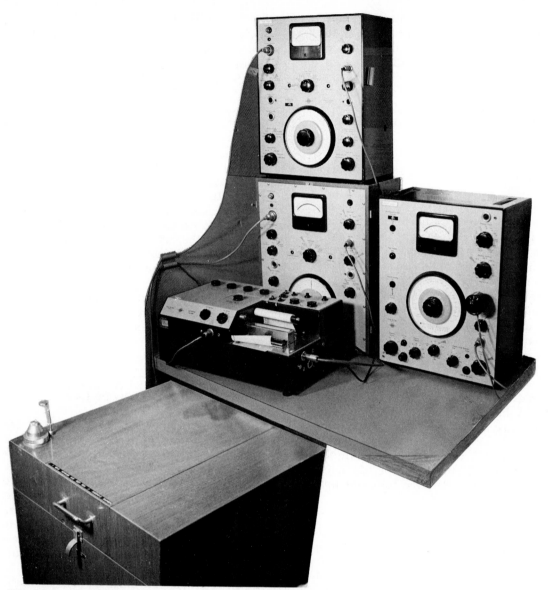

FIG. 36–4. Component parts of the Bruel and Kjaer system for mechanically monitoring hearing-aid performance. It includes the anechoic chamber, frequency analyzer, spectrometer, and graphic level recorder.

lished, a child with amplification should be tested at least annually. These visits should include (after otologic examination) pure tone tests of each ear, speech reception threshold tests of each ear (or speech awareness level if speech recognition is not possible), speech discrimination testing of each ear where possible, sound field tests when the child is wearing a hearing aid, and if binaural amplification is used, both sides should be tested independently as well as together.

A helpful addition to this regimen would be obtaining frequency response information for each hearing aid, including measurement of gain and power output. Figure 36–4 illustrates the Bruel & Kjaer system, but other systems are also available that provide the necessary information about hearing aid performance.

4. Some local test laboratory could be found that would monitor the performance of hearing aid(s) at least 4 times a year if the audiology center cannot provide this service. A child who

daily wears a malfunctioning hearing aid cannot be expected to perform at optimum level. This fact may seem to be too obvious to ignore, but most children never have their hearing aids mechanically monitored, except when they are obviously not working properly. Parents should also be given information about care of a hearing aid and instructed on how to perform a daily check on the hearing aid (4).

SPECIAL MANAGEMENT CONCERNS

School personnel and all other professionals concerned with the total care of the child must be continually informed of the status of the child as seen by the otologist-audiologist team. If a child is seen on a 3-month basis, regular reports should be disseminated to keep other professionals aware of any interesting facts (*i.e.*, whether hearing sensitivity has remained stable or perhaps has begun to decrease and thus will be of concern to all).

There are several types of hearing loss that pose interpretative problems. In these cases it is the responsibility of the otologist-audiologist team to attempt, by every means possible, education of any and all who will come into regular contact with this child.

Among the difficult problems are the following:

1. The child with a unilateral hearing loss. Some of these children have no difficulty functioning in the normal classroom. However, others may require special considerations in the classroom, such as those suggested in the following school report:

In view of the fact that M.R. has normal auditory sensitivity in the left ear, her educational placement should be in the regular classroom with normal-hearing children. Her speech and language skills appear appropriate for her age level. While in the regular classroom, however, certain conditions should be arranged so that M.R. will be in an optimum position for learning: 1) M.R. should have preferential classroom seating (*i.e.*, the teacher's face should be easily visible, and the light should be on the teacher's face and not behind her back); 2) the poor ear should be toward a wall surface rather than toward the center of the classroom. We can expect M.R. will always understand better if she is able to watch the face of the speaker and may also require directions to be repeated for her.

2. The child with a hearing loss of unusual configuration, who often shows awareness for sound at the same levels as the other children in a classroom. Awareness is not comprehen-

sion, although it is easy to assume that this child is unwilling to pay attention. The following paragraphs often help to interpret the problems these children face:

George has a bilateral high-frequency hearing loss. He does have near-normal hearing in the low frequencies. This means that we can expect him to be aware of speech and other environmental sounds at near normal intensity levels. However, the clarity of what he hears will be affected by the greater loss in the high frequencies. This configuration of hearing loss represents a unique problem in educational and rehabilitative planning. The learning of speech and language will be complicated by the fact that he will be able to hear voice and the vowel sounds of speech normally, whereas the consonants (which help to identify words clearly) will be distorted or not heard. For instance, to George the word "pie" may sound like "tie," "die," "my," or "by." "Yes" may sound like "yet" or "jet." Also, because of the decreased speech energy at the end of words, he may fail to hear and thus fail to repeat the final sound. For example, "goal" may sound like "go," and "knees" may sound like "me" or "knee."

Speech-reading will be very helpful. If "pie" and "tie" sound alike, but George is able to see the speaker's lips, he will see the difference. He will always understand best if he is given the opportunity to utilize visual (speech reading) as well as auditory clues.

3. The child with a progressive hearing loss who initially demonstrates a moderate loss and continues to perform as though this degree of loss has remained unchanged. It seems to take quite a long time for performance to show the effect of a reduced hearing threshold. Those who work regularly with such a child often fail to allow for the reduced sensitivity and unconsciously make unreasonable demands upon the child. The following case is a helpful example:

D.C.'s hearing acuity has decreased steadily over the past year. He should still be able to function adequately with amplification in his present educational setting. Despite the fact that he does not demonstrate marked evidence of increased communication difficulty, he can be expected to require more intensive auditory stimulation and additional visual clues to function with the same degree of success and efficiency previously possible. Additional linguistic tutoring and speech therapy may be necessary to assist him in preserving his present skills, and to assist in preventing any reduction in his educational and communicative capabilities.

4. The classroom teacher and all other personnel need to be kept informed about the current status of the child. They need the most recent audiogram, medical information, details re-

garding performance of the hearing aid and its function, the effect of the hearing loss upon communication skills, and other possible classroom considerations. School reports containing this type of information should be sent not only to the school nurse, but also to the teacher and the appropriate office of the school district. A sample report concerning the child with a moderate hearing loss who attends classes for the normally hearing is below.

Pure tone testing reveals that D.B. has a bilateral hearing loss that may be expected to be moderately handicapping. However, because of his excellent response with amplification, we would recommend placement in a classroom for normal-hearing children. These children will be excellent speech models for him.

His speech and language skills appear to be excellent, especially in view of the degree of hearing loss. Speech therapy, however, will certainly need to be considered, in view of the poor articulation noted on the (r) sound and sibilants (s) and (z) in particular.

He may have trouble hearing faint speech at a distance (such as in a noisy classroom) and may miss some of the subtleties of language (prefixes, suffixes, tense, etc.). He should be seated as close to the front of the class as possible. He will still ask for repetition and may need supplementary tutoring in those subject areas that require critical listening abilities (*i.e.*, reading and spelling). We can expect that D.B. will always understand better if he is able to watch the face of the speaker and if directions are repeated for him.

Please feel free to contact us if you have any questions regarding D.B.'s hearing.

REFERENCES

1. Brooks DN: The role of the acoustic impedance bridge in paediatric screening. Scand Audiol 3:99–104, 1974
2. Conference of Executives of American Schools for the Deaf. Total Communication—A Definition. Las Vegas, Nevada, May 5, 1976
3. Gerber S: Introductory Hearing Science—Physical and Psychological Concepts. Philadelphia, WB Saunders, 1974
4. Hanners B, Sitton A: Ears to hear: a daily hearing aid monitor program. Volta Rev 76, 1974
5. McNeill D: The capacity for language acquisition. In Research on Behavioral Aspects of Deafness. Proceedings of a National Research Conference on Behavioral Aspects of Deafness, United States Department of Health Education and Welfare. Washington DC, Vocational Rehabilitation Administration, 1965, pp 11–28

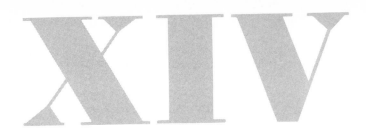

XIV

ADULT
SENSORINEURAL
HEARING LOSSES

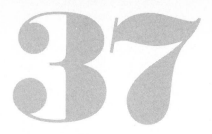

SUDDEN HEARING LOSS SYNDROME

VICTOR GOODHILL
IRWIN HARRIS

Sudden hearing loss is an otologic emergency. A sudden hearing loss may occur as the result of lesions of the external, middle, or inner ear, or as the result of internal auditory meatus, cerebellopontine angle, or CNS lesions. The hearing losses may be mild or moderate in degree, more frequently severe or total, and may be caused by any one of a number of either conductive or sensorineural lesions.

Sudden conductive hearing losses may occur in tympanic membrane or middle ear trauma, in barotrauma, in incus necrosis associated with chronic otomastoiditis, in serous otitis media following acute upper respiratory tract infections, in poststapedectomy complications, and in many other external ear, middle ear, and middle–inner ear interface conditions. Details regarding diagnosis and management of such conductive hearing losses appear in specific chapters.

Sudden sensorineural hearing losses may occur in Meniere's disease, in labyrinthine complications of previous ear surgery, in ear or cranial trauma, in acoustic trauma, in barotrauma, in response to ototoxic drugs, in a number of labyrinthogenic diseases such as syphilis, in sudden edema of an eighth nerve tumor, in multiple sclerosis, Cogan's disease, encephalitis, metastatic carcinoma, and in cerebrovascular lesions. Malingering and psychogenic hearing losses must also be considered in

differential diagnosis. Details concerning specific sudden hearing loss in sensorineural lesions appear in specific chapters.

Sudden mixed conductive–cochlear hearing losses may occur as the result of labyrinthine fistulas in chronic otomastoiditis, after stapedectomy, and in other complications of otologic diseases.

However, the specific term **sudden hearing loss** has acquired a special clinical usage, *i.e.*, to describe syndromes of spontaneous sudden sensorineural hearing loss in patients with presumably unknown previous ear or hearing problems.

Thus, the consideration of sudden hearing loss syndromes in this chapter is limited to the sudden onset of a sensorineural hearing loss (SNHL) in a previously presumably normal ear.

Until recently, all such cases of sudden SNHL were considered to be of idiopathic etiology. Hypothetical and speculative approaches have characterized diagnosis and therapy of presumptive viral, vascular, endocrine, allergic, and other causes. Empiric nonspecific medical treatments and/or surgical approaches have been proposed and used with variable results, since the basic etiopathologic cause is only occasionally verified, since validated temporal bone pathologic findings are rarely available, and since spontaneous recoveries occur frequently. Our recent observations (7, 9) of definite round window membrane and oval window ligament ruptures with perilymph fistulas (in a number of cases associated with barotrauma and physical exertion) are responsible for the need for considering two syndromes of sudden SNHL.

Idiopathic sudden SNHL is presumed to be caused by viral, vascular, endocrine, allergic, or other lesions.

Labyrinth membrane rupture sudden SNHL is caused either by sudden barotrauma, physical exertion, or to other severe stresses (Fig. 37–1).

Management of sudden hearing loss requires not only careful differential diagnosis between conductive hearing loss and SNHL but differentiation between idiopathic sudden SNHL and the sudden SNHL caused by labyrinthine membrane rupture.

ETIOLOGY

IDIOPATHIC SUDDEN SNHL SYNDROME GROUP

Viral Etiology

One viral etiologic cause has been clearly identified —the mumps virus. For many decades it has been known that sudden unilateral severe cochlear hear-

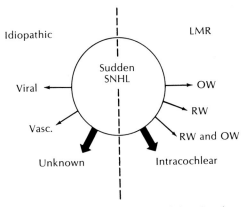

FIG. 37–1. Sudden sensorineural hearing loss: **idiopathic** (viral, vascular, unknown) and labyrinthine membrane rupture **(LMR)** (implosive and explosive) etiologies. **OW,** oval window; **RW,** round window.

ing loss occurs in a small percentage of children and in some adults with epidemic parotitis. Usually, such a hearing loss is not identified until some time after the resolution of the acute mumps, possibly validated by mumps serology titer studies. Temporal bone findings have been described in mumps as well as in rubella, rubeola, and other viral lesions (see Ch. 33, Acquired Congenital Ear Syndromes).

The basic histopathologic findings in specific and presumptive viral lesions consist of atrophy of the stria vascularis, cochlear duct collapse, and displacement and distortion of the tectorial membrane. The mechanism is probably that of viremia with the cochlear stria vascularis as the portal of entry. Although cochlear lesions predominate in the pathologic studies, involvement of the vestibular labyrinth has also been reported.

Vascular Etiology

Vascular factors have been considered etiologic for decades. Various theories advanced include capillary sludging, vascular spasm, small vessel occlusions, massive inner ear hemorrhage related to leukemia, thromboangiitis obliterans (Buerger's disease), serum hyperviscosity syndrome, hypercoagulation, microglobulinemia, inflammatory vasculitis, and microembolism. Gussen (11) (Fig. 37–2) recently reported histopathologic temporal bone findings in a human case of sudden vascular SNHL. Prior histologic evidence for vascular etiology has been based on animal studies.

Hypoxia may play a decisive role in some cases. Experiments in the guinea pig (18) show that the

positive endolymphatic potential is related to ion transport from perilymph across Reissner's membrane, and by special features of the stria vascularis that require oxygen for this function (Fig. 37–3).

Other Idiopathic Etiologies

Although viral and vascular etiologic theories predominate, other causes have been suggested. These include hyperlipidemia, diabetes, drug ototoxicity, allergy, and endocrine causes. The rare lymphocytic meningitis etiology may require diagnostic spinal tap.

LABYRINTH MEMBRANE RUPTURE SYNDROME ETIOLOGY

Schuknecht, Neff, and Perlman (26), in studying the effects of experimental head blows, without fracture of the bony labyrinth, demonstrated perilymph and endolymph space hemorrhages. Behavioral tests showed immediate profound hearing losses. Temporal bone sections revealed not only hemorrhage but also Reissner's membrane tear. Ruptures of Reissner's membrane that can heal were demonstrated in experimental animals (17). The possibility that intracochlear membrane breaks can cause hearing losses was postulated by Simmons (27).

Fee (3) reported three cases of hearing loss following apparently traumatic oval-window fistula, two of which followed head injuries.

Stroud and Calcaterra (28) reported four additional spontaneous oval-window fistulas.

In 1971 three surgically confirmed cases of labyrinthine fistulas were reported by Goodhill (7) in stress-related cases of sudden cochlear hearing loss. Surgical findings showed fistulas in round, oval, or both labyrinthine windows. Since that report, additional studies (4, 6, 9, 13, 19, 23, 29) have confirmed findings of perilymphatic fistulas from one or both labyrinthine windows associated with presumable physical stresses prior to sudden cochlear hearing losses.

Theoretic mechanisms relating to sudden labyrinthine membrane rupture can be considered physiologically.

The labyrinth, with its delicately balanced perilymph–endolymph system, is linked through intimate relationships to hydrodynamic forces in the carotid arterial system, to the intracranial venous-sinus systems, and to cerebrospinal fluid (CSF) pressure gradient fluctuations within the subarachnoid space. A number of rhinopharyngeal

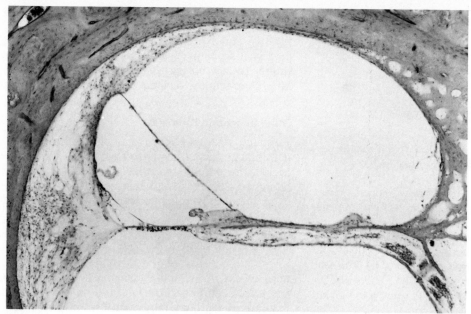

FIG. 37–2. Right cochlea and saccule. Note absence of organ of Corti, degeneration of tectorial membrane, atrophy of stria vascularis, spiral ligament acellularity, nerve fiber loss in bony spiral laminas, and lifted-away lining of outer sulcus. (High-power view of right ascending basal limb.) (H&E, × 75) (Gussen R: Ann Otol Rhinol Laryngol 85:95, 1976)

FIG. 37–3. Oxygen sources in relation to cochlear function. The suprastrial capillaries provide oxygen and plasma filtrate **(PF)** as constituents of perilymph. Positive endolymphatic potential **(EP)** is brought about by ion transport from perilymph across Reissner's membrane and by special features of the stria vascularis that require oxygen for this function. The generation of cochlear microphonics depends upon tunnel oxygen and EP polarization. (Lawrence M, Nuttal A, Burgio P: Ann Otol Rhinol Laryngol 84:499–512, 1975)

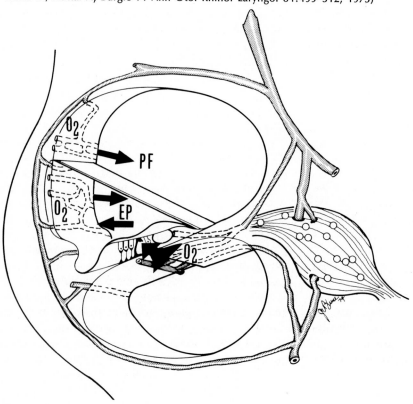

relationships are involved, with aerodynamic factors related to the tubotympanic air-space system. Thus, explosive CSF factors and implosive eustachian-tube–middle-ear factors must be considered.

The intimate hydrodynamic relationship between the subarachnoid space CSF pool, the cochlear aqueduct, the medial vestibular lamina cribrosa, and the labyrinthine perilymph have been studied by a number of investigators (1, 3, 15, 16, 27, 28).

Because of the "barrier membrane" usually present in the human cochlear aqueduct (30), little attention in the past was directed to possible cochlear aqueduct implications in sudden hearing loss. Observations by Palva (20) and Palva and Dammert (21) on anatomic variations in cochlear aqueduct relationships were significant in directing attention to the cochlear-aqueduct–scala-tympani confluence.

Gussen (10) described the potential role of arachnoid villi in the cochlear aqueduct. In two cases, an unusual tract between cochlear aqueduct and internal auditory canal was described. From these findings, it appears that arachnoid villi have a resorptive function within the cochlear aqueduct, which is not normally a free, open passageway between CSF and perilymph systems (Figs. 37–4, 37–5).

Exertion may involve an increase in CSF pressure. The cochlear aqueduct and the cribriform foramens of the internal auditory meatus are both potential pathways for transmission of CSF pressure changes to the perilymph system. Of the two, the cochlear aqueduct seems the more likely primary transmission pathway for change in CSF-perilymph pressure.

In Palva's studies, infant cochlear aqueducts were short (3.5 mm average) and relatively wide. The constant existence of a barrier membrane previously described by Waltner (30) could not be confirmed. By comparison, adult cochlear aqueducts were twice as long (6.2 mm average) although the width remained comparable at the narrowest point (150 μ). A barrier membrane at the junction with scala tympani was demonstrated in only 10% of cases.

Goodhill and associates (9) suggested that an infantile type of cochlear aqueduct may persist in some adults. With a relatively large cross-sectional area, the protective smoothing effect of the longer, relatively narrow adult aqueduct is lost. Stress episodes (Valsalva type) that result in abrupt transient increases in CSF pressure may then be

transmitted with full force to the scala tympani and to vulnerable labyrinthine membranes or to round window membrane and to oval window annular ligament regions. It is also possible that sudden SNHL associated with upper respiratory infections, accompanied by sneezing, coughing, and/or nose blowing, may be attributable to spontaneous labyrinthine membrane ruptures. Such membrane tears may either heal spontaneously, partially or completely, with secondary fibrosis and scarring, or they may remain open.

In a recent clinical study of 25 patients with increased CSF pressures (25), an average hearing loss of 30 dB was found. After appropriate therapy with return of CSF pressure to normal in 16 patients, hearing was significantly improved.

In a study of perilymph displacement by CSF in the guinea pig cochlea, Moscovitch et al. (18a) reported that if an opening is made in the cochlea, all the perilymph in the scala tympani (8.0 μ liter) would be displaced by an equal volume of CSF in approximately 10 min.

Sando et al. (24) did a carbon-particle experiment in a study of perilymph communication routes. When the cochlear aqueducts of guinea pigs were obliterated experimentally, no carbon particles were seen in the inner ear.

In stapedectomy, the surgeon can observe perilymph refilling the vestibule seconds to minutes following intentional or inadvertent suction removal of vestibular perilymph. So-called "perilymph gushers" have been reported occasionally following stapedectomy (see Ch. 19, Otosclerosis). Such observations attest to the intimate relationships between CSF pressures and the vestibular perilymph pool, and the unusual events that may occur in cases with an abnormally patent cochlear aqueduct.

Obviously, the infrequent occurrence of sudden cochlear hearing loss following the pressure changes in ordinary physical exertion or in the barotrauma of diving, etc., suggests the probability that such an episode may be associated with an anomaly in either the cochlear aqueduct or the cribriform foramen boundary in the internal auditory canal. The most likely CSF-perilymph pressure pathway is an anomalous or hyperpatent cochlear aqueduct.

Potential pathways exist from the subarachnoid space to the perilymph pools in the scala vestibuli and scala tympani. The roles of both the cochlear aqueduct and the internal auditory meatus must be considered, with both "explosive" and "im-

FIG. 37–4. A. Tract containing arachnoid fibers and cells opening into internal auditory canal on left. (H&E, × 39) **B.** High power view of tract midway between cochlear aqueduct and internal auditory canal to demonstrate arachnoid cells and fibers. Note fatty marrow. (H&E, × 117) (Gussen R: Arch Otolaryngol 96:565–569, 1972. Copyright 1972, American Medical Association)

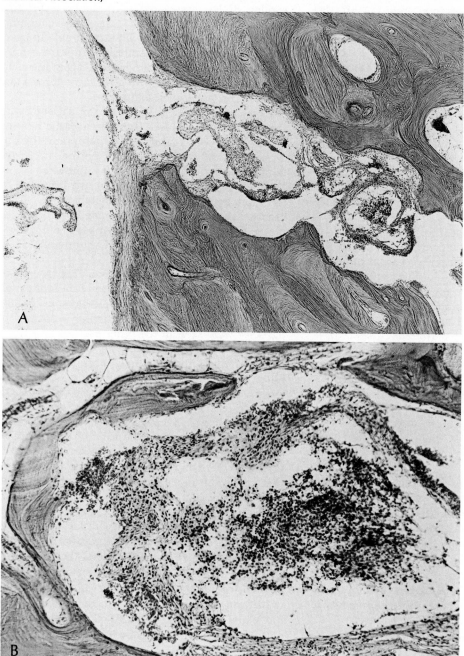

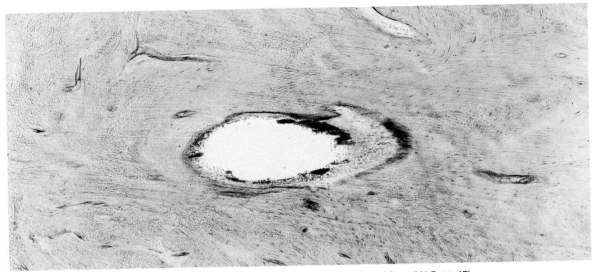

FIG. 37–5. Normal cochlear aqueduct between area of hemorrhage and cochlea. (H&E, × 47) (Gussen R: Arch Ontolaryngol 96:566–569, 1972. Copyright 1972, American Medical Association)

plosive" pathways for membrane ruptures (Fig. 37–6).

The explosive route makes it possible for a sudden increase in CSF pressure, due to physical exertion or barotrauma, to be transmitted through the cochlear aqueduct to the scala tympani, with ensuing rupture of the round window membrane and basilar membrane (Fig. 37–7). In an experimental study in the cat, Harker, Norante, and Ryu (12) showed bulging of the round window membrane as a result of increased CSF pressure in 83% of experimental animals and rupture of the membrane in 39% of experimental animals. A similar mechanism, through the internal auditory meatus, may involve the medial vestibule wall cribriform communication to the scala vestibuli. The ruptured labyrinthine membranes may produce a chain reaction of sequelae in the perilymphatic and endolymphatic systems with hearing loss, vertigo, and tinnitus.

The implosive route from sudden Valsalva forces, involves a sudden increase in tubotympanic pressure with rupture of the round window membrane and/or oval window ligament as sequelae (Fig. 37–8). There may be a similar reverse chain reaction with disruption of internal labyrinthine membranes (basilar and Reissner's), resulting in hearing loss, vertigo, and tinnitus. Friedman and Sasaki (5) recently reported two cases of hearing loss following resuscitation attempts secondary to positive pressure mask ventilation. In at least one patient, excessive pressure transmitted rapidly through the eustachian tube is postulated as an implosive route for damage.

Surgical intratympanic exploration has clearly demonstrated perilymphatic fistulas in a number of cases. In some, the physical exertion or barotrauma history was clear-cut, but in others such a history was vague. Labyrinthine window ruptures with sudden severe cochlear hearing loss with or without vertigo and tinnitus have been observed in deep-sea divers, unrelated to nitrogen embolization. Similar responses to aircraft travel have been noted. Physical exertion such as heavy lifting or unusual exercise have also been reported.

Demonstration of oval window and/or round window fistulas surgically is a definite finding, which can be recorded photographically and is thus a departure from the theoretical aspects of the idiopathic syndrome etiology. However, the presence of a fistula observed through middle-ear exploration *does not* solve the diagnostic dilemma. One knows only of a labyrinthine membrane rupture at the interface of the labyrinthine membrane and middle ear, but there is no recordable objective evidence of possible *critical intralabyrinthine* membrane lesions that are the most likely causes of serious cochlear damage. A limited oval or round window fistula should produce *only* a mild to moderate hearing loss, with little or no evidence of cochlear damage, and with preservation of high speech discrimination scores. But intralabyrinthine fistulas and other lesions undoubtedly cause the severe cochlear losses and vestibular deficits en-

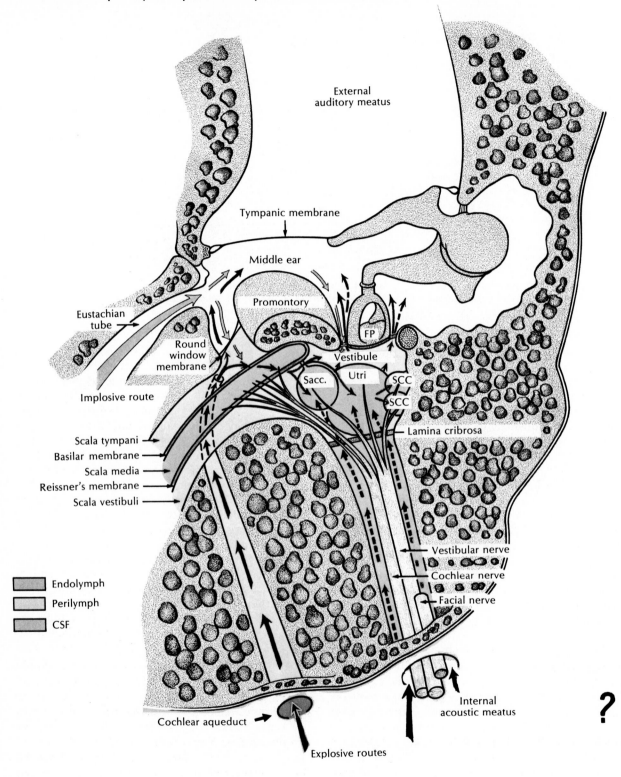

FIG. 37–6. Possible pathways of implosive and explosive forces in inner ear.

External
auditory meatus

Tympanic membrane

Middle ear

Promontory

Eustachian
tube

FP

Round
window
membrane

Vestibule

Implosive route

Sacc.

Utri

SCC

SCC

Scala tympani

Lamina cribrosa

Basilar membrane

Scala media

Reissner's membrane

Scala vestibuli

Vestibular nerve

Cochlear nerve

Facial nerve

Endolymph

Perilymph

CSF

Cochlear aqueduct

Internal
acoustic meatus

Explosive routes

?

Subarachnoid space
CSF

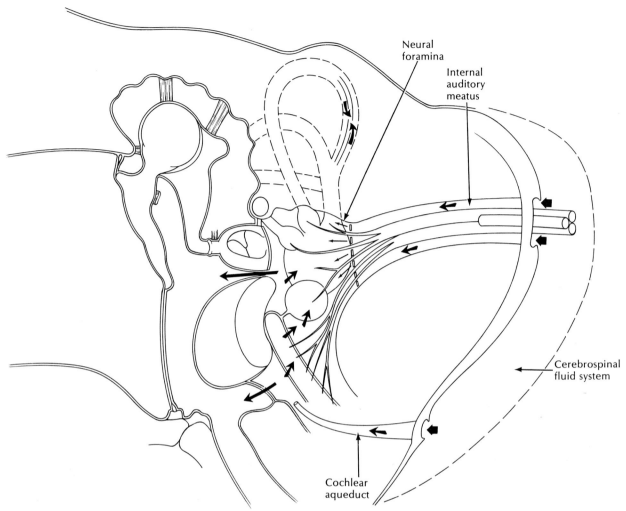

FIG. 37–7. Explosive routes for labyrinthine membrane ruptures from CSF system via cochlear aqueduct or internal auditory meatus. (Goodhill V: Proc Roy Soc Med 69:565–572, 1976)

countered in many cases of sudden SNHL. Thus, the surgical demonstration of fistula does not *per se* complete the etiologic explanation.

CLINICAL ASPECTS

BASIC HISTORY COMMON IN BOTH SYNDROME GROUPS

Spontaneous sudden cochlear hearing loss (usually unilateral) may be mild, moderate, or severe in degree. It may occur alone, or it may be preceded, accompanied, or followed by vertigo. Tinnitus is frequently present. Ataxia has also been reported (13).

The patient with sudden cochlear hearing loss usually requests examination within hours or days of onset. However, a week or more may have elapsed. Occasionally, patients will not be seen for weeks or months following onset.

The term "sudden" may be used by the patient in various ways. It may be described *exactly*, with onset at a precise time (*e.g.*, "I lost my hearing at 12:15 P.M. yesterday"), or the time of onset may be vague (*e.g.*, "I lost my hearing last Tuesday or Wednesday—I think"). In a significant number of patients, the loss comes on at night and is first noted upon arising in the morning. In general, however, the event is rather specifically time-linked.

The patient may emphasize the tinnitus as a

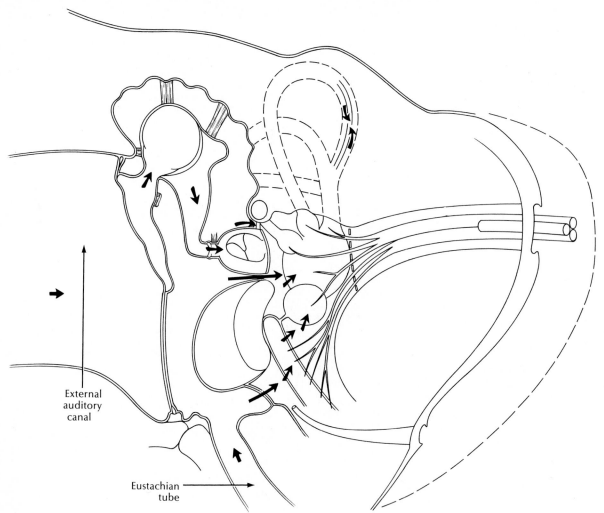

FIG. 37–8. Implosive routes for labyrinthine membrane ruptures from middle ear, eustachian tube, and external ear.

major complaint with secondary reference to the hearing loss, regardless of its severity. Many patients become aware of the hearing loss only after an attempt is made to use the telephone. There is either no response at all to telephone use or severe distortion attributed to the tinnitus by the patient.

Vertigo may accompany the onset of hearing loss and tinnitus, but more often it follows by hours or days. It may be the only symptom. It may vary from a mild "giddy" feeling to severe true vertigo, with spontaneous nystagmus, nausea, and vomiting, or ataxia.

In addition to hearing loss, tinnitus, and vertigo, frequent complaints include a "dead feeling," a "numbness," or a "hollowness" in the affected ear. Slight pain and/or a feeling of itching deep in the

ear occur in some patients. Since clinically the findings are the same, however the patient describes the symptoms, the following additional special syndrome histories are very important.

SPECIAL SYNDROME HISTORIES

Idiopathic Syndrome Histories

In idiopathic syndrome cases there are negative and positive history correlations with labyrinthine membrane rupture syndrome.

In idiopathic (presumably) viral cases, the patient may distinctly give a history of "flu," "cold," upper respiratory infection, sore throat, sinusitis, allergy flare-up, "virus," exposure to family, or work-related contacts with individuals who had "virus infections." The exposure may antedate the hearing loss by several weeks.

In idiopathic (presumably) *vascular* cases the patient may give a history of previous cardiac or hypertensive disease, with or without anticoagulation (heparin or warfarin sodium) therapy. There may be a history of diabetes, arteriosclerosis, hypercholesterolemia, hyperlipidemia, or other systemic disease involving microvasculature.

In other idiopathic cases the patient will give no significant history antedating the onset. There may be nothing to suggest either viral or vascular etiology, and there is no history of barotrauma or physical exertion.

No history of barotrauma (ordinary diving, snorkel or scuba diving, or aircraft flight) is elicited in idiopathic syndrome patients. Such patients will also deny any unusual preceding relationships to physical stress, such as lifting, coughing, sneezing, difficult micturition or defecation, or sexual intercourse. The onset is noted without any preceding stress-related history.

Labyrinthine Membrane Rupture Histories

In most but not all cases of labyrinthine membrane rupture (LMR), there is a clear-cut history of a specific physical event followed immediately or later by a sudden cochlear hearing loss.

The event may be stress or exertion related to barotrauma (swimming, diving, snorkel or scuba diving, or unusual aircraft travel incidents). The hearing loss may have followed lifting, coughing, sneezing, difficult micturition or defecation, intercourse, or any other physical exertion; a severe acoustic trauma episode may have preceded the onset of symptoms.

In sudden SNHL following diving, the differential diagnosis must include consideration of nitrogen embolization, which may pose a difficult problem. However, if there are no constitutional (nonotologic) symptoms of nitrogen sickness ("bends," etc.) a LMR etiology should be strongly considered (22).

The barotrauma, exertion, or physical stress history may not have seemed unusual for the patient, and thus the potential relationship may not be volunteered. The relationship of stress to hearing loss may be clearly remembered by the patient or completely ignored. Careful history and detailed questioning are required to elicit such possible cause-effect relationships. The history described in idiopathic syndrome cases may be identical to that in LMR syndrome cases, thus posing a difficult diagnostic dilemma.

DIFFERENTIAL DIAGNOSTIC STUDIES IN ALL CASES

The clinical findings of sudden SNHL and tinnitus, with or without vertigo or ataxia, may be identical in both types of SNHL syndromes. Because of these great similarities, a definitive clinical diagnosis is not easily made. In general, the clinical impression must be a presumptive one, *primarily in terms of history*.

In some cases the history will be suggestive of idiopathic syndrome SNHL, and in other cases an LMR syndrome SNHL may appear likely. However, such guidelines may not be diagnostic and may even lead to premature false clinical conclusions and inappropriate management.

Specific detailed otologic and general medical histories and physical examinations are necessary.

History

OTOLOGIC HISTORY. A detailed otologic history should be obtained concerning previous ear problems or surgery, previous ear examinations, vertigo, or tinnitus experiences. Inquiry is made into the possibility of trauma or noise exposure, or a family history of deafness.

MEDICAL HISTORY. Medical history-taking should include previous general medical problems, cardio-circulatory disease, anticoagulant drug intake, ototoxic drug use, recent viral, or bacterial upper respiratory infections, related infections or contacts, and recent unexplained fever, chills, or malaise.

Examination

OTOLOGIC EXAMINATION. Complete otologic examination should include otoscopy, standard audiologic tests, special cochlear-retrocochlear auditory test battery, tympanometry, stapedius reflex, and vestibular ENG studies, cranial nerve and basic neurologic examination, as well as screening Schuller and Stenver view radiographs.

MEDICAL EXAMINATION. Medical examination should include special search for bradycardia, arrhythmia, and other cardiac and circulatory problems; bruits; and urine and blood studies, including sedimentation rate, and FTA-ABS tests. Special studies for hypercoagulation, lipidemia, hyperviscosity, and macroglobulinemia and other syndromes may be indicated. The primary purpose of this medical study is to elicit possible clues to idiopathic syndrome etiology.

OTOLOGIC FINDINGS COMMON IN BOTH SYNDROME GROUPS

Otoscopic findings usually show normal tympanic membranes. Audiologic findings usually show moderate, severe, or total SNHL. In most instances of severe loss there is no hearing in the middle and upper ranges, with only a few low-frequency residual responses. If there is sufficient residual hearing for a Bekesy study, a type II or type III Bekesy tracing is found. Very rarely is a type IV Bekesy tracing encountered. Acoustic bridge impedance studies will show normal (occasionally high) impedance, normal tympanometry curves, and positive stapedial reflex on the involved side. There is usually an absent reflex in the opposite (normal ear) side. The audiologic findings are usually cochlear on the differential cochlear-retrocochlear test battery.

Vestibular studies show varied responses. Caloric responses are frequently abnormal. The spectrum may vary from minor labyrinthine preponderance to end-organ paralysis. There may or may not be spontaneous or positional nystagmus. Torsion swing (sinusoidal rotation) studies usually show restricted and asymmetric responses.

Radiographic findings are important in ruling out definitive mastoid or petrous pyramid lesions, but they are usually noncontributory in differentiation between idiopathic and LMR syndromes.

MANAGEMENT

PAST MANAGEMENT APPROACHES

The management of sudden cochlear hearing loss, unrelated to recognizable specific ear lesions, has been based entirely upon idiopathic and presumptive etiologic concepts and on empiric therapeutic theories. Presumptive diagnoses of vascular cochlear accident, viral disease, endocrine, autoimmune, or allergic causes have been made, and empiric nonspecific treatment has been advised. Single or multiple modalities have been in use, including vasodilators, steroids, hyperbaric oxygen therapy, vitamins, IV procaine, IV histamine, adenosine triphosphate, other drugs, and surgical procedures, such as stellate ganglion blocks (2) used on empiric grounds. No single definitive therapeutic approach has been in general use. On the contrary, so-called "shotgun therapy" has been and continues to be normative. In recent years most investigators have been stressing the greater value of steroid therapy in most idiopathic varieties of sudden hearing loss.

SPONTANEOUS RECOVERY AND THE TREATMENT EVALUATION DILEMMA

Among the difficulties in assessing both presumptive diagnoses and empiric therapies are the frequent spontaneous recoveries noted in many patients who have had no treatment. Such recovery may be partial or total and may occur within a matter of hours, days, weeks, or months. Controlled statistics comparing untreated and treated patients are virtually nonexistent. In idiopathic syndrome cases, the etiology must usually be considered presumptive, and only the idiopathic label is realistic. Objective etiology can be confirmed surgically in some LMR syndrome cases, but even in such cases, as in idiopathic syndrome cases, the final definitive answer must await postmortem temporal bone histopathologic studies.

Only in surgically explored LMR syndrome cases does some objective information begin to emerge regarding etiology and therapy. When an otosurgeon sees a definitive oval or round window fistula, or both, in sudden hearing loss cases, and monitors the results of surgery by otologic-audiologic studies, it becomes possible to introduce some objectivity into etiology and therapy. Such data are by no means sufficient for evaluating the total labyrinthine membrane status, which must await adequate postmortem temporal bone histopathologic studies. Needless to say, even marginal objectivity is lacking in the evaluation of etiology and therapy in the larger idiopathic syndrome group.

OUR PRESENT MANAGEMENT APPROACH

The current management approach in our clinic is based upon an evaluation of the history and findings, and on an attempt to divide cases into idiopathic and LMR syndrome groups, primarily on the basis of otologic history and general medical findings. There are no conclusive otologic examination differences between the two syndromes.

The management pattern is based upon 1) those aspects of idiopathic syndrome history and general medical findings that indicate a likely etiology, and 2) those aspects of LMR syndrome history that strongly suggest the possibility of labyrinth membrane rupture.

Every patient with a sudden spontaneous cochlear hearing loss is considered to be an otologic emergency.

MANAGEMENT OF MILD TO MODERATE SUDDEN SNHL CASES

All patients with mild to moderate losses (30–50 dB SRT, 40–80% SDS) with either syndrome possibility are placed at bedrest at home with head elevated 30° and allowed out of bed only for necessary attendance at the clinic for otologic and/or general medical diagnostic studies. No physical stress (exercise, sexual activity, walking, or sports) is allowed. Only bathroom privileges are allowed. No initial medication other than necessary tranquilizers and sedatives are advised during the work up period. In every case of sudden SNHL, complete otologic, radiologic, vestibular and internal medical studies are necessary. Every attempt is made to find a specific otologic cause such as chronic otomastoiditis with fistula, suppurative labyrinthitis, internal auditory meatus or cerebellopontine angle lesions, previous ear surgery, ear trauma, or head trauma. If a definitive otologic cause can be elicited, appropriate management is carried out. If no such otologic cause can be elicited, thorough general medical studies are carried out to elicit possible factors such as viral, vascular, drug, and other "idiopathic" medical causes. Occasionally, unsuspected problems such as clotting defects, bradycardia, auricular fibrillation, vascular occlusions, and other definitive general medical conditions are discovered. If there is no suggestive LMR history, the idiopathic syndrome is suspected, and the presumption is made that there is a relationship between the recognized general medical condition and the hearing loss, and appropriate medical therapies are instituted. In those patients in whom ENT and/or general examination suggests recent viral or bacterial upper respiratory infection, empiric broad-spectrum antimicrobial therapy is started and changed, when possible, to specific antibiotic therapy, if pathogenic bacterial organisms can be cultured from the nasopharynx, nose, or sinuses. If there is no medical contraindication, a course of empiric ACTH or prednisone therapy may be started.

The patient is asked to avoid physical exercise in spite of an apparent systemic etiology. Such systemic lesions may or may not be etiologically related to the sudden SNHL lesion. Conversely, a specific history of barotrauma or physical stress does not necessarily prove a LMR etiologic relationship. When very definitive circulatory upper respiratory diseases, or other possible general medical conditions are discovered and appropriate treatment is instituted, prompt beginning improvement in hearing may be noted in a few days. General supportive therapy includes high vitamin B and C intake, avoidance of tobacco, caffeine, alcohol, salicylates, and the common allergenic foods (milk, chocolate, nuts, shellfish) that might contribute to membrane edema. Audiometric evaluations should be done every 3–4 days to monitor hearing levels. If significant serial audiometric gain is demonstrated, this conservative therapy is continued until audiometric findings show a return of hearing to within normal limits. Thus, if the hearing return reaches a level of 20–25 dB with 70–80% SDS, no further treatment is considered necessary, unless the intensity of vertigo and/or tinnitus continues. Such clinical improvement following nonspecific management may not be accompanied by a precise final etiologic diagnosis.

If there is no spontaneous improvement in hearing in a mild to moderate case of idiopathic syndrome following 7–8 days, a course of empiric corticosteroid therapy is advisable. If the hearing does not remain stable but continues to drop in both SRT and SDS measurements, and/or if there is increased tinnitus intensity and/or if increased vestibular symptoms occur, the management should be changed as follows.

MANAGEMENT OF UNRESPONSIVE OR SEVERE TOTAL SUDDEN SNHL CASES

Idiopathic Syndrome Cases

Those patients with idiopathic syndrome with severe or total losses (80–100 dB SRT, 0–30% SDS), or those with moderate hearing loss who are nonresponsive and show no improvement on empiric medical therapy, including corticosteroid therapy and bedrest at home for 7–10 days, are hospitalized and placed at absolute bedrest with no lavatory privileges, with head elevated 30°. The course of corticosteroid treatment is continued to completion. If there is no beginning hearing gain as measured by bedside audiometry after 3–4 days of such hospitalization (total of 12–14 days), surgical exploration should be considered, in spite of the absence of history suggestive of LMR.

LMR Syndrome Cases

In LMR syndrome cases with severe or total loss (80–100 dB SRT 0–30% SDS), the patient is immediately hospitalized and kept at absolute bedrest with head elevated at 30°. Hospital medical con-

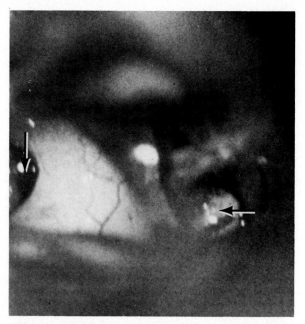

FIG. 37–9. Oval **(horizontal arrow)** and round window **(vertical arrow)** fistulas in same ear, a common occurrence in sudden hearing loss due to LMR. Oval window fistula **(anterior)** is sealed by perichondrium; perilymph and blood are present in round window fistula.

FIG. 37–10. Round window fistula **(arrow).** Niche contains perichondrium supported by absorbable gelatin sponge. Some fluid from accompanying oval window fistula can be seen on promontory; note increased vascularity.

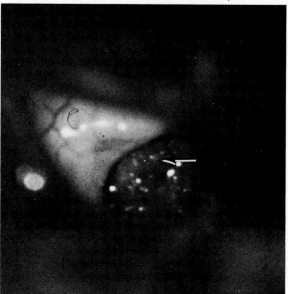

sultation is secured in the search for possible unrecognized vascular, viral, or other systemic diseases. Daily bedside audiograms are done. If the LMR syndrome diagnosis appears tenable on the basis of a significant physical stress history, and if the general medical history and findings are completely negative, the likelihood of membrane rupture is considered to be significant and early surgical exploration is indicated. No absolute guidelines can be laid down for the timing of surgical exploration, but in our experience it seems that it should be considered within the first 10–12 days following the physical stress episode.

SURGICAL TECHNIQUE—LABYRINTH WINDOW EXPLORATION AND REPAIR

Adult patients undergo operation under endomeatal block anesthesia using lidocaine, 1.5% with epinephrine 1,200,000. In children, basal narcosis or general anesthesia is used in conjunction with local anesthesia. An endomeatal tympanotomy in the anterior surgical position (see Ch. 12, Basic Otosurgical Procedures) facilitates visualization of both oval and round window niches.

The oval window exploration is directed first to the incudostapedial joint (partial dislocation may be present), then to the stapes footplate and to the stapedial annular ligament. A slow, patient examination, over a period of several minutes may be necessary to detect a perilymph fistula in some cases. Fibrous webs are frequent clues to the presence of a fistula in the area surrounding the stapedial arch (Fig. 37–9) and should be carefully sectioned. Special attention is then paid to the region of the fissula ante fenestram, the obturator foramen area, the footplate, and the footplate marginal ligamentous region. The appearance of a perilymphatic leak is comparable to that seen in poststapedectomy fistulas (see Ch. 19, Otosclerosis). The fluid may be very copious or extremely scant. Visible clear fluid is gently aspirated with a fine suction tip and the site is observed for refilling with fluid to confirm an active perilymph fistula. In small leaks, observation of the "blotter soaking" effect on dry, compressed, absorbable gelatin sponge squares is useful. If a "leak" is found, the mucoperiosteum surrounding the annular ligament is elevated for placement of tragal perichondrium autograft squares (1 × 1 mm) to cover the fistulous area. Prompt diminution in rate of perilymph flow is usually noted following graft placement, although the flow may continue during the entire exploration.

Exploration of the round window niche also begins with a search for fibrous webs. Gentle sectioning of such webs may be necessary in some cases to demonstrate a definitive fistula. In other cases there may be no webs and the clear fluid will refill within the round window niche very rapidly following suction. Gentle palpation of the stapes to elicit a round window reflex may demonstrate the precise source of the round window membrane fistula. Brief ipsilateral, contralateral, and/or bilateral jugular vein compressions will frequently evoke visualization of a small fistula not otherwise demonstrable. Complete visualization of the entire circumferential area of the round window membrane with its cone-shaped topography is rarely possible. A true hole in the round window membrane is rarely seen and should not be sought, because of danger of great damage to the scala tympani. In grafting the round window niche (Fig. 37–10), usually one large perichondrial graft is used (1.5 × 2.5 mm). Niche bone removal is only rarely necessary.

After completion of the tympanotomy procedure the patient is kept at absolute bedrest with head elevated 30° for a period of 48 hours. Upon returning home, the patient is restricted to sedentary activity for 10 days. Prophylactic broad-spectrum antibiotics are prescribed for 10 days after the operation. The patient is restricted from air travel, from mountain trips, and from strenuous physical activity for at least several months, and diving is completely prohibited. These restrictions are obviously empiric. With longer periods of observation, more precise and realistic guidelines for long-term management will emerge.

RESULTS OF LABYRINTH WINDOW FISTULA SURGERY

In 1973, we reported (9) a total of 21 sudden hearing loss cases that had been explored surgically, in which 15 fistulas were found. In March 1976 (8), I reported a total number of 76 cases, which included 59 surgical explorations; fistulas were found in 47 cases. No fistulas were found in 12 cases. The remaining 17 cases were not explored surgically but were managed medically.

Among the 47 patients with fistulas, all had hearing loss; tinnitus was present in 37, and vertigo in 24.

Of the 47 patients, 29 were males and 18 were females. The age distribution was 3 patients in the 11–20 year group, 13 patients in the 21–40 year group, 23 patients in the 41–60 year group; and 8 patients in the 61–72 year group.

Of great interest is the continued evidence of left ear preponderance, which we described in 1973 (9). Of the 47 fistulas, 14 occurred in right ears and 33 in left ears, a more than 2:1 left ear preponderance.

In the 12 patients without fistulas, 5 had hearing loss in the right ear and 7 in the left ear, with no significant right/left difference.

With reference to site of fistula, only 4 of the 47 were in the round window alone, 19 were in round and oval windows combined, and 24 were in the oval window alone. This is in contrast to some misconceptions that limit fistula consideration to the round window. In our series, the round window was the least significant site appearing alone.

Hearing results in the 47 surgically explored cases with fistulas showed that 12 patients (25%) had SRT gains of more than 30 dB and SDS gains of more than 50%. In 9 patients (18.75%) the gains were only slight, and the majority of patients (26, 62%) showed no gains.

In the 12 patients (25%) with significant gains, explorations were carried out in almost all in the first 13 days. Of the larger group with no gains, the intervals between exploration and onset ranged from 15 days to several years.

Of the 12 patients explored with no fistula, only one showed a significant spontaneous gain.

Among the 47 patients with fistulas, a history of stress was obtained in 29.

Of the 76 in the entire series, 17 patients served as medical management controls.

There were stress histories in 6 of the 17. Because spontaneous hearing improvements in this group were relatively rapid, no surgery was performed. Of these 17 patients, 13 had significant gains, and 4 had no gains. These patients were managed primarily with bed rest. Prednisone was used in 4.

The work on LMR syndrome is still in an early stage. We have found no fistula when a fistula had been expected. In some, there were findings of oval and/or round window fibrosis with no fluid. It is possible that a fistula had healed spontaneously with no improvement in hearing, the hearing loss having been caused by major irreversible intralabyrinthine membrane lesions. In most cases with proven fistulas and surgical repair, there were no hearing improvements, probably also because of coexisting major intralabyrinthine membrane lesions. Time delay was present in almost all of the patients who showed no improvement.

In some patients with clear-cut stress histories and no other positive medical findings, hearing improvements began spontaneously in the hospital before planned surgery. Such patients showed varying degrees of hearing return without any treatment other than bed rest.

Clearly, the problem is complex. The major cochlear hearing losses cannot be explained adequately on the basis of window membrane ruptures alone. We have previously reported recovery of hearing following surgical repair of oval window fistulas in combined conductive-cochlear losses in poststapedectomy oval window fistulas. It is obvious that major cochlear hearing losses must be due to complex intralabyrinthine membrane lesions that accompany oval and/or round window labyrinth membrane ruptures. The observation of a fistula in the round or oval window membrane in a given case does not answer profound questions relating to the fates of basilar membrane, Reissner's membrane, tectorial membrane, hair cells, supporting structures, stria vascularis, and other intracochlear structures (Fig. 37–11).

Recurrent fistulas have occurred in our experience either spontaneously or in response to new physical exertion or barotrauma factors, and have been reexplored and regrafted. What will be the long-range results in these ears which have been diagnosed and successfully grafted surgically? We do not know.

The recognition of the idiopathic syndrome group calls for much investigative work. Studies are now underway to assess relationships between cochlear aqueduct, scala tympani, and round window membrane. It is possible that such membrane ruptures occur slowly or intermittently in previously unrecognized nonspecific cases loosely categorized as SNHL—etiology unknown.

LONG-RANGE FOLLOW-UP CONSIDERATIONS

In all patients in whom no improvement was noted, regardless of management or findings, long-range follow-up is advisable.

The differential diagnosis of sudden cochlear hearing loss idiopathic and LMR syndromes requires repeated considerations of a number of etiologic factors other than the viral, vascular, nonspecific miscellaneous, and labyrinthine window membrane rupture causes. For example, it is possible for an internal auditory meatus or cerebellopontine angle tumor to suddenly enlarge, resulting in an increase from a minimal to a maximal hearing loss. Higgs (14) recently reported sudden hearing loss as the presenting first complaint in 4 of 44 cases of acoustic neurinoma.

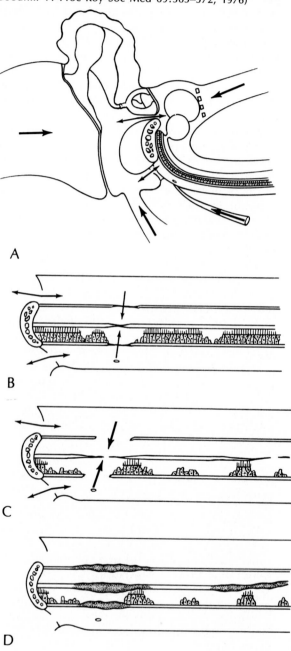

FIG. 37–11. Potential labyrinthine sequelae—theoretic possibilities. **A.** Diagram of explosive-plus-implosive rupture routes. **B.** Minor intralabyrinthine lesion with minimal damage to organ of Corti. **C.** Major ruptures with persistent intracochlear fistulas. **D.** Healed intracochlear lesions. (Goodhill V: Proc Roy Soc Med 69:565–572, 1976)

A

B

C

D

Although, Stenver radiographs of the internal auditory meatus (as well as Schuller mastoid radiographs) are considered part of the diagnostic test battery in the evaluation of every case, it will probably be wise to consider long-range follow-up with polytome radiographs and possibly consider computerized axial tomography (CAT) scans and cerebellopontine angle myelograms in those patients in whom a definitive diagnosis has not been made, following medical or surgical management, and in whom there was no improvement in hearing, tinnitus, or vestibular symptoms.

A patient may actually think that a hearing loss has occurred suddenly when, in effect, a slight loss with no subjective awareness simply became suddenly worse. It is possible that this phenomenon may happen to a patient who had previous cochlear hydrops (Meniere's disease without vertigo) with a very slight subclinical hearing loss which suddenly became worse. A patient with mild, episodic transient ischemic attacks may have a new severe transient ischemic attack with a lesion restricted to a cochlear vessel. These and other facts must be kept in mind in the continuing differential diagnosis of sudden hearing loss in patients who experienced no hearing improvement after either medical or surgical treatment.

Whether other etiologic factors are involved, which may require different managements, only time and further research will tell. It is obvious that the problem of sudden cochlear hearing loss is still in an early stage of study.

The division of the problem into idiopathic and LMR syndrome categories is important in the diagnostic approach to sudden SNHL lesions. The definitive demonstrations of perilymphatic fistulas into the middle ear in sudden hearing loss cases cannot be ignored in sudden cochlear hearing loss, even if the precise intracochlear sequelae cannot be elucidated now. When a fistula is demonstrated, surgical closure of the fistula is mandatory. Closures of perilymphatic fistulas are definitely indicated, regardless of unanswered intralabyrinthine membrane questions, whether spontaneous, due to head injury or ear injury, post stapedectomy, following other ear surgery, and/or other ear diseases. Proven round or oval window fistulas in sudden hearing loss cases require surgical closure with tissue grafts. One cannot ignore the possible dangers of open routes for subsequent transmission of infection to the labyrinth and to the subarachnoid space, as already documented in meningitis following poststapedectomy fistula (see Ch. 19, Otosclerosis).

SUMMARY

1. The patient with sudden spontaneous cochlear hearing loss unrelated to specific demonstrable otologic disease should be considered an otologic emergency.
2. Complete otologic, audiologic, vestibular, and radiologic studies are necessary, accompanied by a complete medical examination.
3. Two basic syndromes may be delineated, idiopathic syndrome (viral, vascular, or unknown) and labyrinthine membrane rupture (LMR) syndrome (labyrinth window membrane ruptures associated with barotrauma, physical stresses).
4. Idiopathic syndrome cases require joint otologic and general medical management.
5. Past empiric therapy for idiopathic syndrome cases must be subjected to critical evaluation; this is impossible with contemporary "shotgun" therapy.
6. Oval and round window labyrinthine membrane fistulas have been demonstrated surgically in a number of LMR syndrome cases.
7. LMR syndrome cases may heal spontaneously with spontaneous hearing improvement; if not, exploratory labyrinthine window surgery is indicated.
8. Surgical fistula repair procedures in LMR syndrome cases must be subjected to long-term critical evaluation.
9. The problem is extremely complex etiologically, pathologically, and therapeutically. Definitive information is only beginning to accumulate. Much further research is necessary.
10. At the present state of our knowledge, if it has been determined that a labyrinthine membrane rupture etiology exists, valuable surgical time should not be lost when there is the possibility of successful repair of the rupture. However, it is not possible to state with certainty what these quantitative time factors are at this early stage of our surgical experiences in dealing with LMR etiology in the sudden SNHL syndrome.

REFERENCES

1. Beentjes BIJ: On the Pressure of the Endolymphatic, the Perilymphatic, and the Cerebrospinal Fluid, with Data on the Endolymphatic Membranes. Experiments on Cats and Guinea Pigs. Haarlem, Henkes Holland NV, 1970, pp 1–68

2. de B Cocks AS: Sudden deafness. J Laryngol 77: 430–436, 1963

3. Fee GA: Traumatic perilymphatic fistulas. Arch Otolaryngol 88:477–480, 1968

4. Fraser JG, Harborow PC: Labyrinthine window rupture. J Laryngol 89:1–7, 1975

5. Friedman SI, Sasaki CT: Hearing loss during resuscitation. Arch Otolaryngol 101:385–386, 1975

6. Freeman P, Edmonds C: Inner ear barotrauma. Arch Otolaryngol 95:556–563, 1972

7. Goodhill V: Sudden deafness and round window rupture. Laryngoscope 81:1462–1474, 1971

8. Goodhill V: Labyrinthine membrane ruptures in sudden sensorineural hearing loss. Proc R Soc Med (Engl) 69:565–572, 1976

9. Goodhill V, Harris I, Brockman SJ et al.: Sudden deafness and labyrinthine window ruptures. Ann Otol Rhinol Laryngol 82:2–12, 1973

10. Gussen R: Arachnoid villi obstruction in the cochlear aqueduct. Arch Otolaryngol 96:565–569, 1972

11. Gussen R: Sudden deafness of vascular origin: A human temporal bone study. Ann Otol Rhinol Laryngol 85:94–100, 1976

12. Harker LA, Norante JD, Ryu JH: Experimental ruptures of the round window membrane. Trans Am Acad Ophthalmol Otolaryngol 78:ORL 448–ORL 452, 1974

13. Healey GB, Friedman JM, Strong MS: Vestibular and auditory findings of perilymphatic fistula. A review of 40 cases. Trans Am Acad Ophthalmol Otolaryngol 82:ORL 44–ORL 49, 1976

14. Higgs WA: Sudden deafness as the presenting symptom of acoustic neurinoma. Arch Otolaryngol 98:73–76, 1973

15. Kerth JD, Allen GW: Comparison of the perilymphatic and cerebrospinal fluid pressures. Arch Otolaryngol 77:581–585, 1963

16. Kobrak H: Untersuchungen uber den Zusammenhang Zwischen Hirndruck und Labyrinthdruck. Beitr Prakt Theoret Hals-Nasen-Ohrenheilk 31:216, 1934

17. Lawrence M, McCabe B: Inner ear mechanics and deafness. Special considerations of Meniere's syndrome. JAMA 171:1927, 1959

18. Lawrence M, Nuttall A, Burgio P: Cochlear potentials and oxygen associated with hypoxia. Ann Otol Rhinol Laryngol 84:499–512, 1975

18a. Moscovitch DH, Gannon RP, Laszlo CA: Perilymph Displacement by Cerebrospinal Fluid in the Cochlea. Ann Otol Rhinol Laryngol 82:53–61, 1973

19. Nedzelski JM, Barber HO: Round window fistula. J Otolaryngol 5:379–385, 1976

20. Palva T: Cochlear aqueduct in infants. Acta Otolaryngol (Stockh) 70:83–94, 1970

21. Palva T, Dammert K: Human cochlear aqueduct. Acta Otolaryngol [Suppl] (Stockh) #246, 1969

22. Pang LQ: Sudden sensorineural hearing loss following diving. Trans Am Acad Ophthalmol Otolaryngol 78:ORL 436–ORL 442, 1974

23. Pullen FW: Round window membrane rupture: a cause of sudden deafness. Trans Am Acad Ophthalmol Otolaryngol 76:1444–1450, 1972

24. Sando I, Masuda Y, Wood RP et al.: Perilymphatic communication routes in guinea pig cochlea. Ann Otol Rhinol Laryngol 80:826–834, 1971

25. Saxena RK, Tandon PN, Sinha A et al.: Auditory functions in raised intracranial pressure. Acta Otolaryngol (Stockh) 68:402–410, 1969

26. Schuknecht H, Neff W, Perlman H: An experimental study of auditory damage following blows to the head. Ann Otol Rhinol Laryngol 60:273–289, 1951

27. Simmons FB: Theory of membrane breaks in sudden hearing loss. Arch Otolaryngol 88:41–48, 1968

28. Stroud MH, Calcaterra TC: Spontaneous perilymph fistulas. Laryngoscope 80:479–487, 1970

29. Tonkin JP, Fagan P: Rupture of the round window membrane. J Laryngol 89:733–756, 1975

30. Waltner JG: Barrier membrane of the cochlear aqueduct. Histologic studies on the patency of the cochlear aqueduct. Arch Otolaryngol 47:656–669, 1948

SUGGESTED READING

Byl P: Thirty two cases of sudden profound hearing loss (SPHL) occuring in 1973: incidence and prognostic findings. Trans Am Acad Ophthalmol Otolaryngol 80:ORL 298–ORL 305, 1975

Donaldson JA: Fossula of the cochlear fenestra. Arch Otolaryngol 88:124–130, 1968

Faltýnek L, Veselý C: Zum Problem du Plötezlich entslantenen ein seitigen Schallempfindungssch—werhörigkeit. Monatsch Ohren Laryngol Rhinol 101:201–208, 1967

Goodhill V: The conductive loss phenomenon in post stapedectomy perilymphatic fistulas. Laryngoscope 77:1179–1190, 1967

Howard M: Complete round window fistula. Ear Nose Throat J 55:382–383, 1976

Lamm H, Klimpel L: Hyperbare Saverstaffth—erapie bei Innenohr—und Vestibularisstörungen. HNO 19:363–369, 1971

McCormick JG, Wever EG, Harrill JA et al.: Anatomical and physiological adaptations of marine mammals for the prevention of diving induced middle ear barotrauma and round window fistula. J Acoust Soc Am [Suppl] 58 (1):88, 1975

McGill T: Carcinomatous encephalomyelitis with auditory and vestibular manifestations. Ann Otol Rhinol Laryngol 85:120–126, 1976

Morrison AW: Sudden deafness. In Management of Sensorineural Deafness. London, Butterworths, 1975, pp 175–216

Nadol JB, Weiss AD, Parker SW: Vertigo of delayed onset after sudden deafness. Ann Otol Rhinol Laryngol 84:841–846, 1975

Nishida H, Kumagami H, Dohi K: Prognostic criteria of sudden deafness as deduced by electrocochleography. Arch Otolaryngol 102:601–607, 1976

Nozue M, Watanabe H, Yamada F: Sudden deafness due to jugular foramen tumor—Its neurological findings. ANLA 1:109–116, 1974

Sasaki CT, Bell D, Levine P: Barotrauma of the inner ear. Conn Med 39:214–215, 1975

Scarpa A: An anatomical observation on the round window. Sellers LM, Anson BJ (trans and ed). Arch Otolaryngol 75:2–45, 1961

Schuknecht HF: Pathology of the Ear. Cambridge, Harvard University Press, 1974, pp 473–479

Sung GS, Kamerer DB, Sung R: Perilymphatic fistula and its interest to audiologists. J Speech Hear Dis 41:540–546, 1976

Wilmot TJ: Sudden perceptive deafness in young people. J Laryngol 73:466–468, 1959

Wright JLW, Saunders SH: Sudden deafness following cardiopulmonary bypass surgery. J Laryngol 89:757–759, 1975

38

SYPHILIS OF THE TEMPORAL BONE

JOEL B. SHULMAN

Syphilis, "the great imitator," has long been recognized as a significant etiologic factor in otologic disease in the late stages of both congenital and acquired infection. The upsurge of diagnosed cases of lues during the 1960's has continued into this decade. Since this has for the most part affected individuals in the child-bearing age group, a corresponding increase of congenital infection can be expected.

Luetic involvement of the temporal bone may produce all varieties of conductive or sensorineural hearing loss and may imitate such diverse clinical entities as otosclerosis, Meniere's disease, toxic or viral labyrinthitis, or intracranial tumors. The subtlety and variability of the early symptoms present a formidable diagnostic challenge.

PATHOLOGY

Temporal bone histopathology in cases of congenital and acquired syphilis has been well documented by several authors (4, 5, 7, 12). The major changes may be summarized as follows:

1. Mononuclear leukocytic infiltration of the cochlea and spiral ganglion (Fig. 38–1).
2. Vascular lesions consisting of obliterative endarteritis in acquired cases and diapedesis in prenatal cases (Fig. 38–2).
3. Proliferative periostitis and osteomyelitis pro-

ducing replacement of endosteum by a thick fibrous connective tissue, followed by tissue invasion and even ossification of perilymphatic and endolymphatic spaces (Figs. 38–3 to 38–6).
4. Endolymphatic hydrops with later atrophy of the auditory and vestibular neuroepithelium.
5. Gummas, occurring more frequently in far advanced lesions
6. Bony abnormalities of the stapes, especially the footplate (Fig. 38–7).

With this constellation of pathologic changes, the protean clinical manifestations of temporal bone lues may be readily understood.

CLINICAL FEATURES

CONGENITAL

Deafness is commonly associated with congenital lues and, along with interstitial keratitis and malformed teeth, is part of Hutchinson's classic triad. Approximately one-third of patients have hearing problems (7). Otologic symptoms may appear any time from the first to the sixth decade and are highly variable with respect to the time of onset, type and degree of hearing loss, severity of vestibular symptoms, and rate of progression. When the onset is before the age of 10 (37%), bilaterally symmetrical profound hearing loss usually appears rather suddenly, unaccompanied by significant vestibular symptoms. Adult onset may be either gradual or sudden and is commonly characterized by asymmetrical fluctuating hearing loss with episodic vertigo indistinguishable from Meniere's disease. In females, hearing losses may be episodic, in association with menses; they may be associated with pregnancy, with dramatic losses during any trimester.

Although physical examination of the ear is usually normal, positive results of brief duration in a fistula test are frequently present without clinical evidence of middle ear disease (Hennebert's sign). In addition, high intensity sound, such as that of the Bárány noise box, may elicit vertigo with nystagmus (Tullio's phenomenon). Hennebert's and Tullio's signs are not limited to lues. They may be elicited in cases of semicircular canal fistula of any etiology, presumably due to perilymph movement between the oval window and the fistula resulting in cupular deviation. However, because Hennebert's sign has also been observed in endolymphatic hydrops resulting from other disorders without fistulas, it has been pro-

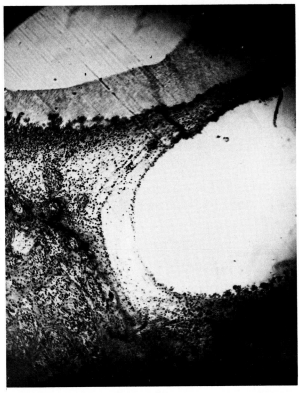

FIG. 38–1. Modiolar region of cochlea, showing lymphocytic infiltration extending along basilar membrane. (Goodhill V: Ann Otol Rhinol Laryngol 48:676–707, 1939)

FIG. 38–2. Hemorrhage into perilymphatic channel of semicircular canal. (Goodhill V: Ann Otol Rhinol Laryngol 48: 676–707, 1939)

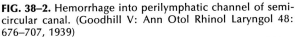

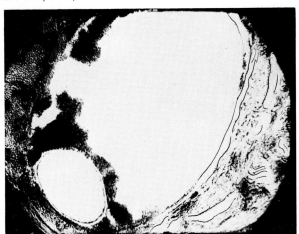

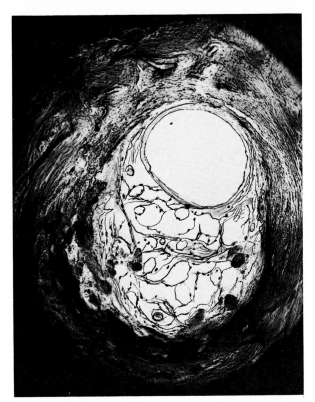

FIG. 38–3. Medial limb of superior semicircular canal showing early fibrosis and bony irregularity of perilymphatic lumen. (Goodhill V: Ann Otol Rhinol Laryngol 48:676–707, 1939)

FIG. 38–4. Medial limb of superior semicircular canal. Note triangular shape, a distortion resulting from luetic bone disease. (Goodhill V: Ann Otol Rhinol Laryngol 48:676–707, 1939)

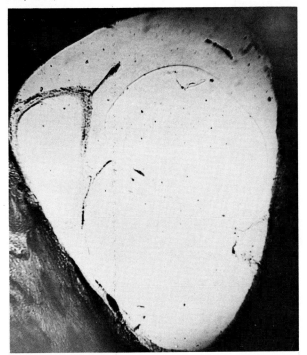

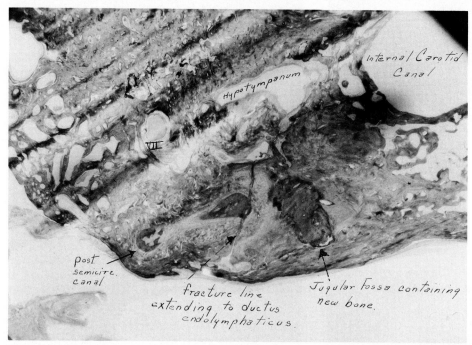

FIG. 38–5. Hypotympanum. The two limbs of posterior semicircular canal solidly cast in new bone, from which fracture line diverges, extending to ductus endolymphaticus. Superior level of jugular fossa also contains new bone. **VII,** seventh nerve. (Goodhill V: Ann Otol Rhinol Laryngol 48:676–707, 1939)

FIG. 38–6. Hypotympanum. Completely ossified ampulla of posterior semicircular canal **(arrow)** causing fracture of surrounding otic capsule. **VII,** seventh nerve. (Goodhill V: Ann Otol Rhinol Laryngol 48:676–707, 1939)

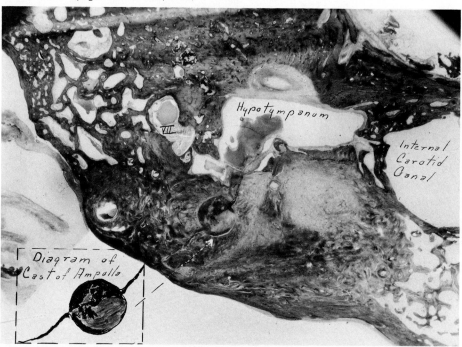

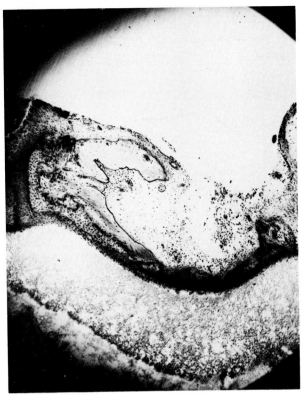

FIG. 38–7. Marked bowing of footplate of stapes with surrounding lymphocytic infiltration. (Goodhill V: Ann Otol Rhinol Laryngol 48:676–707, 1939)

FIG. 38–8. Audiogram of 26-year-old woman with congenital syphilis first diagnosed at age 6. At age 25 she first complained of fluctuating hearing loss and episodic vertigo. The fluctuating sensorineural hearing loss, worse for low frequencies, simulates Meniere's disease. (Karmody CS, Schuknecht HF: Arch Otolaryngol 83:18–27, 1966. Copyright 1966, American Medical Association)

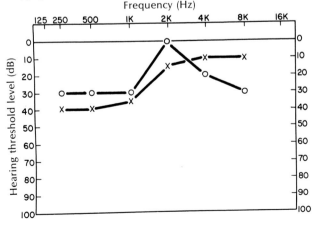

posed that movement of the vestibular membranous labyrinth by fibrous connections to the stapes footplate, rather than erosive fistulas, are responsible for these phenomena (16).

Audiometry typically shows a flat sensorineural hearing loss, although early in the course of the disease the deficit may be greater in the low frequencies. (Figs. 38–8 to 38–12). Middle ear involvement may produce a conductive component. Speech discrimination is usually poor in relation to pure tones and may fluctuate widely. Differential diagnostic audiometric tests most commonly indicate cochlear pathology. There is no characteristic finding on vestibular function tests, although caloric responses are usually depressed. The cerebrospinal fluid is ordinarily normal.

Kerr (8, 9) points out several clinical features that help and distinguish temporal bone lues from Meniere's disease. Meniere's disease is rare in childhood, involvement is unilateral in 80–90% of cases, and progression is usually less rapid. In congenital lues there may be a history of inflammatory eye disease or decreased visual acuity; the family history may contain evidence of decreased hearing, visual problems, miscarriages, or stillbirths; and physical examination often reveals other stigmas of the disease. Nevertheless, it must be emphasized that syphilis can never be ruled out on clinical grounds alone.

ACQUIRED

Otologic manifestations are less common in acquired infections but may occur from meningitis in secondary lues or, more commonly, in late tertiary lues (neurosyphilis). Clinical features are characterized by the same degree of variability as in congenital syphilis, but the cerebrospinal fluid is usually abnormal (pleocytosis, elevated protein, positive serology) (15).

SEROLOGIC DIAGNOSIS

Because of the protean clinical picture, the antemortem diagnosis of temporal bone syphilis depends primarily on serologic tests. Nontreponemal tests, such as the VDRL (flocculation) and Kolmer (compliment fixation) are negative in up to one-third of patients with untreated late or latent lues; therefore, these are of limited use to the otologist who deals with symptoms that occur most often in the late stages of the disease. Of much greater value, because of their specificity and immutability are the treponemal tests, including the *Treponema pallidum* immobilization (TPI) and more recently

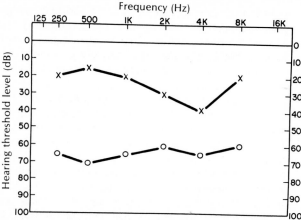

FIG. 38–9. Audiogram of 46-year-old woman, a known congenital syphilitic. At 34 years of age she developed tinnitus and depressed hearing in right ear, together with episodic vertigo. (Karmody CS, Schuknecht HF: Arch Otolaryngol 83:18–27, 1966. Copyright 1966, American Medical Association)

FIG. 38–10. Audiogram of 39-year-old woman. At age 24 she experienced sudden onset of vertigo and hearing loss on both sides. Examination revealed a dry central perforation on left side. Response to caloric tests was diminished. The Hinton test for syphilis was known to have been positive since the age of 12. (Karmody CS, Schuknecht HF: Arch Otolaryngol 83:18–27, 1966. Copyright 1966, American Medical Association)

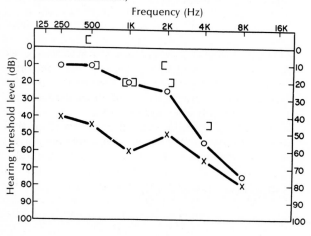

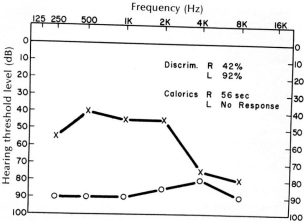

FIG. 38–11. Audiogram of 43-year-old man known to be a congenital luetic since the age of 10. At age 30 he noticed the onset of bilateral throbbing tinnitus, depressed hearing on both sides, and recurrent attacks of incapacitating vertigo. Response to ice-water stimulation was absent on left side—a finding more typical of acoustic neurinoma. (Karmody CS, Schuknecht HF: Arch Otolaryngol 83:18–27, 1966. Copyright 1966, American Medical Association)

FIG. 38–12. Audiogram of 17-year-old girl diagnosed as a congenital syphilitic in childhood. Audiograms show marked fluctuations in auditory thresholds over a 2-month period. (Karmody CS, Schuknecht HF: Arch Otolaryngol 83:18–27, 1966. Copyright 1966, American Medical Association)

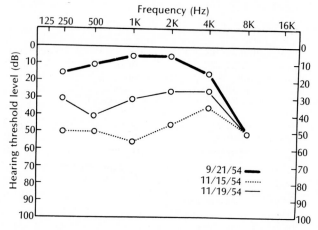

the fluorescent *Treponema* antibody-absorption (FTA-abs) test (Table 38–1).

The FTA-abs is the most sensitive test available in all stages of syphilis, with less than 5% false negative results (6). The TPI is slightly more specific and may be used to confirm the diagnosis in questionable cases, but because this test is technically difficult to perform well, it has been replaced in most laboratories by the FTA-abs (20).

Up to 6% false-positive FTA-abs test results are reported, but almost all these patients have increased or abnormal serum globulins (*e.g.*, collagen-vascular disease, autoimmune hemolytic anemias, alcoholic cirrhosis, and occasionally pregnancy). Thus, if the serologic reaction is 2+ or greater, and if the foregoing conditions can be ruled out, the diagnosis of syphilis should not be

TABLE 38-1. Reactivity of Tests for Syphilis

Stage	Test reactivity (%)	
	FTA-abs	VDRL
Primary	85	78
Secondary	99	97
Late	95	77
Latent	95	74
Presumably normal	1	0
Treated late or latent	95	60

(Sparling PF: N Engl J Med 284:642–653, 1971)

seriously questioned; borderline or 1+ reactions must be repeated (11). Pulec (14) has found a positive FTA-abs in 7% of patients with clinical diagnosis of Meniere's disease. Although the final decision must rest on clinical judgment, a patient with progressive or fluctuating hearing loss and reactive FTA-abs, assuming other conditions leading to false-positive tests have been ruled out, should be considered to have luetic involvement of the temporal bone and be treated accordingly.

TREATMENT

The usual recommended treatment for syphilis involving the central nervous system is 6–9 million units of penicillin in divided doses (3); tetracycline or erythromycin may be substituted in the penicillin-allergic patient. However, the notion that such regimens are invariably effective in eradicating syphilis has recently been challenged. Several investigators have found apparently viable treponemes in the body fluids and tissues of patients with late lues, despite previous intensive antibiotic therapy (2, 17). Spirochetes have been seen in temporal bone sections (10) and recovered from perilymph (21) of patients with congenital lues treated repeatedly with high doses of penicillin. Many of these observations are artifactual, and all are of questionable clinical significance because of the lack of controlled double-blind studies (18); nevertheless, it is alarmingly clear that hearing loss may occur in cases of late syphilis despite massive specific prior therapy, which neither prevents its onset nor retards its progression (13).

Penicillin (19) and ampicillin (8) do seem to reach the perilymph in treponemicidal levels, but the finding of spirochetes in the nearly avascular endochondrial bone of the otic capsule helps to explain the difficulty in treatment. Smith (17) puts forth the theory that treponemes may exist in a dormant state in late lues, multiplying perhaps only once in 60–90 days. Thus drugs such as penicillin, which exert their antibacterial effect only on dividing organisms, may not eradicate the spirochetes unless treatment is continued for at least 3 months.

Although therapy programs recommended for suspected temporal bone lues vary in detail, penicillin (or substitutes) and a corticosteroid administered in combination over a prolonged period seems the most effective (2, 13, 14, 18).

The regimen we have somewhat arbitrarily chosen is penicillin V, 1 g daily in divided doses orally, or weekly intramuscular injections of benzathine penicillin, 2,400,000 units for 3 months, and prednisone, 40 mg daily in divided doses for a minimum of 3 weeks. (Erythromycin or tetracycline is used in equivalent doses for patients allergic to penicillin.)

Audiograms are repeated weekly, and if significant improvement in thresholds or speech discrimination is achieved, the prednisone is slowly tapered to the smallest dose necessary to maintain the hearing level. Steroids are withdrawn if the 3-week trial period fails to bring about sufficient gain in hearing to warrant their continued use. Prior to beginning treatment, all patients must have a general medical checkup to rule out contraindications to the use of long-term steroids and must be prepared to accept the attendant risks.

With treatment, approximately 50% of patients will experience improvement or stabilization of hearing, especially speech discrimination scores; decreased pure-tone thresholds are less commonly achieved (13). Patients with recent deterioration seem to have better chance of amelioration than those with stable audiograms (15).

Serologic responses to treatment are undependable. When the VDRL test is positive, it usually becomes negative in 6–12 months after penicillin therapy, but may take up to 2 years to convert in patients apparently adequately treated with other antibiotics. However, a certain number of patients will never become seronegative, although the titer should be low or decreasing after therapy. As mentioned previously, the FTA-abs test always remains positive in spite of treatment (1).

The most frustrating aspects of the treatment of temporal bone lues are demonstrated in the case reported by Wiet and Milko (21):

A 42-year-old man was admitted to the neurology service of the University of Cincinnati Medical Center in June 1973, for evaluation of headaches, unsteadiness, tinnitus, and hearing loss of 6 weeks' duration. Pertinent past history revealed that the patient was

Ear	SRT	PB max
R	40 dB	12%
L	2 dB	80%

Ear	SRT	PB max
R	95 dB	0%
L	5 dB	90%

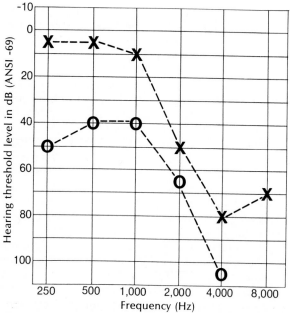

FIG. 38–13. Audiogram of 42-year-old man with congenital syphilis, at time of first admission. O---O, AC, RE; x--x, AC, LE. (Wiet RJ, Milko DA: Arch Otolaryngol 101:104–106, 1975. Copyright 1975, American Medical Association)

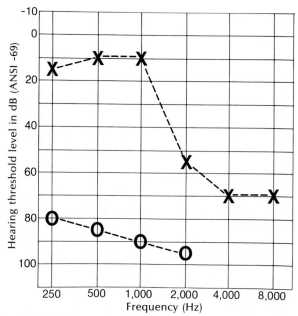

FIG. 38–14. Audiogram of same patient as in Figure 38–13, 1 month later, showing progression in hearing loss. O---O, AC, RE; x--x, AC, LE. (Wiet RJ, Milko DA: Arch Otolaryngol 101:104–106, 1975. Copyright 1975, American Medical Association)

treated with penicillin for congenital syphilis at 15 years of age by a county health department. He was treated again in 1952 at the age of 20 when called for army induction. At both ages 15 and 20 years neurosyphilis was confirmed by a spinal tap.

On examination at this hospitalization, the patient was noted to have an Argyle-Robertson pupil on the left. Tuning-fork tests were interpreted as consistent with a sensorineural hearing loss. Fistula test results were negative. The remainder of his examination was normal.

Laboratory evaluation revealed positive results for VDRL. Findings for skull x-ray films, brain scan, electroencephalogram, and right brachial arteriogram were normal.

An otolaryngology consultation was obtained. Audiometry revealed a bilateral high-frequency sensorineural hearing loss, more severe in the right ear (Fig. 38–13). Tomograms of the petrous bone were normal. An electronystagmogram revealed a hypoactive labyrinth in the right ear.

The patient was discharged from the neurology service and followed in July 1973, when he returned to the otolaryngology outpatient department because of

progression of his hearing loss (Fig. 38–14). Treatment had not been initiated to this date. Because of the rapid progression of his hearing loss, he was readmitted to the otolaryngology service in July 1973. Special audiometric tests were performed on this admission that demonstrated recruitment in the right ear and no auditory fatigue. A posterior fossa myelogram was also performed on this admission to rule out other causes of hearing loss. The right internal auditory canal did not fill with dye. The radiologist's interpretation of this finding was inconclusive. Spinal fluid obtained during the myelogram had a protein content of 59 mg/100 ml.

Because of the strong past history of syphilis, and findings consistent with this condition, the patient was begun on a course of steroid therapy. The patient was also treated with a weekly injection of 2.4 million units of benzathine penicillin for 3 weeks.

During this interval there was improvement in his pure-tone and discrimination scores as recorded by audiometry (Fig. 38–15).

In September 1973, the steroid therapy was discontinued after the onset of epigastric pain and the occurrence of occult blood in stool specimens. X-ray findings were not obtained, but the steroid therapy was discontinued because of the clinical signs of peptic ulcer.

The patient was followed in the otolaryngology outpatient department for several months. During this time, serial audiograms revealed a progression of his hearing loss in the right ear.

In January 1974, the patient was readmitted to the otolaryngology service because of increasing vertigo, profound hearing loss on the right, and progression of hearing loss in his left ear. The patient described his vertigo as so incapacitating that employment was no longer feasible.

Physical examination on this admission was essentially unchanged, except for the progression of the hearing loss in the left ear, confirmed by audiometry. A repeat posterior fossa myelogram was performed, in which filling of the internal auditory meatus was accomplished after extreme manipulation of the patient's head.

FIG. 38–15. Audiogram of same patient in Figures 38–13 and 38–14, 3 months after first admission, revealing improvement in pure-tone and discrimination scores after regimen of cortisone. O---O, AC, RE; **x---x**, AC, LE. (Wiet RJ, Milko DA: Arch Otolaryngol 101:104–106, 1975. Copyright 1975, American Medical Association)

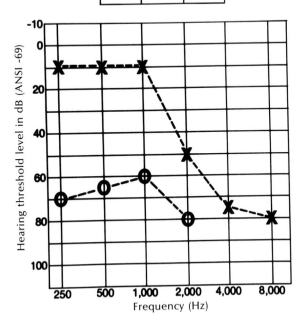

Ear	SRT	PB max
R	60 dB	40%
L	10 dB	64%

Laboratory data were unchanged. The cerebrospinal fluid VDRL test results were negative, but spinal fluid protein determination was elevated to 69 mg/100 ml.

Because of the questionable myelogram, symptomatology comparable with both Meniere's disease and syphilis, a diagnostic labyrinthotomy was performed in February 1974, via an exploratory tympanotomy.

The middle ear was found to be normal during surgery. After an opening into the vestibule was created, the perilymph was aspirated with a micropipet for rapid protein determination and electrolyte determination. Results were as follows: protein, 200 mg/100 ml; Na++ 143, K+ 5 (normal values for perilymph).

Approximately 3 μ liters of perilymph was then aspirated with a microliter syringe (Hamilton, 701–N). This fluid was examined under dark-field illumination, which demonstrated organisms with a characteristic motility and morphology of *Treponema pallidum*. Because of these findings a fluorescent treponemal antibody-absorption test for syphilis was performed. The perilymph fluid was air dried and fixed with acetone. Then a sample of known reactive, pooled, human syphilitic serum was mixed with a FTA-abs sorbent. This known reactive serum was then added to the slide and incubated. After incubation it was combined with fluorescein-conjugated rabbit antihuman globulin. Using this highly specific test, fluorescent treponemes were identified on the slide.

Following detection of spirochetes in the perilymph, the patient was treated with aqueous penicillin G, 20 million units administered intravenously daily for 7 days, according to the regimen of Pulec (13a). Following this course of therapy, the patient has received a weekly injection of 2.4 million units of long-acting penicillin for 3 months. He has also received a course of steroid therapy to prevent further hearing loss in his left ear.

The patient has been followed in the otolaryngology outpatient department for 3 months. He has reported improvement in his vertiginous symptoms but no improvement in his hearing loss, which has been confirmed by serial audiogram.*

CONCLUSION

The diagnosis of temporal-bone syphilis can be made and the otherwise inevitable profound hearing loss prevented only if a high index of suspicion is maintained. The cost of a FTA-abs test is a small price to pay if such a disaster can be avoided in even a few patients. Thus, this test has become an indispensable part of the diagnostic work-up of any patient with an unexplained progressive hearing loss or episodic vertigo.

* Wiet RJ, Milko DA: Arch Otolaryngol 101:104–106, 1975. Copyright 1975, American Medical Association.

REFERENCES

1. Barrett-Conner E: Current status of the treatment of syphilis. West J Med 122:7–11, 1975
2. Collart P: Persistence of Treponema Pallidum in Late Syphilis in Rabbits and Humans Notwithstanding Treatment. Proc World Forum on Syphilis and Other Treponematoses. USPHS Pub #997, 1964
3. Drusin LM: The diagnosis and treatment of infectious and latent syphilis. Med Clin North Am 56:1161–1174, 1974
4. Goodhill V: Syphilis of the ear: a histopathologic study. Ann Otol Rhinol Laryngol 48:676–707, 1939
5. Goodhill V, Guggenheim P: Pathology, diagnosis, and therapy of deafness. In Travis LE (ed): Handbook of Speech Pathology and Audiology. New York, Appleton-Century-Crofts, 1971
6. Hendershot EL: Luetic deafness. Laryngoscope 83:865–870, 1973
7. Karmody CS, Schuknecht HF: Deafness—Congenital syphilis. Arch Otolaryngol 83:18–27, 1966
8. Kerr AG, Smyth GDL, Cinnamond MJ: Congenital syphilitic deafness. J Laryngol 87:1–12, 1973
9. Kerr AG, Smyth GDL, Landau H: Congenital syphilitic labyrinthitis. Arch Otolaryngol 91:474–478, 1970
10. Mack LW, Smith JL, Walter EK et al.: Temporal bone treponemes. Arch Otolaryngol 90:11–14, 1969
11. Miller JN: The value and limitations of nontreponemal and treponemal tests in the laboratory diagnosis of syphilis. Clin Obstet Gynecol 18:191–203, 1975
12. von Nager FR: Die lues hereditaria tarda des innerohres-eine folge chronischer osteomyelitis des felsenbeins. Pract Otorhinolaryngol 17:1–22, 1955
13. Patterson ME: Congenital luetic hearing impairment. Treatment with prednisone. Arch Otolaryngol 87:378–382, 1968
13a. Pulec JL: Vertigo: a natural history and results of treatment. Otolaryngol Clin North Am 6:28–29, 1973
14. Pulec JL: Meniere's disease: results of a 2½ year study of etiology, natural history, and results of treatment. Laryngoscope 82:1703–1715, 1972
15. Rothenberg R, Dancewicz E: Significance of positive FTA-ABS test in Meniere's disease. JAMA 229:707–708, 1974
16. Schuknecht HF: Pathology of the Ear. Cambridge, MA, Harvard University Press, 1974
17. Smith JL: Spirochetes in late seronegative syphilis, despite penicillin therapy. Med Times 96:611–623, 1968
18. Sparling PF: Diagnosis and treatment of syphilis. N Engl J Med 284:642–653, 1971
19. Vrabec DP et al.: A study of the relative concentrations of antibiotics in the blood, spinal fluid, and perilymph in animals. Ann Otol Rhinol Laryngol 74:688–705, 1965
20. Webster B (ed): Symposium on veneral diseases. Med Clin North Am 56:1055–1222, 1972
21. Wiet RJ, Milko DA: Isolation of the spirochete in the perilymph despite prior antisyphilitic therapy. Arch Otolaryngol 101:104–106, 1975

The effects of certain chemicals and drugs on hearing and balance have been recognized for centuries. With the explosive expansion of the modern pharmacopeia, the number of potentially ototoxic medications has become quite large, carrying with it the ever-increasing burden on the physician to be aware of the potential dangers. To illustrate the number and great variety of substances involved, a partial list of agents incriminated in ototoxicity, compiled from several sources, is provided.

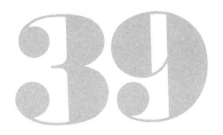

OTOTOXICITY

JOEL B. SHULMAN

Chemicals

Aconite	Gold
Alcohol	Hydrocyanide
Aniline dyes	Iodine
Arsenic	Iodoform
Benzene vapors	Lead
Camphor	Mercury
Carbon disulfide	Nitrobenzol
Carbon monoxide	Oil of chenopodium
Chloroform	Tobacco

Antibiotics

Chloramphenicol	Neomycin
Colistin (polymyxin E)	Pharmacetin
Dihydrostreptomycin	Polymyxin B
Gentamicin	Ristocetin
Kanamycin	Vancomycin
Tobramycin	Viomycin
Minocycline	

Diuretics

Ethacrynic acid	Furosemide

Miscellaneous Drugs

Antipyrine	Morphine
Atropine	Nitrogen mustard
Barbiturates	Novocaine
Caffeine	Quinine
Chlordiazepoxide	Salicylates
Ergot	Strychnine
Hexadimethrine bromide (Polybrene)	

The symptoms and signs of ototoxicity are limited to tinnitus and sensorineural hearing loss, "dizziness" of one description or another, and depressed vestibular function with or without nystagmus. Yet the clinical manifestations may be quite variable, necessitating constant vigilance if otologic disaster is to be avoided. Cochlear and vestibular damage may occur together or separately; they may be heralded by tinnitus and vertigo, or they may progress insidiously; the effects may be transient or permanent or even progressive long after the agent is withdrawn; and they may be unilateral or bilateral, dose-related or idiosyncratic.

The behavior of several of the more important ototoxic agents will be reviewed in some detail, drawing from both clinical reports and animal studies, with pertinent information on histopathology and mechanisms of action (Table 39–1).

ANTIBIOTICS

AMINOGLYCOSIDES

Most of the antibiotics with recognized ototoxic properties belong to the family of aminoglycosides, each consisting of an organic base linked to monosaccharides or disaccharides.

Streptomycin, dihydrostreptomycin, neomycin, kanamycin, gentamicin, and tobramycin are the primary drugs in this group requiring consideration with respect to ototoxicity.

Streptomycin

The first aminoglycoside antibiotic to be isolated (1943), was streptomycin, which is believed to act by interfering with bacterial protein synthesis. Like the other antibiotics in this group, it is largely excreted unchanged in the urine, but 10–30% cannot be accounted for. Although still widely used in the therapy of tuberculosis, its clinical applications have become greatly restricted since the development of other agents with greater effectiveness in gram-negative infections.

TABLE 39-1. Characteristics of Ototoxic Drugs

Agent	Characteristic action				
	Cochleo-toxic	Vestibulo-toxic	Transient	Permanent	Delayed onset
Dihydrostreptomycin	++	+	No	Yes	Yes
Streptomycin	+	++	No	Yes	Yes
Neomycin	++++	+	No	Yes	No
Kanamycin	+++	+	No	Yes	Yes
Gentamicin	+	+++	No	Yes	No
Viomycin	++	+++	No	Yes	No
Vancomycin	++	+	No	Yes	No
Minocycline	–	+	—	—	—
Ethacrynic acid	+	±	Usually	Occas.	No
Furosemide	+	±	Usually	Occas.	No
Quinine	+	–	Usually	Rarely	Occas.
Salicylates	+	+	Always	No	No
Nitrogen mustard	++	++	No	Yes	No

The toxic effect of streptomycin is greater on the vestibular system than on the cochlea, and in susceptible individuals a total dose as small as a few grams may produce vertigo and depressed caloric responses (5). Ordinarily, unless there is renal insufficiency, with daily doses of 1 g or less, toxicity develops only after prolonged therapy, and is related to the total dose administered. If the dose is increased to 2 g per day, 19% of patients will develop abnormal caloric responses within 5–8 weeks, and over 50% will have them in 9–12 weeks (3). The onset of symptoms may be sudden or gradual, usually beginning with slight vertigo upon sudden head movement or when walking in the dark. As the vestibular system becomes quite depressed, vestibular reflex coordination is lost, patients may complain of difficulty walking over uneven ground or down stairs and of diminished ability to recognize others while walking (oscillopsia). Ataxia with tendency to fall when reaching for things may also occur.

Severe vertigo persists for 7–10 days after stopping therapy, and then subsides over the next several months as compensation occurs. If the drug is discontinued immediately upon development of dizziness, partial recovery may occur, especially in children (27, 37). Patients over age 45 seem at greater risk, and there may be a dominant genetic predisposition to streptomycin ototoxicity accounting for the extreme sensitivity of some individuals (57).

The relatively selective ototoxic effect of streptomycin on the vestibular system has led to its therapeutic use for control of intractable vertigo in patients with bilateral Meniere's disease. Disappearance of ice-water caloric response occurs after administering 2–3 g of streptomycin daily for 2–3 weeks (average total dose of 30 g). Hearing is preserved and the marked ataxia becomes minor within several months (51) (Fig. 39–1). Yet despite the cochlear sparing observed in these studies, tinnitus and sensorineural hearing loss, greatest in the higher frequencies, may occur in a few individuals receiving large doses of the drug for prolonged periods (29) (Fig. 39–2).

Dihydrostreptomycin

Dihydrostreptomycin, on the other hand, which was introduced shortly after its congener, was found to have severe, capricious cochlear ototoxicity. The untoward effects were frequently independent of dose with hearing loss progressing after the drug was stopped; irreversible deafness has developed as long as 6 months after cessation of therapy (27, 37). Because it offered no significant therapeutic advantage over streptomycin, the drug was fortunately removed from the market.

Neomycin

Neomycin was the next aminoglycoside antibiotic to be developed (1949), and its ototoxic properties when administered parenterally were soon recognized. Hearing loss may progress after administration of the drug has ceased and is irreversible. Some vestibular impairment also occurs in most cases (27) (Fig. 39–3). Because it is poorly absorbed from the GI tract, neomycin has been used to sterilize the bowel before operation and to reduce blood ammonia levels in patients with liver failure; however, 3% of an oral dose is absorbed. Accordingly, 250 g neomycin given orally achieves

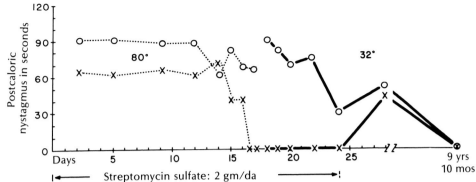

FIG. 39–1. Vestibular test results in a 32-year-old male who was treated with 2 g streptomycin sulfate per day for 24 days for ablation of vestibular function because of bilateral Meniere's disease. For the first 17 days caloric tests performed with 5 cc H_2O at 80° F, and thereafter with 5 cc of ice water. He first noticed dysequilibrium on the 11th day of treatment, following which ataxia increased and vestibular response decreased until termination of treatment. He had no further vertiginous episodes and returned to a full work load at 2.5 months. Tests performed at the U.S. Naval Aerospace Medical Institute, United States Naval Aviation Medical Center, Pensacola, FL, 12 years after treatment, revealed great diminution of canal and otolith function, immunity to motion sickness, and hearing unchanged from pretreatment level. (Schuknecht HF: Pathology of the Ear. Cambridge, Mass, Harvard University Press, 1974)

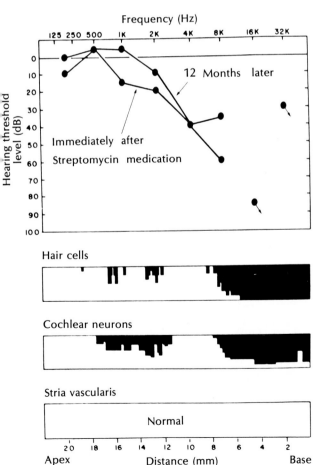

FIG. 39–2. Audiograms and cochlear chart of cat that received streptomycin sulfate, 200 mg/kg/day for 28 days. Post-treatment survival time was 15 months. Behavioral audiograms show a high-frequency hearing loss. Studies of cochlear pathology show loss of hair cells and cochlear neurons in basal 7 mm and in the 12- to 18-mm region. (McGee T, Olszewski J: Arch Otolaryngol 75:295, 1962. Copyright 1962, American Medical Association)

the same degree of systemic absorption as the parenteral administration of 7–8 g, a dose that usually produces ototoxicity (18). In 1970 Ballantyne (1) reported that 6 of 13 patients with liver disease treated with oral neomycin developed irreversible sensorineural hearing loss. He noted that the ototoxicity was not directly dose-related but hearing loss could be produced by total doses ranging from 84–4500 g. By the same token, ototoxicity has been produced by intrapleural and intraperitoneal administration (18), colonic irrigations (14), aerosols, and topical irrigation of wounds and draining sinuses (4, 24). As with other drugs of its type, poor renal function leads to prolonged peaks of serum concentration, more rapid buildup in endolymph, and earlier toxic effects (27).

Kanamycin

Kanamycin, introduced in 1951, is still used widely for severe gram-negative infections, particularly neonatal sepsis. It possesses less vestibular but considerably more auditory ototoxicity than

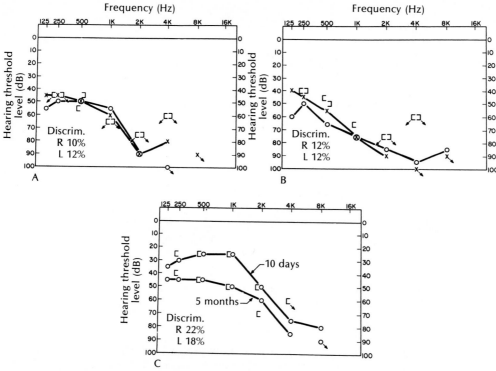

FIG. 39–3. Audiograms of three patients who experienced hearing loss from intramuscular administration of neomycin. Severe loss of speech discrimination suggests that atrophy of the organ of Corti was accompanied by neural degeneration. **A.** This patient received a total of 13.5 g over an 8-day period. She first noticed bilateral deafness and unsteadiness 2 months following administration of the drug. The hearing loss progressed for several weeks. The audiogram was made 5 months after treatment. Caloric response was diminished in left ear only. **B.** This patient received 32.25 g neomycin in 45 days and noticed progressive bilateral hearing loss beginning 1 month after cessation of treatment. Caloric response was diminished in left ear only. **C.** This patient received a total dose of 4 g in 8 days. He developed a diffuse erythematous rash and bilateral symmetrical hearing loss 4 days after completion of therapy. The hearing loss progressed for several months. Caloric tests revealed decreased response in right ear. (Schuknecht HF: Pathology of the Ear. Cambridge, Mass, Harvard University Press, 1974, p 238)

streptomycin. Ototoxicity is almost always heralded by tinnitus. Although recovery of hearing is unusual, progression of hearing loss after discontinuing treatment is rare, unless renal insufficiency is present (Fig. 39–4). The tolerable total dose before hearing loss begins ranges from 32–134 g. Consequently, weekly audiograms are advised, and the drug should be stopped as soon as tinnitus is reported or a hearing deficit is detected (15). Infants treated for neonatal sepsis with the recommended dose of 15 mg/kg/day for 6–10 days experienced no increased incidence of hearing loss over a similar group of patients treated with streptomycin (12). When used for *bowel* sterilization, an oral dose of kanamycin may produce serum levels up to 5μg/ml, and in the presence of renal failure, levels comparable to those

during parenteral therapy may be attained; therefore, the drug cannot be considered nonabsorbable (26).

Gentamicin

Gentamicin is the most widely used aminoglycoside antibiotic, largely because of its effectiveness against most strains of *Pseudomonas*. Its ototoxicity, which is predominantly vestibular, is well recognized. In a report by Meyers (36), 10 of 40 treated patients developed signs of ototoxicity—nine vestibular and one cochlear. Eight of the 10 had compromised renal function, but transient vestibular deficits occurred in two patients with normal renal function. Oddly, the damage was usually unilateral. In patients with normal renal function, 1–3 mg/kg/day, with peak serum levels

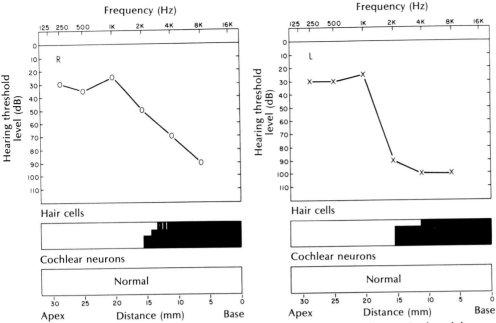

FIG. 39–4. Audiogram of 27-year-old female with severe renal failure, who received an initial dose of 1 g kanamycin followed by 0.25 g every other day for a total of 3 g over 18 days. Tinnitus and high-frequency hearing loss developed on the 18th day, following which there was no further change on repeated testing. She died 2 weeks after completion of therapy. Histologic studies showed severe loss of hair cells in the basal 15 mm of both cochleae. The population of cochlear neurons was normal, and the vestibular sense organs appeared normal. (Schuknecht HF: Pathology of the Ear. Cambridge, Mass, Harvard University Press, 1974, p 280)

not exceeding 12 μg/ml, is considered safe if therapy is not prolonged. There is no evidence that ototoxic damage progresses after the drug is discontinued, but in severely ill bedridden patients, early vestibular signs may not readily be recognized without serial caloric tests.

Tobramycin

Tobramycin is the newest antibiotic of the aminoglycoside family to reach the market. Ototoxicity is qualitatively similar to that of gentamicin, but limited clinical observation suggests that these side effects are less frequent and less severe with tobramycin.

Amikacin

This semisynthetic derivative of kanamycin is effective against most aerobic gram-negative bacteria and ineffective against anaerobes. Most strains of *Pseudomonas* are sensitive to amikacin. Amikacin should be reserved for serious infections caused by bacteria presumed to be resistant to other aminoglycosides. Amikacin can be both ototoxic and nephrotoxic.

MECHANISMS OF AMINOGLYCOSIDE OTOTOXICITY

The pathophysiologic mechanisms by which ototoxic drugs such as the aminoglycosides inflict damage upon the inner ear has been the subject of considerable investigation in experimental animals, with many findings confirmed by microscopic examination of human temporal bones. Toxic substances must first reach the labyrinthine fluids either via the bloodstream, or when applied topically in the middle ear, by direct permeation of the round window or oval window membrane. Early studies concentrated on the striking effects on the sensory epithelium, using light and phase contrast microscopy (Fig. 39–5) and later electron microscopy.

Both kanamycin and neomycin appear to affect the outer hair cells of the basal coil of the cochlea first, with damage progressing toward the apex, thus accounting for the predominantly high-frequency sensorineural hearing loss observed. The outer hair cells most abundantly supplied with large, richly granulated nerve endings seem most vulnerable. Inner hair cells degenerate much later, progressing from the apex toward the base. Degeneration of nerve endings and nerve fibers appears secondarily, soon after loss of the corresponding hair cells, but never occurs alone without loss of sensory cells (25).

Ciges and colleagues (6) found abnormal absorption of supravital stains by hair cells damaged by ototoxic drugs, suggesting a primary effect on cell membrane permeability similar to that seen from anoxic damage. At the ultrastructural level, the nuclei and ribosomes (the protein-synthesizing organelles) are most affected, whereas the nerve endings, which do not synthesize protein, are not damaged. This supports the notion that the toxic effects of aminoglycosides on sensory cells may be the same as their antibacterial effect—*i.e.*, inhibition of protein synthesis (55). It is unclear why the basal region is affected first, although there is evidence that this region has the greatest metabolic activity (1).

As expected, streptomycin and gentamicin exert their most severe effects in the vestibular sensory cells (10, 21, 58) (Fig. 39–6) with degeneration of myelin-figure formation in the mitochondria and swelling of sensory hairs with deformation of cell surfaces. Minor changes in the mitochondria and stereocilia of cochlear hair cells are also observed (11). The explanation put forth for these observations is that these drugs exert a major effect on the plasma membrane and the membrane component of mitochondria, producing damage to the permeability barrier just as they seem to impair bacterial cell membrane function (19). The fact that streptomycin produces immediate depression of the cochlear microphonics, which is reversed by potassium, is further evidence for a primary effect on cell membranes (59).

Hawkins (19) has found that pathologic changes in the sensory cells lag behind those in the stria, spiral ligament, outer sulcus, and Reissner's membrane. The earliest damage appears in the microvasculature of the

FIG. 39–5. A. Phase contrast surface preparation of the organ of Corti from a normal cat, showing the patterns of stereocilia on the row of inner hair cells (**IHC**) and on the three rows of outer hair cells (**OHC**). **IP,** inner pillars; **OP,** outer pillars; **HC,** Hensen cells. (Hawkins JE, Johnsson LG, Aran JM: J Infect Dis 119:417–431, 1969. University of Chicago Press, Publisher) **B.** Gentamicin-damaged organ of Corti, showing loss of many outer hair cells (**OHC**) and normal-appearing inner hair cells (**IHC**). Outer pillars (**OP**) show staining abnormalities. Between the Dieter cells (**DC**) and Claudius cells (**CC**), the Hensen cells have disappeared. (Hawkins JE, Johnson LG, Aran JM: J Infect Dis 119:417–431, 1969. University of Chicago Press, Publisher) **C.** Phase contrast photomicrograph of guinea pig cochlea damaged by kanamycin. All outer hair cells in the first row have been lost, and the second row has been severely damaged, but most of the cells in the third row remain. **White arrows,** two missing inner pillars (**P**); **black arrows,** beginning breakdown of supporting framework of third row. Several inner hair cells (**IHC**) have also collapsed. A "cochleogram" has been constructed from this photomicrograph (**1, 2, 3**) with each remaining cell registered as an open circle and each degenerated cell as a **solid circle.** (Kohonen A: Acta Otolaryngol [Stockh], Suppl 208, 1965)

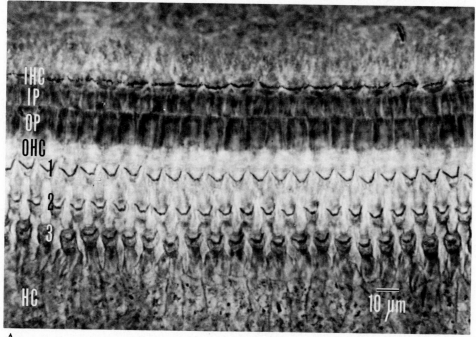

A

FIG. 39–5 (*continued*)

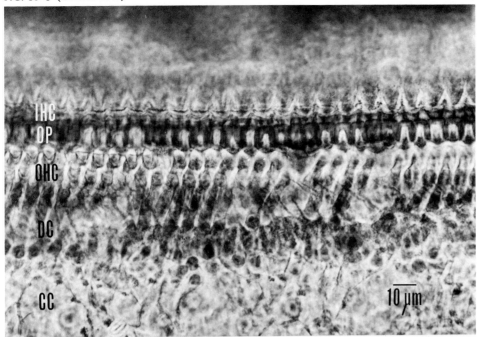

B

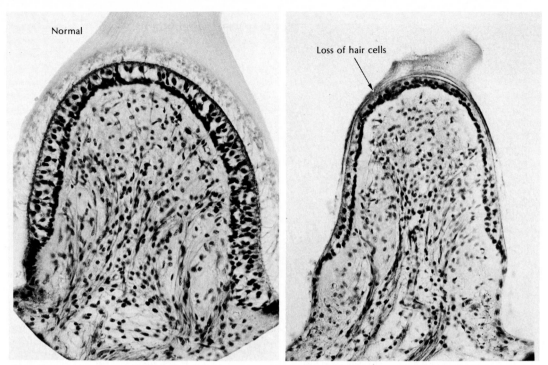

Normal

Loss of hair cells

FIG. 39–6. Cristae of horizontal canals of normal animal **(left)** and an animal exhibiting loss of vestibular function caused by intramuscular administration of streptomycin sulfate, 200 mg/kg/day for 28 days **(right).** In the treated ear the sensory epithelium is flattened, and about 50% of the hair cells are missing. The remaining hair cells appear shrunken and have pyknotic nuclei. Post-treatment survival time was 15 months. (Schuknecht HF: Pathology of the Ear. Cambridge, Mass, Harvard University Press, 1974, p 277)

cochlea, beginning with endothelial swelling, which may be transient, and progressing to capillary occlusion and degeneration (Fig. 39–7). These changes generally precede damage to the organ of Corti in its progression from base to apex. On the basis of these findings, Hawkins proposes the existence of a "blood-ear barrier" maintained by the secretory and absorptive tissues that form an active partition between endolymph and perilymph and help to protect the "microhomeostasis" of the inner ear. He points out that aging, noise trauma, and ototoxic drugs all produce similar changes in the inner ear. It is further implied, but not proved, that the fundamental factor is not a direct assault on the outer hair cells but a breakdown in the "microhomeostatic mechanisms that govern the volume, rate of formation and absorption, and ionic composition of inner ear fluids" (20).

This attractive thesis, however, does not readily explain why the cochlea and vestibular apparatus are differentially affected by many agents. At the biochemical level many questions remain to be answered regarding the precise enzyme systems and metabolic processes affected by the aminoglycosides.

A direct effect on the sensory cells may occur with toxic agents entering the labyrinth via the round window or oval window after topical application (55, 58). Presumably agents may also enter the inner ear from the cerebrospinal fluid via the cochlear or vestibular aqueducts.

OTHER ANTIBIOTICS

Ototoxic properties are not peculiar to the aminoglycoside antibiotics. **Viomycin,** a basic polypeptide antibiotic derived from *Actinomyces*, is an effective antitubercular drug, which may produce both vestibular and cochlear damage (27). The **polymyxins** are also polypeptides used topically or occasionally systemically and have ototoxic potential. The structure of **vancomycin** is not fully characterized except that it contains both sugars and amino acids; it is occasionally used to treat penicillin-resistant staphylococcal infections, and excessive blood levels (80–100 μg/ml) may produce irreversible sensorineural hearing loss which progresses after the drug is discontinued (16).

FIG. 39–7. A. Irregularly swollen and constricted strial capillaries and large vacuoles in marginal cells of gentamicin-treated guinea pig. (Hawkins JE: Adv Otohinolaryngol 20:125–141, 1973. S. Karger AG, Basel, Publisher) **B.** Suprastrial vessels from third turn of gentamicin-treated guinea pig, showing an avascular channel **(right)** and an intervascular strand **(above).** (Hawkins JE: Adv Otorhinolaryngol 20:125–141, 1973. S. Karger AG, Basel, Publisher)

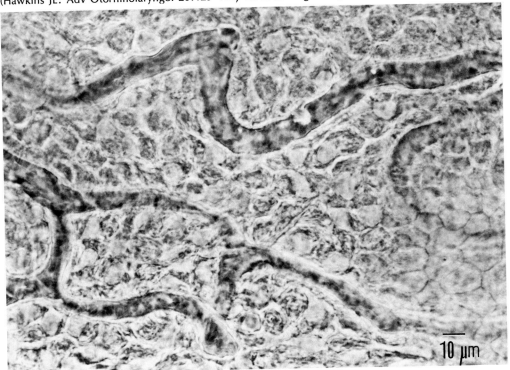

A

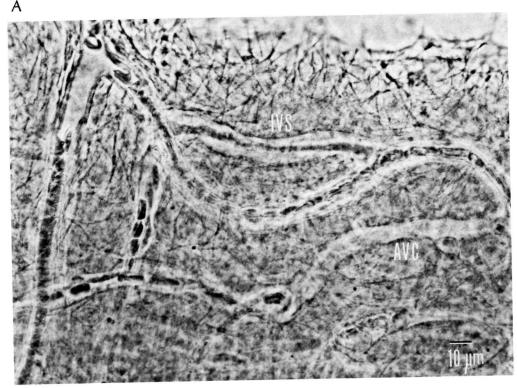

B

Thus, ototoxicity is by no means dependent on any peculiar molecular structure.

Minocycline, one of the newer tetracyclines, may produce transient vertigo, but its ototoxic effects have not been well studied.

TOPICAL PREPARATIONS

Of concern, at least on a theoretical basis, is the effect of ototoxic agents introduced into the middle ear through a tympanic membrane perforation. Although conclusive confirmation in man is lacking, numerous animal studies have demonstrated the deleterious effect on the inner ear of several commonly used topical otologic preparations. For example, chloramphenicol applied directly to the round window membrane of guinea pigs for 30 min produces a depression of the cochlear microphonics that progresses for several hours and recovers only slightly (17, 38). Streptomycin injected into the middle ear produces marked vestibular symptoms within 3–6 hours, with changes observed in the type I hair cells (55). Gentamicin applied topically to the middle ear also produces cochlear hair-cell damage (10). Drugs such as neomycin, polymyxin B, and colistin are ingredients of common topical otic preparations; although designed for use only in the external auditory canal, they are also frequently used in the presence of a tympanic membrane perforation. Theoretically, cochlear and vestibular injury might be expected, but in view of the paucity of such reports, the actual incidence of untoward effects must be extremely low. Perhaps some protection is afforded by inflamed and thickened middle ear mucosa. Even antiseptics and detergents used in preoperative "preps" should not be allowed to enter a tympanic membrane perforation, because of possible inner ear damage.

DIURETICS

The two most potent diuretics now in general use —ethacrynic acid and furosemide—have well recognized ototoxic effects.

Ethacrynic Acid

Rapid intravenous infusion of ethacrynic acid, especially in uremic patients, may produce a sensorineural hearing loss which is usually immediate in onset and transient, lasting a few hours to several days (44, 48, 49). The abnormal retention of toxic breakdown products of ethacrynic acid in uremic patients may be partly responsible for the

hearing loss, but the extremely rapid onset of symptoms suggests a direct toxicity. It should be noted that ototoxicity is reported in patients with normal renal function and may be permanent.

In a report of human temporal bone pathology, Matz, Beal, and Krames (33) described destruction and absence of outer hair cells in the first 20 mm of the basal turn of the cochlea, with preservation of the inner hair cells and supporting cells. Neurophysiologic studies in cats have shown that an intravenous bolus of ethacrynic acid (much in excess of the recommended human dose) produces, within a few seconds, depression of the cochlear microphonic and eighth nerve action potentials and decreased vestibular nystagmus in response to caloric irrigation. Both functions usually return to normal within 1 hour (28, 32). After recovery of the primary depression, a second dose of ethacrynic acid produces a severe secondary depression associated with outer hair cell degeneration in the basal and middle coils of the cochlea. Equivalent doses of chlorothiazide did not produce such changes. Untrastructural changes are most marked in the stria vascularis, with intra- and extracellular edema and destruction of the intermediate cell layer. These abnormalities were noted within 10 min of injection, were dose-related, and were transient (45). The organ of Corti was less affected but showed some degeneration of outer hair cells beginning with degeneration in mitochondria and distortion of stereocilia, which did not recover. In the vestibular system, changes were also noted in type I and type II hair cells, similar to those seen in gentamicin toxicity (41).

Furosemide

A transient cochleotoxic effect, sometimes with vertigo, has been observed after rapid infusion of large doses of furosemide (53). Permanent severe sensorineural hearing loss has also been reported (31, 46).

MECHANISMS IN DIURETIC OTOTOXICITY

The mechanisms for these peculiar side effects remains speculative. They are presumed to be related to acute electrolyte alterations in the endolymph or "cortilymph" brought about by the same mechanism that produces diuresis in the kidneys. However, this does not explain the infrequency of vertigo in association with the hearing loss, nor does it account for the fact that other diuretics with similar metabolic effects are not ototoxic.

At the first sign of hearing loss following the administration of either ethacrynic acid or furosemide, the use of the drug should not be repeated until it has been demonstrated that other diuretics are ineffective (44).

MISCELLANEOUS OTOTOXIC DRUGS AND OTHER DRUGS PRODUCING OTOLOGIC SYMPTOMS

Quinine Derivatives

Quinine derivatives have long been known to produce irreversible sensorineural hearing loss with tinnitus as a prominent symptom. Toxicity usually occurs after prolonged high-dose therapy for malaria or arthritis, but idiosyncratic responses may take place. Toone and co-workers (56) recorded a case of sensorineural hearing loss following the prolonged use of chloroquine; the hearing loss was progressive after discontinuance of the drug. Chloroquine administered to pregnant women during the first trimester has produced severe fetal abnormalities with complete anacusis and marked vestibular paresis as well as other associated congenital anomalies (34). Complete absence of hair cells and of many of the supporting cells throughout most of the organ of Corti was observed.

Salicylates

A peculiar but fortunately remediable example of drug-induced ototoxicity is that produced by salicylates, which are perhaps the most widely consumed medications in the world. Regularly accompanied by tinnitus, high doses of salicylates predictably produce a bilaterally symmetrical, flat sensorineural hearing loss up to 40 dB with a mild decrease in speech discrimination. This effect is not idiosyncratic but closely parallels the salicylate concentration in the plasma. Although the route of administration is generally oral, ototoxicity has been observed following application of salicylates to the skin for psoriasis (43). The magnitude of the hearing loss is directly related to plasma levels between 20 and 40 mg/100 ml, beyond which no further hearing loss occurs (40). In patients with preexisting sensorineural hearing loss, salicylate toxicity tends to flatten the hearing curve by having a relatively greater effect at frequencies with lower thresholds. Special audiometric tests point to intracochlear localization, with no evidence of retrocochlear or central disturbance (2, 35). Universally the hearing loss and tinnitus are completely reversible within 24–72 hours after the drug is discontinued, whether the intoxication is acute or chronic. Sporadic case reports of deafness following aspirin therapy are of questionable validity (22).

The fact that no consistent morphologic or ultrastructural changes have been observed in animals or humans has led to the presumption that the mechanism of salicylate ototoxicity is related to some reversible alteration in biochemical or enzymatic function in the cochlea, probably in the stria vascularis. Patients with preexisting sensorineural hearing loss due to strial atrophy then would be expected to have less additional depression of thresholds from salicylates, thus accounting for the flattening of the audiometric curve (40). In cats with acute salicylate intoxication, malic dehydrogenase in perilymph and endolymph are decreased; glucose levels are increased, reflecting a rise in blood glucose; and sodium, potassium, and protein concentrations remain unchanged. Cochlear microphonics and N_1 action potentials are consistently reduced (54). Yet, the precise mechanism of this unique form of ototoxicity remains speculative.

Antimetabolites

The alkylating agent nitrogen mustard has a well-documented neurotoxic action with a special affinity for the cranial nerves, particularly the facial nerve. Intravenous infusion frequently produces tinnitus, vertigo, and predominantly high-tone sensorineural hearing loss (7, 60). One fatal case observed at pathological examination by Schuknecht demonstrated partial collapse of Reissner's membrane and shrinking of the tectorial membrane, organ of Corti, and neural epithelium of the crista ampullaris (50).

Heterologous Serum

Serum sickness produced by tetanus antitoxin of horse serum origin may be associated with profound and permanent sensorineural hearing loss (52).

OTHER DRUGS PRODUCING OTOLOGIC SYMPTOMS

Many other classes of drugs (oral contraceptive agents, sedatives, tranquilizers, etc.) may have vestibular side effects, but evidence is lacking to classify them properly as directly ototoxic.

CONGENITAL OTOTOXIC HEARING LOSS

Although it is a fundamental principle that no drug should be administered to a pregnant woman without great caution, many ototoxic drugs have unfortunately been shown to produce a constellation of fetal deformities, such as skeletal malformations, cleft palate, dental abnormalities, ocular defects, and anomalies of the cardiovascular system, genitourinary tract, and intestinal tract, as well as ear defects (42). Chloroquine, salicylates, streptomycin, and thalidomide have been the most strongly implicated. The first trimester, especially the sixth or seventh week, appears to be the most vulnerable period for effect on the development of the ear. Streptomycin, for example, passes into the fetus and amnionic fluid in concentrations up to 50% of the maternal levels (39), and in some series, nearly half the children whose mothers received streptomycin had eighth nerve abnormalities, auditory as well as vestibular (8). Others feel that fetal hearing loss is rare following administration of streptomycin during pregnancy (47). This difference of opinion implies that several variables are operant, including the "placental barrier," the duration of treatment, and the stage of development during treatment. Kanamycin, on the other hand, does not appear in the amnionic fluid after injection.

The brief but tragic experience with thalidomide showed that as little as a single dose of 100 mg may produce congenital anomalies, the severity of which is not dose-related (30). Ear defects were among the most commonly observed anomalies, either alone or with limb deformities. Most cases demonstrated labyrinthine abnormalities and multiple cranial nerve palsies as well, but there is no estimate of how many children had only hearing loss (9, 23). Middle ear defects, absence of the seventh and eighth nerves, dysplasia of the organ of Corti, outer and inner hair-cell damage, decrease in the number of spiral ganglion cells, and even complete labyrinthine aplasia have been observed in histopathologic studies (23, 42).

CONCLUSION

The experience with ototoxic drugs has illustrated the importance of considering patient factors as well as drug factors if the tragedy of irreversible hearing loss or vestibular incapacity is to be avoided. It is axiomatic that among the pharmacologic agents effective in a given clinical situation, the one with the least toxicity is to be chosen. Thus ototoxic drugs should be avoided altogether unless essential. When they are necessary, the daily and total dose must be kept to a minimum, with the realization that even oral administration of so-called nonabsorbable drugs or topical applications may achieve toxic blood levels.

Special caution is mandatory if renal or hepatic failure is present. Although reduced dosage schedules calculated from the glomerular filtration rate are useful, they cannot replace frequent monitoring of drug serum levels (26).

Very young and very old patients seem to be at greater risk, and evidence also exists suggesting that prior exposure to ototoxic drugs may render the ear more susceptible to damage from subsequent treatment with other ototoxic agents.

Of course, treatment of pregnant women requires extra consideration of the possible effects on the fetus.

One must always be conscious of potential side effects of any drug and the risk of delayed intoxication. When the patient's condition allows it, serial audiograms and vestibular function tests should be performed at intervals during treatment. Patients should be questioned daily about the presence of tinnitus or imbalance and the offending drug stopped at the first sign of ototoxicity. The careful screening of new drugs in experimental animals, using the surface preparation techniques introduced by Engström, to detect hair-cell damage before clinical trials begin, is likely to reduce the risk of pharmacologic misadventures.

There is no known treatment for cochlear and vestibular damage once it has occurred, and only the vigilance of the physician can help prevent it.

REFERENCES

1. Ballantyne J: Iatrogenic deafness. J Laryngol 84: 967–1000, 1970
2. Bernstein JM, Weiss AD: Further observations on salicylate ototoxicity. J Laryngol 81:915–925, 1967
3. Bignall JR, Crofton JW, Thomas JAB: Effect of streptomycin on vestibular function. Br Med J 1:554–559, 1951
4. Campanelli PA, Grimes E, West ML: Hearing loss in a child following neomycin irrigation. Med Ann DC 35:541–543, 1966
5. Cawthorne T, Ranger D: Toxic effect of streptomycin upon balance and hearing. Br Med J 1:1444–1446, 1957
6. Ciges M, Quesada P, Gonzalez M: Supravital study of guinea pig cochlea referring especially to kanamycin labyrinthotoxy. Acta Otolaryngol (Stockh) 73:270–279, 1972
7. Conrad ME, Crosby WH: Massive nitrogen mustard therapy on Hodgkin's disease with protection of bone marrow by tourniquets. Blood 16: 1089–1103, 1960
8. Conway N, Birt BD: Streptomycin in pregnancy: effect on the foetal ear. Br Med J 2:260–263, 1965
9. D'Avignon M, Barr B: Ear abnormalities and cranial nerve palsies in thalidomide children. Arch Otolaryngol 80:136–140, 1964
10. Dayal VS, Smith EL: Cochlear and vestibular gentamycin toxicity. Arch Otolaryngol 100:338–340, 1974
11. Duvall AJ, Wersall J: Site of action of streptomy-

cin upon inner ear sensory cells. Acta Otolaryngol (Stockh) 57:581–598, 1964

12. Eichenwald HF: Some observations on dosage and toxicity of kanamycin in premature and full-term infants. Ann NY Acad Sci 132:984–991, 1966

13. Engström H, Ades HW, Hawkins JE: Cytoarchitecture of the organ of corti. Acta Otolaryngol (Stockh) 188:92–99, 1964

14. Fields RL: Neomycin ototoxicity. Arch Otolaryngol 79:67–70, 1964

15. Frost JO, Hawkins JE, Daly JF: Kanamycin. II. Ototoxicity. Am Rev Resp Dis 82:23–30, 1960

16. Geraci JE, Heilman FR, Nichols DR et al.: Antibiotic therapy of bacterial endocarditis. VII. Vancomycin for acute micrococcal endocarditis. Mayo Clin Proc 33:172–181, 1958

17. Gulick WL, Patterson WC: The effects of chloramphenicol upon the electrical activity of the ear. Ann Otol Rhinol Laryngol 73:204–209, 1964

18. Halpern EB, Heller MF: Ototoxicity of orally administered neomycin. Arch Otolaryngol 73:675–677, 1961

19. Hawkins JE: Biochemical aspects of ototoxicity. In Paparella M (ed): Biochemical Mechanisms in Hearing and Deafness. Springfield, IL, CC Thomas, 1970

20. Hawkins JE: Comparative otopathology: aging, noise, and ototoxic drugs. Adv Otol Rhinol Laryngol 20:125–141, 1973

21. Hawkins JE, Johnsson LG, Aran JM: Comparative tests of gentamycin ototoxicity. J Infect Dis 119:417–431, 1969

22. Jarvis JF: A case of unilateral permanent deafness following acetylsalicyclic acid. J Laryngol 80:318–320, 1966

23. Jorgensen MB, Kristensen HK, Buch NH: Thalidomide induced aplasia of the inner ear. J Laryngol 78:1095–1101, 1964

24. Kelly DR, Nilo ER, Berggren RB: Deafness after topical neomycin wound irrigation. N Engl J Med 280:1338–1341, 1969

25. Kohohen A: Effect of some ototoxic drugs upon the pattern of innervation of cochlear sensory cells in the guinea pig. Acta Otolaryngol [Suppl] (Stockh) #208, 1965

26. Kunin CM, Finland M: Restrictions imposed on antibiotic therapy by serial failure. Arch Intern Med 104:1030–1050, 1959

27. Leach W: Ototoxicity of neomycin and other antibiotics. J Laryngol 76:774–790, 1962

28. Levinson RM, Capps MJ, Mathod RH: Ethacrynic acid, furosemide, and vestibular caloric responses. Ann Otol Rhinol Laryngol 83:223–229, 1974

29. Linden G: Loss of hearing following treatment with dihydrostreptomycin or streptomycin. Acta Otolaryngol (Stockh) 43:551–572, 1953

30. Livingstone G: Congenital ear abnormalities due to thalidomide. Proc R Soc Med 58:493–497, 1965

31. Lloyd-Mostyn RN, Lord IJ: Ototoxicity of intravenous furosemide. Lancet 2:1156–1157, 1971

32. Mathog RH, Thomas WG, Hudson WR: Ototoxicity of new and potent diuretics. Arch Otolaryngol 92:7–13, 1970

33. Matz GJ, Beal DD, Krames L: Ototoxicity of ethacrynic acid. Arch Otolaryngol 90:152–155, 1969

34. Matz GJ, Naunton RF: Ototoxicity of chloroquine. Arch Otolaryngol 88:370–372, 1964

35. McCabe PA, Dey FL: The effect of aspirin upon auditory sensitivity. Ann Otol Rhinol Laryngol 74:312–325, 1965

36. Meyers RM: Ototoxic effects of gentamicin. Arch Otolaryngol 92:160–162, 1970

37. Meyler L: Streptomycin and not dihydrostreptomycin. Acta Otolaryngol [Suppl] (Stockh) 183:92–94, 1963

38. Morizono T, Johnstone BM: Ototoxicity of topical antibiotics. J Otolaryngol Soc Aust 3:666–669, 1974

39. Moya F, Thorndike V: Passage of drugs across the placenta. Am J Obstet Gynecol 84:1778–1798, 1963

40. Myers EN, Bernstein JM: Salicylate ototoxicity. Arch Otolaryngol 82:483–493, 1965

41. Nakai Y: Electron microscopic study of the inner ear after ethacrynic acid intoxication. Pract Otorhinolaryngol (Basel) 33:366–376, 1971

42. Northern JL, Downs MP: Hearing in Children. Baltimore, Williams & Wilkins, 1974

43. Perlman LV: Salicylate intoxication from skin application. N Engl Med 274:164–167, 1966

44. Pillay V, Schwartz F, Aimi K et al.: Transient and permanent deafness following treatment with ethacrynic acid in renal failure. Lancet 1:77–79, 1969

45. Quick CA, Duvall AJ: Early changes in the cochlear duct from ethacrynic acid: an electron-microscopic evaluation. Laryngoscope 80:954–965, 1970

46. Quick CA, Hoppe W: Permanent deafness associated with furosemide administration. Ann Otol Rhinol Laryngol 84:94–101, 1975

47. Robinson GC, Cambon KG: Hearing loss in infants of tuberculous mothers treated with streptomycin during pregnancy. N Engl J Med 271:949–951, 1964

48. Schmidt P, Friedman IS: Adverse effects of ethacrynic acid. NY State J Med 67:1438–1442, 1967

49. Schneider WJ, Becker EL: Acute transient hearing loss after ethacrynic acid therapy. Arch Intern Med 117:715, 1966

50. Schuknecht HF: The pathology of several disorders of the inner ear which cause vertigo. South Med J 57:1161–1167, 1964

51. Schuknecht HF: Ablation therapy with management of Meniere's disease. Acta Otolaryngol [Suppl] (Stockh) #132, 1957

52. Schuknecht HF: Pathology of the Ear. Cambridge, MA, Harvard University Press, 1974

53. Schwartz GA, David DS, Riggio RR et al.: Oto-toxicity induced by furosemide. N Engl J Med 282: 1413–1414, 1970

54. Silverstein H, Bernstein JM, Davies DG: Salicylate ototoxicity, a biochemical and electrophysiological study. Ann Otol Rhinol Laryngol 76:118–128, 1967

55. Spoendlin H: Zur Ototoxizitat des Streptomyzins. Pract Otorhinolaryngol (Basel) 28:305–322, 1966

56. Toone EC, Hayden D, Ellman HM: Ototoxicity of chloroquine. Arthritis Rheum 8:475–476, 1965

57. Tsuiki T, Murai S: Familial incidence of strepto-mycin hearing loss and hereditary weakness of the cochlea. Audiology 10:315–322, 1971

58. Wersall J, Lundquist P-G, Bjorkroth B: Ototoxicity of gentamycin. J Infect Dis 119:410–417, 1969

59. Wersall J, Flock A: Suppression and restoration of the microphonic output from the lateral line organ after local application of streptomycin. Life Sci 3:1151–1155, 1964

60. Young WG, Lesage AM, Dillon ML et al.: Chemo-therapy of intrathoracic neoplasms employing dif-ferential pelvic perfusion hypothermia. Ann Surg 154:372–385, 1961

SUGGESTED READING

Ballantyne J: Ototoxicity: A clinical review. Audiology 12:325–336, 1973

Gonzalez G, Miller N, Wasilewski V: Progressive neuro-ototoxicity of kanamycin. Ann Otol Rhinol Laryngol 81:127–131, 1972

Hawkins JE: Iatrogenic toxic deafness in children. In McConnell F, Ward PN (eds): Deafness in Child-hood. Nashville, Vanderbilt University Press, 1967, pp 156–168

Hawkins JE: Ototoxic mechanisms. A working hy-pothesis. Audiology 12:383–393, 1973

Holz E, Stange G, Soda T et al.: Decrease of Ototoxicity of Streptomycin Sulfate. Arch Otolaryngol 87:359–363, 1968

Lorian V: Experimental intrabroncheal administration of antibiotics in man and animals. Acta Tuberc Scand 42:149–157, 1962

Musebeck K, Schatzle W: Experimentelle Studien zur Ototoxicitat des Dihydrostreptomycins. Arch Ohr Nas Kehlkopfheilk 181:41, 1962

Pulaski EJ, Tubbs RS: Inhibitory effects of kanamycin and diffusion with various body fluids. Antibiot Med Clin Ther 6:589–593, 1959

Systemic and genetic diseases can produce varied forms of adult sensorineural hearing losses. A number of such diseases are implicated etiologically in pediatric sensorineural hearing losses (see Ch. 32, Hereditary Congenital Ear Syndromes), occurring either before, during, or immediately after birth. Viremias, syphilis, bacterial meningitis, drug ototoxicity, and genetic malformations as well, cause sensory and neural hearing losses in infants and children. Some lesions begin in early childhood, are slowly progressive, and may not give rise to detectable hearing loss until adult life.

Genetic, metabolic, vascular, and other systemic lesions can affect the cochlea or the central auditory neural system in adults in early, middle, or late decades. Slow sensorineural hearing losses that occur in the middle or late decades can be mistakenly attributed either to "premature" or to "normal" presbycusis (hearing loss associated with aging). In many cases, the hearing loss may be recognized first with later recognition of an underlying systemic cause. Systemic or genetic sensorineural lesions in later decades may interact with normal presbycusis (aging) processes resulting in combined hearing loss problems.

(Presbycusis lesions are discussed separately in Chapter 41, Presbycusis.)

PATHOLOGY

Cochlear pathologic lesions produced by genetic and systemic diseases are usually nonspecific. Thus, many of the pathologic cochlear sequelae of genetic malformations, viremias, and other systemic diseases result in similar histopathologic changes. Organ of Corti atrophy with hair cell loss, tectorial membrane deformation, cochlear hydrops, stria vascularis atrophy, and spiral ganglion atrophy are common sequelae. Similarly, cochlear nucleus lesions may be associated with peripheral cochlear lesions. Central nervous system auditory pathway lesions may or may not accompany cochlear and/or cochlear nuclear lesions. There is a need for further research involving neuropathologic studies combined with temporal bone pathology studies to clarify many of the etiopathologic issues in adult sensorineural hearing losses.

CLINICAL ASPECTS

SUBJECTIVE ASPECTS OF HEARING LOSS AND TINNITUS

Clinical aspects are basically confined to subjective hearing losses, which may appear gradually, and in

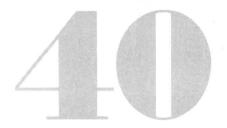

SYSTEMIC ADULT SENSORINEURAL HEARING LOSSES

some patients are accompanied by intermittent or constant episodes of tinnitus. Sociosensory auditory deprivation patterns with accompanying personality changes may occur. The psychosocial isolation of the patient from family and friends can be a serious problem. No one expressed the problems of such hearing loss more poignantly than Ludwig van Beethoven, who described his feelings in a number of letters. He was in his early thirties when he wrote:

My ears whistle and buzz continually, day and night —I am living a wretched life—for two years I have avoided almost all social gatherings because it is impossible for me to say to people: "I am deaf." If I belonged to any other profession, it would be easier, but in my profession, it is an awful state. In order to give you an idea of this singular deafness of mine, I must tell you that in the theatre I must get very close to the orchestra in order to understand the actor. If I am a little distant, I do not hear the high tones of the instruments, or singers, and if I be but a little farther away, I do not hear at all. Frequently, I can hear the tones of a low conversation, but not the words, and as soon as anyone shouts, it is intolerable" (36).

The sad social ostracism which can result in misunderstandings is frequently accompanied by self-imposed secrecy regarding the hearing loss; thus Beethoven described this problem of isolation in classic terms:

I beg of you to keep the matter of my deafness a profound secret to be confided to nobody no matter who it is.

Born with an ardent and lively temperament, ever susceptible to the diversions of society, I was compelled early to isolate myself, to live in loneliness. When I at times tried to forget all this, oh, how harshly was I repulsed by the sad experience of my bad hearing: yet it was impossible for me to say to men, *"speak louder—shout,* for I am *deaf!"* (36).

There are millions of hard-of-hearing people in the world today who secretly harbor fears such as those expressed by Beethoven in the following words:

Forgive me when you see me draw back when I would gladly mingle with you. My misfortune is doubly painful because it must lead to my being misunderstood; for me there can be no recreation in the society of my fellows, no refined intercourse, no mutual exchange of thought, only just as little as the greatest needs command may I mix with society. I must live like an exile. If I approach near to people, a hot terror seizes upon me, a fear that I may be subjected to the danger of letting my condition be observed (36).

OTOLOGIC EXAMINATION

There are no visible abnormalities on either otoscopic or nose/throat examination. Tympanic membrane morphology and mobility and eustachian tube function are usually normal. Tuning fork tests usually show positive Rinne responses and there is rare Weber test lateralization.

AUDIOLOGIC PATTERNS

Varying audiologic patterns occur with any one of a number of hearing loss profiles, including high-frequency losses, middle-frequency dips, straight-line losses, and low-frequency losses. There may be total unilateral or bilateral sensorineural hearing loss (SNHL). Varying changes occur in speech audiometry, impedance, and objective audiometry.

HEREDITARY DEAFNESS SYNDROMES AFFECTING ADULTS

Almost 100 types of hereditary deafness have been recognized through genetic studies in the last few decades. Most of these lesions begin in infancy or are recognized in early childhood A relatively small number of hereditary deafness syndromes are recognized in early or late adult life. Konigsmark (19) described 12 characteristic types of hereditary hearing loss that begin in adult life. They involve either conductive, sensorineural, or mixed losses. The mode of transmission may be dominant, recessive, or sex-linked. Hearing losses may be accompanied by other lesions.

OTOSCLEROSIS

Otosclerosis, a common cause of adult hearing loss, is probably hereditary in the majority of cases. Although conductive lesions predominate, cochlear otosclerosis also occurs (see Ch. 19, Otosclerosis).

DOMINANT LOW-FREQUENCY COCHLEAR HEARING LOSS

Dominant genetic low-frequency cochlear hearing loss can be confused with early otosclerosis because the low-frequency component resembles the air-conduction pattern in otosclerosis. However, this syndrome is entirely sensorineural in character with no conductive (air–bone gap) component (Fig. 40–1). In many cases the hearing loss may be present in the first or second decades in minimal degrees. Clinical recognition may be delayed until the third or fourth decades of life. A later high-frequency component results in eventual flattening of the audiometric pattern in the fifth and sixth decades of life.

Hearing aid use becomes necessary when the overall binaural speech reception thresholds drop below the level of 30–35 dB.

PAGET'S DISEASE OF THE SKULL

Paget's disease of bone affects the skull as well as the extremities.

Temporal bone lesions occur in the middle and inner ears. Stapedial fixation similar to that of otosclerosis can occur in Paget's disease, in which case the hearing loss is purely conductive. In many patients with Paget's disease the hearing loss is mixed or cochlear (see Ch. 21, Temporal Bone Granulomas and Dystrophies).

DOMINANT ANHIDROSIS AND COCHLEAR HEARING LOSS

Among the ectodermal dysplasias, congenital anhidrosis is accompanied by cochlear hearing loss. The disease is characterized by autosomal dominant transmission, congenital anhidrosis, and high-frequency cochlear hearing loss, which usually starts in the middle decades.

FAMILIAL CORNEAL DEGENERATION AND COCHLEAR HEARING LOSS

The syndrome of abnormal calcium metabolism and familial corneal degeneration is accompanied

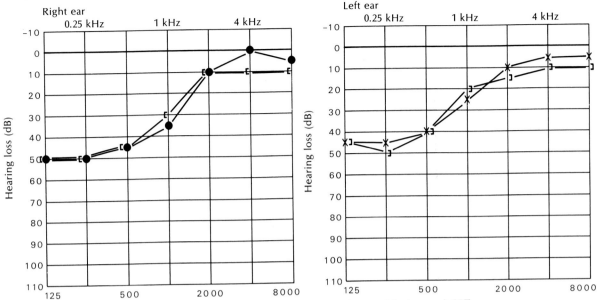

FIG. 40–1. Dominant genetic symmetrical low-frequency SNHL with surprisingly good SRT levels, at age 35. **At left, ●—●,** AC, unmasked, RE; [—[, BC, masked, RE; **At right, x—x,** AC, unmasked, LE;]—], BC, masked, LE; **SRT,** 10 dB RE, 15 dB, LE; **SDS,** 95% RE, 98% LE.

by cochlear hearing loss. It is characterized by autosomal dominant transmission with variable penetrance, ribbon-like corneal degeneration, and delayed, adult onset of cochlear hearing loss.

REFSUM'S DISEASE

This syndrome is characterized by retinitis pigmentosa, polyneuritis, ataxia, and adult cochlear hearing loss. This autosomal recessive disease, characterized by night blindness and ocular nystagmus, is accompanied by progressive cochlear hearing loss in 50% of patients.

VESTIBULAR SCHWANNOMA—FAMILIAL

Schwannoma of the vestibular branch of the eighth nerve (usually called acoustic neurinoma, incorrectly), can be a dominantly inherited disease, accompanied by tinnitus and hearing loss. In that form it occurs primarily in young people and is frequently noted in siblings. Retrocochlear hearing loss is present, due to pressure on the acoustic branch of the eighth nerve in the internal auditory canal (see Ch. 23, Lesions of the Eighth Nerve, Petrous Apex, and Cerebellopontine Angle).

RADICULAR NEUROPATHY AND COCHLEAR HEARING LOSS

This syndrome of peripheral sensory neuropathy is characterized by autosomal dominant transmis-

sion and progressive moderately severe cochlear hearing loss.

DOMINANT PHOTOMYOCLONUS, DIABETES, NEPHROPATHY, AND COCHLEAR HEARING LOSS

This unusual familial syndrome involves the presence of severe diabetes mellitus, dominant photomyoclonus and variable types of nephropathy. This autosomal dominant lesion is characterized first by the onset of photomyoclonic epilepsy in early adult life, and later by diabetes and cochlear hearing loss, usually accompanied by nephropathy. Cerebral cortical degeneration occurs in some patients.

HYPERURICEMIA, ATAXIA, HEARING LOSS SYNDROME

In this syndrome, cochlear hearing loss is first noted in late adolescence or early adult life. A high-tone cochlear loss is accompanied by ataxic gait and associated hyperuricemia.

VAN BUCHEM'S DISEASE

This syndrome is characterized by skull osteosclerosis with involvement of long and short bones. Combined bony constriction of various cranial nerve foramens frequently results in cochlear hearing losses, visual defects, and occasionally in facial paralysis. The most striking finding is an enlarged mandible. Although the disease may first be noted in the second decade, the hearing loss usually occurs in the middle decades.

ALPORT'S DISEASE

The genetic association of renal disease and cochlear hearing loss has gained clinical recognition in the present kidney transplant era. Variable cochlear hearing losses are usually noted in the second and third decades. It is more common in males and is usually characterized by childhood onset of nephritis and ocular lens abnormalities (see Ch. 32, Hereditary Congenital Ear Syndromes).

CIRCULATORY LESIONS

Both unilateral and bilateral adult SNHL are frequently encountered, which are not clearly identified with the specific lesions described in previous chapters. Neither can they be attributed to the normal aging lesions of presbycusis (see Ch. 41, Presbycusis). Since these hearing losses frequently occur in patients with hypertension, arteriosclerosis, or with other circulatory system lesions, etiologic relationships have been assumed but only rarely proved.

Sudden cochlear or retrocochlear SNHL probably can be attributed to circulatory lesions in some cases (see Ch. 37, Sudden Hearing Loss Syndrome). In some experimental animal studies, both behavioral and pathologic observations have demonstrated segmental cochlear changes associated with vascular occlusions.

Fisch, Dobozi and Greig in 1972 (8) reported correlative studies between hearing loss and degrees of arteriosclerosis. Adventitial hyaline thickening was observed in the arteries of the internal auditory meatus.

Schuknecht and colleagues (33) reported necrosis of the membranous labyrinth resulting from anterior inferior cerebellar vessel occlusion. Such infarcts may also produce changes in the central auditory pathway.

Vascular lesions affecting central nervous system pathways can produce specific retrocochlear auditory findings. Noffsinger, Kurdziel, and Appelbaum (26) have recently reported special auditory test findings in the diagnosis of a fluctuating lateromedial inferior pontine syndrome. In a patient with total unilateral retrocochlear hearing loss occurring as part of the syndrome, hearing for pure tones and speech improved following a 2-month period. Retrocochlear findings that per-

sisted were demonstrated by procedures using binaural masking level differences for 500-Hz pure tones and speech, as well as by examination of the amplitude of the acoustic reflex over a 10-sec time period.

The possibility that vascular lesions may be related to sensorineural hearing losses has been advanced by Rosen and co-workers (31) in a number of studies comparing hearing levels of the rural Mabaan tribes with those of inhabitants of urban cities. Relationships between hearing loss, high dietary fat content, and coronary artery disease were analyzed. In 1971, Rosen and Rosen (32) reported a correlation between hypercholesterolemia and hearing loss with the implication of arteriosclerosis as a pathogenic factor. These studies are interesting and call for further investigations.

Much additional research is necessary to clarify circulatory disease/SNHL relationships. There is inadequate scientific evidence to justify the widespread empiric practice of prescribing vasodilators and various anti-hyperlipemic drugs to patients who have SNHL of unproven vascular etiology.

HEMATOLOGIC LESIONS

A number of hematologic lesions can affect the labyrinth primarily by the results of intracochlear and pericochlear nerve hemorrhage. Leukemia, lymphoma, and sickle-cell thalassemia (24) may involve the temporal bone with a number of sequelae, involving both cochlea and cochlear nerve. Hemorrhages can occur throughout the temporal bone with and without infiltration by lymphocytes.

DIABETES

Sensorineural hearing losses have been reported sporadically in diabetics. Since many of the reports have dealt with older people, in whom presbycusis may be a factor, and since many diabetics have concomitant related vascular lesions, it is difficult to attribute specific cochlear lesions to diabetes. There appears to be some type of auditory dysfunction in about 50% of diabetics, comparable with that seen in arteriosclerosis but apparently of greater severity. Igarashi (15) has reported the finding of PAS-positive thickening of capillary walls in stria vascularis in temporal bone studies. In general, diabetic changes are associated with small vessel occlusions. Thus, diabetic auditory dysfunction may be nonspecific and due to the vascular occlusions accompanying the basic metabolic disease.

RENAL FAILURE AND DIALYSIS

Hemodialysis and renal transplantation are frequently accompanied by SNHL and vestibular lesions. Oda and associates (28) reported 290 patients with renal failure seen during a 4-year period, during which 97 of the group showed significant hearing losses during the course of the renal disease. The most likely etiologic factors appeared to be the sequelae of ototoxic diuretics and aminoglycoside antibiotics. The authors studied 26 temporal bones from 8 patients who had chronic renal failure and who underwent hemodialysis and renal transplantations. The findings in these studies suggest that both repetitive hemodialysis and kidney transplantation may affect stria vascularis and vestibular sensory receptor physiology with biochemical changes in inner ear fluids and subsequent audiovascular degenerative changes.

In 1976 Quick (29) reported otologic studies in a total of 602 dialysis and transplant patients. Hearing loss was present in 107 of the 602 patients, either at the time of initial evaluation or during subsequent treatment.

There are anatomic similarities between the kidney and the ear at several levels, including the ultrastructural level. The stria vascularis of the cochlea and the kidney glomerulus are both vascularized epithelial membranes. It is also quite possible that there are immunologic relationships between the stria vascularis and renal glomerular tubules. Structural and immunologic similarities may be related to fluid transport and to electrolyte problems. Auditory deficits and renal disease relationships are complicated by ototoxic drug factors.

Bergstrom and colleagues (1) studied 224 patients with chronic renal disease, 91 of whom had hearing losses. Of illustrative interest is the case of one patient in whom a rapid cochlear loss was noted within 2 weeks following hypotension that occurred during hemodialysis (Fig. 40–2). Temporal bone studies showed endolymphatic hydrops, strial atrophy, and tectorial membrane displacement (Fig. 40–3).

In several cases hearing improvements noted following renal transplantation were probably related to restoration of functional renal systems with improvements in cochlear physiology. Hearing loss in renal disease associated with dialysis

and renal transplantation is rarely due to one cause but stems from the interaction of many factors.

Nephritis and deafness may also be related to concomitant hereditary macrothrombocytopathia, as recently reported by Epstein and co-workers (7). The hearing loss is cochlear in type with primarily high-frequency sensorineural hearing impairments.

BRAIN-STEM AND TEMPORAL-LOBE TUMORS

Brain-stem tumors may produce specific findings of central auditory pathway lesions. Makishima and Ogata (23) recently reported a case with audiometric findings of SNHL. The loss was moderate in one ear and mild in the other. There was evidence of abnormal central vestibular response. Of special note in this study, is the fact that pathologic findings were reported both in temporal bone and in brain. There was a replacement of the right side of the medulla oblongata and pons by an anaplastic astrocytoma. Both cochlear and vestibular nuclei and their connecting fibers were involved. Cochlear changes included organ of Corti atrophy due to flattening, with collapse of Reissner's membrane accompanied by spiral ganglion neural degeneration.

Temporal-lobe tumors are very frequently accompanied by central auditory pathway lesions, which cannot be demonstrated by ordinary pure-tone and speech audiometry. Korsan-Bengsten (20) recently reported the use of distorted speech audiometry. In a study of 11 patients with temporal-lobe tumors that involved the auditory cortex, large differences in performance were noted between ipsi- and contralateral ears, especially in tests with 10 interruptions per second and time-compressed speech. The smallest differences were found for frequency distorted speech. Distorted speech audiometry can reveal lesions involving the auditory cortex and central hearing pathways in early stages.

THYROID DISEASE

The relationship between hypothyroidism and cochlear hearing loss is well documented in the pediatric genetic entity of Pendred's syndrome. Thyroid enlargement may be present at birth or occur at puberty and is associated with a defect in the peroxidase system. The cochlear high-frequency hearing loss is usually severe. This autosomal recessive genetic condition is primarily a

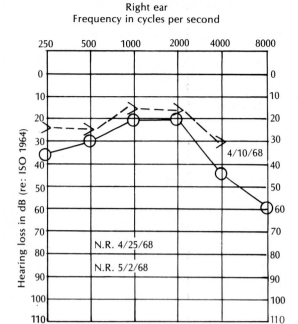

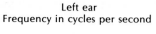

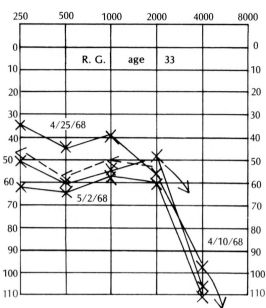

FIG. 40–2. Adult with hearing loss in renal disease. (Bergstrom L, Jenkins P, Sando I et al.: Ann Otol Rhinol Laryngol 82:555–577, 1973)

FIG. 40–3. Right ear of same patient whose audiogram is shown in Figure 40–2. Cochlea, demonstrating filling of fibrous tissue in perilymphatic spaces (**P**), endolymphatic hydrops (**E**), strial atrophy (**S**), and displaced tectorial membrane (**T**) in apposition to Reissner's membrane (**R**). (Bergstrom L, Jenkins P, Sando I et al.: Ann Otol Rhinol Laryngol 82:555–577, 1973)

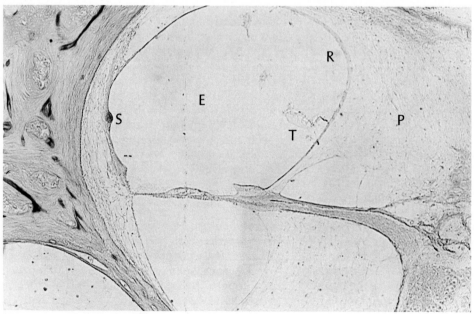

pediatric problem and is not frequently encountered in adults (see Ch. 32, Hereditary Congenital Ear Syndromes).

Empiric relationships between SNHL and thyroid deficiencies in adults require further documentation. There is no definitive proof that hypothyroidism and SNHL are related. However, it is an area that merits careful clinical research.

MALNUTRITION

Multiple nutritional deficiencies, which may or may not be associated with specific thiamine deficiency, such as that found in beri-beri, can produce a number of neuropathies. In Denny-Brown's 1974 report (3) retrobulbar neuritis and the "burning foot" syndrome were accompanied by gradual onset of SNHL. Ironside (16) reported hearing losses in hyperemesis gravidarum, and Spillane (35) reported deafness in nicotinic acid deficiency.

In a recent report on the malabsorption syndrome, Gussen (12) described the temporal-bone findings in a 33-year-old patient with bilaterally progressive severe SNHL. The hearing loss, which started following the onset of gastrointestinal symptoms, became virtually total during hospitalization. Cochlear studies showed marked loss of cellular elements of spiral ligament and spiral prominence and degeneration of the organ of Corti, with no identifiable hair cells. In addition, there was necrosis of the stria vascularis and degeneration of saccular macula, with otolithic membrane displacement. There was bilateral segmental demyelination of vestibular and cochlear nerves, with lesser involvement of the seventh and ninth nerves. Of special interest was the absence of any other peripheral neural involvement (Figs. 40–4, 40–5).

COGAN'S SYNDROME

Cogan's syndrome is a collagen disease characterized by nonsyphilitic keratitis, accompanied by severe cochlear hearing loss. Vestibular lesions may also be present. This uncommon disease occurs primarily in young adults. Ocular and auditory manifestations are variable in terms of onset. The pathologic findings are those of systemic necrotizing angiitis of the polyarteritis type. Endolymphatic hydrops with marked distortion of the vestibular membrane has been described. New bone formation has been noted in the region of a thickened round window membrane. There is also

degeneration of the organ of Corti and cochlear neurons, especially in the basal turn.

Although the use of steroids is of some value in certain cases, no specific therapy has yet been described.

RELAPSING POLYCHONDRITIS WITH LABYRINTHITIS

This rather obscure inflammatory reaction, which may occur in multiple cartilages throughout the body, is accompanied frequently by auricular swelling, and cochlear hearing loss, which is fluctuating in character and frequently accompanied by vestibular symptoms and seventh nerve paralysis. The auricular chondritic lesions can be severe, resulting in sloughing of auricular cartilages. This autoimmune disease frequently responds to steroids or cyclophosphamide therapy. Prompt steroid therapy is indicated and may require repeated administrations (2).

POLYARTERITIS NODOSA

Although hearing losses have been noted in patients with periarteritis nodosa, it was not until 1976 that a temporal bone study was reported. Gussen (13) studied the temporal bone changes of a 66-year-old woman with polyarteritis nodosa, who became deaf in one ear 7 months before death.

There was polyarteritis of the internal auditory artery, with resultant fibrosis and bone formation in the cochlear and vestibular systems. Endolymphatic hydrops of the basal turn of the cochlea was present as well as chronic perforation of the saccule (Fig. 40–6).

It may well be that this example of arterial involvement is a prototype of other varieties of vascular cochlear hearing loss.

WEGENER'S GRANULOMATOSIS

Friedmann and Bauer (9) reported temporal bone involvement by Wegener's granulomatosis in two patients. The mixed hearing loss involved middle and inner ears. Necrotizing granulation tissue in the tympanic cavity included characteristic multinucleated cells. Compact hyperchromatic nuclei formed bizarre patterns, accompanied by pale eosinophilic cytoplasm, differing from the classic findings in Langerhans giant cells. Ossicular and tympanic damage was accompanied by less severe labyrinthine involvement.

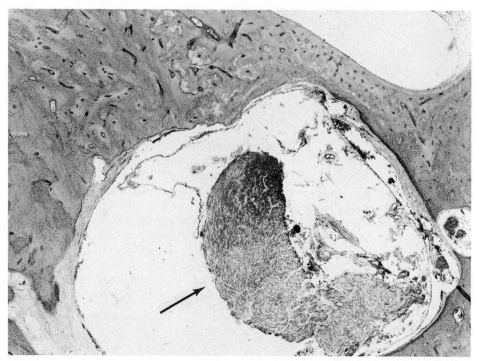

FIG. 40–4. Right cochlear nerve **(arrow)** and inferior vestibular nerve, **(at right).** Note demyelination, more prominent in distal portion. (Gussen R: J Laryngol 88:523–530, 1974)

FIG. 40–5. High-power view, middle turn. Note loss of cellular elements, as in Figure 40–4, plus necrosis of stria vascularis. (Gussen R: J Laryngol 88:523–530, 1974)

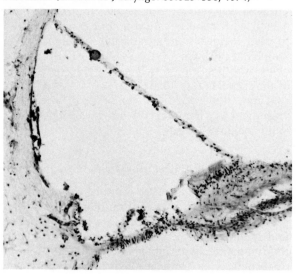

SARCOIDOSIS

Sudden or fluctuating SNHL can occur in temporal bone sarcoidosis. Auditory-vestibular dysfunctions are also accompanied by facial nerve paralysis and other neuropathies.

Sarcoidosis, a systemic granulomatous disease of undetermined etiology is characterized by the histologic appearance of epithelioid tubercles that differ morphologically from those seen in tuberculosis (14).

ANOXIA

Anoxic changes can affect the cochlear nucleus as well as the cochlea, as studied in kernicterus due to Rh factor incompatibilities (see Ch. 33, Acquired Congenital Ear Syndromes). Neonatal asphyxia followed by cerebral palsy can include hearing losses, some of which show high-frequency loss patterns but may include other audiometric profiles. Carbon monoxide asphyxia also causes complex SNHL.

The primary vulnerability is in the CNS auditory system. The major lesions are in the ventral cochlear nucleus, especially in its superior division. The dorsal cochlear nucleus is not affected by

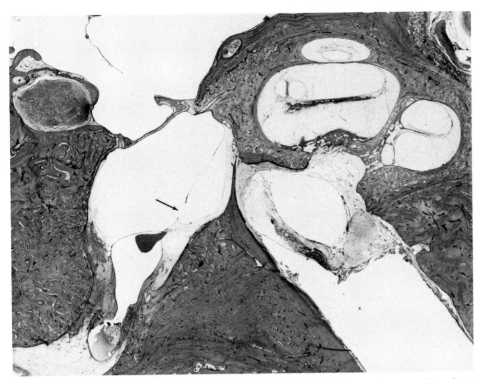

FIG. 40–6. Fibrosis and bone formation of the cochlear and vestibular systems resulting from polyarteritis of internal auditory artery. Note basal cochlear hydrops and chronic perforation of saccule wall **(arrow).** (Gussen R: Arch Otol Rhinol Laryngol [Berlin]. In press)

anoxia. Dublin's studies (5) indicate that the lack of dorsal cochlear nucleus involvement is in keeping with the regressive character of this nucleus (Fig. 40–7).

ALCOHOLIC CIRRHOSIS

The potential relationships between chronic alcoholism and deafness have been subjects of speculation for years. Definitive clinical data, however, have been lacking.

In a recent study by Koff, Oliai, and Sparks (18), it was hypothesized that subclinical hearing impairment might be present in alcoholic cirrhotic patients. In their study, mild, bilateral, high-frequency SNHL were usually noted. Severe SNHL were found only in a group of patients who required surgical shunt procedures, irrespective of whether neomycin therapy had been administered.

Because of potentially complex etiologic aspects it is difficult to state categorically that chronic alcoholism by itself is a cause of severe SNHL. More studies of the type cited will be necessary before a final conclusion can be reached regarding relationships between alcoholism and hearing losses.

MULTIPLE SCLEROSIS

Sensorineural hearing losses in multiple sclerosis are not commonly due to temporal bone involvement. The periphery is usually spared but the CNS auditory pathway is the primary locus of the lesions, which can produce fluctuating hearing losses as well as fluctuating disturbances in the vestibular system. Because of the complex nature of central auditory processing, hearing losses may not always be documented by standard audiometric changes.

Audiometric losses vary in degree and type, either "flat" losses or high-frequency losses. However, there may be no pure tone changes, and the hearing losses may be detectable only by speech audiometry or discovered in some cases by special central auditory pathway testing techniques (SCANS) (see Ch. 6, Audiologic Assessment, Functional Hearing Loss, and Objective Audiometry).

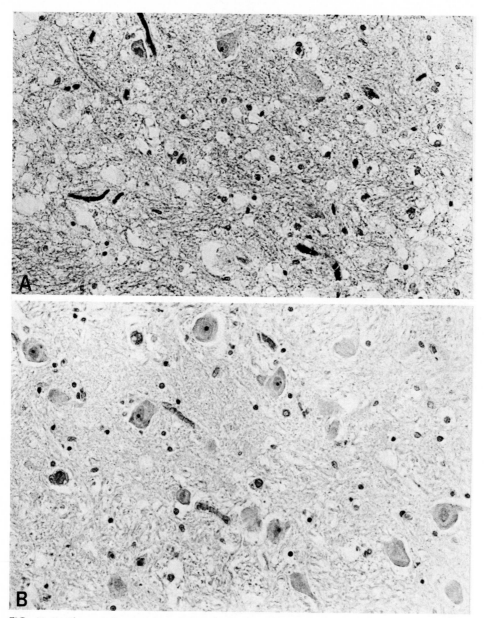

FIG. 40–7. Changes in superior ventral cochlear nucleus, showing severe loss of spheroid cells in upper zone **(A)** and more moderate cell loss in lower zone **(B)**. (Dublin WB: FUNDA-MENTALS OF SENSORINEURAL AUDITORY PATHOLOGY, 1976. Courtesy of Charles C Thomas, Publisher, Springfield, Illinois)

In a study of 61 patients with multiple sclerosis, Noffsinger and associates (27) used a standard audiometric test battery and a series of special tonal and speech tests. The pure-tone tests included the short increment sensitivity index (SISI), adaptation, loudness function, as well as three different tests of binaural auditory function behavior. The speech tests included discrimination of words in the presence of ipsilateral white noise, contralateral competing speech messages in various modes and in various binaural masking situations.

Auditory evaluations demonstrated a marked diversity of auditory aberrations most commonly elicited by tests requiring responses to sustained stimuli, tests requiring discrimination of speech in conditions other than quiet, and by binaural masking tests.

The same group of patients were evaluated from the point of view of the vestibular system utilizing a complex vestibular electronystagmographic test battery.

The most common vestibular abnormalities were abnormal visually induced eye movements, positional nystagmus, and hyperexcitability in response to caloric stimulation.

The study pointed to multileveled lesions of the CNS, especially in the midbrain and brain stem.

The basic pathologic process is one of destruction of myelin by antibody developed against the antigen formed by union of myelin with the virus. Lymphocytes and macrophages proliferate in white matter undergoing demyelination. In late stages there is an absence of myelin, with an increase of glia arranged in dense bands (5) (Fig. 40–8).

MANAGEMENT OF SENSORINEURAL LOSSES OF GENETIC AND SYSTEMIC ETIOLOGY

Medical therapy has been described wherever indicated. Rehabilitation management usually involves consideration of amplification and related approaches (see Ch. 43, Hearing Aids).

"TREATMENT" OF IRREVERSIBLE SENSORINEURAL HEARING LOSS

With the exception of a few systemic conditions associated with SNHL for which specific systemic therapy is available, there is no valid ear treatment for either pediatric or adult SNHL of genetic or systemic origin.

Many futile attempts have been made in the past to stimulate a "weak" or "dead" inner ear or auditory nerve. A careful review of the anatomy and physiology of the ear (see Ch. 1, Clinical Anatomy and Physiology of the Peripheral Ear) and of the central auditory neural pathway (see Ch. 2, Central Representation of the Eight Nerve) will clarify the naiveté involved in "therapies" advocated for restoration of auditory function to a totally degenerated or destroyed cochlea or to the cochlear nerve or cochlear nucleus.

Examples of such proposed ineffectual approaches are 1) transdermal therapy, and 2) acupuncture.

Transdermal Therapy for Sensorineural Hearing Loss

Glattke and Simmons (11) reported a double-blind study to determine the effect of transdermal stimulation on monosyllabic word discrimination scores. The transdermal device was used for stimulation with 20–60 kHz electrical current, modulated with audio frequencies. This was applied via electrodes placed bilaterally on the skin over the zygoma and neck, below the mastoid. Stimulation was ultimately provided across all possible pairs of the electrodes for a total single treatment duration of approximately 1 hour. The treatment periods extended from 12 to 72 episodes.

Following a careful analysis of data on 31 hard-of-hearing subjects, the investigators concluded: "The present study reveals no differences between the control and actively treated patients. Changes in the discrimination scores for some individuals were observed, but these were probably spurious."

In another study of transdermal electrostimulation therapy, Gerken, Glorig, and Roeser (10) studied 16 volunteer subjects with SNHL. They were randomly assigned to treated and placebo groups in a double-blind experiment. These investigators concluded that "no change in word discrimination scores was observed that could be attributed to the treatment. Transdermal therapy is inappropriate for the treatment of sensorineural hearing loss."

Acupuncture as a Treatment of Sensorineural Hearing Loss

Following media publicity of purported cures of SNHL by acupuncture therapy, countless acupuncture clinics have appeared throughout the country, with varying claims regarding the values of such treatments. Regan and Tobin (30) reported data on a random sample of 16 children and adults with medically validated congenital SNHL of unknown etiology, who were treated in an acupuncture clinic. There was no change in post-acupuncture treatment audiograms.

Eisenberg, Taub, and DiCarlo (6) in a similar study of 25 subjects, reported that the hearing tests showed little or no consistent change.

Madell (22), in a study of 40 children (aged 9–16 years) with severe and profound SNHL, who received long courses of acupuncture, found no clinically significant audiometric changes during or following the acupuncture therapy.

My colleagues and I have seen at least 50 patients with documented otologic findings who went to various acupuncture clinics on their own for treatment of sensorineural hearing lesions. Not only did we fail to find even one patient whose hearing was improved, but we had occasion to deal with a number of auricular complications of acupuncture, including chondritis, perichondritis, and auricular abscesses.

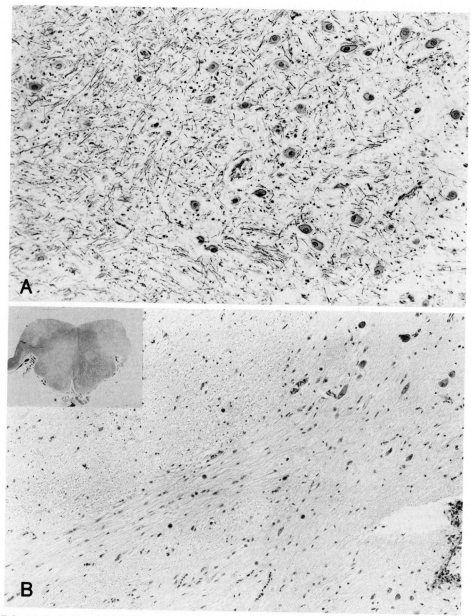

FIG. 40–8. A. Transverse view of right superior ventral cochlear nucleus, Bodian stain, from case of disseminated sclerosis, in which there was no apparent involvement of cochlear nuclear complex. Well-preserved spheroid cells are at right; fibers of trapezoid body sweep diagonally downward to left. **B.** Section from same location as that in Figure 40–8A, from another case of disseminated sclerosis in which there was involvement of cochlear nucleus and trapezoid body. A few remnant spheroid cells appear **(upper right).** A band of gliosis extends down across center to left. **Inset.** Large foci of demyelination, in a section of medulla from same case (Luxol fast blue stain), one of the foci including right cochlear nucleus and trapezoid complex. This type of lesion can produce unilateral SNHL equivalent to that resulting from demyelination of cochlear nerve. (Dublin WB: FUNDAMENTALS OF SENSORINEURAL AUDITORY PATHOLOGY, 1976. Courtesy of Charles C Thomas, Publisher, Springfield, Illinois)

COCHLEAR IMPLANTS FOR IRREVERSIBLE SENSORINEURAL HEARING LOSS LESIONS

In 1800, Volta (37) reported that he was able to create a hearing sensation in his own ears, "not unlike the bubbling of soup" when he discharged about 20 v of direct current through his head by means of electrodes inserted into his ear canals. Since that time, many investigators have attempted to solve the tragic problem of total nerve deafness by implanting electrodes within the inner ear. The basic theory behind these attempts is that such an implant might be able to stimulate intact auditory nerve fibers when the cochlea is completely atrophic and nonresponsive. The methods have usually involved placement of electrodes into the scala tympani via the round window membrane.

In 1957 Djourno and Eyries (4) reported electrical stimulation experiments in both animals and man. Simmons, in 1966 (34), published a landmark classic on the subject in his report of the first careful study of electrical stimulation of a profoundly deaf adult, in whom a multiple electrode array cochlear implant was studied carefully by a number of psychoacoustic methods over a significantly long period of time.

In his concluding remarks, Simmons asked a question: "What is the likelihood that electrical stimulation of the auditory nerve can ever provide a uniquely useful means of communication?"

He pointed out the enormity of the problem of attempting electrical stimulation of the eighth nerve, especially with relationships to such basic questions regarding hearing as that of neural processing of auditory information in the cochlea, in the auditory nerve, and even within the brain stem.

Following this extraordinary study, among his conclusions, Simmons stated: "The chances are small indeed that electrical stimulation of the auditory nerve can ever provide a uniquely useful means of communication. Studies in tactile learning and communication and methods of utilizing and intensively training residual acoustic hearing, especially in children, are more likely to provide generally useful communication" (34).

Since Simmons' work, a number of attempts have been made in the United States and in France to build various types of cochlear implants, a number of which have already been implanted in humans.

At a symposium on the subject of cochlear implants held at the American Otological Society Meeting in 1973, Lawrence and Johnsson (21) stated: "Anything which will disturb the integrity of scala media and its blood supply is likely to cause degeneration of remaining sensory and neural elements." They also pointed out that "when the endosteum of the labyrinth is disturbed, the otic capsule frequently responds with a fairly rapid and extensive bone formation. Such bone formation poses a threat to the effectiveness of the implant by isolating it from the nerve fibers" (21).

In further discussion of this problem Dr. Nelson Y. S. Kiang, of Harvard University and Massachusetts Institute of Technology, stated: "The conclusion to be drawn from the human studies is that stimulating large numbers of fibers synchronously in indiscriminate ways does not provide sufficient cues for the understanding of speech. To be sure there is auditory sensation that may have some value as an aid to lipreading" (17). Dr. Kiang continued: "Let there be no misunderstanding on this point. No existing prosthetic device will make speech intelligible in the absence of visual cues. Since none of the present procedures can be judged to be an adequate treatment for sensorineural deafness, the implantation of electrodes into people must still be regarded as human experimentation."

The First International Conference on Electrical Stimulation of the Acoustic Nerve as a Treatment for Profound Sensorineural Deafness in Man was held in San Francisco under the chairmanship of the chancellor of the University of San Francisco, Dr. Frances A. Sooy (25).

Many issues relating to patient selection, surgical techniques, electrode arrays, integrated circuitry, and other aspects of the problem were considered. Frank discussions concerning otologic, audiologic, and psychoacoustic evaluations of patients who had received cochlear implants revealed the controversial nature of the problem.

It was not demonstrated that cochlear implants could, by themselves, restore useful hearing for speech. Some responses to sound were reported. It appears that Dr. Kiang's comments, which we have quoted, have not been disproved.

Much research of a fundamental nature remains to be done before the use of surgical implants into the cochlea or into the auditory nerve can be prudently advised in humans at the present time.

REFERENCES

1. Bergstrom L, Jenkins P, Sando I et al.: Hearing loss in renal disease: clinical and pathological studies. Ann Otol Rhinol Laryngol 82:555–577, 1973

2. Cody DTR, Sones DA: Relapsing polychondritis: audiovestibular manifestation. Laryngoscope 81: 1208–1222, 1971

3. Denny-Brown D: Neurological conditions resulting from prolonged and severe dietary restriction. Medicine 26:41–113, 1947

4. Djourno A, Eyries C: Prothese auditive par excitation electrique a distance du nerf sensoriel a l'aide d'un bobinage inclus a demeure. Presse Med 35:1417, 1957

5. Dublin WB: Fundamentals of Sensorineural Auditory Pathology. Springfield, IL, CC Thomas, 1976, pp 190–195

6. Eisenberg L, Taub HA, DiCarlo L: Acupuncture therapy of sensorineural deafness: evaluation study. NY State J Med 74:1942–1949, 1974

7. Epstein CJ, Sahud MA, Piel C et al.: Hereditary macrothrombocytopathia, nephritis and deafness. Am J Med 52:229–310, 1972

8. Fisch U, Dobozi M, Grieg D: Degenerative changes of the arterial vessels of the internal auditory meatus during the process of aging. Acta Otolaryngol (Stockh) 73:259–266, 1972

9. Friedmann I, Bauer F: Wegener's granulomatosis causing deafness. J Laryngol 87:449–464, 1973

10. Gerken GM, Glorig A, Roeser RJ: Transdermal electrostimulation therapy. Arch Otolaryngol 100:96–99, 1974

11. Glattke J, Simmons FB: Transdermal therapy and monosyllabic word discrimination. Arch Otolaryngol 100:91–95, 1974

12. Gussen R: Malnutrition and deafness. J Laryngol 88:523–530, 1974

13. Gussen R: Polyarteritis nodosa and deafness. A human temporal bone study. Archotorhinolaryngol (NY) 217:263–271, 1977

14. Hybels RL, Rice DH: Neuro-otologic manifestations of sarcoidosis. Laryngoscope 86:1873–1878, 1976

15. Igarashi M: Pathology of the inner ear end organs. In Minkler J (ed): Pathology of the Nervous System. New York, McGraw Hill, 1972

16. Ironside R: Neuritis complicating pregnancy. Proc R Soc Med 32:588–595, 1939

17. Kiang NYS: Discussion. Trans Am Otolaryngol Soc 61:223–229, 1973

18. Koff RS, Oliai A, Sparks RW: Sensorineural hearing loss in alcoholic cirrhosis. Digestion 8:248–253, 1973

19. Konigsmark BW: Hereditary deafness syndromes with onset in adult life. Int Audiol 10:257–283, 1971

20. Korsan-Bengtsen M: Distorted speech audiometry: methodologic and clinical study. Acta Otolaryngol [Suppl] (Stockh) #310 1973

21. Lawrence M, Johnsson L-G: The role of the organ of Corti in auditory nerve stimulation. Trans Am Otolaryngol Soc 61:176–184, 1973

22. Madell JR: Acupuncture for sensorineural hearing loss. Arch Otolaryngol 101:441–445, 1975

23. Makishima K, Ogata J: Brain stem tumor and otoneurologic manifestations: report of a case with autopsy. Ann Otol Rhinol Laryngol 84:391–400, 1975

24. Marcus RE, Lee YM: Inner ear disorders in a family with sickle cell thalassemia. Arch Otolaryngol 102:703–705, 1976

25. Merzenich MM, Schindler RA, Sooy FA (eds): Proceedings of the First International Conference on Electrical Stimulation of the Acoustic Nerve as a Treatment for Profound Sensorineural Deafness in Man, 1974, (private printing)

26. Noffsinger D, Kurdziel S, Applebaum EL: The value of special auditory tests in the latero-medial inferior pontine syndrome. Ann Otol Rhinol Laryngol 84:384–390, 1975

27. Noffsinger D, Olsen W, Carhart R et al.: Auditory and vestibular abberrations in multiple sclerosis. Acta Otolaryngol [Suppl] (Stockh) #303, 1972

28. Oda M, Preciado M, Quick C et al.: Labyrinthine pathology of chronic renal failure patients treated with hemodialysis and kidney transplantation. Laryngoscope 84:1489–1506, 1974

29. Quick C: Hearing loss in patients with dialysis and renal transplants. Ann Otol Rhinol Laryngol 85:776–790, 1976

30. Regan JB, Tobin J: Acupuncture: effectiveness of acupuncture as treatment of sensorineural hearing loss. RI Med J 57:373–375, 1974

31. Rosen S, Bergman M, Plester D et al.: Presbycusis study of a relatively noise-free population in the Sudan. Ann Otol Rhinol Laryngol 71:727–743, 1962

32. Rosen S, Rosen H: High frequency studies in school children in nine countries. Laryngoscope 81:1007–1013, 1971

33. Schuknecht HF, Watanuki K, Takahashi T et al.: Atrophy of the stria vascularis, a common cause for hearing loss. Laryngoscope 84:1777–1821, 1974

34. Simmons FB: Electrical stimulation of the auditory nerve in man. Arch Otolaryngol 84:2–54, 1966

35. Spillane JD: Nutritional Disorders of the Nervous System. Edinburgh, E & S Livingstone, 1947

36. Thayer AW: The Life of Ludwig Van Beethoven. (trans by HE Krehbiel). New York, The Beethoven Association, 1921

37. Volta A: On the electricity excited by mere contact of conducting substances of different kinds. Trans Roy Soc Phil 90:403–431, 1800

Normal aging processes occur in the auditory system along with aging changes in other organ systems. The catabolic processes involved in senility can affect the middle ear, cochlea, cochlear nucleus, and the central auditory nervous system. Great variations occur in the chronology of such changes, and in individual differences, creating difficulties in attempts to define the characteristics of "normal presbycusis."

"Normal" hearing loss attributable to age alone varies in degree and in auditory patterns, and it has been characterized primarily by degenerative cochlear changes. Such cochlear pathology plays the major role in the aging processes of the auditory system. However, it is now clear that other aging lesions also occur, i.e., in the middle ear, in the auditory nerve, in the cochlear nucleus, and in various levels within the central auditory nervous system.

Pseudopresbycusis is a useful concept for differential diagnostic purposes and includes consideration of all diseases of the ear that can cause hearing losses occurring in the sixth, seventh, eighth, and ninth decades. Thus, genetic diseases, otomastoiditis, otosclerosis, ossicular fixations, temporal bone dystrophies, tumors, direct trauma, barotrauma, acoustic trauma, ototoxic drugs, syphilis, labyrinthine membrane ruptures, viremias, vascular lesions, and other causes must be considered. In addition, differential diagnosis must be concerned with systemic diseases producing hearing losses that can be mistaken for the normal aging patterns of presbycusis (see Ch. 40, Systemic Adult Sensorineural Hearing Loss).

Because of the potential multiple causality inherent in hearing losses, it is important to avoid a simplistic stance in considering diagnostic and management aspects of hearing losses in older people. The label "presbycusis" is tenable only when no other specific cause for older adult hearing loss cases can be found on careful otologic study.

The management of the presbycusis patient is a major medical problem in our constantly aging society. Psychosocial aspects of the sensory deprivation produced by presbycusis require a broad rehabilitation approach to the problem.

PATHOLOGY

Degenerative changes of aging produce middle ear, cochlear (hair cell), and neural (spiral ganglion) lesions. Changes have also been reported in co-chlear nuclei and in higher CNS auditory pathways.

Nixon, Glorig, and High (10) suggested that high-frequency losses can be caused by middle ear lesions, attributable to elasticity losses in tympanic membrane and in ligaments and muscles.

Middle-ear lesions have been identified in ossicular joints and ligaments. Goodhill (6) reported high frequency BC losses in lateral ossicular fixation. Belal and Stewart (1) described arthritic changes in middle ear ossicular joints with fibrous and calcific changes resulting in ankylosis. However, no definitive conclusions have yet been reached regarding relationships between such middle ear lesions and audiometric findings.

The correlation of cochlear lesions with presbycusis has been documented in a number of studies. In 1937 von Fieandt and Saxen (4) reported temporal bone findings in 33 cases of individuals 50 years of age or older. They described senile atrophy of spiral ganglion and angiosclerotic degeneration of cochlear duct epithelial elements.

Four cochlear types of presbycusis lesions were proposed by Schuknecht with definitive relationships to audiometric findings (11):

1. Sensory presbycusis is due to an organ of Corti lesion characterized by losses of basal turn external hair cells and supporting cells. Audiometric studies show high-frequency losses with good discrimination scores.
2. Neural presbycusis is due to a cochlear neuron loss. Audiometric studies show poor discrimination, accompanied by phonemic regression, and a flat, slightly sloping, SNHL pattern.
3. Strial presbycusis is due to patchy atrophy of the stria vascularis in middle and apical turns. Audiometric studies show fairly flat sensori-

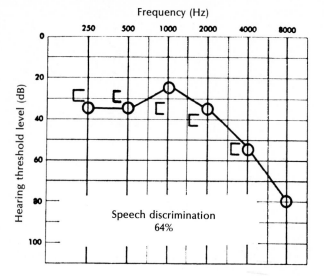

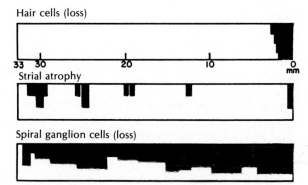

FIG. 41–1. Audiogram and graphic reconstruction of losses of hair cells of the organ of Corti, stria vascularis, and spiral ganglion cells of the right cochlea. **Numbers** below the graph for hair cells indicate distance (mm) along basilar membrane from basal end to cochlear apex. **Black zones** indicate losses of hair cells, stria vascularis, and spiral ganglion cells in percentages. (Suga F, Lindsay J: Ann Otol Rhinol Larnygol 85:169–184, 1976)

neural hearing curves with reasonably good discrimination scores.

4. Cochlear "conductive" presbycusis is theoretically attributed to a disturbance in cochlear partition mobility. Audiometric studies show a descending SNHL curve.

Suga and Lindsay (12), in a report of temporal bone histopathology in 17 aged patients, all of whom had bilateral sensorineural hearing losses, pointed out the primary finding of decrease in the population of spiral ganglion cells. In many cases there was also a diffuse senile atrophy of the organ of Corti and stria vascularis. Of special interest in their findings is the fact that no correlation was

found between the degree of arteriosclerosis and the degree of sensorineural degeneration in the cochlea. Further, their study did not show any consistent correlation between any special type of audiometric curve and localization of lesions to the sensory, the neural, or the vascular elements of the cochlea. They thus concluded that a certain type of audiometric curve does not necessarily indicate a lesion in a specific cochlear location (Figs. 41–1 to 41–4).

Johnsson and Hawkins (8) illustrated both sensory and neural degenerations associated with aging in human inner ear microdissections. When the normal cochlea of a 25-year-old patient (Fig. 41–5) is compared with that of a 92-year-old (Fig. 41–6), there is a dramatic demonstration of degeneration in the myelinated radial nerve fibers in the lower half of the basal turn along with degeneration in the organ of Corti.

Because of the primary attention directed to temporal bone studies in patients with presbycusis, the emphasis has been concentrated on cochlear changes. Undoubtedly these changes represent the major lesions in presbycusis. Yet, since few attempts have been made to correlate middle ear and cochlear pathology with changes in the auditory CNS, our knowledge of the pathology of presbycusis is still incomplete. Relationships of vascular and degenerative changes in the entire auditory CNS must be taken into consideration for a more complete understanding of presbycusis. Such neural pathway changes may occur anywhere from the auditory neurons in the spiral ganglion to the cochlear nuclei and to the entire ascending central nervous system. In addition, it is necessary to consider changes in the auditory cortex, and in other CNS centers relating to auditory memory, attention, and intellectual processing, as related to senile changes.

Degenerative changes in the arteries within the internal auditory meatus begin during the first decade of life in man. Fisch, Dobozi, and Greig (5), in a temporal bone study, report significant changes that consist of progressive thickening of the tunica adventitia, accompanied by an increase of collagenous tissue and loss of fibroblasts. The increasing compactness of the adventitial layer leads to complete acellularity and loss of structure in some specimens. When such changes are related to the normal variations in the arterial system of the internal auditory canal, a number of potentially destructive lesions can be theoretically considered.

Osseous changes can produce compression of auditory nerve bundles in the internal auditory meatus. Krmpotić-Nemanić, Nemanić, and Kos-

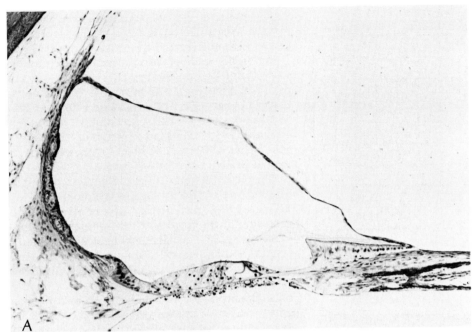

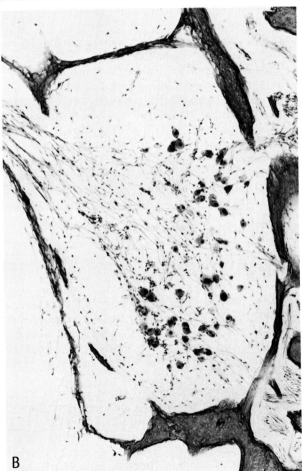

FIG. 41–2. Cochlear duct **(A)** and spiral ganglion **(B)** of midbasal turn of right cochlear. Spiral ganglion cells show marked decrease of population, while hair cells of the organ of Corti and stria vascularis appear normal. (Suga R, Lindsay J: Ann Otol Rhinol Laryngol 85: 169–184, 1976)

tović (9) described increased apposition of bony substances with advancing age, causing compression and atrophy of acoustic nerve fibers and reduction of ganglionic cells. Such hyperostotic changes in the foramens of the osseous lamina cribrosa compress cochlear nerve bundles originating primarily from the basal cochlear turn.

Gussen (7) described plugging of vascular canals in the otic capsule as related to the aging process.

Dublin (2, 3) has described changes in the ventral cochlear nucleus, including a tendency toward dorsal zonal (high frequency) involvement, with specific losses affecting spheroid cells, associated with a reparative gliosis. In the inferior colliculus, there is loss of neuronal elements, nerve cell deterioration, and an increase of glia, which disrupts the laminated pattern. Cellular degeneration also occurs in the medial geniculate body and in the auditory cortex.

Joint temporal bone and cochlear nucleus studies as proposed by Dublin would make possible a total sensorineural mapping pattern for tonotopic combined audiometric, cochlear, and cochlear nucleus study approaches.

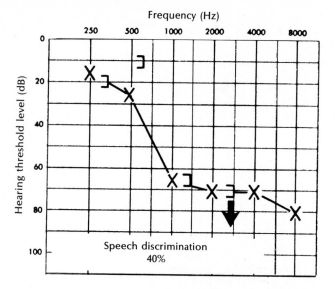

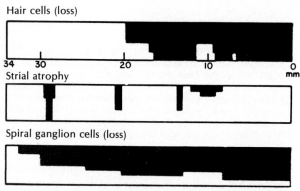

FIG. 41–3. Audiogram and graphic reconstruction of loss of hair cells of organ of Corti, stria vascularis, and spiral ganglion cells of left cochlea of a 74-year-old woman. (Suga R, Lindsay J: Ann Otol Rhinol Laryngol 85:169–184, 1976)

This important correlative plan makes possible a combined audiohistogram taking into consideration temporal bone findings and neuropathologic studies of the superior ventral cochlear nucleus (Figs. 41–7 to 41–9). In addition, auditory cortex findings (Fig. 41–10) may complete a total tissue study plan for clinicopathologic evaluations of degenerative lesions in presbycusis.

AUDIOLOGIC PATTERNS

Sensorineural hearing loss patterns in presbycusis fall into several types. The losses rarely show an air–bone gap. One type of decade pattern for "normal" aging hearing loss is seen in Figure 41–11, but such decade patterns are variable. Pure-tone

SNHL patterns can vary considerably and comprise at least three types—flat, mildly sloping, and severely sloping curves.

Pure-tone audiograms, speech discrimination scores, and Bekesy audiometric patterns are illustrated in Figures 41–12 to 41–15. Occasionally a moderate flat or mixed pure-tone sloping pattern will be combined with exceedingly poor speech discrimination scores as a result of cochlear degeneration and/or phonemic regression, possibly related to CNS pathway lesions.

A serious dilemma is the difficulty of evaluating components of the presbycusis pattern relative to 1) true aging phenomena, which are moderately variable, 2) the results of environmental noise or other causes of noise-induced hearing loss, and 3) results of undiagnosed cochlear lesions that may have nothing to do with age. In clinical practice, rather marked variations are found in the so-called normal hearing levels of individuals in various age groups. Some patients who appear for otologic examination because of vestibular problems with no auditory complaints will frequently show infinitely better audiometric levels than one would expect for age, according to traditional "decade loss" audiometric patterns.

Cochlear and CNS pathway changes responsible for presbycusis produce a broad spectrum of hearing loss patterns that are possibly due to familial genetic traits. Thus, an otherwise unexplained sloping pattern SNHL in the third or fourth decades without other otologic abnormalities may be genetic in origin (see Ch. 40, Systemic Adult Sensorineural Hearing Losses), and masquerade as "premature presbycusis."

DIFFERENTIAL DIAGNOSIS

A number of variants of other SNHL lesions can produce presbycusis-like degenerative patterns. These can be considered pseudopresbycusis lesions. As an example, the fluctuating cochlear hearing losses in bilateral Meniere's disease without vertigo due to endolymphatic cochlear hydrops, occurring in fifth and later decades can reach stable nonfluctuating levels and simulate premature presbycusis.

Phonemic regression in some cases of presbycusis (hearing for speech much poorer than the pure-tone audiogram might suggest) might be the result of reduced cerebral function, rather than to cochlear presbycusis. The emergence of more refined central auditory function tests will be useful in clarifying this hypothesis. Presbycusis patients

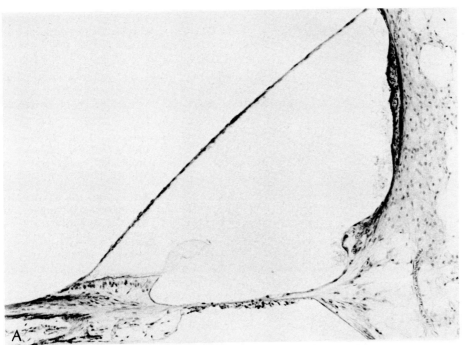

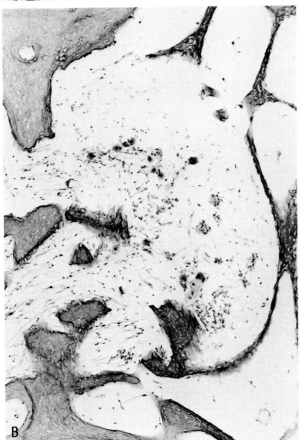

FIG. 41–4. Cochlear duct **(A)** and spiral ganglion **(B)** of mid-basal turn of left cochlea. Loss of hair cells and supporting cells of organ of Corti is total, and stria vascularis is partially atrophied. Despite such severe changes in the organ of Corti, the tectorial membrane appears normal. Atrophy of spiral ganglion is severe. (Suga R, Lindsay J: Ann Otol Rhinol Laryngol 85:169–184, 1976)

with CNS auditory pathway involvement may have greater difficulty with speech in a noisy background.

A presbycusis diagnosis may be mistakenly applied to such lesions as cochleovestibular otosclerosis and/or lateral ossicular fixation.

The lack of an air–bone gap as determined by conventional audiometry may be misleading. More attention must be directed to frontal bone conduction, sound acuity level (SAL), and impedance studies in patients with presumptive presbycusis. An older patient with greater than average decade presbycusic SNHL may have unrecognized mixed stapedial-cochlear otosclerosis and presbycusis. The air–bone gap may not have been detected by conventional mastoid BC studies. The possibility of successful surgical correction of an accompanying stapedial otosclerotic fixation may thus go unrecognized, with denial of needed hearing improvement to such a patient. Discrepancies between mastoid BC studies and SAL, frontal bone, and dental BC studies are now recognizable. The conductive loss test battery including impedance

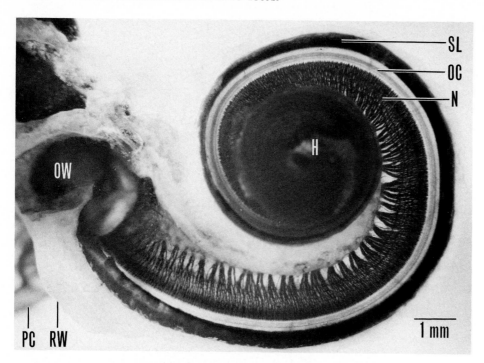

FIG. 41–5. Normal-appearing cochlea from 25-year-old white female. **OW,** oval window; **RW,** round window; **PC,** posterior canal and ampulla; **SL,** spiral ligament, mostly dissected away; **OC,** organ of Corti, seen as a dark band on the translucent basilar membrane, representing inner and outer hair cells separated by the tunnel; **N,** network of myelinated radial and intralaminar spiral nerve fibers; **H,** helicotrema. Right ear, strangulation suicide. Fixation approximately 23 hours post mortem, OsO_4. (Johnsson L-G, Hawkins JE: Ann Otol Rhinol Laryngol 81:179–193, 1972)

FIG. 41–6. Cochlea from a 92-year-old white female. Note degeneration of myelinated radial nerve fibers in lower half of basal turn. Intralaminar spiral fibers are clearly seen in the basal turn. There is some patchy degeneration **(arrow)** of the organ of Corti. Right ear, from a burn patient. Fixation 11 hours post mortem, OsO_4. (Johnsson L-G, Hawkins JE: Ann Otol Rhinol Laryngol 81: 179–193, 1972)

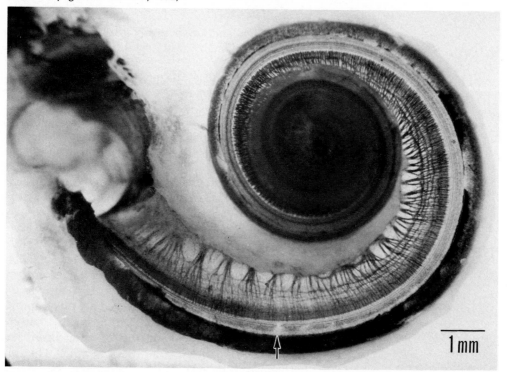

FIG. 41–7. Estimated percentage of injury in different frequency zones represented by height of columns. Spheroid cell loss in superior ventral cochlear nucleus **(svcn).** In various cases, it may range from little or no alteration to virtually complete destruction. In the audiohistogram, the graph for spheroid cell loss in svcn (the frequency zones being delineated according to the logarithmic scale of the audiometric chart) parallels the audiometric curve as well as the graph for loss of spiral ganglion nerve cells. **SV,** stria vascularis; **hc,** hair cells; **sg,** spiral ganglion nerve cells; **svcn,** spheroid cells of svcn. (Dublin WB: Ann Otol Rhinol Laryngol 85:813–819, 1976)

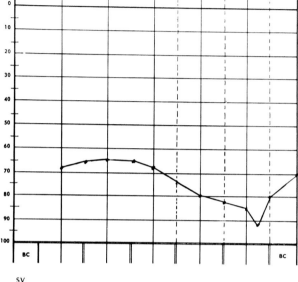

sv

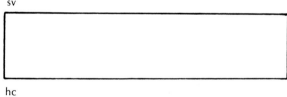

hc

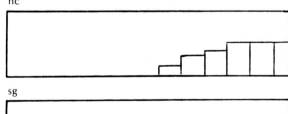

sg

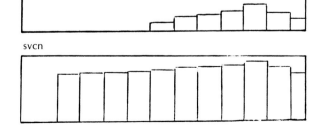

svcn

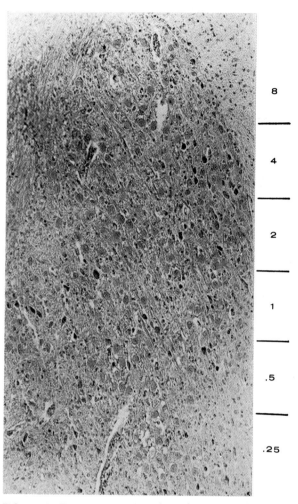

FIG. 41–8. Transverse section through greatest dimension of normal superior ventral cochlear nucleus; frequency levels are indicated in kilohertz. (Dublin WB: Ann Otol Rhinol Laryngol 85:813–819, 1976)

audiometry is of great value in such differential diagnosis dilemmas (see Ch. 7, Acoustic Impedance Tests, and Ch. 8, Conductive Loss and Sensorineural Test Batteries).

Changes in speech discrimination scores in fluctuating hearing loss cases may result in a wrong "routine" diagnosis of presbycusis. A one-time audiogram does not necessarily reflect the true diagnosis in every case. Fluctuating pure-tone and SDS values may be indicative of metabolic, vascular, or CNS problems in which hearing responses fluctuate. Thus, periodic reexamination of the patient with presbycusis is advisable.

The label of presbycusis can be incorrectly applied also to a patient who has a hearing loss of ototoxic nature. For example, the widespread in-

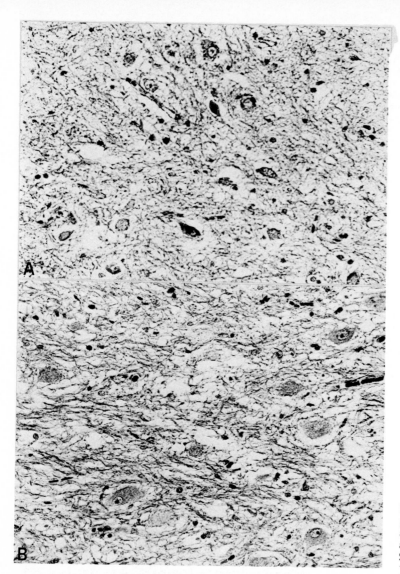

FIG. 41-9. Presbycusis. Microphotographs of superior ventral cochlear nucleus. **A.** At 4 kHz level, loss of spheroid cells is estimated at 90–95%. **B.** At 500-Hz level, loss of spheroid cells is estimated at 65%. (Dublin WB: Ann Otol Rhinol Laryngol 85:813–819, 1976)

FIG. 41-10. Brain from 76-year-old man with presbycusis. Cerebral vertex **(at left)** and two auditory areas **(at right)** show convolutional atrophy. (Dublin WB: FUNDAMENTALS OF SENSORINEURAL AUDITORY PATHOLOGY, 1976. Courtesy of Charles C Thomas, Springfield, Illinois)

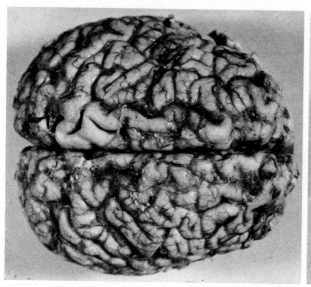
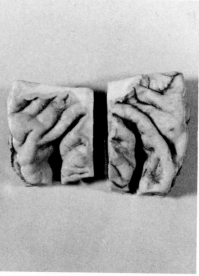

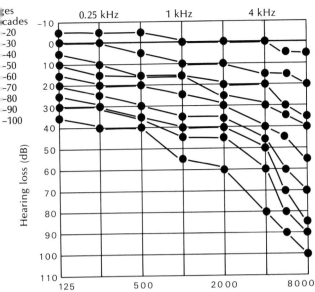

FIG. 41–11. Decade audiogram, illustrating "normal aging." Audiometric patterns encountered in urban otologic practice.

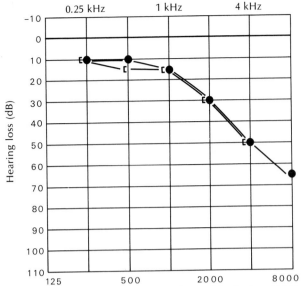

FIG. 41–13. Audiogram representing mild sloping SNHL presbycusis. The SRT (15 dB) reflects normal low-frequency hearing with mildly decreased discrimination ability (70% at 45 dB [+30]; 82% at 55 dB [+40]). ●—●, AC, unmasked, RE; [—[, BC, masked, RE.

FIG. 41–12. Audiogram representing flat SNHL presbycusis. The SRT (35 dB) is consistent with pure-tone average and discrimination ability is good (88% at 65 dB [+30]). ●—●, AC, unmasked, RE; [—[, BC, masked, RE.

FIG. 41–14. Audiogram representing severely sloping SNHL presbycusis. The SRT (15 dB) reflects normal low-frequency hearing with markedly decreased discrimination ability (56% at 45 dB [+30]; 68% at 55 dB [+40]). ●—●, AC, unmasked, RE; [—[, BC, masked, RE.

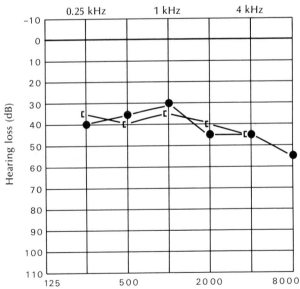

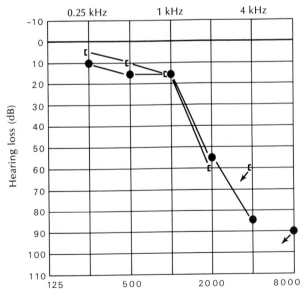

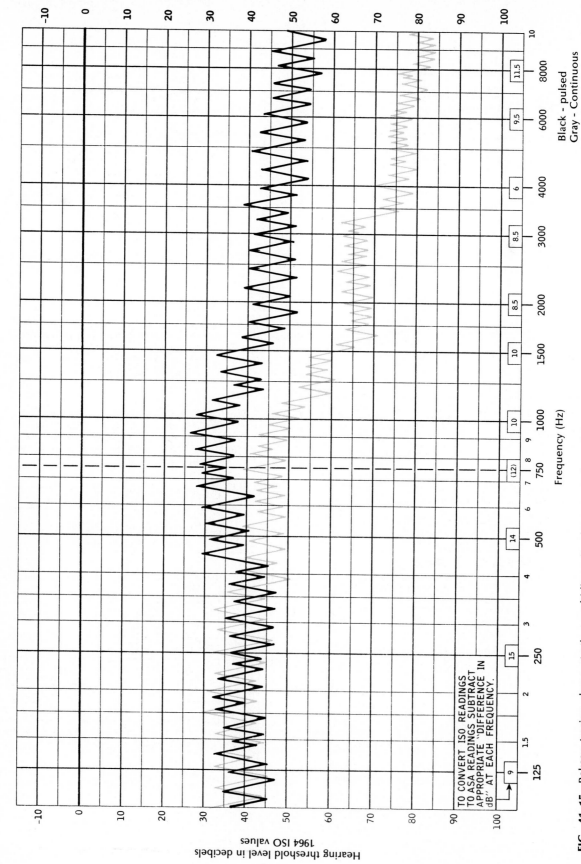

FIG. 41-15. Bekesy tracing demonstrating multidimensional aspects of presbycusis—*i.e.*, peripheral and central components. **Black tracing,** pulsed; **gray tracing,** continuous.

gestion of salicylates is usually unrecognized in the etiology of SNHL. Salicylate ototoxicity superimposed upon a mild subclinical presbycusis is not uncommon.

Mild presbycusis may appear to be more severe than it really is, as the result of other conditions producing intermittent superimposed cellular hypoxia, which can play a role in fluctuating cochlear hearing levels in patients with thyroid disease, diabetes, arteriosclerosis, hypertension, and in other systemic conditions. The roles played by these diseases in hearing losses are not yet clearly defined and must be studied with greater intensity for realistic evaluation.

MANAGEMENT

Once the diagnosis of presbycusis is made, and pseudopresbycusis lesions have been ruled out, the question of treatment arises. Many drugs, vitamins, and other modalities have been suggested in the treatment of presbycusis and for other SNHL lesions.

Patients are frequently advised empirically to take nicotinic acid, other vitamins, and numerous esoteric preparations to prevent further presbycusis hearing losses. Recently, courses of therapy with acupuncture or transdermal stimulation have been advised. The patient with a spontaneous fluctuant hearing loss component superimposed on presbycusis may be convinced that such therapy is of help. **Our clinical experience indicates that there is no effective medical or surgical treatment for presbycusis at the time of this writing** (1977).

Although there is no definitive treatment for presbycusis, the patient with presbycusis requires wise management necessitating a program of rehabilitation.

A glib suggestion to buy a hearing aid and/or attend a lipreading class is not adequate for most patients. Frequently the role of the hearing aid dispenser with presbycusis patients is a pernicious one. Many elderly patients with relatively flat audiometric configurations in the 15–20 dB region, who need no amplification, have been sold hearing aids by door-to-door hearing-aid dealers. Unnecessary hearing aid use not only confuses, baffles, and upsets a patient, but it can convince the patient of the existence of a progressively hopeless hearing loss problem. For most patients with mild presbycusis there is usually no need for anything other than the use of a telephone buzzer and/or amplifier, a loud door buzzer instead of a bell, radio and

FIG. 41–16. Ear cupping can help many patients with minor to moderate hearing losses. **A.** Relatively inefficient cupping technique, since hand is open. **B.** Some improvement in efficiency. **C.** Ideal cupping technique, with the auricle cradled in the closed hand and gently pushed forward slightly. Care must be taken not to occlude the ear canal.

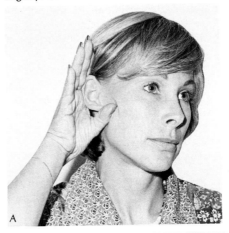

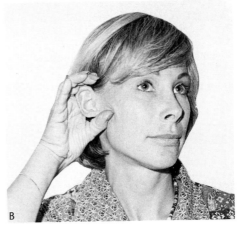

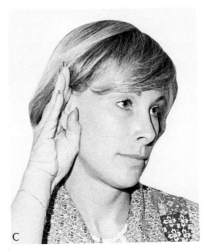

television earphone attachments and, above all, an understanding of the social aspects of mild hearing loss on the part of members of the family. Such understanding, and the uses of ear cupping (Fig. 41–16) and "acoustic strategy" will solve most, if not all, of communicative problems of many older people with mild sensorineural hearing problems.

When indicated, hearing aid selection in patients with presbycusis should be advised by the otologist in collaboration with an audiologist and a skilled and conscientious hearing aid dealer. Newer types of amplification devices are successfully being used by patients with presbycusis, even with sloping high-frequency SNHL. Special details regarding hearing aids and their selection and use are described in Chapter 43.

REFERENCES

1. Belal A, Stewart T: Pathological changes in the middle ear joints. Ann Otol Rhinol Laryngol 83: 159, 1974

2. Dublin WB: The combined correlated audiohistogram. Ann Otol Rhinol Laryngol 85:813–819, 1976

3. Dublin WB: Fundamentals of Sensorineural Auditory Pathology. Springfield, IL, CC Thomas, 1976, pp 173–183

4. Fieandt H von, Saxen A: Pathologic und klinik der altersschwerhorigkeit. Acta Otolaryngol [Suppl] (Stockh) 23, 1937

5. Fisch U, Dobozi M, Greig D: Degenerative changes of the arterial vessels of the internal auditory meatus during the process of aging. Acta Otolaryngol (Stockh) 73:259–266, 1972

6. Goodhill V: External conductive hypacusis and the fixed Malleus syndrome. Acta Otolaryngol [Suppl] (Stockh) #217, 1966

7. Gussen R: Plugging of vascular canals in the otic capsule. Ann Otol Rhinol Laryngol 78:1305–1315, 1969

8. Johnsson L-G, Hawkins JE: Sensory and neural degenerations with aging, as seen in microdissections of the human inner ear. Ann Otol Rhinol Laryngol 81:179–193, 1972

9. Krmpotić-Nemanić J, Nemanić D, Kostović I: Macroscopical and microscopical changes in the bottom of the internal auditory meatus. Acta Otolaryngol (Stockh) 73:254–258, 1972

10. Nixon J, Glorig A, High W: Changes in air and bone conduction thresholds as a function of age. J Laryngol 76:288–298, 1962

11. Schuknecht HF: Pathology of the Ear. Cambridge, MA, Harvard University Press, 1974, pp 389–403

12. Suga F, Lindsay J: Histopathological observations of presbycusis. Ann Otol Rhinol Laryngol 85:169–184, 1976

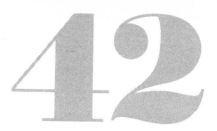

TINNITUS

Everyone may have normal tinnitus in special situations. The healthy person with no ear complaints who goes into an audiometric "soundproof" booth or into an anechoic chamber and sits quietly in an acoustically shielded environment will usually "hear" internal body sounds. This "visceral tinnitus" is normal and represents an awareness of one's own body "at work," of sounds produced by breathing, heart action, blood circulation, middle ear muscle contractions—by living. We subconsciously ignore such sounds. If we deliberately try to hear such body sounds, we usually fail because of the masking effects of environmental sounds. Even in a quiet bedroom at night, there is a constant ambient noise level of at least 25–30 dB. This is sufficient to mask out the ability to hear one's own physiological sounds.

Tinnitus as a symptom occurs when such internal sounds are of higher intensity levels (louder) than the intensity level (loudness) of masking environmental sounds.

Tinnitus can be a troubling human symptom, which may or may not be of ear origin. Tinnitus is not a disease and is not a syndrome. Tinnitus must be considered a *symptom* resulting from any one of a number of lesions.

CLASSIFICATION

Subjective Tinnitus

Subjective tinnitus is an auditory sensation of ringing, humming, whistling, roaring, clicking, or any other sensation of tones or noise. The word "tinnitus" is derived from the Latin "tinnire" which literally means "to jingle." Tinnitus is a subjective symptom in most patients.

Objective Tinnitus—Bruit

Objective tinnitus is a rare phenomenon. The term refers to a tone or sound that can be heard by an examiner (the physician) as well as by the patient. Objective tinnitus may also be described as a bruit and will be discussed in a special section later in this chapter, devoted to bruit.

From the point of view of location, two types of tinnitus must be distinguished: 1) ear tinnitus (tinnitus aurium); and 2) head tinnitus (tinnitus cranii or tinnitus cerebri).

CLINICAL SIGNIFICANCE

Tinnitus is very important from the point of view of otologic and neurologic diagnosis. However, since it is an elusive symptom, which can rarely be measured or quantified accurately, the evaluation of tinnitus as a component of either otologic or systemic diseases is difficult.

Tinnitus is a common symptom, especially in middle and older age groups. Since it may represent a component of a number of diseases, it may be the first symptom to bring the patient to the physician for diagnosis and management. The very elusiveness of tinnitus as a symptom produces a number of functional and psychogenic characteristics. Unfortunately tinnitus is frequently dismissed as being of psychogenic origin when indeed it may be a serious and critical warning of a definitive lesion. For example, unilateral tinnitus may very well be the first symptom of a tumor of the internal auditory meatus or of the cerebellopontine angle. Tinnitus, unilateral or bilateral, may be the first symptom of beginning otosclerosis. Tinnitus may herald the presence of a glomus jugulare tumor. Tinnitus may be the presenting symptom of a vascular lesion in the temporal bone or skull.

A moving subjective description by an unusual "patient" who suffered from tinnitus is that of Ludwig von Beethoven who, in a letter to his good friend Wegeler in 1801, discussed his increasing hearing loss, and had these words to say about his tinnitus: "only my ears whistle and buzz continually, day and night. I can say I am living a wretched life."

ETIOLOGY OF EAR TINNITUS (TINNITUS AURIUM)

Ear tinnitus is usually accompanied by hearing loss. Basically, both of the two classic types of hearing loss, conductive and sensorineural, may be accompanied by tinnitus. Tinnitus may precede hearing loss, the two may appear simultaneously, or tinnitus may follow the onset of hearing loss.

TINNITUS AURIUM IN CONDUCTIVE LESIONS

Any conductive lesion can be accompanied by tinnitus. Simple cerumen in the external ear canal may cause hearing loss with tinnitus. Tympanic membrane perforation, otitis media, and any ossicular lesion may produce hearing loss and tinnitus. Conductive hearing loss tinnitus is due to lesion "block" of ambient room or other environmental noise. Because of this, the patient literally hears visceral tinnitus, comparable to the unmasked visceral tinnitus in the soundproof room. If the middle ear lesion is bilaterally equal (*e.g.*, in symmetrical bilateral otosclerosis), the bilateral ear tinnitus may resemble a nonlocalizing central tinnitus similar to that of tinnitus cranii.

Conductive lesions causing ear tinnitus (tinnitus aurium) may be summarized as follows:

External Ear

1. Auricle diseases, such as perichondritis or tumors resulting in meatal obstruction
2. Cartilaginous ear canal lesions, such as furunculosis and external otitis with soft-tissue occlusion, fibrous atresias, cerumen impactions, and tumors
3. Bony canal lesions, such as occlusive osteophytes (osteomas), tumors, and bony atresias

Middle Ear

1. Tympanic membrane perforations, adhesive fibrosis, atelectasis
2. Intratympanic fluid collections—hemotympanum, serous effusion, purulent exudate, mucoid exudate
3. Tympanic muscular lesions—spasms or tics of stapedius muscle and/or tensor tympani muscles
4. Intratympanic vascular lesions—anomalies of jugular bulb and internal carotid artery, or persistent stapedial artery
5. Tympanic ossicular lesions—lateral ossicular fixation, otosclerosis, ossicular necrosis, ossicular discontinuity
6. Intratympanic tumors—glomus jugulare, hemangioma, carcinoma, cholesteatoma—primary or secondary

TINNITUS AURIUM IN SENSORINEURAL LESIONS

Cochlear and retrocochlear lesions can produce unilateral tinnitus. Unlike conductive-lesion tinnitus, the ambient-noise-masking-effect phenomenon is not significant. In sensorineural hearing loss lesions the tinnitus is more usually attributable to a passive true auditory paresthesia, a subjective phenomenon similar to the phantom limb phenomenon in the amputee, although it may also be due to an active lesion with generation of abnormal bioacoustic signals.

Labyrinthine (endolymphatic) hydrops (Meniere's disease) is frequently accompanied by ipsilateral tinnitus along with hearing loss and vertigo. Such tinnitus has complex acoustic characteristics. It may be steady or pulsating, variable in intensity and frequency, and it fluctuates in relation to the vertigo attacks.

Acoustic neurinoma and cerebellopontine angle tumors are usually characterized by ipsilateral tinnitus as the first symptom prior to hearing loss and vertigo.

Noise-induced hearing loss, with bilateral 4-kHz notch will be accompanied by bilateral tinnitus aurium which may resemble tinnitus cranii because of bilateral cochlear hearing loss symmetry.

Bilateral cochlear presbycusis may be accompanied by bilateral tinnitus aurium.

Sensorineural lesions causing ear tinnitus may be summarized as follows:

Cochlear (Sensory)

1. Bony labyrinth—Paget's disease, otosclerosis, van der Hoeve's syndrome
2. Perilymph diseases—fistulas, infections, hyperpatent cochlear aqueduct
3. Endolymphatic diseases—hydrops (Meniere's disease), viral infections, diseases of the vestibular aqueduct
4. Organ of Corti lesions—ototoxicity, noise damage, atrophy, congenital malformations, edema, allergy, viropathies, and vascular lesions
5. Cochlear ganglion lesions—ototoxicity, noise damage, atrophy, congenital malformations, edema, allergy, viropathies

Eighth Nerve Lesions (Retrocochlear)

1. Internal auditory canal lesions—eighth cranial nerve tumors (acoustic neurinoma or meningioma), inflammation, vascular anomalies
2. Cerebellopontine angle lesions—tumors, vascular anomalies

Central Auditory Lesions

Tumors, vascular anomalies, and focal inflammatory lesions affecting either afferent or efferent auditory nerve fibers, ventral and dorsal cochlear nuclei, lateral lemniscus tract, medial geniculate body, auditory cortex.

ETIOLOGY OF CRANIAL (HEAD) TINNITUS (TINNITUS CRANII)

Nonlocalizing head tinnitus ("in my head") may be either due to true cranial (head) tinnitus or may be confused with bilaterally symmetrical tinnitus aurium, either conductive or sensorineural.

True cranial tinnitus is frequently associated with cerebrovascular and other intracranial lesions. However, since any tinnitus, even though nonlocalizing may be of ear origin, an otologic examination is always indicated.

A definitive discussion of cranial (head) tinnitus will be given later in this chapter.

DIAGNOSTIC APPROACH TO TINNITUS

OTOLOGIC EXAMINATION

The patient with tinnitus, whether unilateral or bilateral, whether tinnitus aurium or tinnitus cranii, must have an otologic examination. The presence of known cerebrovascular disease, for example, does not rule out the possibility of acoustic neurinoma, Meniere's disease, or otosclerosis.

The first step, therefore, in the management of the patient with tinnitus is a complete otorhinologic examination, audiologic examination, and screening mastoid and petrous pyramid x-rays, as described in Chapter 3, Ear Examination.

Obviously, when a specific otologic cause for the tinnitus is found on such studies, specific otologic treatment is indicated.

THE SIGNIFICANCE OF TINNITUS IN DIFFERENTIAL DIAGNOSIS

In conductive lesions, either in external ear or middle ear areas, modern techniques of micro-visualization, audiovestibular tests, and radiologic approaches make a specific differential diagnosis possible in the vast majority of patients without the need for special studies of the tinnitus component.

In sensorineural lesions, however, direct diagnostic accessibility is more difficult than in conductive lesions, and the evaluation of an accompanying tinnitus component of an otologic disease becomes much more significant in differential diagnosis.

In the vast area of "nerve deafness," which comprises many diseases, there are difficulties in topo-diagnosis. The pure-tone and speech audiogram, recruitment tests, the short increment sensitivity index test, the Bekesy audiogram, stapedius reflex, impedance and other studies, and electronystagmographic vestibular studies are important diagnostic tools, along with radiologic information. However, in spite of these recent developments, many differential diagnostic problems in sensorineural hearing loss remain unsolved.

Tinnitus is an important symptom in lesions of the cochlea, auditory nerve, and the central neural auditory pathway. Identification and classification of discrete tinnitus characteristics, when correlated with other otologic data and final postmortem temporal bone and neuropathology findings will undoubtedly increase our knowledge of sensorineural hearing loss differential diagnosis in the future. At the present time, there are only primitive correlations of otologic examination findings with tinnitus analysis data.

METHODICAL ANALYSIS OF TINNITUS

A methodical analysis of tinnitus should be an integral part of the otologic examination. The following method of analysis is suggested as an orderly technique in an attempt to obtain useful data.

Subjective Statements of Patients

When patients with tinnitus are asked for a description, loose indefinite answers are usually obtained. Examples are: "I hear steam escaping"; "I hear a roaring or buzzing in my head"; "I hear a sound like a seashell held up to my ear"; "I hear sounds of a squeaking door"; "I hear the sound of a babbling brook"; "I hear the noise of an ocean roar"; "I hear radio static"; "I hear clicks or rumbles of a dynamo, or a generator."

Subjective Analysis

The patient is questioned for the following specific data:

GENERAL LOCATION OF THE TINNITUS. Is the tinnitus within the patient or does it seem to be somewhere in the room? Occasionally, the patient will insist that the tinnitus is not in the head, not in the ear, but to the right or to the left of the head and apparently projected several inches or feet away.

SOMATIC LOCATION OF THE TINNITUS. Is it in one or both ears and if so, superficially or deeply; or is it in the head, and if so in what part of the head?

SPECIFICITY IN REGARD TO PITCH LOUDNESS. Is the tinnitus high, or low, in pitch? Is it very soft, or loud? Does it "disappear" in the presence of noise? Does it get louder in the presence of noise?

TIME RELATIONS OF TINNITUS. Is the tinnitus louder during certain times of the day? Is it louder at work or at home? Is it louder at certain times of the week. In women, does it vary with menses?

POSITIONAL RELATIONS OF TINNITUS. Does the tinnitus vary with positions of the head or body? Does it increase on stooping? Is it relieved by any specific position of the body or head?

Tinnitus Matching—Acoustic Analysis

If the tinnitus is a pure tone, it may be identified on the audiometer. For these purposes, the ordinary fixed frequency audiometer is not as useful as sweep frequency (Bekesy) audiometer for specific pitch matching. When this type of audiometer is used, the tinnitus intensity and masking intensity may be measured. If the tone is complex, an attempt is made at analysis, in terms of dominant and accessory tones.

The musically articulate or scientifically trained patient may describe tinnitus with great accuracy. A patient with noise-induced hearing loss frequently can localize pitch and intensity characteristics with considerable skill. In the more complex types of tinnitus encountered in otosclerosis, labyrinthine hydrops, and acoustic neurinoma, such a patient may use musical or acoustic terms to describe a preponderance of primary tones with accompanying harmonics, octaves, and overtones.

Further research in tinnitus matching with tinnitus simulation recordings may elicit valuable new diagnostic and prognostic information (1).

COMPENSATED AND DECOMPENSATED TINNITUS

COMPENSATED TINNITUS

Compensated tinnitus is present in much of the population. It accompanies a number of otologic lesions and some constitutional conditions. In most of these instances the tinnitus is not noticeable to the patient except in an extremely quiet environment, therefore not constituting a clinical problem requiring management. Many conductive and sensorineural hearing losses in lesions of varying etiologies may be accompanied by minimal tinnitus. Such patients may not complain at all of the

tinnitus but will acknowledge the presence of the symptom when the history is taken. The complaint of tinnitus is usually not volunteered in patients with compensated tinnitus but can be elicited.

DECOMPENSATED TINNITUS

The term **decompensated tinnitus** describes the tinnitus that is the major ear complaint of the patient. There are two types of otologic problems that will produce decompensated tinnitus. The first is the tinnitus of low acoustic intensity in a patient with significant psychosomatic stress factors. The second is the tinnitus of high acoustic intensity that is measured in a tinnitus-analysis study. In such a patient the complaints are related to the acoustic intensity of the organic ear lesion, and are not related to psychosomatic stress factors.

THE MANAGEMENT OF EAR TINNITUS

BASIC APPROACH

The management of tinnitus aurium is a specific otologic problem in the patient with decompensated tinnitus. This patient seeks help primarily because of the tinnitus. The other otologic symptoms, such as hearing loss, vertigo, ear pain, or otorrhea, are subdued and minimized in the history. The tinnitus itself looms as the chief complaint and is the subject symptom for which otologic management is requested.

As in many medical problems, a double diagnosis must always be considered, eliciting 1) the actual organic etiologic ear lesion, and 2) the psychosomatic status of the patient. However, tinnitus should not be approached primarily as a psychosomatic problem. Crucial etiologic organic disease may be missed if one deals with tinnitus primarily as a psychosomatic problem.

There is no specific treatment for tinnitus aurium.

The goals in the management of the patient with tinnitus aurium are dual. The first goal is specific medical or surgical ear therapy for the underlying condition. If the tinnitus persists despite adequate otologic treatment, the second goal is an attempt to convert decompensated tinnitus into compensated tinnitus.

SPECIFIC OTOLOGIC THERAPY

The specific otologic therapy for the patient with the primary complaint of tinnitus depends on the nature of the lesion. In many conditions specific therapy is available and successful in a large number of cases. In some diseases specific therapy is unknown at the present time. Examples of the former are the following:

1. The patient with tinnitus due to cerumen impaction or a foreign body in the anterior canal sulcus will be immediately relieved upon complete removal of the cerumen or foreign body.
2. The tinnitus accompanying otosclerosis is frequently relieved following a successful stapes operation.
3. The tinnitus accompanying secretory otitis media may disappear the moment the fluid is aspirated from the middle ear.
4. The tinnitus of Meniere's disease may decrease or disappear following such medical treatments as a low-sodium diet, the use of diuretics, or control of allergy.
5. Tinnitus due to cochlear drug ototoxicity (such as that caused by salicylates, quinine, ototoxic antibiotics, etc.) may be relieved by withdrawing the offending drug.
6. Tinnitus due to noise-induced hearing loss or acoustic trauma is usually relieved by the removal of the offending noise source.
7. The pulsating tinnitus due to a tympanic glomus tumor may be completely relieved following surgery, even if the hearing level is unchanged.

There are, however, patients with specific otologic lesions in whom specific otologic therapy is not effective insofar as the tinnitus is concerned as in the following situations:

1. A patient with coexistent cochlear and stapedial otosclerosis may regain considerable hearing following stapedectomy, but the tinnitus may persist because of the cochlear lesion.
2. The patient with tinnitus accompanying Meniere's disease may be relieved of vertigo following medical or surgical therapy, but the tinnitus may persist.
3. The patient whose acoustic neurinoma has been successfully removed may still have persistent tinnitus, even if the entire eighth nerve has been resected.

CONVERSION OF DECOMPENSATED TO COMPENSATED TINNITUS

Reality Reassurance

Regardless of the underlying lesion and the therapy directed to the lesion, the patient whose tinnitus is a major symptom requires special management.

This management should be carried out by the same physician (otologist, or generalist) who has treated the underlying organic cause. It is unwise to relegate such tinnitus management to a psychotherapist unless the patient has clear-cut indications of major emotional or psychiatric disease.

For many patients the symptom of tinnitus is very frightening. Anxieties regarding the tinnitus may not be volunteered by the patient. Among such anxieties are those derived from family, friends, folklore, and other sources. Some patients think that tinnitus is the prelude to total deafness. To others tinnitus implies a sign of a brain tumor. To still others tinnitus means a prelude to a stroke. For some patients tinnitus may be mistakenly interpreted as the beginning of serious mental disease. Although there are remote realities to some of these concerns, for most patients these worries are inappropriate. Such anxieties may even be concealed by the patient.

Simple reassurance as to the real cause and significance of the tinnitus as a component of an ear condition will go far in helping alleviate such anxieties. Inappropriate concerns should be discussed frankly. Reassurance by the physician who carried out the original otologic diagnostic studies and therapy is infinitely more effective than reassurance by another physician or by a psychotherapist.

It is necessary to explain to the patient what ear tinnitus usually represents—that it is real and not imagined, that it is *not* an illusion or a hallucination or a delusion. It is an auditory paresthesia. In this regard it is frequently valuable to give the patient the example of the phantom limb with neuron memory. The amputee with no leg may have "pain" in his absent little toe. The high-pitched tinnitus in a patient with 4-kHz noise-induced hearing loss and a cochlear basal-turn lesion may have a "phantom" neuron memory tinnitus comparable to the phantom limb of the amputee.

The Course of Tinnitus

In the vast majority of patients, the tinnitus accompanying a nonprogressive conductive or sensorineural lesion will become less of a problem with the passage of time. In most patients, such tinnitus may disappear completely, as a symptom, but may return temporarily at times of fatigue, stress, or upper respiratory infections. It is thus appropriate and imperative that an optimistic prognosis be given. Such reassurance per se is necessary and will convert decompensated tinnitus in many patients.

Acoustic "Sedation"

Acoustic "sedation" is very helpful in many cases of tinnitus, especially in regard to difficulty in sleep, which is a great problem for many patients. The reason for greater difficulty at that time is the reduction in ambient masking-noise levels in the quiet of the night, which increases awareness of the ever-present auditory paresthesia. The use of a bedside radio or tape recorder is frequently helpful in providing an artificial source of ambient noise to mask out the subjective tinnitus.

Hearing Aid Use

When there is a lesion for which amplification with a hearing aid is a possibility, even if borderline, such patients should have a hearing-aid consultation. In many cases, a properly fitted hearing aid may be extremely helpful in providing sufficient ambient environmental noise to mask the tinnitus. The hearing aid may also be helpful in reducing the tension that accompanies borderline hearing losses. The hearing aid will be of help as an auditory rehabilitation device as well as a masking device. It is only rarely that a hearing aid accentuates tinnitus rather than masking it.

Medical Therapy of Ear Tinnitus

There is no specific medical therapy for ear tinnitus. The uses of medications such as nicotinic acid, bioflavonoids, or histamine, as specific "treatments" for ear tinnitus are unwarranted. Tinnitus is a symptom, not a disease.

Drug therapy, however, is an important palliative measure, not only for daytime use, but especially for bedtime tinnitus irritability. Drugs such as phenobarbital (0.5 gr = 30 mg), various tranquilizers, and other sedatives in small doses will be helpful. There is no one drug wth specific tinnitus-sedation qualities. No one drug should be used for any long period. It is helpful to alternate the medications so that habituation possibilities are diminished.

Specific Tinnitus Surgery

There is no effective surgery for tinnitus at the present time. Obviously surgery is indicated if there is an underlying otologic disease requiring a surgical procedure. However, when the underlying otologic disease is only a marginal indication for surgery, such surgery should not be recommended specifically for the tinnitus component.

A number of surgical attempts have been made to treat the symptom of persistent tinnitus. Such surgical procedures as tympanic neurectomy, chorda tympani section, labyrinthectomy, and intracranial cochlear nerve section have rarely solved tinnitus problems.

The various surgical procedures that are being experimentally used for Meniere's disease are frequently advocated for the tinnitus component of that disorder. There is *no clear-cut indication* for endolymphatic sac decompressions or shunts, surgical sympathectomy, labyrinth cryosurgery, sacculotomy, labyrinthectomy, eighth nerve section, or other procedures advocated for the treatment of Meniere's disease *if the purpose of the operation is primarily the treatment of the accompanying tinnitus*. Reports of "successes" in "tinnitus surgery" are, of course, entirely subjective, for which no validation is available at the present time.

Biofeedback

Recently, efforts have been made to relieve troublesome tinnitus, when the cause is not otherwise treatable, with relaxation training assisted by biofeedback techniques. Patients are taught a variety of relaxation procedures by which several physiologic parameters of their state of arousal are being monitored: Galvanic skin response, electromyographic activity, and skin temperature have been the most useful measurements. Changes in these parameters are "fed back" to the patient by auditory or visual signals. Skilled technicians or "trainers" assist the patient in developing the ability to voluntarily relax sufficiently to bring about lowering of the galvanic skin resistance, reduction in muscle tension, and elevation of skin temperature, all of which correlate with the degree of relaxation. After several training sessions, most individuals have learned to control the machines, *i.e.,* to regulate their autonomic nervous system and skeletal muscle tension in a way ordinarily thought to be beyond volitional control.

About one-third of patients instructed in this way experience definite reduction in their sensation of tinnitus. Another third report no change in the loudness or quality of the tinnitus when they pay attention to it, but it is somehow much less disturbing to them. The final third notice no significant change in their experience of tinnitus, yet almost invariably they find the training course to have been well worth their while with respect to their general well-being. Patient motivation is very important and the results are entirely subjective. Even in patients who report a reduction in tinnitus, audiometric matching tests fail to show any consistent measurable change.

The connections between the biofeedback instrumentation and training techniques and the symptom of tinnitus (or most other disorders treated with biofeedback, for that matter) is entirely speculative.

UNEXPLAINED EAR TINNITUS

The patient with persistent unexplained tinnitus as an isolated symptom, in whom thorough medical and otologic studies disclose no evidence of disease, requires repeated reexaminations at definite intervals. Tinnitus may be the first symptom in some conditions, long before hearing loss or other findings appear. Reexaminations should include both general medical and otologic studies.

In any patient with a complaint of *increasing tinnitus* in a definitive otologic lesion that has been treated, periodic reevaluation of the organic findings is necessary. There may be a recurrence of the original disease, or there may be another organic cause previously unrecognized.

However, if the patient's complaint of tinnitus becomes inappropriate to the severity of the otologic lesion, and if the physician is certain that there is no organic explanation for the increased intensity of the tinnitus complaint, psychiatric referral is indicated.

AUDITORY HALLUCINATIONS

Many musicians, composers, and music lovers can "hear" entire musical scores as phenomena of normal cerebration. Beethoven "heard" his later compositions when he was totally deaf. Playwrights can "hear" the words of future actors in scenes and acts in conceptual states. These phenomena are certainly not hallucinatory.

Auditory hallucinations are auditory cerebral phenomena unrelated to creative thinking. If they are verbal, they are described as offensive or threatening words or expressions. If they are musical, they are described as uncontrollable auditory experiences, unrelated to a desire to recall a tune or to compose a melody.

Auditory hallucinations have not been shown to be related to peripheral ear disease. Although there have been some reports attempting to connect auditory hallucinations with peripheral temporal-bone lesions (3), no temporal-bone pathology studies have been reported in association with such speculative concepts. Otologic examination is necessary to rule out peripheral disease, however.

The patient with auditory hallucinations, either unformed (tinnitus) or formed (words, sentences, singing, or instrumental music) should be examined neurologically. Formed auditory hallucinations occur in ictal states, temporal lobe seizures, and tumors. If no neurologic etiology can be demonstrated, psychiatric referral is indicated.

CRANIAL (HEAD) TINNITUS (TINNITUS CRANII)

Cranial tinnitus is frequently confused with ear tinnitus, and may actually coexist with it. Cranial tinnitus is a nonlocalized subjective sensation of sound which is usually diffuse in the head and has a nonspecific quality. It is frequently described as a roaring or rushing sound, not directed to the ear region. It may be accompanied by bruits. Its diffuse character may be confused with somatic sensations of the neck and upper thorax and, indeed, may be due to vascular phenomena in these areas as well as intracranially. Usually tinnitus cranii is due to organic or functional intracranial vascular disease and is a medical neurologic problem. Ear tinnitus, on the other hand, is usually localized to one or both ears and is subjectively described with some ear specificity by the patient.

The patient whose primary complaint is that of roaring in the head should have a complete otologic examination in addition to medical and neurologic studies. Both extracranial and intracranial vascular lesions and a number of intracerebral lesions may be accompanied by the symptom of nonlocalizing head tinnitus.

Circulatory problems such as anemia, polycythemia, hypertension, and hypotension may also play etiologic roles in tinnitus cranii.

If otologic disease has been excluded by thorough studies, it is unwise for the patient to be treated for tinnitus as a disease. For example, such drugs as nicotinic acid should not be given indiscriminately to treat tinnitus cranii. They are not only ineffective but they may exacerbate constitutional symptoms. In such problem cases of tinnitus cranii, further medical and neurologic studies should be repeated until a clear systemic diagnosis has been accomplished.

Recent developments in angiography make it advisable to consider carotid and/or vertebral angiography, particularly in patients whose tinnitus cranii is localized to some extent to the right or to the left. It may well be a sign of serious vascular disease, and indeed it may be the only sign. At times it may be accompanied by a distinct bruit heard through a stethoscope. Thus cranial tinnitus may be a signal for further vascular studies of the head and neck.

The management of cranial tinnitus is entirely related to the basic medical or neurologic etiology. If there is no coexistent ear disease with ear tinnitus, there is obviously no indication for any otologic treatment for cranial tinnitus.

EAR BRUITS (OBJECTIVE TINNITUS)

The term **objective tinnitus** is somewhat confusing. Such adjectives as dynamic, vibratory, pseudo-, and extrinsic have been used as synonyms for objective tinnitus. It is preferable to separate tinnitus, a purely subjective symptom, from recordable sound, which can be heard and recorded by an observer as well as by the patient. Such a recordable sound should be termed *bruit.*

A patient may have both tinnitus and a bruit. Just as there is a distinction between tinnitus aurium and tinnitus cranii, so is there a distinction between ear bruit and cranial bruit.

An ear bruit may be detected by the use of a stethoscope which has been modified for use with a plastic or hollow rubber ear plug. The use of an ordinary stethoscope over the ear canal is not as effective. The examiner may well hear a pulsating or a clicking sound through such a converted ear "stethoscope."

A neck bruit or a cranial bruit may be detected by the use of the standard stethoscope.

It is possible to record ear, neck, or cranial bruits with the use of a condensor microphone and a tape recorder or by an audiofrequency spectrometer.

An ear bruit may be of either vascular or muscular origin. The vascular type of ear bruit is usually due to some type of arteriovenous communication producing an audible bruit or murmur (synchronous with the pulse) that can be heard with or without amplification. Muscular types of ear bruits are usually due to contractions of tympanic or tubal muscles, usually in bizarre or atypical rhythm. The mechanism for such contractions is exceedingly complex in etiology. Muscle spasms, functional tics, and other neuromuscular phenomena related to metabolic, neurologic, and psychosomatic states play a part in this relatively rare group of cases.

Among the causes of ear bruits are 1) palatal myoclonus; 2) hyperpatent eustachian tube "autophony"; 3) temporomandibular joint "clicking"; 4) vascular bruits; and 5) pure tone emission bruits.

PALATAL MYOCLONUS

A clicking sound emanating from one or both ears may be heard by the examiner through an ear stethoscope in cases of palatal myoclonus. Examination of the pharynx may disclose the fact that each click is accompanied by a spasmodic tic-like upward movement of the soft palate. There is usually an arrhythmic pattern to these contractions. This condition is usually of psychogenic origin but occasionally may be due to a neurologic lesion.

The presence of palatal myoclonus can be confirmed by the use of the electroacoustic impedance bridge. During an impedance examination of a patient with palatal myoclonus, it is possible to note an actual change in the relative impedance of the ear synchronous with the ticking noises. This can be demonstrated by wide swings on the balance meter.

When palatal myoclonus is a functional condition, it may disappear following corneal or other nonspecific stimulation.

THE HYPERPATENT EUSTACHIAN TUBE BRUIT WITH "AUTOPHONY"

A special type of ear bruit and ear tinnitus is that related to hyperpatency of the eustachian tube. The bruit, which may be heard with an ear canal stethoscope, consists of audible breath sounds. The tinnitus consists of autophonic reverberation of the patient's own voice, associated with the paradoxical feeling of stuffiness. Abnormal patency of the eustachian tube is usually due to loss of peritubal fat that frequently follows sudden weight losses.

Symptomatically this hollow tinnitus may be relieved when the patient lies down because vascular engorgement is induced in the head, and it may recur promptly upon arising. Patients will often sniff compulsively in an attempt to relieve the troublesome pseudostuffy sensations. Objectively the physician can 1) see tympanic membrane motion in response to respiratory movements, and 2) hear respiratory sounds through the use of an ear canal stethoscope.

A number of attempts have been made to deal with this problem surgically. Some otologists have injected Teflon paste in the peritubal area in an attempt to decrease the lumen of the tube. This type of treatment has not yet been evaluated for long periods to judge its ultimate effectiveness. There may be a danger of overclosure of the eustachian tube with subsequent serous effusion (secretory otitis media).

An interesting new approach, which seems to

hold promise, is an operation in which a trans-palatine relocation of one of the eustachian tube muscles provides release of the stretched pharyngeal osteum of the eustachian tube (4).

BRUIT CAUSED BY TEMPOROMANDIBULAR JOINT DISEASES

Some patients with temporomandibular joint problems associated with dental bite imbalance or with temporomandibular joint arthritis may have a bruit and/or tinnitus characterized by clicking. Objective clicking noises may be detected on stethoscopic auscultation of the ear canal and the region of the temporomandibular joint. Such clicking may occur either on opening or closing the jaw, or both, or in voluntary contraction of the mandibular muscles.

VASCULAR BRUITS

A number of patients with extracranial arterial diseases will have subjective tinnitus and objective tinnitus (bruit) of a pulsating character. This type of lesion is usually characterized by stethoscopically ascertained vascular bruits, which can be heard either in the neck or through the "ear stethoscope" placed snugly into the ear canal. They are usually associated with diseases of the carotid or vertebral arterial systems and may be related to arteriovenous lesions, and aneurysms.

PURE-TONE EAR-CANAL BRUIT

An unusual type of pure-tone ear-canal bruit may be audible or inaudible to the patient. A recent report by Huizing and Spoor (2) is that of a patient in whom a continuous high-pitched tone (3400 Hz ± 10 Hz, a 35-dB sound pressure level) was detected and measured.

Neither the cause nor the management of such rare cases of pure-tone bruit has been clarified.

SUMMARY AND CONCLUSIONS

1. Tinnitus, a troublesome symptom of many otologic diseases, exists in several forms.
2. Tinnitus is not a disease but a symptom requiring thorough otologic study.
3. As a symptom, tinnitus occurs in compensated and decompensated forms.
4. The management of the patient with tinnitus as a major symptom requires a dual approach.
5. Auditory hallucinations, cranial tinnitus, and ear bruits must be differentiated from ear tinnitus (tinnitus aurium).

REFERENCES

1. Goodhill V: Tinnitus identification test. Ann Otol Rhinol Laryngol 61:778–786, 1952
2. Huizing E, Spoor A: An unusual type of tinnitus. Arch Otolaryngol 98:134–136, 1973
3. Ross ED, Jossman PB, Bell B: Musical hallucinations in deafness. JAMA 231:620–622, 1975
4. Stroud MH, Spector GJ, Maisel RH: Patulous eustachian tube syndrome. Preliminary report of the use of the tensor veli palatine transposition procedure. Arch Otolaryngol 99:419–421, 1974

SUGGESTED READING

Kalsarkas A, Baxter JD: Cochlear and vestibular dysfunction resulting from physical exertion or environmental pressure changes. J Otolaryngol 5 (1):24–32, 1976
Lyons CD, Melancon BB, Kearby NL et al.: The otological aspects of palatal myoclonus. Laryngoscope 86:930–935, 1976
Mongan E, Kelly P, Nies K et al.: Tinnitus as an indication of therapeutic serum salicylate levels. JAMA 226:142–145, 1973
Ogawa S, Satoh I, Tanaka H: Patulous eustachian tube. Arch Otolaryngol 102:276–280, 1976
Tewfik S: Phonocephalography. An objective diagnosis of tinnitus. J Laryngol 88:869–875, 1974
Watanabe I, Kumagani H, Tsuda Y: Tinnitus due to abnormal contraction of stapedial muscle. Ann Otol Rhinol Laryngol 36:217–226, 1974

43

HEARING AIDS

BARRY S. ELPERN

It is probable that several thousands of years have passed since man first cupped his hand behind his ear to enhance his failing hearing, but it remained for the unprecedented technologic advancements of the present century to spawn the modern hearing aid. Throughout the early part of the century, there were numerous attempts to produce hearing aids that operated on electric power. However, superior though they were to their mechanical predecessors, such as ear trumpets, these instruments were, nonetheless, bulky, nonportable affairs, designed by necessity to utilize large dry-cell batteries that were intended originally for automotive or radio applications. At some time between 1920 and 1930, the rapid proliferation of refinements in radio and telephone design led some unheralded technician to combine certain components of these inventions in such a way as to conduct amplified sound directly to the ear. The significance of this discovery was evident immediately, and shortly thereafter, with the introduction of the miniaturized vacuum tube, the hearing-aid industry was born.

It is of historic interest to note that this new industry, which assumed responsibility for creating a hearing-aid technology from the expanding fund of information in radio and telephone, was guided by individuals whose experience had been confined primarily to merchandising and selling. If it appears illogical that development of a health-related device was left in the hands of "salesmen," it is apparent only through the advantage of hindsight, for otolaryngologists evidenced little interest in hearing aids at that time and the discipline now known as audiology had not yet been conceived. In proper perspective, then, it is clear that the incipient hearing-aid industry had its assignment virtually thrust upon it by default.

Subsequent evolution of the hearing aid has not been without problems, for manufacturer as well as consumer, but there can be little doubt that today's instruments are better than ever. Enthusiastic acceptance by the hearing-impaired population has provided the necessary impetus for industry-conceived innovations as well as application of important peripheral discoveries, such as the mercury battery, the semiconductor and space-age miniaturization of electronic components. In addition, the sophistication of the industry has progressed commensurately, so that industry representatives now collaborate freely with engineering and medical authorities in formulating plans that promise an even more gratifying future for the hearing-impaired.

AUDITORY GOALS OF ACOUSTIC AMPLIFICATION

Electronic amplification systems seldom, if ever, restore normal audition, as various aspects of auditory function remain impaired to some extent even in the most satisfactory cases. On the other hand, in virtually all cases of hearing loss which do not yield to medical or surgical management, an appropriate hearing aid can be a significant element in a comprehensive rehabilitation plan, but only if the patient understands the nature of the structural damage to his ear and the way in which this damage limits the degree of improvement he may realistically expect. Therefore, the establishment of valid goals is a prerequisite to any successful application of a hearing aid.

The goals of amplification may be defined conveniently in terms of auditory discrimination, the ability of the auditory system to analyze and differentiate among the myriad sounds of the environment. The very fine, precise differentiations required to comprehend human speech place the greatest demands on the analyzing system, and, as the required differentiations become more coarse, so the demands on the analyzing system decrease proportionately. At the opposite extreme of the discrimination scale, then, is the mere awareness of the existence of sound, the differentiation only between sound and silence.

Generally speaking, impairment of auditory discrimination is directly related to the degree of sensorineural pathology existing in the auditory mechanism, and the prognosis for restoration of socially adequate discrimination capacity by means of electronic amplification is inversely related to the degree of such pathology. The imposing silence which engulfs those who have sustained profound hearing impairment tends to evoke sensations of isolation and deadness, the emotional reactions to which are only recently becoming understood through experimental studies of sensory deprivation. In all but the most unusual of these extreme cases, a hearing aid can serve to restore auditory reception to the so-called "primitive level," *i.e.,* to recover the significant link between the individual and his acoustic surroundings. In somewhat less extreme cases, where structural damage has not been quite so devastating, appropriate amplification can be instrumental in restoring audition beyond the primitive level to the "signal level," permitting coarse analysis of incoming sounds and, thereby, utilization of certain gross characteristics of these sounds in order to discriminate among them.

Although the auditory faculty referred to as discrimination is the primary means by which we differentiate among the acoustic stimuli that surround us, it is by no means the exclusive determinant of communication ability, nor is it necessarily correlated predictably with communication ability. Each individual brings to the complex process of communication the totality of factors that distinguish him as an individual, and it is the combination of these factors which determines how successfully he will employ his hearing, aided or unaided, for the purpose of verbal communication. These peripheral factors are of such potential power that they can account for paradoxically satisfactory communication in some very severe cases of hearing loss or, conversely, unsatisfactory communication in exceptional cases of moderate or mild loss.

BASIC HEARING-AID COMPONENTS

TRANSDUCERS

The hearing aid microphone and the receiver function to transform one type of physical energy into another, so they are referred to collectively as transducers. The microphone, or input transducer, provides the means for sound entry into the hearing aid. It responds to vibratory sound waves in the vicinity and translates these vibrations into electrical impulses, which are ultimately processed by the hearing-aid circuitry. The receiver, or output transducer, is a subminiature loudspeaker which reverses this process. It converts the electrical impulses back into vibratory sound waves capable of stimulating the ear.

The operational performance of any transducer is determined by its size and various aspects of its physical composition. Limitations imposed by such features preclude any reasonable expectation for any transducer to operate with equal efficiency over an infinite range of sound frequencies and intensities, so there is inherent distortion at any point in the sound processing system at which transduction occurs. However, the transducers used in modern hearing aids have been designed to accomplish the necessary energy conversion with remarkably minimal distortion.

Although sound amplifying systems are susceptible to several different types of distortion, the main types ordinarily considered are frequency distortion, and amplitude distortion. Frequency distortion is the result of resonances and other factors which cause a transducer to respond better to some sound frequencies than to others, and to still others, not at all.

Thus, transducers may be classified with regard to their frequency range, the range of frequencies over which the response of the transducer is relatively equal. Amplitude distortion also occurs as a result of physical limitations that prevent the transducer from responding with equal efficiency to infinite variations in the intensity of the stimulus. The range of amplitudes over which a transducer follows changes in sound intensity with relative fidelity is referred to as the dynamic range of that transducer, and the intensity beyond which it ceases to amplify further is referred to as its saturation level.

AMPLIFIERS

Input sound pressures detected by the hearing-aid microphone are translated into very weak electrical impulses, of magnitudes expressed in thousandths of a volt. Because the amplifier must exaggerate these minute signals in order that they may stimulate the ear adequately, it is the heart of the hearing-aid system. The physical limitations mentioned in conjunction with transducers also apply, at least in part, to amplifiers, for they are not capable of equally efficient operation over an infinite range of sound frequencies or intensities. Restriction with respect to frequency range is, in fact, negligible, for the subminiature amplifiers used in hearing aid circuits function well over remarkably wide ranges. However, they are subject to saturation when they are overdriven by signals having excessive amplitude.

When an amplifier is driven to saturation, the peak sound pressures responsible for the saturation are simply prohibited from passing through the amplifier and, therefore, are not represented as part of the output signal of that amplifier. The result is a form of amplitude distortion referred to as peak clipping, which naturally degrades the quality of the signal, but studies have shown that rather substantial amounts of peak clipping do not reduce the intelligibility of speech that has been amplified in this way. This fact has led some manufacturers to purposefully employ peak clipping in certain cases to limit the output of a hearing aid for patients with decreased tolerance for loud sounds. The subject of output-limiting will be discussed further in a later section, but the more common problem of amplifying without distortion has been met by constructing circuits with several stages of amplification to prevent any single amplifier from being driven to its saturation level. This type of design dramatically reduces total distortion in the system and has been made possible by miniaturized amplifier circuits that are so small they may be viewed clearly only under a microscope.

VOLUME CONTROLS

The volume control provides the means by which the patient may modify the intensity of the amplified sound stimulating his ear. It is mandatory that the control be accessible, for it must be adjusted periodically to meet changing acoustic conditions. In outward appearance, the volume control is usually a small wheel which must be manually rotated in one direction to increase loudness or in the opposite direction to decrease it. In a few hearing aids, volume changes are accomplished by a slide mechanism. In either case, movement of the wheel or slide is mechanically transferred to a variable resistor, altering the electrical resistance and, thus, the voltage developed at that point in the circuit.

Volume controls are usually not linear, *i.e.*, rotation of the control to its half-way point does not ordinarily induce one-half the total amplification of which the instrument is capable, nor does three-fourths rotation induce three-fourths amplification, etc. The correspondence between the position of the volume control and the magnitude of the sound emanating from the output transducer is referred to as the taper of the volume control, and it is a feature of some significance. If the

taper does not comprise a reasonably linear range, then small movements of the control may produce loudness changes at the ear that are too gross to be of practical value. The patient, then, is unable to achieve comfortable loudness levels, but is rather beset by sound that is either too loud or too faint.

Hearing aids, like other sound systems, are not designed to perform optimally at maximum volume, for it is here that distortion is maximized as a result of amplifier and transducer saturation. They should be selected, therefore, to provide a volume reserve for the patient beyond the point at which he hears comfortably in a reasonably normal sound environment.

SWITCHES

Every hearing aid is provided with some means for interrupting the flow of power to the circuit. Whether this is accomplished by a conventional on–off switch or by physically disconnecting the battery from the remainder of the circuit, this function is necessary in order to avoid drainage of the battery when the hearing aid is not in use. Unfortunately, many individuals somehow acquire the belief that reducing the volume control to minimum constitutes turning the hearing aid off, but this is not the case. Ordinarily, battery drainage is just about as great at minimum volume as it is at maximum.

In addition to on–off functions, switches are employed in various hearing aids to provide a selection between telephone or microphone reception, or among two or three tonal qualities, or, possibly, among two or three levels of maximum power. When understood and properly employed by the patient, switching functions can provide a beneficial measure of versatility in his use of the instrument.

POWER SOURCES

As used with regard to today's hearing aids, the term power source is synonymous with battery, for every hearing aid operates on electrical power provided by some type of battery. As implied earlier, the development of the modern hearing aid has been closely associated with refinements in battery design, especially in reduction in size and the significant extension of operating life and storage life (Fig. 43–1).

All batteries function in the same general way. The positive and negative halves are made from two different metals, *i.e.*, zinc and mercury, or zinc and silver, one of which has a tendency to

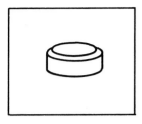

FIG. 43–1. Typical hearing aid battery, 0.445 inch in diameter and 0.165 inch in thickness.

give up electrons and the other to take on electrons in the presence of an electrolyte. Electrical energy flows, therefore, from one metal to the other, and the hearing aid circuit is interposed between the two halves to cause this energy to activate the various components of the circuit.

Batteries represent an ongoing and often significant expense to the hearing-aid user, for they have, after all, a finite operating life and must be replaced periodically. Recognition of this problem has stimulated hearing-aid and battery manufacturers to devise various methods for extending the useful life of batteries. First of all, the design of hearing-aid circuits and components is the subject of continual revision to improve operating efficiency and, thereby, reduce battery drainage to an absolute minimum. A second approach involves batteries that are capable of being recharged by means of ordinary household current. These batteries are made from a nickel-cadmium alloy and may be installed as an integral part of the hearing aid, or they may be insertable cells similar to conventional batteries. In the former case, the entire hearing aid must be connected to a wall outlet via a special transformer supplied with the unit.

In the latter, the batteries are placed, usually two at a time, in a transformer-tray device, which is then plugged into the wall outlet. In either instance, recharging requires a minimum of 10–12 hours each day or, at least every 2 days, a requirement that can present obvious disadvantages in situations where ordinary house current is not available.

There has been considerable interest in the so-called solar battery, which is simply a rechargeable battery connected with a photosensitive transducer. The transducer converts light energy into electricity which, in turn, recharges the battery as it is in the process of being used. The problem here has been one of constructing a photoelectric transducer that is small enough to maintain an acceptable hearing-aid size yet powerful enough to supply the electrical demands of the circuit. This,

combined with the inadequacy of sunlight at various geographic locations, has limited the status of the solar battery to that of an experimental curiosity.

At the present time, battery manufacturers are conducting research related to two entirely new concepts, referred to as the zinc-air system and the silver II system. When perfected, these systems promise as much as a 30% increase in the operating life of the battery or, alternatively, a corresponding reduction in battery size. In either case, the refinement will be of considerable significance in influencing the design of future hearing aids.

ELECTROMAGNETIC DEVICES

Most modern hearing aids incorporate, or are capable of being equipped with an electromagnetic device referred to as an inductance coil. The coil is a metal core wrapped with fine wire and has the capacity to detect magnetic energy in its vicinity. Such coils are installed within hearing-aid circuits solely for the purpose of enhancing hearing via the telephone, and are therefore often referred to as telephone pickups. A telephone receiver emits, in synchrony with its acoustic signal, a magnetic field which is an exact replica of the acoustic signal, and it is this magnetic signal that may be detected by the telephone pickup when the receiver of the telephone is brought into proximity with the hearing aid. As an additional advantage to the patient, coils are ordinarily installed in such a way that the microphone must be switched out of the circuit in order to switch the coil in. Thus, in using the telephone, the patient need not contend with amplified environmental sounds which normally would be brought in via the microphone.

PHYSICAL PARAMETERS OF HEARING-AID PERFORMANCE

GAIN

Gain, in a hearing aid or other sound-amplifying system, is the term used to describe the extent to which the amplitude of the incoming sound is increased by the system. Because the input sound pressure and the output sound pressure are expressed and measured in decibels, the difference between them, the gain, is also expressed in decibels. As an example, given a particular system, if the input sound pressure measured just before the microphone is 60 dB, and the output sound pressure measured just after the receiver is 90 dB, the gain of that system is said to be 30 dB.

To standardize the measurement and expression of gain so that hearing aids may be compared with regard to this factor, the American National Standards Institute (ANSI) has specified a measurement procedure in which a hearing aid is placed in a 60-dB SPL sound field with the volume control set at maximum. The output sound pressure is read for each of three test frequencies, *i.e.*, 1000 Hz, 1600 Hz, and 2500 Hz, and the input sound pressure of 60 dB subtracted from each of the three readings. Finally, the three calculated decibel differences are averaged to yield the average full-on gain of the instrument being tested.

MAXIMUM POWER OUTPUT

Maximum power output is obviously related to the phenomenon of saturation mentioned earlier. Given the maximum amplitude-handling capacities of the various components of the system, there is clearly some finite limit beyond which the hearing aid will not amplify. This limit (expressed in dB SPL) is the maximum power output, the measurement of which has also been standardized by ANSI. The hearing aid, with volume control set at maximum, is placed in a 90-dB SPL sound field and the output sound pressure measured for frequencies of 1000 Hz, 1600 Hz, and 2500 Hz. The three output measurements are averaged to yield a quantity referred to as the average saturation sound pressure level for that instrument.

BANDWIDTH

In evaluating the performance of a hearing aid, it is necessary to determine the range of frequencies over which the instrument may be expected to provide useful amplification. As prescribed by ANSI, the bandwidth is determined by deducting 20 dB from the average full-on gain of a particular instrument, and noting the lowest and highest frequencies at which the gain equals or exceeds the −20 dB level. Consider, for example, a hearing aid with an ANSI gain of 55 dB. Deduction of 20 dB yields a base level of 35 dB. The lowest frequency at which the instrument provides a minimum of 35 dB gain is the lower limit of the bandwidth of that instrument; the highest frequency at which it provides a minimum of 35 dB gain constitutes the upper limit of the bandwidth. Assume that the hearing aid provides 35 dB gain at a frequency of 200 Hz, but at no frequency lower than 200 Hz. Assume further that it provides

35 dB gain at 3800 Hz, but at no frequency higher than 3800 Hz. The calculated bandwidth of this unit is, therefore, 200 to 3800 Hz.

SPECIAL FEATURES IN MODERN HEARING AIDS

OUTPUT LIMITING

Individuals vary widely in their capacity to tolerate amplified sound, and a specific form of hypersensitivity known as loudness recruitment is recognized as an accompanying symptom in certain types of auditory pathology. Limitation of the maximum output of a hearing aid is, therefore, of practical value in precluding discomfort and, possibly, further harm to the ear. One method for limiting output, peak clipping, has been mentioned previously through its relationship to the phenomenon of saturation. Because the distortion resulting from moderate amounts of peak clipping does not interfere significantly with speech intelligibility, it is possible to design circuits in which peak clipping will occur at predetermined sound pressure levels, thus assuring that sound pressures in excess of the predetermined level will not reach the patient's ear.

Compression amplification is another common method for achieving output limiting. This method is analogous to a very rapidly acting volume control, but, in this case, it is the excessively strong sound pressures, themselves, that activate the device which reduces gain. Again, it is possible to design the circuit so that the compression unit is activated at a very precisely specified sound pressure level. Ordinarily, a very short, but measurable, period of time elapses before the compression circuit responds to the excessive sound, and there is another time lapse before the hearing aid returns to normal operation following the reduction of the sound below the predetermined level. These latencies are referred to as attack time and release time, respectively. The net result of a well-designed and executed compression circuit is to afford high amplification of relatively weak input signals, but less amplification of strong signals, thus protecting the patient with a tolerance problem without the penalty of significant distortion.

DIRECTIONAL MICROPHONES

Conventional hearing-aid microphones provide a sound inlet through which all detectable sounds, wanted or unwanted, enter the instrument. To the hearing-aid wearer, noise is the enemy, and his primary complaint often relates to the inability of his hearing aid to discriminate between what he would like to hear and what he would not like to hear at any given moment. Directional microphones are intended to achieve a certain degree of such discrimination by reducing the response of the hearing aid to sounds originating behind the wearer. In addition to the main sound inlet, which faces forward, a second, rearward facing inlet is provided which functions to suppress, rather than amplify sounds coming from that direction. The signal-to-noise ratio is thereby improved in favor of the sound that the user is facing.

NOISE SUPPRESSION

Compression circuits, peak clippers, and directional microphones all contribute to the reduction of environmental sound which the patient perceives as noise, but the problem of unwanted noise is so generalized that the industry has taken advantage of additional concepts to accomplish further suppression of noise. Physical measurement of sounds commonly classified as noise discloses that a significant portion of the power in these sounds is concentrated at the lower end of the audible frequency spectrum. This disclosure, combined with the information that perception of low frequency sound does not contribute substantially to auditory speech comprehension has led to the conclusion that it would be productive to purposefully reduce the sensitivity of a hearing aid to low frequency stimuli. To this end, many hearing aids are now produced with one or two switch-selectable degrees of low frequency suppression. The particular means employed to achieve such suppression are high-pass filter circuits, so called because they permit sounds that are higher than a predetermined frequency to pass on to the remaining circuitry, while sharply reducing the gain for sounds lower than the predetermined frequency.

SYSTEMS FOR CONTRALATERAL ROUTING OF SIGNAL

Until relatively recently, audiologists and otolaryngologists were guided by the assumption that an individual with normal or only mildly impaired hearing in one ear was not a candidate for a hearing aid, even if that individual possessed no useful hearing in the opposite ear. The contralateral routing of signal (CROS) principle was developed after persistent complaints by unilaterally impaired patients made it clear that the foregoing assumption was not true. The original, classic CROS system (Fig. 43–2) incorporated a microphone positioned on the poorer ear and means for transmitting the microphone signal to the opposite, better ear. When properly executed, this system permits the patient to hear not only the sounds he would ordinarily hear via his better ear but also sounds detected on the impaired side.

The classic CROS system is still widely used, as are numerous modifications which have been devised to solve particular types of hearing problems. Bi-CROS systems (Fig. 43–3) have been found useful for persons with significant hearing loss in both ears, one of which is unaidable. A detector microphone is positioned on the side of the poorer ear and is connected to a complete hearing aid (microphone-amplifier-receiver) on the better ear. The addition of the microphone on the better ear results in the combined advantages of a conventional hearing aid on that ear and the CROS amplification of signals detected on the unaidable side.

For patients with profound, but aidable hearing impairment, the power CROS system (Fig. 43–4) has permitted the use of ear-level hearing aids in cases in which only a cosmetically less desirable pocket hearing aid would have been considered previously. Great amplification power, in any hearing aid, always brings with it the potential problem of feedback, an annoying, screeching sound, which occurs when the amplified output of a hearing aid is detected by its own microphone. Separation of the microphone from the remainder of the hearing aid system is, therefore, one method for preventing feedback when dealing with high-gain instruments. The power CROS system is essentially the same as the classic CROS, the exception being that the sound inserted into the aidable ear is contained in that ear by an earmold which occludes the ear. The types of earmolds and their effect on aided hearing will be discussed more completely in a later section.

Many individuals have hearing loss characterized by normal or near-normal hearing for low-frequency sounds, combined with poor hearing for high-frequency sounds. The problem here is to obtain high-gain amplification without feedback and without overloading the ear with low-frequency sounds to which it is already sensitive. The High CROS system (Fig. 43–5) accomplishes these goals by, again, separating the microphone from the remainder of the system and employing a hearing aid that produces high amplification in the high-frequency sound range. As was true in the

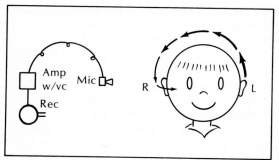

FIG. 43–2. Diagram of CROS hearing aid. **Amp,** amplifier; **w/vc,** with volume control; **Mic,** microphone; **Rec,** receiver; **R,** right ear; **L,** left ear.

FIG. 43–3. Diagram of bi-CROS hearing aid. **w/vc,** with volume control.

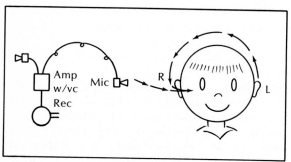

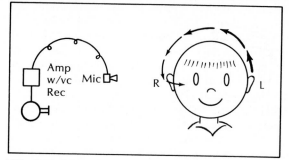

FIG. 43–4. Diagram of a power CROS hearing-aid system. Receiver with closed mold; **w/vc,** with volume control.

FIG. 43–5. Diagram of a high-CROS hearing-aid system. Receiver with closed mold; **w/vc,** with volume control.

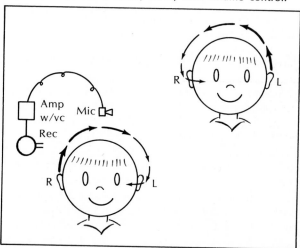

power CROS technique, placement of the microphone on the opposite side of the head causes the head itself to act as a shield to prevent amplified sound from being detected by the microphone. With the elimination of feedback, the patient realizes the advantage of significantly increased useful gain.

VARIABLE CONTROLS

When considered as a basic unit, a hearing aid is a combination of discrete components selected to yield a particular, predefined amplification characteristic. Switching functions, described earlier, add a degree of functional versatility by permitting certain discrete components to be substituted for others, thus altering some parameter of the instrument's performance. Variable-control hearing aids advance the idea of versatile performance a step further, by providing the capability to introduce changes not in discrete steps but rather on a continuum. In this way, the patient receives the benefit of subtle variations in, for example, tonal quality, rather than a restrictive choice of two or three tonal qualities, none of which may be precisely suited to the patient's requirements. Other than tone quality, variable controls have been designed to regulate maximum power output, the amount of compression amplification and even the length of attack time in the compression circuit. In general, the capability for modifying any particular aspect of performance, independently of other aspects, has considerable value in tuning the hearing aid to suit specific, unique needs of the patient and in accommodating changes in these needs as they occur.

AIR-CONDUCTION HEARING AIDS

Air conduction hearing aids are so designated because the signal which has been amplified by the unit stimulates the ear via the external auditory canal. The mode of stimulation is, therefore, the normal one, including the eardrum and middle-ear

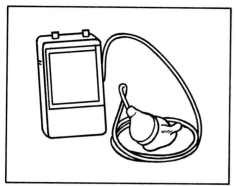

FIG. 43–6. Pocket-type hearing aid, about 50–60% of normal size.

FIG. 43–7. A postauricle hearing aid, approximately normal size.

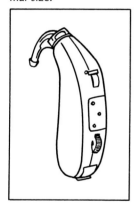

mechanism. There are four styles of air-conduction hearing aids:

POCKET BODY TYPE

The pocket, or body instrument (Fig. 43–6) comprises a small case called the transmitter, an electrical connection cord and a receiver. The transmitter houses the microphone, amplifiers, and all controls, and is connected to the output transducer by means of a cord, which may be 12 to 36 or more inches in length. The capacity for producing acoustic power is greater with the pocket aid than with any other type, so these are often utilized in cases of extremely severe or profound hearing loss.

POSTAURICLE TYPE

The postauricle or behind-the-ear hearing aid (Fig. 43–7) is by far the prevalent style in use today. All components are contained in a case designed to fit behind the ear, in the niche formed by the attachment of the pinna to the temporal area of the skull. A flexible, hollow tube conducts the amplified sound from the instrument to the patient's ear and is usually, but not always, retained in the ear by a molded earpiece. Because the input transducer is located in the vicinity of the ear, and not at chest-level, as it is with a pocket instrument, postauricle, as well as eyeglass and all-in-the-ear aids are often referred to collectively as ear level instruments.

EYEGLASS TYPE

Eyeglass instruments (Fig. 43–8) are electronically identical to their postauricle counterparts, but the components are enclosed within a case designed in the form of an eyeglass temple. Means are provided for attaching the temple to most optical front frames and for accommodating variations

FIG. 43–8. An eyeglass type hearing aid, near normal size.

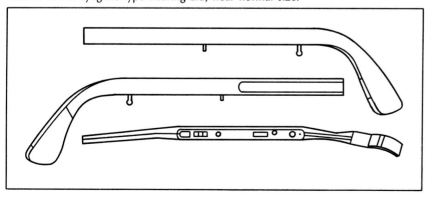

in the required length of the temple from patient to patient. As was true with postauricle instruments, a flexible, hollow tube conducts the amplified signal to the ear, ordinarily via a molded earpiece.

The person who wears glasses only on a part time basis is not a candidate for eyeglass hearing aids, for there may well be situations in which the user would like to wear eyeglasses, or the hearing aid, but not both. Even when glasses are worn full time, the eyeglass hearing aid may not be satisfactory, because the physical connection of the eyeglass to the hearing aid can present problems.

For example, ordinarily the selection in front frames is restricted because of the type of hinge required. Also, if either the glasses or the hearing aid requires repair, the other cannot be used unless a reserve is available. Of particular importance is the difficulty in physical adjustment of the entire assembly if the lenses are trifocals and the precise alignment is critical.

ALL-IN-THE-EAR TYPE

Miniaturization in the construction of components has made it possible to enclose all necessary elements within a hollow earpiece molded to fit the patient's ear (Fig. 43–9). This type of unit ordinarily fills the concha of the external ear and, aside from its cosmetic desirability, sometimes provides the only possible solution in patients with inadequate space behind the ear for a postauricle or eyeglass instrument.

BONE-CONDUCTION HEARING AIDS

The distinctive feature of a bone-conduction hearing aid is the output transducer, commonly referred to as a vibrator or bone oscillator. The vibrator does precisely what its name implies, it vibrates, and when the surface of the vibrator is applied to the skull with firm pressure, its vibrations are propagated through the skull to the cochleas. Regardless of the locus of application on the skull, the vibratory energy reaches each of the two cochleas with approximately equal force. Studies have demonstrated, however, that the most sensitive application point is the apex of the skull. Because of the practical disadvantages of this location, e.g., the abundance of hair, it is common practice to apply the vibrator of a hearing aid to the mastoid process of the temporal bone.

As it is essential to apply the vibrator with some substantial force, at least 400 g, not all types of hearing aids can be adapted to bone transmission. Pocket instruments are especially suitable for bone conduction applications because of their power-generating capacity, as vibrators require considerably more power than air-conduction receivers. The necessary application force is achieved by mounting the vibrator on a spring-steel headband, which is worn across the top of the head. The same type of headband may be used to convert a postauricle instrument to bone transmission, with the instrument mounted on one end of the headband and the vibrator mounted on the other with an electrical connecting cord between the two. Eyeglass units also may be utilized for bone conduction by fitting the temples tightly and situating the vibrator at the rear inner surface of one temple, i.e., against the mastoid surface.

Because bone-conduction hearing aids are worn without any component that occludes the external auditory canal, they provide a practical means for amplification in cases in which such occlusion would precipitate adverse reactions. Patients who have undergone surgery, especially radical surgery, for mastoiditis and those with chronic drainage or a predisposition toward drainage, exemplify cases in this category (see Ch. 36 for a discussion of the application of bone conduction amplification in children).

EARMOLDS

Receivers used with early body type hearing aids were coupled to the ear by means of wooden or hard rubber inserts, the receiver-insert combination being held in position at the ear by wire wrapped around the pinna. This arrangement obviously left much to be desired, and it was not long before the hard rubber inserts were being custom molded from plaster impressions of the ear. The idea of custom molding has persisted as

FIG. 43–9. An all-in-the-ear hearing aid.

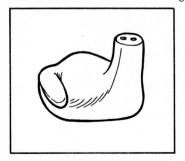

an important aspect of hearing-aid dispensing procedures, but the use of rubber as an earmold material declined rapidly with the emergence of plastic materials following World War II. As the variety and versatility of hearing aids have expanded to accommodate virtually infinite variation in individual requirements, so the diversity of earmolds has expanded (Fig. 43–10). There are now more than a dozen distinct earmold styles, each possessing acoustic and cosmetic features that may be favorable or unfavorable in any particular case.

Once an earmold is attached to a hearing aid, it becomes an integral part of the total transmission system and can have a profound influence on the characteristics of the sound that stimulates the patient's ear. As a general rule, the greater the gain of the hearing aid, the more tightly the earmold must fit into the ear to achieve an acoustic seal. If the acoustic seal is inadequate, the sound pressure developed by a high-gain instrument is not contained within the external auditory canal but rather tends to escape by way of the inadequacies in the seal. One effect of such escape is decreased efficiency of the hearing aid, for only a portion of the amplified sound actually stimulates the ear. Another effect is that of feedback, a phenomenon described earlier in connection with CROS amplification. Both effects are clearly negative, but they can usually be avoided through appropriate earmold fitting techniques.

The practice of fabricating earmolds from an impression of the patient's ear assures that the contours of the mold match the contours of the ear as precisely as possible. This enhances the acoustic seal, comfort in wearing the earmold, and retention within the ear. However, the importance of the acoustic seal diminishes as the need for gain diminishes, as lower-amplitude sound waves are less inclined to escape from the auditory canal. There are, in fact, a number of circumstances under which such escape has a beneficial effect and is actually facilitated through the use of vents. A vent is a hole bored in an earmold in order to establish communication between the air in the auditory canal and the air outside the ear. Through the column of air within the vent, the air pressure within and without the ear is equalized, relieving feelings of occlusion, which can be a source of discomfort for the patient.

In cases of high-frequency hearing loss, venting may provide additional advantages. By facilitating the escape of low-frequency sound, a vent precludes overloading the ear in a sound range to

FIG. 43–10. Three examples of modern earmold styles. **A.** Standard regular mold can be fitted with any type receiver. For body-worn aids with external receivers only. **B.** Standard "perimeter" mold is completely cut out, leaving only the outer ring, excellent for all integral receiver instruments, with best acoustical properties, excellent concealment, and comfort. **C.** Standard "perimeter" mold with outer part of ring eliminated, used when canal mold alone will not suffice. It offers excellent retention along with good concealment and acoustical values. (Courtesy of Westone Laboratories Inc.)

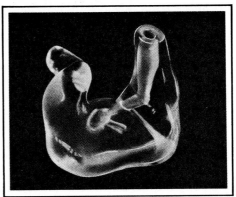

A

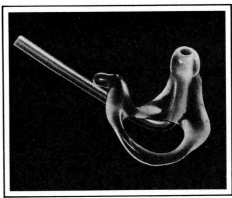

B

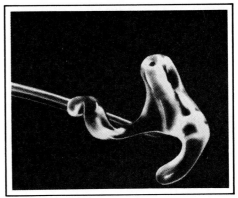

C

which it is already responsive even without amplification, and it also creates an input pathway for environmental sounds which the patient may perceive more naturally with his unimpaired low-frequency hearing. It should be understood from the foregoing discussion that the degree of acoustic seal provided by an earmold may be viewed as a continuum. At one end there is the tight seal required in the application of high-gain instruments; at the other, an extreme instance of venting, in which there is really no earmold at all, but only a tube bent to direct the hearing-aid output into the ear canal.

AUDIOMETRY AND HEARING AIDS

Hearing tests, however primitive or sophisticated, have been administered for centuries in conjunction with physical examination of the ear to facilitate diagnosis and treatment of ear pathology. Clinical audiometry has thus withstood the test of time and is generally considered to be a significant aspect of comprehensive otologic examination. Not long after the emergence of audiology as a formal field of study, published reports began to appear, suggesting that certain audiometric techniques, appropriately modified, might be helpful in placing hearing aid selection procedures on a more scientific foundation.

That there was room for improvement in hearing-aid selection procedures was beyond dispute, and the basic notion possessed substantial face validity in view of the prevailing favorable acceptance of audiometric methods. However, the passing years have not brought forth confirmation of these early ideas. Rather, it has become increasingly evident that auditory test information that is useful for medical objectives is not necessarily adequate in nurturing the successful union of a hearing-impaired patient and a hearing aid.

CANDIDACY FOR A HEARING AID

In consideration of the impressive array of hearing aids presently available, it is no longer reasonable to view audiometric measurements as the ultimate criteria upon which to judge whether an individual is or is not a candidate for a hearing aid. In a very real sense, any individual who reports significant difficulty in auditory reception, and who is not a candidate for medical or surgical treatment, is a candidate for amplification, regardless of the de-

gree of deficit disclosed by test results. This is, of course, a two-sided proposition. Certain patients with quite serious hearing losses, audiometrically established, may be poor candidates for amplification simply because they are not sufficiently motivated to communicate. Conversely, there are individuals with rather mild impairments who are, nonetheless, candidates for amplification because they are personally motivated to exploit their communicative capacities to the maximum level possible.

SPECIFYING FAVORABLE PHYSICAL CHARACTERISTICS

A basic audiometric examination includes measurement of threshold for pure tones via air conduction and bone conduction, measurement of threshold for, and comprehension of appropriate spoken material, and some determination of the intensity of sound that induces physical discomfort. The present discussion is restricted to the use of such test results in the application of hearing aids (see Chs. 1 and 6–8).

In analyzing a patient's audiogram, it is often tempting to conclude that the ideal acoustic remedy would be one whereby the amount of amplification supplied at each frequency is directly related to the measured auditory threshold at that frequency. This idea of selective amplification has waxed and waned in favor for many years, recurring only by virtue of its apparent plausibility. In practice, the system does not produce the anticipated result, primarily because the threshold pattern does not reflect accurately the way in which suprathreshold sounds are perceived.

There is no universally accepted procedure for determining the combination of characteristics in an amplifying device or in the output it produces, which will yield optimum compensation in any specific case of hearing loss. Thus, the fitting of a hearing aid remains more of an art than a science.

Pure-tone audiometry yields measurements of auditory threshold for a variety of sounds within the audio-frequency range. The great majority of patients who take this test are capable of doing so with an acceptable degree of consistency, but the widespread practice of inferring a patient's amplification requirements from the pattern of the threshold measurements is subject to question on theoretic as well as empiric grounds.

It is very common, for example, to assume that a patient whose threshold pattern reveals a high-frequency hearing loss will achieve optimal results through the use of a high-frequency-emphasis hearing aid. On an empiric basis, a significant number of such patients reject these instruments due to the harsh, metallic quality of the amplified sounds, especially speech. If, in fact, the threshold pattern were a valid indicator of the way in which these sounds were heard without aid, and the instrument did, in fact, exaggerate high-frequency sounds, then the expected auditory result would be a more natural, rather than metallic, signal. This expectation is not realized in many cases because of the unavailability of measurements of suprathreshold auditory function and the assumption, completely unjustified, that suprathreshold hearing is related to threshold hearing in some predictable way. The assumption is little more than an expedient. We do not have and cannot obtain directly the information, which is obviously important, so we utilize indirect information whose primary virtue is availability.

Audiometric measurements of uncomfortable loudness levels are the clinician's primary guide for specifying maximum power output requirements. As a first approximation, he must assure that sound levels which might cause discomfort are not transmitted to the ear. On the other hand, the output capability of the hearing aid must be sufficient to allow a useful dynamic range plus some reserve gain. In this regard, the importance of validity in measuring discomfort cannot be overemphasized, for studies have shown that a listener's perception of discomfort is influenced significantly by the manner in which the term is defined for him in pretest instructions. Care must be exercised to differentiate between annoyance and actual physical discomfort, as an individual who has had a hearing loss for some period of time may find relatively normal sound levels truly annoying and, understandably, judge them to be uncomfortable. If, in formulating a set of hearing aid specifications for this individual, the clinician specifies maximum power output on the basis of a spuriously low discomfort threshold, the dynamic range of the instrument will be unnecessarily restricted. This will cause the power of the instrument to seem unsatisfactorily weak after a short period of use, during which the listener adapts to amplified sound input.

The gain of a hearing aid is commonly specified on the basis of audiometric measurements related to the listeners' comfort level. The most comfortable listening level for speech stimuli may be measured directly or deduced by adding from 25–40 dB to the patient's speech reception threshold. The gain may be considered adequate if a comfortable listening level is produced when the volume control is somewhere between one-fourth and three-fourths of its total rotation.

Binaural amplification is advantageous from an auditory standpoint and is advisable when the average threshold loss in each ear is at least 25 or 30 dB. Naturally, the better the speech discrimination score in each ear, the better the overall result. However, poor discrimination in one or both ears, far from being a contraindication, may well constitute a powerful argument in favor of amplification for both ears. The threshold loss in the two ears need not be symmetrical, although it is true that the more extensive the asymmetry, the greater will be the difficulty in achieving the auditory balance between the two ears that is necessary to realize the benefits of binaural hearing.

Obviously, not all patients require or wish to use two hearing aids, so it is often necessary to choose one ear. In general, the most favorable overall result is obtained by applying the hearing aid to the poorer ear, unless that ear is not aidable because of poor speech discrimination, restricted dynamic range, or a disorder such as infection. The effect of using the poorer ear is enhanced if the threshold loss in the better ear is in the mild or moderate range, thus permitting a meaningful contribution by the better ear to the total auditory perception. The benefit is enhanced further, of course, if the poorer ear is capable of good speech discrimination performance and has a broad dynamic range. When one ear is, in fact, not amenable to improvement through amplification, then the clinician may consider options provided by the various forms of CROS amplification. If there are no obvious determining factors favoring one ear or the other, personal preference of the patient, based upon largely intangible factors, may ultimately determine which ear is used.

Anatomic limitations, degree of hearing loss, and aesthetic preferences are all involved in considering the type of hearing aid to be used. The most common anatomic limitations encountered in everyday practice are various forms of atresia and restricted postauricular space. In the former instance, neither a postauricle nor all-in-the-ear instrument may be used; in the latter, a conventional postauricle unit usually cannot be worn comfortably. A bone conduction hearing aid may be considered for any patient with normal or near-normal bone conduction thresholds and, furthermore, may be the only feasible solution for patients with chronic otorrhea due to chronic otitis media—mastoiditis.

When the average threshold loss exceeds 80 dB, a pocket-type instrument may be recommended, although impairments in this range may be successfully managed with a postauricle aid through exceptional attention to the fit of the earmold or through the application of a power CROS unit. Within the hearing loss range between 20 dB and 80 dB, postauricle instruments are ordinarily selected for the inherent advantages of ear-level reception, and in impairments as extensive as 65 dB, all-in-the-ear instruments may provide a workable alternative.

Other factors being equal, it is to the patient's advantage to have the hearing-aid microphone positioned at ear level, but, as mentioned earlier, a pocket instrument is often the only type of instrument capable of producing the power demanded by a particular hearing loss. The resultant shortcomings are clothing noise and a phenomenon referred to as the body-baffle effect. The shearing motion of clothing against the surface of the transmitter, particularly near the microphone, creates a static-like noise, which patients invariably find objectionable. Furthermore, resonances caused by contact between the transmitter and the body tend to augment low-frequency sounds and attenuate high frequencies. This effect is exaggerated by covering the microphone with clothing, which tends to further attenuate high frequencies. The net result is increased amplification of unwanted, noisy sounds and reduction of those sounds which contribute most to speech comprehension.

Ear level instruments are not without disadvantages, as they are subject to wind noise. However, this problem can usually be controlled through the use of specially designed microphone shields.

HEARING-AID SELECTION

Once a general framework of hearing-aid specifications has been determined for a particular patient, it is necessary to select one from among the number of existing instruments which appear to satisfy these specifications. Technical and performance data may be found in catalogs published by the various manufacturers, but a hearing aid cannot be recommended solely on the basis of a catalog description. Even though two or more hearing aids may appear to be identical in every describable respect, there are usually subtle differences among them, which are revealed only when the patient has an opportunity to wear them on a comparative basis. It is the object of a hearing-aid selection procedure, then, to provide such an opportunity

and, in the process, to acquire quantitative and qualitative information upon which to base a specific recommendation.

As a means of control, testing is usually conducted in an enclosure which has been acoustically treated especially for audiometric purposes, i.e., external sounds are largely excluded and reverberation of internally generated sounds is held to a negligible level. The use of a controlled environment is subject to some criticism because it does not represent a real-life listening condition, but real-life listening situations are, themselves, so varied that simulation of one or more of these situations for test purposes would be subject to the same criticism.

The patient is comfortably seated facing a loudspeaker through which speech signals are generated. The speech may be live voice or recorded, but, in either case, is controlled by means of a standard speech audiometer. As the technical details of speech audiometry are beyond the scope of this chapter, it must suffice here to summarize that the patient's speech reception threshold (SRT) and speech discrimination score (SDS) are measured, and subjective reactions noted, for each of a number of hearing aids in turn. Under ordinary circumstances, the instrument that affords the lowest SRT (best sensitivity) and highest SDS (best comprehension) is the one recommended, provided, of course, no adverse subjective reactions were observed during testing with that instrument. Of the two measured quantities, SDS is by far the more significant and is therefore weighted more heavily in arriving at a final recommendation.

Although it was introduced some three decades ago, the foregoing procedure or some modification of it is still widely used. One modification of special interest is referred to as the articulation function method, the term **articulation** being used synonymously with speech discrimination and a throwback to the time when telephone engineers employed speech signals to test transmission equipment. In this procedure, the patient's SDS is measured several times with each hearing aid, each time at a progressively higher intensity. The result is plotted on a graph illustrating the way in which SDS varies as a function of input intensity, and emphasizes the very important point that SDS increases with intensity only to a certain level, beyond which distortion occurs and actually decreases comprehension of speech. Intercomparison of the articulation functions produced by several hearing aids graphically discloses which instrument provides the most desirable combination of dynamic range, high-intensity response, and speech comprehension.

In recent years, there has been a trend either to forego such formalized selection methods entirely, or to temper the results with behavioral observations acquired through a trial period under real-life circumstances.

Selection of a hearing aid on the basis of behavioral observation appears to circumvent some of the problems inherent in doing so through tests only in controlled, clinical environments, as the final recommendation depends not on comparative measurements but rather on patient satisfaction. In the final analysis, it may be said that no single hearing aid selection procedure assures that the instrument ultimately selected is, in fact, the only satisfactory one for a particular patient, as there are too many instruments that must remain untested because of practical considerations. For this reason, patient satisfaction must be the final criterion.

HEARING-AID ORIENTATION

Once a hearing aid has been selected and fitted, it is necessary that the patient learn to use the instrument and make it a part of everyday life. The patient must be taught to insert and remove the earmold, install a fresh battery when required, regulate volume, and manipulate switches and controls to the best advantage. Instruction must be provided concerning the care of the instrument and recognition of malfunction.

The new hearing aid user must learn how to cope with a seemingly hostile environment, filled with noise, unfamiliar sounds, and even familiar sounds, which are not heard in a familiar way. The user must learn that the sound produced by the best of all possible hearing aids must still pass through a pathologic auditory mechanism on its journey to the brain, and that there exists, therefore, an absolute limit to the benefit any instrument can offer.

The skills required to extract the greatest benefit from a hearing aid are not assimilated rapidly, but rather slowly over a period of time, and not without informed guidance. Only a very small fraction of all hearing-aid wearers are ever exposed to a formalized program of aural rehabilitation, including hearing aid use, speech reading, auditory training, and counseling. The necessary skills are ordinarily mastered, therefore, through relentless repetition by the hearing-aid dispensers, and by patiently guiding fingers crippled by arthritis or rendered insensitive by age, in inserting an earmold or locating a volume control; by confronting unrealistic expectations and explaining time and time again why the hearing aid cannot eliminate unwanted sounds and transmit only those sounds which the wearer wishes to hear. For all the vagaries and qualitative nature of the fitting process, and the multiplicity of problems encountered along the way, it is to the everlasting credit of the hearing health team—the otologist, the audiologist, the hearing-aid dispenser—that the great majority of hearing-aid wearers express their gratitude by simply saying: "Why didn't I do this ten years ago? Think of what I've missed."

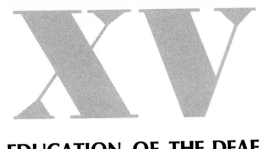

EDUCATION OF THE DEAF

44

THE JOHN TRACY CLINIC APPROACH TO DEAF CHILDREN AND THEIR FAMILIES

EDGAR L. LOWELL

It has been my privilege to serve as the voluntary consulting otologist to the John Tracy Clinic since it was founded. The unique contributions of Mrs. Spencer Tracy and the Clinic have done much to improve the lives of hearing-impaired children and their families, not only in Los Angeles, but throughout the world. Dr. Edgar Lowell, Director of the Clinic, has summarized this program in the following chapter.

VICTOR GOODHILL, M.D.

The John Tracy Clinic approach is a comprehensive program for assisting the young deaf child and his family. It integrates audiology, psychology, education, and parent counseling in a continuing program to meet the needs of the individual family.

The Clinic's program and philosophy is based on the experiences of Mrs. Spencer Tracy with her son John, who was born with a profound hearing loss.

HISTORY

Although the Tracys were able to provide the finest medical and educational help for John, Mrs. Tracy felt that many of her questions were not being answered and that there was much more that she could do to help with John's education. In her quest for additional knowledge, she attended a meeting of speech therapists at the University of Southern California. In the question-and-answer period following the formal presentation, Mrs. Tracy asked the professionals why they were not doing something positive to help parents of young deaf children. The reply came in the form of a challenge: "Why don't you?" Mrs. Tracy accepted that challenge and invited other parents of deaf children present to meet at her home. Mrs. Tracy acknowledges that the 13 families present at the first meeting may have been there in part because of her husband's movie fame. She and the parents soon realized there were genuine benefits to be derived from meeting together to share knowledge and ideas and to discuss their feelings with other parents who were living through the same experience.

Initially the meetings were only for parents and were led by an instructor from the Adult Education Department of the Los Angeles City Schools. Later a nursery school was started on the University of Southern California campus with a trained teacher of the deaf. As a result of publicity about new efforts, Mrs. Tracy began receiving letters from other mothers of young deaf children who wrote to her seeking help or advice. In answering these letters, she used materials from the Wright Oral School that she had used with John. This led ultimately to the establishment of the *John Tracy Clinic Correspondence Course for Parents of Preschool Deaf Children*. The Clinic was formally incorporated in 1942.

PURPOSE

John Tracy Clinic was based then, as it is now, on the belief that education of the young, hearing-impaired child should begin at the earliest possible moment and that parents can play an important role in their child's education.

Perhaps the best statement of the clinic's purpose is contained in the statement by Mrs. Tracy herself:

Communication with our fellow men is possibly the most important single factor in living. The degree to which we understand others and the extent to which we can express ourselves clearly, interestingly, and persuasively determines almost overwhelmingly our successes and our failures.

Anyone with a hearing loss has in some measure a communication problem. But the problems facing a child who is born with a severe loss or a child who through illness loses his hearing before he has acquired speech and language are staggering. A hearing baby learns to understand what people say and to talk simply because he can hear. By being constantly exposed to patterns of voice sounds in association with people, things, actions, and ideas, he soon begins to recognize them and to understand them. Then he begins to imitate them. He begins to talk. A deaf baby does not talk, because not hearing speech he cannot imitate it. He doesn't know he has a voice. He doesn't know that words and language exist. But he can be taught. He can learn to understand what people say by watching the movements of their lips, by lipreading, and he can learn to speak by imitating the formation and movement of his teacher's lips, together with the sound vibrations he feels on her face and the use of any residual hearing he may have.

However, he does not have to wait for a school and a teacher—learning does not wait for schools. Learning, all learning, begins at birth, and everything a child sees and hears, everything he smells, tastes, and touches, everything he experiences contribute toward it. What he learns depends upon his environment and the people in it, that is, usually upon his home and his parents. Acquiring a means of communication is part of the learning process and constitutes a large part of what a hearing child learns during his preschool years.

During this fertile period, a deaf child also can begin to acquire language, lipreading, and speech—words and a means of understanding and expressing them. To do so he will need the love, the understanding, the support, and the knowledge of his parents.

The purpose of John Tracy Clinic is to provide this knowledge at the earliest possible moment. The Clinic is a place where parents may come or may write for information, encouragement, guidance and training. Its program is directed not only to the special skills involved in communication, but toward the total development of the whole child and the attitudes and the feelings of those in his environment which so deeply affect this development (3).

THE EDUCATIONAL PROGRAM

PHILOSOPHY

The John Tracy Clinic follows an oral philosophy, which means that we concentrate on teaching young hearing-impaired children to lipread and to speak. Despite the ancient and often heated dispute over oral versus manual philosophies, the Clinic is not opposed to manual communication. We feel that parents and educators should have the right to elect the method that they believe in. We believe that the oral method is less restrictive, that is, the oral deaf person is not restricted to communicating with people who also understand and use manual communication, and is not dependent upon an interpreter. We recognize that there are other points of view. We staunchly defend the right of manualists to their beliefs and, in fact, provide manual interpretation for deaf parents who use the Clinic's program because they want their children to be oral.

SERVICES

CONSULTATION

The first contact with a family is generally through our consultation service. This includes an audiologic and psychologic evaluation to determine whether the child would benefit from the Clinic's program. The majority of these families are referred by the medical profession.

Testing very young hearing-impaired children is not an easy task, but the Clinic has the advantage of specializing with that age group so that our audiologist and psychologist have the opportunity for a great deal of experience.

Some of the families seen in our consultation service are relieved to find out that their child is not deaf. In some cases, there may be other handicapping conditions that lead the parents to raise questions about their child's hearing.

For those families in which deafness is established, the consultation visit also includes an interview with our psychologist, which gives us some insight into the family structure, provides a preliminary exploration of the parents' feelings and attitudes, and provides them with an orientation to the John Tracy Clinic program.

DEMONSTRATION HOME

One of the first educational services offered the family is an appointment in our Demonstration Home. This is a homelike apartment in the Clinic building where the mother and child meet a teacher on an individual appointment basis. The frequency of these visits depends, in part, on the age of the child. The average is about once a week.

The teacher's goal is to show the parent how the Clinic's communication development program for the young deaf child can be incorporated into everyday household activities. The teacher first demonstrates the activity with the child and then goes into a one-way glass observation booth and coaches the parent as she repeats the activity. The Demonstration Home experience assures us that the parent knows *how* to carry out appropriate activities at home. We believe the Demonstration Home provides much better carryover to the real home than more traditional classroom lectures and demonstration.

Another advantage of the Demonstration Home is that it puts the parent and teacher on a more informal basis than that of the usual student-teacher relationship. We believe that this facilitates communication and the learning process.

PARENT CLASSES

On Tuesday evenings there are 2 hours of classes for parents. We hold them in the evening so that working parents can attend. They are divided into a section on communication training, helping the parents develop communication skills with their child, and a section that deals with the parents' feelings and attitudes.

There is a 4-year curriculum with a fifth year option in communication for those parents who would like to continue with advanced training. While the major emphasis is on the informal or general language development program, there is also an opportunity for work with the more detailed specific language program, which is used by the Clinics' teachers. This range of opportunities allows the parents to elect how deeply they wish to go into the teaching process.

FRIDAY FAMILY SCHOOL

To provide a more complete orientation to the John Tracy Clinic approach, to provide us with an opportunity for additional psychologic and audiologic evaluation, and to provide the children with what for many of them is their first group experience, we have a Friday Family School. The children, along with any hearing siblings, are brought into our Nursery School on Fridays while the parents attend classes that introduce them to the material covered in our Tuesday evening classes.

DEMONSTRATION NURSERY SCHOOL

Twenty-four families are enrolled in our Demonstration Nursery School, which is a 4-year program for children from 2–6 years of age. It provides us with an opportunity to show parents who have just discovered that their child is deaf what can be accomplished by families who follow the Clinic's program. It also provides an opportunity for the general public and particularly college students who are interested in career selection to view the Clinic's educational program and learn more about young deaf children. All of the teaching areas have observation booths with one-way vision mirrors so that observation may be carried out without interrupting the educational program.

The Demonstration Nursery School has twelve 2- and 3-year-olds in one group and twelve 4- and 5-year-olds in the other.

There are four teachers who take the children out of the Nursery School for individual lessons each day. The Nursery School is staffed by a head teacher, an assistant, and three parents who work one day a week in the Nursery School as part of their training. On the day they participate, the parent has an opportunity to observe their child's lesson with the Clinic teacher, and to teach their child under the teacher's supervision.

CORRESPONDENCE COURSE

For families that cannot conveniently come to the Clinic, there is a *Correspondence Course for Parents of Preschool Deaf Children*. This is intended as a 1-year program, although most parents take considerably longer to complete it. There are 12 installments providing parents with instruction about things that they can do at home to help in the communication development process. Each lesson is accompanied by a report form that the parents must complete and return before receiving the next installment. In response to the report forms, a personal letter goes back to the parents from the Clinic, commenting on their child's progress, answering any questions raised in the parents' report, and individualizing the material for their particular child. Parents consistently report that these warm and friendly letters are a great encouragement. Over 42,000 families have been enrolled in this program, and over 2165 are currently enrolled. The course has been translated into 17 languages, and is distributed by the Clinic in both English and Spanish.

The Clinic also offers a second Correspondence Course for Parents of Deaf-Blind Preschool Children. This course is also available in English and Spanish.

SUMMER SCHOOL

For 6 weeks each summer the Clinic offers a program for families and teachers. The parent program gives preference to families living outside the Los Angeles area. The children are enrolled in our Demonstration Nursery School, where the program is similar to the one conducted during the regular year, while parents attend classes every day that cover much of the same material offered in our Tuesday evening program.

The course for teachers is designed for experienced teachers of the deaf who wish to learn about the Clinic's techniques with young children and parents. It provides an intensive professional introduction to the John Tracy Clinic approach.

TEACHER PREPARATION

In cooperation with the University of Southern California, the Clinic offers a 1-year graduate program, which prepares teachers of the deaf who wish to specialize in preschool and parent education with the hearing impaired. Graduates earn California State certification as well as the Council on Education of the Deaf national certificate.

PROGRAM CONTENT

COMMUNICATION DEVELOPMENT PROGRAM

There are three major areas in our communication development program for young deaf children:

language development, speech development, and auditory training. We distinguish language, which is the understanding of our language system, from speech. Auditory training is concerned with the maximum use of residual hearing and with appropriate use of amplification. Obviously, the three are interdependent and interrelated.

Language Development

Language is developed through a multisensory approach: tactile, visual, and auditory. The broad objective is the development of each sense (individually and in combination) to its maximum potential for application in the language areas. The efficiency with which this objective may be attained is dependent on variables, such as amount of residual hearing, age at onset of hearing loss, age at detection of hearing loss, age at beginning of instruction, consistency and quality of instruction, use of amplification, and the individual differences and abilities of each child (2).

We further distinguish between receptive language, which refers to the words that a person understands, and his expressive language or the words he uses in conversation.

Receptive Language

The goal of receptive language teaching is to help the child to develop an understanding of language. Parents are shown how to talk to their child about the things he is interested in, speaking in simple sentences, emphasizing key words, and using declarative sentences instead of questions. We would like, as closely as possible, to approximate the auditory language input experience of the hearing child by bombarding the deaf child, in a meaningful fashion, through all the child's available sensory avenues.

Expressive Language

Expressive language, or how we use our language, is taught with generally the same techniques used in developing receptive language, except that the early expressive words are action verbs—words that cause something to happen and help the child realize the power of language—whereas early receptive words are generally nouns. The development of expressive language goes through four stages: receptive, imitation, reminding, and spontaneous, which represent a continuum from receptive, in which the child is not using language expressively, to the spontaneous stage, in which the child can consistently and spontaneously use the word in an appropriate situation.

Both receptive and expressive language are developed through both general and specific teaching.

1. General receptive language teaching is the talking which goes on with a deaf child throughout his waking hours.
2. Specific receptive language teaching consists of giving planned emphasis to a selected word or words.

The general language program is best typified by Mrs. Tracy's dictum: "Talk, talk, talk to your child, give him something to talk about, someone to talk to, and a desire to talk." There are few rules except trying to talk about what the child is interested in and taking advantage of every possible language input opportunity.

Specific language teaching is generally done in a sit-down lesson with planned and pre-prepared materials.

Speech Development

This is a difficult skill for the young deaf child. It requires the understanding of language and a mastery of his speech mechanism without ever being able to monitor his own efforts. The John Tracy Clinic Approach is both synthetic and analytic. Imitation of whole words and phrases is followed by practice in the elements of speech so that they can be used in correcting the whole. Breath control, rhythm, and stress are taught by exercises in pitch, loudness, and duration.

AUDITORY TRAINING

Since all deaf children have some residual hearing, the goal of auditory training is to develop the best possible listening habits. This is a difficult process for the deaf child because the speech he hears is not meaningful enough to be understood. There are many activities that can be carried out to improve the child's sound awareness and sensitize him to the finer auditory discriminations.

PARENT COUNSELING PROGRAM

As indicated, our parent education program is divided into two parts, one concerned with the development of communication and the other in helping the parents deal with their own feelings about having a child who is different. As Mrs. Tracy has pointed out:

The Clinic believes that, in any program concerned with learning and with parents, feelings are pretty basic. Feelings are responsible for attitudes, for most of what people do or don't do, and for what they are able to take advantage of. For instance, we have a great deal of information and help available, but some-

times parents are unable to use it because of their feelings. Sometimes they cannot even hear what we tell them; they are too absorbed in how they feel. Many of their attitudes are of long standing—legacies from their own childhood, so our program might be said to fall roughly into two parts: Facts and Feelings (4).

The first course, "Child Development and Parent Attitudes," has to do with how any child grows and develops and how the attitudes of his parents affects that development. The advanced class in parent attitudes is group therapy. One major difference, however, is that most participants in group therapy are referred because of difficulty in adjusting to everyday life. The parents in these groups, however, are there primarily because of their child's deafness, but they find many of the same advantages in being able to share their thoughts and feelings in a similarly motivated and understanding group under the leadership of a skilled psychologist.

As Dr. Alathena Smith, the Clinic's first psychologist, said: "Any problem that you can talk about, can talk out, will gradually cease to trouble you. And when you stop worrying about your own adjustment, then you will be able to communicate a feeling of security to your child. Now this you can do for your child" (1).

It is difficult to make generalizations in the field of parent counseling because parental reactions are so different. Although there are theories about grief and crisis reactions, it has been our experience that parents differ widely in their reactions to the discovery that their child is deaf and in their subsequent adjustment to that situation. An extreme example is the deaf parents who may be expecting a deaf offspring and are certainly less distressed than parents with little or no prior knowledge of deafness. It is also likely that the mental health of the family prior to the birth of the child also plays a great role in determining the family's reactions.

Although parental reactions are unpredictable, we find that being available to answer questions and to demonstrate what can be done when parents and professionals work together and having other parents present who have passed through this same experience helps the parents to realize that they are not the only ones to whom this has happened.

We view our parent counseling program with considerable optimism. There are occasionally some parents who are so disturbed that they must receive more intensive individual help elsewhere. We also see parents who have developed an adjustment to having a handicapped child to the point that they do not choose to participate in our parent attitude sessions. In general, however, parents do appear to benefit from these sessions.

One way that we evaluate these group sessions is the extent to which deafness is a focus of the discussion. If it is, we know that our counseling session is not working. Deafness is one of those facts that we cannot change. What we can change is how the parents feel about it. That is where we like to see the group work focus.

REFERENCES

1. Smith A: Listening Eyes (16-mm sound color film about John Tracy Clinic, produced by University of Southern California, 1948)
2. Tidwell MS: John Tracy Clinic Language Guide. John Tracy Clinic, Los Angles, CA, 1976
3. Tracy L: John Tracy Clinic brochure, undated
4. Tracy L: Talk, Talk, Talk to Deaf Children. American Education, January 1965

APPENDIX: GLOSSARY OF ABBREVIATIONS

A–B gap	air–bone gap
AC	air conduction
ANSI	American National Standards Institute
ASA	American Standards Association
BC	bone conduction
CANS	central acoustic nervous system
CNS	central nervous system
CROS	contralateral routing of signals
CSF	cerebrospinal fluid
dB	decibel
DS	Doerfler-Stewart test
EMG	electromyography
ENG	electronystagmography
IAM	internal auditory meatus
ISO	International Standards Organization
MBC	mastoid bone conduction
MLB	monaural loudness balance
NET	nerve excitability test
NIHL	noise-induced hearing loss
OD	right eye
OS	left eye
OW	oval window
PB	phonetically balanced
PT	puretone
PTAC	pure-tone air conduction
PTBC	pure-tone bone conduction
PTS	permanent threshold shift
RW	round window
SAL	sensorineural acuity level
SDS	speech discrimination score
SISI	short-increment sensitivity index
SNHL	sensorineural hearing loss
SOM	serous (or secretory) otitis media
SPL	sound-pressure level
SRT	speech reception threshold
T aurium	ear tinnitus
T cranii	head tinnitus
TD	tone decay
TM	tympanic membrane
URI	upper respiratory infection

INDEX